"This Handbook presents the cutting edge of research, theory, and practice that [illegible] why and how clinical hypnosis is crucial to integrative health care. The editors have gathered the research data and broad-ranging experiences from many international experts to bring our understanding of therapeutic communication — the core of clinical hypnosis — into the 21st century and beyond. I consider this the essential compendium of the field."

Andrew Weil, *MD, Tucson, Arizona*

"This monumental book spans not just the domain of hypnosis but the universe of its history, science, practice and art. While valuable early sections share latest ideas and findings on hypnotic theory, measurement and neuroscience, the heart of the Handbook is its chapters on clinical uses of hypnosis. Leading practitioners working in a range of health care settings offer valuable advice and fresh insights for those already familiar with hypnosis and those new to our field. The Handbook captures and harnesses the power and potential of one of the world's oldest and most storied therapeutic interventions."

Professor Amanda J. Barnier, *PhD, Professor of Cognitive Science and Pro Vice-Chancellor (Research Performance and Development), Macquarie University; Fellow of the Academy of Social Sciences in Australia; Fellow of the Society of Clinical and Experimental Hypnosis*

"This book provides a comprehensive overview of the principles and techniques of hypnosis, along with practical guidance on its use in different medical settings. The authors give clear and concise explanations of complex concepts based on their wealth of experience in the field and extensive references to the literature. It is an invaluable resource for any medical practitioner looking to expand their knowledge and incorporate hypnosis into their practice."

Csaba Dioszeghy, *MD PhD, Honorary Associate Professor, Surrey and Sussex Healthcare NHS Trust, UK*

"Encyclopedic in breadth and depth, with a focus on *SELF*-regulation grounded in evidence-based neuroscience, this 63-chapter handbook frames clinical hypnosis as an integrative *healing* practice for young and old alike."

Richard E. Kreipe, *MD, FAAP, FSAHM, FAED, Professor Emeritus, Golisano Children's Hospital, University of Rochester Medical Center, USA*

"The *International Handbook of Clinical Hypnosis* is a treasure trove for finding everything you always wanted to learn about hypnosis and, even more importantly, about what you didn't think of yet and would benefit from knowing in the rapidly changing, digitally-driven world. The international perspective and variety of the contributors' backgrounds avoid any one school of thought and provide a rich and diverse range of viewpoints for novices and practitioners of hypnosis alike. It is an instructive and greatly enjoyable read for anyone interested in hypnosis and promises to become the definitive reference on the topic."

Elvira V. Lang, *MD, FSIR, FSCEH, Founder and President of Comfort Talk®*

"This handbook does a wonderful job of synthesizing and pushing forward the vibrant field of hypnosis research. It draws together an impressive cast of world experts at the forefront of both the science and practice of hypnosis. The diversity and nuance of these perspectives is testament to the remarkable development of this field in recent years. This volume will be of great interest to anyone who seeks to appreciate the cutting edge of scientific research on hypnosis—one of the oldest and most powerful of the healing arts."

Michael Lifshitz, *PhD, Assistant Professor of Social and Transcultural Psychiatry, McGill University*

THE ROUTLEDGE INTERNATIONAL HANDBOOK OF CLINICAL HYPNOSIS

The Routledge International Handbook of Clinical Hypnosis explores and clarifies the challenge of defining what hypnosis is and how best to integrate it into treatment.

It contains state-of-the-art neuroscience, cutting-edge practice, and future-oriented visions of clinical hypnosis integrated into all aspects of health and clinical care. Chapters gather current research, theories, and applications in order to view clinical hypnosis through the lens of neurobiological plasticity and reveal the central role of hypnosis in health care. This handbook catalogs the utility of clinical hypnosis as a biopsychosocial intervention amid a broad range of treatment modalities and contexts. It features contributions from esteemed international contributors, covering topics such as self-hypnosis, key theories of hypnosis, hypnosis and trauma, hypnosis and chronic pain management, attachment, and more.

This handbook is essential for researchers, clinicians, and newcomers to clinical hypnosis in medical schools, hospitals, and other healthcare settings.

Julie H. Linden, PhD, is a psychologist and past president of the International Society of Clinical Hypnosis. She teaches globally about incorporating hypnosis skills into all aspects of healthcare practice.

Giuseppe De Benedittis, MD, PhD, is an associate professor of Neurosurgery at the University of Milano, Italy. He is internationally recognized as one of the leading experts in pain therapy and as a pioneer in the clinical and experimental use of hypnosis for pain control, contributing to the elucidation of the complex neurophysiological mechanisms of hypnotic analgesia.

Laurence I. Sugarman, MD, is a pediatrician and research professor at the Rochester Institute of Technology's College of Health Sciences and Technology. He studies, writes, and teaches globally about integrating therapeutic hypnosis into clinical care.

Katalin Varga, PhD, DSc, is a psychologist and past president of the Hungarian Association of Hypnosis and a board member of the International Society of Clinical Hypnosis. She is a hypnosis researcher and Ericksonian psychotherapist, as well as a teacher of the application of suggestive techniques in various fields.

THE ROUTLEDGE INTERNATIONAL HANDBOOK SERIES

THE ROUTLEDGE INTERNATIONAL HANDBOOK OF
COMMUNITY PSYCHOLOGY
Facing Global Crises with Hope
Edited by Carolyn Kagan, Jacqui Akhurst, Jaime Alfaro, Rebecca Lawthom, Michael Richards, and Alba Zambrano

THE ROUTLEDGE INTERNATIONAL HANDBOOK OF MORALITY, COGNITION, AND EMOTION IN CHINA
Edited by Ryan Nichols

THE ROUTLEDGE INTERNATIONAL HANDBOOK OF
COMPARATIVE PSYCHOLOGY
Edited by Todd M. Freeberg, Amanda R. Ridley and Patrizia d'Ettorre

THE ROUTLEDGE INTERNATIONAL HANDBOOK OF NEUROAESTHETICS
Edited by Martin Skov and Marcos Nadal

THE ROUTLEDGE INTERNATIONAL HANDBOOK OF
PSYCHOANALYSIS AND PHILOSOPHY
Edited by Aner Govrin and Tair Caspi

THE ROUTLEDGE INTERNATIONAL HANDBOOK OF PSYCHOLINGUISTIC AND COGNITIVE PROCESSES
Edited by Jackie Guendouzi, Filip Loncke and Mandy J. Williams

THE ROUTLEDGE INTERNATIONAL HANDBOOK OF CLINICAL HYPNOSIS
Edited by Julie H. Linden, Giuseppe De Benedittis, Laurence I. Sugarman, and Katalin Varga

THE ROUTLEDGE INTERNATIONAL HANDBOOK OF CLINICAL HYPNOSIS

Edited by Julie H. Linden, Giuseppe De Benedittis, Laurence I. Sugarman, and Katalin Varga

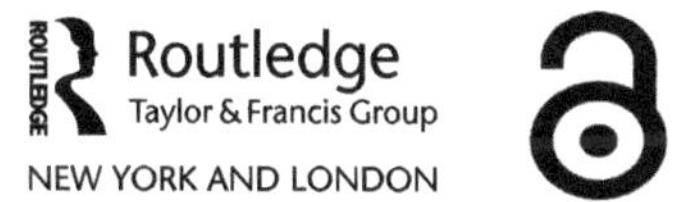

Designed cover image: © Getty Images

First published 2024
by Routledge
605 Third Avenue, New York, NY 10158

and by Routledge
4 Park Square, Milton Park, Abingdon, Oxon, OX14 4RN

Routledge is an imprint of the Taylor & Francis Group, an informa business

© 2024 selection and editorial matter, Julie H. Linden, Giuseppe De Benedittis, Laurence I. Sugarman and Katalin Varga; individual chapters, the contributors

The right of Julie H. Linden, Giuseppe De Benedittis, Laurence I. Sugarman and Katalin Varga to be identified as the authors of the editorial material, and of the authors for their individual chapters, has been asserted in accordance with sections 77 and 78 of the Copyright, Designs and Patents Act 1988.

With the exception of Chapters 4, 35, 62 and 63, no part of this book may be reprinted or reproduced or utilised in any form or by any electronic, mechanical, or other means, now known or hereafter invented, including photocopying and recording, or in any information storage or retrieval system, without permission in writing from the publishers.

Chapters 4, 35, 62 and 63 of this book are available for free in PDF format as Open Access from the individual product page at www.taylorfrancis.com. They have been made available under a Creative Commons Attribution-Non Commercial-No Derivatives (CC-BY-NC-ND) 4.0 license. Chapters 4 and 63 are funded by Roxanna Erickson Klein. Chapter 35 is funded by Oslo Universitetssykehus. Chapter 62 is funded by Department for Child and Adolescent Mental Health in Hospitals, Oslo University Hospital.

Trademark notice: Product or corporate names may be trademarks or registered trademarks, and are used only for identification and explanation without intent to infringe.

Library of Congress Cataloguing-in-Publication Data
Names: Linden, Julie Hope, editor. | Sugarman, Laurence I., editor. | De Benedittis, Giuseppe (Associate professor of neurosurgery), editor. | Varga, Katalin (Psychology professor), editor.
Title: The Routledge international handbook of clinical hypnosis / edited by Julie H. Linden, Laurence I. Sugarman, Giuseppe De Benedittis, and Katalin Varga.
Other titles: International handbook of clinical hypnosis | Routledge international handbooks.
Description: New York, NY : Routledge, 2024. | Series: Routledge international handbooks | Includes bibliographical references and index.
Identifiers: LCCN 2023032315 (print) | LCCN 2023032316 (ebook) | ISBN 9781032311401 (hbk) | ISBN 9781032313238 (pbk) | ISBN 9781003449126 (ebk)
Subjects: MESH: Hypnosis
Classification: LCC RC499.A8 (print) | LCC RC499.A8 (ebook) | NLM WM 415 | DDC 615.8/5122--dc23/eng/20231002
LC record available at https://lccn.loc.gov/2023032315
LC ebook record available at https://lccn.loc.gov/2023032316

ISBN: 978-1-032-31140-1 (hbk)
ISBN: 978-1-032-31323-8 (pbk)
ISBN: 978-1-003-44912-6 (ebk)

DOI: 10.4324/9781003449126

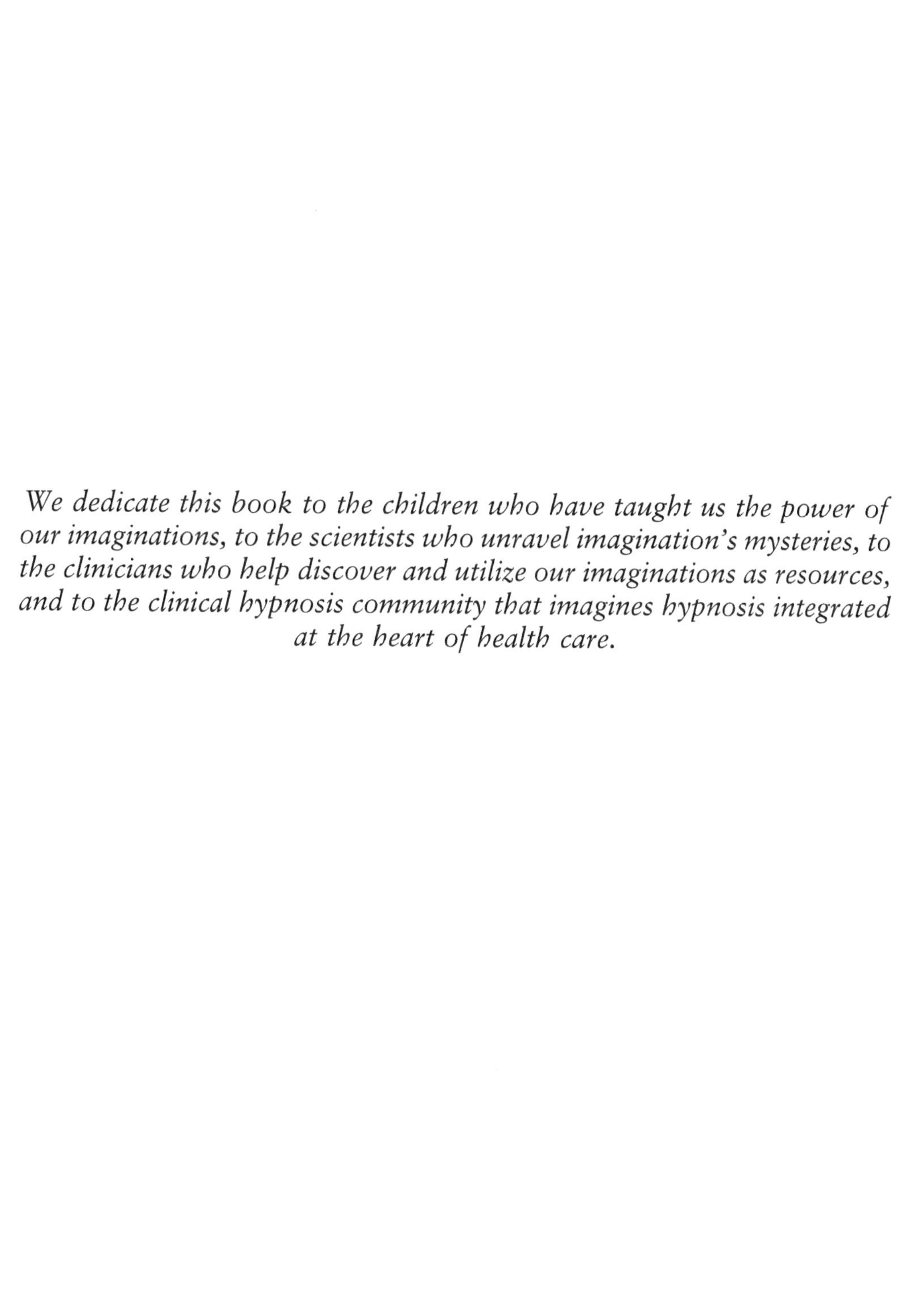

We dedicate this book to the children who have taught us the power of our imaginations, to the scientists who unravel imagination's mysteries, to the clinicians who help discover and utilize our imaginations as resources, and to the clinical hypnosis community that imagines hypnosis integrated at the heart of health care.

CONTENTS

CONTENTS

TABLES

FIGURES

Figures

Chart

ACKNOWLEDGMENT

We would like to acknowledge the long list of teachers, researchers, mentors, and clinicians on whose shoulders we stand. We are grateful to the contributing authors who generously gave their time, energy, expertise, and patience to this project. We also want to thank the many busy colleagues, friends, and family members who supported us throughout the project. Their trust in our mission has been incalculable. And most profoundly, we thank the countless clients and patients from whom we have learned the value of suggestive therapeutics.

INTRODUCTION

Julie H. Linden, Giuseppe De Benedittis, Laurence I. Sugarman, and Katalin Varga

This volume presents a new discourse on how we understand, investigate, and apply clinical hypnosis. Our scope is systemic, integrative, holistic, biopsychosocial, and neuroscientific. We have invited many of the world's expert theoreticians, researchers, teachers, and practitioners to share their reasons to render the skills of hypnosis as an integral and crucial part of health care. Our collective health and well-being are our common purpose. Interpersonal communication is our method. With this handbook, our goal has been to build and improve upon previous volumes by shining a bright light on the central role hypnosis plays philosophically, phenomenologically, and pragmatically in health and health care. This was the aspiration that guided each contributor.

As a form of suggestive communication, hypnosis has been called the oldest therapy. It emphasizes rapport and relationship. Suggestion, trance, and meditation are familiar but enigmatic terms. Over the centuries, the increasing complexity and depth of our biomedical knowledge brought both confusion about what hypnosis is and clarity about what hypnosis can do. In fact, defining hypnosis has been one of the defining characteristics of the study of hypnosis. When we ask, *What is hypnosis?* and *What is trance?* the answers tend to vary with the expertise and orientation of the responder. The experts who have contributed to these pages have an unceasing fascination and curiosity about our minds, consciousness, behaviors, and the neurobiological processes beneath them. They seek to reveal the enigma of clinical hypnosis.

Science is often portrayed as and practiced in silos that separate our biology, psychology, and sociology, and scientists as lone pioneers. These are contrived conceptual boundaries. The "mind-body" gap certainly persists in our biomedical orientation and training, but not in our embodied minds, where each of us lives. Clinical hypnosis is a community endeavor that builds bridges among the scientific disciplines. It is both an experimental probe and a clinical tool across a range of disciplines insistent in its integration of emotions, cognition, behaviors, and relationships. Our handbook reflects this bridgebuilding and confluence.

Section 1 looks at the long history of hypnosis, its past and present theories. It tells the story of the developing links between hypnosis and other disciplines, reminding us that when a theory is punctured with a splinter of evidence, there are holes in every story.

DOI: 10.4324/9781003449126-1

Section 1 sets the stage for contemporary research into and the applications of clinical hypnosis.

The success of science rests on the increasing quality of empirical evidence. The science of hypnosis tackles the long causal chain from molecules to genes through culture to personhood. Long seen as a fringe topic, hypnosis has become surprisingly well established in the cognitive sciences today as a measurable, repeatable set of phenomena. Section 2 presents a compelling examination of what we know (and do not yet know) about the complexity and interactions within the embodied mind, and what has been termed "hypnosis" and "trance." It also exposes the limits of those operational definitions. The chapters in Section 2 explore the neural correlates of expectation, conditioning, positivity, and relationships.

The first two sections anticipate Section 3 in which we experience the varied and productive application of clinical hypnosis in a variety of health care contexts. As we shift our thinking to spectra of possibilities, we delve into suggestive therapeutics applied in the outpatient clinic, hospital inpatient units, emergency department, and dental office. We consider the roles of hypnosis as people prepare for surgery, receive urgent life-saving care, get ready for childbirth, and find comfort at the end of life. The authors offer glimpses of the mostly untapped potential of how we can interact with those in our care to foster better treatment, less pain and anxiety, better self-efficacy, and faster healing. We are left wondering, how to do more?

Section 4 poses some challenges and strategies. It places hypnosis in larger legal and cultural contexts that can limit and enhance its beneficial impact. It details how best hypnosis can be taught to promote effective therapeutic communication for health care and self-care. In contrast to the backward glance of Section 1, Section 4 looks toward the future horizon – urging innovative research frameworks, unconventional thinking, and creativity – to anticipate and propel the evolution of hypnosis. This final section wonders about the future legacy of hypnosis given its established durability. It asks, "How best can our collective abilities integrate hypnosis into worldwide health and care?"

Our discourse has sought to undo the conflation of hypnosis and trance. We have begun a conceptual map with hypnosis at the center. We imagine it as a methodology of interpersonal change and influence. We survey its theoretical models, the linked phenomena of plasticity and hypnotizability, the evolving neuroscience, and unfolding practical usefulness.

We expect this wonderful collection of ideas will open the minds of those unfamiliar with clinical hypnosis and challenge the minds of those within the field. All of the generous contributors to this volume hold that the ongoing integration of clinical hypnosis across the range of health care around the world will lead to better health and improved well-being. We invite you to join the discourse.

SECTION I

The Roots of Contemporary Clinical Hypnosis

Historical Overview and Key Concepts

1
BRIEF HISTORY OF WORLD HYPNOSIS

Gérard Fitoussi

Private Practice, Fontainebleau, France

Interest in hypnosis has waxed and waned in the modern era. However, practices resembling what we now call hypnosis have been around since ancient times. The history of hypnosis can be divided into four eras: trance, animal magnetism, hypnotism, and contemporary hypnosis.

Prehistory and Antiquity: The Trance

Who was the first hypnotist? "God", answered some, referring to a passage from Genesis, "Then the Eternal God caused a deep sleep to fall on the man, who fell asleep [...]" (Bible). For others, such as the neurologist Hippolyte Bernheim (1840–1919), it is the mother who suggests to her child the idea of sleeping who should be considered "the first hypnotist" (Bernheim, 2011).

I begin with this excerpt from the Bible to gesture toward the fact that practices similar to hypnosis have existed since the dawn of humanity. We can speculate that we have long observed that the power of the voice, the fixation on an "object" like fires, stars in the sky, the spectacle of nature or alternating rhythms, chants, and drumbeats had calming and dissociative effects. This spontaneous "natural trance" would later be induced by shamans, healers, priests, and doctors for therapeutic purposes. Later on, incubation rites were used perhaps as early as the Pleistocene in Assyria-Babylonia, Egypt; this entailed going on pilgrimage to a sacred place, lying there, and waiting for a message or a revelation from the divinity (Taffin, 1960). In the temples of Aesculapius, these rites were associated with the Logos, meaning both the discourse and the reason to heal the soul through incantations described as "the beautiful speeches" (Platon, 1967).

Enlightenment, Animal Magnetism, 1750–1815

With modernity came the Viennese doctor, Franz Anton Mesmer (1734–1815) and a new name, "animal magnetism". The old struggle of Hippocrates (480–377) to dissociate medicine from religion and to distance it from "charlatans" continued well into the 18th century

DOI: 10.4324/9781003449126-4

during the period when magnetism appeared upon the scene and priests of Aesculapius could be considered as Mesmer's precursors (Sineux, 2011).

Ancient knowledge about the magnetic force, Luigi Galvani (1737–1798) and Alessandro Volta's (1745–1827) works on animal electricity, and the Montgolfier brothers' hot air balloons are all accredited with shifting mentalities around the existence of imperceptible forces. Isaac Newton (1642–1726) prepared the ground postulating with the *Principia Mathematica* (1687) the existence of an invisible force acting at a distance upon all the celestial bodies. With this, he drew criticism for introducing the idea of "occult forces" to the sciences. It was in this historical context that Mesmer proposed the concept of a "magnetic fluid", a subtle energy circulating in the universe, "serving as an intermediary between man, the earth and the celestial bodies" (Ellenberger, 1965/1994). Mesmer had distant precursors, Marsile Ficino (1433–1499), Paracelsus (1439–1541), Robert Fludd (1574–1637), Jean-Baptiste van Helmont (1579–1644), William Maxwell (1581–1641), and Richard Mead (1673–1754), the latter whom Mesmer partly plagiarized (Pattie, 1994). For his thesis, *De Planetarum Influxu* (1766), Mesmer met Maximilien Hell (1720–1792), director of the Vienna Observatory (Ryerson, 2007) and was inspired by Hell's astronomical observations and his work to relieve pain with "mineral" magnetism; however, Mesmer realized that magnets were not necessary in order for healing to occur (Belhoste, 2018), abandoned them and introduced what he termed "animal magnetism".

In 1775, Mesmer's rising celebrity prompted the Prince-Elector of Bavaria to ask him for a report about the Abbot Johann Joseph Gassner (1729–1779), a Catholic priest and noted exorcist. Gassner was criticized both by the scientific community and the Catholic Church—the clergy stated that "he was not doing exorcism according to the rules" (Peter, 2005, p. 1). Mesmer concluded that Gassner's cures were real but that Gassner "was curing his patients through animal magnetism without being aware of it" (Ellenberger, 1994, p. 87).

Mesmer's practice in Vienna led him to cure the young Maria Theresa Paradis (1759–1824) from blindness. But after an initial success, she relapsed, thus discrediting Mesmer (Lanska & Lanska, 2016) who would then leave Vienna for Paris in February 1778. On March 30, 1779, he published *Memoir on the Discovery of Animal Magnetism* in which he outlined his 27 propositions on animal magnetism (Mesmer, 1781). For Mesmer, the magnetic fluid is a physical reality. The magnetizer uses "his power" to restore its circulation until the occurrence of a spectacular crisis purging the patient of his problem. Faced with an influx of patients, Mesmer built his "famous bucket" (Turbiaux, 2009) where patients sit around. Without touching anyone, Mesmer "established 'connection' through physical rather than emotional contact" (Ryerson, 2007). However, Mesmer did not recognize the importance of dialogue or suggestions in therapeutic cures.

The turmoil caused by these cures led King Louis XVI to appoint on March 12, 1784, a commission chaired by Benjamin Franklin, already famous for his experiments with electricity, another form of energy (1706–1790). The commission refuted the existence of a magnetic fluid and attributed the therapeutic successes solely to the power of the imagination: "imagination without magnetism produces convulsions [...] magnetism without imagination produces nothing" (Chertok, 2002, p. 25). This report was confirmed by that of the French Royal Academy of Medicine (Riguet, 2018), and by a secret report, written by Jean Sylvain Bailly (1736–1793), that would not be revealed until after the Revolution (Ryerson, 2007). It underlined the erotic aspect of magnetic phenomena and proved to be inadvertently prescient about relational aspects of hypnosis 150 years hence, highlighting the complexity of relations between magnetizer and magnetized and the moral and social consequences resulting thereof—effectively condemning magnetism for several decades.

Despite the disfavor he experienced in his lifetime, Mesmer is considered one of the precursors of psychology and the discovery of the unconscious. His great merit is to have been the first to provide a rational explanation for the phenomena observed during "animal magnetism", authorizing their refutation which for the historian of science Karl Popper (1902–1994), in *The Logic of Scientific Discovery* (1934), is characteristic of the scientific approach.

His successors can be divided into three currents. The Fluidists, who advocated the material reality of the fluid; the Animists for whom "will alone" could explain the phenomenon of trance (Waterfield, 2004)—for both these schools, the participation of the subject was negligible (Waterfield, 2004); and finally, the psychofluidists, spiritualists, like the Marquis de Puységur (1751–1825) and Joseph Deleuze (1753–1835), for whom "somnambulism reveals the latent power of the soul" but refused supernatural explanations instead, "claiming reason" (Méheust, 1992).

The Marquis Armand-Marie-Jacques Chastenet de Puységur emulated Mesmer until 1784 when he encountered a young patient, Victor Race who instead of the expected magnetic crisis "falls asleep" and "talks" (Puységur, 2003). As a result, Puységur rejected the fluidic explanation alone and assumed the existence of psychological forces in "somnambulistic sleep" or "artificial somnambulism", a state resembling sleep but during which the patient is able to speak, and may name his illness, its nature, even the day it will be cured (Peter, 2009). Even if Puységur believed the will of the magnetizer still played a role, listening and speaking took on a greater importance, opening the way to the recognition of suggestion and psychology.

Abbé José Custodio de Faria (1755–1819), an Indian-Portuguese priest, departed from the theory of magnetic fluid. For his Imaginationist school, trance phenomena are understood to have a psychological base and nervous sleep, called by Faria *lucid sleep*, can be explained by natural causes (Faria, 1819). For Faria there is no material fluid (Chertok, 1990), and the magnetizer does not enact his will upon the patient (Méheust, 2001). In 1819, Faria set out his ideas in *De la Cause du Sommeil Lucide*. Posterity would only see Faria as a charlatan, "a miracle worker from India" (Binet, 1887), until Hippolyte Bernheim regenerated interest in him and his work (Bernheim, 1886). The doctor Alexandre Bertrand (1795–1831) and François-Joseph Noizet (1792–1885) expanded upon Faria's teachings, which would later be taken up by the School of Nancy (École de Nancy). However, interest in magnetism would decline in France despite the positive reception of Joseph Deleuze's *Histoire Critique du Magnétisme Animal* (1813) and the favorable report (1831) of a commission led by Dr Husson (1772–1853) but which unfortunately was never made public (Hutin, 2014).

Hypnotism (1841–1933)

Hypnosis as we know it today began with the Scottish surgeon James Braid (1795–1860) and a new name hypnotism. On November 13, 1841, Braid attended the French-Swiss magnetizer Charles Lafontaine's (1803–1892) performance in Manchester (Robertson, 2009). Intrigued, Braid repeated the experiments by fixing his gaze on a shiny object. Prolonged concentration and the ensuing tension led to a state of fatigue or "nervous sleep". He used the word "hypnotism" to describe this "artificial sleep", where there is a loss of memory upon awakening but which is remembered by the subject when thrown again "into the same degree of hypnotism" (Robertson, 2009, p. 147). In *Neurypnology* (1843), Braid argued that the effects of hypnotism are neither due to the supposed power of the magnetizer nor to the imagination of the magnetized but to the "physiological and psychological nature" present in the hypnotized subjects (Robertson, 2009, p. 136).

During this same period, in London, doctor John Elliotson (1791–1868) discovered mesmerism, initially in 1829, with Richard Chenevix (1774–1830) one of Faria's followers, then later, in 1837 with Jean du Potet de Sennevoy (1796–1881; Bramwell, 1921). In 1843, Elliotson founded the *Zoïst,* a journal dedicated to the dissemination of mesmerism. His views on mesmerism put him into conflict with *Lancet* creator's Thomas Wakley who accused him of "theatricality and even fraud" (Grey, 2018, p. 88).

In *Mesmerism in India* (1846), surgeon James Esdaile (1808–1859) recounted the hundreds of interventions he performed while his patients were under hypnosis—they did not experience pain, and their mortality rate was reduced from 50% to 5%. However, the discovery of ether in 1846, and chloroform in 1847, dealt a fatal blow to the recognition of Esdaile's work and to the development of mesmerism more generally.

The hypnosis pendulum swung once again toward France. Though the anathema cast around magnetism persisted, there was a major shift in the perceptions of hypnosis when the world renowned doctor, Jean-Martin Charcot (1825–1893),—on February 13, 1882, in a communication to the French Academy of Sciences—compared "the great hypnotism" to the hysterical crisis. This was a turning point, legitimizing the use of hypnotism by doctors. For Charcot and the Parisian Salpêtrière school, hysteria and hypnosis were considered to be the consequences of a neurological pathology (Gravitz, 2004). Opposed to this approach was the School of Nancy including Henri-Étienne Beaunis (1830–1921), Jules Liègeois (1833–1908), Hippolyte Bernheim, and Ambroise-Auguste Liébeault (1823–1904). It was no longer Mesmer's fluid, Faria's imagination, or Braid's physiological action but suggestion that lay at the heart of hypnotism—and suggestion was something that could be practiced upon all individuals and not only hysterical patients. Charcot's international reputation helped legitimize the practice of hypnotism and attracted doctors from all over the world. However, it was the ideas of the School of Nancy that prevailed.

In *Psychological Automatism* (1889), Pierre Janet (1859–1947), who studied with Charcot at La Salpêtrière, sets out his theory of "psychological disintegration" and the process of psychological dissociation that splits consciousness into subparts during the hypnotic process (Ellenberger, 1994). Though without followers in France, Janet would become "one of the main sources of Freud, Adler and Jung" (Ellenberger, 1994, p. 355) as well as the Boston School of Psychotherapy: William James (1842–1910), Morton Prince (1854–1929), Boris Sidis (1867–1923), and others (Green et al., 2014). Later on, Ernest Hilgard (1904–2001) renewed the interest in dissociation by introducing "neo-dissociation" and "hidden observer" (Hilgard, 1977).

In Europe, the interest in hypnosis never disappeared completely. The interest in Germany and Austria continued thanks to a better knowledge of Mesmer's work, while in Spain, Italy, and Russia it was triggered by Charcot's legitimation of hypnotism.

Germany and Austria

While Mesmer was in retirement, he received a visit from Dr Karl Christian Wolfart (1778–1832) who had revived the German interest in animal magnetism founding in 1811 the journal *Askläpeion* (Ellenberger, 1994). This revival was supported by the emergence of Schelling's *Naturphilosophie* and German romanticism (Montiel, 2009).

The School of Nancy would play a major role in the deployment of hypnosis in Germany. Ernest Simmel (1882–1947) used hypnotism to treat war neuroses, while Albert Moll's (1862–1939) *Der Hypnotismus* (1889) would have a considerable influence in the German-speaking world. In addition to Oskar Vogt's (1870–1959) theoretical contributions to hypnotism, he is also famous for having induced a trance in a patient after the 300th session (Chertok, 2002) and for being the inventor of the "fractional hypnosis" method, i.e., going into trance, coming out of trance, and going back into trance again, which has the effect of deepening the trance (Gauld, 1992). His work would inspire Johannes Heinrich Schultz's (1884–1970) autogenic training method (Ellenberger, 1994). Sigmund Freud (1856–1939) also used hypnosis, but ultimately rejected it. His opposition to hypnosis and the tremendous advances in anesthesia and analgesia would, once again, lead to the abandonment of hypnosis in the medical world.

Spain

In Spain, distrust of hypnosis reigned. The Catholic Church "emphasized to the public the loss of the subject's will during hypnotic sleep and the possibility of being involved in a criminal action without being aware of it" (Graus, 2017, p. 3). However, this did not prevent Spanish doctors from taking an interest in hypnosis. From 1880 to 1900, Spanish doctors had only a reading knowledge of hypnotism, which sparked their curiosity and interest in attending hypnosis shows even if they "claimed to be scandalized by the demonstration", a façade of indignation to justify their attendance (Graus, 2017, p. 2).

In 1887, works by Beaunis and Bernheim were translated into Spanish. That same year, the first important works on hypnotism were published by Spanish doctors A. Sánchez Herrero and J. Giné y Partagás (Graus, 2017). Interest in hypnosis decreased in the 1930s until physician Alfredo Caycedo (1932–2017), noting the negative reaction of patients to the term hypnosis, stopped using the term in favor of "another more appropriate one": Sophrology, the science of the harmony of the mind (Cangas &Wagstaff, 2000). In the 2000s, there seems to have been a recent upsurge of Spanish interest in hypnosis (Cangas & Wagstaff, 2000).

Italy

In Italy, hypnotism did not receive good press either. For the Catholic Church, practices of magnetism "would shake society", troubling "the social order" (Edelman, 2009, p. 131). The Church forbade the stage hypnotist Lafontaine from practicing cures, which it considered to be, "blasphemous imitations of the miracles of Christ" (Ryerson, 2007, p. 187). For Italian scientists, impregnated with positivism: "Magnetism, like occultism and popular religious beliefs, were considered a sign of the backwardness of the country" (Brancaccio, 2017, p. 159). It was not until the 19th century that the psychiatrist Bonfanti revealed "that he had been practicing magnetism since the 1850s, but that [...] he hid this practice for fear of being ridiculed by his colleagues" (Brancaccio, 2017, p. 170).

As early as 1879, Giuseppe Seppilli (1851–1939) and Gabriele Buccola (1854–1885) carried out research on the effects of electric currents and magnets. Meanwhile, the translation of Charcot's works (1880) revived interest in hypnosis in Italy. Buccola proclaimed the need for more scientific studies on the topic and even though Enrico Morselli (1852–1929; 1886) cautioned the practice of magnetism, publications and studies multiplied by Lombroso, Castelli, and Vizioli (1885) (Brancaccio, 2017). However, it was the controversy evoked by stage hypnosis that brought hypnosis to the foreground. Morselli would be one of the few doctors to recognize the quality of stage hypnotist Donato's work (Brancaccio, 2017) and the role of hypnosis shows in the emergence of studies on magnetism, and he would refuse their ban (Brancaccio, 2017). In contrast, Cesare Lombroso (1835–1909), Tebaldi, and Gonzales called for its ban, underlining the dangers of hypnosis, especially with vulnerable populations like adolescents and the "nervous" patients.

The Novara Congress in 1889 marked a turning point for hypnosis in Italy. Seppilli, observing the virtual impossibility of inducing hypnosis in subjects suffering from paranoia, melancholy, or mania, concluded that "hypnotism was in fact a dangerous method even [when] used by doctors" (Brancaccio, 2017, p. 166). Interest in hypnosis declined, but the practice continued even if it was not recognized as a proper therapeutic method in psychiatry (Brancaccio, 2017).

Russia

Magnetism would spread from Germany to Russia (Gauld, 1992). Many of the Russian practitioners were of German origin like G.F. von Parrot (1767–1852), who published *Coup d'œil sur le magnétisme animal* in 1816. The following year, the Tsarina's doctor Stoffregen visited Dr Karl Wolfart. However, despite Danilo Velianski's publication *Zhivotniy Magnetizm*, interest in magnetism died out in the mid-1820s (Gauld, 1992). Several decades later, in 1889, 15 or so Russians attended the first International Hypnosis Congress in Paris (Gauld, 1992). Ardalion Tokarsky (1859–1901) inaugurated the first "Course of Hypnosis and Physiological Psychology" in Moscow (Guilloux, 2014) and published *The Therapeutic Use of Hypnotism* in 1890 (Havenaar et al., 1998). The next year, at the 4th Congress of Russian Physicians, Vasily Danielevsky (1852–1939) gave a presentation about the effects of suggestions for the healing of burns (Guilloux, 2014). The interest in hypnosis continued to expand in Russia and, in 1904, neurophysiologist Vladimir Mikhaïlovitch Bechterev (1857–1927) founded the journal *Zeitschrift für Psychologie Kriminal-Anthropologie und Hypnotisus* (Gauld, 1992). Hypnotherapy was a cutting-edge method of Soviet psychotherapy, based on the work of the 1904 Nobel Prize winner, Ivan Petrovich Pavlov (1849–1936), who contributed greatly to the understanding of hypnotic phenomena (Tukaev, 2022). In the 1950s, at the meeting of the Academies of Science and Medicine, the study and the use of hypnosis were advocated by many, who claimed hypnosis "to be a physiologically based psychotherapy" (Chertok, 2002, p. 46). After 1975, the popularity of the Ericksonian school increased in Russia (Havenaar et al., 1998).

Outside Europe

As in Europe, phenomena related to hypnotic trances existed in traditional cultures. However, hypnosis, as we know it today, emerged in the 19th century, in Japan, China, and India under the influence of European scientists such as Charcot and Moll.

Japan

Traditional trances existed in Japanese culture, under the guidance of the Mikos, female shaman and in the Zen tradition (Maeda, 1967). It was during the Meiji era (1868) that hypnotism made its appearance, widely disseminated by a powerful publishing industry. The partial translation of Albert Moll's book "*Der Hypnotismus*" by Takeuchi Nanzō ushered in, around 1903, Japan's golden age of hypnosis. After a long absence, hypnosis disappeared before making a comeback when Dr Gosaku Naruse founded the Japanese Society of Hypnosis in 1956.

China

The history of hypnosis in China remains to be written (Fitoussi, 2021). Sinologist Jean-François Billeter expressed his surprise at "the unexpected association" between the *Zhuangzi dialogues* and Ericksonian hypnosis and "the hypnotic phenomena that are implied in the dialogues in the Zhuangzi" (Billeter, 1995, p. 27). The scholar Akira Otani also drew parallels between Eastern meditation and hypnosis (Otani, 2003; see Otani in this book).

Between 1900 and 1910, there were hypnosis shows, self-hypnosis manuals, how-to books to learn hypnosis, as well as illustrated articles in the popular press in China (Xiao, 2014). Hypnosis was practiced from 1904 onward. Chinese practitioners trained in Japan. The Chinese Institute of Mentalism (Zhongguo Xinling Yanjiuhui), the most important Chinese society devoted to hypnotism, was first established in Tokyo before moving, in 1911, to Shanghai. The institute claimed, in 1933, to have trained more than 60,000 students (Xiao, 2014). Newspapers devoted to topics connected to hypnosis appeared, correspondence courses were given, and debates took place around the various approaches of Charcot, Bernheim, Liébeault, and Braid. Even so, interest in hypnosis waned in the late 1930s—hypnosis was increasingly considered a "pseudoscience" and a "backwards slide" toward occultism (Xiao, 2014). In recent years, however, there has been a renewal of interest in hypnosis. In July 2017, the first Chinese Congress of Clinical Hypnosis took place in Beijing. Faculty included members of the Board of Directors of the International Society of Hypnosis (ISH) and of the Chinese Hypnosis Society. Approximately 1000 professionals in health care attended the conference (ISHNL, 2017).

India

In India, spirituality and mysteries intertwine—gymnosophists, fakirs, mages, yogis, hermits, snake charmers are part of everyday Indian life, and made magic "consubstantial with India" (Padoux, 2006, p. 448). In this context, three names are linked to India: Abbé Faria, Braid, and Esdaile. Faria was noted for his birth, primary education, and as a source of inspiration for young contemporary Indians more than for being an authentically Indian thinker (Khandelwal, 2014). Braid wrote that, after the publication of *Neurypnology* (1843), he was encouraged in his approach after reading works about India and the similarities between its ancestral practices and hypnotism. Lastly, Esdaile gained prominence for the surgical interventions he carried out at the Calcutta Hospital while his patients were under hypnosis, even if his methods are subject to discussion (Sugarman, 2021). It was only in 2003 that the Indian Ministry of Health and Family Welfare recommended the use of hypnosis and the University of Delhi began teaching its first course in 2007 (Sarfare, 2008).

Stage Hypnosis in the 19th Century

In the 19th century, the history of hypnosis became interwoven with that of stage hypnosis. Some condemn stage hypnosis for the dangers it exposes to the public and for the erroneous image it gives of hypnosis. Others praise it for increasing the profile for hypnosis among the general public, especially during historical moments when hypnosis was largely condemned by the scientific community.

Certain stage hypnotists like Lafontaine, Carl Hansen (1833–1897), and Donato (1845–1900) were immensely popular among the general public, and also had an influence on doctors leading some of them "to revise their attitude after having witnessed (some of their) exploits" (Ellenberger, 1994, p. 118). Lafontaine's work interested Elliotson and Braid, and Donato's that of Lombroso (Brancaccio, 2017) and Morselli (Ellenberger, 1994). Freud was influenced by Hansen whose method Bernheim recognizes, "[...] could be studied and used for therapeutic purposes" (Trueman, 2018, p. 6). For others like William Kroger (1906–1995) or André Weitzenhoffer (1921–2005), stage hypnosis was their first encounter with hypnosis (Yapko, 1989).

Professionals are divided. For the Belgian philosopher and psychologist Joseph Delbœuf (1831–1896) "Donato produces phenomena of which no licensed doctor is yet capable, [...]" (Méheust, 1999, p. 529), whereas Paul-Louis Ladame (1842–1919) in Switzerland (Wils, 2017), Lombroso in Italy, Charcot in Paris (Wils, 2017), and Moll in Germany were opposed to hypnosis shows (Graus, 2017). More recently, Michael Yapko (1954-) argues that stage hypnotists implanted the "erroneous conclusions that the hypnotists had some mysterious power that can make people do things they would not do ordinarily" (Yapko, 1989, p. 19). Despite these objections, there have been no laws regulating hypnosis shows except for the 1952 *Hypnotism Act* in the United Kingdom (Heap, 2000) and in Israel where there is a total ban (Kleinhauz et al., 1979).

Critics of stage hypnosis focus on questions of authenticity, on the risks incurred by the subjects on stage, and the spread of misconceptions around hypnosis (Echterling & Whalen, 1995). To this must be added the long-term impact of the "humiliating and embarrassing activities" (Lynn et al., 2000, p. 127) that individuals perform on stage, and "what is the effect of the audience's and friends' behavior during and after the show" (Lynn et al., 2000, p. 130) Hypnosis shows appear to give a negative or, at the very least, a truncated image of hypnosis, but these opinions are principally based on impressions. There have been several studies of the impact of stage hypnosis; William Meeker and Theodor Barber break down what occurs during the hypnosis into "eight principles which do not utilize the concept of hypnotic state or trance" (Meeker & Barber, 1971, p. 61). To this we can add the works of social psychology on submission to authority by Stanley Milgram (1933–1984), Robert Rosenthal (1933-) (Rosenthal & Jacobson, 1968) self-fulfilling prophecy, the group effect, and the concern to look good, described in 1959 by Erving Goffman (1922–1982).

Despite the fact that critics of stage hypnotists claim that hypnosis shows circulate misconceptions and employ deception and tricks, stage hypnosis "does not drive people away from clinical hypnosis. It actually encourages them to consider hypnosis for treatment" (Echterling & Whalen, 1995, p. 20). Similar to in a clinical settings and research, a minority of 8–49% individuals who attended a hypnosis show reported transient negative post-hypnotic experiences (e.g., headaches, dizziness, nausea, stiff necks). In fact, 62–85% individuals reported "positive experience including relaxation" (Lynn et al., 2000).

Can anything be done by health professionals to counterbalance the impact of stage hypnosis? In a study, Lennis Echterling concluded that circulating more reliable information, including lectures by professionals, could help counter and positively modify the public's beliefs and attitudes toward hypnosis (Echterling & Whalen, 1995). However, Steven Lynn argues for an even greater need to study stage hypnosis and that "research is absolutely necessary" (Lynn et al., 2000).

Hypnosis, 1933–1985

In the 19th century, the history of hypnosis crossed the Atlantic, through the east coast and into Louisiana, then a French colony, and arrived with a new name: "hypnosis". Despite the Franklin Commission's negative findings, mesmerism found its way to America. As early as 1815, Joseph du Commun founded a society of animal magnetism (Gauld, 1992). Then it spread through "charlatans, spiritualists, show hypnotists" (Guilloux, 2014), and around 1840, through the "missionaries" like John Bovee Dods (1795–1872) and La Roy Sunderland (1804–1885) founder of *Magnet* in 1842. Missionaries were defined as individuals who "deliberately set out to convert the populace to the gospel of magnetism" (Gauld, 1992, p. 183). It would appear that the religious dimensions prevailed over the clinical aspects. Phineas Parkhurst Quimby (1802–1866) successfully treated Mary Baker Eddy, who believed that faith in healing could cure disease and would go on to found Christian Science.

It was on this American soil that the pharmacist and genius observer Émile Coué de la Châtaignerie (1857–1926) was grafted. The transition was made from suggestion to autosuggestion, "that is to say the implantation of an idea, of oneself by oneself" (Centassi & Grellet, 1990, p. 47). For Lindsay Yeates, Coué's intuitions, observations, and procedural innovations have "greatly influenced hypnotism in the English-speaking world [...]" (Yeates, 2016, p. 2).

From the end of the First World War to the beginning of the 1950s, the use of hypnosis was limited apart from a few pioneers like Morton Henry Prince, a friend of Janet (Ellenberger, 1994). As the "leading representative of the French school of psychopathology in America" (Barresi, 1994), Prince would oppose the Freudian psychoanalytical school. Other pioneers included Henry Sumner Munro, whose 1907 hypnosis manual has been reprinted four times (A.G, 1917) and who inspired lay hypnotist Dave Elman (1900–1967; Guilloux, 2014) as well as Alice Magaw (1860–1928) "the mother of anesthesia" (Vattier & Mercadier, 2018), Paul Campbell Young (1892–1991), Robert Winthrop White (1904–2001), and Boris Sidis (1867–1923).

In 1921, the third edition of Milne Bramwell's book still referred to hypnotism, but times were changing and when Clark Leonard Hull (1884–1952) published his landmark book *Hypnosis and Suggestibility* (1933), he no longer referred to hypnotism but to hypnosis and introduced it to modern research. This marked the first "golden age" of hypnosis research (Kihlstrom, 1999).

The psychiatrist Milton Hyland Erickson (1901–1980) would renew hypnotic practice. With Erickson's hypnotic interventions, the directive becomes permissive and specific to each patient, and the unconscious is no longer a problem but a place of resources, with which it is possible to communicate through confusion, the breaking of patterns, humor, paradoxes, or metaphors. Erickson's fame increased with Jay Haley's publication of *Uncommon Therapy* (1973). Erickson stood at the confluence of many therapies: systemic, family, solution-oriented. He founded both the American Society of Clinical Hypnosis and its periodical, the *American Journal of Clinical Hypnosis*. His students continued his work with the Erickson Foundation and the Milton Erickson institutes. Ernest Lawrence Rossi (1933–2020), a Jungian psychologist, would gather Erickson's articles in the *Collected Papers* (Rossi, 1980). Rossi's numerous personal interests led him to investigate ultradian rhythms, a quantum approach of hypnosis (Rossi, 1972) as well as the links between hypnosis and genomics (Rossi, 2002). His book, *The Psychobiology of Mind Body Healing* (1986) was ahead of its time "summarizing the burgeoning field of mind-body interaction" (Saunders, 1996, pp. 152–153).

For many clinicians, Rossi's name remains associated with the "Rossi mirroring hands technique" (Hill, 2018). Obstetrician/Gynecologist David Bradley Cheek (1912–1996), another of Rossi's mentors, promoted the ideas, controversial at the time, that fetuses are influenced in utero, and that patients remain aware "of ongoing events during their surgeries while under the influence of anesthesia" (Yapko, 1996, p. 2). With Leslie M. LeCron, he suggests "that one can search for very old information in a subject by appealing to unconscious muscular movements" (Yapko, 1989, p. 59).

In the years 1950–2000, the status of hypnosis grew alongside the development of hypnotizability scales, the Stanford Hypnotic Susceptibility Scale, in 1959 by Hilgard and Weitzenhoffer (1921–2005), and the intense research activities in five major laboratories, Hilgard at Stanford, Orne at Harvard, Barber (1927–2005) at the Medfield Foundation, Sarbin at the University of California, and Hammer and Sutcliffe in Sydney (Nash & Barnier, 2008). In 1955, these advances led the British Medical Association to approve the use of hypnosis and in 1958, the American Medical Association decided that hypnosis should be included as a teaching discipline during medical studies.

Hypnosis into the 21st Century, 1985–2022

Three facts mark this first part of the 21st century: the increasing legitimacy of hypnosis and the multiplication of research teams, the extension of hypnotic practice in the world beyond Europe and North America, and a general societal interest in hypnosis.

Throughout the 19th century, scientists searched, without success, for a hypnotic signature, so the advent of imagery was a revolution. Lee Baer was the first, in 1985, to use imagery in the study of hypnosis at the University of Pennsylvania (Baer et al., 1985). Subsequently, scientific publications multiplied. Crawford (Crawford et al., 1993), Faymonville (Faymonville et al., 1995), and Maquet (Maquet et al., 1999) studied hypnosedation. Rainville (Rainville et al., 1997) shed light upon the importance of the anterior cingulate cortex. Szechtman studied auditory hallucinations (Szechtman et al., 1998). Laureys (Laureys et al., 2000) and Kosslyn explored visual hallucinations (Kosslyn et al., 2000). Horton was the first to highlight an anatomical difference in highly hypnotizable subjects (Horton et al., 2004). Finally, Jensen brought a research focus on pain (Jensen et al., 2011; see also Jensen's chapter in this book). Elvira Lang (Lang & Rosen, 2002), using a medico-economic research, showed that hypnosis reduces complications and the length of hospital stay, thus providing an economic incentive for its use.

Despite tremendous technical advances in medicine, health systems are reaching their limits—technical and medical efficiency is no longer enough. Patients are more informed, wish to be agents of their own cures, want to be considered as a whole individual, and not just an illness. In this context, hypnosis has proven to be a powerful tool for care, improving communication between health professionals and their patients as well as reinforcing the practice that each doctor–patient interaction should be adapted to an individual's specific needs.

In order to advance its growing legitimacy in medical and mental health settings and the studies done on the benefits of hypnosis, professionals will have to address two paradoxical concerns: the underutilization of hypnosis (Johnson et al., 2019) and its use by individuals who do not have the appropriate skills. There is a strong tendency by licensed clinicians enthralled by the potential of hypnosis to ignore the oft-cited, motto that "one does with hypnosis only what one knows how to do without". Thus, consent, patient education, and the ethics of hypnosis are becoming a research priority.

Will the 21st century lead to a new and exciting chapter in the practice of hypnosis? Will future discoveries solve "the enigma of hypnosis" of what happens in this particular moment where "something happens but what"? (Chertok, 1992). The long and complex history of hypnosis with its ups and down encourages us to be cautious. The key for the future of hypnosis will be the pursuit of rigorous research and its translation into effective clinical care.

References

A.G. (1917). [Review of the book *Handbook of suggestive! therapeutics and applied hypnotism*, By Henry S. Munro. 4th ed. St. Louis. Mosby Company]. *California State Journal of Medicine*. p. 377.

Baer, L., Ackerman, R. H., & Hackett, T. P. (1985). PET studies during hypnosis and hypnotic suggestion. In P. Pichot , P. Berner , R. Wolf , & K. Thau (Eds),*Biological psychiatry, higher nervous activity* (pp. 293–298). Springer.

Barresi, J. (1994). Morton Prince and B.C.A.: A historical footnote on the confrontation between dissociation theory and Freudian psychology in a case of multiple personality. In R. Klein & B. Doane (Eds.), *Psychological concepts and dissociative disorders: Reverberation and implications* (pp. 85–91). Hillsdale, NJ: Lawrence Erlbaum Associates.

Belhoste, B. (2018). Franz Anton Mesmer: Magnétiseur, Moraliste et Républicain. *Annales historiques de la Révolution française*, *391*(1), 27–56. https://www.revues.armand-colin.com/histoire/annales-historiques-revolution-francaise/annales-historiques-revolution-francaise-no391-12018/franz-anton-mesmer-magnetiseur-moraliste

Bernheim, C. (2011). *Hippolyte Bernheim, un destin sous hypnose*. Paris, France: Jbz & Cie.

Bernheim, H. (1886). *De la Suggestion et de ses applications thérapeutiques* (S. Nicolas (Ed.), 2005). Paris, France: L'Harmattan.

Bible. (1970). *Trad. du Rabbinat Français*. Paris, France: Colbo.

Billeter, J.-F. (1995). Seven dialogues from the Zhuangzi. (M. Elvin, Trans.). *East Asian History*, 9(Juin), 23–46.

Binet, A., & Féré, C. (1887). *Le magnétisme animal*. Paris, France: Félix Alcan.

Bramwell, J. M. (1921). *Hypnotism, its history, practice, and theory* (3rd ed.). London, UK: William Rider & Son.

Brancaccio, M. T. (2017). Between Charcot and Bernheim: The debate on hypnotism in finde-siècle Italy. *The Royal Society Journal of the History of Science*, *71*(2), 20 June, 157–177. 10.1098/rsnr.2017.0008

Cangas, A. J., & Wagstaff, G. F. (2000). The current status of hypnosis in Spain. *Contemporary Hypnosis*, *17*(1), 42–47. 10.1002/ch.191

Centassi, R. et Grellet, G. (1990). *Tous les jours de mieux en mieux. Émile Coué et sa méthode réhabilités*. Paris, France: R. Laffont.

Chertok, L. (1990). *Mémoires d'un hérétique*. Paris, France: La Découverte.

Chertok, L. (1992). *L'Énigme de la relation au cœur de la médecine*. Les Empêcheurs de penser en rond, Chilly-Mazarin, France: Laboratoire Delagrange.

Chertok, L. (2002). *L'hypnose*. Paris, France: Payot.

Crawford, H. J., Gur., R. C., Skolnick, B., Gur, R. E., & Benson, D. M. (1993). Effects of hypnosis on regional cerebral blood flow during ischemic pain with and without suggested hypnotic analgesia. *International Journal of Psychophysiology, 15*, 181–195. 10.1016/0167-8760(93)90002-7

Echterling, L. G., & Whalen, J. (1995). Stage hypnosis and public lecture effects on attitudes and beliefs regarding hypnosis. *American Journal of Clinical Hypnosis, 38*, 13–21. 10.1080/00029157.1995.10403173

Edelman, N. (2009). Un savoir occulté ou pourquoi le magnétisme animal ne fut-il pas pensé « comme une branche très curieuse de psychologie et d'histoire naturelle »?. *Revue d'histoire du XIXe siècle, 38*, 115–132. 10.4000/rh19.3877

Ellenberger, H. F. (1994). *Histoire de la découverte de l'inconscient*. Paris, France: Fayard.

Esdaile, J. (1846). *Mesmérism in India, and its practical application in surgery and medicine*. London, UK: Longman, Brown, Green and Longmans.

Faria Abbé de. (1819). *De la cause du sommeil lucide ou étude de la nature de l'homme* (S. Nicolas (Ed.), 2005). Paris, France: L'Harmattan.

Faymonville, M. E., Fissette, J., Mambourg, P. H., Roediger, L., Joris, J., & Lamy, M. (1995). Hypnosis and adjunct therapy in conscious sedation for plastic surgery. *Regional Anesthesia, 20*, 145–151. PMID: 7605762.

Fitoussi, G. (2021). *Dictionnaire encyclopédique d'hypnose*. Sucy-en-Brie, France: Anfortas.

Gauld, A. (1992). *A history of hypnotism*. New York: Cambridge University Press.

Goffman, E. (1959). *The presentation of self in everyday life*. Garden City, NY: Anchor Books, Doubleday.

Graus, A. (2017). Hypnosis lessons by stages magnetizers: medical and lay hypnotists, in Spain. *Notes Records, The Royal Society Journal of the History of Science, 71*(2), 141–156. 10.1098/rsnr.2017.0009

Gravitz, M. A. (2004). The historical role of transference in the theoretical origins of transference. *International Journal of Clinical and Experimental Hypnosis, 52*(2), 113–131. 10.1076/iceh.52.2.113.28096

Green, J. P., Laurence, J.-R., & Lynn, S. J. (2014). Hypnosis and psychotherapy: from Mesmer to Mindfulness. *Psychology of Consciousness: Theory, Research and Practice, 1*(2), 199–212. 10.1037/cns0000015

Grey, F. L. (2018). *Interdisciplinary perspectives on Mesmer and his legacy: Literature, culture, and science*, Thesis, University of Kent.

Guilloux, C. (2014). Colloque. *Hypnose d'ici et Hypnose d'ailleurs*, 6–8 fév.

Haley, J. (1973). *Uncommon therapy*. New York: W.W. Norton & Company.

Havenaar, J. M., Meijler-Iljina, L., van den Bout, J., & Melnikov, A. V. (1998). Psychotherapy in Russia. Historical backgrounds and current practice. *American Journal of Psychotherapy, 52*(4), 501–513. 10.1176/appi.psychotherapy.1998.52.4.501

Heap, M. (2000). The alleged dangers of stage hypnosis. *Contemporary Hypnosis, 17*(3), 117–126. 10.1002/ch.200

Hilgard, E. R. (1977). *Divided consciousness, multiple controls in human thoughts and action*. New York: John Wiley & Sons.

Hill, R., & Rossi, E. L. (2018). *The practitioner's guide to mirroring hands: A client responsive therapy that facilitates natural problem-solving and mind-body healing*. Bancyfelin, UK: Crown House Publishing.

Horton, J. E., Crawford, H. J., Harrington, G., & Hunter Downs, III, J. (2004). Increased anterior corpus callosum size associated positively with hypnotizability and the ability to control pain. *Brain, 127*, 1741–1747. 10.1093/brain/awh196

Hutin, J. F. (2014). Le docteur Henri Marie Husson (1772–1853) et l'introduction de la vaccine à Reims. *Histoire des sciences médicales, XLVIII*(3), 361–378. PMID: 25966537

International Society of Hypnosis. (2017). *Newsletter, 41*(3).

Jensen, M. P., Ehde, D. M., Gertz, K. J., Stoelb, B. L., Dillworth, T. M., Hirsh, A. T., Molton, I. R., & Kraft, G. H. (2011). Effects of self-hypnosis training and cognitive restructuring on daily pain intensity and catastrophizing in individuals with multiple sclerosis and chronic pain. *International Journal Clinical Experimental Hypnosis, 59*(1), 45–63. 10.1080/00207144.2011.522892.

Johnson, P. J., Jou, J., Rockwood, T. H., & Upchurch, D. M. (2019). Perceived benefits of using complementary and alternative medicine by race/ethnicity among midlife and older adults in the United States. *Journal of Aging Health*. September, *31*(8), 1376–1397. 10.1177/089826431 8780023

Khandelwal, S. K. (2014). Contributions of an Indian to the science and art of hypnosis. *Indian Journal of Psychiatry*, *56*(4), October–December, 415–417.

Kihlstrom, J. F. (1999). Hypnosis research in Australia, Symposium discussion, Australian Psychological Society.

Kleinhauz, M., Dreyfuss, D. A., Beran, B., Goldberg, T., & Azikri, D. (1979). Some after-effects of stage hypnosis: A case study of psychopathological manifestations. *International Journal of Clinical and Experimental Hypnosis*, *27*(3), 219–226. 10.1080/00207147908407563

Kosslyn, S. M., Thompson, W. L., Costantini-Ferrando, M. F., Alpert, N. M., & Spiegel, D. (2000). Hypnotic visual illusion alters color processing in the brain. *American Journal of Psychiatry*, *157*, 1279–1284. 10.1176/appi.ajp.157.8.1279

Lang, E. V., & Rosen, M. P. (2002). Cost analysis of adjunct hypnosis with sedation during outpatient interventional radiologic procedures. *Radiology*, *222*(2), 375–382. 10.1148/radiol.2222 010528

Lanska, D. J., & Lanska, J. T. (2016). Franz Anton Mesmer and the rise and fall of animal magnetism: Dramatic cures, controversy, and ultimately a triumph for the scientific method. *History of Neurology*, 301–320. 10.1007/978-0-387-70967-3_22

Laureys, S., Faymonville, M. E., Moonen, G., Luxen, A., & Maquet, P. (2000). PET scanning and neuronal loss in acute vegetative state. *Lancet*, *355*, 1825–1826; discussion 1827. 10.1016/s0140-6736(05)73084-1

Lynn, S. J., Myer, E., & Mackillop, J. (2000). The systematic study of negative post-hypnotic effects: Research hypnosis, Clinical hypnosis and stage hypnosis. *Contemporary Hypnosis*, *17*(3), 127–131. 10.1002/ch.201

Maeda, S. (1967). The present state of hypnosis in Japan. *Japan Journal of Educational and Social Psychology*, *VII*(1), 65–71.

Maquet, P., Faymonville, M. E., Degueldre, C., Franck, G., Luxen, A., & Lamy, M. (1999). Functional neuroanatomy of hypnotic state. *Biological Psychiatry*, *45*, 327–333. 10.1016/ s0006-3223(97)00546-5

Meeker, W. B., & Barber, T. X. (1971). Toward an explanation of stage hypnosis. *Journal of Abnormal Psychology*, *77*(1), 61–70. 10.1037/h0030419

Méheust, B. (1992). *Somnambulisme et médiumnité, Le défi du magnétisme*. Le Plessis-Robinson, France: Les Empêcheurs de penser en rond.

Méheust, B. (1999). *Somnambulisme et médiumnité*. Le Plessis-Robinson, France: Les Empêcheurs de penser en rond.

Méheust, B. (2001). Balzac et le magnétisme animal: Louis Lambert, Ursule Mirouet, Seraphita. In E. Leonardy (Ed.), *Traces du mesmérisme dans les littératures européennes du XIX° siècle* (Bruxelles, Actes du colloque du 9–11 novembre 1999). Bruxelles: Facultés universitaires Saint-Louis.

Mesmer, F. A. (1781). *Précis historique des faits relatifs au magnétisme animal*, S. Nicolas (Ed.), 2005. Introduction de Serge Nicolas et des écrits de Delon, Horne, Paulet et Bergasse. Paris, France: L'Harmattan.

Milgram, S. (1963). Behavioral study of obedience. *Journal of Abnormal Psychology*, *67*, 371–378. 10.1037/h0040525

Montiel, L. (2009). Une révolution manquée: le magnétisme animal dans la médecine du romantisme allemand, A failed revolution: the animal magnetism in the medicine of German romanticism. *Revue d'histoire du XIXe siècle*, *38*, 61–77, Société d'histoire de la révolution de 1848 et des révolutions du XIXe Siècle. http://journals.openedition.org/rh19/3870

Morselli, E. (1886, April 21). Le esperienze del signor Donato. *Gazzetta letteraria artistica e scientifica, supplement de la Gazetta Piemontese*.

Nash, M. R., & Barnier A. J. (Eds.). (2008). *The Oxford handbook of hypnosis: Theory, research and practice*. Oxford, UK: Oxford University Press.

Otani, A. (2003). Eastern meditative techniques and hypnosis: A new synthesis. *American Journal of Clinical Hypnosis*, *46*(2), October, 97–108. 10.1080/00029157.2003.10403581

Padoux, A. (2006). Magie indienne. In J.-M. Sallmann (Ed.), *Dictionnaire historique de la magie et des sciences occultes.* p. 448. Paris, France: Librairie Générale Française/Livre de Poche.
Pattie, F. A. (1994). *Mesmer and animal magnetism: A chapter in the history of medicine.* Hamilton, NY: Edmonston Publishing Inc.
Peter, B. (2005). Gassner's exorcism – not Mesmer's magnetism – is the real predecessor of modern hypnosis. *International Journal of Clinical and Experimental Hypnosis, 53*(1), 1–12. 10.1080/00207140490914207
Peter, J. P. (2009). De Mesmer à Puységur. Magnétisme animal et transe somnambulique, à l'origine des thérapies psychiques, Savoirs occultés: du magnétisme à l'hypnose. *Revue d'histoire du XIX° siècle, 38*(1), 19–40. 10.4000/rh19.3865
Platon. (1967). *Charmide.* Paris, France: GF-Flammarion.
Popper, K. (1934). *The logic of scientific discovery* (1959). Abingdon-on-Thames: Routledge.
Puységur, A. M. J. de C. de. (2003). *Mémoires pour servir à l'histoire et à l'établissement du magnétisme animal* (1784). Paris, France: Imago.
Rainville, P., Duncan, G. H., Price, D. D., Carrier, B., & Bushnell, M. C. (1997). Pain affect encoded in human anterior cingulate but not somatosensory cortex. *Science, 277,* 968–971. 10.1126/science.277.5328.968
Rapport des commissaires chargés par le roi de l'examen du magnétisme animal, Imprimerie royale, Moutard, Paris (1784) In Chertok (2002). *L'hypnose.* Paris, France: Payot.
Riguet, E. (2018). Le magnétisme animal. *Les Dossiers de l'OZ.*
Robertson, D. (2009). On hypnotism (1860), De l'Hypnotisme. *International Journal of Clinical and Experimental Hypnosis, 57*(2), 133–161. 10.1080/00207140802665377
Rosenthal, R., & Jacobson, L. (1968). Pygmalion in the classroom. *The Urban Review, 3*(1), 16–20. 10.1007/BF02322211
Rossi, E. L. (Eds). (1980). *The collected papers of Milton H. Erickson on hypnosis* (Vol. 1–4). New York: Irvington Publishers.
Rossi, E. L. (1972/2000). *Dreams, consciousness & spirit: The quantum experience of self-reflection and co-creation* (3rd Edition of Dreams & the Growth of Personality). New York: Zeig, Tucker.
Rossi, E. L. (1986). *The psychobiology of mind-body healing: New concepts of therapeutic hypnosis.* New York: W. W. Norton.
Rossi, E. L. (2002). *The psychobiology of gene expression: Neuroscience and neurogenesis in therapeutic hypnosis and the healing arts.* New York: W. W. Norton Professional Books.
Ryerson, H. G. (2007). An evolution of the historical origins of hypnotism prior to the twentieth century: between spirituality and subconscious. *Contemporary Hypnosis, 24*(4), 178–194. 10.1002/ch.341
Sarfare, S. (2008, March 2). Healing through hypnosis. *Indian Times.*
Saunders, T. R. (1996). [Review of the book *The psychobiology of mind-body healing: New concepts of therapeutic hypnosis,* by E. L. Rossi.]. *Psychotherapy: Theory, Research, Practice, Training, 33*(1), 152–153. 10.1037/h0092360
Sineux, P. (2011). La guérison dans les sanctuaires du monde grec antique: de Meibom aux Edelstein, remarques historiographiques. *Anabases, 13,* 1–16. 10.4000/anabases.1713
Sugarman, L. I. (2021). Leaving hypnosis behind? *American Journal of Clinical Hypnosis, 64*(2), 139–156. 10.1080/00029157.2021.1935686
Szechtman, H., Woody, E., Bowers, K. S., & C. (1998). Where the imaginal appears real: A positron emission tomography study of auditory hallucinations. *Proceedings of National Academy of Science,* USA, *95,* 1956–1960. 10.1073/pnas.95.4.195
Taffin, A. (1960). Comment on rêvait dans les temples d'Esculape. *Bulletin de l'Association Guillaume Budé,* 3, octobre, 325–366. 10.3406/bude.1960.3909
Trueman, L. (2018). Progression/regression: Hypnotism and the superstitious in Maupassant's Le Horla. *Romance Notes, 58*(1), 5–15. 10.1353/rmc.2018.0001
Tukaev, R. D. (2022). Ivan O. Pavlov et l'hypnose soviétique (Trad. Thomas Pruvot,). *La Revue de l'hypnose et de la santé,* Juillet, *20,* 89–93.
Turbiaux, M. (2009). À l'occasion de deux expositions sur le tricentenaire de la naissance de Benjamin Franklin, Benjamin Franklin (1706-1790), Antoine Mesmer (1734-1815) et le magnétisme animal. *Bulletin de psychologie, 1*(Numéro 499), 51–65. 10.3917/bupsy.499.0051

Vattier, L., & Mercadier, L. (2018). Le secret d'Alice Magaw. Une pionnière aux commandes d'une anesthésie humaniste et hypnotique. *Transes*, *4*, 9–14.
Waterfield, R. (2004). *Hidden depth: The story of hypnosis*. London, UK: Pan Books.
Wils, K. (2017). From transnational to regional magnetic fevers: The making of a law on hypnotism in late nineteenth-century Belgium. *Notes and Records, The Royal Society Journal of the History of Science*, *71*(2), 179–196. 10.1098/rsnr.2017.0007
Xiao, T. (2014). *Hypnotism and 'pseudoscience' in China*. Department of East Asian Languages and Cultures, Indiana University.
Yapko, M. (1989). *Trancework: An introduction to the practice of clinical hypnosis* (2nd ed.). Bristol, PA: Brunner/Mazel.
Yapko, M. (1996). An interview with David Cheek, M.D. *American Journal of Clinical Hypnosis*, *39*(1), 2–17. 10.1080/00029157.1996.10403360
Yeates, L. B. (2016). Émile Coué and his method (I): The chemist of thought and human action. *Australian Journal of Clinical Hypnotherapy & Hypnosis*, *38*(1), Autumn, 3–27. 10.3316/informit.305951832285241

2

ON THE HARD PROCESS OF UNDERSTANDING HYPNOSIS

Epistemological Issues in the Debate Between State, Trait, and Hypofrontality Theories

Enrico Facco

Department of Neurosciences, University of Padua, Italy; Institute Franco Granone, Italian Center of Clinical and Experimental Hypnosis, Turin, Italy

I would give great praise to the physician whose mistakes are small, for perfect accuracy is seldom to be seen

HIPPOCRATES

The definition of hypnosis is an everlasting work in progress. Its initial definition in late 18th century was restrained by two factors: (1) the intrinsic limits of the inductive process of knowledge in empirical sciences; (2) the dependence of knowledge on the adopted paradigm. These factors have led to hypnosis being misunderstood and rejected a priori despite its outstanding effects. The dominant medical class prioritized interventions supported by increasingly rigorous scientific method and increasingly rejected any shadow of unfounded quackery (Facco et al., 2019; Hajek, 2017). The concern and the prejudice were so strong at that time as to reject facts in order to save adopted axioms, theories, and beliefs.

Given its ostensible oddity, hypnotic phenomenology[1] was described borrowing the psychiatric terminology (e.g., somnambulism, catalepsy, dissociation, hallucination). As a whole, the used terms have helped cast a long shadow of a less-than-normal or even an insane condition until the later 20th century, a shadow not yet fully dispelled. Actually, most of the terms used are ambiguous at best and others are simply wrong (e.g., the concept of negative hallucination) and should be put under scrutiny to check whether they should be replaced by more precise and non-pathological terms.

The main steps in the definition of hypnosis can be summarized as follows:

1 The Mesmer's hypothesis of an animal magnetic fluid;
2 A matter of heated imagination, as judged by the Commission established by Louis XVI in 1784;
3 A sleep-like condition [a fact leading James Braid to name it hypnosis, from the Greek ὕπνος (sleep)];
4 The Charcot's opinion of hypnosis as a sort of experimental hysteria;

DOI: 10.4324/9781003449126-5

5 The Bernheim and Liébeault's theory of suggestion;
6 An altered state of consciousness (ASC);
7 A condition of hypofrontality.

According to the last definition by the APA Division 30 (Elkins et al., 2015), hypnosis is "A state of consciousness involving focused attention and reduced peripheral awareness characterized by an enhanced capacity for response to suggestion". This definition is the last step in the hard process of definition of hypnosis, but it is probably only the next rung on the ongoing ladder of its comprehension. According to the authors, it is purposefully "a concise and heuristic description" emphasizing that hypnosis is a physiological state of consciousness. If this is the case, the report of subjective experience is essential for its understanding. The assessment of behavior is not sufficient to properly measure hypnotic ability, given that different motivations may give rise to the same behavior within and outside hypnotic contexts. For instance, arm levitation may be the result of plain obedience to commands or the ability to turn hypnotic instructions into a change of experience (viz., perception of lightness): only the latter pertains to hypnosis.

Here, the key epistemological points involved in the process of understanding hypnosis and the related flawed interpretations of the past will be outlined; then the debated theories of hypnosis as a state/non-state and state/trait as well as the theories of neodissociation and hypofrontality will be discussed.

Key Epistemological Points

The long-lasting misunderstanding of hypnosis is epistemological in nature – i.e., it reflects the dependence of knowledge on the adopted axioms, theories, and paradigms, a complex issue the analysis of which is beyond the aim of this chapter (the topic has been detailed in Facco, 2022b; Facco et al., 2017). Here, essential key points will be emphasized to identify pitfalls.

The century-old Western rationalism is based on Aristotle's tripartite logic (principle of identity, non-contradiction, and excluded middle). Though valuable, it is not as universal and flawless as deemed by the posterity, who turned it into an established doctrine. Karl Popper considered Aristotle as the "first real dogmatist" for he introduced a positive method of knowledge based on induction (Popper, 2012). In fact, inductive reasoning provides no more than a kind of conjecture or hypothesis based on adopted definitions, where the demonstration of truthfulness is provided by the use of syllogisms. As a result, it entails an overestimation of the power of definition in the attempt to find a way out to its intrinsic limits. In fact, according to Aristotle, definitions specify the essence of phenomena by the description of their necessary features. On the other hand, definitions are not demonstrated in themselves and are hardly (if possible) able to provide a full and an unerring knowledge of the observed entity. As a result, rational knowledge has been based on undemonstrated axioms, hypotheses, and theories, as well as partial and fallible definitions: thus, its results necessarily remain δόξα (*dóxa*, relative knowledge, opinion) as emphasized by Aristotle himself (*Metaphysics* 1005B, 1–5).

The outstanding rationalist revolution of the 17th century led to the birth of the new sciences, but they were born as a compromise with the Church (claiming the exclusive purview on the soul), where Descartes' ontological separation of *res cogitans* and *res extensa* was a smart loophole to allow for the compromise. As a result, the soul (consciousness) was arbitrarily separated from the body and left to the exclusive competence of the Church, while the new sciences were unnaturally limited to the investigation of the physical world. At the same time, Descartes' radical dualism – claiming the incommensurability between soul and matter – favored the separation of the observer from the observed fact in the illusion of his independence and neutrality. Likewise, medicine focused on the Cartesian *earthen body machine* only, as if the soul would be irrelevant in both health and disease.

The new sciences were successfully based on Galileo and Descartes' mathematical-geometrical apriorism, a paradigm unable to properly face the world of subjectivity however, as questioned by Pavel Florenskij:

> The rationalistic understanding of life does not distinguish, and is not able to distinguish, between a person and a thing. More precisely, it has only one category, the category of thingness, and therefore all things, including persons, are reified by this understanding, are taken as a thing, as res. (Florenskij, 2004, p. 58)

Later on, the Western thought has developed through Enlightenment, Empiricism, Positivism, and Materialist Monism, with an increasing inclination to determinism and objectivism. Nevertheless, determinism is an ideology rather than a theory (Popper et al., 1993), while Positivism is based on a metaphysical foundation establishing that the objective, external world is real and exists regardless of human perception. As a result, Positivism has been affected by naive realism, optimism, and faith in science, a *spirit of times* well painted by Max Ernst:

> The belief in occult magic powers of nature has gradually died away, but in its place a new belief has arisen, the belief in the magic power of science. (Mach, 1897, p. 189)

In short, classic Western thought has led to the adopted paradigm and mental categories being inadvertently projected into the reality, and facts being constrained within their limits in the illusion that the resulting observation is "objective". In this regard, it is worth noting that the so-called objectivity cannot trespass the limits of shared subjectivity: scientific knowledge is an intersubjective product of mind living in the world of consciousness and its products are partial models of the world, i.e., they are *Weltbild* (image of the world; Facco, 2022b).

Fortunately, quantum physics has started a huge revolution in early 20th century, leading to the role of subjectivity being reintroduced and Aristotelian logic being dismantled in its foundation by showing the dual nature particle-wave of photons (Merli et al., 1974). Furthermore, it has led to a shift from the deterministic logic of classical physics to a probabilistic formalism (also able to admit some contradictions) and from the ontology of properties to the ontology of relationship, compared and defined as follows:

1 The ontology of properties regards things as separate entities endowed with well-definable features embedded in a local world where they may undergo reciprocal relationships; if so, their essence is knowable through Aristotelian induction.
2 The ontology of relationships establishes that things manifest themselves only through reciprocal interaction, a fact entailing their correlation – i.e., their description can only be the result of their interaction, including the observer–observed relationship – rather than the possibility to define what things are in themselves.

The development of quantum physics has been paralleled by the introduction of para-consistent logics, like fuzzy logic and dialetheism, aiming to exceed the inflexible limits of the classical binary logic [true (1) vs. false (0)]. The former accepts the full range of values between 0 and 1, while the latter admits that some proposition are "true contradictions" – viz., their assertion and negation are both true (Cintula et al., 2021; Priest, 1998). As a result, one must realize that knowledge cannot be as rock-hard and immutable as formerly believed.

The increasing appeal of quantum physics has led to the spread of its paradigm to other disciplines and the introduction of several related neologisms such as quantum economics, quantum finance, quantum cognition, quantum hypnosis, quantum psychology, and quantum medicine (Bien, 2004; Curtis 2004; De Benedittis, 2020; Morstyn, 1989; Orrell, 2018; Robson, 2020). However, one should not simply borrow appealing terms from quantum physics and take them outside the world of particles without knowing their meaning and proper use, in order to avoid unscientific, irrational drifts. The concept of quantum-like can be properly applied to "classic" phenomena when they can be better understood applying the quantum mathematical apparatus, or, at least, when new hypotheses correctly meet the conceptual framework of quantum physics. Otherwise, it is better to avoid quantum-like claims and reappraise the paradigm of pre-Socratic and Eastern philosophies, given their wisdom and compatibility with the paradigm of quantum-physics (Facco & Fracas, 2022). Such an approach has been already adopted in both psychotherapy and hypnosis[2] (Elkins & Olendzkj, 2019; Facco, 2020; Yang, 2017).

The Enduring Misunderstanding of Hypnosis

The above-mentioned arguments may explain the main reasons for the difficult process of understanding hypnosis in the past two centuries. In fact, the ruling third-person perspective (3PP) of science was blind to subjective phenomena, the meaning of which can be assessed only by the first- and second-person perspective. Hypnotic phenomena were also hardly intelligible by a culture that still ignored the unconscious and held the naive century-old idea of man as a monolithic creature beloved by God and endowed with a rational soul. The link between hypnosis, dissociative identity disorders, possession, and clairvoyance, as well as the prejudice of a medical class wishing to get rid of any form of quackery also hampered a proper comprehension of hypnosis (Facco et al., 2019: Facco et al., 2019). Therefore, it was considered absurd or likened to a dysfunctional phenomenon to be described by psychiatric terms.

Mesmer's initial hypothesis of a magnetic fluid and planetary influence on bodies, despite being false, was not implausible at that time; it was compatible with Newton's concept of gravity, suggesting the existence of forces acting at a distance. Modern electrophysiology was at its very beginning in the 18th century: Luigi Galvani introduced the concept of intrinsic animal electricity by observing the frog's muscle contraction following electrostatic stimulation, while Abbe Jean Antoine Nollet discharged the Leyden jar – the first capacitor invented by von Kleist and van Musschenbroek in 1745 – through 700 monks holding hands in a line. Likewise, the nature of heat as energy-work had not been recognized yet and it was considered as a caloric fluid flowing through the pores of matter. As a result, hypnosis might be legitimately hypothesized as the expression of a still unknown magnetic fluid.

According to Kihlstrom,

> There is no doubt that the studies performed by the Franklin Commission are masterpieces of the experimental method ... No one – not even the Franklin Commission – ever doubted that Mesmer's cures were genuine or that he was able to succeed where conventional approaches had failed. But evidence of efficacy was not sufficient for Academic approval. (Kihlstrom, 2002, p. 412)

Thus, the Franklin Commission dismissed Mesmerism as a mere product of imagination in the absence of proofs of its underlying mechanisms, a fact reflecting the above-mentioned desire to adopt a rigorous scientific method free from any shadow of quackery. Nevertheless, this judgment entailed two major flaws:

1 The lack of knowledge of mechanisms does not exclude real effects. Giving more weight to accepted theories than facts especially occurs when a new phenomenon seems alien. For instance, traditional acupuncture and hypnosis have been a priori rejected until the end of 20th century in the West due to their incompatibility with the materialist–reductionist paradigm. On the other hand, salicylates have been used for about 3,500 years as willow bark extracts and as aspirin from 1897 without knowing the existence of prostaglandins (discovered in 1935). In 1972, its mechanism of action was still considered a mystery, but this did not affect its use at all (West, 1972). These facts emphasize the use of a double standard with the related dogmatic drift. Actually, scientific proofs are the endpoint of research, rather than a precondition for acceptance.
2 Imagination has been disparaged by the post-Enlightenment rationalism as a valueless source of illusions. In the early 20th century, it was still considered as a property of the less developed brain of children and "inferior races" (according to the Victorian myth of the superiority of western white man; Thomas, 2010; 2019). Instead, imagery is a valuable mental faculty for cognition, art, science, and therapy. According to Kandinsky, the aim of art is to make visible the invisible, but the same is true for science and philosophy. Both Albert Einstein and Nikola Tesla were gifted with a huge imagination enabling them to conceive new theories and inventions. Furthermore, motor imagery may help rehabilitation following brain disorders like stroke and Parkinson disease (Caligiore et al., 2017; García Carrasco & Aboitiz Cantalapiedra, 2016).

As reported by Gilles de la Tourette, Castel – a member of the Husson Commission at the Académie Royale de Médecine of Paris appointed to reexamine mesmerism in 1831 – strongly opposed its results, claiming that:

> If the majority of facts were real, they would dismantle half of the available knowledge of physiology and, thus, their publication would be harmful. (Tourette, 1887, p. 33)

As a result, Husson's report, which represented a sum of considerable work and sustained efforts undertaken to illuminate the complex phenomena of animal magnetism, remained a dead letter (Tourette, 1887, p. 33).

Likewise, Meynert, a distinguished neuropsychiatrist and anatomist, at a German medical congress stated: “Hypnosis is surrounded by a halo of absurdity. Even recoveries do not prove anything” (Freud, 1889, p. 187).

To summarize, the history of hypnosis has been marked by serious epistemological errors that may be framed within the coherence and correspondence theories of truth. The former establishes that a statement is true if it coheres with the rest of knowledge. The latter establishes that a statement is true if it corresponds to the facts. According to Popper, “the coherence theory is utterly conservative: ‘entrenched’ knowledge can hardly be overthrown” (Popper, 1972, p. 23). Indeed, hypnosis was rejected due to its ostensible incompatibility with previous knowledge and the adopted *Weldbild*. This is to say that when facts contradict the accepted theories, too bad for facts. As a result, hypnosis was a priori rejected, instead of earlier (questionable) knowledge being discarded (as per the Husson Commission).

The most impressive case is that of James Esdaile, who published over 300 surgical interventions in 1846 reporting a huge decrease of pain, stress, and mortality from about 40–50% to 5% (Esdaile, 1846; Hammond, 2008). Despite these outstanding results, the prejudicial opposition from the medical class – paralleled by the introduction of pharmacological anesthesia – led to hypnosis being buried in oblivion until recent years. Only a handful of case reports with hypnosis as stand-alone anesthesia have been published between 1955 and 2015 (Facco, 2016; Kihlstrom, 2001). It is worth mentioning that Esdaile was not a disciple of Mesmer or Braid. He self-taught hypnosis through written descriptions and also included in his practice observations from Hindu fakirs and conjurers showing some similarities with mesmeric techniques. His openness toward Indian practices of healing and the involvement of native assistants also biased the British medical opposition by adding a suspicion of imposture (Hammond, 2008; Schmit, 2010; Sugarman, 2021). Furthermore, his behavior was hardly acceptable by the Victorian imperialist myth of the superiority of white man and the inferiority of indigenous medicines.

The idea of hypnosis as a sleep-like condition stemmed from the deceitful 3PP observation of patients standing still with eyes closed, while ignoring their experience and involved mental processes; at any rate, it helped to leave the theory of magnetic fluid and redefine hypnosis in the field of neurology with related physiological and psychological interpretations. However, this approach resulted in two opposite views, the Charcot’s pathological view and the psychological, non-pathological explanation by Bernheim and Liébeault.

The Charcot’s positivist–objectivist interpretation of hypnosis as a form of experimental hysteria was misleading, in that it only detected some formal similarities between hypnotic induction and hysterical seizures. Furthermore, his charisma and strongly directive experimental approach led his docile, hysteric, highly hypnotizable, and acquiescent patients to follow his orders. As a result, they reproduced hysterical crises, fainting, and epileptic-like symptoms on demand, supporting the illusion of an insane suggestibility ().

Bernheim recognized the role of imagination and hypothesized that hypnosis was a matter of suggestion. He thought that suggestions neither depended on magnetism nor hypnotic state; rather, they were the expression of a physiological property of the brain, regardless of the state of consciousness (Bernheim, 1911). This view anticipated Grinder and Bandler’s opinions that “All communication is hypnosis” and “I disagree, nothing is hypnosis; hypnosis doesn’t exist”, respectively (Grinder & Bandler, 1987, p.1).

Freud endorsed the Bernheim and Liébeault's psychological interpretation, but questioned the theory of suggestion as an unproven claim:

> Later on my resistance took the direction of protesting against the view that suggestion, which explained everything, was itself to be preserved from explanation ... The word is acquiring a more and more extended use and a looser and looser meaning and will soon come to designate any sort of influence whatever, just as in English, where "to suggest" and "suggestion" correspond to our Nahelegen [urge, intimate. Authors' note] and Anregung [offered idea. Author's note]. But there has been no explanation of the nature of suggestion. (Freud, 1921, pp. 36–37)

The term suggestion still remains ambiguous after over a century, while the role of suggestibility in hypnosis remains uncertain at best – a sort of leitmotiv that has been dragged along from the 19th century, slipping into the idea of an impaired critical capacity and free will (Facco, 2022a; Montgomery et al., 2011; Tasso & Perez, 2008). If this is the case, it should be put under scrutiny and be better defined or, perhaps, left behind.

Hypofrontality and Neodissociation Theories

The theory of suggestibility as well as the inclusion of hypnosis in the so-called altered states of consciousness (ASCs) have supported the modern theories of hypofrontality, also corroborated by neurophysiological findings [for a systematic review, see (Landry et al., 2017)]. Gruzelier introduced this theory with the aim of gathering neurophysiological and sociocognitive theories and exceeding the sterile state/trait debate, in order to provide an empirical knowledge of brain processes explaining the phenomenology of hypnosis (Gruzelier, 2000). Accordingly, the process of hypnosis induction and deepening entails a focused attention followed by a selective inhibition of frontal functions, leading to critical evaluation, will, and reality testing being suspended. Dietrich proposed that the transient prefrontal deregulation was the unifying marker of all ASCs, as well as an essential features of anxiety and depression, allowing for phenomena like impairment of initiative, agency, and timelessness being experienced (Dietrich, 2003).

In short, the hypofrontality and neodissociation theories emphasize the decrease of prefrontal activity and/or a disconnection between the central executive (CEN) and the salience networks (SN). They result in top-down changes of cognitive and executive control, and other higher-order activities, in turn leading to an enhanced proneness to suggestions. Nevertheless, these neuropsychological findings may result in two opposite interpretations:

1 Hypnosis as an ASC marked by a less-than-normal condition involving an impairment of control, when data are viewed through the prism of a reductionist perspective and the old leitmotiv of suggestion.
2 An enhanced metacognitive control enabling one to intentionally stop the executive control when deemed useful to one's goal.

For instance, arm levitation and the related loss of agency may be viewed as the result of a plain impairment of prefrontal activity, or a metacognitive process involving inaccurate higher-order thoughts – i.e., a hypnotic response marked by the intention to perform the task while remaining unaware of the intention. This is also suggested by the increase of hypnotic suggestibility following repetitive transcranial stimulation of the dorsolateral prefrontal cortex (DLPFC) (Dienes & Hutton, 2013).

The problem is more complex than a plain matter of impairment, be it sustained by cognitive or metacognitive processes. Actually, the right DLPFC activation with deactivation of the default mode network (DMN) is a feature of decontextualized processes and metacognitive awareness, where decontextualized supervision allows for reasoning about oneself using impersonal, objective rules of inference (Gerrans, 2014). The metacognitive ability for perceptual decisions and memory retrieval involves an enhanced connectivity between lateral regions of prefrontal cortex (PFC) and right dorsal anterior cingulate cortex, and between medial PFC, precuneus, and parietal lobule, respectively (Baird et al., 2013). These brain circuits explain the introspective capacity to manage information coming from perception and memory according to the meaning of what is experienced, improving flexibility in the interaction with the environment. Furthermore, the connectivity between frontal and parietal areas, DMN (involved in self-referential processing), SN, and CEN is related to high-creative thinking ability (Beaty et al., 2018).

The whole of the above data is in line with (a) the increased connectivity between DLPFC and SN in high-hypnotizable subjects (Hoeft et al., 2012) and (b) the changes of DMN activity in hypnosis and its complex interrelationship with CEN and SN (Facco et al., 2019). The latter enables one to guide behavior and modify the neurovegetative balance accordingly. If this is the case, hypnosis is far from being a plain result of an ill-defined suggestibility and hypofrontality. Rather, it entails an enhanced activity of the highest-order processes enabling one to intentionally manage perceptions and memories. This in turn can improve the metacognitive control by blocking or disregarding what is deemed irrelevant or inappropriate to one's goal. As a result, one can improve the control over pain, emotions, stress, and psychological disorders (including anxiety, phobia, depression, and dissociative identity disorders). In other words, hypnosis may result to be a better-than-normal introspective activity allowing for individual's empowerment.

The available data also disprove the theory of neodissociation introduced by Hilgard, who defined hypnotic analgesia as a negative hallucination (Hilgard, 1975; 1977a; 1977b).[3] He described it by positing the concept of a "hidden observer", defined as the capacity of a part of the subject to monitor what had been cancelled by hypnotic suggestion – i.e., to perceive pain during hypnotic analgesia. On the other hand, this was the result of a self-contradictory suggestion asking to do two opposite tasks at the same time. The concept of a hidden observer has raised a lengthy debate (Kihlstrom, 1998; 2003; Kirsch & Lynn, 1998; Laurence et al., 1983; Spanos & Hewitt, 1980), the resolution of which has required a better knowledge of the neurophysiology of both pain – viz., the pain neuro-matrix (Melzack, 2001) – and hypnotic analgesia. Actually, hypnosis-focused analgesia yields the activation of the right DLPFC and a modulation of the pain neuro-matrix leading to both painful inputs and sympathetic stress response being blocked (unlike Hilgard's findings). This allows for surgical analgesia with perfect stability of hemodynamic parameters (Casiglia et al., 2020; Facco et al., 2021).

The theory of hypofrontality also raises the issue of hypnosis as an ASC.

Hypnosis as State or Trait: Both or Neither?

Since the beginning, hypnosis appeared as a condition other than ordinary consciousness, while the central role ascribed to suggestion helped support the idea of hypnosis as a state featured by decreased critical ability and increased proneness to hypnotist's commands. Hull endorsed the concept of hypnosis as a state of hypersuggestibility. However, like Freud, he wisely emphasized the lack of an accurate definition of the principle with the possible risk of its eventual rejection (Hull, 1933). Later, a heated debate on hypnosis as state/non-state took place, where the holders of the latter questioned the role of the formal induction of hypnosis in the responsiveness to suggestion (see Pintar & Lynn, 2009).

Hypnosis has also been included in the classification of ASCs, a fact calling for a short discussion of this concept. The term ASC has been introduced in medicine by Ludwig in 1966 with an open-minded approach to indicate all conditions straying from the so-called normal consciousness (Ludwig, 1966). In 2005, the ASC Consortium classified ASCs adopting an empirical-descriptive-mechanistic stance in the attempt to develop an ASC model, taking into account their triggers and neurocorrelates (Vaitl et al., 2005). On the other hand, the very concept of ASC has been questioned, emphasizing that it may depend on misinterpretation of data, rather than on a condition of altered consciousness or perception per se (Revonsuo et al., 2009).

In the author's opinion, the very term ASC is semantically questionable for three main reasons:

1 The term "altered" is ambiguous, for it could mean both modified and disordered. As a result, it implicitly hints to a less-than-normal condition, especially when pathological and non-pathological conditions are gathered together.
2 Normality is a conventional statistical concept. The definition of "normal" consciousness and its boundaries is very uncertain, if possible, making the concept of "altered state" shaky at best. Therefore, the definition of ostensibly odd non-pathological conditions as ASCs is based on an ill-grounded concept. It is affected by naive realism with the related epistemological implications, for they reflect a deviation from the adopted *Weltbild*.
3 The concept of state – though widely used in science and not being wrong in itself – is an abstract, conventional concept also affected by naive realism. In fact, it pragmatically defines an epoch during which the variables of interest do not change, while all other components of the observed phenomenon are plainly skipped. One should never forget that the observed phenomenon is always much richer than the measured variables, albeit relevant. Furthermore, the concept of state is the product of a static view attempting to freeze the observed phenomenon – a sort of snap-shot useful to understand it – reflecting the need of the ego to create steady pictures of the world in order to find one's bearings and manage the reality. If this is the case, it is pragmatically useful, but remains a conventional, partial abstraction that is subject to flaws. It can be compared to a sort of synecdoche, the figure of speech in which a part of something is used to signify the whole.

Actually, the whole world is never in a state. Instead, it is marked by an unceasing transformation, a fact already well established in the West by Heraclitus and Hippocrates (with his concept of *dynamis*, i.e., the inseparable, dynamic interrelationship of mind-body-world), as well as by Eastern philosophies, especially Taoism. This is remarkably true for both living beings and consciousness, the former liable to continuous change and decline and the latter marked by a ceaseless mind-brain activity and flow of experience. Since consciousness emerges from a ceaseless flux of information and processing, the concept of state of consciousness may only be a convenient descriptive facility not to be ontologized. In this regard, it is worth mentioning that in Indian culture consciousness is not meant as a "thing" but a non-reified, unceasing, intrinsically dynamic functional process. Accordingly, its Sanskrit names are *vṛtti* and *cittavṛtti* (mind activity and wave-vortex of mind activity, respectively).

According to Perlovsky,

> Most of the brain's operations (more than 99%) are inaccessible to subjective consciousness. The mind operates with "islands" of conscious-logical states in an ocean of unconsciousness; it "jumps" among conscious-logical islands over an ocean of unconscious states. And all the while we remain subjectively convinced that we are conscious. Since consciousness deals only with logical states, it is biased toward logic [a fact depending on the rationalist Western stance; Author's note]. (Perlovsky, 2013)

Freud's metaphor of consciousness as the tip of the iceberg remains effective, if one refrains from reifying it. Actually, it entails its inseparability from the part laying under the waterline. Their boundaries remain uncertain – without solution of continuity or changes in their nature – despite that they appear phenomenally different.

Interestingly, sleep and dream have been included in the ASC classification by Vaitl et al. (2005) – a fact probably depending on wakefulness being naively considered as the fundamental human condition allowing for consciousness by Western common sense. But it is a deceptive view. In fact, we spend about one-third of our life sleeping and incessantly shift between different levels of arousal, awareness, absorption, distraction, drowsiness, sleep, and dream (all of them being equally essential for life and health), making their whole an inseparable dynamic process including a non-stop exchange of information between consciousness and the unconscious. When considering the wakefulness–sleep cycle that is embedded in the natural rhythm of night and day, defining sleep as an ASC is comparable to referring to the night as an altered state of the day, which is absurd.

The misleading concept and classification of ASCs has brought about the proposal to replace them with the term non-ordinary mental expressions (NOMEs) – encompassing all non-pathological conditions, including hypnosis and meditation (Facco et al., 2021). The use of the term NOME helps us resist implicit linkage to the idea of a less-than-normal condition and emphasizes the epistemological implications of their definition – i.e., their ostensible oddity, in turn depending on their shift from the adopted *Weltbild* – a fact in line with the wise approach of William James to consciousness:

> It is that our normal waking consciousness, rational consciousness as we call it, is but one special type of consciousness, whilst all about it, parted from it by the filmiest of screens, there lie potential forms of consciousness entirely different. We may go through life without suspecting their existence; but apply the requisite stimulus, and at a touch they are there in all their completeness, definite types of mentality which probably somewhere have their field of application and adaptation. No account of the universe in its totality can be final which leaves these other forms of consciousness quite disregarded. (James, 1917, p. 111)

In the debate state/non-state and state/trait, altered state theorists consider hypnosis (at least what has been named as "deep hypnosis") as a specific psychological and/or physiological condition allowing for hypnotic experience and enhanced suggestibility. However, non-state theorists conceive it as the result of interaction with the hypnotist, involving the subject's motivation, expectancy, desired goal, and, according to Sarbin, the role they consciously or unconsciously take: "The induction is an entrance ritual—an invitation to engage in 'as-if' behavior, an invitation to enact a particular social role" (Sarbin, 2005, p. 130).

In short, the controversy state/non-state swings between the idea of similarity or contrast between hypnotic and non-hypnotic mind processes. It also intertwines with the debate on hypnosis as a state or trait. According to Pintar andLynn (2009), the latter has resulted into three main views:

1 No need for a specific trait or ability, making anyone potentially able to respond to hypnotic suggestions;
2 A mix of trait and state entailing the possibility to improve the response by training;
3 Hypnosis as a stable trait that cannot be improved by training, especially when most difficult tasks are concerned.

There seems to be no reason for excluding the coexistence of both – i.e., a variable blend of trait and non-trait variables, where a given hypnotic ability may reach its full expression by rapport, motivation, expectations, and other context dependent variables. Perhaps, a supposed incompatibility between state and trait positions depends on their "ontologization" and a bad use of Aristotelian logic, a priori constraining them within an inflexible dichotomy (true vs. false) on the basis of the principle of non-contradiction. Furthermore, a different relative weight of trait and state components may be present in medicine and psychotherapy. In the former, especially in dentistry and surgery, a higher performance is needed, making trait components more relevant for a good outcome. Figure 2.1 shows a representative example, where a patient's low hypnotic ability (as predicted by the Hypnotic Induction Profile) led to the intervention being interrupted, notwithstanding a careful training (Facco et al., 2015).

Thus, hypnotic analgesia is a relevant topic in the assessment of the state/trait relationship. It has been claimed in the past that only highly hypnotizable subjects (Highs) – viz., no more than 15–20% of the population – can face surgery with hypnosis as stand-alone anesthesia. Nevertheless, it is only an anecdotal opinion relying on the belief that only hypnotic virtuosos can achieve it, whereas the minimum requested ability has not been established so far. Despite the effectiveness of hypnosis in chronic pain seems to be related to suggestibility (Thompson et al., 2019), hypnotic analgesia may be a more widespread phenomenon depending on a complex set of factors. In fact, significant increases of pain threshold have been seldom reported even in Lows (Benhaiem et al., 2001; Carli et al., 2008). An experimental study has found a full analgesia in 45.1% of subjects and a significant increase of pain threshold in further 19.1% of cases (Facco et al., 2011). Furthermore, patients with a score of 8 in the Stanford Hypnotic Suceptibility Scale Form C (i.e., at boundaries between Mediums and Highs) may undergo surgery in full well-being, analgesia, and cardiovascular stability (Facco et al., 2013). As a result, hypnotic analgesia is not the exclusive epiphenomenon of hypnotizability as defined by suggestibility scales. Other relevant factors should be taken into account such as attention, absorption, motivation, memory, the meaning of pain, the loop between perception and unconscious processing shaping the features of future experience, as well as specific instruction for hypnotic-focused analgesia and neglect (Chapman & Nakamura, 1998; Chaves, 1994; Milling et al., 2010).

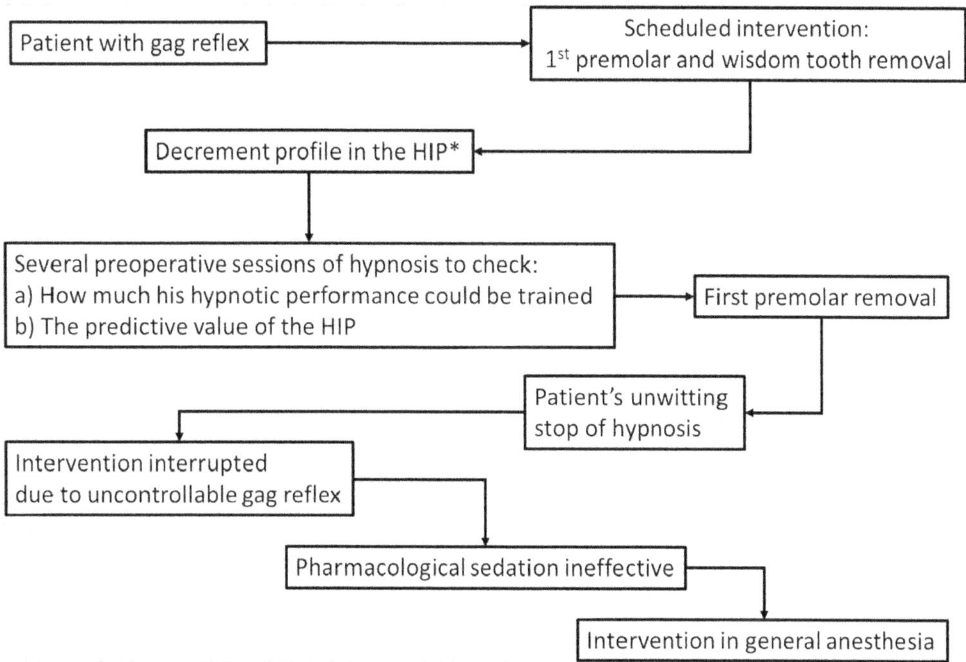

Figure 2.1 Schematic description of a patient with gag reflex and low hypnotic ability submitted to oral surgery: the decrement profile led to the intervention being interrupted, despite the preoperative training performed in the attempt to improve patient's response (*HIP = Hypnotic induction Profile (Spiegel & Spiegel, 2004); the decrement profile discloses the incapacity to maintain the ribbon of attention in the hypnotic task, leading to the patient unwittingly stopping hypnosis in a few minutes).

Conclusions

Hypnosis has a weird history marked by outstanding clinical effects accompanied by prejudicial refusal, a fact highlighting the epistemological issues involved in its comprehension. Its phenomenology, depending on introspective mental processes, could not be easily understood by the paradigm of positive sciences – only adopting a 3PP and observing behavior. Its ostensible oddity led to hypnosis being defined for some two centuries with terms borrowed from psychiatry – all misleading terms casting a long-lasting shadow of less-than-normal or dysfunctional mind-brain activity. Later, this shadow has been endorsed by defining hypnosis in terms of suggestibility, a little-defined term hinting at an impaired control. The modern theories of hypofrontality and neodissociation attempted to provide a better knowledge of the mind-brain correlates of hypnosis. However, skipping their metacognitive implications, they still maintained the same nuance of impaired condition engendered by decreased activity of PFC and executive control.

The controversy on state/non-state and state/trait may be at least partly dependent on the inclination to overestimate the value of the adopted definitions and make them incompatible by a bad use of the principle of non-contradiction. Fortunately, the division between state and non-state started fading away at the end of last century (Pintar & Lynn, 2009) – a fact reflecting the mix of their intrinsic weakness, inflexible stances, and claimed strength – and a biopsychosocial theory of hypnosis has been introduced (Jensen et al., 2015).

The past theories and terms used to to define its phenomenology have been helpful in the hard process of understanding it, but at the same time have engendered a cultural filter a priori constraining its phenomenology within their limits. Fortunately, the wealth of data obtained in the past two decades have provided new food for thought to redefine hypnosis from a physiological standpoint and withdraw the undue implication of a less-than-normal condition. The concept of hypnosis as an "altered state" is at least questionable, for the very concept of altered state is ill-grounded and misleading. Furthermore, what the subject is able to do during hypnosis is at least partly able to do even outside hypnosis and may be enhanced by motivation and other contextual factors.

Hypnosis is the result of a still little-known complex of factors, including imaginative involvement, absorption, ego receptivity, insight, proneness to fantasy and trust, social sensitivity, empathy as well as detachment, openness to experiences, cognitive and emotional flexibility (Balthazard & Woody, 1992; Council & Green, 2004; Dienes et al., 2009; Facco et al., 2017; Flemons, 2020; Testoni et al., 2020). If this is the case, the traditional emphasis on suggestibility is inconsistent; rather than proneness to accept suggestions, hypnosis may be more reasonably defined as the capacity to convert suggestions into plastic monoideism (Facco, 2022a).

In the welcome process of redefinition of hypnosis, it is worth taking into account the above-mentioned James' definition of consciousness, encompassing all its still little-known, non-ordinary expressions as inseparable aspects. The whole of these capacities depend on that unique, inseparable mind-brain-body unit with its manifold, mighty abilities able to perform a wealth of different tasks and experiences - be they conventionally considered as ordinary or non-ordinary and classified as "observed" states or non-states. Among them, hypnosis, meditation, as well as other similar NOMEs have been fruitfully used by humankind since time immemorial to improve the control over mind and body comprehend the reality, adapt to the environment, develop the self and spirituality, and help healing. If the above discussion is correct, the time is now ripe to reexamine the whole topic in order to exceed the limits of past interpretations and adopted terminology. As a result, hypnosis might be described in new entirely physiological terms and redefined as a better-than-normal introspective activity allowing for subject's empowerment, rather than an "altered state".

Notes

1 The term phenomenology is understood here as the study of "phenomena", i.e., of things as they appear in our experience, or the ways we experience them from the first person point of view.

2 It is worth noting that mindfulness meditation, mindful psychotherapy, and mindful hypnosis stem from the Buddhist meditation *Vipassanā* (for further details, see Facco, 2017).

3 It is worth noting that the concept of negative hallucination as meant in the world of hypnosis does not exist in psychiatry, where it indicates adversative auditory hallucinations; therefore, it would be better to leave it behind [see (Facco, 2022a) as a review].

References

Baird, B., Smallwood, J., Gorgolewski, K. J., & Margulies, D. S. (2013). Medial and lateral networks in anterior prefrontal cortex support metacognitive ability for memory and perception. *Journal of Neuroscience*, *33*(42), 16657–16665. 10.1523/JNEUROSCI.0786-13.2013

Balthazard, C. G., & Woody, E. Z. (1992). The spectral analysis of hypnotic performance with respect to "absorption". *The International Journal of Clinical and Experimental Hypnosis*, *40*(1), 21–43. 10.1080/00207149208409644

Beaty, R. E., Kenett, Y. N., Christensen, A. P., Rosenberg, M. D., Benedek, M., Chen, Q., Fink, A., Qiu, J., Kwapil, T. R., Kane, M. J., & Silvia, P. J. (2018). Robust prediction of individual creative ability from brain functional connectivity. *Proceedings of the National Academy of Sciences of the United States of America*, *115*(5), 1087–1092. 10.1073/PNAS.1713532115

Benhaiem, J. M., Attal, N., Chauvin, M., Brasseur, L., & Bouhassira, D. (2001). Local and remote effects of hypnotic suggestions of analgesia. *Pain*, *89*(0304–3959 (Print)), 167–173.

Bernheim, I. (1911). *De la suggestion* (2007). L'Harmattan.

Bien, T. H. (2004). Quantum change and psychotherapy. *Journal of Clinical Psychology*, *60*(5), 493–501. 10.1002/JCLP.20003

Caligiore, D., Mustile, M., Spalletta, G., & Baldassarre, G. (2017). Action observation and motor imagery for rehabilitation in Parkinson's disease: A systematic review and an integrative hypothesis. *Neuroscience & Biobehavioral Reviews*, *72*, 210–222. 10.1016/J.NEUBIOREV.2016.11.005

Carli, G., Suman, A. L., Biasi, G., Marcolongo, R., & Santarcangelo, E. L. (2008). Paradoxical experience of hypnotic analgesia in low hypnotizable fibromyalgic patients. *Archives Italiennes de Biologie*, *146*(0003–9829 (Linking)), 75–82.

Casiglia, E., Finatti, F., Tikhonoff, V., Stabile, M. R., Mitolo, M., Albertini, F., Gasparotti, F., Facco, E., Lapenta, A. M., & Venneri, A. (2020). Mechanisms of hypnotic analgesia explained by functional magnetic resonance (fMRI). *The International Journal of Clinical and Experimental Hypnosis*, *68*(1), 1–15. 10.1080/00207144.2020.1685331

Chapman, C. R., & Nakamura, Y. (1998). Hypnotic analgesia: A constructivist framework. *The International Journal of Clinical and Experimental Hypnosis*, *46*(0020–7144 (Print)), 6–27.

Chaves, J. F. (1994). Recent advances in the application of hypnosis to pain management. *The American Journal of Clinical Hypnosis*, *37*(0002–9157 (Print)), 117–129.

Cintula, P., Fermüller, C. G., & Noguera, C. (2021). Fuzzy logic. In E. N. Zalta (Ed.), *The Stanford encyclopedia of philosophy* (pp. 1–49). Stanford University. https://plato.stanford.edu/archives/win2021/entries/logic-fuzzy/

Council, J. R., & Green, J. P. (2004). Examining the absorption-hypnotizability link: The roles of acquiescence and consistency motivation. *The International Journal of Clinical and Experimental Hypnosis*, *52*(0020–7144 (Print)), 364–377.

Curtis, B. D., & Hurtak, J. J. (2004). Consciousness and quantum information processing: Uncovering the foundation for a medicine of light. *Journal of Alternative and Complementary Medicine*, *10*(1075–5535 (Print)), 27–39.

De Benedittis, G. (2020). From quantum physics to quantum hypnosis: A quantum mind perspective. *International Journal of Clinical and Experimental Hypnosis*, *68*(4), 433–450. 10.1080/00207144.2020.1799380

Dienes, Z, Brown, E., Hutton, S., Kirsch, I., Mazzoni, G., & Wright, D. B. (2009). Hypnotic suggestibility, cognitive inhibition, and dissociation. *Consciouness and Cognition*, *18*(1090–2376 (Electronic)), 837–847.

Dienes, Z. & Hutton, S. (2013). Understanding hypnosis metacognitively: rTMS applied to left DLPFC increases hypnotic suggestibility. *Cortex*, *49*(2), 386–392. 10.1016/J.CORTEX.2012.07.009

Dietrich, A. (2003). Functional neuroanatomy of altered states of consciousness: The transient hypofrontality hypothesis. *Consciousness and Cognition*, *12*(2), 231–256. 10.1016/S1053-8100(02)00046-6

Elkins, G., & Olendzkj, N. (2019). *Mindful Hypnotherapy: The Basics for Clinical Practice*. Springer.

Elkins, G. R., Barabasz, A. F., Council, J. R., & Spiegel, D. (2015). Advancing research and practice: The revised APA Division 30 definition of hypnosis. *International Journal of Clinical and Experimental Hypnosis*, *63*(1744–5183 (Electronic)), 1–9.

Esdaile, J. (1846). *Mesmerism in India, and its practical applications in surgery and medicine*. Longman, Brown, Green, and Longmans.

Facco, E. (2016). Hypnosis and anesthesia: Back to the future. In *Minerva Anestesiologica* (Vol. 82, Issue 12, pp. 1343–1356). Edizioni Minerva Medica.

Facco, E. (2017). Meditation and hypnosis: Two sides of the same coin? *International Journal of Clinical and Experimental Hypnosis*, *65*(2), 169–188. 10.1080/00207144.2017.1276361

Facco, E. (2020). Hypnosis for resilience. *OBM Complementary and Alternative Medicine*, *5*(3), 1–20. 10.21926/obm.icm.2003032
Facco, E. (2022a). Hypnosis and Hypnotic ability between old beliefs and new evidences: An epistemological reflection. *American Journal of Clinical Hypnosis*, *64*(1), 20–35. 10.1080/00029157.2020.1863181
Facco, E. (2022b). A neurophenomenological theory of the three worlds. *Theory & Psychology*, *32*(5), 733–753. 10.1177/09593543211068426
Facco, E., Bacci, C., & Zanette, G. (2021). Hypnosis as sole anesthesia for oral surgery: The egg of Columbus. *The Journal of the American Dental Association*, *152*(9), 756–762. 10.1016/J.ADAJ.2021.04.017
Facco, E., Casiglia, E., Masiero, S., Tikhonoff, V., Giacomello, M., & Zanette, G. (2011). Effects of hypnotic focused analgesia on dental pain threshold. *International Journal of Clinical and Experimental Hypnosis*, *59*(4), 454–468. 10.1080/00207144.2011.594749
Facco, E., Fabris, S., Casiglia, E., & Lapenta, A. M. (2019). Moving beyond the narrow icon of criminal atavism: Cesare Lombroso as physician-philosopher and hypnotist in the sociocultural context of 19th century. *General Medicine Open*, *3*, 3–10. 10.31234/osf.io/yxze7
Facco, E., & Fracas, F. (2022). De Rerum (Incerta) Natura: A tentative approach to the concept of "quantum-like". *Symmetry*, *14*(3), 1–13. 10.3390/sym14030480
Facco, E., Fracas, F., & Tressoldi, P. (2021). Moving beyond the concept of altered state of consciousness: The non-ordinary mental expressions (NOMEs). *Advances in Social Sciences Research Journal*, *8*(3), 615–631. 10.14738/ASSRJ.83.9935
Facco, E., Lucangeli, D., & Tressoldi, P. (2017). On the science of consciousness: Epistemological reflections and clinical implications. *EXPLORE: The Journal of Science and Healing*, *13*(3), 163–180. 10.1016/j.explore.2017.02.007
Facco, E., Mendozzi, L., Bona, A., Motta, A., Garegnani, M., Costantini, I., Dipasquale, O., Cecconi, P., Menotti, R., Coscioli, E., & Lipari, S. (2019). Dissociative identity as a continuum from healthy mind to psychiatric disorders: epistemological and neurophenomenological implications approached through hypnosis. *Medical Hypotheses*, *130*(109274), 1–11. 10.1016/j.mehy.2019.109274
Facco, E., Pasquali, S., Zanette, G., & Casiglia, E. (2013). Hypnosis as sole anaesthesia for skin tumour removal in a patient with multiple chemical sensitivity. *Anaesthesia*, *68*(9), 961–965. 10.1111/anae.12251
Facco, E., Testoni, I., Ronconi, L., Casiglia, E., Zanette, G., & Spiegel, D. (2017). Psychological features of hypnotizability: A first step towards its empirical definition. *International Journal of Clinical and Experimental Hypnosis*, *65*(1), 98–119. 10.1080/00207144.2017.1246881
Facco, E., Testoni, I., & Spiegel, D. (2015). Ipnotizzabilità e Hypnotic Induction Profile. In E. Casiglia (Ed.), *Ipnosi e altri stati modificati di coscienza* (pp. 271–287). CLEUP.
Flemons, D. (2020). Toward a relational theory of hypnosis. *American Journal of Clinical Hypnosis*, *62*(4), 344–363. 10.1080/00029157.2019.1666700
Florenskij, P. (2004). *The pillar and ground of the truth: An essay in orthodox theodicy in twelve letters*, B. Jakim (Ed.). Princeton University Press.
Foucault (1975). La Casa della follia. In Basaglia F. , & Basaglia Ongaro F. (Eds), *Crimini di pace. Ricerche sugli intellettuali e s ui tecnici come addetti all'oppressione*(kindel Edition, pp. 233-261). Einaudi.
Freud, S. (1889). Recensione a "L'Ipnotismo" di August Forel. In C. Balducci & A. Ravazzolo (Eds.), *Il Sogno e Scritti su Ipnosi e Suggestione* (2008). Newton Compton Editori.
Freud, S. (1921). Group psychology and the analysis of the ego. In J. Strachey (Ed.), *The standard edition of the complete psychological works of Sigmund Freud* (Volume XVIII, 1949). The Hogarth.
García Carrasco, D., & Aboitiz Cantalapiedra, J. (2016). Effectiveness of motor imagery or mental practice in functional recovery after stroke: A systematic review. *Neurologia (Barcelona, Spain)*, *31*(1), 43–52. 10.1016/J.NRL.2013.02.003
Gerrans, P. (2014). Pathologies of hyperfamiliarity in dreams, delusions and déjà vu. *Frontiers in Psychology*, *5*(article 97), 1–10. 10.3389/fpsyg.2014.00097
Grinder, J., & Bandler, R. (1987). *Trance-formations neuro-linguistic programming and the structure of hypnosis*, A. Connirae (Ed.). Real People Press.

Gruzelier, J. H. (2000). Redefining hypnosis: Theory, methods and integration. *Contemporary Hypnosis*, *17*, 51–70.
Hajek, K. M. (2017). 'A portion of truth': Demarcating the boundaries of scientific hypnotism in late nineteenth-century France. *Notes and Records of the Royal Society of London*, *71*(2), 125–139. 10.1098/rsnr.2017.0010
Hammond, D. C. (2008). Hypnosis as sole anesthesia for major surgeries: Historical & contemporary perspectives. *American Journal of Clinical Hypnosis*, *51*(0002–9157 (Print)), 101–121.
Hilgard, E. R. (1975). The alleviation of pain by hypnosis. *Pain*, *1*(0304–3959 (Print)), 213–231.
Hilgard, E. R. (1977a). *Divided consciousness: Mutiple controls in human thought and action*. Wiley & Sons.
Hilgard, E. R. (1977b). The problem of divided consciousness: A neodissociation interpretation. *Annals of the New York Academy of Sciences*, *296*, 48–59. http://www.ncbi.nlm.nih.gov/pubmed/279254
Hoeft, F., Gabrieli, J. D., Whitfield-Gabrieli, S., Haas, B. W., Bammer, R., Menon, V., & Spiegel, D. (2012). Functional brain basis of hypnotizability. *Archives of General Psychiatry*, *69*(1538–3636 (Electronic)), 1064–1072.
Hull, C. L. (1933). *Hypnosis and suggestibility: An experimental approach*. Appletone-Century.
James, W. (1917). *The varieties of religious experience. A study in human nature* (Kindle edition). Longmans, Green, & Co.
Jensen, M. P., Adachi, T., Tomé-Pires, C., Lee, J., Osman, Z. J., & Miró, J. (2015). Mechanisms of hypnosis: Toward the development of a biopsychosocial model. *International Journal of Clinical and Experimental Hypnosis*, *63*(1), 34–75. 10.1080/00207144.2014.961875
Kihlstrom, J. F. (1998). Dissociations and dissociation theory in hypnosis: Comment on Kirsch and Lynn (1998). *Psychological Bulletin*, *123*(2),186–191. American Psychological Association. 10.1037/0033-2909.123.2.186
Kihlstrom, J. F. (2001). Hypnosis in surgery: Efficacy, specificity, and utility. In *Institute for the Study of Healthcare Organizations & Transactions* (pp. 1–9). http://socrates.berkeley.edu/~kihlstrm/ISHOTWeb/hypnosis_pain_utility.htm
Kihlstrom, J. F. (2002). Mesmer, the Franklin Commission, and hypnosis: A counterfactual essay. *The International Journal of Clinical and Experimental Hypnosis*, *50*(0020–7144 (Print)), 407–419.
Kihlstrom, J. F. (2003). The fox, the hedgehog, and hypnosis. *The International Journal of Clinical and Experimental Hypnosis*, *51*(2), 166–189. 10.1076/iceh.51.2.166.14611
Kirsch, I., & Lynn, S. J. (1998). Dissociation theories of hypnosis. *Psychological Bulletin*, *123*(0033–2909 (Print)), 100–115.
Landry, M., Lifshitz, M., & Raz, A. (2017). Brain correlates of hypnosis: A systematic review and meta-analytic exploration. *Neuroscience & Biobehavioral Reviews*, *81*(1873–7528 (Electronic)), 75–98.
Laurence, J. R., Perry, C., & Kihlstrom, J. (1983). "Hidden observer" phenomena in hypnosis: An experimental creation? *Journal of Personality & Social Psychology*, *44*(0022–3514), 163–169.
Ludwig, A. M. (1966). Altered states of consciousness. *Archives of General Psychiatry*, *15*(0003–990X (Print)), 225–234.
Mach, E. (1897). *Popular scientific lectures*. The Open Court Publisching Co.
Melzack, R. (2001). Pain and the neuromatrix in the brain. *Journal of Dental Education*, *65*(0022–0337 (Print)), 1378–1382.
Merli, P. G., Missiroli, G. F., & Pozzi, G. (1974). Electron interferometry with the Elmiskop 101 electron microscope. *Journal of Physics E: Scientific Instruments*, 7(9), 729–732. 10.1088/0022-3735/7/9/016
Milling, L. S., Coursen, E. L., Shores, J. S., & Waszkiewicz, J. A. (2010). The predictive utility of hypnotizability: The change in suggestibility produced by hypnosis. *Journal of Consulting and Clinical Psychology*, *78*(1939–2117 (Electronic)), 126–130.
Montgomery, G. H., Schnur, J. B., & David, D. (2011). The impact of hypnotic suggestibility in clinical care settings. *The International Journal of Clinical and Experimental Hypnosis*, *59*(1744–5183 (Electronic)), 294–309.
Morstyn, R. (1989). Quantum metaphors in deep psychotherapy. *Australian and New Zealand Journal of Psychiatry*, *23*(4), 483–490. 10.3109/00048678909062615

Orrell, D. (2018). *Quantum economics: The new science of money*. Icon Books.
Perlovsky, L. (2013). Learning in brain and machine-complexity, Godel, Aristotle. *Frontiers in Neurorobotics*, 7(1662–5218 (Linking)), 23.
Pintar, J., & Lynn, S. J. (2009). *Hypnosis: A brief history*. John Wiley & Sons, Ltd.
Popper, K. R. (1972). *Objective knowledge*. Oxford University Press.
Popper, K. (2012). *The world of parmenides. Essays on the presocratic enlightenment*, A. F. Petersen (Ed.), 2nd ed. Routledge Classics.
Popper, K. R., Lindahl, B. I., & Arhem, P. (1993). A discussion of the mind-brain problem. *Theoretical Medicine*, *14*(0167–9902 (Print)), 167–180. 10.1007/BF00997274
Priest, G. (1998). What is so bad about contradictions? *Journal of Philosophy*, *95*(8), 410–426. http://www.jstor.org/stable/2564636
Revonsuo, A., Kallio, S., & Sikka, P. (2009). What is an altered state of consciousness? *Philosophical Psychology*, *22*(2), 187–204. 10.1080/09515080902802850
Robson, B. (2020). Extension of the quantum universal exchange language to precision medicine and drug lead discovery. Preliminary example studies using the mitochondrial genome. *Computers in Biology and Medicine*, *117*, 1–30. 10.1016/J.COMPBIOMED.2020.103621
Sarbin, T. R. (2005). Reflections on some unresolved issues in hypnosis. *The International Journal of Clinical and Experimental Hypnosis*, *53*(0020–7144 (Print)), 119–134.
Schmit, D. T. (2010). The mesmerists inquire about "Oriental mind powers": West meets East in the search for the universal trance. *Journal of the History of the Behavioral Sciences*, *46*(1520–6696 (Electronic)), 1–26.
Spanos, N. P., & Hewitt, E. C. (1980). The hidden observer in hypnotic analgesia: Discovery or experimental creation? *Journal of Personality & Social Psychology*, *39*(0022–3514 (Print)), 1201–1204.
Spiegel, H., & Spiegel, D. (2004). *Trance and Treatment* (2nd edition). American Psychiatric Association Publishing.
Sugarman, L. I. (2021). Leaving hypnosis behind? *The American Journal of Clinical Hypnosis*, *64*(2), 139–156. 10.1080/00029157.2021.1935686
Tasso, A. F., & Perez, N. A. (2008). Parsing everyday suggestibility: What does it tells us about hypnosis? In M. R. Nash & A. J. Barnier (Eds.), *The Oxford handbook of hypnosis* (Issue 11, pp. 283–309). Oxford University Press.
Testoni, I., Facco, E., Ronconi, L., Alemanno, F., & D'Amico, M. (2020). The role of flexibility and other factors associated with hypnotizability: Second step towards its definition. *Contemporary Hypnosis & Integrative Therapy*, *34*(1), 7–24.
Thomas, N. J. T. (2010). Supplement to mental imagery. European responses: Jaensch, Freud, and Gestalt psychology. *Stanford encyclopedia of philosophy*. Stanford University. http://plato.stanford.edu/entries/mental-imagery/european-responses.html (pp. 1–3).
Thomas, N. J. T. (2019). Mental imagery. In *Stanford encyclopedia of philosophy* (pp. 1–345). https://plato.stanford.edu/archives/sum2019/entries/mental-imagery/
Thompson, T., Terhune, D. B., Oram, C., Sharangparni, J., Rouf, R., Solmi, M., Veronese, N., & Stubbs, B. (2019). The effectiveness of hypnosis for pain relief: A systematic review and meta-analysis of 85 controlled experimental trials. *Neuroscience and Biobehavioral Reviews*, *99*, 298–310. Elsevier Ltd. 10.1016/j.neubiorev.2019.02.013
Tourette de la, G. (1887). *L'hypnotisme et les états analogues au point de vue médico-légal*. K. Plon.
Vaitl, D., Birbaumer, N., Gruzelier, J., Jamieson, G. A., Kotchoubey, B., Kubler, A., Lehmann, D., Miltner, W. H., Ott, U., Putz, P., Sammer, G., Strauch, I., Strehl, U., Wackermann, J., & Weiss, T. (2005). Psychobiology of altered states of consciousness. *The Psychological Bulletin 131*(0033–2909), 98–127.
West, G. B. (1972). Aspirin and the prostaglandins. *The Chemist and Druggist*, *198*, 196–197. https://pubmed.ncbi.nlm.nih.gov/12262561/
Yang, M. C. (2017). *Existential psychology and the way of Tao*. Routledge.

3

SUGGESTIBILITY AND HYPNOTIZABILITY MEASURES OF HYPNOSIS AND HYPNOTIZABILITY

Burkhard Peter

MEG-Stiftung.de, Munich, Germany; www.Burkhard-Peter.de

Introduction

As founding president of the Milton Erickson Society for Clinical Hypnosis Germany (MEG), I have been involved with clinical hypnosis/hypnotherapy in therapeutic application and training since 1978. As organizer of hypnosis congresses and editor of a German-language hypnosis journal since 1984, as well as author of books and articles on hypnosis, I follow with concern the controversial international discourse on the meaning and definition of hypnosis and hypnotherapy. Other therapeutic procedures such as cognitive behavioral therapy have adopted methods and techniques of hypnosis, often without explaining them or their background as genuinely hypnotic. With such erosion, what is left for hypnosis itself? I think we should concentrate again, especially in clinical research and therapy, on what constitutes the essence of hypnosis. This includes, among other things, hypnotizability scales.

The experimental-scientific literature on suggestibility and hypnotizability is almost impossible to survey. The following presentation can only deal with a very small part of this extensive field.

First, some basic preliminary remarks and definitions: people differ in many ways, also in different abilities like intelligence or musicality. It would be strange if they did not also differ in suggestibility and hypnotizability.

Hypnotizability is defined here as the inherent, *intra*-individual ability of a person to engage in the experience of hypnotic phenomena or to demonstrate them after a hypnosis induction. *Hypnotic suggestibility* is understood as the *inter*-individual ability to demonstrate this intra-individual ability in response to a suggestive communication. *Suggestion* is the name given to a communication when it prompts a behavior (e.g., arm-levitation) or experience (e.g., hallucination) that is not or cannot usually be realized voluntarily in everyday life – as opposed to an *instruction* that can be followed arbitrarily (Weitzenhoffer, 1974).

Franz Anton Mesmer (1775, p. 28) and some of his followers noted interindividual differences in susceptibility to animal magnetism. Bernheim (1888, p. 20) reported figures of 1,011 patients of his medical colleague Liébeault, and Hilgard (1965, p. 75) the figures

DOI: 10.4324/9781003449126-6

of 19,534 patients of another 14 hypnotic practitioners of the 19th century, whose percentage distributions regarding hypnotizability are similar to those of today. However, experimental investigation and systematic observation of suggestibility and hypnotizability began only in the previous century with Hull (1933), Friedlander & Sarbin (1938), Barber (1964), and Hilgard et al. (1961).

Theory

The terms suggestibility and hypnotizability are often used synonymously, but they do not denote the same. The term suggestibility must also be differentiated because it refers to quite different forms of response, of which hypnotic suggestibility is only one, namely suggestibility following hypnosis induction, also referred to as hypnotizability. In a survey conducted by Christensen (2005), the majority decided to primarily use the term "hypnotizability". However, this consensus was preceded by decades of discourse about the proper understanding of suggestion and hypnosis or suggestibility and hypnotizability.

Non-Hypnotic Suggestibility

Suggestibility in general is the ability to react spontaneously to a suggestive communication without having checked its content for correctness or with regard to possible alternatives. Such general suggestions do not require hypnosis to be effective. This non-hypnotic, imaginative, or waking suggestibility also includes sensory and interrogative suggestibility and placebo responses. One aspect of nonhypnotic suggestibility concerns people in situations of absolute personal helplessness in which they are dependent on others. Prototypical of such situations of heightened suggestibility are many medical situations. Recently, Ernil Hansen has made a point of emphasizing the importance of this aspect of medical hypnosis or medical communication (Nowak et al., 2020).

Hypnotic Suggestibility

At the end of the 19th century, suggestibility had been closely associated with hypnosis. Hippolyte Bernheim had invented the suggestion-theory of hypnosis. He stated that a more or less naturally existing suggestibility could be enhanced by hypnosis, because in the state of hypnosis the controlling consciousness was switched off, so that the suggestions were accepted and carried out "in an unconscious manner with evasion of volitional activity" (Bernheim, 1888, p. 125). This idea of "hypnotic suggestibility" as kind of "hyper-suggestibility" was followed by Clark Hull and others: "The only thing which seems to characterize hypnosis as such and which gives any justification for the practice of calling it a 'state' is its generalized hyper-suggestibility" (Hull, 1933, p. 391).

Hypnotizability

As waking suggestibility correlates with hypnotic suggestibility quite well Braffman and Kirsch (1999) used a regression analysis to separate both of them: 29% of subjects showed no change after hypnosis induction, 46% showed an increase, and 25% showed a decrease in suggestibility. These data were – and still are – frequently used to argue that hypnosis induction does not significantly increase existing suggestibility – and that hypnosis induction can therefore be dispensed with. However, it is rarely pointed out that an increase in almost 50% of the subjects was found. Obviously, for non-hypnotizable persons, a hypnosis induction has no effect. For highly hypnotizable persons, it probably has a large effect.

Weitzenhoffer (1980a) had already pointed out that the term hypnotizability could not be used to refer to the ability to respond to suggestions, but only to the ability to achieve a hypnotic state. The first hypnotizability scale by Friedlander and Sarbin (1938), on which the Stanford scales by Weitzenhoffer and Hilgard (1959) were based, was called "Scale for measuring hypnotic depth". Because "depth of hypnosis" could also be understood as the ability in execution of increasingly difficult hypnotic tasks, this would correspond to the definition given at the beginning: hypnotizability is the inherent, intra-individual capacity of a person to engage in or demonstrate the experience of hypnotic phenomena following a hypnosis induction.

Because human beings are social – and if one disregards cases of auto-hypnosis – it is difficult to imagine hypnosis taking place entirely without suggestion in practice, for already Bernheim (1888, p. 190) had stated: "The sick person is put to sleep by suggestion, by having the idea of sleep impressed upon his brain; he is now also treated by suggestion, by having the idea of cure imposed upon his brain". This sentence points to the interpersonal aspect of hypnotic suggestibility. At least the induction of hypnosis requires verbal instructions, which by definition are called "suggestions" because they refer to involuntary processes (Peter, 1996).

However, even after hypnosis induction, further suggestions are given to alter physiology, sensory, emotion, cognition, and behavior. So, can hypnosis be measured as a pure state of consciousness, and can the communicative-interactive act that is suggestion be disregarded? This approach has been pursued by only a few since the beginning of the 21st century, for example by a Finnish-Swedish group of researchers (Tuominen et al., 2021). McGeown et al. (2009, p. 848) have shown "a distinctive and unique pattern" in form of deactivation of anterior parts of the default mode network (DMN). Lipari et al. (2012) also addressed this question by inducing "pure hypnosis" in a hypnotic virtuoso and giving no other suggestions. Replications of these findings are, to my knowledge, still pending. (For further brain-physiological studies, see Section 2 of this book.)

The hope to be able to unambiguously determine hypnotizability on the basis of identifiable brain states has thus not yet been fulfilled and the ambiguities remain. This is evident, for example, in the revised version of a definition of hypnosis (Elkins et al., 2015, p. 6) and in the attempt at a consensus statement by Kirsch et al. (2011): proponents of a "narrow definition" see the induction of hypnosis as a prerequisite for speaking of hypnosis and hypnotizability. Others still prefer a "broader definition" in which a preceding hypnosis induction or the presence of a hypnotic state is negligible. The seeds for such an argumentation had already been sown by Bernheim with the provocative sentence *"Il n'y a pas d'hypnotisme, il n'y a que de la suggestibilité"* ("There is no hypnotism, there is only suggestion") (Bernheim, 1917, p. 47). Weitzenhoffer (1980b, p. 252) had tried to set the record straight – Bernheim "clearly did not mean by this that he was rejecting the existence of hypnosis as a state" – but the idea that a formal induction ritual to produce a state of hypnosis was negligible still has its adherents today.

On the basis of the two terms, suggestibility and hypnotizability, one could determine the demarcation line that divided the community of hypnosis researchers from the 1960s on into two camps: the so-called state theorists (e.g., Ernest Hilgard, 1991) concentrated on proving hypnosis as a special state of consciousness. They thus placed emphasis on the aspect of hypnotizability. This was contradicted by the social-psychologically or later the sociocognitively oriented theorists (Lynn & Sivec, 1992): they argued that it is not the nonexistent *special* state of hypnosis that is responsible for the hypnotic phenomena exhibited, but rather the particular internal and external "suggestive" conditions such as task motivation, expectation, or context, and the general sociocultural "response set" (Kirsch, 2001) in which the suggestions are embedded. This extreme position has only recently been revised, conceding on the basis of brain-physiological data the obvious differences in hypnotizability. With this recognition, sociocognitive theorists now "contend that hypnosis produces genuine changes in consciousness"; hypnosis however should not be considered as "a special state or 'trance' somehow divorced from the operations of day-to-day consciousness" (Lynn et al., 2015, p. 315).

Milton H. Erickson

Outside of this academic discourse, but based on vast hypnotherapeutic experience, is Milton H. Erickson's position, which could be located across the continuum between suggestion and hypnosis or suggestibility and hypnotizability, i.e., among both social psychologists and consciousness researchers. Lankton (2020, p. 4) reports that Erickson always explained hypnosis to him as a *state*. This could place him in the camp of the state theorists. If the traditional view was to understand hypnosis as a kind of "sedative for consciousness" (Peter, 2009) and to use it to achieve a state of hyper-suggestibility that would make it easier for the hypnotist to succeed with his/her suggestions, Erickson's understanding of the function of hypnosis diverged decidedly from this. His attention was directed to the particular intra-individual conditions of the patient. By this, however, he meant not only cognitive sets of expectations and attitudes as the sociocognitive theorists but also the "unconscious resources" of a person that could be actualized with the help of hypnosis. For this purpose, he made use of the metaphor of the "unconscious as therapeutic tertium" (Peter, 2002) to shift the locus of control or self-efficacy expectation from an external hypnotherapist back into the patient. Erickson became known especially for the multitude of creative, so-called indirect induction and suggestion techniques (Zeig, 1995), with which he made it possible for even the many medium hypnotizables to experience hypnosis. The application of principles for the "construction of reality" (Peter, 2015b) describes only a very small part of his hypnotherapeutic skills. However, he thus shifted the focus from the hypnotizability of the patient to the skills of the hypnotherapist. This utilization approach is one of the core elements of Ericksonian hypnotherapy (Short, 2021) which does not refer to the hypnotizability of patients, but to the hypnotizing ability of hypnotherapists. With regard to hypnotizability of the patient, only a few explicit statements can be summarized according to Havens (1985) as follows: hypnosis is a normal and general experience and can be evoked in practically all people, if only the circumstances are adequate and a skilled hypnotherapist carries out the appropriate inductions. With this opinion, Erickson goes far beyond what social psychologists have advocated, namely that hypnotizability is trainable.

Enacting and Vivid Imagining or: Is Hypnotizability Modifiable?

An explicit program to modify hypnotizability was developed by Spanos (1986), the Carleton Skills Training Program (CSTP). Subjects learn that hypnotic responding is an active process. They are not passively waiting for something to happen on its own. With the CSTP, progress in hypnotizability was achieved, but only to a limited extent (Gorassini & Spanos, 1986), which was later explained by Lynn et al. (2015, p. 323) with brain-physiological factors. Woody et al. (1997) were able to demonstrate gains only for easier hypnotic phenomena, but not for more difficult ones. Kihlstrom (2008, p. 31) does not attribute these increases to hypnotizability as genuine ability, but suspects simple compliance factors. Laurence et al. (2008, p. 234f) distinguish between "natural" and "trained" high-suggestibles. "Natural" high-suggestibles differ from these "trained" ones in that they exhibit the hypnotic phenomena spontaneously, i.e., without prior training, and report complete involuntariness, without any action on their part. This spontaneous experience of involuntariness is called the "classical suggestion effect" by Weitzenhoffer (1974) and is referred to as a reduction of the sense of agency (Polito et al., 2015).

Is There One Hypnotizability or Several?

It was long assumed that hypnotizability was a unitary construct and as such could be measured with the known scales. Various factor analyses showed that the classic Stanford and Harvard scales did not contain a single factor, but up to three (Hilgard, 1965, p. 218f; Piesbergen & Peter, 2006). These three factors have often been referred to as "direct-motor" (e.g., head falling), "challenging-motor" (e.g., arm immobilization), and "perceptual-cognitive" (e.g., hallucination of a fly). Woody et al. (2005), identified a fourth factor "posthypnotic amnesia", a purely "cognitive" factor. From the correlations of these four factors, they inferred the presence of a latent underlying general factor "hypnotizability". This multicomponent theory of hypnosis is discussed in summary by Sadler and Woody (2021). The result of Zahedi and Sommer (2022) is in the same direction. Structural equation modeling of latent factors revealed that the challenging-motor factor predicted the other two secondary factors, suggesting that challenging-motor suggestions (e.g., you can no longer move your arm) may require more basic processes than the other types of suggestions.

The fact that challenging-motor tasks appear to be quite central to the HGSHS:A for measuring hypnotizability was also demonstrated by Riegel et al. (2021). From the original version of the HGSHS:A, they distilled, via factor analysis, a shortened version containing only the five challenging-motor tasks of the original version with a high loading on this one factor. The reliability of this shortened version HGSHS-5, which takes only 30 minutes to complete, is comparable to the original version, which is twice as long, and the correlation of both versions with each other is high. It is interesting to note that the five challenging-motor tasks of this short version measure a person's basic willingness to set aside his/her everyday "I", to give up the normal sense of agency (Polito et al., 2015), and to allow another "author" access, at least to control the body and motor behavior. This corresponds to Weitzenhoffer's (1974) "classical suggestion effect" and is the "minimal phenomenal selfhood (MPS)" of a person. MPS is "the conscious experience *of being a self* [...] capable of global self-control and attention, possessing a body and a location in space and time" (Blanke & Metzinger, 2009, p. 7). In a state-like understanding of the nature of hypnosis, at least this MPS should be changed in order for someone to feel hypnotized (Peter, 2015c). The change in selfhood is tested by these five challenge items of the HGSHS-5.

The question of whether there is only one hypnotizability or several was also raised by Peter (2015d), and systematically checked later on (Peter & Roberts, 2022): in 66 norming tests, of a total of 33,338 subjects, 58.57% were college and university students, and of these the majority were psychology students. Because 83.08% of these subjects had been informed in advance that they were to participate in a hypnosis study, self-selection bias must be assumed in addition to sampling bias. It is therefore not unreasonable to assume that because of the non-representativeness of the normalization samples, the hypnotizability "out there" in the general population – among farmers, workers, but also bankers, engineers, or lawyers – may show a quite different distribution pattern than the generally accepted "normal distribution" established in previous studies, which refers mainly to the well-educated, economically well-off, and mostly humanistically oriented middle class. Ernil Hansen has as yet unpublished data from hospital patients that show a clearly left-skewed distribution.[1] In contrast, data from hypnosis using dentists show a clearly right-skewed distribution (Wolf et al., 2022). Thus, despite the many studies, our knowledge of hypnotizability is still incomplete.

Hypnotizability and Other Personality Variables

Children's hypnotizability is particularly high between 9 and 12 years and slowly decreases with age, showing an inverted U-shape; females often scored higher than males (Riegel et al., 2021). Twin studies showed that hypnotizability has a heritable component (Morgan, 1973), as does high retest reliability over a period of up to 25 years (Piccione et al., 1989). This suggests a biological basis for hypnotizability. In light of the remaining ambiguities about the "true nature" of hypnotizability, the following results about whether hypnotizability is related to intelligence or other personality variables should be viewed with caution. These results have long been inconsistent. At least for intelligence, recent data suggest a correlation with hypnotizability that is moderated by the gender variable: in women, intelligence correlates with hypnotizability, but not in men (Geiger et al., 2014). At least moderate correlative relationships could be found with personality traits that are already in the conceptual shadow of hypnosis or have been developed from it such as "absorption" (Tellegen & Atkinson, 1974), "imaginative involvement" (J. R. Hilgard, 1970), "fantasy proneness" (Wilson & Barber, 1982), "imagery vividness" (Terhune & Oakley, 2020), "emotional contagion" (Cardeña et al., 2009), and "self-transcendence" (Cardeña & Terhune, 2008). However, attempts to relate hypnotizability to personality traits that are independent of hypnosis, such as the "Big Five" (Costa & McCrae, 1992), have long proved not very fruitful (Nordenstrom et al., 2002). It was not until later that Milling et al. (2013) were able to demonstrate a relationship between hypnotizability and openness to experience. However, this trait is not specific to hypnosis, as higher scores have also been found in studies of therapists with a psychodynamic orientation (as opposed to a cognitive-behavioral orientation; Taubner et al., 2014).

Terhune et al. (2011) found two distinguishable groups among high hypnotizables, a "dissociative" and an "imaginative" subtype: highly hypnotizable/highly dissociative subjects showed a greater degree of involuntariness in hypnosis, more dissociative symptoms, and reported stressful life events more often than highly hypnotizable/lowly dissociative subjects; the latter had better visual imaginative abilities.

Another possible link is that between hypnotizability and schizotypy. Jamieson and Gruzelier (2001) were the first to report associations, among others Polito et al. (2015) confirm them. Our research group also found associations with schizotypy, but in the studies to date, first among individuals *interested in hypnosis* in general, and specifically among psychotherapists and dentists using hypnosis (Peter & Böbel, 2020; Wolf et al., 2022). This concerns the personality variables of those persons who use hypnosis, i.e., the hypnotizing ability.

The Person of the Hypnotherapist

At the time of orthodox mesmerism (from 1775) and romantic somnambulism (until about 1820) (Gauld, 1992; Peter, 2015a), the person of the magnetizer was crucial, because only he could serve as an accumulator for the energy of animal magnetism, and only he possessed the ability to transfer it to other persons via the "magnetic rapport".

It took a long time for serious consideration to be given again to this hypnotherapist variable, first under the psychoanalytic notion of countertransference and later as theoretical considerations (Peter & Revenstorf, 2018b). The first investigation of German-speaking hypnotherapists (Peter et al., 2012a) showed a personality profile which differed significantly from the norm and revealed a characteristic trait that consistently appeared in follow-up studies whenever the label hypnosis or hypnotherapy was mentioned in the acquisition of subjects, and was absent when any reference to hypnosis was intentionally avoided. An initial summary of the research series (Peter & Böbel, 2020) and further studies (Peter et al., 2018; Peter & Wolf, 2022; Wolf et al., 2022) showed that hypnosis practitioners had high scores in the personality style intuitive/schizotypal. Peter (2015d) had coined the term *homo hypnoticus* referring to "hypnophiles", i.e., people who are interested in hypnosis in general; these primarily include hypnotherapists or all those who use hypnosis professionally. Schizotypy as a main characteristic, however, does not yet allow any statement about the hypnotizing ability of these persons, i.e., about how well these professionals can use hypnosis. By which abilities and skills "hypno-shrinks" are characterized, whether and how they can be trained, still has to be researched. So far, we can only say that people who are generally interested in hypnosis show high scores on the personality style schizotypy. Furthermore, there is preliminary evidence that the degree of schizotypy correlates with the level of hypnotizability (Peter & Böbel, 2020, p. 349). And, as noted above, the distribution of hypnotizability among hypnophilic professionals is clearly right skewed, i.e., there are few low-hypnotizables but many medium- and even more high-hypnotizables among them (Wolf et al., 2022). For the scientific recognition of hypnosis and hypnotherapy, unfortunately, this personality trait is rather problematic. The four items with which this style is surveyed are:

- I believe others sometimes feel my emotions even if they are far away.
- I sometimes feel the presence of a far-away person, as if he or she were really standing next to me.
- I believe in thought transfer via psychic means.
- There are supernatural forces.

Science-oriented people such as students of STEM subjects and most professionals in the medical and human sciences deny these statements and therefore have low scores in the personality style schizotypy (Bochter et al., 2014; Wolf et al., 2022). Ominous-intuitive abilities, as expressed in the first two statements, may well be useful for hypnosis and hypnotherapy (c.f. Varga & Kekecs, 2014). However, they can also degenerate into esoteric extremes via the last two statements and then scare off sober scientists. This is not beneficial for the scientific recognition of hypnosis and hypnotherapy. Against this background, the intensive and persistent efforts of the so-called non-state hypnosis researchers to keep hypnosis away from such esoteric speculations and to give it a solid place in social and cognitive psychology are well understandable.

Measurement

There are several instruments for measuring non-hypnotic suggestibility (Gheorghiu et al., 1989). In the following, only the measurement of hypnotic suggestibility or hypnotizability is of interest. Barely used is the Carleton University Responsiveness to Suggestion Scale (CURSS) by Nicholas Spanos et al. (1983) and the Hypnotic Induction Profile (HIP) by Herbert Spiegel et al. (1976). Other, less frequently used scales are also not discussed in detail such as the Revised Stanford Profile Scales of Hypnotic Susceptibility: Forms I and II (Weitzenhoffer & Hilgard, 1967) or the Phenomenology of Consciousness-Hypnotic Assessment Procedure (PCI-HAP) (Pekala, 1995), although the PCI is occasionally used in research, but not in hypnotherapeutic practice. Omitted are also hypnotizability tests for children such as Children´s Hypnotic Susceptibility Scale by London (1963) or The Stanford Hypnotic Clinical Scale for Children by Morgan and Hilgard (1978). These are discussed in detail in the textbook by Kohen and Olness (2022). Similar to the assessment of intelligence or musicality, hypnotizability is measured by operationalizing hypnotic tasks that are hypnotic phenomena of increasing difficulty. The degree of hypnotizability is calculated by adding up single scores. For example, on a 12-point scale, 0–4 is considered being low-hypnotizable, 5–8 medium-hypnotizable, and 9–12 high-hypnotizable.

Measurement of Hypnosis Depth

In the form of hypnotizability discussed above as "depth of hypnosis", it is quite relevant not only in research but also for hypnotherapeutic practice to determine it because it may be crucial for the patient to experience himself as hypnotized, which in turn may influence his/her expectation (Kirsch, 2001). Field's (1965) Inventory Scale of Hypnosis Depth has long been available for this depth measurement. For everyday hypnotherapeutic practice, however, no explicit measurement needs to be made, because here the patient's general subjective expression is crucial.

Measurement of "Hypnotic" Imagination: The Creative Imagination Scale

The Creative Imagination Scale (CIS) (Barber & Wilson, 1978) can be applied in clinical as well as experimental contexts, in individual or group settings. It is found in studies or even in practices whenever the word "hypnosis" is to be avoided or replaced by "imagination". Barber and his associates found in various studies that "task-motivational instructions" were as effective as "hypnotic suggestions". Although the CIS contains some of the same and some similar tasks as the Stanford and Harvard scales discussed below, it is explicitly called an imagination scale. Accordingly, there are no introductory suggestions for hypnosis induction, but rather a very brief instruction to focus on the task.

Measurement of Hypnotizability I: The Stanford Hypnotic Susceptibility Scales for Individual Testing

The most commonly used hypnotizability measurement instruments to date trace back to the original Stanford Hypnotic Susceptibility Scale, Forms A and B (SHSS:A, B) (Weitzenhoffer & Hilgard, 1959) and Form C (SHSS:C) (Weitzenhoffer & Hilgard, 1962).

They start with easier ideomotor tasks such as "arm lowering" or "moving hands apart" which are passed by about 90%. The following motor challenge tasks of SHSS:C are more difficult and correspond to "loss of voluntary control" (Piesbergen & Peter, 2006). Similarly difficult are the easier olfactory sweet/sour hallucination and the dream and age regression items. Even more difficult is the amnesia item as well as the negative-hallucinatory (not smelling, not seeing) and the positive-hallucinatory tasks (hearing something that is not audible), which are only passed by a few.

Measurement of Hypnotizability II: The Harvard and Walterloo-Stanford Scales of Hypnotic Susceptibility for Group Testing

For group testing, the Harvard Group Scale of Hypnotic Susceptibility, Form A (HGSHS:A) (Shor & Orne, 1962) was developed from the SHSS:A, the Waterloo-Stanford Group Scale of Hypnotic Susceptibility, Form C (WSGC) (Bowers, 1998) from the SHSS:C. The most translated and normed scale in other languages worldwide is the HGSHS (with at least 20 norming studies, followed by the SHSS:C with at least 11 norming studies) (Peter & Roberts, 2022). In WSGC, the ammonia item of the SHSS:C has been replaced by a posthypnotic suggestion. The HGSHS also contains 12 items, but only one is from the perceptual domain (perception of a fly) and two are from the cognitive domain (posthypnotic suggestion and amnesia). All other items of the HGSHS originate from the motor-kinesthetic domain. Because the original HGSHS takes very long to administer, Riegel et al. (2021), via factor analysis, proposed a shortened version HGSHS-5 containing only the five motor challenging tasks and reduces the administration time to 30 minutes.

These scales have been criticized for some disadvantages: their scoring is dichotomous with "fulfilled" or "not fulfilled" and does not allow intermediate scores, and they, with the exception of HGSHS-5, take more than one hour to complete. The SHSS:C also includes an unpleasant task with the ammonia item and a problematic task with the age regression item.

Measurement of Hypnotizability III: The Elkins Hypnotizability Scale

As a more recent scale, the Elkins Hypnotizability Scale (EHS) (Elkins, 2014) sought to compensate for these drawbacks. Instead of the ammonia and age regression items, it has suggestions for flower garden and rose scent, so performance is experienced as distinctly positive. Unlike the other scales, whose items are not strictly presented by difficulty, in the EHS the individual tasks are actually ordered by difficulty and well balanced in terms of item category from the easier motor to various sensory-cognitive items to the purely cognitive amnesia item. The scoring is not dichotomous but ordinal, i.e., for most items both behavioral reactions and subjective experiences are asked. For example, it is asked whether the heaviness (or lightness) of the arm was not only subjectively felt, but whether the arm was actually also cataleptic (or actually went up), whether the scent of roses was only vaguely imagined or really hallucinated. Thus, the subjective sensation (e.g., of lightness in the arm) is also counted, although only with one point; the objective behavioral response of hand levitation counts with 2 points, and 3 points are awarded if the elbow also lifts involuntarily. The psychometric criteria of the EHS (similar to those of the Stanford/Harvard scales) are very good.

The Introductory Hypnosis Inductions

T.X. Barber's CIS does not intend to induce a state of hypnosis in order to test "hypnotic" phenomena thereafter but it tests subjects' compliance to engage in imagining such phenomena. Thus, instead of first presenting suggestions to induce hypnosis for about 20 minutes as in the SHSS and HGSHS, the CIS begins immediately after a very brief instruction to focus on the task.

In contrast, the original hypnosis induction texts of the Stanford scales (SHSS:A, B, C) and their group versions WSGC or HGSHS, and HGSHS-5 are very detailed and last 15–20 minutes. The key words in these texts are relaxation and sleep, which are associatively linked with the term hypnosis and thus are supposed to introduce the state of hypnosis. With these time-consuming suggestions about relaxation and sleep, the traditional reference in the understanding of hypnosis as a kind of sleep is very clearly established.

The hypnosis induction of the EHS is not quite as short as the task-based instruction of the CIS, but it is also not as long as in the Stanford/Harvard scales; this is one of the reasons why the EHS takes only about 25 minutes to complete. In its hypnosis induction, terms for sleeping are missing; instead, the suggestions are primarily directed to a systematic relaxation of all muscles of the body with hints that this leads to a state of hypnosis. As a theoretical background of Elkins' EHS, it can be assumed that increasing muscular relaxation changes proprioception so that the "body ego" increasingly dissolves and hereby also the "minimal phenomenal selfhood (MPS)" of a person (Blanke & Metzinger, 2009). This, in turn, alters authorship or sense of agency.

If Braffman and Kirsch (1999) found an increase in hypnotizability in almost 50% of the subjects after a hypnosis induction, what is the reason of not performing a hypnosis induction? The answer follows from the tenor of what has been said so far: through a hypnosis induction, a person is to be guided to construct an "alternative reality" (Peter, 2015b; Peter, 2015c): the person is supposed to temporarily take leave of his/her current reality orientation, to leave his/her present-oriented and location-based reality, which he/she usually perceives with awake senses, consciously recognizes, and in which he/she acts in the knowledge of her own authorship (sense of agency). An explicit hypnosis induction leads to a state of motor restriction and sensory deprivation as an aid or even a prerequisite for the temporary relaxation of the general reality orientation. Motor restriction and sensory deprivation are prerequisites for classical conditioning à la Pavlov, i.e., learning outside conscious or voluntary control. This is an excellent concern of hypnotherapy – in contrast to behavior therapy, for example – and should therefore not be neglected.

Imagination or Hallucination?

With regard to hypnosis, one can distinguish between imagination and hallucination using the criterion of "authorship" or "sense of agency" (Peter, 1994; Peter, 2015c). Such a distinction is useful because it is the only way to distinguish hypnotherapy from other psychotherapeutic methods such as cognitive behavior therapy, which also make extensive use of imaginations without calling this "hypnotic" or inducing hypnosis specifically for this purpose. In imagination, strictly speaking, there is still an acting "I" or an active author ("I" imagine), and the imagination has a lesser or no reality character as in hallucination, where the "I" is passive or receptive or the authorship/agency feeling has disappeared ("it" happens) and the hallucinated object has the character of "verisimilitude". Of course, an imagination can turn into a hallucination and the experience then has "hypnotic" qualities. Whether and under which conditions this may happen is still open to research. If, in the sense of the definitional distinction between imagination and hallucination above, one can understand CIS as a measuring instrument for the imaginative capacity of an active author and the Stanford/Harvard scales as a measuring instrument for involuntariness (Weitzenhoffer's "classical suggestion effect"), then the EHS would stand in between and would cover the whole range of what is broadly understood by hypnosis today.

Phenomena of Identity Delusion

In none of the existing instruments for measuring hypnotizability tasks on phenomena of identity delusions are included. These are occasionally shown in stage hypnosis. Identity delusions have been intensively researched by the Australian research group of Barnier, Connors, and Cox (Connors et al., 2014). These are hypnotic analogues of clinical symptoms of illusions found in psychopathology, in neurological or psychotic disorders. Because they are produced by hypnosis, such phenomena are temporary and reversible and may contribute to the understanding of such disorders. However, when they are elicited in stage hypnosis without selecting participants according to criteria of contraindication (Revenstorf & Peter, 2023), significant problems can arise (Kleinhauz et al., 1984; Peter, in press).

Meaning and Purpose of Hypnotizability Testing

Frankel (1978, p. 210) cited several reasons for measuring hypnotizability, especially in the clinical context. The first reason, he said, is "meaningful communication" among ourselves, the researchers and clinicians – so that we know what we are talking about when we use the term hypnosis. Unfortunately, our community is still a long way from this – if only in the internal dialogue. In the external dialogue with professionals of other disciplines and especially other psychotherapeutic approaches, the dissent makes the positioning of hypnosis much more difficult. Today, there are well-established techniques of relaxation such as progressive muscle relaxation or autogenic training, as well as well-known methods of imagination that are extensively used by recognized behavior therapy and psychodynamic approaches. If hypnosis is nothing more than these techniques, its *raison d'être* is at stake. Then, we find ourselves in the same situation as Mesmer in 1784, when two scientific commissions proved to him that the demonstrated phenomena had nothing to do with the animal magnetism he claimed, but were simply the result of imagination (and imitation) – and thus scientifically worthless as well as therapeutically useless. Hypnotizability tests help to prove that the effects in clinical studies are due to hypnosis. The same is true for hypnotherapeutic practice.

Note

1 Data obtained using the HGSHS-5 (Riegel et al., 2021) are available from 275 of the 385 patients in the multicenter study by Nowak et al. (2022): 118 scored 0, 33 scored 1, 33 scored 2, 34 scored 3, 35 scored 4, and 23 scored 5 on the HGSHS 5:G (Riegel et al., 2021); i.e., 43% of patients were not hypnotizable at all and only 8% were very highly hypnotizable (data kindly provided by Ernil Hansen, 2022).

References

Barber, T. X. (1964). Hypnotizability, suggestibility, and personality: V. A critical review of research findings. *Psychological Reports*, *14*(1), 299–320.

Barber, T. X., & Wilson, S. C. (1978). The barber suggestibility scale and the creative imagination scale: Experimental and clinical applications. *American Journal of Clinical Hypnosis*, *21*(2-sup-3), 84–108.

Bernheim, H. (1888). *Die Suggestion und ihre Heilwirkung (übers. von Sigmund Freud)*. Franz Deuticke.

Bernheim, H. (1917). *Automatisme et suggestion*. Alcan.

Blanke, O., & Metzinger, T. (2009). Full-body illusions and minimal phenomenal selfhood. *Trends in Cognitive Sciences*, *13*(1), 7–13. 10.1016/j.tics.2008.10.003

Bochter, B., Hagl, M., Piesbergen, C., & Peter, B. (2014). Persönlichkeitsstile von Psychologiestudierenden im Vergleich zu Studierenden sogenannter MINT-Fächer [Personality styles of students of psychology in contrast to STEM students]. *Report Psychologie*, *39*(4), 154–165.

Bowers, K. S. (1998). Waterloo-Stanford group scale of hypnotic susceptibility, Form C. Manual and response booklet. *International Journal of Clinical and Experimental Hypnosis*, *46*(3), 250–268.

Braffman, W., & Kirsch, I. (1999). Imaginative suggestibility and hypnotizability: An empirical analysis. *Journal of Personality and Social Psychology*, *77*, 578–587.

Cardeña, E., & Terhune, D. B. (2008). A distinct personality trait? The relationship between hypnotizability, absorption, self-transcendence, and mental boundaries. *The Parapsychological Association Convention 2008*.

Cardeña, E., Terhune, D. B., Lööf, A., & Buratti, S. (2009). Hypnotic experience is related to emotional contagion. *International Journal of Clinical and Experimental Hypnosis*, *57*(1), 33–46. 10.1080/00207140802463500

Christensen, C. (2005). Preferences for descriptors of hypnosis: A brief communication. *International Journal of Clinical and Experimental Hypnosis*, *53*(3), 281–289. 10.1080/00207140590961358

Connors, M. H., Barnier, A. J., Langdon, R., Cox, R. E., Polito, V., & Coltheart, M. (2014). Delusions in the hypnosis laboratory: Modeling different pathways to mirrored-self misidentification. *Psychology of Consciousness: Theory, Research, and Practice*, *1*(2), 184–198. 10.1037/css0000001

Costa, P. T., & McCrae. (1992). *NEO personality inventory-revised (NEO-PI-R) and NEO five-factory inventory (NEO-FFI) professional manual*. Psychological Assessment Resources.

Elkins, G. R. (2014). *Hypnotic relaxation therapy: Principles and applications*. Springer Publishing.

Elkins, G. R., Barabasz, A. F., Council, J. R., & Spiegel, D. (2015). Advancing research and practice: The revised APA Division 30 definition of hypnosis. *International Journal of Clinical and Experimental Hypnosis*, *36*(1), 1–9.

Field, P. B. (1965). An inventory scale of hypnotic depth. *International Journal of Clinical and Experimental Hypnosis*, *13*(4), 238–249.

Frankel, F. H. (1978). Scales measuring hypnotic responsivity: A clinical perspective. *American Journal of Clinical Hypnosis*, *21*(2–3), 208–218. 10.1080/00029157.1978.10403972

Friedlander, J. W., & Sarbin, R. T. (1938). The depth of hypnosis. *Journal of Personality and Social Psychology*, *33*, 281–294.

Gauld, A. (1992). *A history of hypnotism*. Cambridge University Press.

Geiger, E., Peter, B., Prade, T., & Piesbergen, C. (2014). Intelligence and hypnotizability: Is there a connection? *International Journal of Clinical and Experimental Hypnosis*, *62*(3), 310–329. 10.1080/00207144.2014.901083

Gheorghiu, V. A., Netter, P., Eysenck, H. J., & Rosenthal, R. (Eds.). (1989). *Suggestion and suggestibility: Theory and research*. Springer.

Gorassini, D. R., & Spanos, N. P. (1986). A cognitive skills approach to the successful modification of hypnotic susceptibility. *Journal of Personality and Social Psychology*, *50*, 1004–1012.

Havens, R. A. (Ed.). (1985). *The Wisdom of Milton H. Erickson. Vol. I: Hypnosis & hypnotherapy*. Irvington.

Hilgard, E. R. (1965). *Hypnotic susceptibility*. Harcourt, Brace & World.

Hilgard, E. R. (1991). A neodissociation interpretation of hypnosis. In S. J. Lynn & J. W. Rhue (Eds.), *Theories of hypnosis: Current models and perspectives* (pp. 83–104). Guilford.

Hilgard, E. R., Weitzenhoffer, A. M., Landes, J., & Moore, R. K. (1961). The distribution of susceptibility to hypnosis in a student population: A study using the Standford Hypnotic Susceptibility Scale. *Psychological Monographs: General and Applied*, *75*(8), 1–22.
Hilgard, J. R. (1970). *Personality and hypnosis. A study of imaginative involvement.* University of Chicago Press.
Hull, C. L. (1933). *Hypnosis and suggestibility: An experimental approach.* D. Appleton-Century Company.
Jamieson, G., & Gruzelier, J. H. (2001). Hypnotic susceptibility is positively related to a subset of schizotypy items. *Contemporary Hypnosis*, *18*(1), 32–37.
Kihlstrom, J. F. (2008). The domain of hypnosis, revisited. In M. R. Nash & A. J. Barnier (Eds.), *The Oxford handbook of hypnosis. Theory, research and practice* (pp. 21–52). University Press.
Kirsch, I. (2001). The response set theory of hypnosis: Expectancy and physiology. *American Journal of Clinical Hypnosis*, *44*(1), 69–73.
Kirsch, I., Cardeña, E., Derbyshire, S. W., Dienes, Z., Heap, M., Kallio, S., Mazzoni, G., Naish, P. L., Oakley, D. A., Potter, C., Walters, V., & Whalley, M. (2011). Definitions of hypnosis and hypnotizability and their relation to suggestion and suggestibility: A consensus statement. *Contemporary Hypnosis and Integrative Therapy*, *28*(2), 107–115.
Kleinhauz, M., Dreyfuss, D. A., Beran, B., & Azikri, D. (1984). Some after-effects of stage hypnosis: A case study of psychopathological manifestations. *International Journal of Clinical and Experimental Hypnosis*, *27*, 219–226.
Kohen, D. P. & Olness, K. N. (2022). *Hypnosis with children.* Routledge.
Lankton, S. (2020). What Milton Erickson said about being Ericksonian. *American Journal of Clinical Hypnosis*, *63*(1), 4–13. 10.1080/00029157.2020.1754068
Laurence, J.-R., Beaulieu-Prévost, D., & du Chéné, T. (2008). Measuring and understanding individual differences in hypnotizability. In M. R. Nash & A. J. Barnier (Eds.), *The Oxford handbook of hypnosis. Theory, research and practice* (pp. 225–253). University Press.
Lipari, S., Baglio, F., Griffanti, L., Mendozzi, L., Garegnani, M., Motta, A., Cecconi, P., & Pugnetti, L. (2012). Altered and asymmetric default mode network activity in a "hypnotic virtuoso": An fMRI and EEG study. *Consciousness and Cognition*, *21*(1), 393–400. 10.1016/j.concog.2011.11.006
London, P. (1963). *Children's Hypnotic Susceptibility Scale.* Consulting Psychologists Press.
Lynn, S. J., Laurence, J.-R., & Kirsch, I. (2015). Hypnosis, suggestion, and suggestibility: An integrative model. *American Journal of Clinical Hypnosis*, *57*(3), 314–329. 10.1080/00029157.2014.976783
Lynn, S. J., & Sivec, H. (1992). The hypnotizable subject as creative problem-solving agent. In E. Fromm & M. R. Nash (Eds.), *Contemporary hypnosis research* (pp. 292–333). Guilford.
McGeown, W. J., Mazzoni, G., Venneri, A., & Kirsch, I. (2009). Hypnotic induction decreases anterior default mode activity. *Consciousness and Cognition*, *18*, 848–855.
Mesmer, F. A. (1775). Letter from M. Mesmer, doctor of medicine at Vienna, to A.M. Unzer, doctor of medicine, on the medical usage of the magnet. In *Mesmerism. A translation of the original scientific and medical writings of F.A. Mesmer"* (G. Bloch (translated and compiled by)) (1980 ed., pp. 25–38). W. Kaufmann.
Milling, L. S., Miller, D. S., Newsome, D. L., & Necrason, E. S. (2013). Hypnotic responding and the five factor personality model: Hypnotic analgesia and openness to experience. *Journal of Research in Personality*, *47*(1), 128–131. 10.1016/j.jrp.2012.10.006
Morgan, A. H. (1973). The heritability of hypnotic susceptibility in twins. *Journal of Abnormal Psychology*, *82*, 55–61.
Morgan, A. H., & Hilgard, J. R. (1978). The Stanford Hypnotic Clinical Scale for children. *American Journal of Clinical Hypnosis*, *21*(2–3), 148–169. 10.1080/00029157.1978.10403969
Nordenstrom, B. K., Council, J. R., & Meier, B. P. (2002). The "big five" and hypnotic suggestibility. *International Journal of Clinical and Experimental Hypnosis*, *50*(3), 276–281.
Nowak, H., Zech, N., Asmussen, S., Rahmel, T., Tryba, M., Oprea, G., Grause, L., Schork, K., Moeller, M., Loeser, J., Gyarmati, K., Mittler, C., Saller, T., Zagler, A., Lutz, K., Adamzik, M., & Hansen, E. (2020). Effect of therapeutic suggestions during general anaesthesia on postoperative pain and opioid use: Multicentre randomised controlled trial. *BMJ*, *371*, m4284. 10.1136/bmj.m4284
Pekala, R. J. (1995). A short, unobtrusive hypnotic-assessment procedure for assessing hypnotizability level: I. Development and research. *American Journal of Clinical Hypnosis*, *37*(4), 271–283. 10.1080/00029157.1995.10403156

Peter, B. (1994). Zur Relevanz hypnotischer Trance und hypnotischer Phänomene in Psychotherapie und Psychosomatik [On the relevance of hypnotic trance and hypnotic phenomena in psychotherapy and psychosomatic]. *Verhaltenstherapie*, *4*(4), 276–284.

Peter, B. (1996). Normale Instruktion oder hypnotische Suggestion: Was macht den Unterschied? [Normal instruction or hypnotic suggestion: What makes the difference?]. *Hypnose und Kognition*, *13*(1+2), 147–163. www.MEG-Stiftung.de

Peter, B. (2002). The "therapeutic tertium": On the use and usefulness of an old metaphor. In B. Peter, W. Bongartz, D. Revenstorf, & W. Butollo (Eds.), *Munich 2000. The 15th international congress of hypnosis* (pp. 247–258). www.MEG-Stiftung.de

Peter, B. (2009). Zur Ideengeschichte des Unbewussten in Hypnose und Psychoanalyse [On the history of ideas of the unconscious in hypnosis and psychoanalysis.]. *Hypnose-ZHH*, *4*(1+2), 49–78. www.MEG-Stiftung.de

Peter, B. (2015a). Geschichte der Hypnose in Deutschland [History of hypnosis in Germany]. In D. Revenstorf & B. Peter (Eds.), *Hypnose in Psychotherapie, Psychosomatik und Medizin. Ein Manual für die Praxis* (3rd ed., pp. 817–851). Springer.

Peter, B. (2015b). Hypnose und die Konstruktion von Wirklichkeit [Hypnosis and the construction of reality]. In D. Revenstorf & B. Peter (Eds.), *Hypnose in Psychotherapie, Psychosomatik und Medizin. Ein Manual für die Praxis* (3rd ed., pp. 37–45). Springer.

Peter, B. (2015c). Hypnosis. In J. D. Wright (Ed.), *International encyclopedia of the social & behavioral sciences* (2nd ed., pp. 458–464). Elsevier. 10.1016/B978-0-08-097086-8.21069-6

Peter, B. (2015d). The hypnosis-prone personality. *Paper presented at the American Psychological Association 2015 Annual Convention, August 6–9, Toronto, Canada*, 246.

Peter, B. (in press). Hypnotische Phänomene und psychopathologische Symptome [Hypnotic phenomena and psychopathological symptoms]. In D. Revenstorf, B. Peter & B. Rasch (Eds.), *Hypnose in Psychotherapie, Psychosomatik und Medizin*. Springer.

Peter, B., & Böbel, E. (2020). Does the homo hypnoticus exist? Personality styles of people interested in hypnosis. *International Journal of Clinical and Experimental Hypnosis*, *68*(3), 348–370. 10.1080/00207144.2020.1756294

Peter, B., Böbel, E., Hagl, M., Richter, M., & Kazén, M. (2018). Unterschiede in den Persönlichkeitsstilen von psychotherapeutisch Tätigen in Deutschland, Österreich und der Schweiz in Abhängigkeit vom psychotherapeutischen Verfahren und der Verwendung von Hypnose [Differences in personality styles of psychotherapists in Germany, Austria and Switzerland in relation to the applied psychotherapeutic techniques and the use of hypnosis]. *Hypnose-ZHH*, *13*(2), 169–192. www.MEG-Stiftung.de

Peter, B., Bose, C., Piesbergen, C., Hagl, M., & Revenstorf, D. (2012a). Persönlichkeitsprofile deutschsprachiger Anwender von Hypnose und Hypnotherapie [Personality styles of German-speaking practitioners of hypnosis and hypnotherapy]. *Hypnose-ZHH*, *7*(1+2), 31–59. www.MEG-Stiftung.de

Peter, B., & Revenstorf, D. (2018b). Rapport und therapeutische Beziehung in der Hypnotherapie [Rapport and therapeutic alliance in hypnotherapy]. In P. Fiedler (Ed.), *Varianten psychotherapeutischer Beziehung. Transdiagnostische Befunde, Konzepte, Perspektiven* (pp. 119–142). Pabst.

Peter, B., & Roberts, L. (2022). Hypnotizability norms may not be representative of the general population: Potential sample and self-selection bias considerations. *International Journal of Clinical and Experimental Hypnosis*, *70*(1), 49–67. 10.1080/00207144.2021.2003694

Peter, B., & Wolf, T. G. (2022). Personality styles of hypnosis-practicing dentists: A brief report. *International Journal of Clinical and Experimental Hypnosis*, *70*, 314–324. 10.1080/00207144.2022.2097082

Piccione, C., Hilgard, E. R., & Zimbardo, P. G. (1989). On the degree of stability of measured hypnotizability over a 25-year period. *Journal of Personality and Social Psychology*, *56*(2), 289–295.

Piesbergen, C., & Peter, B. (2006). An investigation of the factor structure of the Harvard Group Scale of Hypnotic Susceptibility, Form A (HGSHS:A). *Contemporary Hypnosis*, *23*(2), 59–71.

Polito, V., Langdon, R., & Barnier, A. J. (2015). Sense of agency across contexts: Insights from schizophrenia and hypnosis. *Psychology of Consciousness: Theory, Research, and Practice*, *2*(3), 301–314. 10.1037/cns0000053

Revenstorf, D., & Peter, B. (2023). Kontraindikationen, Bühnenhypnose und Willenlosigkeit [Contraindications, show hypnosis, and lack of willpower]. In D. Revenstorf, B. Peter, & B. Rasch (Eds.), *Hypnose in Psychotherapie, Psychosomatik und Medizin. Ein Manual für die Praxis* (4th ed., 135–162). Springer.

Riegel, B., Tönnies, S., Hansen, E., Zech, N., Eck, S., Batra, A., & Peter, B. (2021). German norms of the Harvard Group Scale of Hypnotic Susceptibility (HGSHS-A) and proposal of a 5-Item short-version (HGSHS 5:G). *International Journal of Clinical and Experimental Hypnosis*, *69*(1), 112–123. 10.1080/00207144.2021.1836645

Sadler, P., & Woody, E. Z. (2021). Multicomponent theories of hypnotizability: History and prospects. *International Journal of Clinical and Experimental Hypnosis*, *69*(1), 27–49. 10.1080/00207144.2021.1833210

Shor, R. E., & Ome, E. C. (1962). *Harvard Group Scale of Hypnotic Susceptibility Form A*. Consulting Psychologists Press.

Short, D. N. (2021). What is Ericksonian therapy: The use of core competencies to operationally define a nonstandardized approach to psychotherapy. *Clinical Psychology: Science and Practice*, *28*, 282–292. 10.1037/cps0000014

Spanos, N. P. (1986). Hypnosis and the modification of hypnotic susceptibility. In P. L. N. Naish (Ed.), *What is hypnosis* (pp. 85–120). Open University Press.

Spanos, N. P., Radtke, H. L., Hodgins, D. C., Stam, H. J., & Bertrand, L. D. (1983). The Carleton University responsiveness to suggestion scale: Normative data and psychometric properties. *Psychological Reports*, *53*, 523–535.

Spiegel, H., Aronson, M., Fleiss, J. L., & Haber, J. (1976). Psychometric analysis of the Hypnotic Induction Profile. *International Journal of Clinical and Experimental Hypnosis*, *24*(3–4), 300–315. 10.1080/00207147608416210

Taubner, S., Munder, T., Möller, H., Hanke, W., & Klasen, J. (2014). Selbstselektionsprozesse bei der Wahl des therapeutischen Ausbildungsverfahrens: Unterschiede in therapeutischen Haltungen, Persönlichkeitseigenschaften und dem Mentalisierungsinteresse. [Self-selection processes in the choice of the therapeutic training approach: Differences in therapeutic attitudes, personality traits, and attributional complexity]. *Psychotherapie, Psychosomatik, Medizinische Psychologie*, *64*(6), 214–223.

Tellegen, A., & Atkinson, G. (1974). Openness to absorbing and self-altering experiences ("absorbtion"), a trait related to hypnotic susceptibility. *Journal of Abnormal Psychology*, *83*, 268–277.

Terhune, D. B., & Oakley, D. A. (2020). Hypnosis and imagination. In A. Abraham (Ed.), *The Cambridge handbook of the imagination* (pp. 711–727). Cambridge University Press. 10.1017/9781108580298

Terhune, D. B., Cardeña, E., & Lindgren, M. (2011). Dissociated control as a signature of typological variability in high hypnotic suggestibility. *Conscious and Cognition*, *20*(3), 727–736.

Tuominen, J., Kallio, S., Kaasinen, V., & Railo, H. (2021). Segregated brain state during hypnosis. *Neuroscience of Consciousness*, *7*(1), niab002. 10.1093/nc/niab002

Varga, K., & Kekecs, Z. (2014). Oxytocin and cortisol in the hypnotic interaction. *International Journal of Clinical and Experimental Hypnosis*, *62*(1), 111–128. 10.1080/00207144.2013.841494

Weitzenhoffer, A. M., & Hilgard, E. R. (1959). *Stanford Hypnotic Susceptibility Scale, Forms A and B*. Consulting Psychologists Press.

Weitzenhoffer, A. M., & Hilgard, E. R. (1962). *Stanford Hypnotic Susceptibility Scale Form C*. Consulting Psychologists Press.

Weitzenhoffer, A. M., & Hilgard, E. R. (1967). *Revised Stanford Profile Scales of Hypnotic Susceptibility: Forms I and II*. Consulting Psychologists Press.

Weitzenhoffer, A. M. (1974). When is an "instruction" an "instruction"? *International Journal of Clinical and Experimental Hypnosis*, *22*(3), 258–269.

Weitzenhoffer, A. M. (1980a). Hypnotic susceptibility revisited. *American Journal of Clinical Hypnosis*, *22*(3), 130–146.

Weitzenhoffer, A. M. (1980b). What did he (Bernheim) say? A postscript and an addendum. *International Journal of Clinical and Experimental Hypnosis*, *28*(3), 252–260.

Wilson, S. C., & Barber, T. X. (1982). The fantasy-prone personality: Implications for understanding imagery, hypnosis, and parapsychological phenomena. In A. A. Sheikh (Ed.), *Imagery: Current theory, research, and application* (pp. 340–387). Wiley.

Wolf, T. G., Baumgärtner, E., & Peter, B. (2022). Personality styles of dentists practicing hypnosis confirm the existence of the homo hypnoticus. *Frontiers in Psychology*, *13*, 835200. 10.3389/fpsyg.2022.835200

Woody, E. Z., Barnier, A. J., & McConkey, K. M. (2005). Multiple hypnotizabilities: Differentiating the building blocks of hypnotic response. *Psychological Assessment*, *17*(2), 200–211. 10.1037/1040-3590.17.2.200

Woody, E. Z., Drugovic, M., & Oakman, J. M. (1997). A reexamination of the role of nonhypnotic suggestibility in hypnotic responding. *Journal of Personality and Social Psychology*, *72*(2), 399–407.

Zahedi, A., & Sommer, W. (2022). Can hypnotic susceptibility be explained by bifactor models? Structural equation modeling of the Harvard group scale of hypnotic susceptibility – Form A. *Consciousness and Cognition*, *99*, 103289. 10.1016/j.concog.2022.103289

Zeig, J. K. (1995). Direct and indirect methods: Artifact and essence. In M. Kleinhauz, B. Peter, S. Livnay, V. Delano, & A. Iost-Peter (Eds.), *Jerusalem lectures on hypnosis and hypnotherapy* (pp. 17–30). www.MEG-Stiftung.de

Theoretical Models

4

THE CONTRIBUTIONS OF MILTON ERICKSON TO MODERN CLINICAL HYPNOSIS

Roxanna Erickson-Klein[1] *and Dan Short*[2]

[1]The North Texas Society of Clinical Hypnosis; [2]The Milton H. Erickson Institute of Phoenix

Roxanna Erickson-Klein, Ph.D., has a lifelong interest in health care inspired by her father, Milton Erickson. She learned both as a subject of his hypnotic explorations and from his mentorship of her own clinical career. Since 1982, she is on the board of directors for the Milton H. Erickson Foundation and an active member of the American Society of Clinical Hypnosis. Erickson-Klein is a Registered Nurse and Licensed Professional Counselor in private practice who has authored books and articles about Ericksonian therapy. She is currently engaged in the digitization of her father's primary written works for dissemination at www.erickson-rossi.com.

Dan Short, Ph.D., has been interested in suggestion and interpersonal psychology since childhood, when he developed intense interest in the hypnotic effects of certain childhood games. His introduction to two of Erickson's daughters, and subsequently the Milton H. Erickson Foundation, occurred shortly after college graduation, resulting in close connections with others who have been key contributors to the exploration of Erickson's works. Short served as Editor of the *Milton H. Erickson Foundation Newsletter* for five years and was selected as project manager to preserve the holdings of the Milton H. Erickson Foundation Archives. While transferring the audio content from reel-to-reel to digital format, Short was immersed in hundreds of hours of analysis. The 1500 hours of unique recordings of Erickson involved two years, working eight hours a day to organize materials. During this time, Short watched videos of Erickson's hypnotic demonstrations, listened to Erickson's words, transcribed many recordings, and made connections between the overarching ideas.

Erickson's Theoretical Framework

Erickson's fascination and bold exploration into the nature of hypnosis were both innovative and expansive. A hallmark of his long career as a psychiatrist, spanning an interval of over half a century, was his ongoing inquiries, investigations, and communications about the potential of hypnosis to promote therapeutic change. The methodology pioneered by Erickson was instrumental in the transformation of paradigms of clinical practice, helping to usher in new eras of both brief therapy and modern hypnosis.

DOI: 10.4324/9781003449126-8

This chapter has been made available under a CC BY-NC-ND 4.0 license.

During this period, there was a great deal of progress in societal values, in the arts, and in science. A metaphor Erickson often alluded to was that during his lifetime (1901–1980) man's ability to fly progressed from the Kitty Hawk (1903) to men walking on the moon (1969). When he made this statement to students, Erickson's intent was for listeners to automatically engage in self-reflective orientation. The strategic use of comments and circumstances to stimulate experiential inner search was part of the way Erickson taught hypnosis.

While his deep interest in human behavior began in childhood, Erickson's explorations into hypnosis began in college, an era in which Sigmund Freud's ideas held a dominant influence on psychology and psychiatry. Erickson was additionally influenced by the writings of William James (Short, 2020) and the work of Arthur Noyes (1940), whose textbook, *Modern Clinical Psychiatry,* he kept on his office shelf throughout his career. Noyes emphasized that psychiatry must recognize man as a "unitary reacting biological organism" (p. 7). Erickson's ambition to bring hypnosis into the practice of medicine was a commitment made early in life and from which he never deviated. While repeatedly at odds with researchers, at no time did he waver from his respect for scientific methodology as the optimal tool to advance professional understanding.

Looking at his work from the perspective of his publications, various trends are revealed. Within his first decade of practice, Erickson began to challenge the central ideology of psychoanalytic practice. His explorations into suggestive therapeutics and the advancement of clinical hypnosis continued from the mid-1920s until his death. Erickson's own style of practice gradually shifted from a traditional style of direct suggestion to development of open-ended, permissive techniques (Erickson & Erickson-Klein, 1991).

Though he enjoyed teaching throughout his career, during the final decade of his life (1970–1980), Erickson sought to engage the interest of younger psychotherapists who could continue investigations into the nature of hypnosis. Following his death, a large number of professionals who had studied with him emerged as "Ericksonians" and began to teach their own perspectives of key ideas central to his work (Hilgard, 1992).

Hypnotic Rapport and Therapeutic Alliance

Contemporary meta-analytic studies have shown that the quality of the therapeutic alliance, empathetic capacity, and genuineness are predictive of successful outcomes in psychotherapy (Ardito & Rabellino, 2011). The same emphasis on quality of relationship is reflected in Erickson's attention to hypnotic rapport, which was manifested as a deeply felt connection – experienced by his patients and students alike.

Erickson's ability to establish strong rapport is shown as his daughter-in-law, Helen, described meeting him as "an experience that altered my way about thinking about learning, about my potential and about myself" (Erickson et al., 2006, p. 17). In this nursing textbook, Helen Erickson explicitly describes the way Milton Erickson entered her world (modeling) and facilitated her own growth into a broader world view (role-modeling). Erickson's innovative approach to building a strong therapeutic alliance is further detailed in numerous sections throughout this chapter.

Integration of Hypnosis in Therapy

Erickson distinguished between the waking state and the hypnotic state, and intentionally integrated both into his therapeutic work (Erickson, 1958/2008). He advocated for professionals to learn to identify naturalistic trance states and to strategically capitalize on these moments. In a 1966 lecture, Erickson stated that, "the [hypnotic] technique in itself serves no other purpose than that of securing and fixating the attention of patients, creating then a receptive and responsive mental state, and thereby enabling them to benefit from unrealized or only partially realized potentials for behavior of various types" (Erickson, 1966). Thus, Erickson emphasized the goal of hypnotherapy is to move beyond the limitations of the conscious mind to the creativity of the unconscious mind (Gilligan, 2002).

Framing hypnosis as a distinct phenomenon, Erickson (1961/2010) wrote a six-page definition of hypnosis for the Encyclopedia Britannica. Within, Erickson states, "hypnosis is a unique complex form of unusual but normal behavior which can probably be induced in all normal persons under suitable conditions" (p. 27). When asked to define hypnosis in teaching seminars, author Roxanna remembers he frequently offered a succinct explanation, "Hypnosis is a dissociation of the conscious mind from the unconscious mind." In a later discussion with Ernest Rossi, Erickson expresses that trance is "a deep state of inner absorption ... resorted to in order to cope with a problem that was apparently overwhelming for his conscious mind" (Erickson & Rossi, 1977/2008, p. 197).

Trance and Suggestion

Noting that Ernest Rossi was Erickson's closest collaborator, author Dan Short asked Rossi which written work best summarized Erickson's views on hypnosis. Rossi replied that *Hypnotic Realities* was the greatest exposition of Erickson's ideas. This work states that the purpose of trance is to focus an individual's attention inwardly to help alter habitual attitudes and belief systems associated with "everyday consciousness" (Erickson & Rossi, 1976/2010, p. 225). Throughout, Erickson repeatedly identifies therapeutic trance as being characterized primarily by feelings of comfort, limited awareness, and heightened expectancy. Recent neurobiological research suggests that comfort and relaxation help facilitate sudden insights, solving problems without use of conscious deliberation. As insight researcher John Kounios puts it, "If you want to encourage insights, then you've got to also encourage people to relax" (Lehrer, 2008, p. 40).

The relevance of relaxation to trance, and learning in general, is of interest to researchers and clinicians alike. Even so, the field of hypnosis remains polarized by the "state versus non-state" debate, which traces back to disagreements between T.X. Barber and Milton Erickson over the meaningfulness of trance behavior. While a majority of clinicians view Erickson as the person who set the standards of modern hypnosis (Baker, 1988; Rodolfa et al., 1985), many researchers argue that distinction should go to Barber (Gauld, 1992). To better understand their differences, we turn to a transcript of a face-to-face debate between Erickson and Barber.

During this panel discussion, Barber's basic argument was that if trance is a defining feature of hypnosis, then trance phenomena should not occur outside of trance. However, his research had shown hypnotic phenomena can be easily obtained with unhypnotized individuals (no trance) given sufficient motivation and positive expectancies (Barber, 1961). For example, Barber posited that hypno-catatonic behavior is nothing more than giving a special label to a person sitting rigidly in a chair. In Barber's words, "The only research we need to do on 'catalepsy' is to show that it can readily be duplicated by a motivated person, and hypnotic subjects are usually very motivated" (Erickson, 1960/2010, p. 329). Barber's implication was clear – clinicians, such as Erickson, were unwittingly manipulating their client's motivations, attitudes, and expectancies with trance having no bearing on responsiveness to suggestion. In Barber's words, "I am bothered by Dr. Erickson's formulations because I get the impression that there is magic being attributed here that does not promote scientific understanding or investigation" (Erickson, 1960/2010, p. 328).

To address this criticism, Erickson replied, "I believe that the hypnotic subject can, in the trance state, do something besides please Dr. Barber. I think he can use his own behavior for his own purposes and do it in his own way. He doesn't lose his capacity to behave to please himself" (Erickson, 1960/2010, p. 329).

Three decades prior, Erickson had reported a lack of relationship between depth of trance and suggestibility. To the contrary, Erickson found that individuals demonstrating deep trance behavior were sometimes more resistant to suggestion (Erickson, 1932/2010). What Barber failed to recognize was that Erickson did not use trance to achieve greater compliance, but rather to stimulate unconscious intelligence (Short, 2022).

Furthermore, Erickson rejected the premise that positive outcomes achieved with hypnosis must be exclusive to hypnosis. As Erickson had already explained, "I have known people who *never went into hypnosis*, but who went to a movie because they had a severe headache, forgot their headache during the course of an interesting movie ... and perhaps didn't remember the headache until the next day" (Erickson, 1960/2010, p. 321). Again, to explain that amnesic behavior is not exclusive to hypnosis, Erickson stated, "I believe that the hypnotic subject can do in a trance state the same sort of things he can do in the waking state. I might introduce someone to a dozen other people. At the end of that time, by virtue of having directed this person's attention first to Mr. Jones then to Mr. Green, to Mr. Brown, etc., and after I had finished the 15th or 16th introduction, I could ask him, 'Tell me, what was the name of the first man, the second man, the third, the fourth, the fifth?' We would readily appreciate how rapidly a person can forget something, especially when his attention is constantly redirected" (Erickson, 1960/2010, p. 326).

Recognizing that for researchers in attendance, the term "trance" was often associated with mystical ideology, Erickson sought to explain his position using different terminology, "You alter a person's state of awareness by the conditions associated with, and the character of, the stimulation which you offer along with the inner behavior of potentials in that person. I do not think that I am in error to give the general term 'state of awareness' to the memories, ideas, and emotions characterizing a person at a given time, nor do I consider this a 'mystical appellation'" (Erickson, 1960/2010, p. 326). Succinctly, Erickson later wrote, "Of significant importance to the author in furthering his awareness that waking state realities were quite different from the realities of the hypnotic state" (Erickson, 1967/2008, p. 89). Returning to the book mentioned earlier in this section, *Hypnotic Realities*, it is reasonable to conclude that Erickson was less concerned with altered states of consciousness than with altered states of reality.

Philosophical Underpinnings

The argument has been made that Erickson's use of hypnosis to advance the flourishing of human consciousness has deep roots in the psychology and philosophy of William James (Short, 2020). This is reflected in Erickson's pragmatic approach to problem-solving as well as his embrace of dynamic dualism. At the center of this perspective is the belief in an unconscious mind and a conscious mind that possess different resources and serve different functions, any of which can and should be utilized in therapy. These Jamesian psychodynamics involve embracing unseen processes of reorganization, reassociation, and adaptation – the opposite of Freudian psychodynamics. Above all else, Erickson insisted that therapy should recognize a person's capacity for innate healing and growth. Thus, he taught that the use of hypnotic suggestion should be permissive enough to address the human need for freedom and the exercise of self-determination. These ideas can be traced back to James who argued that freedom of choice must be the starting point in any attempt to influence others. In James's own words, "The first thing to learn in intercourse with others is noninterference with their own peculiar ways of being happy, provided those ways do not assume to interfere by violence with ours" (Short, 2020, p. 2).

In the interval after Erickson's death, an echo of his ideas emerged which inspired students expressing differing viewpoints to define his innovative approaches. Despite a series of attempts among Ericksonians to reach a concordance, perspectives remain as individualized as the approaches Erickson promoted. While some key elements have been generally agreed upon and even operationalized (Short, 2021a), the very nature of his work is a non-standardized and highly individualized experiential process.

Erickson's Top Six Contributions to Hypnosis Practice and Theory

Attempts to encapsulate Erickson's approaches in definable or operationalized concepts are as elusive as working with a translucent Rubik's cube. Efforts to isolate principal contributions become a perceptual window, seen from many different perspectives, each interconnected to other aspects of Erickson's work. Leading Ericksonian scholars (e.g., Lankton, 2010; Zeig, 2019) have identified the concept of utilization as central to Erickson's ability to generate a strong therapeutic alliance. Accordingly, Erickson describes utilization as the integration of the "subject's own attitudes, thinking, behaviors and aspects of their of the reality situation, variously employed [within therapeutic interactions]" (Erickson, 1959/2008, p. 301).

This chapter focuses on central areas in which Erickson's contributions influenced broader structures; we offer descriptions of six fundamental building blocks from which Erickson's unique explorations clearly impacted the way hypnosis is understood and practiced today. Along with the innovations, new paradigms began to emerge, all of which revolve around a fulcrum of utilization by engaging the client's subjective and situational resources.

Naturalistic Approach

One of Erickson's most celebrated innovations in hypnosis is his method of conversational hypnosis, essentially the practice of hypnosis without the use of formal trance induction or awakening (Short, 2018). Erickson operated from the premise that hypnotic states are a common information processing capability containing universal value for learning and problem-solving.

What Erickson called "the naturalistic approach to hypnosis" differs significantly from traditional premises of hypnotizability (i.e., not everyone is responsive to hypnosis). In Erickson's words, "there is an imperative need to accept and to utilize those psychological states, understandings, and attitudes that each patient brings into the situation. To ignore those factors in favor of some ritual of procedure may and often does delay, impede, limit, or even prevent the desired results. The acceptance and utilization of those factors, on the other hand, promotes more rapid trance induction, the development of more profound trance states, the more ready acceptance of therapy, and greater ease for the handling of the total therapeutic situation" (Erickson, 1958/2008, p. 269).

As demonstrated in the following case example, trance states are a spontaneous, natural response to collaborative engagement when (1) both parties agree on the problem to be solved, and 2) existing response tendencies are given structure through highly appealing hypnotic suggestions. In this case, the parents brought Erickson their own opinions about the problem of their angry, enuretic son. Erickson recognized that the boy had been dreaming of owning a dog. So, he utilized the desire to design his approach, telling the young boy to "see a dog over there." The child responded, "But there is no dog over there." Erickson then increased his "intensity of expectation," by simply stating, "Yes, that is right. But I want you to just SEE the dog, over there," as he pointed to an empty spot. This induced a visual hallucination (Erickson, 1952). Connecting this altered state of reality to a larger therapeutic agenda, Erickson told the child, "I don't think that you or I have to tell your parents anything. In fact, maybe it would serve them just right for the way they brought you here if you waited until the school year was almost over. But one thing is certain, you can just bet that after you've had a dry bed for a month, they will get you a puppy just about like little Spotty there, even if you never say a word to them about it. They just have to!" (Erickson, 1958/2008, p. 267). The actual puppy was delivered by the boy's father 31 days later.

With Erickson's naturalistic approach, the qualities of spontaneity and individual uniqueness are integrated into the methodology of hypnosis. One of clinical psychology's most recent paradigm shifts is the slow transition away from mechanistic models of logical positivism which prioritize technique and standardization, over a wholistic model prioritizing human connection. In support of this shift, studies have shown that the quality of relationship is the greatest predictor of success in psychotherapy (Ardito & Rabellino, 2011).

Individualization

Clark Hull, a distinguished behaviorism researcher, published the first textbook on controlled hypnotic experimentation (Hull, 1933). As an undergraduate, Erickson was invited to present his own research to Hull's graduate hypnosis seminar. As a young student, Erickson initially accepted Hull's structured procedural approach (Fromm & Shor, 1979, p. 33). However, as Erickson's exploration of hypnosis broadened, a schism emerged between Erickson's commitment to individualization and Hull's commitment to logical positivism and standardized treatment procedures.

Weitzenhoffer (1957) observed that, "According to Erickson hypnosis is a highly individualistic process because it is a function of intrapersonal (or intrapsychic) relationships and of the interpersonal relationships, they themselves are contingent and dependent upon the former. Every individual has a unique personality, and his behavior, including that of the trance-inducing situation, is a function of his personality, the time, the situation, and the purposes which are served. Thus, it is invalid to assume that under identical conditions of administration, identical suggestions must invariably yield identical responses in different subjects or in the same subject at different times" (pp. 269–270). Likewise, Short (2019, p. 27) comments, "Because each person is an individual, each session is a unique creation. When therapist and client first meet, they create a relationship that did not exist before. In this new system, each will influence the other in potentially unexpected way." The information Erickson gathered during communication (both verbal and non-verbal) was utilized in an individual manner specific to the person and his or her needs at that specific point in time.

Unfortunately, individualized care does not lend itself well to operationally defined, evidenced-based approaches to treatment. Erickson's commitment to the necessity of activating unique individual inner resources created stumbling blocks to clinicians who seek reimbursement in a field dominated by evidence-based therapies as well as for researchers needs for standardized protocols. It is only during the last five years that the development of operationally defined evaluations of Ericksonian approaches has begun to bridge the gap between the pragmatic needs of research and the individual attention and creativity required for tailored approaches to hypnosis (Short, 2019).

Experiential Arousal

Erickson's experiences as an adolescent, rehabilitating from ravages of polio, led to a thousand-mile Mississippi River canoe journey which challenged the limits of his physical capacity. This odyssey served as a benchmark for the powerful combination of conscious aspirations and unconscious capabilities (Erickson, 1922/2018). Erickson challenged himself to restrain from directly requesting assistance using a multitude of indirect ways to stimulate curiosity in others. His indirect communication methods attracted the attention of volunteers to assist him in individually unmanageable portages. Erickson's determination to overcome limitations imposed by polio served as an experiential metaphor that helped frame his future. This journey modeled the process of discovering hidden potential as one seeks to exceed apparent limits of immediate circumstances.

Erickson's subsequent undergraduate research with Clark Hull involved investigations of automatic writing, hand levitation, and kinesthetic imagery as various means of trance induction. Each technique involved direct or imagined physical activity (Erickson, 1961/2008). Erickson continued his investigations into the nature of the mind body interface in the 1940s, publishing articles in the *Journal of Psychosomatic Medicine.* His pioneering exploration of hypnotic deafness and hypnotic color blindness increased his appreciation for inextricable links of the body and mind (Erickson, 1943/2010).

Having demonstrated hand levitation techniques in his college studies, Erickson continued using hand levitation with frequency. In the 1950s, he went on to develop the My Friend John technique in which a positive hallucination involved hand levitation in a hallucinated companion. His own explanation about hand levitation techniques emphasize its utility for induction, trance ratification, and in particular to enhance dissociation (Erickson, 1961/2008).

A dramatic demonstration at Stanford Laboratory of Hypnosis Research during the 1960s clarified that experience is an intrapersonal process. Erickson's demonstration involved a man who reported no sensation in his hand when touched. Also, while positioned in front of him, he hallucinated his hand to be resting in his lap (Hilgard, 1992, p. 72). In a discussion about ideomotor feedback, Erickson notes that the key element of initiating motor activity, real or imagined, is a means of fixating and focusing the individual's attention on inner experiential learnings and capabilities. Erickson (1945/2008) explains:

> ... the subject is told that, as he goes to sleep, his hand will gradually and involuntarily begin to lift up in the air. This he may not notice at first, but when he does become aware of it, he will find himself tremendously interested and absorbed in

> sensing and enjoying that effortless, involuntary movement of his hand and arm. Thus, the subject is given the opportunity of observing his hypnotic response as a personal experience that is occurring within himself. There follow suggestions that soon the direction of the hand movement will change, that he is to be greatly interested in discovering what the new direction may be. This suggestion does result in an alteration of the hand movement, an alteration recognized by the subject as not determined in direction by specific hypnotic suggestions but determined by the continuing processes within himself as a hypnotic subject. This gives him a growing realization of his active participation in a progressive intrapsychic experience in which he plays an undefined but definite directive role governed by forces within him. (p. 39)

While hypnosis is by nature experiential, the utilization of physical activity within the trance state amplifies the opportunity for dissociative effects that can then be integrated into therapeutic objectives. Over the years, Erickson developed a reputation for assigning tasks to his clients that sometimes involved moderate to intensive physical exercise, including hiking up a nearby mountain. As suggested in the discussion of Erickson's canoe journey, the integration of vigorous activity into personal improvement began early in his life. As he developed his professional style, with hypnosis at the center, he also explored incorporation of numerous ways to engage physical and emotional responses.

Shock and surprise are techniques liberally integrated into Erickson's repertoire of approaches. While there are distinctions between physical movement, and emotional responses, they may serve a similar stimulation. Erickson describes his work eliciting surprises in this way, "all that I hope to know in most such experimental situations that I devise is the possible general variety of psychological processes and reactions I would like to elicit, but do not know if I shall succeed in so doing, nor in what manner this will occur. Thus, as the subjects respond in their own fashion, I promptly utilize that response" (Erickson, 1961/2008, p. 328).

In his clinical explorations, Erickson found that various physiological interrelationships and interdependencies seemed to vary substantially between individuals without a direct relationship to hypnotic suggestion. Erickson posited that, "it may be that the primary task in the therapy of various psychopathological conditions may be dependent on an approach seemingly unrelated to the actual problem" (Erickson, 1943/2010, pp. 17–18).

Seeding and Incubation

Some of Erickson's most striking contributions to the practice of hypnosis continue to germinate beneath the field's collective awareness. While most who study Ericksonian hypnosis are familiar with the concept of seeding (gradual exposure and subsequent elaboration of new ideas in advance of utilizing them for therapeutic purposes), few fully appreciate the value of incubation – the strategic practice of patiently waiting for ideas to grow outside of conscious awareness. Both constructs relate to the element of time, an essential component of growth and maturity.

In Erickson's case studies, there are examples of him patiently waiting 1–2 hours in silence, as the patient sits motionless in a trance state (Erickson, 1954). This makes no sense within the context of traditional hypnosis, where the hypnotic procedure depends on repetitiously suggesting new attitudes, beliefs, or behaviors to the client. Erickson expanded hypnosis from suggestive applications to include process work (Short, 2021b). As stated by Erickson, "I don't think the therapist does anything except provide the opportunity to think about your problem in a favorable climate" (Zeig, 1980, p. 219).

Using the analogy of a gardener: Erickson planted seeds in the form of evocative ideas that were intentionally obscured from conscious review during an incubation period. As unconscious processing of these ideas took place, Erickson patiently waited to see what would grow. Erickson's pause enabled clients to create their own solutions – in their own way, in their own good time (Rossi, 1973). As Erickson put it, "You should enjoy the process of waiting ... There is nothing more delightful than planting flower seeds and not knowing what kind of flowers are going to come up" (Erickson & Rossi, 1979/2014, p. xiv).

An essential point made by Erickson is that, "it is possible that hypnotherapy can take place entirely at an unconscious level without the patient (and sometimes even the therapist) knowing the 'why' of the cure" (Erickson & Rossi, 1979/2014, p. 165). This Ericksonian principle seems strange and unrealistic from a Freudian perspective. Freud's approach was founded on the philosophies of the 18th- and 19th-century enlightenment, which squarely equates conscious reason with human progress.

Though not opposed to conscious insight, Erickson relegates it to a secondary position, emphasizing the value of unconscious incubation. As Erickson states, "And then the results of that unconscious functioning can become conscious. But first they have to get beyond their conscious understanding of what is possible" (Erickson & Rossi, 1976/2010, p. 10). Similarly, cognitive scientists now argue that successful performance on tasks that require creative recategorization is best accomplished by downregulation of the cognitive control regions. One study found that when individuals were induced to allow their minds to wander, they showed an improvement of 40% compared to their baseline level of creative performance. This was achieved by simply saying, "move the problem to the back of your mind" (Baird et al., 2012). When considering the value of a relaxed, self-absorbed trance state, it is interesting to look at the neurological studies of Bowden and Jung-Beeman who argue that effortful thought interferes with insight because focused concentration favors the left hemisphere, causing the right to become less active (Bowden et al., 2005; Bowden & Jung-Beeman, 2003).

In addition to conscious surrender and relaxation, a third crucial element in preparation for insight is time. At least one study found that longer unconscious thought has led to better decisions than brief unconscious thought (Dijksterhuis, 2004). Though this line of research remains controversial due to small sample size (Nieuwenstein et al., 2015), using the greater power of meta-analysis, Sio and Ormerod (2009) found that longer preparation periods gave a greater incubation effect and that incubation works best for problems that require creative solutions (divergent thinking).

From a competency-based perspective, growth-oriented change is achieved by inviting the client to exercise choice and creative problem-solving – often at unconscious levels. Whether it is the problem-solving step of defining the problem, identifying a solution, or solution implementation, at all stages of the process, Erickson sought the involvement of the client's unconscious intelligence (Short, 2021b).

Utilizing Resistance

Erickson broadened the identification of meaningful hypnotherapeutic responses to include resistance to suggestion. To help others understand this critical paradigm shift, Erickson used the analogy of a car stuck in a ditch. He pointed out that only by rocking backward can you obtain the momentum needed to move forward (Erickson & Haley, 1985, p. 306). While logic tells us that to achieve success we must avoid failure, history shows that only those who have willingly embraced failure go furthest in accomplishments. Similarly, to succeed at hypnosis the clinician must be willing to fail.

Viewing resistance as a legitimate starting point for progress, Erickson found ways to get his clients to commit to "discharging" their resistance. For example, one individual announced that he wanted to be treated with hypnosis but then insisted that he could not be hypnotized. This position represents a contradictory attitude not only to hypnosis but also to the whole of therapy – otherwise the client would have requested a form of therapy that he thought would work well. For this reason, we should recognize that Erickson's response was not only limited to the process of induction but also to the client's responsiveness to therapy as a whole.

Erickson (1976/2010, p. 221) commented to the patient, "There is, of course, a possibility that you can be hypnotized." Then he predicted, "There is more possibility that you can't be hypnotized." Paradoxically, Erickson seems to be suggesting failure rather than success. Next, Erickson observed that there were three additional chairs in the office. Again, he speculated that if hypnosis were attempted in each of these chairs, the induction would probably fail more times than it succeeded. For the induction, Erickson, indicating a different chair, said, "Now let's try this chair. If you fail in this one, there is still the possibility that you can go into trance." After trying three chairs, unsuccessfully, the patient entered a spontaneous trance in the fourth chair. In other words, Erickson removed all performance pressure and turned failure into an asset (Erickson & Rossi, 1976/2010, p. 221).

This same strategy could be applied to posthypnotic suggestion. Imagine that you had a client struggling with sleep issues who after sleeping easily, in response to hypnosis, expressed tenacious concerns that he would not be able to achieve the same results at home. The expectation of failure can be accommodated by saying, "This is a learning process. I will give you therapeutic suggestions each visit. However, it may not work until after the third or fourth visit. But with each failure, I believe you will come closer and closer to success." This sounds easy. But for most of us it is reflexive to resist resistance, perhaps politely countering the previous client's concern with, "After doing so well here, I'm sure you can do it at home." Such a well-intended statement does not accept the client's position. In contrast, when you are willing to account for failure in the predictions you make, two important things occur: (1) performance pressure is greatly diminished, and (2) a process of unconscious goal striving is initiated (Short, 2021b). Just as happiness is not obtained by avoiding unhappiness, confidence is not obtained by avoiding risks.

Erickson role-modeled enthusiastic discovery as he observed person's real-time responses. With his astute observations, he integrated what he learned about the individual, their motivation, their readiness, and their participation in the hypnotic process to individualize his approach with them. Fully accepting the individual's doubts and uncertainty, he utilized that energy to gradually shift to a process of discovery by offering confidence, enthusiasm, hope, and just enough guidance to mobilize and sustain adaptive internal processes.

Individuation

Reinforcement of self-organizing change is a pillar seen in Erickson's earliest case comments and amplified as therapeutic brevity and present/future orientation emerged as hallmarks of his work. The idea of individuation involves assumptions of self-responsibility and a capacity for ongoing adjustments over time. Favoring individualized, self-defined, assessments of health and functionality, Erickson's clinical approach departed from a standard-based system of compliance with societal norms.

Rather than seeking understandings or explanations that make rational sense, Erickson focused on creating an atmosphere within which the client could successfully adapt to living life in a meaningful and satisfactory manner, specific to their individual needs. The therapeutic style that evolved over Erickson's decades of clinical work was above all else pragmatic and highly efficient. Tangible progress was often achieved without insight. Erika Fromm and Ronald Shor (1979), known for their psychoanalytic approaches to hypnotherapy, described Erickson's work figuratively, "Erickson enters the world of the patient's neuroses with him and with clinical artistry and intuitive understanding of non-rational dynamics rearranges definitions and symptoms to make the neuroses more successfully adaptive" (p. 33).

In a paper titled, *The Burden of Effective Psychotherapy*, Erickson describes three cases in which hypnosis rapidly and effectively brought resolution to problems that these patients had already failed to resolve using traditional psychotherapy. These cases illustrate that it is each person's creative inner work that brings forth adaptive growth. Self-direction, reinforced by Erickson's suggestions, fostered the acceptance of self-responsibility for needed changes (Erickson, 1964/2008).

In some of Erickson's case stories, he is very specific such as this suggestion made to an athlete, "I told him in a trance state to feel all of his muscles, to get acquainted with his body" (Erickson, 1979/2014, p. 62). Sometimes, his suggestions were so elusive the listener didn't recognize the activity as being an assignment such as looking for the boojum tree in the botanical garden. The commonality is that Erickson had a deep trust in the patient's unconscious mind to work through what was needed in a personalized way and in the service of the individual personality.

Whereas many of Erickson's case consultations were time-limited in nature, he did not shy away from working with severe mental illness. The case of John (Zeig, 1985) is an example of guidance of one of Erickson's long-term clients through major life adjustments. The patient, having spent a significant part of his youth confined to mental hospitals, set his own goal at living alone in an apartment. After several years of adapting to the responsibilities of independent living, which included daily check-ins with Erickson, John was encouraged to adopt a pet dog. Arrangements included the dog residing at Erickson's home/office with John assuming responsibilities for daily care. Thus, John's (scarce) happy childhood memories of walking a pet were utilized. In addition to promotion of social contacts, the responsibilities demonstrated John's capacity to care for a living being and develop a friendship. Related assignments included John working with someone to construct a doghouse and periodic vet visits. Over the years, these activities broadened John's base of friendships. Despite a significant underlying mental disorder, John adapted successfully to satisfactory self-care and independent living.

Cases, such as this one, are outside of mainstream practice but emphasize the degree of dedication Erickson brought to his work with clients. Whereas the standards of confidentiality are more pronounced today, Erickson communicated a profound respect for the safety and integrity of patients' needs that also went beyond the mainstream. Erickson stipulated, "The essential necessity of safety of the patient remains paramount. It is essential that the subject feel protected if his full participation in hypnotic work is expected.

The subject has a strong need for protection of infringement of his rights and privacy" (Weitzenhoffer, 1957, pp. 272–273).

Erickson's ability to work within each person's own frame of reference required a deep sense of respect for individual integrity and freedom of choice. He also had solid commitments to the welfare of society and to the advancement of knowledge. Having done studies in criminal behavior (Erickson, 1927/2008), and having participated in war efforts to interrogate enemy soldiers, Erickson debated with colleagues that hypnosis cannot be used to suggest criminal behavior contrary to the individual's internal self-directives (Estabrooks, 1943, p. 189). Erickson took a definitive stand that such directives would be impossible, stating, "I feel strongly that you can get a person to do in the trance state at most only what he is willing to do in the waking state, but usually even not that much in the manner of offensive behavior" (Erickson, 2000, p. 204).

Erickson focused his work in hypnosis on the responsibilities of professionals in healing arts and on the process of healthy adaptation to individual needs and circumstances. His prolific writings of case consultations and his clinical exploration illustrate that all health professionals have a role in advancing science by challenging what is known and not yet known, continuing to work in the direction of promoting health and well-being with resources available today.

Core Competencies in Ericksonian Therapy

In support of Erickson's work as a conceptually distinct therapeutic approach, the *Principles and Core Competencies of Ericksonian Therapy* was spearheaded by Dan Short in 2016 to establish whether Ericksonian therapy is based on a coherent and consistent set of principles. The goal of this undertaking was to provide researchers and practitioners with a practical skill set most closely associated with performance as an Ericksonian therapist.

In collaboration with an international assembly of experts on Erickson's work, Short conducted a qualitative study (with subsequent quantitative validation) that resulted in a series of foundational principles for practitioners seeking mastery in Ericksonian therapy. The core skill sets that were able to reliably distinguish a competent Ericksonian therapist from other practitioners include tailoring, utilization, strategic, destabilization, experiential, and naturalistic (Short, 2021a). An operationalized treatment manual and accompanying teaching videos made by leaders in Ericksonian therapy are freely available (Short, 2019).

As with Erickson's overall influence on hypnosis, these core elements can be adapted to most individual circumstances and to a host of cultural differences. They can be taught and objectively measured in clinical practice. Ericksonian Core Competency principles position professionals to further investigate and practice the ideas central to Erickson's work in a changing cultural climate.

Future Implications for Training and Professional Development

A worldwide communication network today brings opportunities to share knowledge and compile information from others in an unprecedented manner. With this opportunity comes challenges associated with expanding expectations and responsibilities. Mental health concerns are rising in urgency around the world related to the COVID pandemic aftermath and risks of future uncertainties. The availability of technology fostered rapid adaptation to internet-based delivery of hypnotherapeutic services (Palsson et al., 2022). Not only did internet-based teaching become popular but it was also demonstrated that virtual global outreach is feasible, achievable, and rewarding.

The last few years of communication development have enabled individuals and organizations to build relationships in other countries, offering extensive and unique forums for us to learn about cultural as well as regulatory differences. Professional organizations, such as the International Society of Hypnosis (ISH), have succeeded in bringing together divergent perspectives with recognition for the value of working together and a convergence of energy and resources. For example, recently the Milton H. Erickson Foundation joined with the American Society of Clinical Hypnosis, the Society for Clinical and Experimental Hypnosis, the ISH, and other major hypnosis organizations to form a task force for establishing efficacy standards for clinical hypnosis. Nine selected researchers from Hungary, the United States, the United Kingdom, and Italy developed ten specific recommendations and up-to-date guidelines for applied practice (Kekecs et al., 2022).

Clearly, we need to utilize cultural developments, resources, and circumstances of today, which offer glimpses of what will be needed for future adaptation. The most capable learners reach back in time to foundations of knowledge, while seeking to address immediate challenges and anticipate needs of the future. Erickson's innovations, struggles, and triumphs, expressed through his own primary works, offer a multifaceted perspective of working with clients in an individualized manner.

As beneficiaries of the past, each of us must do our own small part to advance the works of our predecessors. Milton Erickson was clearly dedicated to an ongoing effort, over the fullness of his career, to promote and advance a better understanding of clinical psychology's oldest healing tradition – hypnosis. In studying his primary works, in the context of time, we gain appreciation for the magnitude and breadth of his contributions. As one reflects upon his communication with professionals, colleagues, mentees, and students, the legacy he left is considerable. At the time of his death, Erickson had created what Jeffrey Zeig, Director of the Milton Erickson Foundation, refers to as streams of intellectual heirs that continue to influence upcoming generations of psychotherapists (Zeig, 2019, p. xiii). In other words, each student of Erickson has a unique perspective – a constellation of personal knowledge, culture, experiences, and circumstances.

A close examination of Erickson's works reveals a consistent pattern of carefully crafted integration of experiential activities, changing frames of reference, and intrapersonal self-reinforcement in service of amplification of each person's own ability to self-determine a path to healing (Gilligan, 2002). Similarly, the co-creation of outcomes is an ongoing process within the client that is only partially guided by the therapist. This approach involves utilization of the client's unique perspectives, behaviors, and resources to facilitate needed or desired change (Lankton, 2010, p. 353).

Erickson's great faith in the ability of people to draw upon personal resources was one of his greatest attributes. In his own words, Erickson stated, "It isn't so much what the therapist does, it's what he gets his patients to do" (Cheek, 1994, p. 16). Central in Erickson's writings is the idea that nurturing clients to take self-responsibility for their own growth and development is not only an element of therapeutic necessity but also of successful hypnotic suggestions (Gilligan, 2002). As we join our colleagues from different backgrounds, from different nations, from different perspectives, and together learn from the legacy of this singular contributor, Milton Erickson, we enter the opportunity to co-create an experience that will benefit us all. Working together as an international community, uniting differing cultures, and historical efforts, we are given the opportunity to express our doubts, differences, and hesitations. Now is the time for us to ponder shared understandings as we appreciate the natural evolution of hypnosis as it finds its own place in the art and science of medicine.

References

Ardito, R. B., & Rabellino, D. (2011). Therapeutic alliance and outcome of psychotherapy: Historical excursus, measurements, and prospects for research. *Frontiers in Psychology*, *2*(270), 1–11. 10.3389/fpsyg.2011.00270

Baird, B., Smallwood, J., Mrazek, M. D., Kam, J. W., Franklin, M. S., & Schooler, J. W. (2012). Inspired by distraction: Mind wandering facilitates creative incubation. *Psychological Science*, *23*(10), 1117–1122. 10.1177/0956797612446024

Baker, E. L. (1988). The contributions of Milton Erickson: Reflections on the forest and the trees. *International Journal of Clinical and Experimental Hypnosis*, *36*(3), 125–127. 10.1080/0020714 8808410502

Barber, T. X. (1961). Physiological effects of hypnosis. *Psychological Bulletin*, *58*(5), 390–419. 10. 1037/h0042731

Bowden, E. M., & Jung-Beeman, M. (2003). Aha! Insight experience correlates with solution activation in the right hemisphere. *Psychonomic Bulletin & Review*, *10*(3), 730–737. 10.3758/BF03196539

Bowden, E. M., Jung-Beeman, M., Fleck, J., & Kounios, J. (2005). New approaches to demystifying insight. *Trends in Cognitive Sciences*, *9*(7), 322–328. 10.1016/j.tics.2005.05.012

Cheek, D. B. (1994). *Hypnosis: The application of ideomotor techniques*. Allyn and Bacon.

Dijksterhuis, A. (2004). Think different: The merits of unconscious thought in preference development and decision making. *Journal of Personality and Social Psychology*, *87*(5), 586–598. 10. 1037/0022-3514.87.5.586

Erickson, B. A., & Erickson-Klein, R. (1991). Milton Erickson's increasing shift to less directive hypnotic techniques illustrated by work with family members. In S. R. Lankton, S. G. Gilligan & J. K. Zeig (Eds.), *Views on Ericksonian brief therapy* (1st ed., Vol. 8). Brunner/Mazel.

Erickson, H. L., Erickson, M., & Clayton, D. (2006). *Modeling and role-modeling: A view from the client's world*. Unicorns Unlimited.

Erickson, M. H. (1922/2018). *The Canoe Diary of Milton H. Erickson: Audiobook*. Milton H. Erickson Foundation. https://catalog.erickson-foundation.org/category/the-canoe-diary

Erickson, M. H. (1927). *Some aspects of abandonment, feeblemindedness and crime*. [Unpublished Bachelor of Arts degree thesis]. University of Wisconsin.

Erickson, M. H. (1932/2010). Possible detrimental effects of experimental hypnosis. In E. L. Rossi, R. Erickson-Klein & K. L. Rossi (Eds.), *Collected works of Milton H. Erickson: General & historical surveys of hypnosis* (Volume 8, pp. 47–52). Milton H. Erickson Foundation Press.

Erickson, M. H. (1943/2010). Hypnotic investigation of psychosomatic phenomena: Psychosomatic interrelationships studied by experimental hypnosis. In E. L. Rossi, R. Erickson-Klein, & K. L. Rossi (Eds.), *Collected works of Milton H. Erickson: Basic hypnotic induction and suggestion* (Volume 7, pp. 5–18). Milton H. Erickson Foundation Press.

Erickson, M. H. (1945/2008). Hypnotic techniques for the therapy of acute psychiatric disturbances in war. In E. L. Rossi & R. Erickson-Klein (Eds.), *The collected works of Milton H. Erickson, Basic hypnotic induction & suggestion* (Volume 2, pp. 35–41). Milton H. Erickson Foundation.

Erickson, M. H. (1952). *A teaching seminar by Milton H. Erickson. An archival recording of a seminar taught in Chicago*. Milton H. Erickson Foundation Archive.

Erickson, M. H. (1954/2008). Special techniques of brief hypnotherapy. In E. L. Rossi & R. Erickson-Klein (Eds.), *The collected works of Milton H. Erickson: Opening the mind* (Volume 3, pp. 5–29). Milton H. Erickson Foundation.

Erickson, M. H. (1958/2008). Naturalistic techniques of hypnosis. In E. L. Rossi, R. Erickson-Klein & K. L. Rossi (Eds.), *The collected works of Milton H. Erickson: The nature of therapeutic hypnosis* (Volume 1, pp. 261–270). Milton H. Erickson Foundation Press.

Erickson, M. H. (1959/2008). Further clinical techniques of hypnosis: Utilization techniques. In E. L. Rossi, R. Erickson-Klein, & K. L. Rossi (Eds.), *The collected works of Milton H. Erickson: The nature of therapeutic hypnosis* (Volume 1, pp. 271–306). Milton H. Erickson Foundation Press.

Erickson, M. H. (1960/2010). Explorations in hypnosis research. In E. L. Rossi, R. Erickson-Klein & K. L. Rossi (Eds.), *The collected works of Milton H. Erickson* (pp. 305–332). Milton H. Erickson Foundation.

Erickson, M. H. (1961/2010). Definition of hypnosis. In E. L. Rossi, R. Erickson-Klein & K. L. Rossi (Eds.), *The collected works of Milton H Erickson: General & historical surveys of hypnosis* (Volume 8, pp. 27–34). Milton H. Erickson Foundation Press.

Erickson, M. H. (1961/2008). Historical note on the hand levitation and other ideomotor techniques. In E. L. Rossi, R. Erickson-Klein, & K. L. Rossi (Eds.), *The collected works of Milton H. Erickson: The nature of therapeutic hypnosis* (Volume 1, pp. 223–228). Milton H. Erickson Foundation Press.

Erickson, M. H. (1964). The burden of responsibility in effective psychotherapy. In E. L. Rossi, R. Erickson-Klein, & K. L. Rossi (Eds.), *The collected works of Milton H. Erickson: Opening the mind* (Volume 3, pp. 67–72). Milton H. Erickson Foundation Press.

Erickson, M. H. (1966). *A lecture by Milton H. Erickson, Houston, TX. February 18, 1966. (Audio Recording No. CD/EMH.66.2.18).* The Milton H. Erickson Foundation Archives.

Erickson, M. H. (1967/2008). Further experimental investigation of hypnosis: Hypnotic and non-hypnotic realities. In E. Rossi, R. Erickson-Klein & K. L. Rossi (Eds.), *The collected works of Milton H. Erickson: The nature of therapeutic hypnosis* (Volume 1, pp. 89–160). Milton H. Erickson Foundation Press.

Erickson, M. H. (1979/2017). *In the Room with Milton H. Erickson, M.D.: October 3rd–5th, 1979.* Parsons-Fein Press.

Erickson, M. H. (1939/2000). Letter to G. H. Estabrooks. In J. K. Zeig & B. B. Geary (Eds.), *The letters of Milton H. Erickson.* Zeig, Tucker & Theisen, Inc.

Erickson, M. H., & Haley, J. (1985). *Conversations with Milton H. Erickson, M.D.: Changing individuals* (Vol I). Triangle Press.

Erickson, M. H., & Rossi, E. L. (1976/2010). Hypnotic realities: The induction of clinical hypnosis and forms of indirect suggestion. In E. L. Rossi, R. Erickson-Klein, & K. L. Rossi (Eds.), *The collected works of Milton H. Erickson* (Volume 10). Milton H. Erickson Foundation Press.

Erickson, M. H., & Rossi, E. L. (1977/2008). Autohypnotic experiences of Milton H. Erickson. In E. L. Rossi, R. Erickson-Klein, & K. L. Rossi (Eds.), *The collected works of Milton H. Erickson: The nature of therapeutic hypnosis* (Volume 1, pp. 189–217). Milton H. Erickson Foundation Press.

Erickson, M. H., & Rossi, E. L. (1979/2014). Hypnotherapy: An exploratory casebook. In E. L. Rossi, R. Erickson-Klein, & K. L. Rossi (Eds.), *The collected works of Milton H. Erickson* (Volume 11). The Milton Erickson Foundation Press.

Estabrooks, G. H. (1943). *Hypnotism.* Dutton.

Fromm, E., & Shor, R. E. (1979). *Hypnosis: Developments in research and new perspectives.* Aldine Publishing.

Gauld, A. (1992). *A history of hypnotism.* Cambridge University Press.

Gilligan, S. G. (2002). *The legacy of Milton H. Erickson: Selected papers of Stephen Gilligan.* Zeig, Tucker & Theisen, Inc.

Hilgard, E. R. (1992). Dissociation and theories of hypnosis. In E. Fromm & M. Nash (Eds.), *Contemporary hypnosis research* (pp. 69–101). Guilford Press.

Hull, C. L. (1933). *Hypnosis and suggestibility: An experimental approach.* Crown House Publishing, LLC.

Kekecs, Z., Moss, D., Elkins, G., De Benedittis, G., Palsson, O. S., Shenefelt, P. D., Terhune, D. B., Varga, K., & Whorwell, P. J. (2022). Guidelines for the assessment of efficacy of clinical hypnosis applications. *International Journal of Clinical and Experimental Hypnosis, 70*(2), 104–122. 10.1080/00207144.2022.2049446

Lankton, S. (2010). A basic footprint of Milton H. Erickson's process of change. In E. L. Rossi, R. Erickson-Klein, & K. L. Rossi (Eds.), *Collected works of Milton H Erickson: Classical hypnotic phenomena* (Volume 6, Part 2). Milton H. Erickson Foundation Press.

Lehrer, J. (2008). The Eureka Hunt. *The New Yorker* (July 28). https://www.newyorker.com/magazine/2008/07/28/the-eureka-hunt

Nieuwenstein M. R., Wierenga T., Morey R. D., Wicherts J. M., Blom T. N., Wagenmakers E.-J., & Rijn H. (2015). On making the right choice: A meta-analysis and large-scale replication attempt of the unconscious thought advantage. *Judgment and Decision Making*, *10*(1), 1–17.

Noyes, A. P. (1940). *Modern clinical psychiatry* (2nd ed.). Saunders.

Palsson, O. S., Kekecs, Z., De Benedittis, G., Moss, D., Elkins, G., Terhune, D., Varga, K., Shenefelt, P., & Whorwell, P. (2022). Current practices, experiences, and views in clinical hypnosis: Findings of an international survey. *International Journal of Clinical and Experimental Hypnosis*. http://real.mtak.hu/149906/

Rodolfa, E. R., Kraft, W. A., & Reilley, R. R. (1985). Current trends in hypnosis and hypnotherapy: An interdisciplinary assessment. *American Journal of Clinical Hypnosis*, *28*(1), 20–26. 10.1080/00029157.1985.10402627

Rossi, E. L. (1973). Psychological shocks and creative moments in psychotherapy. *American Journal of Clinical Hypnosis*, *16*(1), 9–22. 10.1080/00029157.1973.10403646

Short, D. (2018). Conversational hypnosis: Conceptual and technical differences relative to traditional hypnosis. *American Journal of Clinical Hypnosis*, *61*(2), 125–139. 10.1080/00029157.2018.1441802

Short, D. (2019). *Principles and core competencies of Ericksonian therapy: 2019 edition* [PDF]. The Milton H. Erickson Institute of Phoenix. http://www.iamdrshort.com/PDF/Papers/Core%20Competencies%20Manual.pdf

Short, D. (2020). *From William James to Milton Erickson: The care of human consciousness*. Archway Publishing from Simon & Schuster. https://www.bokus.com/bok/9781480891623/from-william-james-to-milton-erickson/

Short, D. (2021a). What is Ericksonian therapy: The use of core competencies to operationally define a non-standardized approach to psychotherapy. *Clinical Psychology: Science and Practice*, *28*(3), 282–292. 10.1037/cps0000014

Short, D. (2021b). *Making psychotherapy more effective with unconscious process work*. Routledge. 10.4324/9781003127208

Short, D. (2022). The aim of clinical hypnosis—Intelligence or compliance? *American Journal of Clinical Hypnosis*, *64*(4), 283–289. 10.1080/00029157.2022.2039637

Sio, U. N., & Ormerod, T. C. (2009). Does incubation enhance problem solving? A meta-analytic review. *Psychological Bulletin*, *135*(1), 94–120. 10.1037/a0014212

Weitzenhoffer, A. M. (1957). *General techniques of hypnotism*. Grune & Stratton.

Zeig, J. K. (1980). *Teaching seminar with Milton H. Erickson, M.D.*. Routledge.

Zeig, J. K. (1985). *Experiencing Erickson*. Brunner/Mazel.

Zeig, J. K. (2019). *Evocation*. Milton H. Erickson Foundation.

5

ATTACHMENT AND HYPNOSIS

Revisiting Our Evolutionary Past to Reconstruct Our Future

David S. Alter

Partners in Healing of Minneapolis, MN, United States

Introduction

Sometime in the 1990s, an enchanter, a wandless wizard, and a necromancer of nuance guided this author through his first advanced level training in clinical hypnosis. Kay Thompson, DDS, left me with more than an appreciation of our mouths as our "emotional learning centers" (Kane & Olness, 2004). She imprinted on my mind, and rewired into the neural networks of my brain, that language, our predominant form of communication expressed through the mouth, rarely means *only* what spoken semantics state. Language is a multi-leveled conveyor of meaning, connection, influence, surprise, and affection. Too often, clinical hypnosis, as currently taught, is stripped of its inherent elegance for influencing and evoking change in favor of its surface level message, conveyed as a scripted denotation, thereby bypassing its connotative potential. The trajectory of my clinical life was forever altered through my encounters with Dr. Thompson.

My definition of clinical hypnosis, incorporating what I learned from Dr. Thompson and many others, is both evolutionarily grounded and ultimately future oriented. My training in neuropsychology and health psychology is influenced by my view of what makes hypnosis and trance so potent when directed to healing efforts. Specifically, I view hypnosis as an interactive, relationally attuned process by which I evoke clients' capacity for ongoing neuroplastic adaptation through curiosity-driven inquiries and interactions with clients in a spirit of collaborative uncertainty and wonder. This chapter aims to alter your perception of hypnosis and to ultimately influence your utilization of it. This effort will be pursued in relation to the neuroscience of attachment, the fertile subsoil upon which clinical hypnosis is constructed.

Clinical hypnosis may well be a nonsensical construct except in terms of a distinctive environment in which relationally attuned interaction patterns oriented to evoking nascent client capacities are utilized (Alter, 2020; Sugarman, 2021; Sugarman et al., 2020). The progressive steps to be undertaken herein include: (1) a review of the evolutionary endowments that led to emergence of attachment; (2) re-consideration of attachment in relation to the neuro-sculpting of the brain and mind; (3) attachment-based prerequisites for changing one's mind; (4) the role that trance plays, when utilized in hypnotic

DOI: 10.4324/9781003449126-9

encounters, in mind-changing activities; and (5) the sweeping ramifications for hypnosis teaching and clinical application of attachment-based hypnosis practices.

Delving into the neuroscience of attachment and its relevance to clinical hypnosis invites the reader on a multi-directional journey. The engaged reader, possessing a current passport and a sense of wonder, will visit foreign lands to unexpected ports of call replete with both timeless and contemporary discoveries. The curious traveler will come away with an altered view of the mind, the social brain, embodied cognition, emergent potentials, the nature of change, and how clinical hypnosis, intentionally and unwittingly, instantiates these constructs in ways that facilitate the client–clinician dyad's capacity to foment and facilitate positive change.

This chapter, then, seeks to corral divergent lines of research about attachment. It funnels them toward the elucidation of the lifespan developmental role through which attachment patterns, channeled through client–clinician encounters within our extant system of healthcare, potentiate the emergence of enhanced adaptive flexibility (i.e., health and healing). In addition, I highlight the unique role that clinical hypnosis can play in facilitating improved health in the individuals who make use of hypnotic processes in the course of the forms of care in which they participate.

Evolution of Attachment

To commence our journey, let's posit the obvious: attachment patterns exist, arising among earth's varied denizens even before the arrival on earth of social mammals, including humans. Attachment has been observed to operate during critical periods early in the life of non-human animals (Hoffman, 1987; Lorenz, 1935; Tzschentke & Plagemann, 2006). In other words, while the observable and biologically driven behaviors to attach endure throughout many creatures' lives, it is during time-limited periods of heightened sensitivity to environmental contexts that the specific permutations and elementally constructed mosaics of attachment patterns come to be established. Alongside seeking security and enhanced survival odds associated with successful attachment, there also exists its evolutionary converse: fear conditioning. LeDoux (2012) cites the precursors to the discrimination between safe vs. dangerous environments as present even in single-celled animals. With time and evolutionarily driven enhancements to brain development, structures such as the amygdala, hippocampus, and prefrontal brain regions, which include the insula, cingulate, and medial prefrontal cortex, emerged. Along with them (or perhaps enabled by them), the palette of social engagement behaviors that could be expressed by mammals that eventually included homo sapiens expanded exponentially.

Success with attachment and avoidance of threat are expressions of behavior driven in part by the neural circuitry of the amygdala, which is specialized for its capacity to determine stimulus relevance (Olsson & Phelps, 2007; Sander et al., 2003). After all, little is more evolutionarily *relevant* than survival! Increasingly finer and more sophisticated brain-circuit determiners of stimulus relevance expanded as did the sophistication of the brain in which those circuits were housed. The ability to weigh relative risk/reward potentials for engaging with a fickle or historically volatile social group member entails far greater processing complexity than does a mere go-no-go, approach-avoid decision tree characteristic of amphibians (Goodall, 1986; Panksepp & Biven, 2012; Porges, 2011).

That attachment patterns, which are established early on in humans, persist over a lifetime is not news either (Cozolino, 2006; Frith, 2007; Feinberg, 2009; Siegel, 2012).

A current terrain where the field of attachment is traveling involves the nature of varied facets of "attachment" of body-to-brain, brain-to-body, and mind-to-brain. Maturana and Varela (1987) overtly and sometimes implicitly emphasize that attachment occurs between embodied human beings and is a central underpinning for social lives and much that such lives experience and produce. Beginning in primary subcortical and cortical neural circuits involved with sensing and the expression of early motor behavior in the first few years of life, Sydnor et al. (2021) trace the ontogenetic path along which social attachment environments become fortified (but not fixed) biological structures. Depending upon the character and quality of the nurturing environment to which the individual is exposed, the maturing brain follows different formative paths. Ontogenesis grooms later-developing, higher-order association cortices of the brain to rigidify developing neural circuits, thereby sculpting preferred neural pathways for activation of variations of fear responding when pronounced environmental stressors persist. Alternatively, ontogenesis, under the sculpting influence of safer, more attentive caregiving environments, prolongs neuroplastic maleability such that the individual can maintain for a longer time greater adaptive capacity in the face of an ambiguous external environment. That capacity is characterized by greater tolerance of uncertainty, a propensity for curiosity-driven exploratory behaviors, and diminished prevalence of various forms of psychopathology (Cicchetti & Curtis, 2015; Davidson, 2000; Sydnor et al., 2021). The later-maturing tertiary association cortices are where the individual particularities of attachment circuit learnings manifest via the dynamic choreography that occurs between and among the mind-brain-bodies of different individuals across their lifespans (Stanton et al., 2014). Contemporary clinicians recognize these particularities of attachment, originally described by Bowlby in the 1960s, as *secure, avoidant, ambivalent,* and *disorganized* in children (Belsky, 2002), or as *autonomous (secure), dismissing (avoidant), preoccupied (anxious),* and *unresolved (fearful-avoidant)* in adults (Sperling et al., 1992). A wide range of therapeutic interventions were built off of the foundational and formative work of early attachment researchers. Mary Main, the co-developer of the Adult Attachment Interview (George et al., 1986), deepened and expanded our understanding of the clinical relevance of attachment patterns such as the disorganized attachment subtype. The psychotherapeutic benefits of this understanding permeate multiple therapeutic approaches (Levy et al., 2010) and Sue Johnson's *Emotionally Focused Therapy* (Johnson et al., 2008).

Neuro-Sculpting the Social Brain

It was just a few short decades ago that Bowlby (1969, 1973) and Ainsworth (1969) engaged in healthy debate regarding the functional parameters within which observed attachment behaviors in infants operated. Through their intellectual tussles, and those of many others that followed, there emerged recognition that early attachment behaviors both confer and enable numerous emergent developmental benefits to humans that extend far beyond enhancement of the odds of infants' survival. Examples include internalization of infants' interpersonal attunement skills essential to brain-based empathy development (Cozolino, 2006; Ranson & Urichuk, 2008; Schore, 2019); learning how attachment patterns impact upon the cultivation of an effective and adaptable social brain (Cozolino, 2006; Frith, 2007; Siegel, 2012); and the transmission of culture across generations through the acquisition of civilizing socio-culture-specific interpersonal behavioral expectations (Granqvist, 2021). Clearly, the expanding trajectories of lines of research involving attachment amply demonstrate the profoundly diverse domains of human functioning subsumed to one degree or another by the early and continuous influences on humans' patterns of attachment.

With notable exceptions, the field of attachment has adopted a unidirectional focus: Distinct adults possess established patterns of attachment, which then, through their social interactions with infants, shape the nascent and immature attachment patterns possessed by the infant. Fonagy and Target (2005) eloquently emphasize how processes such as gene expression and receptor density changes in the infant unfold through a sequential process that theoretically optimizes pro-social relatedness. Gillath et al. (2008), Bryant et al. (2012), and Zelinka et al. (2014) explicate the genetic roots of adult attachment and the role of oxytocin that function as modulators of relational attachment patterns. More recently, Long et al. (2020) formulated a neurobiological model (the neuro-anatomical model of human attachment, or NAMA) that posits that innate attachment pathways become modified through subsequent attachment experiences (e.g., orienting the individual toward secure vs. insecure attachment styles).

These authors' works harbor important implications for clinical hypnosis. Genetic, hormonal, and neuro-anatomical bases of attachment are shown to be modifiable through experience (i.e., subject to epigenetic influences). Oxytocin, known to mediate patterns of attachment and social bonding, appears to impact hypnotizability (Zelinka, 2014). Thus, clinical hypnosis may offer clients a powerful means by which the maleability of their attachment styles may be positively modified in the direction of neuroplasticity-driven enhanced adaptiveness.

Numerous authors have explicated how social connections and contexts shape the immature brain (Feinberg, 2009; LeDoux, 2002; Sporn, 2011; Sueng, 2012). In the case of parent–child interactions, for example, the child and parent are simultaneously the organizers and the ones being organized. One implication of this is that whether operating within immature or mature brains, attachment patterns remain plastic. The potency of this mutually self-reorganizing capacity is especially important in the client–clinician encounter. Erickson (1980) emphasized how therapy generally and hypnosis specifically utilize the self-reorganizing capacity relationally operating "in the in between," as described by Baker and Spiegel (2019), of the therapeutic encounter to enable the client "to use his own thinking, his own understandings, his own emotions in the way that best fits him in his scheme of life" (Erickson, 1980, p. 223).

The prominence, if not predominance of the prevailing view that attachment occurs between interacting but ultimately separate beings (i.e., caregiver–infant; intimate partner–intimate partner; client–clinician), prefigures how we understand what transpires in the therapeutic process, how we conceptualize hypnosis, and how hypnosis is taught. From a neuroscientific perspective, attachment binds us to a conceptual framework in which separate entities regularly come into contact with other independent entities.

But there is more going on than meets the casual eye. In their meeting, a transductive change occurs through multiple layers of interaction. Sharma (2015) offers a metaphor. Molecules released from a baker's freshly baked bread waft through the air and contact the mucosal surface of a passers-by nasal membrane. There, they transduce the scent molecule into an electrical signal carried to the individual's olfactory bulb, which rapidly and somewhat non-consciously precipitates a behavioral change in the passing pedestrian, who then changes course to make a quick stop in the bakery on the way to the bus stop (Sharma, 2015). The key interactive elements are literally floating in the atmosphere *between* the baker's bread and the pedestrian.

Thus, beyond the social interpenetration of two distinct selves that arise via their relational interactions and the intersection of their embodied attachment patterns emerges uncertainties as to whether the concept of *two entirely separate selves interacting* is even a best fit framework (Siegel, 2017) through which to consider attachment. As Stolorow and Atwood (1996, p. 181) described, perhaps "interacting subjectivities" is a more apt framework. For your consideration I offer: *My ever-shifting subjective experience, continuously influenced by your ever-shifting subjective experience, which is subject to the evolving influence of the spatial context within which we are both embedded and embodied, is forever in the process of becoming.*

The implications of this dynamic mutuality of influence are quite profound as it extends to the therapeutic relationship and into a special role for hypnotic processes when they are utilized within a wide range of therapeutic approaches. In other words, perhaps the whirlpool or vortex from which change arises does not only or even primarily take place *between* client and clinician but also concurrently *within* each party to the therapeutic environment's co-creative process as each attunes to the other emotionally, cognitively, energetically, and behaviorally. Going a step further, perhaps the capsule of time, space, and energy surrounding the interacting parties is actually the plasma within which change arises. Like the air surrounding the bakery, the parties are exchanging within that space what each of them breathes in and out, which is dynamically and simultaneously impacting both. Therapeutically, what each party to the dyadic process brings is in constant flux, shaping and being shaped, evoking and being evoked, suggesting and being suggested to, the result not predetermined but emerging in and through this attuned and attuning process. The therapist's pre-eminent skill may be in channeling conscious awareness of the potential inherent in this state of flux to evoke through verbal and non-verbal means iterative shifts in the client's receptivity to change. The process of clinical hypnosis is particularly well suited to achieving this.

The multi-level merger of client and clinician is captured by Stern (2010), who said, "*Even in the absence of other people, we learn about ourselves by listening to our own thoughts about ourselves through the ears of the other. We need an emotionally responsive witness ... We need a witness to become a self; and later in life, in similar fashion, we need a witness to heal ourselves*" (my italics, p. xvii). Kahn and Fromm's (2001) edited collection of clinician reflections on how each author was changed through the therapeutic dyad tenderly highlights the unavoidable "self" permeability that arises between parties to the change process. Perhaps this melding of two beings into a shared meta-being is a shorthand for the process of *utilization* consistently cited as a key element of the hypnotic process (Flemons, 2022). Flemons (2022) adopts a mentalized relational framework when he describes hypnosis as based upon "shared-mind-attunement" or "connected knowing," that "unfolds in the mutuality, the synergy, of the relationship between hypnotist and client" (p. xix).

Thus, attachment, whether in the realm of the biochemically synthesized glue that links together separate creatures in life, or, especially in the domain of human beings, the diaphanous strands joining one person to another across time, defines the basis of formative and lasting connections between individuals. Clinically, this is enacted by helping clients respond to their life circumstances more adaptively and flexibly, a process arising through iterative modifications to pre-existing attachment that manifest in the dyadic therapeutic space. In so doing, we assist clients to transcend a stimulus-response-bound existence. One benefit of hypnosis rests in its capacity to insert deliberative and reflective pauses between stimulus and response. In this manner, clients become less bound by historically rooted responses and can instead express a wider range of future-oriented explorations for new ways of being and behaving (Alter, 2020), and manifest cultivation of positive expectancy (Yapko, 2021).

Stephen Porges (2003, 2011) highlighted the existence of attachment circuits in non-human, mammalian species as he was developing the foundations for what became known as the *Polyvagal Theory*. Humans share neuroendocrine and neurotransmitter molecules with pre-human species. No wonder, then, that Carter et al. (2017, 2011) and Perkeybile et al. (2019), for example, describe how neuroendocrine molecules such as oxytocin and vasopressin exert powerful effects on social bonding patterns in non-sapien mammals that are preserved in humans. These findings build on the foundational work of Panksepp and Biven (2012). They researched how brain circuitry drives attachment and bonding pattern formation in social mammals. This circuitry is a prerequisite for rapid *neuroception* (Porges' term) of environmental safety and the rapid activation of behavioral survival strategies, or social approach/engage behaviors that cultivate group connection, cohesion, and cooperation.

As this author contends, a common denominator of social engagement and attachment across species is its dependence upon and expression through a physical body. The body is not merely the vehicle enabling attachment to be exhibited. Lakoff (2012) and Johnson (2007) argue compellingly that the physical body actively shapes the essential form of the sensory stimuli that are perceived, consequently determining the actions undertaken by the embodied being. The field of embodied cognition is involved with exploring the manner in which mind, brain, and body intersect and interact to shape cognition and, in turn, behavior. For our purposes, incorporation of the evolving states of the clinician and client's bodies into the therapeutic encounter, especially when hypnotic attunement is actively utilized, can result in far-reaching clinical impact for clients and their goals.

Evan Thompson orients us to several salient points in regard to humans' predilection for attachment (Thompson, 2010). Summarily, human perception occurs in and through our physical bodies, which *can't not* use the sensorimotor skills with which they are endowed to initiate actions in the external world in which they reside. The particular actions undertaken by an individual, which range from reflexive responses to complex, thoughtful, and planful strategies, emerge in and through social contexts (Gallese & Cuccio, 2015). The responses are adaptive, moving toward ever-evolving, future-oriented, but not necessarily conscious outcomes, that are concurrently non-predictive (not determined by existing circumstances in a formulaic, pre-scripted fashion) and non-reductive (not able to be anticipated through a study of the deconstructed elements comprising a given response).

Thus far, the ubiquity of attachment patterns' existence across eons of time and across life's diverse species has been emphasized. With the evolutionary emergence of social mammals, however, which coincided with increased interconnectivity of brain circuits and the outfolding of the prefrontal brain regions, the sophistication of neuroceptive circuits and their behavioral response correlates multiplied. Nevertheless, at its core, attachment remains an umbrella construct that subsumes the primal drive to rapidly extract from the external environment cues that identify what is safe, what is not, and hence, what form of engagement or disengagement is requisite in the moment-to-moment unfolding of an interactive encounter. The relevance of this to interactions in a clinical context will be addressed next.

Attachment, Intention, and Decision-Making

While attachment seeking is not optional, it is also not reflexive. Attachment is anything but invariant. Brown (2016) cites extensive evidence that regards attachment as an ongoing "best-fit dyadic correspondence" (Sander & Julia, 1966) forever engaged in relationship-building. Brown (2016, p. 77) references research by Cassidy (2008) emphasizing that the attachment system, replete with strong motivational drives akin to those for feeding and sex, endows the attachment seeker with the capacity to "respond flexibly to environmental changes while attempting to attain a goal," that goal being, according to Brown, the reduction of states of internal distress. The deceptively innocuous and simple goal of alleviating "internal distress" masks the far-ranging anthology of variations in human relationality.

Much variability and potentiality of expression is embedded within a goal of alleviation of internal distress. Achieving the goal begs the following questions.

1 What constitutes *distress* (e.g., subjective report or validated index)?
2 What factors influence *variations in individual tolerance* of distress (e.g., individual differences in pain sensitivity (Cortade et al., 2023))?
3 Can similar levels of externally defined distress (e.g., fixed decibel level, cold water temperature, pressure using forceps on a subject's thenar webspace) result in variations in a person's response patterns oriented toward its alleviation, implying that distress must work in tandem with environmental contingencies that activate response A vs. response B?
4 Is there evidence that a specific distress alleviation response by someone at Time A evolves with experience such that at Time B a more effective or adaptive response pattern is exhibited by that individual to a similar distress triggering circumstance?

The research consensus of these questions points toward attachment behaviors getting triggered throughout the human lifespan when a perceived threat to a person's felt sense of safety or comfort, initially internalized to one degree or another in infancy, is subsequently retriggered when salient perceptual elements of the original experience are again present (Brown, 2016). The perception being discussed here need not be and frequently does not entail conscious awareness. What constitutes distress to a given individual, regardless of age, depends, according to Brown (2016), on the extent to whether general factors such as a good enough caregiver was *physically present*, with sufficient *consistency* in their caregiving behavior, that the caregiver was *reliable* in their provision of this care, and they exhibited perceptible *interest* in the needs of the care recipient.

The shaping of the infant's attachment template is influenced by five primary caregiver affectively charged behaviors that include: how well the infant was *protected*, whether affective *attunement* to the infant's dynamic needs was present, the extent to which responses to the infant's distress included both transmission of *soothing* responses and comforting *reassurance*, and that *expressions of delight* in the infant's behavior and in the mere existence of the infant's *"beingness"* were conveyed (Brown, 2016, pp. 86–87).

The infant's understanding of *receptive* language is followed by the emergence of facility with expressive language beginning in the 12- to 18-month-old period. This does not negate but becomes intertwined with the continuing influence of non-verbal, primarily right-hemisphere influences (Schore, 2019). As Lindell (2006) reminds us, the right hemisphere is actively involved in non-semantic aspects of both language reception and expression. Nevertheless, McGilchrist (2009) cogently notes the culturally pervasive risks to mental health when left hemisphere processing assumes a disproportionately dominant role in the world of interpersonal relating, which he concludes is the Western way. He goes on to indict our Western culture's deification of left hemisphere processing at the expense of the right in numerous aspects of our societal rituals, rules, and regulations, and as their being causally implicated in a range of today's societal ills (e.g., detached, transactional evaluation vs. empathic engagement; over-valuation of the material, quantifiability of the external world vs. the qualitative subjectivity of one's internal phenomenology and that of the actively reading of the "other"; and the worship of the individual over the individual's role in the collective whole) (McGilchrist, 2009).

Studies of hemispheric specialization have much to offer clinicians, regardless of the therapeutic tradition in which they may have been trained. The spoken word is the universal currency used in the majority of therapies. However, over-reliance on words, especially when conveyed while detached from the intentional utilization of the clinician's body, is akin to interacting with another person while both are gazing through the wrong end of a pair of binoculars; the images may be accurate as far as they go, but the breadth and context of the information flow are sorely restricted.

If therapeutics fundamentally entails facilitation of the clients' capacities to *change their minds* (Sugarman et al., 2020), it is important to appreciate how quickly and largely non-consciously peoples' minds arrive at decisions (Klein & O'Brien, 2018). As previously noted, prior to and operating beneath conscious awareness, attachment patterns are central to the person's assessment of social safety that titrates the engagement behavior that follows. While this is certainly true for children, even otherwise self-aware adults often act on habit patterns ingrained in cognitive, affective, social, and behavioral neural circuits that still arise from non-conscious levels of the multi-layered brain without reaching conscious awareness despite exerting a strong influence on consciously mediated actions (Bierman, 2004; Mullaney & Regan, 2019). As this pertains to clinical hypnosis, Erickson's experience with limited paralysis during his post-polio recovery sensitized him to the critical role of non-verbal and gestural aspects of communication, which he later incorporated into his trance evocation philosophy and practices (Havens, 2003).

Studies on embodied cognition are therefore important in part because they remind clinicians to deliberately embody the therapeutic interaction, to enliven it with gesture, bodily movement, alterations in inflection, pace, and other prosodic aspects of vocalization. Cook and Goldin-Meadow (2006) demonstrated the importance of intentional use of gestures (e.g., using our hands, leaning in, or sitting back) when conveying information to children, in tandem with prosodic aspect of speech, and how much improved their learning rate and volume was. Moreover, the authors found that when it comes to *changing their mind* about what they are learning, inclusion of gestures, that is, utilizing embodied communication, enriched the learning process for the learner (Cook & Goldin-Meadow, 2006).

Changing one's mind, regardless of the relative contribution of each cerebral hemisphere, depends upon the emergence of various metacognitive functions through childhood, adolescence, young adulthood, and beyond. One of them is called *Theory of Mind* (ToM) and involves the ability to predictively mentalize what another is thinking or believes (Flavell, 2004; Shahaeian et al., 2011). This capacity is central to the ability to *"read"* the other. Effective interpersonal interactions depend upon it. The mechanism enabling *theory of minding*, the capacity to imagine, understand, and feel what another may be thinking, arises in and through the architecture of the brain during development

(Leslie et al., 2004). Theory of minding is wired into our neuroanatomy as part of complex relationally oriented neural networks. The emphasis on belief in ToM research is important because when faced with a choice between observed reality and a belief held about it, the belief trumps the perception: People act in accord with their beliefs, and changing their beliefs, when consciously held and even more so when grounded in attachment-based presuppositions out of which beliefs are fashioned, takes emotional, energetic, and experiential effort. Cognitive dissonance is but one example of the inertia persons encounter when their prevailing *theory of mind* conflicts with encountered reality (Wellman, 2018). To change one's mind, especially under conditions of personal challenge, as is largely the case in clinical settings, entails transcending the observable facts; alteration of emotionally charged experiences with the inculcated and presumed facts is needed. As noted earlier, plasticity of attachment patterns persists throughout life, which is a hopeful tone to strike when considering the far-reaching potential of therapeutically attuned interactions between clients and their clinicians.

The ToM neural circuits are attuned to significant others and enable mentalization of what the other may be thinking or feeling by activating within the self, various sensations and emotions ascribed to the other. The research into the mirror neuron system (Rizzolatti & Craighero, 2004) has explored this domain extensively, searching for the biological/neurological roots of empathy, compassion, as well as various motor learning and problem-solving skill acquisition. The system enables reflective functioning and in-the-moment attitudinal and behavioral course corrections that fine tune social engagement (i.e., approach/avoid) and interaction. This highly calibrated interpersonal attunement depends in part on the role of interneurons within the brain (Cardin, 2018) that provide perpetual feedback to the brain's social networks, assuring divergence from fixed, reflexive social behaviors toward nuanced and emotional intimacy-promoting connections and actions. The interneurons within the brain's mirroring system also enable self-aware reflection. These circuits act as a type of mirroring of the self to other aspects of the self as the existence and capabilities of the self-aware self gradually emerge (Fonagy & Allison, 2016). Conclusions about the mirror neuron system's existence, function, and role in empathy acquisition are not universally accepted, however (Hickok, 2009).

Nevertheless, as we move ever closer to discussing the clinical applications of attachment and metacognition in all its varied forms, a central point stands out. The experience of the "other" becomes inextricably bound up in the experience of the self. As we alluded to earlier when discussing Thompson's contributions to understanding *mind*, there is ultimately a blurring of the distinctions necessary to characterize attachment as occurring between separate selves, and more toward deep states of multi-level intersubjectivity (i.e., *You and I are an I-You*) (Spiegel & Baker, 2019). This constitutes embodied and interactive fulfilment of Martin Buber's *I-Thou* relationship (Buber, 1971).

Attachment, mentalization, and theory of mind are all examples of reflective functioning capacities of the human brain. It is important to note that the reflection need not be mediated consciously. Given the primal nature of attachment and human mentalization capacity, that these functions can occur without the intercession of conscious mediation is a blessing and a curse. The non-conscious, subcortical regions of the brain rely very heavily on associative conditions to hone the neural circuits that enable numerous facets of perception, motor responding, and physiologic response patterning. This includes the patterning involved in attachment styles that vary across individuals or within individuals across time and shifting contexts.

As Baker and Spiegel (2019) note, it's a central goal of the psycho-emotionally-charged physical space in which therapies take place, especially when optimized by the power of hypnotic processes, to utilize both regression and attuned attention to cultivate and evoke "developmentally focused interventions" that are key to helping clients change their minds, their bodies, and their lives. This work involves both bottom-up and top-down re-channeling of patterns of associative learning toward alterations in cognitive expectancy (Davidson, 2012). The well-attuned clinician facilitates a process whereby the client encounters reactivation of what has been *learned*, in a therapeutically and iteratively disorienting *unlearning* context, which facilitates a new and more adaptive *re-learning* to arise. Spiegel and Baker (2019) describe this past-present-future process as one of *internalization* of the novel learning, so that it becomes *incorporated* into the pre-reflective domain of the client's revised sense of self and where that self-sense becomes accessible to and recurrently used by the self to guide future behavior, especially in the interpersonal realm. The goal of this relearning process is *integration* in which those aspects of a fragmented or at least multi-faceted self are able to open an internal dialogue of sorts in which the various components of the self-operate more effectively as a complex, communicative, and cooperative whole (Spiegel & Baker, 2019).

A powerful example of the disruptive nature of the unlearning and relearning, or internalization, incorporation, and integration, is found in Akira Kurosawa's film, *Red Beard* (Kurosawa, 2002). In it, a young teen girl is brought to the hospital having been rescued from a brothel. Red Beard, the senior physician, leaves Yasumoto, the medical resident to "work her up," as she seems feverish, possibly delusional, and certainly uncooperative. After numerous unsuccessful attempts to elicit her cooperation with the examination, during which the girl repeatedly pushes away Yasumoto's outstretched hand in which he was balancing a spoonful of sticky, syrupy medicine, thereby spilling it and covering Yasumoto with the medicinal goo, he gives up. Red Beard re-enters and continues to offer the medicine to her, but in a careful, attuned, and evocatively engaging manner that iteratively gains the girl's behavioral cooperation: She opens her mouth and swallows the medicine, whereupon Red Beard leaves the scene. At that moment, speaking for the first time in the film, the girl asks of Yasumoto, *"Why didn't he slap me?"*

We all bring our acquired associations to our daily encounters. Particularly powerful are attachment-based associations that become, to one degree or another, anticipatory expectations that assure that the world conforms to client expectations, too often in seemingly maladaptive actions that run counter to idealized pro-social forms, even as the client's deepest desires are for them to change.

Attachment and Hypnosis

We are nearing the end of our journey. It is time to link the neuroscience of attachment research to the process and practice of clinical hypnosis. To date, we have mined the riches of the domains we have visited. We have established that attachment is an imperative of all life forms for their survival. The specific pattern of that attachment that gets exhibited is both highly variable, across and within species, and remains, to a greater or lesser extent, malleable, even within an individual across time. Much of what determines people's struggles in life, at least within clinical contexts, contains significant dollops of attachment-based difficulties. To draw upon statistical process called factor analysis, much of the variance in what ails people loads along a range of attachment variables.

Clinical hypnosis can be a formal and structured process. That is not an imperative, however, as much informal hypnotic influence (i.e., naturally occurring interpersonal suggestions such as placebo or nocebo) clearly demonstrates. Clinical hypnosis, whether overtly acknowledged or implicitly present, and even when explicitly denied, has always depended for its impact and efficacy on attachment-based variables, within the client, but especially in the intersubjective space encompassing client and clinician. Though he may have been loath to acknowledge it, Jean-Martin Charcot, working at the Saltpêtrière with Blanche, his famous client, as depicted in Brouillet's painting, *A Clinical Lesson*, (1887) was indirectly demonstrating the ineluctable presence of the attachment process that arises between client and clinician (Ropper & Burrell, 2019). Charcot actively explored the use of hypnosis in his efforts to treat her. Charcot believed that what rendered hypnosis effective was its similarity to hysteria, which he believed arose from bona fide neurological lesions in the brain. Looked at through our current understanding of the neuroscience of attachment, both Charcot's view and those of Hippolyte Bernheim and others at the Nancy School, who contemporaneously argued that *suggestion* and even *autosuggestion* operated to generate the observed results of hypnosis (*ibid*), were arguing that the relationship between client and clinician was an important variable in the results they observed. The point is that both theoretical camps were essentially unwittingly arguing that variations in attachment patterns were coursing through the hypnotic processes that were being utilized.

This review of the neuroscientific underpinnings of attachment, which operates within and between individuals who interact, whether in their actual external social environments, or when attachments are imaginally re-vivified within a given person's mind (Nachmanovitch, 2019), is action oriented (Baker & Spiegel, 2019; Kihlstrom 2013; Neufeld et al., 2016; Rossi, 2005). Attachment patterns operate to guide *how* social interactions unfold. Attachment patterns are agonists that activate psycho-biologically based social behavior. Clinical hypnosis is a *process* (Sugarman et al., 2020) through which those agonistic activators are channeled. Clinical hypnosis is but one *process* among many (peak performance states, meditative moments, experiences of awe and wonder, etc.) that are evocative of what flows beneath and enables the *processes* in question to emerge. What flows beneath them is the capacity for *trance*. Trance is rooted in the experiential space between the known and the unknown; the expected and the disorienting surprise; the certain and the ambiguousness of unrealized possibilities. In short, trance exists in the momentary disorienting space within which we can become "unattached" from what was and engage a host of neuroceptive circuits that search and discover what best-fit social engagement potential can be cognitively, affectively, and behaviorally formed, engaged in, and attached to, and then reactivated in the future through memorization mechanisms.

Viewed this way, clinical hypnosis is a process that channels trance toward its neuroplastic potential. Evoking uncertainty, curiosity, and discovery constitutes a triad of neuroplastic agonistic activators that support people's ability to change their minds. Moreover, moving beyond the traditional view of clinical hypnosis as comprising an *induction*, followed by *deepening*, to a point of sufficient mental depth whereupon *suggestions* get offered, and before *re-alerting* of the client commences in preparation for *debriefing* of the experience, a wholesale shift grounded in attachment processes comes into focus (Alter & Sugarman, 2017). Attachment shapes action. Actions shape attachment. Hypnosis, which is grounded in the attachment patterns that circulate in the intersubjective space of the client-clinician interaction, entails a shift in attachment within subconsciously encoded and sometimes consciously remembered history in preparation for modified attachment via new learning. For Rossi (1987), state-dependent learning, memory, and behavior (SDLMB), were descriptors for what went on within the cortico-limbic-hypothalamic system that enables people to change their minds. Given the action-orientation of hypnosis that these various authors posit, perhaps a different lexicon describing what hypnosis entails could better capture for students and practitioners of hypnosis what this social-relational therapeutic process involves.

The "shared-mind-attunement" and "connected knowing" view of hypnosis (Flemons, 2022) invites immersion in the intersubjective space that connection and sharing occupy. Within this space, the hypnotic ramifications of intentional empathizing as described by Flemons (2022) become clear. Descriptively, nouns do not cut it. Verbs, which are language structures that describe actions, states, and occurrences, are more appropriate. Broadly speaking, hypnosis is a process of deliberate and intentional empathic " ... *ing-ing,*" where this action-based, process-oriented suffix serves as a re-organizing map for hypnotic interacting. Defining empathy as "a projective curiosity, a desire to develop a body-based understanding of the other from within their world" (Flemons, 2020, p. 67), each " ... *ing*" stands as a teachable, trainable, interactive, elemental hypnotic enactment that resists becoming reductive or prescriptive. Hypnosis, in the opinion of the author, hews most closely with contemporary psychobiological discoveries when it retains the dual qualities of wondering and wandering while iteratively exploring the field of possibilities inherent in evoking a change of mind (Alter & Sugarman, 2017) in the co-creative space that incorporates the client and clinician. Hence, this author concludes with a description of the attachment-based process of hypnosis as that which emerges when client and clinician are jointly and continuously immersed in *attending, noticing, relating, respiring, reviewing, re-orienting, empathizing, influencing, modifying, re-regulating, exploring, re-discovering, evolving, incorporating,* and ultimately *integrating* the moment-to-moment phenomenology of their joint capacity to change their minds, and hence, their lives.

References

Ainsworth, M. (1969). Object relationships, dependency, and attachment: A theoretical review of the infant-mother relationship. *Child Development*, *40*, 969–1026. 10.2307/1127008

Alter, D. S. (2020). In the intersubjective space: Hypnosis through a neuropsychological lens. *American Journal of Clinical Hypnosis*, *65*(1–2), 74–94. 10.1080/00029157.2019.1581049

Alter, D. S., & Sugarman, L. I. (2017). Reorienting hypnosis education. *American Journal of Clinical Hypnosis*, *59*(3), 235–259. 10.1080/00029157.2016.1231657

Baker, E. L., & Spiegel, E. B. (2019). Dancing in the in-between: Hypnosis, transitional space, and therapeutic action. *American Journal of Clinical Hypnosis*, *62*(1–2), 31–59. 10.1080/00029157.2019.1585328

Belsky, J. (2002). Developmental origins of attachment styles. *Attachment & Human Development*, *4*(2), 166–170. 10.1080/14616730210157510

Bierman, D. J. (2004). Non conscious processes preceding intuitive decisions. *5th Bial foundation symposium: Behind and beyond the brain* (pp. 1–13). Research Gate Publication. http://www.researchgate.net/publication/254898676

Bowlby, J. (1969). *Attachment and loss. Attachment* (Vol. 1). New York: Basic Books.

Bowlby, J. (1973). *Attachment and loss. Separation: Anxiety and anger* (Vol. 2). New York: Basic Books.

Brown, D. & Elliott, D. S. (2016). *Attachment disturbances in adults: Treatment for comprehensive repair*. New York: W. W. Norton & Company, Inc.

Bryant, R. A., Hung, L., Guastella, A. J., & Mitchell, P. B. (2012). Oxytocin as a moderator of hypnotizability. *Psychoneuroimmunology*, *37*(1), 162–166. 10.1016/j.psyneuen.2011.05.010

Buber, M., & Kaufmann, W. (Translator). (1971). *I and Thou*. New York: Charles Scribner's Sons.

Cardin, J. (2018). Inhibitory interneurons regulate temporal precision and correlations in cortical circuits. *Trends in Neurosciences*, *41*(10), 689–700. 10.1016/j.tins.2018.07.015

Carter, C. S. (2017). The role of oxytocin and vassopressin in attachment. *Psychodynamic Psychiatry*, *45*(4), 499–517. 10.1521/pdps.2017.45.4.499

Carter, C. S., Harris, J., & Porges, S. W. (2011). Neural and evolutionary perspectives on empathy. In J. Decety, & W. Ickes (Eds.), *The social neuroscience of empathy* (pp. 241–262). Cambridge: The MIT Press.

Cassidy, J. (2008). The nature of child's ties. In J. Cassidy, & P. R. Shaver (Eds.), *Handbook of attachment: Theory, research, and clinical applications* (2nd ed., pp. 3–220). New York: Guilford Press.

Cicchetti, D., & Curtis, W. (2015). The developing brain and neural plasticity: Implications for normality, psychopathology, and resilience. In D. Cicchetti, & D. J. Cohen (Eds.), *Developmental psychopathology: Volume Two: Developmental neuroscience* (2nd ed., pp. 1–64). New York: John Wiley & Sons, Inc.

Cook, W. S., & Goldin-Meadow, S. (2006). The role of gesture in learning: Do children use their hands to change their minds? *Journal of Cognition and Development*, 7(2), 211–232. 10.1207/s15327647jcd0702_4

Cortade, D. L., Markovitz, J., Spiegel, D., & Wang, S. X. (2023). Point-of-care testing of enzyme polymorphisms of predicting hypnotizability and postoperative pain. *The Journal of Molecular Diagnostics*. 10.1016/j.jmoldx.2023.01.002

Cozolino, L. (2006). *The neuroscience of human relationships: Attachment and the developing social brain*. New York: W. W. Norton & Co., Inc..

Davidson, R. (2012). *The emotional life of your brain: How its unique patterns affect the way you think, feel, and live, and how you can change the;m*. New York: Penguin Publishing.

Davidson, R. J. (2000). Affective style, psychopathology, and resilience: Brain mechanisms and plasticity. *American Psychologist*, *55*(11), 1196–1214. 10.1037/0003-066X.55.11.1196

Erickson, M. H. (1980). The collected papers of Milton H. Erickson on hypnosis. In E. Rossi (Ed.), *Innovative hypnotherapy (Volume IV)*. New York: Irvington Publishers, Inc.

Feinberg, T. E. (2009). *From axons to identity: Neurological explanations of the nature of the self*. New York: W.W. Norton & Co., Inc.

Flavell, J. H. (2004). Theory-of-mind development: Retrospect and prospect. *Merrill Palmer Quarterly*, *50*(3), 274–290. https://www.jstor.org/stable/23096166

Flemons, D. (2022). *The heart and mind of psychotherapy: Inviting connection, inventing change*. New York: W. W. Norton & Company, Inc.

Fonagy, P., & Allison, E. (2016). Psychic reality and the nature of consciousness. *International Journal of Psychoanalysis*, *97*(1), 5–24.

Fonagy, P. & Target, M. (2005). Bridging the transmission gap: An end to an important mystery of attachment research. *Attachment & Human Development*, 7(3), 333–343. 10.1080/14616730500269278

Frith, C. D. (2007). The social brain? *Philosophical Transactions of the Royal Society B: Biological Sciences*, *363*(1480), 671–678. 10.1098/rstb.2006.2003

Gallese, V., & Cuccio, V. (2015). The paradigmatic body: Embodied simulation, intersubjectivity, the bodily self, and language. In T. Metzinger, & J. Windt (Eds.), *Open Mind* (pp. 1–22). Frankfurt am Main: Mind Group.

George, C., Kaplan, N., & Main, M. (1986). Discovery of an insecure-disorganized/disoriented attachment pattern. In T. B. Brazelton, & W. Yogman (Eds.), *Affective development in infancy* (pp. 95–124). Washington, DC: Ablex Publishing.

Gillath, O., Shaver, P. R., Baek, J.-M., & Chun, D. S. (2008). Genetic correlates of adult attachment style. *Personality and Social Psychology Bulletin*, *34*(10), 1396–1405. 10.1177/0146167208321484

Goodall, J. (1986). Social rejection, exclusion, and shunning among the Gombe chimpanzees. *Ethology and Sociobiology*, 7(3–4), 227–236. 10.1016/0162-3095(86)90050-6

Granqvist, P. (2021). Attachment, culture, and gene-culture co-evolution: Expanding the evolutionary toolbox of attachment theory. *Attachment and Human Development*, *23*(1), 90–113. 10.1080/14616734.2019.1709086

Havens, R. (2003). *The Wisdom of Milton H. Erickson: The complete volume.*Crown House Publishing, Ltd.
Hickok, G. (2009). Eight problems for the mirror neuron theory of action understanding in monkeys and humans. *Journal of Cognitive Neuroscience, 21*(7), 1229–1243. 10.1162/jocn.2009.21189
Hoffman, H. (1987). Imprinting and the critical period for social attachments: Some laboratory investigations. In M. H. Bornstein (Ed.), *Sensitive periods in development* (pp. 99–123). Washington, D.C.: Psychology Press.
Johnson, M. (2007). *The meaning of the body: Aesthetics of human understanding.* Chicago: University of Chicago Press, Ltd.
Johnson, S. M., Wiebe, S. A., & Allan, R. (2008). Emotionally focused couple therapy. In J. L. Lebow, & D. K. Snyder, *Clinical handbook of couple therapy* (pp. 107–137). New York: Guilford Press.
Kahn, S., & Fromm, E. (2001). *Changes in the therapist.* Mahwah: Lawrence Erlbaum Associates, Publishers.
Kane, S., & Olness, K. (2004). *The art of therapeutic communication: The collected works of Kay F. Thompson.* Carmarthen, UK: Crown House Publishing.
Kihlstrom, J. F. (2013). Neuro-hypnotism: Prospects for hypnosis and neuroscience. *Cortex, 49*(2), 365–374. 10.1016/j.cortex.2012.05.016
Klein, N., & O'Brien, E. (2018). People use less information than they think to make up their minds. *Psychological and Cognitive Sciences, 115*(52), 13222–13227.
Kurosawa, A. (2002). *Red Beard.*
Laberge, F., Muhlenbrock-Lenter, S., Grunwald, W., & Roth, G. (2006). Evolution of the amygdala: New insights from studies in amphibians. *Brain, Behavior and Evolution, 67*(4), 177–187. 10.1159/000091119
Lakoff, G. (2012). Explaining embodied cognition results. *Topics in Cognitive Science, 4*(4), 773–785. 10.1111/j.1756-8765.2012.01222.x
LeDoux, J. (2002). *Synaptic self: How our brains become who we are.* New York: Viking: The Penguin Group.
LeDoux, J. E. (2012). Chapter 21 – Evolution of human emotion: A view through fear. In M. A. Hofman, & D. Falk (Eds.), *Progress in brain research: Evolution of the primate brain* (Vol. 195, pp. 431–442). Amsterdam: Elsevier.
Leslie, A. M., Friedman, O., & German, T. P. (2004). Core mechanisms in 'theory of mind'. *Tremds in Cognitive Sciences, 8*(12), 528–533. 10.1016/j.tics.2004.10.001
Levy, K. N., Ellison, W. D., Scott, L. N., & Bernecker, S. L. (2010). Attachment style. *Journal of Clinical Psychology, 67*, 193–203. 10.1002/jclp.20756
Lindell, A. K. (2006). In your right mind: Right hemisphere contributions to language processing and production. *Neuropsychology Review, 16*(3), 131–148. 10.1007/s11065-006-9011-9
Long, M., Verbeke, W., Ein-Dor, T., & Vrticka, P. (2020). A functional neuro-anatomical model of human attachment (NAMA): Insights from first- and second-person social neuroscience. *Cortex, 126*, 281–321. 10.1016/j.cortex.2020.01.010).
Lorenz, K. (1935). Der kumpan in der umwelt des vogels. Der artgenosse als auslosendes moment socialer verhaltensweisen. *Journal fur Ornithologiie, 83*(137–215), 289–413.
Maturana, H. R., & Varela, F. J. (1987). *The tree of knowledge: The biological roots of understanding* (revised edition). Boston: Shambhala Publications, Inc.
McGilchrist, I. (2009). *The master and his emissary: The divided brain and the making of the Western world.* New Haven: Yale University Press.
Mullaney, K., & Regan, M. (2019). One minute in Haditha: Ethics and non-conscious decision-making. *Journal of Military Ethics, 18*(2), 75–95. 10.1080/15027570.2019.1643593
Nachmanovitch, S. (2019). *The art of is: Improvising as a way of life.* Novato: New World Library.
Neufeld, E., Brown, E. C., Lee-Grimm, S.-I., Newen, A., & Brune, M. (2016). Intentional action processing results from automatic bottom-up attention: An EEG-investigation into the Social Relevance Hypothesis using hypnosis. *Consciousness and Cognition, 42*, 101–112. 10.1016/j.concog.2016.03.002
Olsson, A., & Phelps, E. A. (2007). Social learning of fear. *Nature Neuroscience, 10*, 1095–1102. 10.1038/nn1968
Panksepp, J., & Biven, L. (2012). *The archaeology of mind: Neuroevolutionary origins of human emotions.* New York: W. W. Norton & Co.

Perkeybile, A. M., Carter, C. S., Wroblewski, K. L., Puglia, M. H., Kenkel, W. M., Lillard, T. S., Connelly, J. J. (2019). Early nurture epigenetically tunes the oxytocin receptor. *Psychoneuroimmunology*, *99*, 128–136. 10.1016/j.psyneuen.2018.08.037

Porges, S. W. (2003). Social engagement and attachment. *Annals of the New York Academy of Science*, *1008*(1), 31–47. 10.1016/S0031-9384(03)00156-2

Porges, S. W. (2011). *The polyvagal theory: Neurophysiological foundations of emotions, attachment, communication, and self-regulation*. New York: W.W. Norton & Co., Inc.

Ranson, K. E., & Urichuk, L. J. (2008). The effect of parent-child attachment relationships on child biopsychosocial outcomes: A review. *Early Child Development and Care*, *178*(2), 129–152. 10.1080/03004430600685282

Rizzolatti, G., & Craighero, L. (2004). The mirror neuron system. *Annual Review of Neuroscience*, *27*, 169–192. 10.1146/annurev.neuro.27.070203.144230

Ropper, A. H., & Burrell, B. D. (2019). *How the brain lost its mind: Sex, hysteria, and the riddle of mental illness*. New York: Penguin Random House.

Rossi, E. L. (1987). From mind to molecule: A state-dependent memory, learning, and behavior theory of mind-body healing. *Advances*, *4*(2), 46–60.

Rossi, E. L. (2005). The ideodynamic action hypothesis of therapeutic suggestion: Creative replay in the psychosocial genomics of therapeutic hypnosis. *European Journal of Clinical Hypnosis*, *6*(2), 2–12.

Rossi, E. L. (1980). *The collected papers of Milton H. Erickson on hypnosis: The nature of hypnosis and suggestion* (p. 223). Irvington, NY: Irvington Publishers, Inc.

Sander, D., Grafman, J., & Zalla, T. (2003). The human amydala: An evolved system for relevance detection. *Reviews in the Neurosciences*, *14*(4), 303–316.

Sander, L. W., & Julia, H. L. (1966). Continuous interactional monitoring in the neonate. *Psychosomatic Medicine*, *28*(6), 822–835. 10.1515/REVNEURO.2003.14.4.303

Schore, A. N. (2019). *Right brain psychotherapy*. New York: W. W. Norton & Co., Inc.

Seung, S. (2012). *Connectome: How the brain's wiring makes us who we are*. Boston: Houghton Mifflin Harcourt.

Shahaeian, A., Peterson, C. C., Slaughter, V., & Wellman, H. M. (2011). Culture and the sequence of steps in theory of mind development. *Developmental Psychology*, *47*(5), 1239–1247. 10.1037/a0023899

Shamay-Tsoory, S. G. (2011). Empathic processing: Its cognitive and affective dimensions and neuroanatomical basis. In J. Decety, & W. Ickes (Eds.), *The social neuroscience of empathy* (pp. 305–322). Cambridge: The MIT Press.

Sharma, K. (2015). *Interdependence: Biology and beyond*. New York: Fordham University Press.

Siegel, D. J. (2012). *The developing mind: How relationships and the brain interact to shape who we are* (2nd ed.). New York: The Guilford Press.

Siegel, D. J. (2017). *Mind: A journey to the heart of being human*. New York: W.W. Norton & Co., Inc.

Singer, T., & Frith, C. (2004). Introduction: The study of social interactions. In C. Frith, & D. Wolpert (Eds.), *The neuroscience of social interaction: Decoding, imitating, and influencing the action of others* (pp. 133–135). New York: Oxford University Press.

Sperling, M. B., Berman, W. H., & Fagen, G. (1992). Classification of adult attachment: An integrative taxonomy from attachment and psychoanalytic theories. *Journal of Personality Assessment*, *59*(2), 239–247. 10.1207/s15327752jpa5902_2

Spiegel, E. B. (2016). Attachment-focused hypnosis in psychotherapy for complex trauma: Attunement, representation, and mentalization. *International Journal of Clinical and Experimental Hypnosis*, *64*(1), 45–74. 10.1080/00029157.2016.1163658

Spiegel, E. B., & Baker, E. L. (2019). The generative presence of relatedness. *American Journal of Clinical Hypnosis*, *62*(1–2), 1–11. 10.1080/00029157.2019.1609840

Spiegel, E. B., Baker, E. L., Daitch, C., & Diamond, M. J. (2019). Hypnosis and the therapeutic relationship: Relational factors of hypnosis in psychotherapy. *American Journal of Clinical Hypnosis*, *62*(1–2), 118–137. 10.1080/00029157.2019.1599319

Sporns, O. (2011). *Networks of the Brain*. Cambridge: The MIT Press.

Stanton, M. A., Lonsdorf, E. V., Pusey, A. E., Goodall, J., & Murray, C. M. (2014). Maternal behavior by birth order in wild chimpanzees (Pan troglodytes): Increased investment by first-time mothers. *Current Anthropology*, *55*(4), 483–489. 10.1086/677053

Stern, D. B. (2010). *Partners in thought: Working with unformulated experience, dissociation, and enactment*. New York: Routledge Taylor & Francis Group.
Stolorow, R., & Atwood, G. (1996). The intersubjective perspective. *The Psychoanalytic Review*, *83*(2), 181–194.
Sueng, S. (2012). *Connectome: How the brain's wiring makes us who we are*. New York: Houghton Mifflin Harcourt Publishing.
Sugarman, L. I. (2021). Leaving hypnosis behind? *American Journal of Clinical Hypnosis*, *63*(1), 139–156. 10.1080/00029157.2021.1935686
Sugarman, L. I., Linden, J. H., & Brooks, L. W. (2020). *Changing minds with clinical hypnosis: Narratives and discourse for a new health care paradigm*. New York: Routledge Taylor & Francis Group.
Sydnor, V., Larsen, B., Bassett, D. S., Alexander-Bloch, A., Fair, D. A., Liston, C., Satterthwaite, T. D. (2021). Neurodevelopment of the association cortices: Patterns, mechanisms, and implications for psychopathology. *Neuron*, *109*(18), 2820–2846. 10.1016/j.neuron.2021.06.016
Thompson, E. (2010). *Mind in life: Biology, phenomenology, and the sciences of mind*. Cambridge: Harvard University Press.
Tzschentke, B., & Plagemann, A. (2006). Imprinting and critical periods in early development. *World's Poultry Science Journal*, *62*(4), 626–637. 10.1017/S0043933906001176
Varela, F. J., Thompson, E., & Rosch, E. (2016). *The embodied mind*. Cambridge: The MIT Press.
Wellman, H. M. (2018). Theory of mind: The state of the art. *European Journal of Developmental Psychology*, 15, 728–755. 10.1080/17405629.2018.1435413
Yapko, M. D. (2021). *Process-oriented hypnosis: Focusing on the forest, not the trees*. New York: W.W. Norton & Co., Inc.
Zelinka, V., Cojan, Y., & Deseilles, M. (2014). Hypnosis, attachment, and oxytocin: An integrative perspective. *International Journal of Clinical and Experimental Hypnosis*, *62*(1), 29–49. 10.1080/00207144.2013.841473

6

MIND, SELF, AND HYPNOSIS

A Relational Theory

Douglas Flemons

Nova Southeastern University, Asheville, Context Consultants Arden, NC, USA

The relational theory of hypnosis developed in this chapter draws not from Freud's psychoanalytic ideas (cf. Bonshtein, 2012; Diamond, 1987; Kubie, 1972), but, rather, from Gregory Bateson's (2000, 2002) cybernetic conceptions of communication and mind (Flemons, 1991); from research in neuroscience and the field of embodied cognition (e.g., Barrett, 2020; Siegel, 2017; Varela et al., 1991), and from mind-body practices such as mindfulness meditation (e.g., Harris, 2014; Suzuki, 2006; cf. Elkins & Olendzki, 2019; Yapko, 2011). The theory attends not only to the interactive dynamic between hypnotist and client (a key concern of a psychoanalytic approach, though approached differently) but also, more fundamentally, to the nature of perception and conscious awareness; to the properties of certain language/thought constructions (classification, metaphor, irony, and negation); and to the self-defining and problem-enduring effects of judging and othering.

From a relational perspective, clinical hypnosis is distinguished as both a context and a method for altering the perceived boundaries of the client's sense of self. These boundaries shift in concert with the evocation and focusing of the client's avolitional agency – a phenomenon central to hypnotherapeutic change. Hypnosis provides the medium and means for the therapist to utilize such agency, inviting changes in the sensations, perceptions, thoughts, images, emotions, actions, and/or communications that constitute and define the client's problem.

Hypnosis can be usefully understood as a form of what the psychologist Mihaly Csikszentmihalyi (1990) called *flow*: "Concentration is so intense that there is no attention left over to think about anything irrelevant, or to worry about problems. Self-consciousness disappears, and the sense of time becomes distorted" (p. 71). Hypnosis transitions clients from self-conscious scrutiny and conscious effort to unselfconscious (selfless) absorption and effortless engagement. To make sense of how such a shift is possible, it is necessary to understand something of the nature of mind and the self.

Mind

The 17th-century French philosopher René Descartes famously believed that his mind was "entirely and absolutely distinct" from his body and could "exist without it" (1641/1911, p. 28). Contemporary philosophers and neuroscientists have established that Descartes's

DOI: 10.4324/9781003449126-10

dualistic proposition was all wrong. "Cognition depends upon the kinds of experience that come from having a body with various sensorimotor capacities" (Varela et al., 1991, p. 173). This means that "what we call 'mind' is really embodied" (Lakoff & Johnson, 1999, p. 266) and that our bodies think: "There are neural networks ... in the intrinsic nervous system of our heart and intestines. We're seeing that we have a head-brain, heart-brain, and gut-brain" (Siegel, 2017, p. 153).

Mind "extends beyond the physical cortex of the brain's flesh" (Beilock, 2015, p. 210), but it also extends beyond the physical boundaries – beyond the "skin sack" (Norris, 2012, p. 258) – of the *body's* flesh. According to the cybernetic epistemologist Gregory Bateson (2000), mind is not separate from, but rather is immanent in, the body. But "it is immanent also in pathways and messages outside the body" (p. 467): "The mental world – the mind – ... is not limited by the skin" (p. 460). Given this, it is relevant to ask, "Where does the mind stop and the rest of the world begin" (Clark & Chalmers, 1998, p. 7)?

Barrett (2020) said that mind "emerges from a transaction between your brain and your body while they are surrounded by other brains-in-bodies that are immersed in a physical world and constructing a social world" (p. 100). Siegel (2017) offered a similar observation: "Our minds are a part of an interacting, interconnected system that involves our bodies and brains, as well as the environment in which we live, including our social relationships" (p. 42). Bateson (1977) also viewed mind not as individually possessed but as interpersonally shared:

> My mind is not something confined inside me. A good deal of it is inside me. But a good deal of it is outside. ... With that view of self, if I begin to say, "Well, now what happens when you and I talk?" Obviously all the things that I do, which are picked up by your perceptions, are a part of you. And things that you do, which are picked up by my perceptions, are a part of me. And there's an enormous overlap in our two minds. So that it is not unreasonable to speak of a "shared mind." This is not a miraculous phenomenon; it is a commonsense phenomenon. (p. 144)

The view of mind as embodied, extended, and shared makes possible the illumination of qualities and processes of hypnosis that would otherwise be obscured or distorted by theories that conflate minds and brains and/or that implicitly and dualistically treat mind and body, as well as hypnotist and client, as distinct things. Descartes's legacy is alive and well in such characterizations. For Descartes, "mind and body, subject and object, were radically disparate entities" (Berman, 1984, p. 21). Such dualism, lying "at the heart of the Cartesian paradigm" (p. 23), inhered not only in the split between mind and body but also in the gap between self and world.

Traditionally (dualistically) understood, the hypnotist unilaterally produces a circumscribed state of consciousness (a hypnotic trance) in the circumscribed mind of the client through the execution of a delimited stand-alone scripted induction. The hypnotist's induction renders the client more "suggestible," that is, avolitionally responsive to the hypnotist's control. Such a view is in evidence in Christensen and Gwozdziewycz's (2015) description of hypnosis as involving "the influence of the *mind over the body* at the unconscious level" (my italics; p. 449). It can also be seen in Zimbardo et al.'s (1972) description of hypnosis as a "process in which the issues of *control* become salient, since it enables new forms of *control* to be created and old forms to be suspended or destroyed" (my italics, p. 540).

As Wendell Berry (1987) pointed out,

> the root meaning of the word *control* is to roll against, in the sense of a little wheel turning in opposition. The principle of control, then, involves necessarily the principle of division: One thing may turn against another thing only by being divided from it. ... One wheel can turn another wheel outside itself only in a direction opposite to its own. (p. 69)

Striving for control, whether of oneself or another person, is grounded in the Cartesian assumption of there being a fundamental division between mind and body, between observer and experience, and between self (client) and other (hypnotist).

If, instead, you make the non-Cartesian assumption that there are fundamental *connections* within and between the mindful bodies and the embodied and shared minds of clients and hypnotists, then instead of striving for control, your hypnotic goal will be to invite *coordination* (from the Latin *co-* "with, together" + *ordinatio* "arrangement": "to arrange together"). A relational approach to hypnosis thus orients toward facilitating coordination in hypnotist-client and mind-body communications. To explain how this happens, I need first to say a few more words about the communicational nature of mind, and then I'll turn to the curious boundary-shifting nature of the self.

All communications of embodied, extended, and shared minds – perceptions, sensations, ideas, memories, emotions, imaginings – involve the processing of information, and all information processing (i.e., cognition) involves the recognition and classification of *difference*. Bateson (2002) defined information as "news of difference" (p. 64). What a "sensory end organ responds to is a *difference* or a *change*" (p. 89), and this "perception of difference is limited by threshold. Differences that are too slight or too slowly presented are not perceivable" (p. 27). A descriptive illustration of this fact can be found in the opening scene of Virginia Woolf's (1931) *The Waves*:

> *The sun had not yet risen. The sea was indistinguishable from the sky, except that the sea was slightly creased as if a cloth had wrinkles in it. Gradually as the sky whitened a dark line lay on the horizon dividing the sea from the sky and the grey cloth became barred with thick strokes moving, one after another.* (italics in the original, p. 7)

In predawn murkiness, sea and sky remain indistinguishable – as one – until a difference in illumination produces a line of demarcation, "a dark line ... dividing" (p. 7) one from the other.

We assume that we are perceiving and cognitively processing bounded objects or things – a tree, a birdsong, an idea, the texture of a scarf, the scent of lemon, an imagined scene – but these entities are all derived from perceived relationships, from contrasts and associations: "While I can know nothing about any individual thing by itself," said Bateson, "I *can* know something about *relations between things*" (Bateson & Bateson, 1987, p. 157). But if a relation between things – a difference – is to become information, if it is to be known and acted upon, it has to be both discernible *and* meaningful. In other words, it has to be a "difference that makes a difference" (Bateson, 2002, p. 212), that is, a difference that is *classified within a context*.

My wife and I have two dogs, Tally and Layla. The most important object in Tally's universe is a soft, flexible flying disk, which, every day at the park, she races to catch in mid-air. The disk itself clearly makes a difference to her, but so does the word we use to name it.

Whenever she hears someone say "frisbee," she snaps to attention. If I bring the same disk to Layla's attention, she will register its existence (from the Latin *ex-* "out" + *sistere,* "to stand": "to stand out"), but, perhaps disappointed that it isn't edible, she'll then wander away. For her, both the perception of and the name for the disk are not differences that make a difference; they are differences about which she is decidedly *in*different.

An understanding of context, difference, and indifference is helpful in teasing out the nature of our everyday sense of self and what happens to it during hypnosis.

Self

As you go throughout your day, you maintain varying levels of conscious awareness of what you're doing or attending to from moment to moment. If at some point you turn your focus to the *fact* of your awareness, that is, if your awareness turns back on itself, then you become aware that you're aware. Such self-referentiality spins a sense of self: *You* are aware that *you, yourself,* are aware.

This self-conscious self of yours feels real, but it is not the entity you assume it to be (Harris, 2014). If you try to grab hold of it, you'll come up empty handed. This is because your sense of self takes shape always and only *in relationship*, in contradistinction to something *other*. The contrast creates a differentiating boundary, which defines your self vis-à-vis what it is not; however, the border is more sharply etched when you stand in judgment of, and/or are contending with, this other. Depending on what or who you're up against, the encircling line of demarcation will shift, rendering your circumscribed self more or less encompassing, more or less inclusive.

For example, if you're driving and someone veers into your lane, you yell, "You cut *me* off!" Your circumscribed self feels inclusive of your vehicle. If you're walking outside in the cold, experiencing the otherness of the air temperature, you think, "*I* am freezing!" Your sense of self is now more restricted in scope, inclusive of just your body. Later, if your stomach is hurting, the enclosing circumference of the boundary may shrink still further, such that you construe your body not as *a part of* you but, rather, as *apart from* you, as other: "*I* am so over this stupid pain; my stomach keeps betraying *me*." And then if you start ruminating about betrayal, your circumscribed self will consider not only your body as other but also your thinking: "*I* can't turn off these intrusive thoughts. They're driving *me* crazy." This can lead to your reifying and othering a "worried self," distancing from it by referring to it in second person: "What's wrong with you?!"

Flow

Because your sense of being a self comes into existence in contrast to something or someone you're experiencing as other, then when the contrast is minimized (by the difference becoming indifferentiated, by its no longer making a difference), the circumscribing boundary delineating you as *you* dissipates. This is what happens during flow experience (Csikszentmihalyi, 1990). When you get thoroughly absorbed in an engaging activity, you lose yourself in the doing of it. Hypnosis is an interactive method for developing such flow by dissipating the boundary of the circumscribed self; meditation accomplishes boundary dissolution and creates flow *intra*-actively.

A mindfulness approach to meditation involves bringing your full attention to your body, often to the process of breathing. As breathing happens, in and out, your awareness moves in unison with the rhythm of it. You don't think *about* breathing, you attend *alongside* – or, better, *inside* – it, in sync with its unfolding. This has the effect of indifferentiating the difference between mind and body, which serves to dissolve the boundary delineating the circumscribed self. The Zen teacher Shunryu Suzuki described the process and effect recursively: "If you are concentrated on your breathing you will forget yourself, and if you forget yourself you will be concentrated on your breathing" (2006, p. 139).

Such absorbed attention tends not to last; before long, you're distracted by and caught up in a thought, sound, sensation, memory, or anticipation. As soon as you realize you've lost track of your breath, you patiently come back to it. The act of judging separates the judge from the judged, so by reorienting to the breath without self-admonishment, you're better able to get back in sync with it, effortlessly renewing your mind-body attunement, again and again.

The rhythmic pairing of awareness and breath can be considered a process of *entrainment*: "the synchronization of two or more rhythmic systems into a single pulse" (Nachmanovitch, 1990, p. 99).

> It is entrainment that provokes the trance states in the *samä* dances of the Sufis. When improvisers play together, they can rely on this natural phenomenon to mesh the music so that they breathe together, pulse together, think together. ... In entrainment, the voices are not locked in exactly; they are always slightly off from each other, finding each other again and again in micromoments in time, weaving in and out of each other's rhythms. (pp. 99–100)

Hypnosis involves entrainment between the therapist and client and between the client's awareness and experience.

Transitioning into Hypnosis

The hypnotic induction is traditionally conceived of as stand-alone set of instructions and injunctions. Intoned as a kind of charm, it is designed to transport the client from everyday awareness into "trance." Indeed, some clinicians

> deceive themselves into thinking that hypnosis is somehow to be found in the script they read to the client. Some apparently believe that unless you say this magical incantation, these words in this scripted sequence, you are not really doing hypnosis. (Yapko, 2014, p. 237)

Treating the induction as the isolable source or localized cause of the client's moving into flow experience misconstrues the process in linear and monologic terms. Nondualistically understood, the client's transition is the result of a dialogic, recursive interplay of call and response, oriented not toward the creation of an individual *state of trance* but, rather, toward *relationships of attunement*:

> When we attune to others we allow our own internal state to shift, to come to resonate with the inner world of another. This resonance is at the heart of the important sense of "feeling felt" that emerges in close relationships. (Siegel, 2010, p. 27; cited in Yapko, 2019, p. 75)

Attunement develops interactively, as a form of conversation (from the Latin *com-*, "with, together" + *versare* "to turn": "to turn together"). It is generated in the shared-mind dialogic interplay between client and therapist, as well as in the conversational connection between the client's embodied mind and mindful body (cf. Bányai, 1991).

Developing hypnotic attunement with some clients takes time, patience, and deft skill; however, with others, such as the woman featured in the clinical example later in the chapter, both inter- and intrapersonal rapport and boundary dissolution come quickly. This is often the case with children, whose creative capacity for full-on imaginative, body-engaged play is often just half a dance-step away (cf. Kohen & Olness, 2011; Sugarman & Wester, 2014).

Entrainment supports and intensifies hypnotic attunement. You make rhythmic connections between what you say and your clients' embodied experience when you cluster, emphasize, and alter the tempo of your words so they sync up with your clients' breathing; when you make mention of words such as "relaxing," "letting go," "slowing down," or "feeling heavier" in time with clients' exhales; and when you refer or allude to other client actions (e.g., blinking, itching the face, shifting position) as they are happening (see Flemons, 2022, ch. 5). But, as you'll see in the clinical illustration below, entrainment is also enhanced when you endorse your clients' verbal and non-verbal responses to your offerings.

With hypnosis, you create a context of trust and connection, a context for in-differentiating the typical self-other boundaries that define and maintain the circumscribed self of everyday conscious awareness. As Kubie (1972) put it, "The essence of the relationship of hypnotist to subject consists of [a] blurring of the boundaries between the two, which occurs regularly during the process of induction" (p. 215).

You invite your clients into flow experience by facilitating a meeting of minds, an interactive collaboration involving their active and absorbed engagement in the process. This allows their sense of self to shift from being circumscribed and exclusive (i.e., defined in contradistinction to and in judgment of whatever at the moment they are experiencing as other) to being expansive and inclusive. And their experience of you shifts from assessing you as an outsider to accepting you as an insider. They determine that your comments, stories, and suggestions needn't be judgmentally scrutinized and gingerly kept at arm's length (cf. Diamond, 1987). Instead, your contributions can become insider communications to be freely considered and played with, and, when they resonate, safely taken to heart. With no circumscribed self in evidence, identifying itself as responsible for initiating or steering (i.e., controlling) what is unfolding, the changes that arise – changes in what the clients are perceiving, imagining, thinking, feeling, and/or doing – are experienced as avolitional.

Utilization

Dualistically understood and practiced, hypnosis becomes something you do *to* passively receptive clients – you *hypnotize* them. Such an approach lends itself to directive or injunctive communication styles; the hypnotist unilaterally determines what will happen and what the client will experience. For example,

> I want you to look upward at a spot on the ceiling and to fixate your eyes on it. ... You are becoming sleepy. ... You will pay attention to nothing but the sound of my voice. You will not awaken until I tell you to. (Weitzenhoffer, 1957, pp. 206–207)

If your clients are comfortable complying with such exhortations, they may let go of their circumspect awareness and purposeful intent and thus be able to experience an indifferentiation of the boundary distinguishing their circumscribed self. In such cases, avolitional responsiveness can follow. But if they are put off by your tone or your insistence, or if they are distracted by their surroundings or by doubt or fear or some other personal experience, then there will be no interactive attunement and no hypnosis.

Clients who won't, don't, or are unable to accept your invitation into attunement have traditionally been understood as resistant. Stage hypnotists typically dismiss resistant volunteers from their show; traditional clinicians look for ways to "overcome" resistance, to "break it down" (e.g., Weitzenhoffer, 1957, p. 401) so the patient will become compliant and cooperative.

Milton Erickson (2008) reversed the formulation of what's required to establish a hypnotic relationship. Rather than requiring his patients to cooperate with *him*, he took it upon himself to cooperate with *them*, to get in sync with whatever they were doing, saying, and experiencing. He called this commitment and practice *utilization.*

Commanding your clients to "pay attention to nothing but the sound of my voice" (Weitzenhoffer, 1957, p. 207) is an *exclusion*-based approach to protecting the hypnotic context. You entreat clients to guard against interruptions by directing them to focus entirely on you and what you tell them to do. Utilization, in contrast, is a commitment to *inclusion*: It takes care of interruptions not by disallowing or trying to prevent them but by welcoming them as contributions. The hypnotist becomes like a stand-up comic weaving hecklers' provocations into the routine: Threats to the relationship or the process are transformed into enhancements.

The inclusivity of utilization means that nothing that happens, and nobody who is involved – neither the client nor you – is singled out as wrong or problematic. Any response is legitimate. By eschewing judgment, you prevent unhelpful self-other boundaries from getting inadvertently inscribed – boundaries of opposition between the client and the setting, between the client and the hypnotist, or between the client's circumscribed self and the client's body and/or unconscious experience.

The avoidance of inadvertent boundary creation can be further aided through the use of Milton Erickson's *permissive language* practices (e.g., O'Hanlon & Martin, 1992). If you tell your clients what *will* happen and what they *will* do and experience (or are already experiencing), and your predictions and claims are borne out, then the resonance between your words and their experience will contribute to the indifferentiation of the boundary of their circumscribed self. This, along with your clients' feeling like you are determining what's happening to them, will support or even intensify the avolitional quality of their experience. If, however, your predictions and claims are doubted or inaccurate, then your clients' confidence in you, as well as in their ability to experience hypnosis, will be undermined, and the boundaries of their circumscribed self will be more definitively inscribed.

If, instead of imposing certainties, you float *possibilities* of what *might* or *could* happen, or what clients *may* find themselves noticing, you ensure that whatever unfolds, no one is at fault and every response is acceptable. Rather than predicting and determining what will happen, you create the opportunity for your clients to actively *discover* it, and, in the process, you preclude the formation of judgment- or failure-based circumscribing boundaries.

Avolitional Agency

We are all familiar with the feeling of volitional agency: We consider options and make a choice, and once we make a decision, we intentionally implement it. But according to neuroscientists, this feeling, this "impression of agency" (Harris, 2014, p. 90), this sense that our circumscribed self is in charge, is inaccurate:

> Your brain is wired to initiate your actions before you're aware of them. ... In everyday life, you do many things by choice, right? At least it seems that way. ... But the brain is a predicting organ. It launches your next set of actions based on your past experience and current situation, and it does so outside of your awareness. (Barrett, 2020, p. 76)

This means that "all actions, mundane or novel, planned or unplanned, hypnotic or otherwise, are at the moment of activation initiated automatically, rather than by a conscious intention" (Lynn et al., 2008, p. 126). As the novelist Michael Crichton (2008) wryly put it, our "human sense of self-control and purposefulness, is a user illusion. We don't have conscious control over ourselves at all. We just think we do" (p. 135).

Hypnosis creates the conditions for eschewing the delusional beliefs and circumventing the controlling efforts of the circumscribed self while initiating and developing experiential change. You accomplish this through the invitation and support of *avolitional agency* (Flemons, 2022).

The most direct way of encouraging avolitional agency is to appeal to "the unconscious" as an instigator of action:

> "While your *conscious mind* is still wondering how you'll first recognize the feeling, the experience, of hypnosis, your *unconscious mind* can already be preparing the ground, can already be implementing hypnotic changes – changes in your comfort, changes in your perception, changes in your focus, changes in your body's ability to relax all the way into the chair."

In keeping with the non-Cartesian assumption about the mindfulness of the body, you can also invite avolitional agency by invoking the capacity for body components and/or systems to participate in coordinated (not controlled), thoughtful action and change. Possibilities for such coordination can be outlined by referencing the brain-and-body's potential for *avolitional emulation*:

> "*Just as* your right hand and left foot move in sync as you walk, *so too* your imagination and curiosity can interweave as you drift into hypnosis, facilitating an image or even a dream to begin to develop and play out as effortlessly as strolling down a path. As you get a glimmer of what beginning to take shape, let me know what you're noticing."
>
> or
>
> "*Just as* your lungs and heart effortlessly collaborate in the circular process of delivering oxygen and removing carbon dioxide, *so too* your muscles and brain can collaborate in releasing tension and delivering endorphins. And because it's all so interconnected, so circular, I don't know if you'll recognize the *physical* feeling of

relaxation preceding or following a developing *emotional* sense of comfort and ease. ... As you tune in, what are you sensing?"

The idea of avolitional emulation follows from a more encompassing recognition of the associational nature of hypnotic communication and experience. In a context of connection – between hypnotist and client and between the client's embodied mind and mindful body – change is initiated and developed through the logic of *correspondence*:

"if *that* can happen *there*, then *this* can happen *here*"

or

"as *that* happens *there*, *this* can happen *here*"

The Context of Hypnosis

Not unlike chess, soccer, meditation, and music performance, hypnosis is a context and method for facilitating flow experience – that is, for focused absorption accompanied by changes, to varying degrees, in perception, time-sense, physical sensation, sense of self, avolitional agency, and so on. Such experiential changes contribute to the client's marking the context as a definable event or process (e.g., "This change in how I am feeling/thinking/acting is not normal for me; it must be a sign that I am actually experiencing hypnosis"). But the reverse is also true. When you frame what you and the client are doing as hypnosis (or an analogous mind-body form of engagement such as guided meditation), you define the parameters of, and create and reinforce expectancies (Kirsch, 1985, 1990) for, what can and may happen. Marking the context as hypnosis orients both you and the client toward acknowledging avolitional agency and discovering avolitional change.

Vance (2016) described the way the "theater of medicine" puts "us in the frame of mind that we are receiving treatment[,] and [it builds] our confidence in it" (p. 38). The doctor's manner ("a kindly hand on your shoulder, eye contact, a sense of confidence and authority") is a context marker for this theater, as are "all the accoutrements, such as the white coat, the fancy tools, the jars of Q-tips and gauze" (p. 38). The same is true for hypnosis, albeit without the white coat and Q-tips. We mark the context of hypnosis physically, temporally, metaphorically, and experientially.

Physical context cues are established if you conduct the hypnotic portion of your sessions in a set-off part of your office or in what you designate, say, as the "hypnosis chair." Relocating for hypnosis implies that something uniquely different happens there.

You create *temporal* context cues anytime you verbally distinguish hypnotic from non-hypnotic awareness, relative to whichever one your client is currently experiencing:

- Hypnotist: Before you begin moving into hypnosis, I have one more question.
- H: Ready to embark?
- H: Welcome back!

It is common to ascribe *metaphoric* dimensionality to hypnotic experience. There is of course no actual physical "depth" or "location" to hypnosis, but familiar spatial cues provide useful three-dimensional coordinates for distinguishing inside from outside and for graphically capturing clients' degree of absorption and imaginative engagement.

- H: As I count backward from 10 to 1, you can, each step of the way, find yourself going deeper and deeper down into hypnosis.
- H: Before you start reorienting to regular awareness, take a moment to get your bearings and pin your location so you can easily find your way back here the next time.

The *experiential* framing of hypnosis is accomplished through both entrainment and endorsement. Entrainment, you'll recall, involves, in part, matching what you say and how you say it with your clients' automatic behaviors – their breath, gestures, and physiological changes (such as physical relaxation). This inevitably creates noticeable, unexpected pauses, as well as demonstrable shifts in pace, pitch, and tone. Such an altered communication style paralinguistically marks the context (i.e., the nature of your interaction and the meaning attributed to it) as different from what was happening only a few minutes earlier.

Endorsement, or what in the Ericksonian hypnosis literature is called *ratification* (e.g., Zeig, 2014), involves mentioning or acknowledging avolitional changes you and/or your clients are noticing:

- H: In the last few minutes, your facial muscles have relaxed and your breathing has slowed and deepened.

Such comments make explicit hypnosis-defining indicators that avolitional change is underway. Something analogous occurs when you warmly confirm, mid-hypnosis, the experiences your clients report to you:

- H: And what's happening now?
  Client: I can't feel my hands.
  H: No, you can't, can you?

By endorsing what clients report, you provide insider confirmation of the details and significance of their experience. In doing so, you highlight and contextually mark the uniqueness of what's transpiring, which enhances your clients' expectancy and allows you to bring forth and utilize its hypnotherapeutic potential.

Throughout the chapter, I've been probing the theoretical and practical implications of adopting a relational understanding of mind, self, and hypnosis. It's now time to turn to some clinical ramifications of this orientation.

Hypnotherapy

With hypnosis, you invite avolitional change in various forms of avolitional experience – actions, sensations, perceptions, conceptions, and/or imaginations. With hypno*therapy*, you invite avolitional change in avolitional *problems*:

> By definition, both hypnosis and symptoms occur, to some extent, "out of conscious control." Some of the effectiveness of hypnosis perhaps stems from the possibility that the problem is addressed at the level of experience from which it is generated. (Zeig, 2014, p. 77)

We all generally conceive of, talk about, and experience avolitional – "out-of-conscious-control" – problems as if they were stand-alone, othered entities, or malevolent forces intent on taking us down. Addiction, anxiety, anger, depression: We say they "hijack" us, "attack" us, "get the better" of us, "suck the life" out of us. Once you've reified and othered a problem in this way, relating to it as decidedly *not* part of *you*, it follows that you would incline toward *countering* it, whether by attempting to deny or escape from it, or by doing your best to contain, control, manage, or eradicate it. But all such negation-infused efforts to find relief are doomed to fail. Because of the way negation works (see Flemons, 1991, 2002), countering efforts further differentiate the boundary of the circumscribed self and heighten the significance and intransigence of whatever it is battling.

An avolitional problem doesn't exist *apart from* you; it is, in fact, *a part of* you, a part of the interactive relationships patterning – constituting – your sense of self. In the relational world of mind, actively attempting to sever a relationship is itself a relational act. Failing to effect the free-and-clear relief so decidedly desired, such severing attempts succeed only in producing *separated connections* (see Flemons, 1991, 2002) – ongoing alienated relationships with the problem that resemble the sour interactions of a bad divorce.

This is where hypnotherapy comes in, offering a radical alternative to your clients' contrarian approach to problem-solving. Rather than stoke their entrenched opposition *to* the problem, thereby unintentionally underscoring the defining boundaries of both it and their circumscribed self, you evoke and develop avolitional agency for resourcefully engaging *with* it and for altering the experiential strands composing it. Through shared-mind curiosity, acknowledgment, utilization, and pattern reconfiguration, you and your clients create the conditions for the significance and defining characteristics of their problem to dissipate, as they discover and learn new ways of orienting to their experience.

To illustrate a few of the ways these ideas can be put into practice, I'd like to walk you through part of a demonstration I recorded in a graduate hypnosis class in 2018 with one of my PhD students, Kathy. Although she "had always been skeptical of hypnosis" and had had a previous experience with a hypnotherapist that resulted in "no positive outcome," Kathy volunteered for the class demonstration because she wanted to stop feeling "very squeamish about anything to do with 'medical stuff' – hospitals, needles, blood, all of that." For as long as she could remember, she would "cringe," get "sweaty and hot," and "nauseous and sometimes lightheaded" if she looked at needles or IVs or "open wounds," even on TV. Typically, she would look away or close her eyes so she wouldn't have to see it, but this strategy wasn't practical when she was working. She had a job at the time as an in-home therapist, and one of her clients was recovering from a tracheostomy. Kathy found it anxiety provoking to maintain eye contact with her client, as she couldn't avoid seeing her throat.

As a context-marking preparation for beginning the hypnotherapeutic process, I asked Kathy what she anticipated as a possible outcome of our demonstration and what she thought she might experience during the hypnosis itself. She hoped, she said, to be able to "just function like everyone else, ... not to have to cringe or turn [away] or feel nauseous, ... or [to] hesitate to walk into a hospital or [to] be afraid to stop and help someone who's had a car accident." We touched on possibilities for what she might experience during the demonstration, and I noted that as she got absorbed, my voice might fade in and out, and she might, as well, lose track of the presence of the other students, even as they "join us in their curiosity." Acknowledging the presence of something can be helpful in letting it go.

I listed a few things Kathy didn't have to bother doing, and as I mentioned them and the possibility that she could daydream, her eyes defocused, and her eyelids started to close.

I utilized what was avolitionally happening to contextually mark the beginning of hypnosis and to develop our interactive attunement. I offered nothing that resembled a traditional induction – I simply got in sync with what she was telling me and what her body was doing.

Douglas: Now that's a good way to start, as you can just let your eyes do that. Because your eyes are just basically catching up to where you've already begun to move.

I posited a relationship between what her eyes were doing and what was already happening avolitionally elsewhere in her embodied mind.

Kathy had mentioned that she'd been affected by "medical stuff" from early on in her life. This suggested the possibility of framing the hypnosis as an opportunity for developmental learning, for making it possible for a reactivity established in childhood to evolve and resolve in keeping with the rest of her adult way of being.

I prepared the ground for avolitional emulation by establishing the idea of communication channels opening up between different areas of her mindful body and brain:

D: There can be a movement that begins in one [place] and makes that learning available to other [areas].

Noticing that one of Kathy's hands had started to slide sideways on her leg, I asked her to fill me in on what was going on. So informed, I could better maintain our attunement, ensuring that what I was saying resonated with what was occurring for her.

Kathy: [as her other hand also begins to move] My hands are sliding.

Most hypnosis theorists would describe the avolitional sliding of Kathy's hands, along with her ability to divvy up her experience so that she could verbally report on something that was happening independently of conscious intention, as examples of dissociation (e.g., Hilgard, 1991; Yapko, 2019). It certainly feels that way to clients – as if this or that body part or chunk of experience has an autonomous mind of its own. However, such responses only become possible as a function of the attunement between hypnotist and client. Given that hypnosis is fundamentally a context of *connection*, it is more accurate to view them as *associated* dissociations or *connected* separations (Flemons, 1991, 2002).

I endorsed what Kathy reported –

D: Your hands are sliding, that's right. ...

– and then, a little later, I remarked on her capacity to closely attend to particularities:

D: I wonder about the vividness of your ability to perceive and that sensitivity you have to notice small details, fine-grained details, like texture, situation, shades of color.

I made the assumption that Kathy's sensitivity to medical stuff was heightened by her natural ability to home in on specifics – the color of blood, the shape and colors and textures of an open wound, and so on. A non-therapeutic intervention would have involved a suggestion that she become less sensitive, that she prevent or negate her tendency to become hyper-focused on what for her were gross details associated with suffering. The hypnotherapeutic alternative was to accept and endorse her tendency as a *skill* that could be utilized as an essential component of a hypnotic correspondence:

> "if you can focus *microscopically*, then you can also focus *macroscopically*"

D: As your hands continue to slide their way into their own discoveries, what else are you noticing?
K: Odd.
D: It *is* odd, isn't it? Yeah. Isn't it interesting that depending on proximity you can notice different grains of texture. That's it. There are just different ways of encountering whatever it is that you're noticing. If you bring yourself to closely notice, you can notice fine-grained details that would escape your notice if you were to be further away. And if you move further away, you open up the possibility of seeing a large picture, and ... the grain of texture is blurred in some way as you gain a wider perspective. And how effortless that can be to move between a microscopic clarity and a telescopic clarity. That you can move closer to whatever it is that you're noticing and develop an appreciation for the finer details. And that taking a step back, finding a perspective above or further away, you see a very different, a bird's eye, view.

What happened next was a testament to the kind of synergistic creativity that becomes possible in a context of shared-mind attunement:

D: What are you noticing now, Kathy?
K: I saw my client.
D: You saw your client. Uh huh. And as you looked at her what did you notice happening within you?
K: I wasn't focused on the trach[eostomy].
D: You weren't focused on the trach[eostomy]. Uh huh. You were able to see it without being focused there?
K: Uh huh.
D: And as your focus shifted – that's right – what happened to your experience in your body?
K: I wasn't squeamish.
D: You weren't squeamish, were you?
K: No.
D: You could see it without focusing there.

Without my directly suggesting it, Kathy found herself test-driving her ability to shift from microscopic to telescopic clarity, discovering in the process that a shift in perspective and distance altered her automatic body response. We weren't mounting a campaign *against* a "phobia"; we were engaging with, utilizing, and discovering possibilities for change in the experiential strands that had been weaving it.

The demonstration continued for another 28 minutes, during which I told a story about a student whose fear of seeing her very first client dissipated when she started relating to the client as a *whole* person, shifting her focus so that she could take in *all* of her. We conducted some experiments that involved Kathy practicing her ability to (utilizing the movement in her hands) *glide* effortlessly back and forth between fine-grained details and a bird's-eye view of whatever came into her awareness. We then expanded this from the visual to the kinesthetic realm, playing with altering her focus on a sensation or temperature by an analogous process of gliding from a position of close proximity to one with enough distance to take in the whole of what she was encountering.

I suggested that the learning she was undertaking could be felt in her heart, allowing it to be distributed throughout her body by her cardiovascular system. This offered an opening to talk in some detail about veins and arteries and blood being so essential in delivering this newly developed learning – a learning, of course, about not being bothered by veins and arteries and blood. Therapeutic irony is a nice complement to the paradoxical quality of so much symptomatic experience (see Flemons, 2022; Flemons & Charlés, 2019).

Finally, I asked Kathy to glide into the future, where she could explore and develop the same capacity to shift focus. When I checked in with her, Kathy told me she was helping people in the hospital. She felt a tingling in her hands, and her feet had lost touch with the floor. I noted how interesting it is that feeling grounded is accompanied by the sensation of floating. Soon after, she floated back into the present, where, before reorienting, she memorized the texture of the learning in her heart and in her bones.

When I followed up with Kathy in 2022, she remembered that when she reoriented to the room, she felt like she was emerging from "a deep sleep." For a week or so after, she continued to feel "dazed": "very calm (internally), which was unusual," and "no agitation." The "many daily stressors that had previously affected" her "no longer did." Discovering "that a non-anxious Kathy actually exists," it felt "unbelievable to feel so at ease." She had "no issues being around the client" and no longer "avoid[ed] looking at open wounds or IVs." As of 2022, the ability to feel "comfortable seeing wounds and helping if someone gets injured" were still in place.

Making a Difference

Informed by an understanding of the embodied- and shared-mind nature of experience, a relational orientation to clinical hypnosis articulates a collaborative approach to inviting clients' avolitional agency and developing therapeutic shifts in their experience of avolitional symptoms. Rather than attempting to unilaterally induce hypnosis and implant suggestions to contradict (from the Latin *contra* "against" + *dicere* "to speak": "to speak against," "voice opposition to") the client's problem, you instead coordinate with the client's embodied mind to dissolve (indifferentiate) the boundaries of the circumscribed self and invite non-willful changes in the intra- and interactive patterns of relationship that have been constituting, defining, and maintaining the problem.

References

Bányai, É. (1991). Toward a social-psychobiological model of hypnosis. In S. J. Lynn & J. W. Rhue (Eds.), *Theories of hypnosis* (pp. 564–598). Guilford.

Bateson, G. (1977). Epistemology of organization. *Transactional Analysis Journal*, 27(2), 138–145. 10.1177/036215379702700210

Bateson, G. (2000). *Steps to an ecology of mind*. University of Chicago Press.

Bateson, G. (2002). *Mind and nature: A necessary unity*. Bantam Books.

Bateson, G., & Bateson, M. C. (1987). *Angels fear: Towards an epistemology of the sacred*. Hampton Press.
Barrett, L. F. (2020). *Seven and a half lessons about the brain*. Houghton Mifflin Harcourt.
Beilock, S. (2015). *How the body knows its mind*. Atria Books.
Berman, M. (1984). *The reenchantment of the world*. Bantam Books.
Berry, W. (1987). *Home economics*. North Point Press.
Bonshtein, U. (2012). Relational hypnosis. *International Journal of Clinical and Experimental Hypnosis*. 10.1080/00207144.2012.700613
Clark, A., & Chalmers, D. (1998, January). The extended mind. *Analysis*, *58*(1), 7–19. 10.1093/analys/58.1.7
Crichton, M. (2008). *Prey*. Harper.
Christensen, C., & Gwozdziewycz, N. (2015). Revision of the APA Division 30 definition of hypnosis. *American Journal of Clinical Hypnosis*, *57*, 448–451. 10.1080/00029157.2015.1011498
Csikszentmihalyi, M. (1990). *Flow: The psychology of optimal experience*. Harper Perennial.
Descartes, R. (1641/1911). Meditations on first philosophy. In E. S. Haldane (Trans.), *The philosophical works of Descartes*. Cambridge University Press.
Diamond, M. J. (1987). The interactional basis of hypnotic experience: On the relational dimensions of hypnosis. *The International Journal of Clinical and Experimental Hypnosis*, *35*(2), 95–115. 10.1080/00207148708416046
Elkins, G. R., & Olendzki, N. (2019). *Mindful hypnotherapy*. Springer.
Erickson, M. H. (2008). Hypnosis: Its renascence as a treatment modality. In E. L. Rossi, R. Erickson-Klein, & K. L. Rossi (Eds.), *The collected works of Milton H. Erickson. Basic hypnotic induction and suggestion* (Vol. 2, pp. 61–85). The Milton H. Erickson Foundation Press.
Flemons, D. (1991). *Completing distinctions*. Shambhala.
Flemons, D. (2002). *Of one mind: The logic of hypnosis, the practice of therapy*. W. W. Norton.
Flemons, D. (2022). *The heart and mind of hypnotherapy: Inviting connection, inventing change*. W. W. Norton.
Flemons, D., & Charlés, L. (2019). Transvision: Unknotting double binds in the fog of war. In L. Charlés & G. Samarasinghe (Eds.), *Family systems and global humanitarian health: Approaches in the field* (pp. 123–141). Springer.
Harris, S. (2014). *Waking up*. Simon & Schuster.
Hilgard, E. R. (1991). A neodissociation interpretation of hypnosis. In S. Lynn & J. Rhue (Eds.), *Theories of hypnosis: Current models and perspectives* (pp. 83–104). Guilford.
Kirsch, I. (1985). Response expectancy as a determinant of experience and behavior. *American Psychologist*, *40*, 1189–1202. 10.1037/0003-066X.40.11.1189
Kirsch, I. (1990). *Changing expectations*. Brooks/Cole.
Kohen, D. P., & Olness, K. (2011). *Hypnosis and hypnotherapy with children* (4th ed.). Routledge.
Kubie, L. S. (1972). Illusion and reality in the study of sleep, hypnosis, psychosis, and arousal. *International Journal of Clinical and Experimental Hypnosis*, *20*(4), 205–223. 10.1080/00207147208409293
Lakoff, G., & Johnson, M. (1999). *Philosophy in the flesh*. Basic Books.
Lynn, S. J., Kirsch, I., & Hallquist, M. N. (2008). Social cognitive theories of hypnosis. In M. R. Nash & A. J. Barnier (Eds.), *The Oxford handbook of hypnosis: Theory, research, and practice* (pp. 111–139). Oxford University Press.
Nachmanovitch, S. (1990). *Free play: Improvisation in life and art*. Tarcher/Putnam.
Norris, C. (2012). Further thoughts: On the extended mind hypothesis. *Southern Humanities Review*, *46*(3), 243–269.
O'Hanlon, B., & Martin, M. (1992). *Solution-oriented hypnosis: An Ericksonian approach*. W. W. Norton.
Siegel, D. J. (2017). *Mind: A journey to the heart of being human*. W. W. Norton.
Sugarman, L. I., & Wester, W. C. (Eds.). (2014). *Therapeutic hypnosis with children and adolescents* (2nd ed.). Crown.
Suzuki, S. (2006). *Zen mind, beginner's mind*. Shambhala.
Vance, E. (2016). *Suggestible you: The curious science of your brain's ability to deceive, transform, and heal*. National Geographic.

Varela, F. J., Thompson, E., & Rosch, E. (1991). *The embodied mind: Cognitive science and human experience*. MIT Press.
Weitzenhoffer, A. M. (1957). *General techniques of hypnotism*. Grune & Stratton.
Woolf, V. (1931). *The waves*. Harcourt.
Yapko, M. (2011). *Mindfulness and hypnosis: The power of suggestion to transform experience*. W. W. Norton.
Yapko, M. D. (2014). The spirit of hypnosis: Doing hypnosis versus being hypnotic. *American Journal of Clinical Hypnosis*, *56*, 234–248. 10.1080/00029157.2013.815605
Yapko, M. D. (2019). *Trancework* (5th ed.). Routledge.
Zeig, J. K. (2014). *The induction of hypnosis: An Ericksonian elicitation approach*. The Milton H. Erickson Foundation Press.
Zimbardo, P., Maslach, C., & Marshall, G. (1972). Hypnosis and the psychology of cognitive and behavioral control. In E. Fromm & R. E. Shor (Eds.), *Hypnosis: Research, development, and perspectives*. Aldine Transaction.

7

FROM PHENOMENOLOGY TO NOETIC ANALYSIS

The Use of Quantitative First-Person Self-Reports to Better Understand Hypnosis

Ronald J. Pekala[1] *and Adam J. Rock*[2]

[1]Private Practice, West Chester, PA, USA; [2]School of Psychology, University of New England, Armidale, Australia

Quantifying Phenomenological Experience

A famous philosophical conundrum postulates: "Epistemology precedes metaphysics:" ***what we know*** is a function of ***how we know what we know***. Epistemology, "the study ... of the nature and grounds of knowledge especially with reference to its limits and validity" (Webster's Seventh New Collegiate Dictionary, 1970, p. 280), it is argued, must necessarily precede metaphysics, which concerns itself with the nature of being and existence. This is supported by the recent individual differences article of Milton et al. (2021), where extreme differences in visual imagery vividness (very low vs. very high) were associated "with measurable implications for psychological functioning" (p. 2): how such individuals perceived and interacted with their world, and what they believed about that world. Why is this important?

How we "see" the world will determine what we believe about that world, as microscopic and telescopic technologies have demonstrated. We have a level of analysis to study brain neurophysiology, and a cognitive-behavioral level of analysis to study human behavior and cognition. We need a noetic level of analysis (the Greek word for mind is "*nous*") to study those first-person, phenomenological aspects of the embodied brain, typically called the mind, from an empirical, quantitative perspective.

Just as physics comprehensively quantifies objective, physical reality, we need a methodology to comprehensively quantify subjective, or phenomenological, reality. Furthermore, we are not going to find the subjective experience of mind (the qualia, Shoemaker, 1991, of human consciousness) beneath a scalpel or lifted from an fMRI (functional magnetic resonance imaging), i.e., the "hard problem" of human consciousness (Chalmers, 2007):

> The hard problem of consciousness is the problem of experience. When we think and perceive, there is a whirl of information-processing, but there is also a subjective aspect. ... Then there are bodily sensations, from pains to orgasms; mental images

DOI: 10.4324/9781003449126-11

> that are conjured up internally; the felt quality of emotion, and the experience of a stream of conscious thought. (p. 226)

To make significant progress in better understanding hypnosis and its relationship to consciousness and the brain, we need a comprehensive quantitative phenomenology to scientifically investigate the mind. This was echoed over two decades ago: "A growing number of cognitive scientists now recognize the need to make systematic use of introspective phenomenological reports in studying the brain basis of consciousness" (Lutz & Thompson, 2003, p. 31).

More recently, Lifshitz (2016) stated that "whereas scientists have access to a plethora of advanced methods for investigating brain and behavior, they face a dearth of techniques for the empirical analysis of phenomenology" (p. 9). Physics became queen of the natural sciences because it wedded mathematical analysis to the observation and description of natural phenomena. This model from physics has since been applied to the other natural and social sciences with tremendous success. The same model, we believe, can and should be applied to the mind via noetic analysis.

Phenomenology and Its Quantitative Development

In philosophy, the concept of phenomenology is a rather fuzzy one; that is, there are "as many phenomenologies as there are phenomenologists" (Laughlin & Rock, 2013, p. 265). For Heidegger, phenomenology refers to what humans learn through reflection upon their own lived experience (Gelven, 1970). In contrast, Husserl's (2013) "pure" phenomenology, for example, is a "the disciplined application of single-minded and undistracted concentration upon the object of consciousness over sustained durations" (Laughlin & Rock, 2021, p. 44). We, however, in this chapter, are using the term phenomenology to simply denote first-person reports of the qualia of consciousness.

The scientific methodology used to investigate phenomenology via quantification has been previously described (Forbes & Pekala, 1993; Pekala, 1980, 1985a, 1995a, 1995b, 2010, 2011, 2015, 2016; Pekala & Creegan, 2020; Pekala & Forbes, 1997; Pekala & Kumar, 1984, 1986, 1987, 2000, 2007; Pekala & Nagler, 1989; Pekala et al., 2010a, 2010b; Pekala & Wickramasekera, 2007).

The methodology involves a **quantitative** phenomenological approach for mapping the various structures and patterns of consciousness. By consciousness, we mean the awareness of one's subjective experience which includes the various processes and contents of that awareness, i.e., the noeses (the processes) and the noema (the content) of phenomenological consciousness (Kockelsmans, 1967). The approach, called retrospective phenomenological assessment (RPA), involves the retrospective completion of a self-report, phenomenological state instrument in reference to a preceding stimulus condition (Pekala, 1991b).

In addition, noetic analysis can be used to quantify the "state of consciousness," a la Tart (1975), associated with a particular stimulus condition (e.g., hypnosis), by mapping the intensity and/or pattern of organization of those aspects of mind. The methodology generates a reliable and valid "snapshot" of the state of consciousness associated with a particular stimulus condition, be it hypnosis (Pekala & Kumar, 1986, 1989), a spiritual/religious experience (Wildman & McNamara, 2010), or an anomalous experience/event (Rock & Beischel, 2008).

The use of such a quantitative, phenomenological analysis, or noetic analysis (Pekala, 2015, 2016), is distinguished from the descriptive, non-quantitative phenomenological analyses of the psychological phenomenologists (Giorgi, 2009; Moustakas, 1994) and also neurophenomenology (Laughlin et al., 1990; Lutz, 2002; Varela & Shear, 1999).

Noetic Analysis

Noetic Analysis vis-à-vis Phenomenological Psychology and Neurophenomenology

Phenomenological psychology, as described by phenomenological psychologists such as Giorgi (2009) or Moustakas (1994), does not empirically quantify the processes and contents of consciousness in such a way as to make the approach statistically useful in correlating such processes with the brain, human behavior, and individual differences factors (e.g., extraversion, dissociation, transliminality) (although their approaches do furnish us with very rich, descriptive data about the mind).

Neurophenomenology, on the other hand, is a scientific research approach that combines neuroscience with phenomenology to better understand consciousness and human experience, especially as it is embodied by the human brain. The term was coined by neuroanthropologist Charles Laughlin in 1988 (see Rock & Laughlin, 2021), and appropriated and popularized by cognitive neuroscientist Varela (1996).

Laughlin's original formulation of the neurophenomenological method paired neuropsychological research with the methods of Husserlian transcendental phenomenology (Laughlin & Rock, 2013), with the latter "focused upon, describing and analyzing the essential structures of 'pure experience'" (Laughlin & Rock, 2021, p. 43). Neurophenomenology, as defined by Lutz and Thompson (2003), uses "first-person methods," which are:

> disciplined practices subjects can use to increase their sensitivity to their own experiences at various time-scales. ... These practices involved the systematic training of attention and self-regulation of emotion. (p. 33)

Such trained introspection was used in classical introspectionism over 100 years ago. This approach resulted in different laboratories "training" introspectionists in different ways: "laboratory atmosphere crept into the descriptions, and it was not possible to verify, from one laboratory to another, the introspective account of the consciousness of action, feeling, choice, and judgment" (Boring, 1953, p. 174).

In contrast, noetic analysis uses "untrained" introspectionists, i.e., individuals with no specific training in introspection. Such training is not necessary since individuals retrospectively rate their subjective experience in reference to relatively short stimulus intervals/conditions via standardized questionnaires and specific instructional sets.

Future research is needed to determine whether noetic analysis or the "trained" phenomenological analysis of the neurophenomenologists (as defined above) gives a less biased window into the human brain–mind interface. However, regardless as to its relationship to neurophenomenology, noetic analysis is a separate discipline: an empirical, quantitative phenomenological methodology to map human subjectivity (see Pekala, 1980, 1991b, 2015, 2016; Pekala & Creegan, 2020).

Noetic Analysis and its Underlying Presuppositions

In summary, noetics uses standardized self-report questionnaires that measure dimensions of phenomenological experience (such as imagery, absorption, volitional control, positive affect) in a reliable and valid manner. To do this, participants retrospectively rate the items of such questionnaires in reference to a preceding short stimulus condition; thus, the act of introspection is not reactively influencing their stream of consciousness, as might be the case with concurrent observation.

This methodology is based on the assumption of stimulus-state specificity:

> across groups of randomly selected individuals, the same behaviors in the same stimulus setting (the same stimulus conditions), will be associated with the same intensities and patterns of phenomenological experience (the same phenomenological state), while different stimulus conditions will be associated with different intensities and/or patterns of phenomenological experience. (Pekala & Wenger, 1983, p. 255)

This assumption presupposes that subjective consciousness or the mind can be reliably, and validly, quantified. (See Pekala, 1991b, for a review of the methodological and statistical assumptions behind this approach.) Psychophysiological isomorphism (Scheerer, 1994) posits "a one-to-one correspondence between mind and brain states" (Fell et al., 2010, p. 222). The principle of "stimulus-state specificity" (Pekala & Wenger, 1983) was posited as a means to relate quantifiable phenomenological (mental) experiences with their corresponding behavioral and stimulus settings and environments.

Noetic Analysis Questionnaires

The two main questionnaires that have been developed with RPA include the Phenomenology of Consciousness Inventory (PCI; Pekala, 1980, 1982, 1991d) and the Dimensions of Attention Questionnaire (DAQ; Pekala, 1985b, 1991c). These instruments, respectively, quantify consciousness, in general, and attention, in particular.

The PCI[1] is a 53-item retrospective phenomenological assessment questionnaire that quantifies "both the major contents of consciousness, and the processes or means by which these contents are 'illuminated,' cognized, perceived, and so forth by consciousness" (Pekala, 1991b, p. 82). That is, "the PCI quantifies temporal patterns in phenomenological characteristics available to conscious awareness" (Rock et al., 2013, p. 117), which consists of 12 major dimensions (e.g., altered experience, positive affect, vivid imagery) and 14 minor dimensions (e.g., time sense, perception, absorption).

The PCI has been especially useful in mapping the subjective experience of hypnosis, and has been shown to have adequate construct, discriminant (Kumar & Pekala, 1988, 1989; Kumar et al., 1996; Pekala, 1991a, 1991b; Pekala & Forbes, 1997; Pekala & Kumar, 1986, 1989; Pekala et al., 2006; Pekala & Nagler, 1989; Pekala et al., 1986), and predictive validity (Forbes & Pekala, 1993; Hand et al., 1995; Pekala & Kumar, 1984, 1987) for measuring phenomenological experiences associated with hypnosis.

In addition, the PCI has also been used to quantify such stimulus conditions (besides hypnosis) as meditation (Venkatesh et al., 1997), fire-walking (Hillig & Holroyd, 1997/1998;

Pekala & Ersek, 1992/1993), an out-of-the-body experience (OBE) within a near death experience (NDE; Maitz & Pekala, 1991), shamanic-like trances (Rock et al., 2008), charismatic leadership (Churches, 2015), religious/spiritual narratives (Wildman & McNamara, 2010), a virtual reality environment (Huang et al., 2000), drumming (Maurer et al., 1997), ostensible mediumship (Beischel et al., 2021), schizophrenia (Roussel & Bachelor, 2000/2001), epilepsy (Johanson et al., 2011), music perception (Nagy & Szabo, 2004), poker-machine gambling (Dale et al., 2020; Tricker et al., 2016), and psi phenomena (Rock & Storm, 2010; Rock et al., 2013). Whereas the PCI has been translated into 14 languages, the DAQ has been translated into four. (See the website: www.quantifyingconsciousness.com.)

The following sections will demonstrate how noetic analysis has been used to quantify and illustrate states and altered states of consciousness; better map the "domains" of hypnosis; briefly summarize a case study in which noetic analysis was used to understand the similarities and differences between hypnosis and sidhi meditation from a neurophenomenological perspective; and finally, document the usefulness of this approach for assessing your client's/participant's hypnotic talents.

Using Noetics to Quantify States of Consciousness

The Model

C. T. Tart (1972, 1975) is the theoretician and researcher who has developed an influential theoretical model for defining states of consciousness. Tart (1972) described a "state of consciousness" as

> a unique configuration or system of psychological structures or subsystems, a configuration that maintains its integrity or identity as a recognizable system in spite of variations in input from the environment and in spite of various (small) changes in subsystems. (p. 62)

Tart's approach highlights the importance of the pattern of relationships among dimensions of consciousness in determining a state of consciousness: "A unique, dynamic pattern or configuration of psychological structures" (1977, p. 170). Singer (in Zinberg, 1977), on the other hand, suggested that intensity effects were also important and need to be considered in determining if a(n) (altered) state of consciousness is evident: "Are alternate states of consciousness discrete states, to use Tart's words, or are differences among alternate states of consciousness merely differences of degree, as Singer insists?" (p. 9).

Several decades ago, drawing upon the theorizing of Tart, Singer, and Mandler (1985), a "state of consciousness" was defined as "the particular intensity and pattern of associated phenomenological parameters that characterize one's subjective experience during a given time period (Pekala & Wenger, 1983, pp. 252–253)". (Pekala, 1991b, p. 83)

Quantifying States of Consciousness

A person's scores for those questionnaire items making up a particular (sub)dimension of consciousness are averaged to arrive at an intensity score for the various (sub)dimensions of consciousness, allowing for the intensity parameters of subjective experience to be assessed and quantified. By administering the PCI to many individuals in reference to a particular stimulus condition, a Pearson correlation matrix of the scores can be computed for the various dimensions of consciousness. The intercorrelation matrix represents a quantification of the pattern of relationships among the various dimensions per Tart's (1972, 1975, 1977) criteria for his pattern approach to defining states of consciousness.

The correlation matrices associated with different stimulus conditions (e.g., hypnosis vs. relaxation) or differing participant groups (e.g., low vs. high hypnotizables) can then be compared and statistically evaluated via the Jennrich (1970) test, assessing for differences in correlations or patterns of organization among the various dimensions (Pekala, 1991b).

Diagramming States of Consciousness: Pips and Psygrams

The PCI can be used to not only quantify states of consciousness associated with hypnosis, meditation, and other stimulus conditions; the results can also be visually diagrammed. A phenomenological intensity profile (pip) can be used to visually illustrate the 26 PCI major dimensions and subdimensions of a client/participant or group for a particular stimulus condition. Intensity scores can also be visually diagrammed via radar graphs vis-à-vis EXCEL for individuals and groups of individuals.

A psygram (Pekala, 1985a) represents a "snapshot," as assessed across a group of individuals, of the *psychophenomenological* state of consciousness associated with the stimulus condition/participant group assessed. As an example, by illustrating the differences in patterns of connectivity among PCI dimensions for individuals of low and high hypnotic susceptibility during hypnosis, researchers can use this methodology to determine how hypnosis may differentially affect the patterns of association (for the PCI dimensions) among low and high hypnotizables.

Pekala and Kumar (1986) assessed the pattern of relationships among phenomenological subsystems of consciousness across low and high hypnotically susceptible individuals by means of the PCI. Participants experienced a baseline condition (eyes closed sitting quietly) and then retrospectively completed the PCI in reference to that condition. They then experienced the induction procedure of the Harvard Group Scale of Hypnotic Susceptibility: Form A (HGSHS:A; Shor & Orne, 1962), and retrospectively completed the PCI in reference to the sitting quietly period embedded in that induction.

These procedures were replicated in a later study (Pekala & Kumar, 1989), with data from the two studies combined to increase the sample size and reported in Pekala and Bieber (1989/1990). Participants were divided into four susceptibility groups based on their HGSHS:A scores: lows, low-mediums, high-mediums, and highs. Correlation matrices were constructed for the susceptibility groups using the 12 major PCI dimensions for the hypnotic induction conditions. The matrices were compared with the Jennrich (1970) test. The pattern differences between the low and high susceptible groups were significant. By converting the correlations to coefficients of determination (which indicate the percentage of variance in common between PCI dimensions), psygrams were constructed for the low and high susceptible participants for the hypnosis condition.

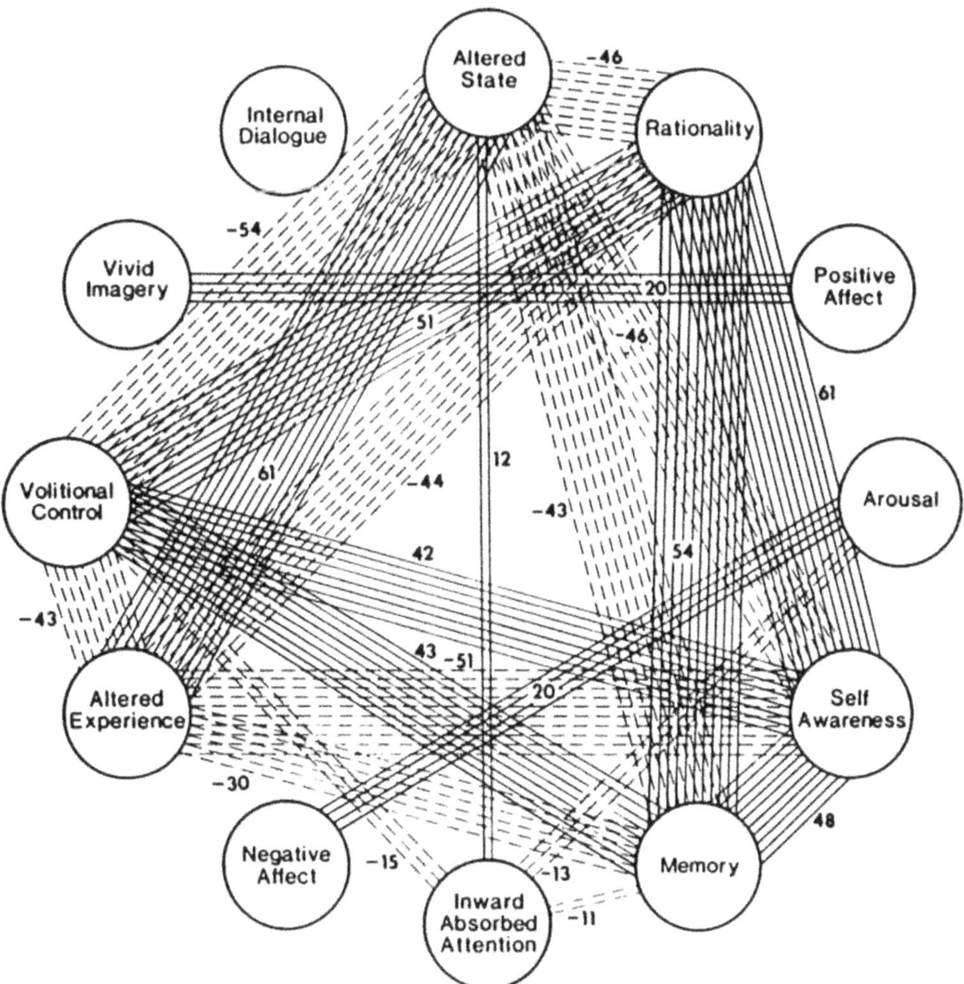

Key: Each line represents approximately 5 percent of the variance in common. (All variance percentages represent correlations significant at alpha less than approximately .001.) $n = 111$.

Figure 7.1 Psygram: Low hypnotizables during hypnosis.

From: Pekala, R. J., & Bieber, S. L. Operationalizing Pattern Approaches to Consciousness: An Analysis of Phenomenological Patterns of Consciousness among Individuals of Differing Susceptibility. *Imagination, Cognition and Personality* 9(4), pp. 303–320. Copyright © 1990, Baywood Publishing Co., Inc. Reprinted by permission of SAGE Publications, Inc.

Figures 7.1 and 7.2 show the patterns of association for low and high susceptibles during hypnosis, respectively. Each line represents 5% of the variance in common. The coefficients of determination are listed besides the lines, with negative correlations (from which the coefficients of determination were computed) listed with a negative number (and dashed lines). Huge differences in the patterns of association are evident between the two groups.

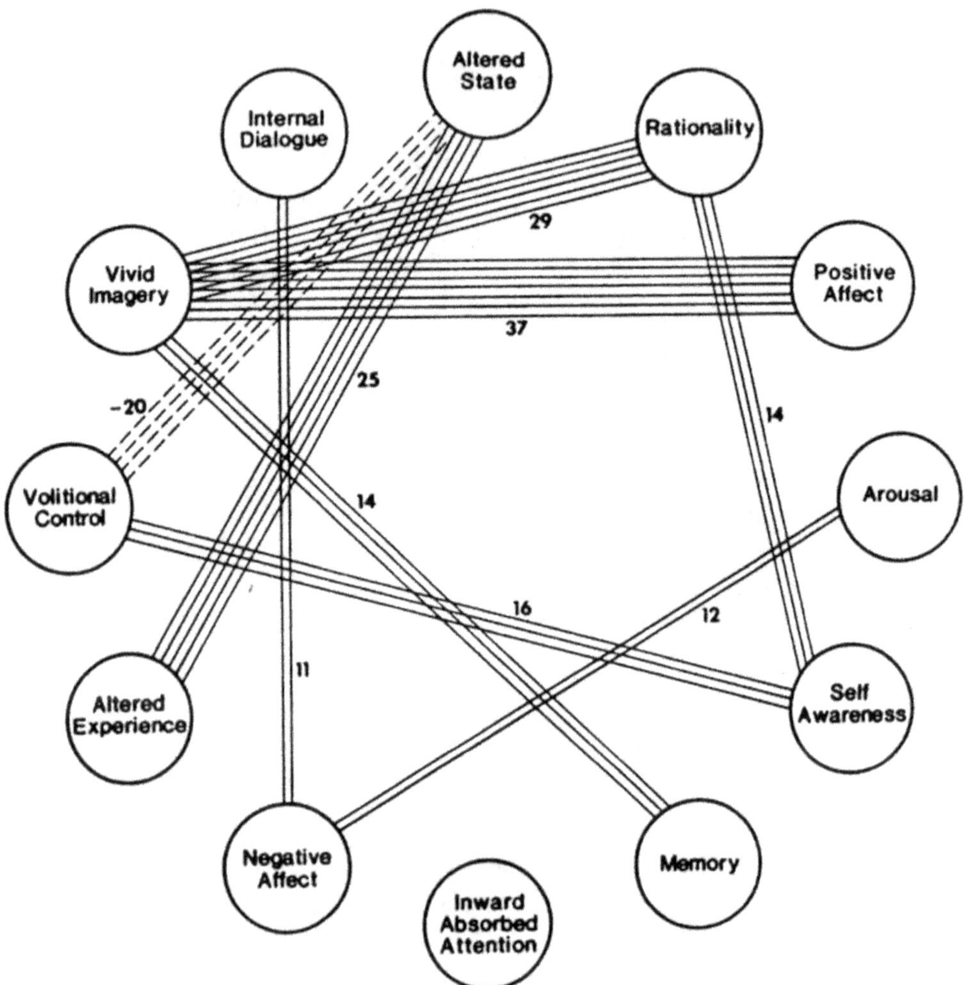

Key: Each line represents approximately 5 percent of the variance in common. (All variance percentages represent correlations significant at alpha less than approximately .001.) $n = 106$.

Figure 7.2 Psygram: High hypnotizables during hypnosis.

From: Pekala, R. J., & Bieber, S. L. Operationalizing Pattern Approaches to Consciousness: An Analysis of Phenomenological Patterns of Consciousness among Individuals of Differing Susceptibility. *Imagination, Cognition and Personality* 9(4), pp. 303–320. Copyright © 1990, Baywood Publishing Co., Inc. Reprinted by permission of SAGE Publications, Inc.

Increased magnitude and frequency of associations among subsystems may make it much more difficult for lows to experience a hallucinated fly or to dissociate the perceptual experience of one's arm levitating, since a change in one particular subsystem is associated with changes in other subsystems. This would make it quite difficult for lows to modify the phenomenological contents of a particular subsystem of consciousness without affecting other subsystems concurrently.

Research into the relationships between hypnosis and dissociation (Kluft, 2003), as measured by various questionnaires like the Dissociative Experiences Scale (DES), has found only weak correlations at best (Carlson & Putnam, 1992). The above psygram results suggest a way of quantitatively operationalizing dissociation, not as a function of the *various contents of consciousness*, as is usually assessed with such instruments as the DES, but rather as an association or disassociation among the subsystems of consciousness for high, vis- à-vis, low susceptibles during hypnosis. Such "dissociative" effects have been replicated by Cleveland et al. (2015).

Using Noetic Analysis to Assess Hypnotic Responsivity: The Phenomenology of Consciousness Inventory: Hypnotic Assessment Procedure (PCI-HAP)

The experience of hypnosis for the client or the research participant is a very subjective event (Spiegel & Spiegel, 2004). Hence, it seems that trying to better understand the mind of the client/participant during hypnosis, via quantification, may be an important piece of the puzzle in helping to decipher the mystery of hypnosis.

Mind, or the state of consciousness of the client/participant, occupies an important position in Holroyd's (2003) theorizing concerning the three major domains that contribute to a person's hypnotic responsivity: trance or altered state of consciousness, imagination/ suggestibility, and expectancy. She posited that imagination/suggestibility and altered state effects combine with expectancy to account for how individuals experience hypnotism: "Suggestion without an altered state is just an invitation to use imagination and fantasy. An altered state without suggestion is just trance or meditation. Not only are altered states and suggestibility interactive contributors, but they also interact with expectancy" (p. 121) to produce hypnotic phenomena.

These are the major domain variables that many theorists and researchers (Barabasz & Watkins, 2005; Barber, 2000; Cardeña, 2005; Elkins, 2014; Gruzelier, 2000; Kihlstrom, 2003, 2005; Kirsch, 1985, 1991; Lankton, 2015; Lynn & Kirsch, 2006; Shoemaker, 1991; Weitzenhoffer, 2002; among others) have also posited as significant components of hypnotic responsivity. The PCI-HAP[1] was developed (Pekala, 1995a, b) to not only measure these major hypnotic domains but also quantify 26 (sub)dimensions of subjective experience associated with hypnosis.

Major Domains Assessed by the PCI-HAP

Trance/altered state effects: Weitzenhoffer (2002) distinguished between hypnosis and hypnotism:

> I will otherwise generally reserve the term hypnosis for the "state" and the term hypnotism, for the production, study and use of suggestion with the state of hypnosis presumably being present, whether or not it adds anything tangible to the situation. (p. 210)

Hence, hypnotism, according to Weitzenhoffer (2002), implies the giving of suggestions, via imagination, fantasy, and/or other means, and the acceptance of those suggestions by individuals whether or not they are in the "altered state" of hypnosis. Additionally, Weitzenhoffer (2002) wrote that the term "trance" has been used interchangeably with the term hypnosis since Braid (1843) but especially in modern times. He suggested that "trance," however, appears to be an older and much broader concept than hypnosis:

> [Trance] denotes various states of being that have the appearance of consciousness but seem to differ from normal consciousness [...] as being a sleeplike, or a half-awake, half-asleep state. (Weitzenhoffer, 1989, p. 298)

Suggestibility: Suggestibility is usually defined in terms of responsiveness to suggestions (because suggestibility means different things to different theorists, see Schumaker, 1991, for a comprehensive review of these differing viewpoints). Kirsch and Braffman (1999) distinguished two main types of suggestibility: "[I]f 'hypnotic suggestibility' is responsiveness to suggestions given after hypnosis has been induced" (p. 226) then "nonhypnotic suggestibility" may be used "to denote responsiveness to suggestions administered without the prior induction of hypnosis" (p. 226). They emphasized the role of imagination in suggestibility. They defined "imaginative suggestions" as "requests to experience an imaginary state of affairs as if it were real" (Kirsch & Braffman, 2001, p. 59) and "imaginative suggestibility" as the "degree to which the person succeeds in having the suggested experiences" (p. 59), whether such experiences occur within, or outside of, hypnosis.

Expectancy: Kirsch (1991) has made expectancy a central concept in his theorizing concerning hypnosis, considering it the "essence" of hypnosis and defining it as "the capacity of people's beliefs and expectations to bring about changes in experience" (p. 461). In particular, Kirsch stated that the "attempts to eliminate expectancy as 'artifact' may be doomed to failure" (p. 461) and felt that therapist-directed changes in expectancy can lead to changes in hypnotic experience and behavior and, hence, therapeutic change.

In response to the American Psychological Association (APA) Division 30 definition of hypnosis (Elkins et al., 2015), the sociocognitive group (Lynn et al., 2015) affirmed the importance of expectancy in understanding hypnotism: "[M]easures of expectancy ... are better and more consistent predictors of hypnotic responding than are trait measures of hypnotic suggestibility ... " (Lynn et al., 2015, p. 394).

Operationalizing the Model via the PCI-HAP

The PCI has been combined with a hypnotic induction procedure to generate the PCI-HAP. The Phenomenology of Consciousness Inventory: Hypnotic Assessment Procedure (PCI-HAP; Pekala, 1995a; 1995b) is a phenomenologically-based assessment instrument that was developed to measure hypnotic responsivity from a more phenomenological, and state-based, perspective than traditional, cognitive-behavioral trait assessments like the Harvard Group Scale of Hypnotic Susceptibility (Shor & Orne, 1962) or the Stanford Scale of Hypnotic Susceptibility: Form C (Weitzenhoffer & Hilgard, 1962). The PCI-HAP includes a pre-assessment, hypnotic induction, and a post-assessment, along with retrospective completion of a 53-item self-report inventory, the PCI, in reference to a sitting quietly period during hypnosis.

The PCI-HAP generates a "hypnoidal state" score (Pekala, 2002; Pekala & Nagler, 1989) that may be construed as a "general measure of trance" (see Pekala & Kumar, 2000, for a review of that concept). In addition to the hypnoidal state score, the PCI-HAP assessment protocol includes a measure of "imagoic suggestibility," an aspect of imagination and fantasy as defined by Sheehan (1979), or "imaginative suggestibility" as defined by Kirsch and Braffman (2001). The PCI-HAP also includes self-report measures of two types of expectancies (Kirsch, 1985): pre-hypnotic estimated hypnotic depth and pre/posthypnotic therapeutic efficacy.

The PCI-HAP allows participants to estimate their hypnotic depth in the spirit of LeCron (1953): the self-report hypnotic depth (srHD) score. The post-assessment form also assesses responses to several other items. In addition, the PCI HAP generates an average summary and percentile score for the client's overall hypnotic responsivity, called the hypnotic responsivity index (HRI).

The HRI is the average of the four main domain variables assessed by the PCI-HAP: the hypnoidal state score, the imagoic suggestibility score, the average total expectancy score, and the posthypnotic self-reported hypnotic depth (srHD) score. Values for the HRI index score range from 0.0 to 10.0, with associated percentile scores. The HRI allows the clinician and researcher to assign a client or participant a percentile score concerning their hypnotic responsivity (Pekala, 2014a, 2014b), and most importantly, allows for the clinician/researcher to tailor hypnotic suggestions to the clients'/participants' hypnotic talents (Pekala, 1995a, b).

Using Noetic Analysis for Better Understanding the Brain/Mind/Behavior Interface during Hypnosis

Using the PCI-HAP to Differentiate the Component Processes Underlying Self-Reported Hypnotic Depth

Several studies (Pekala et al., 2006; Pekala et al., 2010a; 2010b; Pekala et al., 2017) have assessed how well the srHD score could be predicted from the PCI/PCI-HAP variables. Participants from the earlier studies were chronic drug and alcohol individuals residing at an in-patient program who were involved in using self-hypnosis training for relapse prevention post-discharge. Pekala et al.'s (2017) study involved 95 Italian participants.

Table 7.1 Predicting Self-Reported Hypnotic Depth from the PCI-HAP Variables

Subscale	R	R^2	*Unstandardized Coefficient*	*Standardized Coefficient*	F *Value*[a]	p *Value*[b]
Hypnoidal State[c] (pHGS Score)	0.742	0.550	0.773	0.446	113.71	0.000
Total Combined Expectancy	0.773	0.598	0.293	0.230	10.85	0.001
Eye Catalepsy (Numeric)	0.797	0.635	0.296	0.220	9.34	0.003
Imagoic Suggestibility	0.804	0.647	0.126	0.129	3.00	0.087
Constant			-2.668			

Reproduced with permission from: Pekala, R., Baglio, F., Cabinio, M., Lipari, S., Baglio, G., Mendozz, L., Cecconi, P., Pugnetti, L., & Sciaky, R. (2017). Hypnotism as a function of trance state effects, expectancy, and suggestibility: An Italian replication. *International Journal of Clinical and Experimental Hypnosis, 65*(2), 210–240.

Notes

a *F* and *p* are initial values for independent variables left in the regression equation, respectively.
b $n = 95$.
c Items not included in the regression equation were pre-hypnotic estimated hypnotic depth, pre-hypnotic visual imagery vividness, pre-hypnotic kinesthetic imagery vividness, pre-hypnotic estimated therapeutic efficacy, post-hypnotic expected therapeutic efficacy, the finger response item, negative affect, and the sleep state item.

Since the 2017 study essentially replicated the results of the earlier studies, this study's results will be summarized. In a step-wise multiple regression equation predicting srHD (Pekala et al., 2017), trance as measured by the hypnoidal state score, and expectancy (as measured by total combined expectancy) accounted for about 60% of the relative variance (standardized coefficients), generating an *R* of 0.804, predicting 65% of the total variance (the eye catalepsy item and imagoic suggestibility were the only other items left in the regression equation) (see Table 7.1). What these results illustrate is that one's srHD was found to be a function of trance, expectancy, and imagoic suggestibility, results consistent with the theorizing of Holroyd (2003), and other major hypnosis theorists and researchers (Kirsch, 1991; Kirsch & Braffman, 1999; Weitzenhoffer, 2002).

Table 7.2 Predicting Self-Reported Hypnotic Depth Only from the PCI Major Dimensions

Subscale	R	R^2	*Unstandardized Coefficient*	*Standardized Coefficient*	F *Value*[a]	p *Value*[b]
Altered State of Awareness	0.702	0.493	0.777	0.439	90.52	0.000
Positive Affect	0.762	0.581	0.565	0.228	19.33	0.000
Visual Imagery	0.784	0.614	0.339	0.219	7.72	0.007
Volitional Control	0.795	0.632	−0.282	−0.165	4.35	0.040
Constant			1.220			

Reproduced with permission from: Pekala, R., Baglio, F., Cabinio, M., Lipari, S., Baglio, G., Mendozz, L., Cecconi, P., Pugnetti, L. & Sciaky, R. (2017). Hypnotism as a function of trance state effects, expectancy, and suggestibility: An Italian replication. *International Journal of Clinical and Experimental Hypnosis, 65*(2), 210–240.

Notes

a *F* and *p* are initial values for independent variables left in the regression equation, respectively.
b $n = 95$.

The srHD score was also predicted from the PCI major dimensions. Table 7.2 demonstrates those results. Left in the regression equation were altered state of awareness, positive affect, visual imagery, and volitional control, generating an *R* of 0.795 for an R^2 of 0.632. These are dimensions of consciousness that many hypnosis clinicians would attest to being important in understanding what aspects of consciousness are modified with hypnosis.

The PCI-HAP, as mentioned, also generates a HRI score. It gives "an overall estimate of the client's hypnotic responsivity from a more state perspective" (Pekala et al., 2017, p. 224). It was also predicted from the various PCI major dimensions in Pekala et al.'s (2017) study. The regression analysis results generated an *R* of 0.922 and an R^2 of 0.85. (see Table 7.3). Left in the regression equation were altered state of awareness and imagery, accounting for about half of the relative variance (as measured by the standardized regression coefficients). Also included in the regression equation were positive affect, volitional control, attention, and internal dialogue.

The standardized regression coefficients listed in each of the three tables shows the relative variance associated with each coefficient. Because the standardized regression coefficients partial out the variance associated with the other variables left in the regression equation (Grimm & Yarnold, 1995), the aforementioned analyses suggest that one's srHD appears to be a function of several relatively different domains (when using the PCI-HAP), or several specific PCI dimensions. As Wagstaff (1981) suggested over 40 years ago, hypnotism appears to be a "domain" phenomenon, with hypnosis subsuming several

Table 7.3 Predicting the Hypnotic Responsivity Index from the PCI Major Dimensions

Subscale	R	R^2	*Unstandardized Coefficient*	*Standardized Coefficient*	F *Value*[a]	p *Value*[b]
Altered State of Awareness	0.738	0.545	0.449	0.365	111.22	0.000
Imagery	0.878	0.771	0.418	0.387	90.96	0.000
Positive Affect	0.901	0.811	0.393	0.228	19.26	0.000
Volitional Control	0.914	0.835	-0.206	-0.173	13.35	0.000
Attention	0.918	0.843	0.195	0.122	4.23	0.043
Internal Dialogue	0.922	0.851	−0.100	−0.096	4.78	0.031
Constant			2.326			

Reproduced with permission from: Pekala, R., Baglio, F., Cabinio, M., Lipari, S., Baglio, G., Mendozz, L., Cecconi, P., Pugnetti, L. & Sciaky, R. (2017). Hypnotism as a function of trance state effects, expectancy, and suggestibility: An Italian replication. *International Journal of Clinical and Experimental Hypnosis, 65*(2), 210–240.

Notes

a *F* and *p* are initial values for independent variables left in the regression equation, respectively.

b $n = 95$.

different domains or dimensions of subjective experience. The research supports Woody and McConkey's (2003) theorizing concerning hypnosis as requiring "different combinations of underlying component abilities."

Using the PCI-HAP to Evaluate Hypnosis vis-à-vis Sidhi Meditation in a Single Case Study

In a case study by Pekala and Creegan (2020), qEEGs were obtained during a hypnotic assessment with the PCI-HAP, and also during sidhi meditation of a long-term TM meditator (see pdf for details: http://www.lidsen.com/journals/icm/icm-05-02-019). The PCI was retrospectively completed in reference to the PCI-HAP and also in reference to sidhi meditation.

On the PCI-HAP, the participant obtained a HRI percentile score suggesting moderate hypnotic responsivity. Concerning noetic differences between hypnosis and sidhi meditation, meditation was associated with higher scores on self-awareness, altered awareness, and altered experience (altered body image and meaning), in addition to greater feelings of love. Sidhi meditation was also associated with more alpha and higher beta activity than hypnosis, with greater high beta in the left pre-frontal cortex.

How such qEEG differences between hypnosis and meditation may relate to differences in noetic experience were explored in Pekala and Creegan's (2020) paper. The case study suggests that, when quantifying the brain with the qEEG, and the mind with the PCI, a "noetic snapshot" of the mind can be obtained that may be used to better quantify the brain/mind interface, and augment the ability of neurophenomenology to unravel the mystery of hypnosis, meditation, and possibly other (altered) states of consciousness.

Hypnotic Assessment and Subsequent Hypnotic Intervention via the PCI/PCI-HAP

By being able to ***quantify*** the major domains of hypnosis, as measured by the PCI-HAP, and 26 PCI (sub)dimensions of subjective experience, the researcher and clinician have a methodology to not only assess their participant's/client's hypnotic abilities and talents but also tailor hypnotic suggestions/interventions to those talents (Pekala, 2016). (See the interpretative manual to the PCI-HAP, Pekala, 2009.)

We believe that such an approach can, in turn, lead to an increased ability to artfully apply hypnotic interventions to your particular client's hypnotic abilities and presenting symptoms (see Pekala, 2002). The PCI-HAP EXCEL programs generate a five-page report concerning those hypnotic domains and (sub)dimensions of consciousness activated by hypnosis. Such data can then be used to tailor hypnotic interventions congruent with the client's own hypnotic phenomenology.

Conclusions

The aforementioned review demonstrates that "the mind can be quantified, as can quarks, the economy, or a neutron star: *precise descriptive first-person reports about subjective experience* can be obtained in a reliable and valid manner." (Pekala, 2015, pp. 404–405). Given the current lack of approaches to quantify and analyze phenomenology (Lifshitz, 2016), we believe that noetic analysis provides not only a comprehensive methodology for the quantitative analysis of phenomenological experience but also a way to define, quantify, and diagram states and altered states of consciousness (Tart, 1975). Noetic analysis furnishes a methodology that may be especially useful in helping decipher not only the mysteries of hypnosis but also the hypnotic mind/brain/behavior interface, especially when combined with cognitive-behavioral and neurophysiological methodologies (Pekala & Creegan, 2020).

Note

1 Copies of the PCI (Pekala, 1991d) and the user's manual and EXCEL scoring protocols for the PCI (Pekala, 2019) are available at www.quantifyingconsciousness.com. Copies of the PCI-HAP (Pekala, 1995a; 1995b), the therapist and self-report pre- and post-assessment forms, the administration (Pekala et al., 2009) and interpretive (Pekala, 2009) manuals, and the EXCEL scoring program are available at www.quantifyingconsciousness.com.[Please note: while anyone can download and procure a copy of the PCI and its EXCEL scoring sheet; you must be a clinician or researcher with validated experience in hypnosis to download the PCI-HAP and its accessories.]

An earlier version of this paper was presented to the American Psychological Association by the first author for the Annual Meeting in August, 2023, Washington, DC.

The authors wish to thank Daniel Kaufmann, PhD for his helpful comments on an earlier version of this paper.

References

Barabasz, A., & Watkins, J. G. (2005). *Hypnotherapeutic techniques* (2nd ed.). Brunner-Routledge.

Barber, T. X. (2000). A deeper understanding of hypnosis: Its secrets, its nature, its essence. *American Journal of Clinical Hypnosis*, *42*, 208–272. 10.1080/00029157.2000.10734361

Beischel, J., Rock, A. J., Pekala, R. J. Boccuzzi, M. (2021). Survival psi and somatic psi: Exploratory quantitative phenomenological analyses of blinded mediums' experiences of communication with the deceased and psychic readings for the living. *Journal of Near-Death Studies*, *39*(2), 61–102.

Boring, E. G. (1953). A history of introspection. *Psychological Bulletin*, *50*, 169–189. 10.1037/h0090793

Braid, J. (1843). *Neurypnology: Or the rationale of nervous sleep considered in relation with animal magnetism.* John Churchill.

Cardeña, E. A. (2005). The phenomenology of deep hypnosis: Quiescent and physically active. *International Journal of Clinical and Experimental Hypnosis*, *53*, 1–12. 10.1080/002071404 90914234

Carlson, E. B., & Putnam, F. W. (1992). *Manual for the dissociative experiences scale*. [Unpublished manuscript, Department of Psychology Beloit College].

Chalmers, D. (2007). The hard problem of consciousness. In M. Velmans & S. Schneider (Eds.), *The Blackwell companion to consciousness* (pp. 225–235). Blackwell Publishing.

Churches, R. M. (2015). *The followership effect: Charismatic oratory, hypnoidal and altered states of consciousness* [Doctoral dissertation, University of Surrey].

Cleveland, J. M., Korman, B. M., & Gold, S. N. (2015). Are hypnosis and dissociation related? New evidence for a connection. *International Journal of Clinical and Experimental Hypnosis*, *63*(2), 198–214. 10.1080/00207144.2015.1002691

Dale, G., Rock, A. J., & Clark, G. I. (2020). Cue-reactive imagery mediates the relationships of reward responsiveness with both cue-reactive urge to gamble and positive affect in poker-machine gamblers. *Journal of Gambling Studies*, 36, 1045–1063.

Elkins, G. (2014). *Hypnotic relaxation therapy: Principles and applications*. Springer.

Elkins, G., Barabasz, A. F., Council, J. R., & Spiegel, D. (2015). Advancing research and practice: The revised APA Division 30 definition of hypnosis. *International Journal of Clinical and Experimental Hypnosis*, *63*, 1–9. 10.1080/00207144.2014.961870

Fell, J., Axmacher, N., & Haupt, S. (2010). From alpha to gamma: Electrophysiological correlates of meditation-related states of consciousness. *Medical Hypotheses*, *75*, 218–224.

Forbes, E., & Pekala, R. J. (1993). Predicting hypnotic susceptibility via a phenomenological approach. *Psychological Reports*, *73*, 1251–1256. 10.2466/pr0.1993.73.3f.1251

Gelven, M. (1970). *A commentary on Heidegger's being and time*. Harper & Row.

Giorgi, A. (2009). *The descriptive phenomenological method in psychology: A modified Husserlian approach*. Duquesne University Press.

Grimm, L. G., & Yarnold, R. R. (1995). *Reading and understanding multivariate statistics*. American Psychological Association.

Gruzelier, J. H. (2000). Redefining hypnosis: Theory, methods, and integration. *Contemporary Hypnosis*, *17*(2), 51–70. 10.1002/ch.193

Hand, J., Pekala, R. J., & Kumar, V. K. (1995). Prediction of Harvard and Stanford scale scores with a phenomenological instrument. *Australian Journal of Clinical and Experimental Hypnosis*, *23*, 124–134.

Hillig, J. A., & Holroyd, J. (1997/1998). Consciousness, attention, and hypnoidal effects during fire walking. *Imagination, Cognition, and Personality*, *17*, 153–163. 10.2190/2G9W-QHA2-R2T5-EFY

Holroyd, J. (2003). The science of meditation and the state of hypnosis. *American Journal of Clinical Hypnosis*, *46*, 109–128. 10.1080/00029157.2003.10403582

Huang, M. P., Himle, J., & Alsip, N. E. (2000). Vivid visualization in the experience of phobia in virtual environments: Preliminary results. *Cyber Psychology & Behavior*, *3*, 315–320.

Jennrich, R. I. (1970). An asymptotic $\chi 2$ test for the equality of two correlation matrices. *Journal of the American Statistical Association*, *65*, 904–912.

Johanson, M., Valli, K., & Revonsuo, A. (2011). How to assess ictal consciousness? *Behavioural Neurology*, *24*, 11–20. 10.1155/2011/874295

Kihlstrom, J. (2003). The fox, the hedgehog, and hypnosis. *International Journal of Clinical and Experimental Hypnosis*, *51*, 166–189. 10.1076/iceh.51.2.166.14611

Kihlstrom, J. F. (2005). Is hypnosis an altered state of consciousness or what? *Contemporary Hypnosis*, *2*, 34–38. 10.1002/ch.20

Kirsch, I. (1985). Response expectancy as a determinant of experience and behavior. *American Psychologist*, *40*, 1189–1202. 10.1037/0003-066X.40.11.1189

Kirsch, I. (1991). The social learning theory of hypnosis. In S. J. Lynn & J. W. Rhue (Eds.), *Theories of hypnosis: Current models and perspectives* (pp. 439–465). Guilford.

Kirsch, I., & Braffman, W. (1999). Correlates of hypnotizability: The first empirical study. *Contemporary Hypnosis*, *16*, 224–230. 10.1002/(ISSN)1557-0711

Kirsch, I., & Braffman, W. (2001). Imaginative suggestibility and hypnotizability. *Current Directions in Psychological Science*, *10*, 57–61. 10.1111/cdir.2001.10.issue-2

Kluft, R. P. (2003). Current issues in dissociative identity disorder. *Bridging Eastern and Western Psychiatry*, *1*, 71–87.
Kockelsmans, J. J. (Ed.). (1967). *Phenomenology: The philosophy of Edmund Husserl and its interpretation*. Doubleday and Company.
Kumar, V. K., & Pekala, R. J. (1988). Hypnotizability, absorption, and individual differences in phenomenological experience. *International Journal of Clinical and Experimental Hypnosis*, *36*, 80–88. 10.1080/00207148808409332
Kumar, V. K., & Pekala, R. J. (1989). Variations in phenomenological experience as a function of hypnotic susceptibility: A replication. *British Journal of Experimental and Clinical Hypnosis*, *6*, 17–22.
Kumar, V. K., Pekala, R. J., & Cummings, J. (1996). Trait factors, state effects, and hypnotizability. *International Journal of Clinical and Experimental Hypnosis*, *44*, 232–249.
Lankton, S. (2015). A SoC model of hypnosis and induction. *American Journal of Clinical Hypnosis*, *57*, 367–377. 10.1080/00029157.2015.1011461
Laughlin, C. D., McManus, J., & d'Aquili, E. G. (1990). *Brain, symbol and experience: Toward a neurophenomenology of human consciousness*. Columbia University Press.
Laughlin, C. D., & Rock, A. J. (2013). Neurophenomenology: Enhancing the experimental and cross-cultural study of brain and experience. In H. L. Friedman & G. Hartelius (Eds.). *The Wiley-Blackwell handbook of transpersonal psychology* (pp. 261–280). Wiley-Blackwell
Laughlin, C. D., & Rock, A. J. (2021). Transpersonal phenomenology: The cosmological and spiritual dimensions of the Husserlian epoché. *Transpersonal Psychology Review*, *23*(2), 41–62.
LeCron, L. M. (1953). A method of measuring the depth of hypnosis. *Journal of Clinical and Experimental Hypnosis*, *1*, 4–7. 10.1080/00207145308409812
Lifshitz M. (2016). Contemplative experience in context: Hypnosis, meditation, and the transformation of consciousness. In A. Raz & M. Lifshitz (Eds.), *Hypnosis and meditation: Towards an integrative science of conscious planes* (pp. 3–16). Oxford University Press.
Lutz, A. (2002). Toward a neurophenomenology as an account of generative passages: A first empirical case study. *Phenomenology and the Cognitive Sciences*, *1*, 133–167.
Lutz, A., & Thompson, E. (2003). Neurophenomenology: Integrating subjective experience and brain dynamics in the neuroscience of consciousness. *Journal of Consciousness Studies*, *10*, 31–52.
Lynn, S. J., Green, J. P., Kirsch, I., Capafons, A., Lilienfeld, S. O., Laurence, J.-R., & Montgomery, G. H. (2015). Grounding hypnosis in science: The "new" APA division 30 definition of hypnosis as a step backward. *American Journal of Clinical Hypnosis*, *57*, 390–401. 10.1080/00029157.2015.1011472
Lynn, S. J., & Kirsch, I. (2006). *Essentials of clinical hypnosis: An evidence-based approach*. American Psychological Association.
Maitz, E. A., & Pekala, R. J. (1991). Phenomenological quantification of an out-of-the-body experience associated with a near-death event. *Omega*, *22*, 199–214.
Mandler, G. (1985). *Consciousness: An essay in cognitive psychology*. Lawrence Erlbaum.
Maurer, R. L., Kumar, V. K., Woodside, L., & Pekala, R. J. (1997). Phenomenological experience in response to monotonous drumming and hypnotizability. *American Journal of Clinical Hypnosis*, *40*, 130–145. 10.1080/00029157.1997.10403417
Milton, F., Fulford, J. Dance, C., Gaddum, J., Heuerman-Williamson, B., Jones, K., Knight, K., MacKisack, M, Winlove, C., & Zeman, A. (2021). Behavioral and neural signatures of visual imagery vividness extremes: Aphantasia versus hyperphantasia. *Cerbral Cortex Communications*, *2*, 1–15. 10.1093/texcom/tgab035
Moustakas, C. E. (1994). *Phenomenological research methods*. Sage Publications.
Nagy, K., & Szabo, C. (2004). Differences in phenomenological experiences of music-listening: The influence of musical involvement and type of music on musical experiences. *Proceedings of the 8th International Conference on Music Perception & Cognition*, Evanston, IL.
Pekala, R. J. (1980). *An empirical-phenomenological approach for mapping consciousness and its various "states* [Doctoral dissertation], Michigan State University.
Pekala, R. J. (1982). *The phenomenology of consciousness inventory*. Psychophenomenological Concepts. (Now published by Mid-Atlantic Educational Institute. See Pekala, 1991b).
Pekala, R. J. (1985a). A psychophenomenological approach to mapping and diagramming states of consciousness. *Journal of Religion and Psychical Research*, *8*, 199–214.

Pekala, R. J. (1985b). *The dimensions of attention questionnaire*. Psychophenomenological Concepts. (Now published by Mid-Atlantic Educational Institute. See Pekala, 1991d).

Pekala, R. J. (1991a). Hypnotic types: Evidence from a cluster analysis of phenomenal experience. *Contemporary Hypnosis*, *8*, 95–104.

Pekala, R. J. (1991b). *Quantifying consciousness: An empirical approach*. Plenum Press.

Pekala, R. J. (1991c). *The dimensions of attention questionnaire*. Mid-Atlantic Educational Institute.

Pekala, R. J. (1991d). *The phenomenology of consciousness inventory*. Mid-Atlantic Educational Institute.

Pekala, R. J. (1995a). A short unobtrusive hypnotic induction for assessing hypnotizability level: I. Development and research. *American Journal of Clinical Hypnosis*, *37*, 271–283. 10.1080/00029157.1995.10403156

Pekala, R. J. (1995b). A short unobtrusive hypnotic induction for assessing hypnotizability: II. Clinical case reports. *American Journal of Clinical Hypnosis*, *37*, 284–293. 10.1080/00029157.1995.10403157

Pekala, R. J. (2002). Operationalizing "trance": II. Clinical application using a psychophenomenological approach. *American Journal of Clinical Hypnosis*, *44*, 241–255. 10.1080/00029157.2002.10403484

Pekala, R. J. (2009, October). *Therapist's manual: Interpretation of the phenomenology of consciousness inventory: Hypnotic assessment procedure (PCI-HAP)*. MAEI.

Pekala, R. J. (2010). Reply to "methodological and interpretative issues regarding the phenomenology of consciousness inventory-hypnotic assessment procedure: A comment on Pekala et al. (2010a, 2010b)." *American Journal of Clinical Hypnosis*, *53*, 119–132. 10.1080/00029157.2010.10404334

Pekala, R. J. (2011). Reply to Wagstaff: "Hypnosis and the relationship between trance, suggestion, expectancy, and depth: Some semantic and conceptual issues." *American Journal of Clinical Hypnosis*, *53*, 207–227. 10.1080/00029157.2011.10401758

Pekala, R. J. (2014a, May). *Phenomenological snapshots of the hypnotic mind: An overview*. [Invited address]. The Greater Philadelphia Society of Clinical Hypnosis.

Pekala, R. J. (2014b, August). *Quantifying the mind to better understand your client's hypnotic talents*. [Paper presentation]. American Psychological Association Annual Convention.

Pekala, R. J. (2015). Hypnosis as a "state of consciousness:" How quantifying the mind can help us better understand hypnosis. *American Journal of Clinical Hypnosis*, *57*, 402–424. 10.1080/00029157.2015.1011480

Pekala, R. J. (2016). The "mysteries of hypnosis": Helping us better understand hypnosis and empathic involvement theory (EIT). *American Journal of Clinical Hypnosis*, *58*, 274–285. 10.1080/00029157.2015.1101679

Pekala, R. J. (2019) *Using the phenomenology of consciousness inventory (PCI) to quantify the mind: User's manual*. MAEI.

Pekala, R., Baglio, F., Cabinio, M., Lipari, S., Baglio, G., Mendozzi, L., Cecconi, Pugnetti, L., & Sciaky, R. (2017). Hypnotism as a function of trance state effects, expectancy, and suggestibility: An Italian replication. *International Journal of Clinical and Experimental Hypnosis*, *65*(2), 210–240.

Pekala, R. J., & Bieber, S. L. (1989/1990). Operationalizing pattern approaches to consciousness: An analysis of phenomenological patterns of consciousness among individuals of differing susceptibility. *Imagination, Cognition, and Personality*, *9*, 303–320. 10.2190/V89B-F4X2-5HLW-R0E4

Pekala, R. J., & Creegan, K. (2020). Hypnotic states of consciousness, the qEEG, and noetic snapshots of the brain/mind interface. *OBM Integrative and Complementary Medicine*, *5*(2), 1–35. 10.21926/obm.icm.2002019

Pekala, R. J., & Ersek, B. (1992/1993). Fire walking versus hypnosis: A preliminary study concerning consciousness, attention, and fire immunity. *Imagination, Cognition, and Personality*, *12*, 207–229. 10.2190/J703-N7H8-KMGL-0DLG

Pekala, R. J., & Forbes, E. J. (1997). Types of hypnotically (un)susceptible individuals as a function of phenomenological experience: Towards a typology of hypnotic types. *American Journal of Clinical Hypnosis*, *39*, 212–224. 10.1080/00029157.1997.10403386

Pekala, R. J., & Kumar, V. K. (1984). Predicting hypnotic susceptibility by a self-report phenomenological state instrument. *American Journal of Clinical Hypnosis*, *27*, 114–121. 10.1080/00029157.1984.10402867

Pekala, R. J., & Kumar, V. K. (1986). The differential organization of the structures of consciousness during hypnosis and a baseline condition. *Journal of Mind and Behavior*, *7*, 515–539.

Pekala, R. J., & Kumar, V. K. (1987). Predicting hypnotic susceptibility via a self-report instrument: A replication. *American Journal of Clinical Hypnosis*, *30*, 57–65. 10.1080/00029157.1987.10402723

Pekala, R. J., & Kumar, V. K. (1989). Patterns of consciousness during hypnosis: Relevance to cognition and individual differences. *Australian Journal of Clinical and Experimental Hypnosis*, *17*, 1–20.

Pekala, R. J., & Kumar, V. K. (2000). Operationalizing "trance": I. Rationale and research using a psychophenomenological approach. *American Journal of Clinical Hypnosis*, *43*, 107–135. 10.1080/00029157.2000.10404265

Pekala, R. J., & Kumar, V. K. (2007). An empirical-phenomenological approach to quantifying consciousness and states of consciousness: With particular reference to understanding the nature of hypnosis. In G. Jamieson (Ed.). *Towards a cognitive-neuroscience of hypnosis and conscious states: A resource for researchers, students, and clinicians* (pp. 167–194). Oxford University Press.

Pekala, R. J., Kumar, V. K., & Maurer, R. (2009, October). *The phenomenology of consciousness inventory: Hypnotic assessment procedure (PCI-HAP)*. Administrator's manual. MAEI.

Pekala, R. J., Kumar, V. K., Maurer, R., Elliott-Carter, N., & Moon, E. (2006). "How deeply hypnotized did I get?" Predicting self-reported hypnotic depth from a phenomenological assessment instrument. *International Journal of Clinical and Experimental Hypnosis*, *54*, 316–339. 10.1080/00207140600691344

Pekala, R. J., Kumar, V. K., Maurer, R., Elliott-Carter, N., Moon, E., & Mullen, K. (2010a). Suggestibility, expectancy, trance state effects, and hypnotic depth: I. Implications for understanding hypnotism. *American Journal of Clinical Hypnosis*, *52*, 271–286.

Pekala, R. J., Kumar, V. K., Maurer, R., Elliott-Carter, N., Moon, E., & Mullen, K. (2010b). Suggestibility, expectancy, trance state effects, and hypnotic depth: II. Assessment via the PCI-HAP. *American Journal of Clinical Hypnosis*, *52*, 287–314.

Pekala, R. J., & Nagler, R. (1989). The assessment of hypnoidal states: Rationale and clinical application. *American Journal of Clinical Hypnosis*, *31*, 231–236. 10.1080/00029157.1989.10402777

Pekala R. J., Steinberg J., & Kumar V. K. (1986). Measurement of phenomenological experience: Phenomenology of consciousness inventory. *Perceptual and Motor Skills*, *63*, 983–989.

Pekala, R. J., & Wenger, C. F. (1983). Retrospective phenomenological assessment: Mapping consciousness in reference to specific stimulus conditions. *Journal of Mind and Behavior*, *4*, 247–274.

Pekala, R. J., & Wickramasekera, I. (2007). An empirical phenomenological approach to hypnotic assessment: Overview and use of the PCI-HAP as an assessment instrument. *Psychological Hypnosis: Society of Psychological Hypnosis*, *16*, 15–19.

Rock, A. J., & Beischel, J. (2008). Quantitative analysis of mediums' conscious experiences during a discarnate reading versus a control task: A pilot study. *Australian Journal of Parapsychology*, *8*, 157–179.

Rock, A. J., Friedman, H. L., & Jamieson, G. A. (2013). Operationalizing psi-conducive altered states: Integrating insights from consciousness studies into parapsychology. In S. Krippner, A. J. Rock, J. Beischel, H. L. Friedman, H. L., & C. L. Fracasso (Eds.), *Advances in parapsychological research* (volume 9, pp. 110–125). McFarland.

Rock, A. J., & Laughlin, C. D. (2021). The advancement of transpersonal psychological science: A neurophenomenological trajectory. In D. A. MacDonald & M. Almendro (Eds.), *Transpersonal psychology and science: An evaluation of its present status and future directions* (pp. 6–13). Cambridge Scholars Publishing.

Rock, A. J., & Storm, L. (2010). Shamanic-like journeying and psi: II. Mental boundaries, phenomenology, and the picture-identification task. *Australian Journal of Parapsychology*, *10*, 41–68.

Rock, A. J., Storm, L., Harris, K., & Friedman, H. L. (2013). Shamanic-like journey and psi-signal detection: II. Phenomenological dimensions. *Journal of Parapsychology*, *77*, 249–270.

Rock, A. J., Wilson, J. M., Johnston, L. J., & Levesque, J. V. (2008). Ego boundaries, shamanic-like techniques, and subjective experience: An experimental study. *Anthropology of Consciousness*, *19*, 60–83. 10.1111/j.1556-3537.2008.00003.x

Roussel, J. R., & Bachelor, A. (2000/2001). Altered state and phenomenology of consciousness in schizophrenia. *Imagination, Cognition and Personality*, *20*, 141–159. 10.2190/QUTK-Q833-69XH-FG4Q

Scheerer, E. (1994). Psychoneural isomorphism: Historical background and current relevance. *Philosophical Psychology*, *7*, 183–210.

Schumaker, J. F. (Ed.). (1991). *Human suggestibility: Advances in theory, research, and application.* Routledge.

Sheehan, P. W. (1979). Hypnosis and the processes of imagination. In E. Fromm & R. E. Shor (Eds.), *Hypnosis: Developments in research and new perspectives* (2nd ed., pp. 381–411). Aldine.

Shoemaker, S. (1991). Qualia and consciousness. *Mind*, *100*, 507–524.

Shor, R. E., & Orne, E. C. (1962). *The Harvard group scale of hypnotic susceptibility*. Consulting Psychologists Press.

Spiegel, H., & Spiegel, H. (2004). *Trance and treatment: Clinical uses of hypnosis* (2nd ed.). American Psychiatric Press.

Tart, C. T. (1972). *Altered states of consciousness*. Wiley.

Tart, C. T. (1975). *States of consciousness*. Dutton.

Tart, C. T. (1977). Discrete states of consciousness. In P. R. Lee, R. E. Ornstein, D. Galin, A. Deikman, & C. T. Tart (Eds.), *Symposium on consciousness* (pp. 89–175). Penguin.

Tricker, C., Rock, A. J., & Clark, G. I. (2016). Cue-reactive altered state of consciousness mediates the relationship between problem-gambling severity and cue-reactive urge in poker-machine gamblers. *Journal of Gambling Studies*, *32*(2), 661–674.

Venkatesh, S., Raju, T. R., Shivani, Y., Tompkins, G., & Meti, B. L. (1997). A study of structure of phenomenology of consciousness in meditative and non-meditative states. *Indian Journal of Physiology and Pharmacology*, *41*, 149–153.

Varela, F. J. (1996). Neurophenomenology: A methodological remedy for the hard problem. *Journal of Consciousness Studies*, *3*(4), 330–349.

Varela, F. J., & Shear, J. (1999). First-person methodologies: What, why, how. *Journal of Consciousness Studies*, *6*, 1–14.

Wagstaff, G. (1981). *Hypnosis, compliance, and belief*. St. Martin's Press.

Webster's Seventh New Collegiate Dictionary. (1970). G. & C. Merriam.

Weitzenhoffer, A. M. (1989). *The practice of hypnotism: Traditional and semi-traditional techniques and phenomenology* (Vol. 1). John Wiley and Sons.

Weitzenhoffer, A. M. (2002). Scales, scales, and more scales. *American Journal of Clinical Hypnosis*, *44*, 209–220. 10.1080/00029157.2002.10403481

Weitzenhoffer, A. M., & Hilgard, E. (1962). *Stanford Hypnotic Susceptibility Scale: Form C.* Consulting Psychologists Press.

Wildman, W. J., & McNamara, P. (2010). Evaluating reliance on narratives in the psychological study of religious experiences. *The International Journal for the Psychology of Religion*, *20*, 223–254. 10.1080/10508619.2010.507666

Woody, E. Z., & McConkey, K. M. (2003). What we don't know about the brain and hypnosis, but need to: A view from the Buckhorn Inn. *International Journal of Clinical and Experimental Hypnosis*, *51*, 309–338.

Zinberg, N. E. (1977). The study of conscious states: Problems and progress. In N. E. Zinberg (Ed.), *Alternate states of consciousness* (pp. 1–36). Free Press.

8

STATES OF CONSCIOUSNESS MODEL AND ERICKSONIAN APPROACHES TO HYPNOSIS

Stephen R. Lankton

PRIVATE PRACTICE, PHOENIX, AZ, USA

States of Consciousness and Ego State

Hypnosis is not a treatment. It is a context for delivering therapeutic interventions just as are individual, group, and family therapy. In each case, the interpersonal field is a key element. That interpersonal field has been shown to "correlate more highly with client outcome" (Lambert & Barley, 2001, p. 357). This chapter examines that field as intertwined states of consciousness and suggestive communication. To be clear, hypnosis is a context in which (usually) two individuals (a therapist and a client) engage in communication that initiates and constructs an optimal state of consciousness (SoC) to be used for therapeutic change.

Attempts to understand, inventory, or investigate states of consciousness from various frames of reference are numerous. These include structural states of consciousness (Lankton, 1985; Tart, 1975); stimulus conditions (Pekala & Levine, 1981); neodissociation (Hilgard, 1980), phenomenological (Pekala, 1991); and various schemas for mapping higher and mystical states (Assagioli, 1965; Bucke, 1991; Lilly, 1972), and more. However, this chapter avoids the expansive range of considerations and concentrates on commonly experienced states of consciousness including hypnosis, and its induction.

Tart's Definition

Foundations for understanding a SoC were proposed by Charles Tart. Tart described the contents or "stuff" of the SoC as psychological structures with active subsystems. He writes, "Our ordinary or 'normal' state of consciousness is a tool, a structure, a coping mechanism for dealing with a certain agreed-upon social reality – a consensus reality" (Tart, 1975, p. vii). He explains that a state is, " … a unique, dynamic pattern or configuration of psychological structures, an active system of psychological subsystems" (Tart, 1975, p. 5).

A SoC is induced by the stimulation provided by sensory and chemical input and once induced, it is maintained or "stabilized" by feedback created by "mental monitoring" (Tart, 1975, p. 5). He adds that the channels for induction and stabilization of a SoC are the sounds (words), sights, feelings, smells, tastes, and also reactions to internalize chemical

DOI: 10.4324/9781003449126-12

substances for the duration of time during which the continuance of those stimuli prevails. SoCs maintain an awareness of experiences which are subtly monitored, usually without distracting consciousness, so as to ensure critical experiences remain within an acceptable range of tolerance. For example, in most SoCs, heart rate, oxygen levels, fatigue, hunger, elimination needs, etc., are constantly monitored outside of awareness unless reaching a certain "concerning" limit. Most SoCs comprise numerous experience monitors.

Experiential Resources and Ego States

Emphasizing the concept of a unique amalgam of "human potentials," Tart equates his concept of "discrete" SoCs with the more familiar term "ego state" (Tart, 1975, pp. 60–61). One of the comprehensive discussions of ego states is the work of Eric Berne. Berne states, "The term 'ego state' is intended merely to denote states of mind and their related patterns of behavior ..." (Berne, 1961, p. 30). They function as "a coherent system of feelings, and operationally as a set of coherent behavior patterns" (Berne, 1964, p. 23). Citing Penfield and Roberts (1959), Berne also clarifies that an ego state is more than just the stimulated auditory and visual cortex that comprises the memory of speech and words: An ego state includes the potential re-experiencing of the complete memory (Berne, 1961, p. 18).

"Today, we can also conceptualize them as the manifestations of specific neural networks in the brain" (Allen, 2011, p. 12). A useful working model is that ego states or SoCs are complex neural net bundles of memory composed of thinking, feeling, and behaving. Some aspects of each SoC may be conscious while other aspects remain outside of consciousness and stay unconscious for any given length of time. These phenomena and their operational characteristics have been described by others, not as ego states, but as "sub-personalities."

> William James dealt with this concept of sub-personalities - which he called "the various selves." The functions of an individual, in whom various psychological traits are not integrated, form what we consider to be sub-personalities ...
> people shift from one to the other without clear awareness, and only a thin thread of memory connects them ... – they act differently, they show very different traits. (Assagioli, 1965, p. 75)

These are not cases of dissociative personality disorders but rather the day-to-day or minute-by-minute shifting of SoCs. These account for acts of daily living, creativity, and general survival in society (Assagioli, 1965; Frederick, 2016; Lowen, 1967; Watkins & Watkins, 1997). For this discussion, the term SoC is used as it seems to convey a more malleable phenomenon than the term ego state.

As mentioned, each SoC is composed of experience monitors. Specific experience monitors may be shared with or isolated from other SoCs. Each person's monitors develop unique tolerances for their various bodily experiences regardless of the specific SoC (e.g., hunger, pain, pressure). Differences in sensitivity are created from genetics, social learning, modeling, trial and error, conditioning, and deliberate training. When an experience rises above or drops below a learned threshold, monitoring brings it into consciousness. That is, we suddenly become hungry, uncomfortable, cold, feel pain, and so on. In some SoCs, individuals deliberately attend to a certain monitor (e.g., heart rate during aerobic exercising).

I'm using the term *experiential resources* to refer to <u>sets</u> of monitors. Experiential resources are the building blocks of therapy. Erickson often helped a client elicit what he referred to as "pride" or "joy" or "confidence" by heightening their memory of early learning accomplishments like learning to tie shoelaces. He referred to these early learnings as experiential resources or a clients' "experiential life" (Erickson, 1948, p. 576). As a child, the client would have executed and monitored several experiences when first learning how to tie his shoes. The child would have to monitor gripping, hand position, balance, eye-focus, breathing, and so on, to accomplish the learning. An experiential resource, like how to tie your shoes, is a <u>set</u> of monitored experiences. Each person learns labels for these sets of experience monitors and in my experience, those labels remain fairly constant throughout life. Even though experiential resources comprise complex sets of monitored affects, cognitions, and perceptions and so on, on a daily basis people simply refer to them by names such as "confident," "weary," "happy," "frightened," "affectionate," "angry," and "focused." Going forward, experiential resources will be abbreviated as ER or ERs. Not all of an individual's ERs are included in any single SoC.

An ER is remembered by a verbal label or a sensory image. This label or image is associated with memories of historical events during which they occurred. Research on learning and modeling illustrates that symbolized or coded image representations (auditory, visual, olfactory, etc.), or words, function as mediators for subsequent response retrieval and reproduction of the learned experience. If experiences "are repeatedly elicited a constituent stimulus acquires the capacity to evoke images ... the associated stimulus event ..." (Bandura, 1969, p. 133). That is, ERs may be remembered by means of verbal labels or sensory representations (for instance, a certain smell can trigger a memory of a previous life event). Just as with most experiences awareness of an ER fluctuates over time. Memory and conscious access to experiences may fade or be suppressed over time rendering them an unconscious resource. That is, people experience more or less courage, confidence, belonging, etc., throughout time. This is, partially, due to the fact that as people age they have more elaborate existing SoCs and develop additional SoCs. In differing contexts, people will have a different SoC and each state will have its own unique ERs. Some ERs will exist in several SoCs (e.g., alertness, joy, sadness) and in each SoC there will be limited access to certain ERs (e.g., a competitive swimmer's SoC is unlikely to find an available pathway to the ER of doing long-division).

Paths of Connectivity

Various ERs are the building blocks of each SoC. Some SoCs have access to shared ERs, and some do not. For instance, people often use the experience of daydreaming to shift from one state to another. An example of this would be that in one moment the person might chuckle at the content of the daydream (i.e., a potential shift to Berne's Child ego state), then in self-talk say, "that's interesting and explains a lot" (i.e., a potential shift to another SoC – Berne's Adult ego state), and the next moment emphasize, "it's a damn shame more people don't realize this" (i.e., a potential shift to another SoC – Berne's Parent ego state). ERs, such as daydreaming, that are shared with multiple SoCs provide avenues for switching states and recombining with other ERs contained within them.

If some external or internal stimulus triggers an ER beyond the customary limits, it may involuntarily and suddenly signal that it is out of bounds and the person may shift SoCs.

For instance, when a person is happily running on a beach and becomes aware that she stepped on something that cut her foot, she suddenly shifts from a SoC of carefree exercising to a concerned self-care SoC triggered by pain. If concern and caution ERs are not among the components of her exercising SoC, she will suddenly shift to another SoC where they are available. In so doing, her path to the previous ERs (and therefore previous SoC) may no longer be available. Thus, the avenue back to the carefree jogging in the previous SoC is temporarily impossible. This is an example of "paths of connectivity" that govern switching from one set of experience to another.

Some paths may be biologically determined but in many cases they are learned. That is, therapeutic opportunities exist when people can't acquire the experiences needed in the context in which they are required. As Erickson explained it, "psychological problems exist precisely because the conscious mind does not know how to initiate psychological experience and behavior change to the degree that one would like" (Erickson & Rossi, (1979, p. 18). As a consequence, "The therapist is needed to facilitate the emergence of untapped potentials and response systems that the patient's own ego has not been able to utilize in a voluntary and intentional way. The purpose of Erickson's *indirect approach* was to circumvent the patient's learned limitations so that previously unrealized potentials may become manifest" (Rossi, 1980, p. 97). The induction process helps bypass boundaries of the conventional waking state and locate required ERs (i.e., confidence, comfort, courage, tenderness, success) from other SoCs and finally reassociating them to occur within the client's needed situation.

To summarize, states of consciousness are identifiably different collections of *sets* of perceptions, thoughts, feelings, behaviors, monitoring processes, and the capacity for consciousness. It is important to note four factors in defining a SoC:

a There must be awareness at some level (e.g., the sights, smells, and proprioception of running on a beach, as well as possibly unconscious awareness tracking temperature, hunger, blood flow, and so on);
b The SoC will contain experience monitors for health, comfort, safety checking, etc., using feedback from motor skills, perceptions, cognitions, bodily function monitors, affects, etc. (i.e., breathing, fatigue, bleeding, pain);
c Most *sets* of experience monitors, called experiential resources (ERs), will have labels (e.g., joy, confidence, courage, determination, persistence, confused);
d Within and between SoCs are paths for connectivity connecting and limiting movement between ERs (e.g., after the painful cut to the foot, the runner can't immediately return to joyful jogging).

These concepts can now be applied in the context of induction and hypnosis. Induction and stabilization of hypnosis deal with eliciting and reorganizing ERs located in other SoC. The following emphasizes an indirect communication approach within an empathic interpersonal field as they pertain to evoking and organizing ERs within and between SoCs.

Hypnosis and Induction

The most recent definition of hypnosis from the American Psychological Association stated that hypnotizability or hypnotic susceptibility is observed to be an ability to experience suggested alterations in physiology, sensations, emotions, thoughts, or behavior during hypnosis (Elkins et al., 2015). That is a definition of what may occur during hypnosis. Erickson wrote, “It [hypnosis] is, in simple terms, nothing more than a *special state of conscious awareness* in which certain chosen behaviors of everyday life is manifested in a direct manner, usually with the aid of another person” (Erickson, 1970, p. 72) [italics mine]. Hypnosis is a SoC created from ERs that comprise other SoC and the induction process illustrates how they are retrieved and assembled. While Erickson was an innovator of many aspects of hypnosis, there was an evolution of his induction process (Lankton, 2021). The importance of his later work is the focus as it is in contrast to the induction outlined by Tart. Erickson’s earlier authoritarian induction approach is most similar to that discussed by Tart.

Tart’s Seven Steps of Induction

Chart 8.1 summarizes Tart’s (1975) view of an induction process and how it affects consciousness to culminate in a hypnotic state. It illustrates his reliance on the traditional authoritarian model of exposing the subject to redundant suggestions for sleep, drowsiness, and reliance upon the hypnotist.

	Suggesetions	Purpose
1.	sit or lie comfortably	to help “kinesthetic receptors adapt out, as in going to sleep” (p. 78).
2.	listen only to the hypnotist’s voice	to stop “subsystems active in the waking state“ (p. 78.)
3.	don’t think about what the hypnotist is saying	to stop “evaluative and decision-making activity and ... subsystems” (p. 78.)
4.	focus attention on some particular thing	to “reduce further your scanning of the environment” (pg. 78-79.)
5.	fall into sleep or get drowsy	to "elicit a variety of memory associations ... as a disruptive force" (p. 79)
6.	this “sleep” allows you to hear the hypnotist	to “produce a passive sleep like state” (p. 80)
7.	for simple motor procedures	so your "sense of self begins to include the hypnotist" (p. 80)

Chart 8.1 Tart’s Seven-Step Induction Process.

The suggestions in Chart 8.1’s “suggestion” column illustrate the traditional induction pattern still often used by many in the healthcare profession. Designing a SoC model that correctly includes a nonauthoritarian, non-redundant, non-“sleep”-oriented approach demonstrated by Erickson in the last two decades of his career, requires aspects of Tart’s explanation to be recast, modified, and expanded.

Ambiguity

One essential facet of an Ericksonian approach is that it is nonauthoritarian with an emphasis on stimulating clients' mental activity to evoke and reassociate needed experiences. "His techniques for induction evolved from being largely direct and authoritarian to egalitarian and indirect - matching his approach to therapy and healing" (Lankton, 2021, p.11). Erickson explains that he "offers" ideas and suggestions and explicitly states, "*I don't like this matter of telling a patient I want you to get tired and sleepy*" (Erickson & Rossi, 1981, p. 1–4) [italics mine]. Erickson's definition of a cure is utilitarian, "It is ... re-associating and reorganizing his own experiential life that eventuates in a cure ..." (Erickson, 1948, p. 576). His interventions introduce clients to a tolerable amount of light confusion and ambiguity. The mental action of resolving that ambiguity and identifying personal meaning from the communication is precisely what an SoC model must explain.

Sociocognitive Factors and Expectancy

Placebo effects and expectancy influence the induction process. Expectancy generally refers to a patient's belief that treatment will be successful (Kirsch & Weixel, 1988). Expectancy is evoked by means of language and social factors like practitioner prestige, promised improvement, waiting lists, therapy approach, and demand characteristics. Subjects' responses to those factors depend upon their learning history associated with those received cues. Research on these sociocognitive factors affecting induction has been extensive (Lynn et al., 2008). Several studies showing the effect of expectancies (Milling et al., 2005) suggest patients become predisposed to conflate treatment with remembered incidences of hope, desire, anticipation, unexpected or surprising relief. In fact, Kirsch (1994) posits that the entire experience of hypnosis is essentially a non-deceptive placebo.

This is an appropriate encapsulation of the process since what is referred to as expectancy may be the activation of an unconscious search for meaning (Erickson & Rossi, 2008; Sternberg, 1975), that is, a "transderivational search" (Lankton, 1980/2003, pp. 193–194). People require frames of reference to understand their experience (Goffman, 1969). Specifically, positive expectancy is the byproduct of mental searching to locate fuzzy (i.e., approximate) matches for similar favorable past circumstances. When initiated, the search process traverses the boundary of the current SoC and is receptive to finding common experiences residing in others. It is successful when the process frames the event by giving it meaning of a favorable outcome.

Hypnosis and Induction in the SoC Model

An understanding of hypnosis, induction, and hypnotherapy can be recast as follows.

a *Hypnosis* occurs when a SoC is created by retrieving and stabilizing a group of specific required experiences that are customarily uncombined in the customary waking state.
b *Induction* is the process of evoking and associating required experiences so as to assemble and stabilize the state.

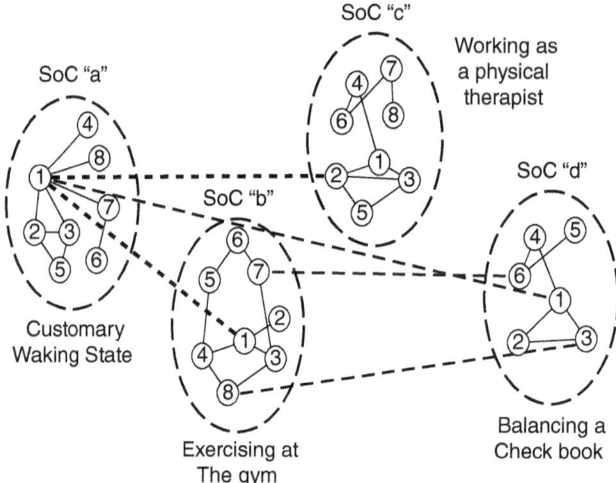

Figure 8.1 Experiential resources distributed within states of consciousness.

c *Hypnotherapy* can be defined as using an induction process to create and stabilize a SoC of hypnosis as a context for subsequently delivering therapeutic interventions.

Figure 8.1 illustrates a simplified imaginary example of four SoCs and several ERs within each of them. Each oval represents a different SoC and within each are a few circled numbers. The numbered circles represent experiential resources. Labels for the ERs can be found in Table 8.1. (These representations are only meant as helpful aids for the following discussion. They do not make any attempt to depict the complexity of SoCs.)

Some of these ERs are not connected to one another. The disconnect between some ERs represents what may be learned limitations that bring people to therapy (e.g., a client can't get comfortable in a crowd). Highly connected ERs may be related by sharing common experience monitors or similar learning history (e.g., relaxation during reading, meditating, and watching TV). Each SoC is likely to share several ERs with other SoCs: For the sake of simplicity, such overlapping geometry is not shown in Figure 8.1. The key aspects represented in Figure 8.1 can be summarized by these four elements.

1 SoCs have boundaries which are represented here by a dashed enclosure.
2 Experiential resources (ERs) are represented with numbered circles.
3 Paths or associations between ERs are learned limitations and opportunities represented by dotted lines.
4 Paths that exist from an ERs in one SoC to an ER within another SoC are represented by heavy dotted lines.

The numbered experiences in Figure 8.1 can be further elaborated by the following brief descriptions presented in Table 8.1. Hypothetical examples of various ERs will be referenced throughout this chapter.

Table 8.1 Experiential Resources in the SoCs of Figure 8.1

Description of the contents of SoC "a:" This is the individual's hypothetical SoC that we'll call her customary waking state.

a1 is "feeling alert and awake."
a2 is "relaxing."
a3 is "ignoring other stimuli."
a4 is "being able to explain."
a5 is "weighing situations."
a6 is "daydreaming."
a7 is "falling asleep."
a8 is "feeling relaxed."

Description of the contents of SoC "b:" This is the individual's hypothetical SoC that exists when she is exercising at the gym.

b1 is "preparing" - warming up.
b2 is "self pep-talk."
b3 is "dissociating."
b4 is "planning" – (used determining next exercise).
b5 is "experiencing second wind."
b6 is "withdrawn and thinking."
b7 is "feeling like giving up."
b8 is "feeling exhaustion."

Description of of the contents of SoC "c:" This is the individual's SoC that exists when on the job as a physical therapist.

c1 is "assessing" – used evaluation patients' range of motion.
c2 is "analyzing" – used when planning for a patient's recovery.
c3 is "being articulate" – used giving clear exercise assignments.
c4 is "confidence" – used forming a recovery plan to a patient.
c5 is "withdrawing" – used to clear her mind;"
c6 is "being responsible" – used checking paperwork, procedures, and signed forms.
c7 is "enjoying" – accompanying seeing patient improvement.
c8 is "being firm" – used enforcing exercise assignments.

Description of of the contents of SoC "d:" In this illustration "d" is shown to represent any other distinct SoC, but it could possibly be named the SoC used when balancing a check book.

d1 is "determination."
d2 is "curiosity."
d3 is "concentration."
d4 is "forgetting."
d5 is "disappointment."
d6 is "frustration."

Why Hypnosis Is a Valuable SoC

By bypassing the conscious mind's learned limitations, hypnosis can amplify a subject's capability to elicit experiences often unavailable in the standard waking state (Erickson et al., 1976). Some needed ERs cannot be directly reached within an existing SoC and others may be difficult to elicit due to their location in other SoCs. This has to do with connectivity of the learned pathways between experiences.

In Figure 8.1, it's possible to move from experience a1 to several other experiences – a2, a3, a4, a7, or a8. But the diagram illustrates it's not possible to move directly from a1 to a6 or to move from a6 to a8 or to a4, etc. The example represents being unable to directly move from feeling awake and alert to falling asleep. This is not a big revelation; yet it clarifies that movement between experiences is governed by learned connections. Since they are learned, they can be changed.

If a person in this hypothetical example is having the experience of a1 (feeling awake and alert) she can't directly move to b6 (withdrawn and thinking) which is part of an different SoC. But she can most easily achieve this by the path of a1 shifting to b1 (preparing – warming up) – a connected path to a different SoC. Then from b1 (preparing – warming up) to b3 (dissociating), to b7 (giving up), and finally to b6 (withdrawn and thinking). When these shifts happen in everyday life, people are largely unconcerned – it just happens. But movements to desired ERs for which there are no learned paths do not "just happen."

What happens when the subject wants a feeling of confidence to ask for an employment promotion? If that confidence is not a part of his SoC and he doesn't have experience getting from point A to point B, so to speak, he can't consciously produce the needed confidence. Therein lies an example of what brings people to therapy: Lack of connectivity to resources is often learned by factors of psychosocial development or even the sequelae of trauma. One effect of trauma is to create a *pervasive* oversensitive experience monitor or several experiences being bearishly monitored from multiple SoCs.

Oversensitive monitoring can prevent appropriate movement between other SoCs and ERs. This occurs, for example, when a child, physically punished for receiving low test scores, subsequently can't feel confidence taking a test. Sitting for an exam can then trigger over-sensitive monitoring and anticipation of pain. To the extent that consciousness is flooded with anticipation, the child's ability to evoke the resource of confidence is inhibited. The ongoing anxiety could stabilize a SoC far different from the one needed to pass exams. These experience monitors which are meant to protect the person from the reoccurrence of an unpleasant or painful situation may be easily triggered by benign environmental cues which in some way resemble the trauma that created it.

Illustrating pervasive experience monitoring, two research studies compared the neuroimaging of hypnotically induced and physically induced pain responses. Derbyshire et al. (2004) studied several subjects scoring 8 or more on the Harvard Group Scale of Hypnotic Suggestibility: Form "A" with findings later replicated by Raij et al. (2005) using participants who scored 8 or higher on the Stanford Hypnotic Suggestibility Scale: Form "C." Their studies found "widespread brain activation throughout the brain circuitry associated with the mediation of pain" in the thalamus, anterior cingulate, insula, prefrontal and parietal cortices "with the additional observation that source monitoring by medial prefrontal cortex may contribute to the subjective reality of pain in both cases" (Oakley, 2008, p. 369). Such widespread brain excitement would seem to illustrate that multiple SoCs learn pervasive hyper-sensitive monitoring.

This is why the increased suggestibility available during hypnosis becomes extremely helpful for therapy. When subjects display increased hypnotic susceptibility during hypnosis, they have a heightened ability to experience suggested alterations in experience (Elkins et al., 2015). One of the valuable aspects of therapy are times when it helps relax the boundaries between SoCs and previously difficult to evoke ERs (such as bypassing limits created by oversensitive monitoring so that a client can retrieve experiences of confidence such as needed in the above example). However, during therapy, easy access to needed experiences may rely on the successful use of expectancy and empathy in the induction or treatment process.

Empathy and Boundaries

When there is a perceived difference, there is a boundary. Interpersonally, a client may perceive their therapist as "different" and conclude, "This therapist can't understand my situation." In a similar manner, intrapsychically, a momentary uncommon feeling of success may seem so "different" to a client's current state of mind he or she may conclude, "I can't ever feel that way again."

Empathy and empathic rapport make it possible to relax differences and to evoke and reassociate experiences. Empathy is not merely having a cognitive understanding of another person's situation and feelings. It refers to a felt understanding of another person's situation, feelings, thoughts, and desires (Rogers, 1961). "The state [of hypnosis] is also characterized by a quality called rapport, a functioning of the Sense of Identity subsystem *to include the hypnotist as part of the subject's own ego*" (Tart, 1975, p. 81) [italics mine]. That is, the subject believes the hypnotist has a shared sense of his or her situation and thus blurs boundaries between self and other, and between SoCs.

Regarding how a person blends identity with another, Bateson explains, "perception operates only upon difference. ... [and] ... Differences that are too slight or too slowly presented are not perceivable" (Bateson, 1979, p. 29). The more the therapist's "conversation capture essential elements of, and resonate with, the client's experience, the more the client finds the differences between him or herself and the therapist to be irrelevant – in-differentiated [unnoticed]. The borders of the client's self are able, for the time being, to become unremarkable, making it possible for the therapist to become accepted as an insider" (Flemons, 2020, p. 349).

There is a colloquial understanding that, "A good therapist intuitively judges the subject's situation." "Judgments [mental impressions] can be made with the help of clues whose formulation have not yet become or may never become conscious, but which nevertheless are based on sense impressions, including smell ... such intuitions are synthesized from discrete sensory elements ('subliminal perception') whose perceptions and synthesis both take place below the threshold of consciousness" (Berne, 1977, p. 2). Kempt (1921) also observed that intuition is reflex imitation through similar brief muscle tensions. Such imitation is derived partially through a "psychological function which transmits perceptions in an unconscious way" (Jung, 1946, pp. 567–568).

This has been born out in research by Varga et al. (2014) as they monitored changes in both subjects and hypnotists along several dimensions, including susceptibility, attention, arousal, positive affect, and more. Among their findings, they noted a large number of similarities in test results endorsed by both groups. They concluded that hypnotists and subjects had shared in creating the experience of hypnosis: "Our results provide tentative support for theories of hypnosis that conceptualize hypnosis as a reciprocal, two-way process, an intersubjective rather than an intrapsychic event, and as constructed rather than caused" (Varga et al., 2014, p. 9). These findings provide support for the conclusion that hypnotist and subject can intuitively form mental impressions of each other's experience. This occurs by means of careful observation and unconscious cues leading to empathic rapport, dissolving perceived differences, and blurring the sense of mental boundaries. The process facilitates clients bypassing habitual paths of connectivity between their usual waking state and allowing the elicitation of experience sets from other SoC to emerge and be rearranged.

Induction and Ulterior Transactions

It has been noted that hypnosis may be induced without an empathic relationship as seen with 'stage hypnotists,' who appear to induce hypnotic states without an empathic connection (Reid, 2016). Two dynamics may be at work in these cases – expectancy and ulterior communication. There is a category of ulterior communication, called "angular transactions," that stimulates involvement by appealing to vulnerabilities in the listener (Berne, 1961, p. 104). These vulnerabilities are unfulfilled desires such as to belong, to be considered strong, beautiful, talented. Communications that appeal to these vulnerabilities plant seeds of hope that desires will be fulfilled. They stimulate involvement of multiple SoCs. In Berne's terms, these angular transactions "involve multiple ego states" (Berne, 1964, p. 33). Stage hypnotists often make statements such as "When you awaken, you'll be the strongest man anyone has ever met, in trance you'll feel you are never wrong," etc. This is a communication that stimulates a transderivational search throughout multiple SoCs for possible favorable memories or fantasies containing the excitement of fulfilling those desires. The affective component of such searching can be referred to as "enchantment" (Lankton & Lankton, 1989). The subject's enchantment is likely to continue as long as the relationship with the hypnotist continues and, as such, it becomes the context for responding to further suggestions.

Induction in a Clinical Setting

The reassociation and stabilization of certain experiences into a novel SoC are accomplished by an induction process. The SoC of hypnosis is the result of stimulating, associating, and temporarily stabilizing the combined experiential components. The experiential content of one person's state of clinical hypnosis will only be approximately similar to the experiential content in a different person's state of hypnosis. This is to be expected since experiences from each person's learning history is unique. After all, even something as universal and common as the experience of breathing varies for each person. Nevertheless, socialization provides everyone in a given culture a similar vocabulary for these fairly similar phenomenological events. For example, consider the term "relaxation." While it refers to the bodily event of muscle laxity, the set of relaxed muscles and degree of fatigue is not identical between any two individuals. Yet, the label is tossed about in discussion as if it refers to an identical experience.

This may be why some hypnotists rely upon a technique of systematic muscle tensing and relaxing with clients, and in so doing, are likely to achieve a more standardize phenomenological outcome for "relaxation." Consequently, for each person's unique variation for experiences (e.g., concentration, relaxation, absorption, deepening, remembering, forgetting), there is no agreed upon set of experiential components making up the composition of clinical hypnosis. Each person's state of hypnosis should comprise experiences unique to them and relevant to the therapy goals being sought.

Establishing an Empathic Relationship

The process of establishing an hypnotic state may begin by establishing an empathic relationship. This provides the hypnotist with a deep understanding of the client's situation and helps the client sense that the hypnotist has that understanding. Figure 8.3 uses a wavey line to highlight the two-way communication that occurs both consciously and unconsciously throughout the exchange. Consequently, such a relationship creates a lack of "difference" or a lack of boundary as discussed previously. This allows for more easy movement between experiences within the customary SoC as well as the elicitation of experiences found in states outside of the current SoC.

The initiation of induction may include suggestions, statements, questions, anecdotes, stories, or requests for eye fixation, relaxation, etc., depending upon the hypnotist's training. The list of all possibilities may be endless. While it is not necessary, it is still common practice once the process has begun to facilitate experiences of relaxation, eye closure, comfort, and so on. Some will begin with anecdotes or stories about desired experiences needed to meet the client's goals. For instance, with a client seeking to overcome test anxiety, an Ericksonian oriented hypnotist might begin discussing various ways children develop confidence by learning to walk, hold eating utensils, tie their shoes, button buttons, learn the letters of the alphabet, and so on. Those memories are customarily outside a client's standard waking state. However, the context of empathic rapport facilitates a client's wondering and mental searching beyond the normal waking state into other SoCs to attach meaning to those ideas. Of course, one of the meanings those learnings have in common is the development of confidence. Erickson (1958) called this a naturalistic approach because the client's own mental activity is employed to come upon his or her unique experience of confidence.

If a chosen avenue of discourse is not eliciting ideomotor indicators, or "minimal cues," referred to by Erickson et al. (1976), favoring the desired goal, the therapist's presentation can easily be altered. For instance, the hypnotist may suggest that remembering comes more easily when people close their eyes. Again, the choices for personalizing the induction are endless. Regardless, in these scenarios, there is no need for an authoritarian role vis-à-vis the client or for directly suggesting a particular named experience. In fact, the very opposite is true when attempting to have the client do the mental activity of searching and finding a personally meaningful memory.

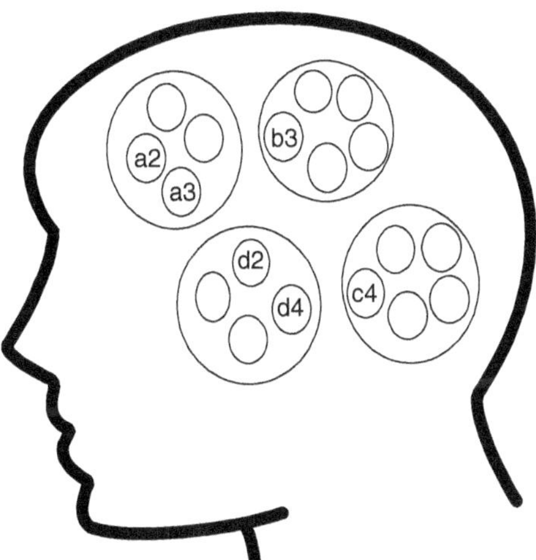

Figure 8.2 Experiences desired for inducing hypnosis often reside in differing SoCs.

The SoCs shown in example (Figure 8.1) have sets of numerous specific experiences identified with names in Table 8.1. Those in SoC "a," "b," "c," and "d" are delineated below.

a2 is "relaxing."
a3 is "ignoring other stimuli."
b3 is "dissociating."
c4 is "confidence."
d2 is "curiosity."
d4 is "forgetting."

This set of six experiences (Figure 8.2) will comprise the SoC of hypnosis in this imaginary example of induction. The hypothetical hypnotic state being assembled in Figure 8.2 requires using experiences from four different SoCs, "a" through "d."

The representation in Figure 8.3 uses a wavy line to represent the empathic two-way exchange wherein the self-other boundary is relaxed access to these six experiences.

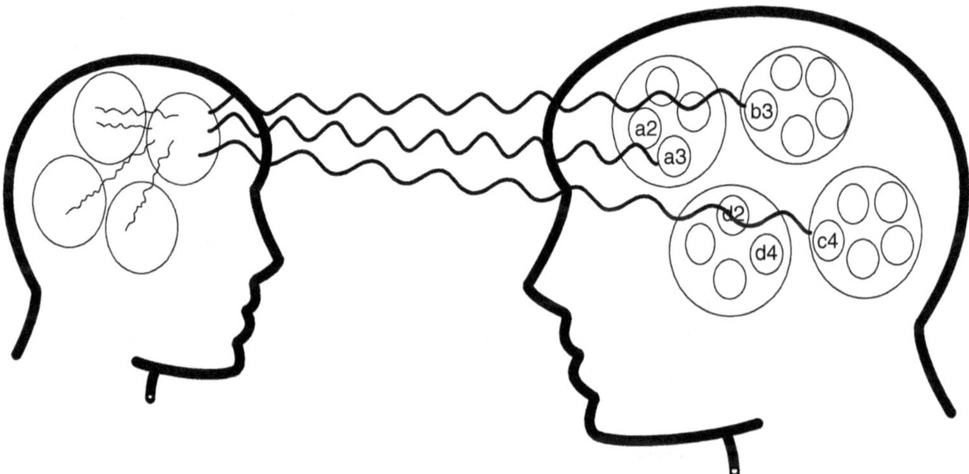

Figure 8.3 Eliciting experience within SoCs with relaxed boundaries.

Depotentiating Boundaries and Retrieving Experience

As Flemons succinctly stated, "Clients recognize themselves in what the therapist says and how it is said. In receiving confirmation of their experience, they find the boundaries of the self are redrawn, becoming inclusive, in some sense, of both themselves and the therapist. This makes it possible for the therapist's suggestions for hypnotic and hypnotherapeutic experience to be experienced as insider ideas, rather than rejected as outsider impositions" (Flemons, 2020, pp. 349–350). As induction proceeds, the transderivational search process increases and may become more efficient (e.g., the greater the length of time spent trying to recall a song, the larger the number of lyrics will be remembered). Clients will locate experiences that seem to have a higher "goodness of fit" for increasing amounts of ambiguous content offered by the hypnotist. Each meaningful experience that is evoked in turn increases internal absorption.

In the above example, the experiences of "relaxing," "ignoring other stimuli," "dissociating," being "confident," having "curiosity," and "forgetting" have been presented as ERs to be brought together for a SoC of hypnosis. Indirect suggestions, binds, anecdotes, and so on which evoke and combine those experiences one after another create associational conditioning that results in their respective neurons firing together. Of course, acceptance of this sort of communication can become increasingly easier to the degree that the empathic relationship continues or intensifies. This remains a crucial factor for evoking ERs when they are located in other SoCs.

For example, consider the following suggestions of stimulating the client to recognize processes across states of consciousness where the different experiences may lie. "As you sit there ignoring stimuli around you [a3], you might begin to relax [a2]. And people relaxing don't know how they do it, but often become curious [d2] even as they begin dissociating from some bodily feelings [b3]. And as your conscious mind notices that, you may be curious [d2] about your how your unconscious can recall feeling confident [c4] and wonder if you are able to remember how to forget [d4] other things – like what had made you anxious in the past?"

This example uses only one sentence for stimulating each of the various ERs. In real life, however, that task would be accomplished using several indirect and direct suggestions. Those communication techniques are elaborated elsewhere (Erickson & Rossi, 2008; Lankton & Lankton, 1983/2008). Yet, once these experiences have been individually evoked, the above example illustrates how they could be associated together. Repeatedly associating several resources produces a conditioned pairing.

> Associating suggestions in such interlocking chains creates a network of mutually reinforcing directives that gradually form a new self-consistent inner reality called "trance." It is construction of such interlocking networks of associations that gives "body" or substance to trance as an altered state of consciousness with its own guideposts, rules, and 'reality. (Erickson & Rossi, 2008, p. 194)

Ratifying and Stabilizing the SoC of Hypnosis

As experiences are expressed together or in near temporal proximity, they tend to become conditioned. This observation is referred to as Hebb's Rule of "assembly theory" in the field of neuropsychology (Hebb, 1949) and noted by the often-repeated slogan – neurons that fire together, wire together. The combination of experiences, even when originating from different SoCs, become conditioned to express themselves at the same time. Stating this neurological event in such terms may seem like overstatement since all that is being said is that associational learning and conditioning occur as normal. The only difference between learning during a state of hypnosis and learning a poem or chord shapes on guitar is that the conscious mind is not usually as involved. "The depotentiation of a subject's limited and habitual frames of reference ... facilitate new possibilities of creativity, healing, and learning" (Erickson et al., 1976), p. 295). The *therapeutic* consequence of depotentiating of conscious sets in this manner, in my clinical experience, is that reassociating of ERs occurs more quickly and requires less effort than in waking state. This is probably why numerous research studies have shown interventions done in the context of hypnosis to be more effective than when delivered in conventional therapy (Figure 8.4).

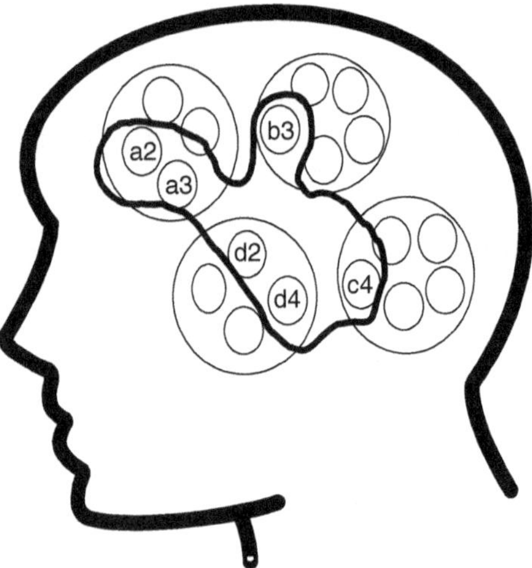

Figure 8.4 Assembled experiences by repeated association.

A SoC of hypnosis is, initially, a temporarily arranged grouping of experiences – a grouping whose combination can be learned. Once this novel SoC is identified and labeled, the neurons that relate to the retrieved resources which created the hypnosis can also fire and wire together due to the aid of the client's own monitoring process. Encouraged to do so, clients may create a self-monitoring positive feedback stabilization. Once that has been established, subjects can report when they are in or when they are out of trance. This awareness may be accomplished if a hypnotist directs a client's attention to uncommon events such as how much time has passed and how heavy or light an arm feels. A client's realization that some aspect of an ER has exceeded the high or low limits of its normal range of functioning reinforces an understanding that a novel state exists. The combined experiences then begin to be recognized as a stabilized unique state. After the state is ratified (that is, a boundary is recognized), it can operate as an independent SoC. This is depicted as the solid boundary line around the experience cluster in Figure 8.5.

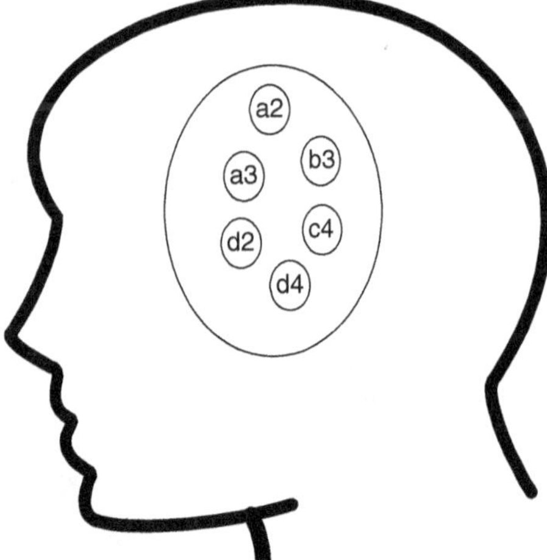

Figure 8.5 Ratified experiences becomes an independent hypnotic state.

The common way to begin stabilizing the hypnosis SoC is to simply call it "hypnosis." This may seem so obvious that it need not be mentioned. However, if the newly assembled set of experiences is *not* labeled or called to the attention of the subject, he or she may not recognize the boundaries of the state or the newly grouped ERs. Further, without labelling or recognizing it, after the hypnosis session, clients may report that they are unsure or doubtful that they were hypnotized. This situation was often used by Erickson when the *only* goal of the therapy was to evoke needed experiences and make them available for the client's use (e.g., having confidence and mental acuity when taking an exam). When the hypnosis state is not ratified, clients may leave a successful session and report they don't know what occurred during the therapy but that they feel they achieved their desired goals. This often empowers clients to conclude they solved their problem by themselves.

Hypnosis is not itself a therapy, but rather a context for doing therapy. It can be helpful for both therapist and subject if the SoC is recognized as hypnosis and that the continuance of other interventions constitutes the therapy. For example, "And now you know that you have established a depth of hypnosis that is appropriate for you to use. So, you can continue to stay in the state of hypnosis as we work on solving the problems that brought you here today." Statements such as that help demystify the difference between hypnosis and the actual therapy that occurs in that context. Also, knowing how to recognize it can help the clients develop a bridge back to the state so they can do their own self-hypnosis at a later time. It is important to note from the start of the induction process that appropriate idea should be introduced as seeds from which the therapy can grow. There need be no distinction between the induction and the beginning of therapeutic interventions.

The ease of establishing subsequent hypnosis will depend upon the degree to which the hypnotist stabilized it. Since the ERs were evoked together, there can be several pathways for reestablishing it. The more often an association of experiences is repeated, the easier they connect. In a meta-analysis of the efficacy of self-hypnosis, Eason and Parris (2018) looked at 22 studies that met the criteria for randomized controls. They concluded that learning self-hypnosis over three or more practice sessions resulted in effective clinical results in various areas including pain, anxiety, stress, and childbirth experiences. The results improved when the number of training sessions increased.

Conclusion

This chapter illustrates a model of states of consciousness, their component experiences, and how those experiences can be evoked and reassociated. This SoC model unites: (1) the impact of language, prestige, social, and transactional cues on subjects; (2) responses of transderivational searching (usually called "expectancy"); (3) empathic relationships that evoke experiential resources; and, (4) the reorganizing of experiential resources from different SoCs into a state of hypnosis. Highlighting the two-way unconscious communication between the hypnotist and subject in this model illustrates an unmistakable union between the sociocognitive and state theory of hypnosis. The "issues dividing the field can no longer be portrayed as simple dichotomies, such as state vs nonstate or trait vs situation" (Kirsch & Lynn, 1995, p. 846). Components of each theory are a required nexus on the same continuum when considering hypnotic induction. They are a unified procedure that create the context of hypnosis. In totality, these ideas form a workable model of the context of hypnosis as a treatment modality and hopefully contribute to a productive direction of future research.

References

Allen, J. (2011). New introduction: As if suddenly a door. In E. Berne (Eds.), *Games people play: The basic handbook of transactional analysis* (pp. 11–23). Old Daybrook, CT: Tantow Media, Inc.

Assagioli, R. (1965). *Psychosynthesis*. New York: Viking.

Bandura, A. (1969). *Principles of behavior modification*. New York: Holt Rinehart and Winston.

Bateson, G. (1979). *Mind and nature: A necessary unity*. New York: Dutton.

Berne, E. (1961). *Transactional analysis in psychotherapy*. Secaucus, NJ: Castle Books.

Berne, E. (1964). *Games people play*. New York: Grove.

Berne, E. (1977). *Intuition and ego states*. San Francisco, CA: TA Press.

Bucke, R. (1991). *Cosmic consciousness: A study in the evolution of the human mind*. New York: Random House.

Derbyshire, S., Whalley, M., Stenger, V., & Oakley, D. (2004). Cerebral activation during hypnotically induced and imagined pain. *NeuroImage*, *23*, 392–401. 10.1016/j.neuroimage.2004.04.033

Eason, A., & Parris, B. (2018). Clinical applications of self-hypnosis: A systematic review and meta-analysis of randomized controlled trials. *Psychology of Consciousness: Theory, Research, and Practice*, *6*(3), 262–278. 10.1037/cns0000173

Elkins, G. R., Barabasz, A. F., Council, J. R., & Spiegel, D. (2015). Advancing research and practice: 285 The revised APA division 30 definition of hypnosis. *American Journal of Clinical Hypnosis*, *57*(4), 378–385. 10.1080/00029157.2015.1011465

Erickson, M. (1958). Naturalistic techniques of hypnosis. *American Journal of Clinical Hypnosis*, *1*, 3–8. 10.1080/00029157.1958.10401766

Erickson, M. (1948). Hypnotic psychotherapy. *Medical Clinics of North America*, *32*(3), 571–583. 10.1016/S0025-7125(16)35675-9

Erickson, M. (1970). Hypnosis: It's renaissance as a treatment modality. *American Journal of Clinical Hypnosis*, *13*(2), 71–89. 10.1080/00029157.1970.10402085

Erickson, M., & Rossi, E. (1979). *Hypnotherapy: An exploratory casebook*. New York: Irvington.

Erickson, M., & Rossi, E. (1981). *Experiencing hypnosis: Therapeutic approaches to altered states*. New York: Irvington.

Erickson, M., & Rossi, E. (2008). Indirect forms of suggestion. In E. Rossi, R. Erickson-Klein, & K. Rossi (Eds.), *The collected works of Milton H. Erickson: Basic hypnotic induction and suggestion* (Volume 2, pp. 181–208). Phoenix, AZ: The Milton H. Erickson Foundation.

Erickson, M., Rossi, E., & Rossi, S. (1976). *Hypnotic realities*. New York: Irvington.

Frederick, C. (2016). Beyond empathy: The tree of compassion with malevolent ego states. *American Journal of Clinical Hypnosis*, *58*(4), 331–346. 10.1080/00029157.2015.1103203

Flemons, D. (2020). Toward a relational theory of hypnosis. *American Journal of Clinical Hypnosis*, *62*(4), 344–363. 10.1080/00029157.2019.1666700

Goffman, E. (1969). *Frame analysis*. Chicago, IL: Double Day.

Hebb, D. (1949). *The organization of behavior: A neuropsychological theory*. New York: John Wiley & Sons.

Hilgard, E. (1980). Consciousness in contemporary psychology. *Annual Review of Psychology*, *31*, 1–28. 10.1146/annurev.ps.31.020180.000245

Jung, C. (1946). *Psychological types*. New York: Harcort, Brace.

Kempt, E. (1921). *The autonomic functions and the personality*. New York: Nervous and Mental Disease.

Kirsch, I. (1994). Clinical hypnosis as a nondeceptive placebo: Empirically derived techniques. *American Journal of Clinical Hypnosis*, *37*(2), 95–106. 10.1080/00029157.1994.10403122

Kirsch, I., & Lynn, S. (1995). The altered state of hypnosis: Changes in the theoretical landscape. *American Pyschologist*, *50*(1), 846–858. 10.1037/0003-066X.50.10.846

Kirsch, I., & Weixel, L. (1988). Double-blind versus deceptive administration of a placebo. *Behavioral Neuroscience*, *102*(2), 319–323. 10.1037/0735-7044.102.2.319

Lambert, M. J., & Barley, D. (2001). Research summary on the therapeutic relationship and psychotherapy outcome. *Psychotherapy: Theory, Research, Practice, Training*, *38*(4), 357–361. 10.1037/0033-3204.38.4.357

Lankton, S. (1980/2003). *Practical magic: A translation of basic neuro linguistic programming into clinical psychotherapy* (Rev. ed.). White Plains, NY: Crown House.

Lankton, S. (1985). A states of conscious model of Ericksonian hypnosis. In S. R. Lankton (Ed.), *Ericksonian monographs number: Elements and dimensions of an Ericksonian approach* (Vol. 1, pp. 26–41). New York: Brunner/Mazel.

Lankton, S. (2021). What Milton Erickson said about being Ericksonian. *American Journal of Clinical Hypnosis*, *63*(1), 4–13. 10.1080/00029157.2020.1754068

Lankton, S., & Lankton, C. (1983/2008). *The answer within: A clinical framework of Ericksonian hypnotherapy*. Williston, VT: Crown House.

Lankton, C., & Lankton, S. (1989). *Tales of enchantment: Anthology of goal directed metaphors*. Levittonwn, PA: Taylor & Francis/Brunner-Routledge.

Lilly, J. (1972). *The center of the cyclone*. New York: Julian.

Lowen, A. (1967). *The betrayal of the body*. New York: Macmillan.

Lynn, S. J., Kirsch, I., & Hallquist, M. (2008). Social cognitive theories of hypnosis. In M. R. Nash & A. J. Barnier (Eds.), *The Oxford handbook of hypnosis: Theory, research, and practice* (pp. 111–139). Oxford, England: Oxford University.

Milling, L., Kirsch, I., Allen, G., & Reutenauer, E. (2005). The effects of hypnotic and nonhypnotic imaginative suggestion on pain. *Annals of Behavioral Medicine: A Publication of the Society of Behavioral Medicine*, *29*(2), 116–127. 10.1207/s15324796abm2902_6

Oakley, D. (2008). Hypnosis, trance and suggestion: Evidence from neuroimaging. In M. R. Nash & A. J. Barnier (Eds.), *The Oxford handbook of hypnosis: Theory, research, and practice* (pp. 365–392). Oxford, UK: Oxford University.

Pekala, R. (1991). *Quantifying consciousness: An empirical approach*. New York: Plenum. 10.1007/978-1-4899-0629-8

Pekala, R, & Levine, R. (1981). Mapping consciousness: Development of an empirical-phenomenological approach imagination. *Cognition and Personality*, *1*, 29–47. 10.2190/GAUY-R0PM-XLNQ-E93G

Penfield, W. & Roberts, L. (1959). *Speech and brain mechanisms*. Princeton, NY: Princeton University.

Raij, T., Numminen, J., Narvarnen, S. Hiltunen, J. & Hari, R. (2005). Brain correlates of subjective reality of physically and psychologically induced pain. *Proceedings of the National Academy of Sciences*, *102*, 2147–2151. 10.1073/pnas.0409542102

Reid, D. (2016). Hypnosis without empathy? Perspectives from autistic spectrum disorder and stage hypnosis. *American Journal of Clinical Hypnosis*, *58*(3), 304–320. 10.1080/00029157.2015.1103204

Rogers, C. (1961). *On becoming a person: A therapist's view of psychotherapy*. Boston, MA: Houghton Mifflin.

Rossi, E. (1980). Indirect approaches to symptom resolution. In E.L. Rossi (Ed.), The collected papers of Milton H. Erickson on hypnosis: Vol. 4. Innovative hypnotherapy (pp. 97–98). Irvington.

Sternberg, S. (1975). Memory scanning: New findings and current controversies. *Quarterly Journal of Experimental Psychology*, *22*, 1–32. 10.1080/14640747508400

Tart, C. (1975). *States of consciousness*. New York: E. P. Dutton & Co.

Varga, K., Józsa, E., & Kekecs, Z. (2014). Comparative analysis of phenomenological patterns of hypnotists and subjects: An interactional perspective. *Psychology of Consciousness: Theory, Research, and Practice*, *1*(3), 308–319. 10.1037/cns0000013

Watkins, J., & Watkins, H. (1997). *Ego states: Theory and therapy*. New York: W.W. Norton.

9

THE FOUNDATION OF AN ECOLOGICAL MODEL OF HYPNOTHERAPY

The Base for Defining the Structural Dimensions of Hypnotherapy

Matthias Mende

Psychotherapy-Center, Salzburg, Austria

My Relationship to This Topic

My professional background as a psychologist lies in social psychology. Without being aware of it when I wrote my doctoral dissertation (Mende, 1984), I did experimental research on pacing and leading. I was not familiar with these concepts at the time while following the lead of Jones and Gerard (1967) who distinguished between communication that was contingent upon internal stimuli like inner thoughts, sensations, moods (i.e., leading), and communication that was contingent upon external stimuli like specifics of behaviors shown by the interacting partner (i.e., pacing). Also, the authors distinguished between symmetrical interactional patterns where both partners showed identical communicational styles and asymmetrical interactional patterns where the partners exhibited different communicational styles (Jones & Gerard, 1967).

I conducted an experiment with this classification where the subjects were listening to an audio recording of a conversation by an interacting dyad (the stimulus persons). I created six conditions with two independent variables: the communication style (just pacing vs. pacing followed by leading vs. just leading) and the interactional pattern of the dyad (symmetrical vs. asymmetrical). I examined the effects of the type of communication style and the type of interactional pattern might have on observers (the subjects) who rated the stimulus persons on a questionnaire measuring the extent to which personality traits were attributed to the stimulus persons.

The results were stunning: In the symmetrical conditions where both actors showed the same behavior, no personality traits other than average were attributed to the actors. However, as soon as the communication styles of the stimulus persons were different from one another in the asymmetrical conditions, there was an extreme readiness to make conclusions regarding the personalities of the actors. Greater dissimilarity between the actors in the asymmetrical conditions prompted more extreme trait attributions. When one actor was pacing while the other was leading, the actor showing leading behavior was rated

 DOI: 10.4324/9781003449126-13

as being socially competent, likable, resonating in a positive way, good-humored, spontaneous, and dominant. In contrast, the actor showing pacing behavior was rated as being socially incompetent, unattractive, resonating in a negative way, depressed, excessively self-controlled, and subdued. These findings were very robust, indicating strong simultaneous contrast phenomena being highly significant cues in interpersonal perception as well as for the resulting inferences.

I concluded that observers use responses of other people toward an actor as cues for attributing personality traits, much more than the actor's behavior itself. If the other person is basically ignored by an actor who is solely leading, negative personality traits are attributed to the one who is ignored. On the other hand, if the other person is closely mirrored and responded to by an actor who is solely pacing, positive personality traits are attributed to the one who is attended to.

Only years later when I had become familiar with hypnosis and hypnotherapy, it occurred to me that what I had examined were the effects pacing and leading had on interpersonal perception. What I had labelled "internally contingent communicational behavior" was nothing else than leading, and what I had called "externally contingent communicational behavior" was actually pacing. I realized that establishing rapport in the hypnotherapeutic relationship by pacing meant for the therapist to assume a one-down-position on purpose, thus lifting the patient to a one-up-position. Thus, a hypnotherapeutic relationship is created in which narcissistic needs of the patient are inherently replenished. At the same time, an asymmetrical relationship is created, resembling the early mother–child connection, easily giving rise to regression in the service of the ego (Gill & Brenman, 1959) allowing the addressing of conflict-oriented issues (Brown & Fromm, 1986), or promoting of structural nourishing (Baker, 2000).

Conceptual Clarifications

Hypnosis and Trance

In the past decades, the debate whether hypnosis was a distinguishable state of consciousness created a lot of unrest among professionals in the field of hypnosis. The concepts of hypnosis and trance become a lot clearer if "hypnosis" is used as a term signifying a mode of communication that allows a person to access a certain state of awareness labeled as "(hypnotic) trance". But then: is there anything as a "state" of consciousness? When we speak of the "waking state" or sleeping state" we rarely question the concept of "state" to signify these phenomena. Taking a closer look, we must admit that these phenomena are better described as processes, characterized by typical fluctuations of brain processes that allow telling these phenomena apart from one another.

Trance and Links between Neurobiology and Experience

During the past two decades, overwhelming evidence was gathered by researchers of various scientific backgrounds, indicating that in a trance, brain functions show significant patterns typical for this mode of neurophysiological functioning. Ulrike Halsband and her scientific team in Freiburg, Germany showed that it was even possible to discriminate between different trance states like meditational trances and hypnotic trances. Specific activation patterns could be observed, typical for a specific trance mode (Halsband, 2015).

Moreover, it was possible to link those specific alteration patterns of brain functioning to certain modes of experiencing: The robust finding of hypofrontality during a hypnotic trance reflects experiencing a reduced reality proneness (Dietrich, 2003). The reduced activity of the amygdala (Gruzelier, 1998) in a hypnotic trance is helpful when focusing on trauma-related materials and corresponds with the experience of dissociation between trauma-related imagery and affect, facilitating the stress reduction necessary for reprocessing the traumatic experience.

The discovery of the default mode network (DMN) (Greicius et al., 2003) led to a deeper understanding of dissociation – the predominant psychophysiological feature of both, the hypnotic trance and trauma. Researchers showed (Greicius et al., 2008) that in a relaxed waking state without externals task requirements, a neurophysiological network becomes active: the DMN. This network includes a circuit of nodes connected to one another by brain fibers. An increased interconnectivity between the DMN-nodes is associated with unintentional thoughts or ruminations wandering around in one's head in the absence of an external task. In a trance, the nodes of the DMN themselves remain active. However, the interconnectivity is significantly decreased or ceases altogether (Deeley et al., 2012). The experiential equivalent is relaxed absorption, reduced distractibility, and a feeling of being dissociated from ruminations and irrelevant stimuli.

Hypnotherapy: The Neurobiology of the Hypnotherapeutic Relationship

Whenever therapy studies are conducted to assess and compare the effectiveness of certain therapeutic methods, there is overwhelming evidence that therapeutic effects depend mostly on unspecified factors like characteristics of the therapist, the patient, and the quality of the therapeutic relationship. Only a small portion of the variance is explained by the specifics of the therapeutic method (e.g., Barkham & Lambert, 2021). A very special feature of hypnotherapy is that it places emphasis on the formation of the hypnotherapeutic relationship, utilizing the subjective reality models of patients as much as possible to facilitate trust and cooperation for the good of the therapeutic progress. Pacing patients means mirroring them intentionally in all aspects of their verbal, paraverbal, and nonverbal self-expressive behavior. Pacing also includes mirroring more complex cognitive, emotional, and social aspects of their personalities. Thus, rapport is created, an intense form of exclusive relatedness, leading to a strong activation of the mirror neuron system (MNS). The discovery of mirror neurons in primates (Rizzolatti et al., 1996) firing when a behavior is performed as well as when it is merely observed turned out to be groundbreaking for understanding many processes involved in hypnotherapy. Marco Iacoboni gathered evidence showing how the MNS paradigm can easily be transferred to humans and all aspects of human experience including emotions, affect, and pain (Iacoboni, 2009). The MNS theory delivers the neurobiological basis for understanding the ideodynamic principle: mirror neurons form the neurobiological bridge between an idea and its dynamic realization – in motor activities, sensory activities, or emotional/effective responses. The MNS also explains the experience of safe proximity seen when strong rapport exists between therapist and patient. Attuning to the patient's subjective reality as much as possible by applying the utilization principle further activates the MNS, maximizing responsiveness to therapeutic leadings and readiness to engage in conscious and unconscious learning. Pacing optimizes the patient's attention, supports positive transference, and induces two-way mirroring typical for the early mother–child relationship, facilitating hypnotic age regression.

The Development of Hypnotherapy

After the schism following the rejection of hypnosis by Freud in favor of the psychoanalytic cure, hypnosis was relinquished by most psychotherapists/analysts of the time (Peter, 2015b). Hypnotherapy was reborn as hypnoanalysis in the psychodynamic tradition, when it became legitimate to overcome the demand for the analyst to remain completely abstentious, in favor of utilizing specific hypnotherapeutic interventions within the domain of psychoanalysis. In their groundbreaking work, Erika Fromm and Dan Brown (Brown & Fromm, 1986) devised a framework for hypnotherapy and hypnoanalysis meant to be psychotherapeutic modalities in their own rights. They confirmed the finding that transference is highly salient in a hypnotherapeutic relationship. Typically, transference and countertransference are analyzed and/or managed in psychodynamic therapies. Hypnotherapy can go beyond managing transference by utilizing it in line with the therapeutic goal. In operational terms, hypnotic transference can be described by expectations and fantasies patients hold concerning hypnosis and the role of the hypnotherapist (Brown & Fromm, 1986).

Gill and Brenman (1959) discovered another feature of hypnosis valuable for hypnotherapy: In a hypnotic trance, patients readily regress to earlier stages of their lives. Gill and Brenman found that age regressions could be utilized therapeutically "in the service of the ego". Thus, they set the groundwork for all hypnotherapeutic applications in the trauma-related work that make use of age regressions to support younger selves in need.

Milton Erickson revolutionized hypnotherapy by introducing the utilization principle (Erickson, 1959). The idea of utilizing disturbing symptom characteristics to promote emotional and physical well-being and turning aspects of the disorder into resources gave hypnotherapy a boost in popularity. Even though Erickson also conducted long-term therapies with slow therapeutic progress (Erickson, 1980), followers were concentrating on the solution-oriented hypnotherapeutic applications aiming for quick success with structurally quite mature patients showing concise psychic symptoms. This describes the traditional realm of "hypnotherapy" as it is applied by most clinicians and taught by most hypnotic societies around the globe. With these restrictions, hypnotherapy blends easily as an adjunct with other psychotherapeutic modalities like CBT, Gestalt-therapy, systemic family therapy, psychodynamically oriented and humanistic therapeutic approaches.

Hypnosis-Psychotherapy

What is neglected by many hypnotherapists is that there are a vast number of patients on a medium level of structural integration. Those patients suffer from excruciating inner conflicts that need to be repressed for an individual to maintain homeostasis – at the expense of constricting symptoms. Another group of patients on a lower level of structural integration have suffered early developmental deficits resulting in vulnerable self-boundaries and an instable sense of the self. Primitive defense mechanisms like splitting, denial, or projection are meant to protect the self and maintain homeostasis – at the cost of very constricting symptoms.

It was Elgan Baker who expanded the scope of applicability of hypnotherapy by adapting the different modes of interventions to different levels of structural integration (Baker, 2000). Hypnotherapeutic interventions can be designed to deal with inner conflicts and the defense mechanism keeping them alive on a medium level of structural Integration. For patients at an early stage of developmental arrest, resulting in a low level of structural integration, a hypnotherapeutic approach may be chosen which is solely based on offering a nurturing hypnotherapeutic relationship, replenishing the deficits from neglect or abuse suffered in early childhood.

With such a comprehensive methodology, applicable on all levels of structural integration and a method-specific theoretical foundation integrating psychodynamic, behavioral, systemic, and perceptional aspects of experiencing reality, we are able to claim that hypnosis-psychotherapy is a psychotherapeutic modality in its own right (Kanitschar, 2009). In a few countries in Europe, namely Austria, Italy and Sweden, hypnosis-psychotherapy is listed as a lawful psychotherapeutic modality integrated in the public health system.

The Foundation of an Ecological Model of Hypnotherapy

If hypnotherapy is conceived and perceived as a very effective approach to attain personal change, we must ask what aspects of the personality and symptomatology will undergo the change and how will the changes affect other aspects of perception, communication, behavior, and meaning. How can we guarantee that only the intended change takes place and that the therapeutic change is integrated in the self without raising new, unforeseen conflicts with other parts of the personality?

Inspired by Gregory Bateson's work describing steps to an ecology of mind (Bateson, 2000), the above question led me to develop the ecological model of hypnosis. The ecological model reflects the fact that any change in an ecosystem will affect other elements in this ecosystem – for the worse or the better. This concerns natural environments like forests and waters, and emotional and cognitive environments of the human mind. To be ecologically sound, any therapeutic change must be somehow integrated in the existing mental, behavioral, emotional, and social environment of the client. When an agoraphobic patient overcomes her anxiety, several questions arise: What effect will this have on her relationship with the partner, if the patient does not depend on being accompanied away from home, anymore? Moreover, how will the patient utilize her newly acquired freedom to move around? Will she use it to embrace more responsibilities, taking on tasks and obligations, and running errands? Or will she devote her new freedom to leisure and social activities? These new options may create inner or interpersonal conflicts the client did not become aware of, while she was agoraphobic.

For a therapeutic change to be ecologically sound, the newly acquired abilities, resources, and liberties must fit into the existing team of inner parts or ego states. They have to be integrated, for a new homeostasis to emerge, in which none of the existing resources and capabilities are compromised (Mende, 2006).

The Ecological Nature of Hypnotherapy

Hypnotherapy is ecological by nature, for it combines two essential features. First, it embraces the constructivist approach of hypnotherapy (Fourie, 1991). In clinical practice, it is extremely helpful to construe the unconscious mind as a wise, benevolent entity full of resources. Following Erickson's approach (Erickson, 1980), in my model many helpful skills and qualities are attributed to the unconscious, in a way that it is experienced by the client as acting and responding autonomously and unmanipulated by the conscious mind. These reality constructions help to tap resources previously unknown to the client. Communication can be established with the unconscious, and upon realizing its good intentions and taking its messages seriously, deals and agreements can be reached. As a result, existing symptoms are reduced or dissolved, because they have become dispensable.

The second ecological feature of hypnotherapy is rooted in working with trances accessible by a special way of hypnotic communication. This model defines trance as an intended and enhanced learning process involving somatic, emotional, behavioral, and social changes. It is an ecological safeguard against unintended learning processes or ones that might occur against the will of the patient, if profound learning processes are only accessible upon purposefully entering a special state of mind (Mende, 1998) which the use of hypnosis skills facilitates.

The Ecology of the Basic Emotional Needs

Researchers in the field of social psychology have produced a wealth of material pertaining directly to hypnosis. A valuable approach is Edwards Deci's work on intrinsic motivation (Deci & Flaste, 1995). The authors discovered that motivation can be named "intrinsic", if it is driven by three basic needs: The need to feel autonomous, the need to feel related, and the need to feel competent. Since the existence of autonomy is a philosophical question, Deci found it more appropriate to address the subjective feeling of being autonomous, related, and competent. When I learned about this approach, it became clear to me that these emotional needs are not only relevant for intrinsic motivation. They are also key factors for a sound, balanced emotional homeostasis. When I discussed this idea with colleagues, it became evident that there was one need missing: The need to feel oriented, meaning the need to experience a sense of purpose, meaning, and clarity regarding one's values and priorities and the need for predictability of future events and other people. And there they were, the four Basic Emotional Needs: The need to feel autonomous, related, competent, and oriented. Moreover, I found that emotional stability can be defined operationally as an experience in which (1) all four basic emotional needs are sufficiently accommodated (2) with none of the needs being overemphasized or neglected, (3) and no major conflicts (4) or perceived incompatibilities between these needs exist (Mende, 2006).

Psychic, somatoform, and psychosomatic disorders can be described in terms of a perceived imbalance of those needs. Take for example a patient with OCD. Driven by the need to feel competent, the patient has perfect control over tiny bits and pieces of his daily life. But what exactly is it good for? The need to feel oriented is compromised, in favor of the need to feel competent and having control. The need to feel autonomous is captured by the symptom. The obsessions and compulsions occur in a compelling, nonvolitional manner, no matter what the circumstances are or what other people might say. The need to feel related is also jeopardized, as relatives and friends have the choice of adjusting to the obsessions of the patients or leaving the relationship.

The relevance basic emotional needs have regarding emotional stability becomes evident looking at trauma. The severity of a trauma affecting both the psyche and soma can be operationally defined as the suspension and unavailability of the basic emotional needs. In a trauma, the victim is at least temporarily cut off from all four needs. For example, if a 12-year-old boy is sexually abused by a priest, the need to feel oriented and the belief in a predictable world is upset. This can trigger feelings of acute helplessness and being incapacitated. The needs to experience competence and control are suspended. The relation to the priest is traumatically altered. If the boy dares not to tell the parents due to feelings of shame, guilt, or fear of not being believed, the relation to them is affected as well. The need to feel autonomous is devastated. There is nothing the boy can decide for himself. The abuse is traumatic in that all four needs are impacted.

After illustrating the significance of the basic emotional needs for psychological disorders on one hand and emotional well-being on the other, it was a fascinating discovery for me that all four basic emotional needs are taken care of implicitly in hypnotherapy, even if the therapist is not aware of it. The need to feel autonomous is satisfied by working with the unconscious – the most autonomous part of a person that cannot be manipulated. The need to feel related is supported by establishing rapport in the hypnotherapeutic relationship, building trust and proximity without interfering with the need to feel autonomous. The need to feel competent is supplied in hypnotherapy by focusing on resources and trance phenomena evolving with ease, in a way that the therapeutic relationship is not jeopardized by a "failure" at a certain hypnotic task. Finally, the need to feel oriented is met in hypnotherapy by working with suggestions given in a way that does not interfere with the need to feel autonomous. To the contrary, suggestions are utilized to elicit autonomous inner search processes directed by the unconscious that will eventually lead to a solution. Thus, hypnotherapy implicitly nourishes and balances the basic emotional needs (Mende, 2006). Additionally, hypnotherapeutic interventions can be devised, explicitly addressing perceived conflicts or incompatibilities between certain needs or negative effects of overemphasizing one of the needs at the expense of others or neglecting one of them.

Hypnosis-Psychotherapy as a Comprehensive Psychotherapeutic Modality

As Burkhard Peter noted, for a psychotherapeutic modality to be comprehensive, it must cover all reality levels of human experience in the course of the psychotherapeutic process (Peter, 2015a). Psychotherapeutic modalities can be distinguished by identifying the reality level they are primarily concerned with. Cognitive behavior therapy is primarily focusing on the *actions* the patient takes. Psychodynamically oriented therapies put the emphasis on detecting the *meaning* of a psychological disorder and its origin. Systemic family therapy is primarily engaged in *communication* and interactional patterns present in the family system or within the person.

As I will show, hypnotherapy covers all reality levels. To begin with, however, hypnotherapy focuses on the *perception* of the self, others, and the environment, and ways of modifying perceptions (Peter, 2015a). The plasticity of sensory perceptions and the profound ways of altering and modifying them always belonged to the most fascinating phenomena of hypnosis. In a therapeutic context, trance phenomena utilizing perception modifications build the base for new ways of experiencing. This can result in the generalized experience that things can be different than we assumed them to be previously. Thus, rigid ways of perceiving and thinking may become more flexible.

Hypnosis-psychotherapy, as a complete psychotherapeutic modality, touches directly on all four reality levels of human experience as they are directly linked to the basic emotional needs. (1) The perceptional level is related to the need to feel autonomous. The most prominent feature of autonomy lies in the ability to direct one's perceptual attention to where it really matters and ward off irrelevant or misleading perceptions. (2) The reality

Table 9.1 The Ecological Model of Hypnotherapy in the Nutshell

Experiential Reality Level	*Corresponding Basic Emotional Need*	*In Hypnotherapy Realized By …*
Perception	Autonomy	Unconscious
Communication	Relatedness	Rapport
Action	Competence	Resources/trance phenomena
Meaning	Orientation	Suggestions

level of communication is linked to the need to feel related to significant others and the entire social environment. (3) The reality level of action corresponds with the emotional need to feel competent and have sufficient control, for instance in the sense of self-efficacy. (4) Finally, the reality level of meaning corresponds with the basic emotional need to feel oriented about the nature and composition of the outer and inner world, as well as one's values, goals, and priorities (Table 9.1).

The Structural Dimensions of Hypnotherapy

A Model for Planning, Shaping, and Reflecting the Hypnotherapeutic Process

In the often-chaotic world of our patients, our task is to provide the structures along which patients can orient themselves when working on their therapeutic issues. In this part of the chapter, I examine hypnotherapy itself on the structural level and present a model providing hypnotherapists with criteria to plan, shape, and reflect the hypnotherapeutic process – e.g., for training purposes or supervision. The model describes which therapeutic decisions will have to be made during the hypnotherapeutic process. These decisions may be made implicitly on an intuitive level or based on thoughtful planning and reflecting along the structural dimensions. They are hierarchical in the sense that decisions made on a more specific dimension build on decisions made on the more basic structural dimensions. The model of the structural dimensions of hypnotherapy results in a pyramid structure with the reality levels of human experiencing at its base, building up to the specifics of actual trancework options at the top. This is a revised and expanded version of a publication in German (Mende, 2021) (Figure 9.1).

Reality Levels and Therapy Goals: The Basic Structural Dimensions of Hypnotherapy

Building on the ecological model of hypnotherapy with the reality levels as the most basic structural dimension, it becomes obvious that any truthfully therapeutic goal affects the way reality is experienced on the levels of perception, communication, action, and meaning. Based on these levels of reality, all therapy goals may be allocated to one or more basic emotional needs. In many cases, the goal is to strengthen the feeling of *autonomy*, the fulfillment of the desire to experience oneself as being self-determined, independent, and free. The common denominator of many psychopathologies is that they disrupt the feeling of autonomy, when at the same time the inner part that produces the symptoms acts autonomously. Thus, the need to feel autonomous is transferred to the part of the personality expressing the symptoms when at the same time the patient is afflicted by the loss of autonomy. This is obvious in OCD where the compulsions lead a life of their own. It is

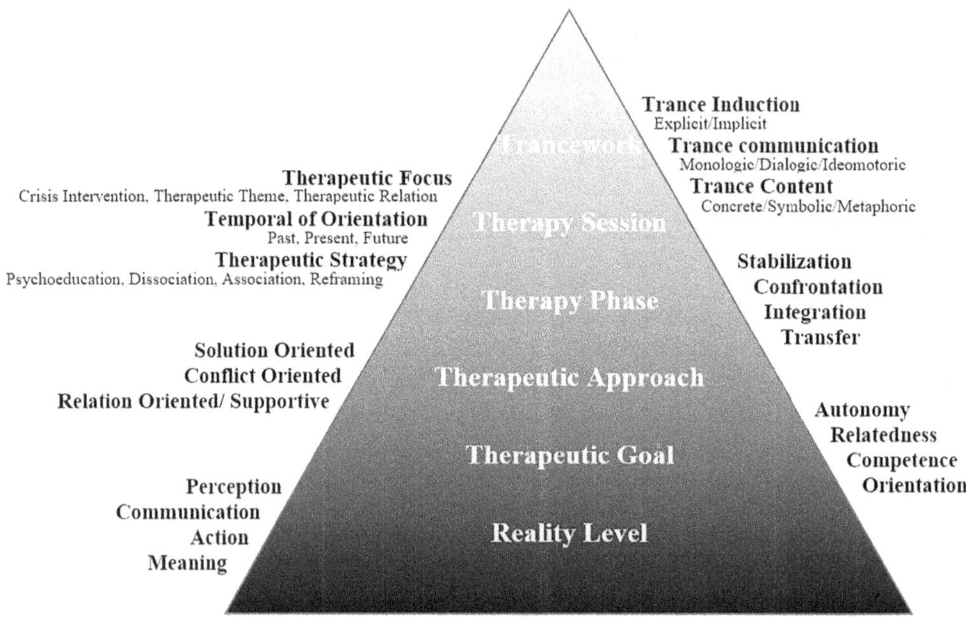

Figure 9.1 The structural dimensions of hypnotherapy.

also true for anxiety disorders like agoraphobia or social phobias, that restrict the freedom to move around or engage with others.

Other therapy goals represent the wish to feel security and proximity in a stable relationship. This is especially true for general anxiety disorders where the need for feelings of *relatedness* is secured by being dependent on the physical presence of someone else. Severe depressions and psychosomatic disorders may create the same intense kind of dependency. This can be addressed by both modeling security and encouraging autonomous behaviors within the hypnotherapeutic relationship.

For other cases in anxiety, psychosomatic disorders, and trauma, the need for a feeling of *competence* and self-efficacy and regaining a sense of control is the core goal. In trauma, OCD, and depression, the need for feeling of *orientation* and making sense of oneself and the world is often damaged and needs to be reinvigorated.

When defining therapy goals, possible interactions between the basic emotional needs must be considered. The resolution of a generalized anxiety disorder might strengthen the feelings of competence and autonomy. This empowerment may be a threat to an existing relationship because the dependency on the partner caused by the constraining symptoms no longer exists. Focusing on the basic emotional needs when formulating therapy goals is an obvious thing to do, especially in hypnotherapy, since accommodating these needs is integral to this therapeutic method.

Building psychotherapeutic interventions on explicit therapy goals is paramount in any psychotherapeutic modality. For hypnotherapy, this is especially true, since we are working with suggestions in a state of reduced reality orientation occurring during a hypnotic trance. Thus, we are ethically obliged to reassure the patient that everything we do as hypnotherapists is in line with the agreed therapeutic goal, even though the patient may not see how the intervention relates to a specified therapy goal.

The Hypnotherapeutic Approach: Solution-oriented, Conflict-oriented, Relation-oriented/Supportive

Based on the therapy goals, further structural dimensions of hypnotherapy may be derived, as a base for the therapeutic decisions that will be made one way or another as the hypnotherapeutic process evolves. Once the therapeutic goal is defined, the task is to choose a hypnotherapeutic approach to reach this goal. Depending on the nature of the goal and most of all on the level of structural integration of the patient, the approach will be solution-oriented, conflict-oriented, or relational-supportive (Kanitschar, 2009).

For simple cases, a solution-oriented approach promoting the availability of unconscious or neglected resources or evoking new ones is sufficient. The solution-oriented approach is especially suitable for the treatment of stress-related disorders involving depression or anxiety, or conditioned disorders like certain phobias for patients on a *higher level of structural integration.*

Patients on a *medium level of structural integration* often profit in a sustainable way only if the psychodynamic conflict that evoked the symptoms has been resolved. Conflict-oriented hypnotherapy aims at uncovering and modifying childlike coping strategies by utilizing the resources of the more mature adult self. Subsequently, strategies for coping with stress and interventions for ego-strengthening can then be devised utilizing the solution-oriented approach.

For patients on a lower *level of structural integration* with more pronounced structural deficits in their personal development, it is often futile to work with hypnotherapeutic interventions in the narrower sense. In these cases, the relation-oriented/supportive approach aims at structural maturation in the sense of re-parenting within the hypnotherapeutic relationship. Patients with severe personality disorders, for example, profit from the capability of the hypnotherapist to maintain stable rapport and utilizing countertransference feelings therapeutically, regardless of the patient exhibiting hostility, affective lability, and immature defense mechanisms like projective identification (Mende, 2009). For some patients, the experience of being endured by another person, in this case the therapist, with a stable, attentive, and respectful demeanor can be a rare, valuable experience.

The Therapy Phases: Stabilization, Confrontation, Integration, Transfer

The *stabilization phase* marks the beginning of any hypnotherapy. Stabilization occurs by experiencing the hypnotic trance itself as a resourceful state. Significant aspects are focused while feeling secure and pleasantly relaxed. Irrelevant disturbing perceptions or activities fade out. The availability of an imagined safe place signifies successful stabilization.

In the treatment of PTSD, it is fundamentally significant to have reached sufficient emotional and psychophysiological stabilization before confronting trauma content (Frederick & Phillips, 2007). A general rule for hypnotherapeutic work, regardless of the clinical picture, is that stabilization takes precedence over confrontation, and confrontation only makes sense if it is done within an acceptable stress level, because excessive stress blocks new learning (Sandi & Pinelo-Nava, 2007).

Within the *confrontation phase*, the crucial hypnotherapeutic moment lies in the corrective emotional experience. Due to the reduction of psychophysiological stress attained by successful stabilization and encouraged by stable rapport within the hypnotherapeutic relationship, it becomes perceptible in a trance, on all levels of sensory and emotional experience, that the feared negative consequences of a confrontation with anxiety or trauma content are absent. Instead, feelings of joy or pride come with the coping experiences. In moments like this, the potential of hypnotherapy as an experiential therapeutic modality becomes evident (Bongartz & Bongartz, 2000).

During the *integration phase*, the therapeutic task is to put the authorship for therapeutic success in the hands of the patients. This can be done by the therapist pointing out the merits of the work done by the patient's unconscious, and its capacity to mobilize the inner resources to reach the therapy goal. Trancework is done verifying the extent to which the basic emotional needs have been integrated. Has the therapy succeeded in accommodating deficient or neglected needs for feelings of autonomy, relatedness, competence, or orientation? Has it succeeded in calming overemphasized needs, or solving conflicts and perceived incompatibilities and interdependencies that existed between the needs? Finding answers to these questions serves as an operational criterion for the therapist and the patient to decide when to end the therapy.

During the *transfer phase*, the therapeutic success is validated. To what extent does reaching the therapy goals yield an improvement in the everyday life of the patient on the four levels of reality. Has the change become noticeable by perceiving oneself and others differently? Does the patient feel more liberated and mindful in the way he or she is communicating with oneself and others? Has the patient overcome confining impulses to avoid, while accessing existing potential and resources freely? What meaning does the patient attribute to the previously existing problems and the fact that they could be resolved in the context of the therapy?

The Therapy Session

Therapeutic Focus: Crisis Intervention, Therapeutic Theme, Therapeutic Relationship

At the beginning of each therapeutic session, a mutual decision must be made about what the focus of this session might be. Depending on the current physical/mental state and urgency, it may be necessary to work hypnotherapeutically doing *crisis-intervention*. In this case, the general therapeutic goal must take a back seat in favor of stabilization. In the absence of acute emotional turmoil, the *therapeutic theme* can be addressed. Transference, countertransference, and defense mechanisms may direct the focus on daily actualities instead of the therapeutic topic. The hypnotherapist should be aware that patients tend to utilize their defense mechanisms to guide therapists into areas where the patient's defense mechanisms work best (Mende, 1998). Most patients benefit from being gently reminded of the therapeutic theme, even in the face of everyday problems. When therapy falters or rapport breaks down, it may be necessary to address the *therapeutic relationship* itself.

Temporal Orientation: Past, Present, Future

In every therapeutic approach and every phase of therapy, there is the possibility of working on different temporal levels (Revenstorf, 2015). The therapy session may focus on the present, the past, or the future. In the treatment of social phobia for example, hypnotherapeutic imaginary work can be done *in the present*, where the patient experiences being surrounded by a protective shield inside of which it is safe to relax in the face of social stimuli, before engaging in the feared social encounter. Subsequently, a time progression into a concrete social situation *in the future* can be utilized as a future pacing, leading to an experience of self-confident coping which in turn – by hypnotherapeutic work – may attain the status of a memory of something that was experienced. Especially on a medium level of structural integration, conflict-oriented work is devoted to access the origins of the social phobia, for instance addressing early experiences *in the past* when the younger self felt insecure in the presence of others, out of fear of being rejected.

The choice of the temporal level ought to follow the utilization principle. As such it can be based as much as possible on the patient's model of reality and his or her subjective assumptions about the causes of the problem and the conditions for its solution (Schmid, 2011).

Therapeutic Strategy: Psychoeducation, Dissociation, Association, Reframing

In every therapy session, there are several therapeutic strategies (Revenstorf, 2015) available to address the therapeutic theme. With appropriate disorder-specific *psychoeducation*, decisive points for the successful course of therapy are set first. Education about the psychophysiological processes involved also satisfies the need for orientation. When trauma is the focus, patients benefit from understanding the underlying trauma dynamics (Reddemann, 2016). When these dynamics are explained early on, rapport is strengthened enormously. For the patients, it may seem like "mind reading", since the trauma dynamics follow very predictable patterns across most affected persons. Subsequently, they feel recognized and acknowledged in their suffering. Patients with other stress-related disorders (e.g., panic disorders, burnout, or somatoform disorders) benefit from understanding the psychophysiological impacts of stress on body and mind, as it helps them to think of their problem not as a personal failure, but as a protective measure of the unconscious against a self-overloading lifestyle.

Dissociation is an essential feature of the hypnotic trance experience. It is a common denominator across most theories of hypnosis (Spiegel, 2007; Woody & Sadler, 2008). The human ability to become detached from overwhelming body sensations, thoughts, and affective states enables cohesive actions even in life-threatening situations. In hypnotherapy, dissociation is utilized as a resource for reprocessing constrictive or harmful patterns of perceiving, thinking, feeling, and acting. The temporary dissociation of certain aspects of perception and experience (Revenstorf, 2015) is a strategy of choice, for instance, in symptom-oriented hypnotherapy for pain relief. By gradually lifting the therapeutic dissociation in the solution-oriented treatment of phobias, trancework can take on the character of systematic desensitization. In conflict-oriented work, dissociation enables experiencing that it is safe to give up constricting defense mechanisms, thus revealing new degrees of freedom in experiencing and acting. In the relational/supportive approach, the task frequently is to dissolve dissociation, e.g., to promote a coherent body scheme.

In other cases, it is useful to use *association* as a therapeutic strategy by connecting a problem with a resource. For example, an imagined fear-evoking encounter could be hypnotherapeutically associated with ego-strengthening feelings of competence the patient experiences in other social situations or with feelings of being accepted by significant others regardless of social performance.

The possibilities of *reframing* (Gerl, 2015) are based on the plasticity people show when it comes to the attribution of meaning to perceptions and experiences. Typically, patients view their symptomatology as annoying, or even hostile. However, it is often easy to see from the outside that the symptomatology serves an important function in the patient's mental and emotional household. Reframing then may be done by pointing out that positive intention of the symptom. Thus, for most people suffering from a somatoform pain disorder, it is easy to acknowledge that, without digging any deeper, a part of the message of the symptom is the order: "Look after yourself". The pain symptom succeeds in forcing the patient's attention inward in a negative way. In this case, it is safe to predict that the symptom will be relieved once the patient volunteers to find positive ways of self-care.

The Trancework

Trance Induction: Explicit, Implicit

Within each therapy session, decisions must be made when and how actual trancework will be done. There are several criteria for choosing to work with explicit or implicit trances: *Explicit trances*, which are announced and include an induction ritual, correspond to patients' classical expectations of hypnosis. An explicit trance induction places the patient in an inwardly focused, concentrated, and relaxed state.

Sometimes it is useful or even necessary to work with *implicit trances* developing during the therapeutic conversation, without any induction ritual. In some disorders – such as OCD, certain trauma sequelae, or with over-controlled patients or children – it is often advisable to work with such *conversational trances*. The resulting trance states are rarely registered as such by the patients but are sufficient to stimulate therapy-relevant unconscious search processes.

Some people cannot operate within a trance. Others are unable to do so due to the nature and severity of their mental illness. Sometimes there is a contraindication to hypnotic work because the therapeutic contact is unstable and fragile and communication patterns are inconsistent. This is often the case in borderline personality disorders or psychotic disorders (Revenstorf & Peter, 2015). Hypnotherapeutic work can still be done, provided the therapy is limited to the use of *hypnotic communication*. Pacing and leading structures are utilized for stabilizing rapport achieving a therapeutically helpful position on the proximity–distance axis. Hypnotic communication techniques are shaped to attain basic psychophysical and emotional stabilization, to strengthen the ties to reality, to enhance the connection to the body, and to distinguish between the inner and outer world.

Trance Communication: Monologic, Dialogic, Ideomotoric

For the actual trancework, there are several options to design the hypnotic communication. It can be monologic, dialogic, or ideomotor. In the beginning, many patients find it easier to go into trance if the trance is induced in a *monologic* way, with only the therapist talking. In trances for resource activation or several indirect techniques such as the proxy technique, it is also often sufficient to work monologically.

However, most patients easily succeed in speaking while in trance without subjectively disturbing their trance experience. *Dialogic* communication opens countless options for hypnotherapeutic interventions, especially for doing conflict work. In dialogue, the hypnotherapeutic rapport is also more stable and intense. This is especially important doing trauma work when it is necessary to protect the patient from a malignant regression and trauma-induced pathological dissociation.

Often to their own surprise, most patients find it easy to give *ideomotor signals* for communicating with the "unconscious" when exploring the roots of a problem or a viable solution. Ideomotor communication can also be utilized for indicating the beginning or end of an unconscious therapeutic process and for building trust in the intuition and the resources of the unconscious (Kaiser-Rekkas, 2013).

Trance Content: Concrete, Symbolic, Metaphoric

Trancework can refer to experiencing specific past, present, or future *concrete situations* and experiences in which new ways of perceiving and acting are tested and anchored. A typical example of this type of work is the therapy of simple phobias, where the feared exam situation, for example, is imagined and mastered in a hypnotic trance.

Most of the hypnotherapeutic trauma work is concerned with concrete situations of the past where the victimized younger self is provided with shelter, care, and healing. The symptom-oriented part in the hypnotherapeutic treatment of OCD also focuses on imagined concrete situations in which the impulse to engage in compulsive behavior can fade while feeling safe and relaxed.

Hypnotherapy develops a special power when working with *symbolizations* provided by the patient in a dialogic trance. Inviting the patient to visualize the inner part responsible for the symptom, e.g., as a person, a fantasy figure, an animal, or even a plant creates a therapeutically useful distance between the conscious and the unconscious – especially regarding the emotional attitude the patient takes toward the symptom. In the hypnotic dialogue, the resources of the symbolization representing the symptom and its messages can be explored. If an IBS symptom is experienced by the patient simply as disturbing, restricting, and unpleasant, the symbolization of the part responsible for the symptom may well have sympathetic features (e.g., a salamander that simply feels comfortable in a boggy swamp that is difficult to access for other people). During the therapeutic process, appreciating the resources of the symptom then becomes possible in the long run.

Trancework with *metaphors*, usually provided by the therapist in a monologic trance, opens wide spaces for creativity evolving during the hypnotherapeutic process, especially in the generalized definition of the term that includes analogies, anecdotes, and fairy tales. Utilizing metaphors triggers unconscious search processes accompanied by the patient's curious question what this meaningfully presented story could possibly have to do with her own problem. Resistance that could be generated if a therapeutic message was expressed directly is minimized. If the indirect message of the metaphor evokes resistance nonetheless, it was just another story.

Conclusion

I developed the ecological model of hypnotherapy as a tool for describing psychopathological disorders in terms of emotional imbalances, conflicts, and perceived incompatibilities that go along with them. The ecological model identifies four basic emotional needs: the need to feel autonomous, related, competent, and oriented. Hypnotherapy inherently accommodates all four basic emotional needs by working with the unconscious, by establishing stable rapport within the therapeutic relationship, by working with resources and suggestions meant to enhance feelings of competence, control, and autonomy. In practice, the paradigm of the basic emotional needs has proven to be applicable and helpful for defining therapy goals. It also delivers operational criteria for timing the ending of a successful hypnotherapy.

Based on the ecological model of hypnotherapy, the structural dimensions of hypnotherapy can be defined as a roadmap for essential decisions made during hypnotherapy. The structural dimensions are hierarchical, as the more specific decisions e.g., regarding the type of trancework done during the therapy session, depend on more basic decisions regarding the type of hypnotherapeutic approach that was chosen to reach the therapy goals. This can help novices in hypnotherapy to recognize various treatment alternatives and to make sound decisions for choosing an appropriate path for a particular case. Those with long experience doing hypnotherapy understandably tend to use their often tried and well-tested hypnotherapeutic treatment strategies repeatedly. For them, the model could be a stimulus to look at the structures behind intuitive therapeutic decisions, to remember existing hypnotherapeutic alternatives, and in this way to bring more variety into the therapeutic routine.

The paradigm of the basic emotional needs and the innate accommodation and alignment of these needs through hypnotherapy lends itself to be validated by outcome research, e.g., by developing a pre-post questionnaire assessing the relative prevalence of these needs and detecting possible conflicts between them and changes resulting from hypnotherapy.

Neurobiological research of hypnosis has proliferated and is exploring the mechanisms of trance and hypnosis. Many of the therapeutic perspectives and benefits of working with the hypnosis skills and the trance process that I have outlined in my model of ecological hypnotherapy are being corroborated with this research. It is validating of the historic and ongoing use of hypnosis skills. For me, the research support of clinical treatment is most encouraging.

References

Baker, E. L. (2000). Reflections on the hypnotic relationship: Projective identification, containment, and attunement. *International Journal of Clinical and Experimental Hypnosis*, *48*(1), 56–69. 10.1080/00207140008410361

Barkham, M., & Lambert, M. (2021). The efficacy and effectiveness of psychological therapies. In M. Barkham, W. Lutz, & L. G. Castonguay (Eds), *Bergin and Garfield's Handbook of Psychotherapy and Behavior Change*, pp. 225–262.

Bateson, G. (2000). *Steps to an ecology of mind: Collected essays in anthropology, psychiatry, evolution, and epistemology*. University of Chicago Press.

Bongartz, W., & Bongartz, B. (2000). *Hypnosetherapie*. Hogrefe, Verlag für Psychologie.

Brown, D., & Fromm, E. (1986). *Hypnoanalysis and hypnotherapy*. Lawrence Erlbaum Associates.

Deci, E. L., & Flaste, R. (1995). *Why we do what we do: The dynamics of personal autonomy*. GP Putnam's Sons.

Deeley, Q., Oakley, D. A., Toone, B., Giampietro, V., Brammer, M. J., Williams, S. C., & Halligan, P. W. (2012). Modulating the default mode network using hypnosis. *International Journal of Clinical and Experimental Hypnosis*, *60*(2), 206–228. 10.1080/00207144.2012.648070

Dietrich, A. (2003). Functional neuroanatomy of altered states of consciousness: The transient hypofrontality hypothesis. *Consciousness and Cognition*, *12*(2), 231–256. 10.1016/s1053-8100(02)00046-6

Erickson, M. H. (1959). Further clinical techniques of hypnosis: Utilization techniques. *American Journal of Clinical Hypnosis*, *2*(1), 3–21. 10.1080/00029157.2009.10404314

Erickson, M. H. (1980). Collected papers. In E. Rossi (Ed), *Rossi*. Ervington.

Fourie, D. P. (1991). The ecosystemic approach to hypnosis. In S. J. Lyn , & W. Rhue (Eds), *Theories of hypnosis: Current models and perspectives* (pp. 467–484). Guilford Publications.

Frederick, C., & Phillips, M. M. (2007). Handbuch der Hypnotherapie bei posttraumatischen und dissoziativen Störungen. *Heidelberg: Carl Auer*, *2*.

Gerl, W. (2015). Reframing. In D. Revenstorf , & B. Peter (Eds), *Hypnose in Psychotherapie, Psychosomatik und Medizin* (pp. 253–263). Springer.

Gill, M. M., & Brenman, M. (1959). *Hypnosis and related states: Psychoanalytic studies in regression*. International University Press.
Greicius, M. D., Kiviniemi, V., Tervonen, O., Vainionpää, V., Alahuhta, S., Reiss, A. L., & Menon, V. (2008). Persistent default-mode network connectivity during light sedation. *Human Brain Mapping*, *29*(7), 839–847. 10.1080/00029157.2009.10404314
Greicius, M. D., Krasnow, B., Reiss, A. L., & Menon, V. (2003). Functional connectivity in the resting brain: A network analysis of the default mode hypothesis. *Proceedings of the National Academy of Sciences*, *100*(1), 253–258. 10.1073/pnas.0135058100
Gruzelier, J. (1998). A working model of the neurophysiology of hypnosis: A review of evidence. *Contemporary Hypnosis*, *15*(1), 3–21. 10.1002/ch.112
Halsband, U. (2015). Neurobiologie der Hypnose. In D. Revenstorf , & B. Peter (Eds), *Hypnose in Psychotherapie, Psychosomatik und Medizin* (pp. 795–816). Springer.
Iacoboni, M. (2009). *Mirroring people: The new science of how we connect with others*. Farrar, Straus, and Giroux.
Jones, E., & Gerard, H. (1967). *1967: Foundations of social psychology*. Wiley.
Kaiser-Rekkas, A. (2013). *Klinische Hypnose und Hypnotherapie: Praxisbezogenes Lehrbuch für die Ausbildung*. Carl-Auer Verlag.
Kanitschar, H. (2009). Hypnosepsychotherapie, ein integratives, tiefenpsychologisch fundiertes Verfahren. *Hypnose-ZHH*, *4*(1+2), 1–23.
Mende, M. (1984). *Die Wahrnehmung sozialer Interaktion* [Doctoral dissertation], Wien.
Mende, M. (1998). Hypnotherapeutic responses to transference in the face of therapeutic change. *Hypnos*, *25*, 134–144.
Mende, M. (2006). The special effects of hypnosis and hypnotherapy: A contribution to an ecological model of therapeutic change. *International Journal of Clinical and Experimental Hypnosis*, *54*(2), 167–185. 10.1080/00207140500528281
Mende, M. (2009). Die Utilisierung von Übertragung und Gegenübertragung in der lösungsorientierten Hypnotherapie. *Hypnose-ZHH*, *4*(1), 2.
Mende, M. (2021). Die strukturellen Dimensionen der Hypnotherapie: Ein Modell für die Planung, Gestaltung und Reflexion des hypnotherapeutischen Prozesses. In D. Revenstorf , & B. Peter (Eds), *Hypnose und Hypnotherapie: Manual für Praxis, Fortbildung und Lehre* (pp. 45–50). Carl-Auer Verlag.
Peter, B. (2015a). Hypnose und die Konstruktion von Wirklichkeit. In D. Revenstorf, & B. Peter (Eds), *Hypnose in Psychotherapie, Psychosomatik und Medizin* (pp. 37–45). Springer.
Peter, B. (2015b). Geschichte der Hypnose in Deutschland. In Revenstorf D. , & Peter B. (Eds), *Hypnose in Psychotherapie, Psychosomatik und Medizin* (pp. 817–851). Springer.
Reddemann, L. (2016). *Imagination als heilsame Kraft (Imagination als heilsame Kraft. Zur Behandlung von Traumafolgen mit ressourcenorientierten Verfahren): Ressourcen und Mitgefühl in der Behandlung von Traumafolgen* (Vol. 288). Klett-Cotta.
Revenstorf, D. (2015). Trance und die Ziele und Wirkungen der Hypnotherapie. In D. Revenstorf , & B. Peter (Eds), *Hypnose in Psychotherapie, Psychosomatik und Medizin* (pp. 13–35). Springer.
Revenstorf, D., & Peter, B. (2015). Kontraindikationen, BühnenhypnoseBühnenhypnose und Willenlosigkeit. In D. Revenstorf, & B. Peter (Eds), *Hypnose in Psychotherapie, Psychosomatik und Medizin* (pp. 125–151). Springer.
Rizzolatti, G., Fadiga, L., Matelli, M., Bettinardi, V., Paulesu, E., Perani, D., & Fazio, F. (1996). Localization of grasp representations in humans by PET: 1. Observation versus execution. *Experimental Brain Research*, *111*(2), 246–252. 10.1007/BF00227301
Sandi, C., & Pinelo-Nava, M. T. (2007). Stress and memory: Behavioral effects and neurobiological mechanisms. *Neural Plasticity*, *2007*, 1–20. 10.1155/2007/78970
Schmid, G. B. (2011). *Selbstheilung durch Vorstellungskraft*. Springer-Verlag.
Spiegel, H. (2007). The neural trance: A new look at hypnosis. *International Journal of Clinical and Experimental Hypnosis*, *55*(4), 387–410. 10.1080/00207140701506367
Woody, E. Z., & Sadler, P. (2008). Dissociation theories of hypnosis. In M. Nash , & A. Barnier (Eds), *The Oxford handbook of hypnosis: Theory, research, and practice*. Oxford University Press.

10

AN EMPIRICALLY-INFORMED INTEGRATIVE THEORY OF HYPNOSIS

Clinical Implications

Steven Jay Lynn[1], *Joseph P. Green*[2], *Anoushiravan Zahedi*[3], *Clément Apelian*[4], *and Irving Kirsch*[5]

[1]Psychology Department, Binghamton University, NY, USA; [2]Ohio State University, Lima, Ohio, USA; [3]Humboldt-Universitat Ze Berlin and Neuroscience Research Center, Charité-Universitätsmedizin, Berlin, Germany; [4]ARCHE Formation, Paris, France; [5]Harvard University Medical School, Program in Placebo Studies, Boston, MA, USA

Lynn et al. (2022) recently proposed a multi-variate integrative theory of hypnosis that updates and extends response set theory (Kirsch, 2000; Kirsch & Lynn, 1999) and earlier integrative models of hypnosis (Lynn & Rhue, 1991; Lynn et al., 2015a). Herein, we present clinical implications of our theory and the empirical basis of variables germane to clinical practice. We first summarize our model and supportive research and then discuss interventions that we extrapolate from the theory. Our clinical recommendations derive not only from theory and a large corpus of experimental studies but also from our clinical observations.

A cornerstone of our theory is that hypnosis unfolds independent of a background "trance" or special state of consciousness unique or specific to hypnosis. We argue that such a state is rendered irrelevant by findings that different hypnotic suggestions (i.e., direct imaginative suggestions) elicit diverse experiences and attendant alterations in consciousness (e.g., sensations, cognition, emotions, perceptions, memories), behaviors, and psychophysiological responses (Landry et al., 2017; Lynn et al., 2007), and no special state is required to experience a gamut of suggestions.

Additionally, in and apart from hypnosis, consciousness falls along a wide spectrum from alert wakefulness at one end to mind wandering in the middle and deep sleep and analgesia at the other end, with different experiences often shading into and overlapping subtly into one another (Monti, 2012). Hypnotic suggestions can be utilized to aggregate and direct spontaneous and evanescent experiences to virtually any point on this continuum of consciousness for research and treatment purposes. Suggestions thus elicit highly diverse states of consciousness with innumerable nuances and manifestations to facilitate adaptive experiences and responses.

 DOI: 10.4324/9781003449126-14

Although the definition of "hypnosis" is controversial (see, Lynn et al., 2015b), Lynn and Green (in press) contend that a strand of agreement exists across different definitions that suggestions can alter the spontaneous and contextually activated flow of thoughts, feelings, action tendencies, and behaviors in situations defined as hypnosis by an external agent (e.g., clinician, researcher) or as construed by the participant. A broad culture-based expectancy is that hypnosis produces significant shifts in subjective experiences. In fact, the potency of hypnosis to capitalize on the inherent malleability of consciousness is what potentially advantages hypnosis relative to other methodologies.

We view conscious experience as akin to a virtual reality simulation in which individuals construct meaningful and unique heuristic models of the self and the world (Miskovic & Lynn, 2023). We conceptualize hypnosis as a simulation within a simulation in which participants mentally model suggested events with varying degrees of conviction and verisimilitude. Hypnotic suggestions, related experiences, and goal-directed imaginings shape responses that reflect and facilitate response sets and behaviors with an assortment of clinical applications (Lynn et al., in press).

Response sets are expectancies and intentions that are coherent, dynamically emergent networks of mental associations, or representations that affect experiences, physiological functions, and behaviors (Lynn et al., in press). They are temporary states of readiness to respond in particular ways to particular stimuli, including hypnotic suggestions. Functionally, they prepare cognitive-behavioral-affective schemas, personal narratives, roles, and scripts for automatic (or at least highly efficient) activation when triggered.

Response sets vary from general (e.g., broad set to experience hypnosis) to specific (e.g., hand levitation, amnesia suggestions). When response sets form based on expectancies, they constitute expectations that a predicted event will occur nonvolitionally. In contrast, when intentional response sets form, the anticipated act is initiated with conscious awareness and agency. Intentions can be engaged to amplify motivation to attend to and imagine suggested events, discern suggestion-related cues and demands, and enact the role of a responsive hypnosis participant. Intentions can initiate actions perceived to be non-volitional based on demand characteristics (e.g., actions during hypnosis are nonvolitional), the passive wording of certain suggestions, and the automatic nature of behavior that marks much human action (see Kirsch & Lynn, 1999; Lynn et al., in press).

According to Erickson et al. (1976), the "therapeutic aspect of trance" occurs when "the limitations of one's usual conscious sets and belief systems are temporarily altered so that one can be receptive to an experience of other patterns of association and modes of mental functioning ... that are usually experienced as involuntary by the client" (p. 20). When adaptive sets are activated, they can be utilized to achieve important clinical objectives, including accessing personal resources, creating new perspectives, enhancing psychological flexibility, promoting motivation and engagement in novel behavioral repertoires, exploring value-based solutions to problems, and de-automatizing habitual ego-dystonic responses. According to our model, responsive participants strive to create cognitive-affective representations of suggested events that activate response sets and prime suggested behaviors. Successful responses reinforce a general positive response set toward hypnosis and positive expectancies regarding specific suggestions.

Our updated theory differs from previous integrative models in that it is based on the predictive coding model (Friston, 2010; Lynn et al., 2022), also called the Bayesian brain model (Clark, 2013). According to this model, we constantly compare predictions (aka expectations; De Lange et al., 2018) with information from multiple sources. When predictions and sensory information, for example, do not accord, it constitutes a prediction error: the difference between what is expected and actual occurrences. To build adaptive heuristic models, which achieve intended outcomes, humans are motivated to reduce prediction errors to better approximate the "true" (i.e., perception) or desired state of affairs (i.e., action) and thereby enhance adaptation, problem-solving, and goal attainment. In this view, participants integrate information from personal and interpersonal experiences and salient aspects of the environment to form a reliable predictive model of the external world. This model will be constantly evaluated based on sensory input (i.e., exteroceptive), proprioceptive, and interoceptive feedback.

Let's consider an example to clarify the previous point. If a participant expects to be responsive to every hypnotic suggestion, but sensory feedback does not confirm expectations with regard to, for instance, a difficult suggestion, such as a negative auditory hallucination, there would be a prediction error that should be resolved. When this occurs, we suggest that it alters response expectancies regarding that specific suggestion and general intentions to respond to suggestions as a person revises "downward" predictions of hypnosis. However, this might happen in multiple ways; for instance, the participant might modify their model regarding the capability of the hypnotist to offer a safe environment or an effective procedure, or alternatively, they might change their expectation regarding the vividness of hypnotic hallucination or their ability to respond to suggestions in general. When positive predictions and outcomes match, it reinforces positive expectancies. Whereas expectancies affect responsivity, responsivity, in turn, affects expectances recursively (Benham et al., 2006), often with minimal or no conscious awareness, perceived volition, or knowledge of response determinants. Moreover, response sets can be influenced by implicit and explicit beliefs, attitudes, and attributions, as they shape and are themselves shaped by expectancies (Schenk et al., 2017).

In clinical situations, adept practitioners are sensitive to participants' subtle and more obvious responses (Lynn et al., 2019). Skilled hypnotists scrupulously observe nuances in participants' verbal and nonverbal responses (e.g., breathing, affect, posture) and tailor interventions to participant feedback to enhance positive expectancies and facilitate attributions that hypnosis was successful, thereby promoting generalization of treatment gains.

Empirical Foundations

Ample evidence exists to conclude that hypnosis is an efficient and cost-effective intervention in treating a diversity of psychological and health-related maladies and in alleviating pain (Elkins, 2016; Lynn & Kirsch, 2006; Thompson et al., 2019). Fortunately, there exists a substantive theoretical and empirical base to guide practitioners. Defining the context as hypnosis, in itself, strengthens positive expectances, improves therapy outcomes, and increases hypnotic suggestibility to a small extent in research contexts (Gandhi & Oakley, 2005; Kirsch et al., 1995; Lynn & Kirsch, 2006). Kirsch and colleagues' (Kirsch et al., 1995) meta-analysis of 18 studies compared nonhypnotic cognitive-behavioral treatments with the same treatment conducted in a hypnotic context: Participants who received cognitive-behavioral hypnotherapy fared better than up to 90% of those who received the identical nonhypnotic treatment (Kirsch, 1994). Earlier in accounting for scant differences in the effectiveness of different hypnotic inductions (e.g., long vs. short, permissive vs. authoritative; suggestions ordered from easy to difficult or vice versa; Lynn et al., 2017; Terhune & Cardeña, 2016), Kirsch (1991) wrote: "The effectiveness of a hypnotic induction appears to depend entirely on people's beliefs about its effectiveness, and highly hypnotizable subjects respond in accordance with their beliefs about hypnotic responding" (p. 460).

Kirsch and Lynn's response set theory (1999), alongside Kirsch's earlier response expectancy theory (see Kirsch, 1997), contends that expectancies play an influential, if not a determinative, role in hypnotic responsiveness. Kirsch et al. (1995) reported that expectancies were the most robust predictor of hypnotic suggestibility among variables that spanned motivation, fantasy-proneness, and absorption. Later studies support a similar conclusion. A three-item expectancy measure correlated at $r = 0.53$ with hypnotic responsiveness, with more predictive power than measures of attitudes toward hypnosis, absorption, and fantasy proneness, and Braffman and Kirsch (1999) documented a similar correlation ($r = 0.59$) between expectancies and hypnotic suggestibility. Kirsch has argued that the generally small advantage of hypnotic suggestions over nonhypnotic suggestions might be attributable to enhanced expectancy and motivation elicited by the context of hypnosis (see Kirsch & Braffman, 2001 ; Terhune & Cardeña, 2016).

Clinical Applications

We have argued that enhancing positive expectancies regarding hypnosis is a viable empirically supported target of clinical intervention. According to Michael Yapko (2003): "If you were to ask me what single stage of the interaction most influences the rest, the overall success of the hypnosis session, I'd say it's the stage of deliberately building response sets" (p. 283). In contrast, the relevance of general personality characteristics to hypnosis is far less certain. Personality measures traits such as the "Big Five" (agreeableness, conscientiousness, openness to experience, extraversion, neuroticism) account for only 6% of the variability in hypnotic suggestibility (Green, 2004). Moreover, trait dissociation is not consistently or highly correlated with hypnotic responsivity (Kirsch & Lynn, 1998).

Still, our integrative theory contends that clinicians should consider other variables in addition to expectancies. A comprehensive account of hypnosis should encompass trait-like propensities that are more pinpointed to hypnotic experiences such as absorption, fantasy-proneness, and imaginative involvement, which typically are linked with hypnotic suggestibility in the range of $r = 0.2$ to $r = 0.4$ (e.g., Green & Lynn, 2008, 2011; Council et al., 1996). Hypnosis practitioners should encourage participants to get fully absorbed in suggested events and to imagine and fantasize along with suggestions, as low levels of imaginative ability and involvement are associated with low responsivity (see de Groh, 1989; Spanos, 1991).

Our theory also considers participant attitudes, beliefs, and motivation. Participants are rarely highly responsive—and may intentionally resist suggestions—if they possess strong negative attitudes and beliefs about hypnosis, which often originate in misleading media characterizations of hypnosis (Spanos et al., 1987). Clinicians should routinely assess for and debunk myths and misconceptions rather than assume that individuals—even those eager to be hypnotized—hold accurate views of hypnosis (Lynn & Green, in press).

Myths we suggest therapists target include beliefs that hypnotic suggestions cannot be resisted or opposed, that people lose touch with surroundings, that hypnosis produces temporary amnesia, and that individuals lose control of their experiences and actions. Attitudes and beliefs typically account for small (5–12%, Green, 2003, 2012) but significant variability in hypnotic responding. Nevertheless, very negative attitudes suppress hypnotic responsiveness and thereby underscore the imperative for therapists to address them.

We add the recommendation that hypnosis not be presented as a trance state, as doing so depresses responsivity (Lynn et al., 2002). Describing hypnosis in such vague general terms (a) is inconsistent with manifold cognitive, affective, and psychophysiological responses to suggestions and (b) increases participant uncertainty regarding whether such an ill-defined state can be achieved, thereby potentially mitigating positive expectations and strongly held response predictions.

Negative attitudes, beliefs, and an inability to imagine suggested events also dampen motivation, an important component of our model. Braffman and Kirsch (1999) found that the combination of expectancy, motivation, and responsivity to similar nonhypnotic suggestions accounted for more than half the variability in hypnotic suggestibility. Motivation enfolds into a broad set to be open to suggestions and can be facilitated by positive rapport with the hypnotist, which is another component of our theory (Gfeller et al., 1987; Lynn et al., 1991). High rapport promotes motivation to attune to role demands and please the hypnotist. In contrast, low rapport minimizes hypnotic involvement, increases distractibility and concerns regarding negative evaluation by the hypnotist, and decreases salience and potency of positive expectancies (Lynn et al., in press). Establishing positive rapport is especially important in enhancing responsivity among low responsive individuals (see Lynn et al., 1991). Clinicians can increase rapport by setting collaborative goals and modifying them, as appropriate; providing a credible rationale for hypnosis based on scientific findings; co-constructing suggestions; and expressing warmth, caring, and empathy for the participant.

We have suggested that a multifaceted response set—a composite of abilities and responses to hypnotic suggestions—underlies high hypnotic suggestibility and warrants recognition on the part of practitioners. Our theory extends observations (e.g., Lynn et al., in press) regarding a *readiness response set* (RRS) marked by a cognitive-affective-behavioral commitment or preparedness to respond to suggestions (Sheehan, 1991; Sheehan & McConkey, 1982; Tellegen, 1981). The finding that highly responsive participants continue to be highly responsive, even when hypnotic rapport is low, implies that they exhibit a distinctively high response readiness (Lynn et al., 1991).

We have observed that individuals who possess high hypnotic ability and enact the RRS maintain positive response expectances and "predictive certainty" regarding their hypnotic ability, despite confrontation with distracting thoughts, sensations, and emotions that would undermine responsiveness absent such a set. When individuals who possess a RRS become distracted, for example, they flexibly redeploy their attention to suggestions and/or ascribe greater salience to suggestions relative to critical thoughts. Moreover, they tend to not introspect or exhibit meta-cognitive awareness (Dienes & Perner, 2007; Lynn et al., 1991; Zahedi & Sommer, 2022; Zahedi et al., 2020, 2023), while they become immersed in suggestions and transform suggested events into felt sensations. Spanos and colleagues (Katsanis et al., 1989; Spanos et al., 1991) highlighted an active rather than a passive set in maximizing hypnotic responsivity. They found that interpreting suggestions as requiring active responding, rather than passively waiting for a suggestion to "happen," increased hypnotic suggestibility compared with not doing so. Further, adopting such a set afforded greater ability to predict hypnotic suggestibility compared with considering expectancies alone.

We suggest that an RRS can be created and facilitated in predisposed individuals. Clinicians can do the following to accomplish this goal: (a) provide accurate information about hypnosis; (b) invite participants to think, imagine, and absorb themselves in suggestions; "go with the flow"; and adopt an active response set; (c) exhort individuals to "feel suggested sensations" to the best of their ability; (d) suggest that participants redeploy attention to suggested events if their focus strays; (e) indicate that successful responses can entail a mix of voluntary and involuntary experiences; (f) implement permissive, indirect suggestions to elicit experiential resources (Lankton, 2021) and diminish feelings of "loss of control," as such suggestions are often experienced as voluntary (Lynn et al., 1993); (g) modify or contravene negative with positive self-suggestions (i.e., self-talk) and thereby deautomatize and depotentiate negative habitual response sets (Lankton, 2021; Yapko, 2003); and (h) set attainable "performance standards" for interpreting a suggested response as successful (e.g., "You don't have to create a perfectly lifelike hallucination in your imagination," see Lynn et al., 2003) to confirm and promote positive expectancies (Lynn et al., 2003).

To bypass unattainable performance standards, Milton Erickson, in his utilization approach, capitalized on participants' learnings "acquired through the process of living itself" (Erickson & Rossi, 1981, p. 8). He leveraged their attitudes, cognitions, emotions, behaviors, response sets, and resources to reinforce perceptions of success (Erickson, 2009). Moreover, stories and metaphors (e.g., see Casula chapter in this handbook) are a highly permissive nondirective method to seed therapeutic change and activate concepts and response sets consistent with treatment goals (Haley, 1973; Lankton, 2015, 2021).

To further optimize gains and bolster positive expectancies, clinicians can establish a positive rapport, as we noted earlier; determine what "worked in the past" (or did not succeed) if participants were hypnotized previously and modify their tactics accordingly; acknowledge and verbally and nonverbally reinforce even minor indications of responsiveness (e.g., eye closure, breathing changes); present "failsafe" suggestions and inductions to promote perceptions of success (see Lynn et al., 1996), especially when loss of control issues are salient; provide choices regarding inductions; tailor suggestions prior to and during hypnosis; and use posthypnotic suggestions to generalize and maintain gains (see Lynn & Kirsch, 2006).

We encourage clinicians to freely and creatively intermingle hypnotic and nonhypnotic suggestions and instructions and to shape response sets via embedding implementation intention instructions in treatment (Gollwitzer, 1999). Doing so breaks down a goal (e.g., responding to suggestions) into smaller steps, linking discrete goal-directed events or actions (e.g., imagining an event, accessing a personal resource) with specific hypnotic responses (e.g., relaxation, feelings of mastery). The clinician thus establishes "if-then" relations such that *if* a participant engages with a particular suggestion in a particular way, then the client will experience a desired outcome (Gollwitzer, 1999). Thus, the skilled clinician uses suggestions to create or augment response sets in a thoughtful stepwise manner to achieve desired goals in hypnosis such as thought suppression (see Gallo et al., 2012) or smoking cessation (Green & Lynn, 2017, see section 3 in this handbook).

Our perspective acknowledges individual differences in hypnotic abilities required to respond to different suggestions successfully (Barnier et al., 2022; Woody et al., 2005, Zahedi & Sommer, 2022). Some individuals, for example, might be more adept at creating visual images and responding to imaginative suggestions than to experiencing suggested sensations. Furthermore, highly suggestible individuals who are also highly dissociative experience hallucination suggestions more so than less dissociative individuals (Terhune et al., 2011), and some participants direct attention more inwardly than others (Terhune & Cardeña, 2010). Knowledge of such differences can help in customizing suggestions with a higher probability of attainment and thereby reinforce positive expectancies.

It is important that participants ascertain the cognitive requirements of passing suggestions and also be motivated to implement their abilities. For example, Wallace (1990) reported that some low-responsive individuals possess the capacity to imagine suggested events yet fail to do so because they do not choose to use imagery. Hypnotic suggestibility modification programs geared to enhance hypnotic suggestibility (Gorassini & Spanos, 1986; Carleton Skill Training Program) have capitalized on intention sets by (a) enhancing positive attitudes and beliefs about hypnosis, instructing participants regarding how to interpret suggestions, and (b) encouraging them to imagine along with suggestions, get absorbed in them, and adopt an active response set.

Conclusion

Our model is one iteration in our evolving understanding of hypnosis, the determinants of hypnotic responding, and the derivation of empirically supported methods to assist participants in achieving their potential in clinical contexts. Our intention is that the model be "open" to accommodate new findings and amenable to clarification and revision and that it stimulates interest in hypnosis in scientific and professional communities. We suggest that hypnosis will gain increasing acceptance and traction to the extent that it is tied to theory that is testable, linked to psychological processes and mechanisms of change, and is supported by a convincing body of evidence. We believe that our theory succeeds in many of these respects. Still, we look forward to future advancements in the study of hypnosis to enhance the potential to refine our theory and alleviate human suffering.

References

Barnier, A. J., Terhune, D. B., Polito, V., & Woody, E. Z. (2022). A componential approach to individual differences in hypnotizability. *Psychology of Consciousness: Theory, Research, and Practice*, 9(2), 130–140. 10.1037/cns0000267

Benham, G., Woody, E. Z., Wilson, K. S., & Nash, M. R. (2006). Expect the unexpected: Ability, attitude, and responsiveness to hypnosis. *Journal of Personality and Social Psychology*, *91*(2), 342–350. 10.1037/0022-3514.91.2.342

Braffman, W., & Kirsch, I. (1999). Imaginative suggestibility and hypnotizability: An empirical analysis. *Journal of Personality and Social Psychology*, *77*(3), 578–587. 10.1037/0022-3514.77.3.578

Clark, A. (2013). Whatever next? Predictive brains, situated agents, and the future of cognitive science. *Behavioral and Brain Sciences*, *36*(3), 181–204. 10.1017/S0140525X12000477

Council, J. R., Kirsch, I., & Grant, D. L. (1996). Imagination, expectancy, and hypnotic responding. In R. Kunzendorf, N. Spanos, & B. Wallace (Eds.), *Hypnosis and imagination* (pp. 41–65). Baywood Publishing.

de Groh, M. (1989). Correlates of hypnotic susceptibility. In N. P. Spanos & J. F. Chaves (Eds.), *Hypnosis: The cognitive-behavioral perspective* (pp. 32–63). Prometheus Books.

De Lange, F. P., Heilbron, M., & Kok, P. (2018). How do expectations shape perception? *Trends in Cognitive Sciences*, *22*(9), 764–779.

Dienes, Z., & Perner, J. (2007). Executive control without conscious awareness: The cold control theory of hypnosis. In G. A. Jamieson (Ed), *Hypnosis and conscious states: The cognitive neuroscience perspective* (pp. 293–314). Oxford University Press.

Elkins, G. R. (2016). *Handbook of medical and psychological hypnosis: Foundations, applications, and professional issues*. Springer Publishing Company.

Erickson, M. D. (2009). Further techniques of clinical hypnosis: Utilization techniques. *American Journal of Clinical Hypnosis*, *5*(14), 3–21.

Erickson, M. H., & Rossi, E. L. (1981). Experiencing hypnosis. Irvington.

Erickson, M. H., Rossi, E. L., & Rossi, S. I. (1976). *Hypnotic realities: The induction of clinical hypnosis and forms of indirect suggestion*. Irvington Publishers.
Friston, K. (2010). The free-energy principle: A unified brain theory? *Nature Reviews: Neuroscience*, *11*(2), 127–138. 10.1038/nrn2787
Gallo, I. S., Pfau, F., & Gollwitzer, P. M. (2012). Furnishing hypnotic instructions with implementation intentions enhances hypnotic responsiveness. *Consciousness and Cognition*, *21*(2), 1023–1030.
Gandhi, B., & Oakley, D. A. (2005). Does "hypnosis" by any other name smell as sweet? The efficacy of "hypnotic" inductions depends on the label "hypnosis". *Consciousness and Cognition*, *14*, 304–315.
Gfeller, J. D., Lynn, S. J., & Pribble, W. E. (1987). Enhancing hypnotic susceptibility: Interpersonal and rapport factors. *Journal of Personality and Social Psychology*, *52*(3), 586–595.10.1037/0022-3514.52.3.586
Gollwitzer, P. M. (1999). Implementation intentions: Strong effects of simple plans. *American Psychologist*, *54*, 493–503.
Gorassini, D. R., & Spanos, N. P. (1986). A social-cognitive skills approach to the successful modification of hypnotic susceptibility. *Journal of Personality and Social Psychology*, *50*(5), 1004.
Green, J. P. (2003). Beliefs about hypnosis: Popular beliefs, misconceptions, and the importance of experience. *International Journal of Clinical and Experimental Hypnosis*, *51*(4), 369–381. 10.1076/iceh.51.4.369.16408
Green, J. P. (2004). The five factor model of personality and hypnotizability: Little variance in common. *Contemporary Hypnosis*, *21*(4), 161–168. 10.1002/ch.303
Green, J. P. (2012). The Valencia scale of attitudes and beliefs toward hypnosis (Client) version and hypnotizability. *International Journal of Clinical and Experimental Hypnosis*, *60*(2), 229–240. 10.1080/00207144.2012.648073
Green, J. P., & Lynn, S. J. (2008). Fantasy-proneness and hypnotizability: Another look. *Contemporary Hypnosis*, *25*(3-4), 156–164. 10.1002/ch.360
Green, J. P., & Lynn, S. J. (2010). Hypnotic responsiveness: Expectancy, attitudes, fantasy proneness, absorption, and gender. *International Journal of Clinical and Experimental Hypnosis*, *59*(1), 103–121. 10.1080/00207144.2011.522914
Green, J. P., & Lynn, S. J. (2017). A multifaceted hypnosis smoking cessation program: Enhancing motivation and goal attainment. *International Journal of Clinical and Experimental Hypnosis*, *65*, 308–335.
Haley, J. (1973). *Uncommon therapy: The psychiatric techniques of Milton H. Erickson, M.D.* New York: Norton.
Katsanis, J., Barnard, J., & Spanos, N. P. (1989). Self-predictions, interpretational set and imagery vividness as determinants of hypnotic responding. *Imagination, Cognition and Personality*, *8*(1), 63–77.
Kirsch, I. (1991). The social learning theory of hypnosis. In S. J. Lynn, & J. W. Rhue (Eds.), *Theories of hypnosis: Current models and perspectives* (pp. 439–465). Guilford Press.
Kirsch, I. (1994). Clinical hypnosis as a nondeceptive placebo: Empirically derived techniques. *American Journal of Clinical Hypnosis*, *37*(2), 95–106. 10.1080/00029157.1994.10403122
Kirsch, I. (1997). Response expectancy theory and application: A decennial review. *Applied and Preventive Psychology*, *6*(2), 69–79. 10.1016/S0962-1849(05)80012-5
Kirsch, I. (2000). The response set theory of hypnosis. *American Journal of Clinical Hypnosis*, *42*(3-4), 274–292. 10.1080/00029157.2000.10734362
Kirsch, I., & Braffman, W. (2001). Imaginative suggestibility and hypnotizability. *Current Directions in Psychological Science*, *10*, 57–61.
Kirsch, I., & Lynn, S. J. (1998). Dissociation theories of hypnosis. *Psychological Bulletin*, *123*(1), 100–115. 10.1037/0033-2909.123.1.100
Kirsch, I., & Lynn, S. J. (1999). The automaticity of behavior and clinical psychology. *American Psychologist*, *54*(7), 504–515. 10.1037/0003-066X.54.7.504
Kirsch, I., Montgomery, G., & Sapirstein, G. (1995). Hypnosis as an adjunct to cognitive-behavioral psychotherapy: A meta-analysis. *Journal of Consulting and Clinical Psychology*, *63*(2), 214–220. 10.1037/0022-006X.63.2.214

Landry, M., Lifshitz, M., & Raz, A. (2017). Brain correlates of hypnosis: A systematic review and meta-analytic exploration. *Neuroscience & Biobehavioral Reviews*, *81*(Part A), 75–98. 10.1016/j.neubiorev.2017.02.020

Lankton, S. R. (2015). *The answer within: A clinical framework of Ericksonian hypnotherapy*. Routledge.

Lankton, S. R. (2021). What Milton Erickson said about being Ericksonian. *American Journal of Clinical Hypnosis*, *63*(1), 4–13. 10.1080/00029157.2020.1574068

Lynn, S. J., & Green, J. P. (in press). An introduction to evidence-based practice in clinical hypnosis. In L. Milling (Ed.), *Evidence-based practice in clinical hypnosis*. American Psychological Association.

Lynn, S. J., Green, J. P., Jaquith, L., & Gasior, D. (2003). Hypnosis and performance standards. *International Journal of Clinical and Experimental Hypnosis*, *51*(1), 51–65. 10.1076/iceh.51.1.51.14062

Lynn, S. J., Green, J. P., Kirsch, I., Capafons, A., Lilienfeld, S. O., Laurence, J-R., Montgomery, G. H. (2015b). Grounding hypnosis in science: The "new" APA Division 30 definition of hypnosis as a step backwards. *American Journal of Clinical Hypnosis*, *57*(4), 290–301. 10.1080/00029157.2015.1011472

Lynn, S. J., Green, J. P., Polizzi, C. P., Ellenberg, S., Guatam, A., & Aksen, D. (2019). Hypnosis, hypnotic phenomena, and hypnotic responsiveness: Clinical and research foundations – A 40-year perspective. *International Journal of Clinical and Experimental Hypnosis*, *67*(4), 475–511.

Lynn, S. J., Green, J. P., Zahedi, A., & Apelian, C. (2022). The response set theory of hypnosis reconsidered: Toward an integrative model. *The American Journal of Clinical Hypnosis 65*, (pp. 1–25). Advance online publication. 10.1080/00029157.2022.2117680

Lynn, S. J., & Kirsch, I. (2006). *Essentials of clinical hypnosis: An evidence-based approach*. American Psychological Association. 10.1037/11365-000

Lynn, S. J., Kirsch, I., Knox, J., Fassler, O., & Lilienfeld, S. O. (2007). Hypnosis and neuroscience: Implications for the altered state debate. In G. A. Jamieson(Ed.), *Hypnosis and conscious states: The cognitive neuroscience perspective* (pp. 145–165). Oxford University Press.

Lynn, S. J. E., Kirsch, I. E., & Rhue, J. W. (1996). *Casebook of clinical hypnosis*. American Psychological Association.

Lynn, S. J., Laurence, J. R., & Kirsch, I. (2015a). Hypnosis, suggestion, and suggestibility: An integrative model. *American Journal of Clinical Hypnosis*, *57*(3), 314–329. 10.1080/00029157.2014.976783

Lynn, S. J., Maxwell, R., & Green, J. P. (2017). Hypnotic induction in the broad scheme of hypnosis: A sociocognitive perspective. *American Journal of Clinical Hypnosis*, *59*, 363–384.

Lynn, S. J., Neufeld, V., & Maré, C. (1993). Direct versus indirect suggestions: A conceptual and methodological review. *International Journal of Clinical and Experimental Hypnosis*, *41*(2), 124–152.

Lynn, S. J., & Rhue, J. W. (1991). An integrative model of hypnosis. In S. J. Lynn & J. W. Rhue (Eds.), *Theories of hypnosis: Current models and perspectives* (pp. 397–438). Guilford Press.

Lynn, S. J., Vanderhoff, H., Shindler, K., & Stafford, J. (2002). Defining hypnosis as a trance vs. cooperation: Hypnotic inductions, suggestibility, and performance standards. *American Journal of Clinical Hypnosis*, *44*(3-4), 231–240. 10.1080/00029157.2002.10403483

Lynn, S. J., Weekes, J., Brentar, J., Neufeld, V., Zivney, O., & Weiss, F. (1991). Interpersonal climate and hypnotizability level: Effects on hypnotic performance, rapport, and archaic involvement. *Journal of Personality and Social Psychology*, *60*(5), 739–743. 10.1037/0022-3514.60.5.739

Miskovic, V., & Lynn, S. J. (2023). *Dreaming reality: Meditations on human consciousness*. Unpublished manuscript.

Monti, M. M. (2012). Cognition in the vegetative state. *Annual Review of Clinical Psychology*, *8*, 431–454. 10.1146/annurev-clinpsy-032511-143050

Schenk, L. A., Sprenger, C., Onat, S., Colloca, L., & Büchel, C. (2017). Suppression of striatal prediction errors by the prefrontal cortex in placebo hypoalgesia. *The Journal of Neuroscience*, *37*(40), 9715–9723. doi:10.1523/jneurosci.1101-17.2017

Sheehan, P. W. (1991). Hypnosis, context, and commitment. In S. J. Lynn and J. W. Rhue (Eds.), *Theories of hypnosis: Current models and perspectives* (pp. 520–541). Guilford Press.

Sheehan, P. W., & McConkey, K. M. (1982). *Hypnosis and experience: The exploration of penomena and process*. Routledge.
Spanos, N. P., Brett, P. J., Menary, E. P., & Cross, W. P. (1987). A measure of attitudes toward hypnosis: Relationships with absorption and hypnotic susceptibility. *American Journal of Clinical Hypnosis*, *30*, 139–150.
Spanos, N. P. (1991). A sociocognitive approach to hypnosis. In S. J. Lynn and J. W. Rhue (Eds.), *Theories of hypnosis: Current models and perspectives* (pp. 324– 361). Guilford Press.
Spanos, N. P., Gabora, N. J. & Hyndford, C. (1991). Expectations and interpretations in hypnotic responding. *Australian Journal of Clinical and Experimental Hypnosis*, *19*, 87–96.
Tellegen, A. (1981). Practicing the two disciplines for relaxation and enlightenment: Comment on "Role of the feedback signal in electromyograph biofeedback: The relevance of attention" by Qualls and Sheehan. *Journal of Experimental Psychology: General*, *110*(2), 217–226. 10.1037/0096-3445.110.2.217
Terhune, D. B., & Cardeña, E. (2010). Differential patterns of spontaneous experiential response to a hypnotic induction: A latent profile analysis. *Consciousness and Cognition*, *19*, 1140–1150.
Terhune, D. B., Cardeña, E., & Lindgren, M. (2011). Dissociated control as a signature of typological variability in high hypnotic suggestibility. *Consciousness and Cognition*, *20*(3), 727–736. 10.1016/j.concog.2010.11.005
Terhune, D. B., & Cardeña, E. (2016). Nuances and uncertainties regarding hypnotic inductions: Toward a theoretically informed praxis. *American Journal of Clinical Hypnosis*, *59*(2), 155–174.
Thompson, T., Terhune, D. B., Oram, C., Sharangparni, J., Rouf, R., Solmi, M., ... Stubbs, B. (2019). The effectiveness of hypnosis for pain relief: A systematic review and meta-analysis of 85 controlled experimental trials. *Neuroscience & Biobehavioral Reviews*, *99*, 298–310. 10.1016/j.neubiorev.2019.02.013
Wallace, B. (1990). Imagery vividness, hypnotic susceptibility, and the perception of fragmented stimuli. *Journal of Personality and Social Psychology*, *58*(2), 354–359. 10.1037/0022-3514.58.2.354
Woody, E. Z., Barnier, A. J., & McConkey, K. M. (2005). Multiple hypnotizabilities: Differentiating the building blocks of hypnotic response. *Psychological Assessment*, *17*(2), 200–211. 10.1037/1040-3590.17.2.200
Yapko, M. D. (2003). *Trancework: An introduction to the practice of clinical hypnosis* (3rd ed.). Routledge.
Zahedi, A., Lynn, S.J., & Sommer, W. (2023). How hypnotic suggestions work – A systematic review of prominent theories of hypnosis. PsyArxiv Preprints[MOU1]. https://doi.org/10.31234/osf.io/mp9bs[jl2]
Zahedi, A., & Sommer, W. (2022). Can hypnotic susceptibility be explained by bifactor models? Structural equation modeling of the Harvard group scale of hypnotic susceptibility–Form A. *Consciousness and Cognition*, *99*, 103289. 10.1016/j.concog.2022.103289
Zahedi, A., Sturmer, B., & Sommer, W. (2020). Can posthypnotic suggestions boost updating in working memory? Behavioral and ERP evidence. *Neuropsychologia*, *148*, 107632. 10.1016/j.neuropsychologia.2020.107632

From Theory to the Art of Practice

11
RAPID HYPNOTIC INDUCTIONS

Gabor Filo
DENTISTRY870, HAMILTON, ON, CANADA

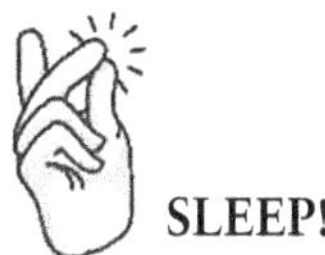

SLEEP!

When most of us imagine a rapid hypnotic induction what comes to mind is the hypnotist intently staring into the subject's eyes, a snap of the fingers and a forceful command of sleep whereupon the subject drops into a deep trance. This is a long-standing cultural meme. Films, broadcast television and YouTube are replete with examples (Barrett, 2006a). Is this not anathema for a clinical hypnosis practitioner?

Would it surprise you to learn that Milton Erickson was not averse to demonstrating rapid inductions in his workshops? His famous handshake induction was not only rapid, but he also did it as pantomime (Erickson, 1961, 1964)!

As a dentist of 40 years experience in venues ranging from private and group to hospital practice, the need for rapid inductions became apparent to me. Dental practice constraints such as scheduling, treatment time, the economics of hypnodontics amongst many daily underscore the need, hence my long-standing quest for the grail of clinically useful rapid or instantaneous inductions.

Yet today, most clinicians are rarely taught rapid or instantaneous inductions. Perhaps this is due to the connotations of stage hypnosis, the influence of Ericksonian hypnosis, or the shift of hypnosis as a therapeutic modality from the "hands-on" medical and dental clinicians to preponderantly mental health professionals. I am going to make a case that this knowledge is valuable and should be familiar to all clinicians using hypnosis.

Before venturing any further, we have to define the parameters of rapid and instantaneous inductions. Ralph Harry Vincent defined the timing of inductions in 1893 stating, "By a skillful operator a large proportion will be hypnotized in times varying from fifty seconds to four minutes" (Vincent, 1893). Note that he did not specifically refer to rapid inductions, but to the whole art of induction. We will address the possible underlying reasons for this span as we progress.

Barber's Rapid Induction Analgesia is the most notable rapid induction by name; however, it is not rapid (Barber, 1977). The format of the induction involves 20 minutes to achieve analgesia which in the hands-on professions is untenable for a variety of reasons from time management considerations to the economics of practice.

DOI: 10.4324/9781003449126-16

So, we need a graspable definition for rapid inductions and the one that makes the most sense to me is based on a well-known induction sequence created by Dave Elman. The entire sequence can be administered in three minutes with the potential of achieving hypnoanesthesia and the Esdaile coma, explained shortly (Elman, 1964). It has successfully been used to ameliorate pain in austere back country environments in patients with second degree burns to dislocated shoulders.

Instantaneous inductions are those that take less than 60 seconds. Many of these are used in the entertainment hypnosis world. They can also be used clinically by the astute clinician in the appropriate context. Vincent's (1893) 130-year-old definition is germane today.

Let me outline Elman's induction. He administered this in a very authoritarian manner, though it can be done permissively. The process begins with a deep breathe followed by eyelid catalepsy, i.e., the eye lids are suggested to be so relaxed as to be non-functional, glued together. There are three series of suggestions for this with a challenge of "*try*" to open them after the suggestion of "*when you are sure that they do not work*" ending each series. With each series the eyes are to double in relaxation and the inability to function. At the end of the third series of suggestions, the challenge is omitted.

Next the patient is asked to develop an amnesia by starting to count backward from 100, slowly, and with each number the relaxation should double each time ... and when they reach the number 98, they can forget the numbers. They are asked if they have forgotten the numbers. If the answer is yes, then the next step is to evoke a glove anesthesia by way of three strokes of the hand with suggestions between strokes to induce the sensation change. To validate this to the patient, an eyes-open state follows in which they are told "*to stay just the way they are and open their eyes*". At this point, they can be asked to notice the difference between hands or a more definitive test of anesthesia can be demonstrated – pinch of the skin or a needle through the skin (something from the past, rarely done today in a clinical context). Once ratified, the anesthesia can be resolved and the therapeutic work can begin.

If, however, a much more profound state is required, then the patient can be asked while still in trance, "*since you have experienced physical relaxation, would you like to experience mental relaxation as well*"? If they answer in the affirmative, then an elevator descent of three floors to the "basement of relaxation" can be started with appropriate imagery for entering the elevator and pushing the down button. Each floor doubles the state of relaxation, until finally the basement is reached. I usually have the patient exit the elevator and go to a safe room. This state is known as the Esdaile coma (Elman, 1984; Filo, 2012).

Pros and Cons

Time

Time is a limited commodity in healthcare professions: medicine, dentistry, first responders, etc. and as such, a protracted induction is not ideal. Not only is the time available for care a limiting factor, but this is also heavily influenced by the economics of healthcare. "The milieu is busy and noisy, such as in emergency rooms or pre-operative suites, or when the patient is experiencing acute stress, anxiety, fear, or pain" (Sunnen, 2011). Acute situations that could lead to serious morbidity do not favor conventional inductions. This may also apply in the mental health context.

Another perspective that underscores the concept of efficiency is offered by Gerald Kein. Let me quote him directly, "for many years the use of clinical instant and rapid inductions was unheard of by the hypnosis practitioner. Instructors were never taught the advantages of using these inductions, how to use them or they were simply ignored ... Many issues that normally require two sessions can be cut to one, with the use of these rapid inductions. If clients are scheduled every hour, just imagine how much more time can be allocated to work with client issues if they are in deep hypnosis within ten minutes from the time they walk into the session" (Kein, 2016). Perhaps there is an ethical issue to consider in this perspective as well.

Time translates into money both as the costs to the patient and the overhead associated with supplying care. In the day and age of brief therapies and third-party payers dictating care, caregivers are constrained to look for clinical efficiencies.

The cons of using rapid inductions are revealed in a study done by Casiglia and cow-orkers. They noted "a cardiovascular response to hypnotic deepening, underlying the stimulating, stressing effect of every technique, particularly of those performed without suggesting relaxation" (Casiglia et al., 2012, p. 351). Hence, one should carefully consider using a rapid technique in a cardiovascular compromised patient. The careful selection of the patient and the type of induction is important. Many rapid inductions are physical in nature and not appropriate for all patients or contexts.

What Are the Prerequisites for Rapid Inductions?

Rapid inductions, like the more protracted methods, have several conditions that need fulfilling to be effective. Without these prerequisites, rapid inductions will likely fail. They can be divided into those pertaining to the patient and to the clinician.

Patient Requirements

To be truly effective, the patient must have a need, be motivated, and believe (Ewin, 1979). In the clinical context, the need must be compelling. That is, hypnosis may be the "last port in the storm" or at that moment nothing else will offer the same solution as efficaciously.

Motivation must be present (White, 1966). Hypnosis must be appealing to the patient, not acquiescing to someone else's agenda. In obstetrics, natural childbirth always has the fallback position of the epidural. Societal trends are such that the "magic pill" will instantly solve the problem. So why have a personal investment of time, money, energy, or accountability for self-help? A wave of the magic wand will let it be someone else's problem, not mine. If the axiom, "all hypnosis is self-hypnosis" is true, then the patient must be vested.

Belief is paramount either in the clinician or the hypnotic procedure, but preferentially both. Trance validation which is a component of inductions is predicated on convincing of the conscious mind. Placebo works because of belief and a relationship with the practitioner (Kaptchuk, 2010). Placebo is an example of what Elman and others have referred to as walking or waking hypnosis (Elman, 1964; Wells, 1966). It is an instruction that is believed and efficacious.

Belief is facilitated if there is rapport between the clinician and the patient. Rapport is a complex concept. Shaw (1958) contends that it is an interplay composed of a ratio of the subject's mindset and the operator's prestige.

The subject's mindset should be one of positive expectancy. Clinicians, as well as entertainers, devote some time to creating this in the subject. Obviously, the stage hypnotist has an easier time of this than the clinician since most audience members and potential participants in the show are expecting an entertaining time compared to a clinical care visit – especially if it's the dentist. The counterbalance, the prestige factor, is paramount. If the clinician is known as "the" clinical hypnotist, "the go to clinician," then the likelihood of the subject's expectancy being high is greater.

Clinician Requirements

To be effective with rapid inductions, one must have a broad base of them stored away in one's repertoire. As much as scripts are frowned upon in general, the clinician should have the gist of many and varied inductions at their command. Each will have a central phrase or maneuver that is the catalyst of the induction. The clinical literature – contemporary or historical – does not refer to many rapid inductions, nor for that matter does the lay literature. Space precludes describing them, but Filo (2012) has collected many from various sources, and demonstrates them in a DVD.

The clinician should be able to segue from one to another in response to the patient. This is the norm in conventional inductions; yet with rapid inductions, it is even more important to be able to do this for full effect. Generally, many of the rapid and instantaneous inductions have points at which the clinician will have only moments to achieve the trance or lose the opportunity altogether. These moments are those that occur when a startle has been affected or a pattern interrupted in which the patient has turned inward to find the correct response. To aid in this momentary "freeze" the clinician offers the solution with a suggestion.

This returns us to Shaw's concept of rapport. In the novice clinician's career, it is more about technique than about prestige. Hence, you must present confidence and "fake it 'til you make it"! Your repertoire must be broad, having many induction techniques. Once you have the reputation and the experience, it is the prestige factor that carries weight with the patients. Whether one wishes to accept it or not, this is synonymous with the entertainer – the stage hypnotist. Shakespeare was quite right when he said all the world's a stage. Metaphorically, a clinical encounter is theatrical in substance and the performance is more important.

There are always exceptions to rules. There are four situations in which rapport is not necessary. These are emergencies, covert hypnosis, street hypnosis, and stage hypnosis. Dabney Ewen said it best about emergencies; you don't need rapport, just credentials (Ewin, 2009). Covert hypnosis is a broad field for which there is limited space here, but the writings of Kevin Hogan (2001) should offer much food for thought. Street hypnosis varies from mere entertainment to nefarious activities (Temple, 1989). As with covert hypnosis, space precludes an in-depth discussion. Suffice it to say that it is a form of covert hypnosis and its induction ranges from instantaneous to rapid in nature.

So just how there is an equivalency between the clinical world and the entertainers? Let us consider that both work within a proscenium arch – the entertainer literally, the clinician metaphorically. Our clinical contexts have a defined setting, scenery – the contents of a dental operatory or a hospital emergency room with beds and equipment, protagonists, and auxiliary players all interacting as defined by their specific roles, along with a cacophonous background "musical score."

There is expectancy and trepidation on the part of the patient. They may already be in a self-induced altered state when arriving to the clinical setting (Hope & Sugarman, 2015). This is especially true of those arriving by ambulance with serious life-threatening conditions (Ewin, 2009). Entertainers utilize this expectancy and mild self-induced altered states of the audience to their advantage. This altered state is also enhanced by the theatrical circumstances, similar to the stage setting of the clinical milieu. Thus, the work of the hypnotist is to apply technique to deepen the existing altered state; of course one must be able to recognize it!

Many of the techniques of the stage inductions are quite pervasive. To illustrate, Capafons (1998) describes a rapid self-hypnotic induction that Arons wrote about (Aarons, 1953) in the 1950s and is derived strictly from the stage. Elman's induction (Elman, 1964), known far and wide, is a derivative of his theatrical days and many of the components of it are widely dispersed throughout clinical use. Components of the hypnotizability scales can find their antecedents on the stage. Ultimately, we must remember that clinical hypnosis in its infancy was largely disseminated by public demonstrations. James Braid, Scottish surgeon and pioneer of hypnosis, first became interested in magnetism after having witnessed Charles Lafontaine's public demonstration at the Manchester Athenæum on Saturday, 13 November 1841. These demonstrations had features of the theatrical while attempting to introduce the laity and the clinician to the wonders of hypnosis.

Stage hypnotists leverage time to be repetitive and emphatic (there is the utilization of fractionation in the candidate selection process). A show must be well paced and the climactic routines take place toward the end of the performance with the most responsive audience members. They cannot waste time. This is not unlike most dental practices, medical offices, and hospitals. Economics demands a well-managed schedule excluding any treatment activity that is not an intentional loss leader.

Thus, to sum up the comparison of clinical and stage hypnosis: leverage time, set the stage figuratively and literally create expectation and anticipation, and control all aspects of the performance (clinical interaction) from the external to the internal by careful preparation and selection.

Induction Types

There are many types of rapid inductions which I have categorized into the following groupings in Table 11.1.

Most of the category names are self-evident as to what generally transpires in the induction. As stated elsewhere, these are not pristine categories as they usually have intermingled components. The listed categories may also not be completely addressing the most frequently encounter types.

Table 11.1 Types of Rapid Inductions

Handshake	Pantomime/non-verbal
Hand clasp	Imaginational
Balance based	Alert
Catalepsy	Miscellaneous
Eye fixation/fascination	Shock
Kinetic	Never use – dangerous /no clinical use

There are two categories that warrant mention: shock and the never-use. The shock induction that I first encountered more than 50 years ago was a description of a severely burned patient entering the emergency department. The physician on duty lunged at him with outstretched arms and commanded sleep. This patient would have been in a sympathetic nervous system-driven hypnoidal state from the trauma of the burns, so the sleep command offered an escape from the life-threatening situation.

Shock inductions rarely have utility, but to speak a language fully, the entire vocabulary should be known – even words your mother would not have approved! One never knows when it may be a useful technique in a less dramatic form than the one described.

The *never-use* category includes ethically questionable ones such as the use of toothache suggestions while tapping of the patient's jaw which is attributed to X. Lamotte Sage (Aarons, 1953) and distinctly dangerous techniques such as Alexander Canon's occidental method where pressure is applied to the whites of the eyes (Edmonston, 1986) or carotid artery pressure techniques (Boris, 1963; Edmonston, 1986; Hartland, 1972; McGill, 1996).

Mechanisms

The underlying mechanism of rapid inductions consists of one or more of the following either individually or in a combination: (1) a startle or surprise, (2) a pattern interruption, (3) postural reflex utilization, physiological phenomena, (4) emotional regression, (5) imagery, (6) non-verbal communications, gestures, or pantomime, and (7) waking hypnosis.

Most of the listed mechanisms are all essentially a startle, a surprise, or even a shock. The startle response is "a largely unconscious defensive response to sudden or threatening stimuli, such as sudden noise or sharp movement, and is associated with negative affect. Usually the onset of the startle response is a startle reflex reaction. The startle reflex is a brainstem reflectory reaction (reflex) that serves to protect vulnerable parts, such as the back of the neck (whole-body startle) and the eyes (eyeblink) and facilitates escape from sudden stimuli. It is found across the lifespan of many species. A variety of responses may occur depending on the affected individual's emotional state, body posture, preparation for execution of a motor task, or other activities" (Startle response, 2022).

Usually with a startle, there is an automatic momentary freeze, a catalepsy, while we internally attempt to search out the appropriate response to the startle stimulus. Cheek considered this catalepsy as a part of the spontaneously occurring animal survival mechanism (Cheek, 1994). It is in that moment that given a command that resolves our catalepsy by offering the answer for which the internal scans are looking, that the induction starts and must be immediately deepened. The axiom is "rapid in, rapid out!" meaning that unless deepening is pursued instantly, the subject will reorient straightaway.

A confounded handshake is an example of a pattern interruption. Elman, (1964), Erickson, (1964), and others have variations on the handshake induction. At the heart of this pattern interruption is essentially a startle, "what's next?" that causes the momentary catalepsy which can then be deepened either verbally, kinesthetically, or both.

Many of the postural reflex-based inductions are all physical in nature usually from a standing position. Once the subject is positioned to be unknowingly slightly off balance, that precarious position is pushed to be fully off balance by some means outside of the subject's awareness. This is the moment of startle or surprise and the inserted direct command of sleep starts the induction followed by an immediate deepening. These types of physically disorienting inductions do not have clinical utility, but you never know when it may be useful.

Emotional regressions as inductions generally do not have a startle. They may have a surprise that is gently elicited. My favourite induction of this sort is a derivative of a stage induction I refer to as the Golden Moment (Angel, 2006; Filo, 2012). It consists of asking the patient to take a deep breathe and let it out slowly while getting comfortable. Then to remember a moment from their life that they consider to be a golden moment, that they would wish would last an eternity. Once they have the memory, they are instructed to go there now. If you have a dental chair, as I do, with an automatic recline feature, the chair is activated to recline as they are instructed to "go back there now." The kinesthetic action of the backward moving dental chair is a non-verbal deepening suggestion. Once reclined, further appropriate deepening instructions are given.

Imagery offers a broad tapestry of possibilities. Novelty within the imagery may be the surprise, though it is not needed. My favorite such induction I experienced at my first formal workshop 40 years ago. It was delivered by my colleague Victor Rausch. The essence involves imagining a color transition from blue, purple to violet. The object is to have each color experienced with the entire sensorium through each of the transitions. Pleasant associations should be chosen. The only instruction given to the patient about the colors is not to worry if one color is harder to experience than another. The elegance of this induction is that the imagery is totally generated by the patient. Once the violet is reached, it can be morphed into a protective white envelope or the patient may be directed to their happy place or safe room (Filo, 2012).

Non-verbal communications, gestures, or pantomime can also be very rapid. Erickson's handshake induction combines the "hypnotic stare" and a very cunning pattern interruption in the handshake itself (Erickson, 1964). Non-verbal suggestions for eye closure are given by defocusing one's eyes and slowly half-closing them as you stare into the eyes of the patient (actually the bridge of their nose), and the handshake is experienced as indistinctive and featureless when compared to a conventional handshake. Since the patient is perplexed by the experience, this is where the startle or surprise hides. The patient is confused by the irregular handshake so in that surprised state the easiest escape from their confusion is to retreat inward from the confusion. It should lead to an arm catalepsy when you remove your hand from their's.

Another favourite induction of mine is an arm catalepsy that may be done verbally or totally non-verbally. The induction was used by Hartland almost exclusively (Matheson & Grehan, 1979). In my non-verbal derivation, it involves holding the patient's wrist while their arm is outstretched. Gentle tugging on the wrist with a slightly upward angle from the horizontal of the arm aids in establishing an arm rigidity. When you sense the catalepsy, mesmeric passes as they are known, moving hands without contact, an inch above the subject's skin, from the head down to the finger tips until you notice that moment when eye closure in the subject can be elicited by a downward pass in front of their eyes (Filo, 2012). At this point, verbal deepening or intensification is followed and may be done by gently pushing the head downward and pressing down on their shoulders.

Wesley Raymond Wells described a method of induction which is called waking hypnosis (Wells, 1966). Though known since 1923, it is infrequently discussed. It can be debated whether it is merely direct suggestion or a form of alert hypnosis. Elman defined it as, "when hypnotic effects are achieved without the use of the trance state. In every case, it involves a bypass of the critical faculty and implanting of selective thinking" (Elman, 1964, p. 67).

Waking hypnosis works best when the patient is already in a hypnoidal state – this would be the phobic dental patient or the patient in the emergency room. Recognizing their slightly altered state and giving direct suggestions for the desired outcome should allow for deepening and the establishing of a conventional trance state.

Physiology and Phenomenology

Discussing the physiology and phenomenology of hypnotic inductions and rapid inductions specifically is challenging. Woody and Sadler (2016) give a very nice overview of the inherent problems in their discussions about what a hypnotic induction can do. They refer to conventional inductions specifically and do not address rapid inductions. Their observations would likely be appropriate for rapid inductions if we accept Vincent's statement.

In discussing the definitions of hypnosis and their shortcomings, the one point that is most salient from a phenomenological perspective is that "in genuine hypnotic phenomena, the person's experience is not that he or she is imagining things, but that there is an alteration of the sense of agency, a feeling of involuntariness called the "classic suggestion effect" (Woody & Sadler, 2016, p. 140). The traditional rapid inductions all underscore this alteration in the sense of agency.

Rainville and Price examined hypnosis phenomenology and the neurobiology of consciousness addressing the issue of agency, among others, and the underpining neurology. Their aim was to determine whether hypnosis is indeed an altered state of consciousness. The salient point to our discussion is their determination that the feeling of being in hypnosis involves "dimensions of experience including mental ease, absorption, and the altered sense of self characterized by changes in orientation and self-agency" (Rainville & Price, 2003, p. 123). Unfortunately, they utilized conventional relaxation-based inductions, so it is difficult to extrapolate their findings to the rapid induction.

Cardeña delved into the phenomenology of deep hypnosis employing quiescent and physically active hypnosis inductions. He concluded that the "results suggest that hypnotic virtuosos have alterations of consciousness that can be better conceptualized as distinct states rather than being on a continuum" (Cardeña, 2005, p. 37). Similarly, he did not address rapid inductions and used exclusively highly hypnotizable subjects.

Landry and Raz offer a relatively current summation of the neurophysiology (Landry & Raz, 2017) of induction, that is, conventional induction as studied in highly hypnotizable subjects. Various forms of brain imaging elucidated areas predominantly involved in induction are the default mode network and the prefrontal attentional network. There is a fluctuating interplay between these and other brain areas involved in higher cognitive functions.

Rapid inductions have a paucity of research in general and specifically in terms of phenomenology and the underlying neurological mechanism. One could reasonably extrapolate that if it applies in conventional inductions, it likely applies for rapid inductions.

Suggestibility Testing

It behooves me to discuss hypnotic suggestibility or hypnotizability tests. Most hands-on clinicians rarely use hypnotizability tests. The reasons vary from they are too time consuming to they may prejudice the patient or the clinician as to the patient's abilities. They do, however, have two discernable uses in the human touch clinical world. Patients may perceive them as validation of their ability to receive and successfully comply with suggestions (with well-worded encouragement from the clinician) and from the lens of the rapid induction, they can all be artfully altered to segue into rapid inductions.

Included amongst the hypnotizability scales (Cheek, 1968; McGill, 1996; Yapko, 2019), such as the Stanford Hypnotic Suggestibility Scales (Weitzenhoffer & Hilgard, 1959), and in many stage performances, the "tests" put forward to the subjects include the postural sway, eye closure and or catalepsy, eye ball set, hand lowering, finger lock, hand clasps, and magnetic hands, to name a few. There are many more, all of which can be utilized as the beginning of an induction.

As an example, the hand clasp test involves the patient holding their arms out in front of them and interlacing their fingers. Suggestions are given to the effect that the fingers and palms are stuck together and can't be separated. When the clinician is of the opinion that the patient has succeeded, a challenge is usually made to *try* to separate them. The success or failure of the test is at this point. Should the patient not be able to undo their hands, then the induction continues something to the effect of, "… very good, now let them relax and as they do so, let yourself be loose and limp … while allowing your hands to slowly lower to your sides … become more and more comfortable, where nothing disturbs, nothing bothers, and nothing concerns … ."

Using any of the suggestibility tests as a stand alone or in combination that segues into an induction takes very little time. Concurrently, they are also acting as a reinforcement to the patient about their ability to be hypnotized, a trance validation, and can be used as a trance reinduction cue for the patient's home practice.

Ethics

We have already touched upon the question of ethics with Gerald Kein's perspective. He considered it unethical to use protracted induction techniques when rapid ones permit treating the patient's problem more expeditiously and offering the patient cost-effective care.

Rapid and instantaneous inductions engender other concerns. In certain presenting clinical situations, there is either insufficient time for informed consent discussions when a rapid induction may alleviate the situation or by communicating "therapeutically" (a synonym for hypnotic language use, especially since there is no universally accepted definition of hypnosis) a prompt resolution may be had.

Hypnosis is used both formally and informally in clinical practice. Formal utilization has the usual discussions required for informed consent, while informal utilization generally lubricates the wheels of an intervention expeditiously in less time than the informed consent discussion would take place. We could debate the pros and cons of these situations at length. Ultimately, the discussions would involve the clinician's intentions, the patient's intentions, and their agency. Each of us must muse on these and other ethical considerations arising for hypnosis utilization in general and rapid inductions specifically and arrive at our own conclusions.

My Favorite Induction

Before we end this brief sojourn, I would like to share my favorite induction. I refer to it as Instant Meditation (Filo, 2012). It is derived from the work of Rick Barrett, a western Tai Chi master (Barrett, 2006b). This technique has many uses that are determined by the context in which it may be used. Personally, I have used it to manipulate my own back pain as a toggle switch. I teach it as a stress management tool for use during the day in any context for no more than a minute or two. Similarly to Stein's Clench Fist technique (Hammond, 1990 p. 145), it is more hidden. It can be used at the grocery store check out line without raising concerns. It is also a very elegant reinduction cue for home practice or post hypnotic suggestion (which of course is the fastest of all inductions).

The aim of this technique is to shut down the chattering monkey mind. The patient is instructed to raise one or both index fingers just enough from the other digits so that they can be aware of it. Their hands may be on their thighs, on a table, or at their sides. They are to focus on the actual physical sensations in the finger(s) keeping their eyes open or closed as they wish. The sensations to have them focus on include ligament and tendon stretches, circulation and the concomitant thermal sensations, muscle tensions, air circulation about the finger, and proximity to their other digits. When their entire field of awareness is restricted to these sensations, they have to then move their awareness one centimeter beyond their finger tip. At this point, you can describe how their chaotic thoughts will have lessened or ceased altogether, and how comfortable they are. A deepening may continue or they may be left in silence. Creativity is the only limit to the use of this induction.

Paradoxically, there are no rapid and instantaneous inductions, merely inductions. If one has a hammer, everything looks like a nail. Having a full toolbox offers more opportunities. Thus, an awareness of rapid and instantaneous inductions similarly enhances our clinical capabilities.

References

Aarons, H. (1953). *Speed hypnosis*. Irvington, NJ: Power Publishing.

Angel, C. (2006, May 10). *Criss Angel levitation*. Retrieved from http://www.youtube.com/: http://www.youtube.com/watch?v=3HoTKXwXDHw.

Barber, J. (1977). Rapid induction analgesia: A clinical report. *American Journal of Clinical Hypnosis*, *19*(3), 138–147. 10.1080/00029157.1977.10403860

Barrett, D. (2006a). Hypnosis in film and television. *American Journal of Clinical Hypnosis*, *49*(1), 13–30. doi: 10.1080/00029157.2006.10401549.

Barrett, R. (2006b). *Taijiquan through the western gate*. Berkeley, CA: Blue Snake Books/Frog, Ltd.

Boris, K. T. (1963). Some dangerous techniques of hypnotic induction. *Journal of Clinical Hypnosis*, *5*(3), 171–176.

Capafons, A. (1998). Rapid self-hypnosis: A suggestion method for self-control. *Psicothema*, *10*(3), 571–581.

Cardeña, E. (2005). The phenomenology of deep hypnosis: Quiescent and physically active. *International Journal of Clinical and Experimental Hypnosis*, *53*(1), 37–59.

Casiglia, E., Tikhonoff, V., Giordano, N., Regaldo, G., Facco, E., Marchetti, P., Schiff, S., Tosello, M. T., Giacomello, M., Rossi, A. M., De Lazzari, F., Palatini, P., & Amodio, P. (2012). Relaxation versus fractionation as hypnotic deepening: Do they differ in physiological changes? *International Journal of Clinical and Experimental Hypnosis*, *60*(3), 338–355. 10.1080/00207144.2012.675297

Cheek, D. B. (1968). *Clinical hypnotherapy*. Orlando, FL: Grune& Sratton.

Cheek, D. B. (1994). *Hypnosis*. Needham Heights, MA: Allyn and Bacon.

Edmonston, J. W. (1986). *The induction of hypnosis*. Toronto, ON: John Wiley & Sons, Inc.

Elman, D. (1964). *Hypnotheraapy*. Glendale, CA: Westwood Pub.Co.

Erickson, M. H. (1961). *The practical application of medical and dental hypnosis*. New York: The Julian Press, Inc.

Erickson, M. H. (1964). Pantomime techniques in hypnosis and the implications. *American Journal of Clinical Hypnosis*, *7*(1), 64–70.

Ewin, D. (1979). Hypnosis in burn therapy. In G. Burrows (Ed.), *Hypnosis* (p. 282). Amsterdam: Elsevier.
Ewin, D. (2009). *101 things I wish I'd known when I started using hypnosis*. Bancyfelin, Carmarthen: Crown House Publishing Ltd.
Filo, G. (2012). *Rapid hypnotic inductions: Demonstrations and applications [DVD]*. Carmarthen, UK: Crown House Publishing Ltd.
Hammond, D. (1990). *Handbook of hypnotic suggestions and metaphors*. New York: W. W. Norton & Company.
Hartland, J. (1972). *Medical and dental hypnosis (2nd ed.)*. London, UK: Balliere Tindall.
Hogan, K. (2001). *Covert hypnosis: An operator's manual*. Eagan, MN: Network 3000 Publishing.
Hope, A. E., & Sugarman, L. I. (2015). Orienting hypnosis. *American Journal of Clinical Hypnosis*, 212–229. doi:10.1080/00029157.2014.976787
Kaptchuk, T. (2010, December 22). *Placebos without deception: A randomized controlled trial*. Retrieved from PLoS ONE 5(12): e15591. doi:10.1371/journal.pone.0015591: http://www.plosone.org/article/info:doi/10.1371/journal.pone
Kein, G. F. (2016). *The ethics of utilizing instant and rapid*. Retrieved 2017 May 8 from www.omnihypnosis.com.: www.omnihypnosis.com.
Landry, M., & Raz, A. (2017). Neurophysiology of hypnosis. In G. R. Elkins (Ed.), *Handbook of medical and psychological hypnosis* (pp. 19–28). New York: Springer Publishing Company.
Matheson, G., &.Grehan (1979). A rapid induction technique. *American Journal of Clinical Hypnosis*, *21*(4), 297–299. 10.1080/00029157.1979.10403987
McGill, O. (1996). *The new encyclopedia of stage hypnotism*. St. Clears, Carmarthen, Wales: The Anglo American Book Company Ltd.
Rainville, P., & Price, D. D. (2003). Hypnosis phenomenology and the neurobiology of consciousness. *International Journal of Clinical and Experimental Hypnosis*, *51*(2), 105–129. 10.1076/iceh.51.2.105.14613
Shaw, S. I. (1958). *Clinical applications of hypnosis in dentistry*. Philadelphia: W.B.Saunders Co.
Startle response (2022, May 1). Retrieved 2021 Nov. 4 from Wikipedia: https://en.wikipedia.org/wiki/Startle_response
Sunnen, G. V. (2011). *Speed hypnosis vs meditative hypnosis in clinical care*. Retrieved 2021 Nov. 4 from http://www.triroc.com: http://www.triroc.com/sunnen/topics/speedhypnosisvclinical.htm
Temple, R. K. (1989). *Open to suggestion: The uses and abuses of hypnosis*. Northhamptonshire, UK: Aquarian Press.
Vincent, R. H. (1893). *The elements of hypnotism*. London: Kegan Paul, Trench, Trubner & Co., Ltd.
Wells, W. R. (1966). Experiments in waking hypnosis. In l. Kuhn (Ed.), *Modern hypnosis* (pp. 45–55). Hollywood, CA: Wilshire Book Company.
Weitzenhoffer, A. M. , & Hilgard, E. R. (1959). *Stanford Hypnotic Susceptibility Scales, Forms A & B*. Palo Alto: Consulting Psychologists Press.
White, R. W. (1966). An analysis of motivation in hypnosis. In L. Kuhn (Ed.), *Modern hypnosis* (pp. 204–224). Hollywood, CA: Wilshire Book Company.
Woody, E., & Sadler, P. (2016). What can a hypnotic induction do? *American Journal of Clinical Hypnosis*, *59*(2), 138–154. 10.1080/00029157.2016.1185004
Yapko, M. D. (2019). *Trancework (5th ed.)*. New York: Routledge.

12
SELF-HYPNOSIS

Balázs Nyiri[1,2] *and Steven Jay Lynn*[3]

[1]Doctoral School of Psychology, ELTE Eötvös Loránd University, Budapest, Hungary;
[2]Institute of Psychology, ELTE Eötvös Loránd University, Budapest, Hungary;
[3]Department of Psychology Binghamton University (SUNY), Binghamton

Introduction

Yapko (1993) keenly observed that how we see ourselves and the world can be altered dramatically by changing how we talk to ourselves. In this chapter, we will consider "talking to ourselves" in a very specific and literal sense, as we embark on a journey to develop a deeper understanding of self-hypnosis. At the outset, it is important to note that our chapter presupposes that readers will be familiar with how to induce hypnosis, formulate suggestions, and utilize them for therapeutic purposes. Our primary focus will be on self-hypnosis, which we conceptualize as autosuggestions, that is, self-induced suggestions that are initiated in a context perceived or defined as hypnosis. We will illustrate how the use of self-hypnosis in treatment can be taught to clients to maximize and generalize treatment gains to everyday life, review research on self-hypnosis, and provide suggestions for future research and advances in the field of self-hypnosis.

Definitions and Overview

To provide needed context for our discussion, we will begin with a consideration of definitional matters and present a brief overview of the history of self-suggestion in and apart from hypnosis. Halligan and Oakley (2014) contend that, in recent decades, the scientific community has largely neglected the domain of suggestion and suggestibility. They consider this outcome surprising given the historical importance of these constructs in the broader field of psychology (see Gheorghiu & Kruse, 1991). To underscore this point, Halligan and Oakley (2014) refer to Sidis (1898) who, much earlier, contended that "the fact of suggestibility existing in the normal individual is that of the highest importance in the theoretical fields of knowledge, in psychology, sociology, ethics, history as well in practical life in education, politics and economics" (p. 17). We will suggest herein that self-suggestion and self-hypnosis, in particular, deserve much greater attention and can make substantial contributions to the lives of people in need of effective psychological interventions.

 DOI: 10.4324/9781003449126-17

Self-suggestion, including autosuggestions apart from the context of hypnosis, reside well within the broader arena of suggestion and suggestibility and recently have been defined as an "instantiation and reiteration of ideas or concepts by oneself aiming to actively influence one's own perceptual, brain or interoceptive states, as well as the valence of perceived sensations" (Myga et al., 2022, p. 383). A century before this definition, Coué (1922) posited that suggestion, or as we would call it today "heterosuggestion," is an "act of imposing an idea on the brain of another person," whereas autosuggestion is "implanting an idea in one's self through one's self" (p. 21). Halligan and Oakley (2014) describe suggestion as "a form or type of communicable belief capable of producing and modifying experiences, thoughts and actions" and add that "suggestions can be (a) intentional/nonintentional, (b) verbal/nonverbal, or (c) hypnotic/nonhypnotic" (p. 111). Varga (2013) similarly stresses that suggestions can be non-verbal as well as verbal. Building on these definitions, we define autosuggestion as a mental process which – based on verbal and non-verbal information – possesses the ability to shape beliefs and experiences. When suggestions that are utilized in the context of hypnosis are self-induced, we can say that the procedure can accurately be described as "self-hypnosis."

We will henceforth refer to hypnosis and self-hypnosis in terms that Green et al. (2005) put forward in which hypnosis is described as a situation in which "one person (the subject) is guided by another (the hypnotist) to respond to suggestions for changes in subjective experience, alterations in perception, sensation, emotion, thought, or behavior," and self-hypnosis is described as "the act of administering hypnotic procedures on one's own (p. 262). We suggest that self-hypnosis possesses the ability to (a) create and alter beliefs about the self and the world; (b) crystallize and channel spontaneous thoughts, images, emotions, and action tendencies for therapeutic purposes; (c) mobilize psychological resources, and deautomatize negative self-suggestions that are, for example, implicated in anxiety and depression; and (d) maintain and transfer therapeutic gains achieved with heterohypnosis to everyday live.

Historical Background

Awareness of the power of words can be traced to ancient Egyptian culture thousands of years ago (Gunn, 1916). Some medical papyri provide texts to be recited by patients that can be considered as antecedents of autosuggestions, as exemplified by examples culled from three different texts:

1 The burdens are relaxed, and the weakness departs that is located in my belly …;
2 Come remedy, come who removes (bad) things in this my heart and in the parts of my body;
3 I am under the protection of Isis; my rescue is the son of Osiris (Grapow et al., 1958, as cited in Zucconi, 2007, p. 32).

Centuries later, Franz Anton Mesmer, who discovered so-called "animal magnetism," was probably the first person to use self-hypnosis (or "self-magnetization") around 1778–1779, which he employed to treat problems in his lower body (Gravitz, 1994; Pintar & Lynn, 2009). Amand-Marie-Jacques de Chastenet – the Marquis de Puységur, another key figure of early hypnosis and a student of Mesmer – likewise believed that it was possible to perform magnetization on oneself (Pintar & Lynn, 2009).

The fact that suggestion and self-hypnosis have strong historical connections to the field of hypnosis is evident from one of its early definitions: "hypnotism [is recommended to] be defined as the science dealing with phenomena explained by suggestion and autosuggestion" (Section de l'Hypnotisme, 1890, as cited in Alvarado, 2010, p. 52). Jones (1923) describes autosuggestion as a phenomenon mentioned as early as in the middle of the 19th century by Baragnon (1853) and referred to it as "automagnétisation." However, Jones acknowledges that traces of the phenomenon can be found as early as the 16th century when Cardan (1550, as cited in Jones 1923) used it to cure his gout. Jones (1923) notes, and we concur, that it is challenging to isolate "pure" self-hypnosis from "ordinary" hypnosis and that it is also difficult to draw a clear line between heterosuggestion and autosuggestion. As an example, he discusses a patient taught how to use autosuggestions, but whenever he would do so, he would also be affected by the "physician in his mind" who taught him.

Émile Coué, a French pharmacist, who was trained in hypnosis by Liébault, and credited with discovering the placebo effect, called attention to autosuggestions in enhancing the efficacy of medications (Short, 2015). He is known for the now famous self-affirmation/self-suggestion (Pintar & Lynn, 2009): "Every day, in every way, I am getting better and better" (Coué, 1922, p. 72). Coué further contended that although the body and mind are controlled unconsciously through autosuggestions, self-control and personal goals could be achieved using autosuggestions on a conscious basis.

Coué believed that autosuggestion could exert a negative as well as a positive effect on the psyche and stated: "Every thought, good or bad, becomes concrete; It materializes and becomes a reality, provided such is within the realm of possibility" (ibid., pp. 73–74). Of course, he was by-and-large on target, as negative self-suggestions are prominent in depression and anxiety, as well as in other distressing conditions (see Lynn & Kirsch, 2006). He also contended that every suggestion first needs to be an autosuggestion to have an impact. The same idea was expressed 15 years prior to his writings in the Japanese suggestion literature, which noted that ideas do not have power on their own and can exert an effect only if attention is allocated to them (Ueno, 1907, as cited in Wu, 2019).

In 1913, during the first sport psychology congress, a professional cyclist presented a lecture titled [the] "Record holder's state of mind" (Müller, 1997, as cited in Kornspan, 2007) and stated that, by using autosuggestions, athletes could manage their emotions and fatigue. Kornspan (2019) notes that until the middle of the 20th century autosuggestion was still taught to professional athletes and finds this approach similar to the use of self-talk and positive affirmations in the training of athletes nowadays.

The idea that the power of thought, and by extension, self-suggestions, could play a role in treating medical conditions has been the subject of speculation. In 1978, Carl Simonton published *Getting Well Again,* in which he described how he helped "incurable" cancer patients by "self-awareness and imagery techniques," although he provided no convincing evidence that the techniques he advocated succeeded in eliminating cancer. Nevertheless, self-hypnosis and autosuggestions could potentially play a role in treating anxiety and depression that accompany serious illnesses, for example, even in the absence of a causal relation between self-suggestions and the actual disease process. In 1986, Ernest Rossi published *The Psychobiology of Mind-Body Healing* about how thinking and believing can affect diseases, much in line with Simonton's writings (Alman, & Lambrou, 1993), although his claims have not been evaluated in systematic fashion to date.

The American Psychological Association Division of Psychological Hypnosis conducted a poll on two occasions (1997 and 2004–2005) to explore expert opinions regarding hypnosis. Based on the results, next to pain control, cancer research, surgical interventions, and the treatment of mental health conditions, self-hypnosis was among the most prominent topics of interest among researchers and clinicians (Pintar & Lynn, 2009). Finally, 2023 marks another important milestone for self-hypnosis and autosuggestion as they are featured not just as parts of individual chapters in this volume, but they are discussed in this chapter devoted to the topic exclusively.

Theory and Practice

Eason and Parris (2019) differentiated self-hypnosis from heterohypnosis in stating that the latter typically is employed in the presence of a hypnosis practitioner or researcher who guides the hypnotic process, whereas in case of self-hypnosis, suggestions are self-generated. As hypnosis may be effective, even in the physical absence of the hypnotist, self-hypnosis was rightfully included in the definition of hypnosis advanced by the Executive Committee of the APA Division of Psychological Hypnosis in 2004 (see Pintar & Lynn, 2009). Fromm and her colleagues (Fromm, 1985; Fromm et al., 1981) conducted perhaps the most extensive investigation of self-hypnosis to date. She found that although heterohypnosis and self-hypnosis are similar in certain respects, some aspects appeared to be unique to each. For example, absorption and the fading away of general reality orientation are common elements across both methodologies. However, free-floating attention and ego receptivity, which derive from internal stimuli (e.g., imagination, sensations, primary process mentation), are more specific to self-hypnosis, whereas concentrated attention and receptivity to a single and focal outside source (the hypnotist) are more specific to heterohypnosis. She also found that imagery that is somewhat realistic, imbued with personal meaning, and rich and vivid (even more so than in heterohypnosis) plays an influential role in self-hypnosis (see also Ruch, 1975). However, this line of research bears replication, as Fromm's intensive studies were based on a selected sample of motivated and well-trained individuals who were highly responsive to heterohypnosis suggestions, which potentially accentuated differences between self and heterohypnosis (Hannigan, 2000).

Fromm highlighted the need for clients to be flexible and adapt to self-hypnosis when beginning to learn the technique, which can be accompanied early on by self-doubt and anxiety. Research subjects reported greater difficulty in experiencing hypnosis during the first week when no hypnotist was present to guide them, which might be linked to skepticism regarding their ability to experience hypnosis in the absence of a hypnotist. However, anxiety and skepticism faded, while experiential involvement increased and reality orientation decreased, as individuals became increasingly comfortable with the process. Fromm (1985) also noted that responsivity to suggestions can differ among individuals across heterohypnosis and self-hypnosis contexts. Finally, she posits that although the depth of the hypnotic experiences fluctuates more in self-hypnosis, relative to hetero-hypnosis, self-consciousness, self-doubt, and embarrassment are generally reduced in self versus heterohypnosis.

In the clinical arena, Trenkle (2017) suggested that teaching clients self-hypnosis prior to heterohypnosis can be beneficial, especially if the clients experience problems in relinquishing control to the hypnotist and in relaxing during heterohypnosis. In these cases, instead of starting with heterohypnosis, he recommends teaching self-hypnosis as a "safe" and generally reliable way to increase clients' comfort with hypnosis and gradually transitioning to heterohypnosis. Trenkle (2017) thus offers self-hypnosis training to most clients as a first hypnosis experience. However, from an empirical standpoint, researchers have not yet established the most effective order of training in self versus heterohypnosis among diverse individuals and across different personal and interpersonal contexts. Self-hypnosis may be an effective and efficient intervention insofar as it may facilitate therapeutic involvement with suggestions and produce treatment gains, require fewer therapy sessions to address treatment goals, and enhance perceptions of personal control as well as self-esteem and self-efficacy, although these possibilities await more controlled empirical confirmation. Readers should consult Trenkle (2017) for a detailed description of his self-hypnosis methodology accompanied by a transcript of a training session.

Peter (2018) states that self-hypnosis can also help clients in practicing and deepening the techniques they have learned in heterohypnosis. He emphasizes the importance of teaching the induction part of self-hypnosis in a way that is comprehensible and easy to follow; for example, incorporating eye fixation, eyelid closure, a staircase metaphor to deepen the experience, and arm levitation. Just as in heterohypnosis, many inductions can potentially be used to establish the context of hypnosis, or in this case self-hypnosis, ranging from simple eye closure and breath counting to deepen involvement, to progressive relaxation. However, scant evidence exists to date to indicate that one induction type or method is superior to another, although comparative studies of diverse inductions are worth pursuing.

We provide the modified steeple technique (or one of its forms) as one illustrative example of an induction that is reportedly effective even when a person is not highly responsive to heterohypnosis and that can be taught within 5–10 minutes (Cyna, 2017). Notably, a single session is usually sufficient to reach the necessary level of proficiency for home use. The technique is based on a physical "truism," that is, a naturally occurring physiological response, linked with self-suggestions, which can be employed even in treating anxious participants. The physiological response occurs when the hands are positioned in a "steeple" position (see description below) in which the flexor tendons of the index fingers pull them together automatically (McCarthy, 2021).

Cyna (2017) provides a detailed description of this procedure, which we summarize as follows. Clients are first asked whether they would like to learn a method for self-hypnosis that can usually be taught in five minutes and are informed that the simple technique can engender a perceived light or even a deep experience of hypnosis. The client response should be the basis for the pace and formulation of suggestions that will follow. The technique can be taught in three phases: demonstration, practice together, and practice alone. The induction begins with the hypnotist demonstrating how to do the induction while the client observes. Next, the client experiences the method as the therapist demonstrates. Finally, the client completes the procedure without assistance.

For the induction, the hands need to be clasped, holding the palms against each other, with the fingers interlocked and the thumbs folded. The client is then asked to extend their index fingers to a parallel position while holding everything else at the previous position. As the final step, the client is asked to gaze at the space between the fingertips of the index fingers, with them 2–3 cm apart in the beginning. The two index fingers will seem to come together all on their own without thinking about it, as if there is a magnetic attraction between a "north pole" finger and "south pole" finger ... As soon as the tips of the index fingers touch ... Close the eyes ... take a deep breath in and hold it for 5 seconds and then ... as you breathe out you can feel yourself blowing away tension into the atmosphere ... as if a balloon is collapsing ... as you breathe out ... Each time you breathe out from now on you will relax even more ... breathe in some strength and control you didn't even know that you had and ... each time you breathe out blow away anything you don't like into the atmosphere as you feel yourself relax ... nothing you need to think about ... nothing you need to try and do ... as it just seems to happen all on its own ... (pp. 234–238).

After the eye closure, the hypnotist can suggest that the client rest their hands on their lap (or abdomen if in a lying position). To deepen the experience, the hypnotist may utilize diverse techniques, for example, progressive relaxation or imagining a favorite place. Following the three phases, the client can also be informed that more they practice the easier and faster it will be to become immersed in self-hypnosis. Therapists might also suggest, when the client gains proficiency in the method, that the client skip interlocking the fingers, as the physical part of this technique will no longer be required: Simply imagining the action will be sufficient to relax and experience hypnosis. It is also helpful to suggest that the technique be used when it is likely to benefit the client: "You now know that you will be able to use this technique any time you want to ... be it at home or wherever or whenever the need arises ... Like anything, when we practice something, it becomes easier to use and more effective for you" (p. 240). From McCarthy's (2021) description, it is clear that after the deepening, with any preferred method, the process can continue with the intervention phase and completed via reorientation and self-suggestions to terminate the experience.

Review of Evidence

According to Eason and Parris (2019), the study of heterohypnosis has received substantial attention that far eclipses the empirical research concerning self-hypnosis. To underline the importance of the often neglected topic of self-hypnosis, the authors reiterated Orne and McConkey's (1981) statement that "Given the popularity and therapeutic potential of self-hypnosis, further research is desirable to establish a scientific data-base concerning its actual clinical use" (p. 314).

To address this research gap, Eason and Parris (2019) conducted a systematic meta-analytic review regarding clinical applications of self-hypnosis that focused exclusively on randomized control trials. The authors analyzed 22 studies that met their selection criteria and reported a medium-to-large treatment effect size across studies. Generally, their findings supported their claim that self-hypnosis was at least as effective as alternative treatment options such as relaxation or mindfulness. More specifically, they reported that in 18 of the studies (82%), self-hypnosis proved to be an effective treatment, and in 14 (64%) cases it also surpassed the active comparison conditions (e.g., active control waiting list control, standard care, conventional treatment; therapeutic methods such as relaxation and mindfulness, CBT, biofeedback) in efficacy. The four studies that found no evidence for the superiority of self-hypnosis did not teach self-directed or self-regulation skills at all to participants, and self-hypnosis was limited to listening to recordings of heterohypnosis. Moreover, including heterohypnosis in the self-hypnosis treatment protocol was not prerequisite for a positive outcome.

The review included studies of pain, childbirth, stress, anxiety, and hypertension, as well as other conditions mentioned below. All of the pain studies succeeded in reducing pain. Interestingly, audio recordings were not necessary to achieve positive results, although practice at home was included in every study. Jensen (2011) also states that practicing self-hypnosis is a key component of hypnotherapies of patients with chronic pain. In the case of childbirth, self-hypnosis did not prove to be efficient. However, all such studies used audio recordings only, which might account for the lack of positive results. The review suggests that "live" teaching of self-hypnosis might be a key component of the protocols in cases where self-hypnosis was employed successfully.

The authors highlight (a) the potential positive impact of self-hypnosis including enhanced self-efficacy (Fromm et al., 1981; Handelsman, 1984; Olness, 1975) and self-esteem (Olness et al., 1987); (b) posit that it is possible that self-hypnosis can be effective even when heterohypnosis is not successful; (c) foster autonomy across circumstances and conditions; and (d) be applicable in noisy conditions such as labor and birthing. The review also indicates that self-hypnosis shows promise in treating stress, anxiety, and hypertension, but also in improving immune functioning, tinnitus, asthma, hemophilia, mental health, and well-being in breast cancer, and insomnia among cancer survivors.

Another intriguing aspect of the studies reviewed pertains to the number of self-hypnosis training sessions in the protocol. The review indicated that, generally, at least three practice sessions optimized effectiveness when it preceded participation in the trial. However, Tan et al. (2014) determined that repetition in sessions might not necessarily play a significant role in outcome. The researchers compared four conditions to treat chronic low back pain: (1) eight self-hypnosis training sessions (no recording, no recommendation to practice alone); (2) eight self-hypnosis training sessions (with recording and recommendation to practice alone); (3) two self-hypnosis training sessions (with recording, recommendation to practice alone and weekly reminder calls); (4) eight sessions of biofeedback-assisted relaxation training.

The researchers determined that self-hypnosis training eventuated in a greater reduction of pain intensity compared to the biofeedback condition, although the positive changes in pain intensity, pain interference, and sleep quality did not differ among the three hypnosis conditions. The results obtained suggested that as few as two sessions of self-hypnosis training might be as effective as eight sessions and that using audio recordings might not be necessary to produce treatment gains. However, the findings could also be interpreted to mean that home practice is redundant, although the researchers note that the direction of the results, albeit not significant statistically, suggests that home practice may actually have an even more beneficial effect. Clearly, as the authors note, further research is a priority.

Suggestions and Recommendations

Given that the research base is promising, yet not extensive or conclusive in evaluating the treatment efficacy and efficiency of self-hypnosis, much more empirical work remains to be done. Additional randomized controlled trials are an imperative that include attention and wait-list control, placebo, heterohypnosis, and treatment as usual comparison conditions. Clear operational definitions of self-hypnosis (and heterohypnosis), alongside developing detailed treatment manuals and procedures, including novel standardized self-hypnosis responsiveness scales, are a high priority, as are studies that replicate promising findings with large samples.

Research on different self-hypnosis inductions and moderator variables to evaluate in future studies encompasses the frequency and intensity of practice, prior experience with heterohypnosis, the sequencing of hetero and self-hypnosis, and the influence of hypnotic suggestibility on outcomes of self-hypnosis interventions. Clinical research would benefit from determining whether (a) responsiveness to suggestions is enhanced when participants play a part in co-creating suggestions with a hypnotist; (b) certain self-hypnotic suggestions are differentially effective depending on the condition treated (e.g., anxiety vs. depression); (c) autosuggestions administered in a nonhypnotic context are as effective as the same suggestions administered in a hypnotic context; and (d) whether mastery and ego strengthening suggestions are more effective than targeted/and or tailored suggestions in modifying negative self-talk or achieving symptom relief.

Additionally, little is known regarding what enhances responsiveness to self-hypnosis, as well as the biological/neurological correlates of self-hypnosis versus heterohypnosis. Mechanistic studies that assess variables researchers have linked with responsiveness to heterohypnosis are worthwhile targets of future studies. These variables include expectancies, attitudes and beliefs about hypnosis/self-hypnosis, motivation, responsivity to nonhypnotic imaginative suggestions, personality variables (e.g., fantasy-proneness, absorption), rapport with the training hypnotist, and response sets (see Lynn et al., 2023). Finally, we agree with Myga et al. (2022) that, despite its potential significance, the available literature on autosuggestion is very limited and deserves more extensive research in its own right.

These concerns and recommendations aside, the research and literature on clinical applications is promising. Indeed, self-hypnosis should be a high priority for researchers for many reasons, not the least is that integrating self-hypnosis and autosuggestions into treatment is entirely consistent with cognitive-behavioral approaches to treating psychological conditions (e.g., anxiety, depression, eating disorders) that modify negative "self-talk" and well-entrenched core beliefs (e.g., "I am unlovable." "I am worthless."). Indeed, such negative cognitions might well be amenable to restructuring with empirically supported "portable" and cost-effective self-hypnosis methodologies, which could be combined with well-established interventions or implemented on a stand-alone basis to promote the transfer and maintenance of treatment gains to everyday life. We hope that our recommendations and suggestions applicable to the future of self-hypnosis will be realized over the coming decades.

References

Alman, B. M., & Lambrou, P. T. (1993). *Self-hypnosis: The complete manual for health and self-change*. Souvenir Press.

Alvarado, C. S. (2010). Nineteenth-century suggestion and magnetism: Hypnosis at the International Congress of Physiological Psychology (1889). *Contemporary Hypnosis*, 27(1), 48–60.

Baragnon, P. P. (1853). *Etude du magnétisme animal sous le point de vue d'une exacte pratique: suivie d'un mot sur la rotation des tables*. Germer-Baillière.

Cardan: De Subtilitate (1550), lib. XXI.

Coué, E. (1922). *Self Mastery through conscious autosuggestion*. Malkan Publishing Company.

Cyna, A. M. (2017). The modified steeple technique and the GR Wicks induction. In M. P. Jensen (Ed.), *The art and practice of hypnotic induction: Favorite methods of master clinicians* (pp. 230–245). Denny Creek Press.

Eason, A. D., & Parris, B. A. (2019). Clinical applications of self-hypnosis: A systematic review and meta-analysis of randomized controlled trials. *Psychology of Consciousness: Theory, Research, and Practice*, 6(3), 262. 10.1037/cns0000173

Fromm, E. (1985). The essential aspects of self-hypnosis. In D. Waxman, P. C. Misra, M. Gibson, & M. A. Basker (Eds.), *Modern trends in hypnosis* (pp. 209–214). Plenum.

Fromm, E., Brown, D. P., Hurt, S. W., Oberlander, J. Z., Boxer, A. M., & Pfeifer, G. (1981). The phenomena and characteristics of self-hypnosis. *International Journal of Clinical and Experimental Hypnosis*, 29(3), 189–246. doi:10.1080/00207148108409158

Gheorghiu, V. A., & Kruse, P. (1991). The psychology of suggestion: An integrative perspective. In J. F. Schumaker (Ed.), *Human suggestibility: Advances in theory, research, and application* (pp. 59–75). Taylor & Francis/Routledge.

Grapow, H., von Deines, H., & Westendorf, W. (1958). *Übersetzung der Medizinischen Texte: Erläuterungen*, 4(2) [Translation of the medical texts: Explanations]. Akademie-Verlag.

Gravitz, M. A. (1994). The first use of self-hypnosis: Mesmer mesmerizes Mesmer. *American Journal of Clinical Hypnosis*, *37*(1), 49–52. 10.1080/00029157.1994.10403109

Green, J. P., Barabasz, A. F., Barrett, D., & Montgomery, G. H. (2005). Forging ahead: The 2003 APA Division 30 definition of hypnosis. *International Journal of Clinical and Experimental Hypnosis*, *53*(3), 259–264. 10.1080/00207140590961321

Gunn, B. (1916). The religion of the poor in ancient Egypt. *The Journal of Egyptian Archaeology*, *3*(1), 81–94. 10.1177/030751331600300124

Halligan, P. W., & Oakley, D. A. (2014). Hypnosis and beyond: Exploring the broader domain of suggestion. *Psychology of Consciousness: Theory, Research, and Practice*, *1*(2), 105–122. 10.1037/cns0000019

Handelsman, M. M. (1984). Self-hypnosis as a facilitator of self-efficacy: A case example. *Psychotherapy: Theory, Research, Practice, Training*, *21*(4), 550–553. doi:10.1037/h0086001

Hannigan, K. (2000). Self-hypnosis revisited: Much ado about nothing. *Australian Journal of Clinical and Experimental Hypnosis*, *28*(2), 148–149.

Jensen, M. P. (2011). *Hypnosis for chronic pain management: Therapist guide*. Oxford University Press.

Jones, E. (1923). The nature of auto-suggestion. *International Journal of Psychoanalysis*, *4*, 293–324.

Kornspan, A. S. (2007). The early years of sport psychology: The work and influence of Pierre de Coubertin. *Journal of Sport Behavior*, *30*, 77–93. https://www.researchgate.net/publication/266327149

Kornspan, A. S. (2019). Autosuggestion. In D. Hackfort, R. J. Schinke, & B. Strauss (Eds.), *Dictionary of sport psychology: Sport, exercise, and performing arts* (pp. 30–31). Academic Press.

Lynn, S. J., Green, J. P., Zahedi, A., & Apelian, C. (2023). The response expectancy theory of hypnosis reconsidered: Toward an integrative model of hypnosis. *American Journal of Clinical Hypnosis*, *65*, 128–210.

Lynn, S. J., & Kirsch, I. (2006). *Essentials of clinical hypnosis: An evidence-based approach*. American Psychological Association.

McCarthy, P. (2021) The special place of bliss technique. In M. P. Jensen (Ed.), *Handbook of hypnotic techniques, Vol. 2: Favorite methods of master clinicians (voices of experience)* (pp. 305–325). Denny Creek Press.

Myga, K. A., Kuehn, E., & Azanon, E. (2022). Autosuggestion: A cognitive process that empowers your brain?. *Experimental Brain Research*, *240*(2), 381–394. 10.1007/s00221-021-06265-8

Olness, K. (1975). The use of self hypnosis in the treatment of childhood nocturnal enuresis. *Clinical Pediatrics*, *14*(3), 273–279. 10.1177/000992287501400316

Olness, K., MacDonald, J. T., & Uden, D. L. (1987). Comparison of self-hypnosis and propranolol in the treatment of juvenile classic migraine. *Pediatrics*, *79*(4), 593–597. 10.1542/peds.79.4.593

Orne, M. T., & McConkey, K. M. (1981). Toward convergent inquiry into self-hypnosis. *International Journal of Clinical and Experimental Hypnosis*, *29*(3), 313–323. doi:10.1080/00207148108409164

Peter, B. (2018). Transforming the Gestalt and carrier of chronic pain: Two hypnotherapeutic approaches. In M. P. Jensen (Ed.), *Hypnotic techniques for chronic pain management: Favorite methods of master clinicians* (pp. 179–202). Denny Creek Press.

Pintar, J., & Lynn, S. J. (2009). *Hypnosis: A brief history*. John Wiley & Sons.

Rossi, E. L. (1986). *The psychobiology of mind-body healing*. W.W. Norton & Company, Inc.

Ruch, J. C. (1975). Self-hypnosis: Result of heterohypnosis or vice versa. *International Journal of Clinical and Experimental Hypnosis*, *23*(4), 282–304. 10.1080/00207147508415952

Short, D. (2015). Erickson-derived or–influenced theories: Overview. In E. Neukrug, (Ed.), *The SAGE encyclopedia of theory in counseling and psychotherapy* (pp. 351–357). SAGE Publications, Inc.

Sidis, B. (1898). *The psychology of suggestion: A research into the subconscious nature of man and society*. Appleton & Company. doi:10.1037/10578-000

Simonton, C., & Simonton, S. (1982). *Getting well again*. Bantam Hooks.

Tan, G., Rintala, D. H., Jensen, M. P., Fukui, T., Smith, D., & Williams, W. (2014). A randomized controlled trial of hypnosis compared with biofeedback for adults with chronic low back pain. *European Journal of Pain*, *19*, 271–280. doi:10.1002/ejp.545

Trenkle, B. (2017). Training in self-hypnosis as a first induction. In M. P. Jensen (Ed.), *The art and practice of hypnotic induction: Favorite methods of master clinicians* (pp. 206–228). Denny Creek Press.

Varga, K. (2013). Suggestive techniques connected to medical interventions. *Interventional Medicine and Applied Science*, *5*(3), 95–100. 10.1556/imas.5.2013.3.1

Weitzenhoffer, A. M. (2000). *The practice of hypnotism* (2nd ed.) John Wiley & Sons.

Wu, Y. C. (2019). The moral power of suggestion: A history of suggestion in Japan, 1900–1930. *Journal of the History of the Behavioral Sciences*, *55*(1), 21–39. 10.1002/jhbs.21944

Yapko, M. (1993). Foreword. In B. M. Alman, & P. T. Lambrou (Eds.) (1993). *Self-hypnosis: The complete manual for health and self-change*. Souvenir Press.

Zucconi, L. M. (2007). Medicine and religion in ancient Egypt. *Religion Compass*, *1*(1), 26–37. 10.1111/j.1749-8171.2006.00004.x

13
HYPNOSIS
A Developmental Perspective

Daniel P. Kohen[1] *and Karen Olness*[2]

[1]National Pediatric Hypnosis Training Institute, MN, USA; [2]Professor Emerita of Pediatrics, Global Health and DIseases Case Western Reserve University, Ohio, USA

Introduction

Just as effective human interaction and communication requires, depends upon, and revolves around careful observation, so it is that a hypnotic relationship – interdependent and interactional – begins and of course has its differences and nuances according to traditions within families and cultures and their associated beliefs and practices. Most specifically the relationship and the emergence of rapport is dependent upon the clinician's initial and ongoing attention to the developmental realities of their client/patient, in an ongoing cycling recycling of learning through all senses, being fully present with the patient, and coming to know and respect them and their perceptions of their concerns, problems, issues (Kohen & Kaiser, 2014).

It seems clear that it is essential for all healthcare professionals that we begin from a knowledge base and position that informs, understands, and honors the fundamental concepts of what normal human psychobiological development entails. Thus, how normal maturation develops from infancy through early and middle childhood, and into adolescence, young adulthood and beyond into older adulthood and the elderly, must always be in our awareness as we meet, get to know, learn from, and develop therapeutic strategies uniquely suited to, and tailored for, each individual. While this may seem to be a "given", too often not considering or integrating principles of development in connecting with individual children or adults results in apparent "failure" of a well-intended therapeutic approach.

Understanding and integrating the reality that each individual person – and each encounter with that person – is new, unique, and different is foundational to developing meaningful rapport. Rapport is essential to recognizing elements of hypnosis and evolving an effective and mutually beneficial therapeutic hypnotic approach.

Hypnosis for habits – for example – must be considered and approached differently and, therefore, "hypnotically", *depending* upon the level of development, nature, and meaning of the habit to the child (i.e., Do they want to be "over" it? Or is the "problem" that of the parents?) versus to the parent (Kohen, 1991; Kohen & Olness, 2023c).

 DOI: 10.4324/9781003449126-18

Knowledge and Skills That Benefit Child Health Professionals Who Are Teaching Hypnosis

In addition to knowing about child developmental changes, it is important to relate this to knowledge about their favorite toys, games, music, and popular characters. With respect to individual children, child health professionals should inquire about specific interests and hobbies, sports and music activities, likes and dislikes. It is helpful to get information from parents about a child's strengths. It is helpful to know what cultural norms may impact a child's interests or life. For example, if one learns that a child is bilingual, one might relate this language fluency to the capacity to develop other new skills. With respect to adolescents, it is especially important to make a judgment about whether he/she has developed the capacity for abstract reasoning ability and to recognize that many adolescents who appear and sound mature do not yet have abstract reasoning ability.

Knowledge about child development and about individual children facilitates the acquisition of skills in communicating with children of different ages, children with different personality types, and with their parents. A child health professional may see many children and adolescents each day and change communication approaches with each individual, depending on developmental level and personality type. Child health professionals need skills in shifting their communication approaches as they recognize developmental advances in children whom they have followed over time. They also need skills in recognizing sadness in a child who has previously seemed happy, and then be sensitive in determining how best and when to address this change. All child health professionals should have skills in a trauma-based approach and know when it should be used (Brown et al., 2017).

Example: The Pre-school – Early Verbal age child

Because preschool age children have limited though ever-increasing vocabulary and have less direct and more non-verbal communication behaviors and skills about feelings, hypnosis approaches must be carefully matched (as with any age) to their maturational level. Accordingly, the use of play is essential – and equivalent and analogous to – hypnosis as a means of engaging, focusing attention, and facilitating the desired behavior change. This is easily accomplished through storytelling, pop-up books, favorite toys/stuffed animals, speaking to the child *through* their favorite doll or stuffed animal (Kohen & Olness, 2023a; Kuttner, 1991a, 1991b). A simple example might well be the habit behavior of hair-pulling, not unusual in preschool aged and school-aged children, increasingly common in adolescents, and most common in late adolescence and young adults, primarily so in young women where occurrence is nine times more common than in boys or men (Kohen, 1991, 1996).

Young children three or four years of age may well start pulling their (scalp) hair and quickly develop a habit of so doing. One such three-and-a-half-year-old [patient of ours] began doing this about the same time as the birth of her newborn baby brother. Though her parents had made every effort to appropriately prepare her for the new arrival to the family and presented the "big sister" role to her with enthusiasm, she was nonetheless stressed by this change in her life, in her environment, in her parents, and the clear change in amount of attention paid to her while they attended to the newborn. She regressed some in her toilet training, returned to having more "temper tantrums", and also seemed to have developed the hair-pulling as an additional non-verbal expression of clear anxiety about the arrival of the new member of the family. She also pulled at the hair on her mother's arms, and the hair of the family dog. While the parents' pediatrician referred them specifically for hypnosis, a developmentally appropriate approach without any hypnosis per se was effective in resolving the problem. Parent counseling and guidance was provided to allow the parents to understand the likely "cause" of hair pulling to be their child's inability to verbally express feelings of being "left out" or "ignored" by the appearance of the new baby. Modeling ways to talk with their daughter and discussion of this allowed them to move from previous well-meaning but ineffective "Stop that!" and pulling her hand away from her scalp, to comforting and distracting play and personal attention from parents. No discussion of hypnosis took place nor was indicated. The "habit" problem of hair pulling quickly resolved.

By hypnosis we mean a state of focused attention and absorbed attention, occurring or evolving spontaneously or upon invitation and/or guidance. We explain to pediatric patients and families, and colleague learners that hypnosis is "a state or feeling like when you are pretending, daydreaming, imagining, or 'zoning out'". For the preschool child their engagement in pretending and imaginative play is the equivalent of hypnosis, and our approach and positively expectant language must join with them to facilitate change through their play. The specificity and uniqueness of working hypnotically with preschool children is reflected in a Preschool Family Asthma Program, which incorporates hypnosis and hypnotic language (Kohen & Wynne, 1997; Kuttner & Catchpole, 2013).

School Age Development

Growth and development in the school age or middle years occurs in discontinuous spurts and changes may seem sudden. Parents, teachers, and child health professionals learn to adapt to these changes. A boy manifests greatly improved neuromotor control and a girl's hand-eye coordination is suddenly much better. Children at this stage improve in their ability to handle and process information as they move from strictly concrete ideas to more conceptual understanding. Metalinguistic skills develop. Children use more complex sentences and become more flexible in their thinking. They improve in their ability to manipulate symbols. Children become aware of their own feelings and experiences as private and distinct from those of others at about 7–8 years. This is also the time when they recognize the permanency of death. Most school age children are very interested in making friends, and peer acceptance and conformity become important (Kohen & Olness, 2023a).

Child health professionals who teach hypnosis to school age children will find that they usually are enthusiastic, learn quickly, and enjoy the sense of control. In speaking with school age children, it is important to consider whether they are still close to all concrete thinking or have begun to develop the capacity to understand metaphors. As at any age, awareness and assessment of the child's developmental age and trajectory will be essential to evolving a therapeutic hypnosis plan (Kuttner & Catchpole, 2013). Since how we talk is how we think is how we feel, we strive to pay careful attention to language before, during, and after formal hypnotic "work". The context of where the child is developmentally will inform what we say and how we say it, with or without formal hypnosis. In a therapeutic relationship driven by our rapport, children are listening carefully. Therefore, we must speak carefully *because* spontaneous hypnosis is occurring throughout our conversation. Attention to this reality potentially increases the therapeutic value of our hypnotic relationship, knowing that so-called "informal" or conversational hypnosis is occurring all the time, and not only during something more "formalized" (see Kohen & Olness, 2023b).

Case History: School Age

Heidi was 9 years old. She had an 11-year-old brother and a 4-year-old sister. She did well in school, had several friends, and especially enjoyed riding her bicycle, playing the piano, and baking with her mom who was a nurse. Her dad was a teacher and she enjoyed going on bike rides with him. Her mother said that they were a happy family with no significant problems until Heidi began to have difficulty changing to clean clothes. This began shortly after Heidi and her siblings had upper respiratory infections and missed some schooldays. Heidi's reluctance to change clothes progressed to the point that she was wearing only one dress. Heidi could not explain this to her parents and was upset by their pleadings to change. Her mother would go into Heidi's bedroom when she was asleep, carefully remove the dress, wash and dry it, and put it back on Heidi. Heidi began to manifest more obsessive compulsive disorder (OCD) type symptoms, insisting that she use the same plate at meals, riding her bike over a fixed route, and having difficulty with any change in school routines. Her parents made a self-referral, asking that Heidi learn hypnosis.

After taking a careful history the pediatrician suggested that Heidi might have PANDAS (Pediatric autoimmune neuropsychiatric disorders associated with streptococcus). However, recognizing that Heidi was herself puzzled and anxious about her symptoms and that she still enjoyed bike riding (albeit in a fixed manner), the pediatrician suggested that Heidi might enjoy using her imagination to ride even better. She praised Heidi for getting exercise in this way and told her about famous athletes who used their imagination to improve skills in all types of sports, including bike racing. She invited Heidi to think about riding her bike and it might be a new bike or the same bike and she could imagine her control of the bike handlebars and the pedals to go where she wanted, in the direction she wanted. Parents and siblings and teachers had been coaxing Heidi to be more flexible and Heidi perceived this as their effort to control her. The pediatrician thought it important to offer Heidi something that she could control. Heidi could use the bike in her imagination exactly as she wished. She suggested that Heidi could enjoy this use of her imagination every day if she wished or perhaps on some days and not on others.

During the next week, one of her siblings had a throat culture positive for streptococcus and Heidi had an elevated ASO (antistreptolysin O) titer. She had received oral penicillin for a week. At the next visit, Heidi said she enjoyed her imaginary bike rides and she seemed calmer. The pediatrician invited her to demonstrate her imagination skill and asked where she would like to go on her bike. She said she would like to ride to a department store and look at bikes and clothes! The pediatrician encouraged her and said that Heidi could share what she was buying if she wished to do so. Heidi bought a new bike, a dress, jeans, and a t-shirt. She said she would like to use the jeans for biking and the dress for school. At the conclusion of the visit, the pediatrician complimented her skill in using her imagination and said she could tell her mom about her purchases if she wished. Heidi said she didn't know if they could afford the bike but she thought they could afford the clothes. This statement represented more concrete thinking.

At the third visit, Heidi was wearing jeans and a t-shirt. She told the pediatrician that she would be getting the bike for her birthday. It is unclear whether her improvement related to the penicillin or to the self-hypnosis. Follow up with Heidi thereafter was by phone for six months. Heidi said that she was happy that her friends were no longer making fun of one dress. She said she was still going on imaginary bike rides. Her parents said she was back to "normal".

Early Adolescent Development

That an adolescent is not an adult seems obvious, but this is sometimes overlooked in hypnosis. If an adolescent is to achieve the goal of mastery of some problem through a successful response to therapeutic strategies and invitation to hypnosis, language must be adapted to the level and interests of the young adolescent, notably being neither too simplistic as with a younger child, nor too complex. Perhaps more than with the young child or adults, it is imperative that clinicians working with an adolescent indeed like teenagers. This (or its absence!) will be spontaneously evident to most teens, and will drive (or hinder) the rapport, which is essential to any clinician's success in introducing and facilitating a therapeutic hypnosis approach with a young adolescent. Perhaps even more importantly for a young adolescent, the clinician teaching and guiding hypnosis must be careful to not treat the adolescent "like a little kid", and rather take into account their natural grappling with and adjustment to puberty, and their overall perceptual and conceptual skills with respect to problems and possible solutions. In this case, more than with younger children, being able to SEE and physically experience differences in hypnosis may be a very useful strategy and hypnotic experience. For example, in addition to suggestions for favorite place imagery, the clinician may find that teaching ideomotor signaling and/or the "magnetic fingers" (fingers "automatically" coming together), or arm catalepsy may allow for appreciation that changes can "happen" and they can become engaged with the process. Such a strategy was useful in the following case example and went a long way toward ratifying trance behavior and driving hypnotic rapport for the young adolescent who was previously hesitant/skeptical.

By contrast with the earlier example of a 3-year-old, a 12-year-old girl – Maria - with an "official" label of "Trichotillomania" was referred for pulling out the hair of eyelashes, eyebrows, and scalp. The history revealed a rather abrupt onset but no known history of either preceding associated obsessive-compulsive behaviors or streptococcal infection. There was no family history of hair pulling. Rapport with Maria and history taking at the first visit revealed – to the surprise of her parents – that she was very upset about the fact that one of her best friends had started to like other girls more and was not talking as much with Maria as she had in the past. She had not (yet) spoken with the friend or her parents or anyone else about her sadness and stress about this. She expressed anger at herself at the feeling that she "had to" pull her eyelashes, eyebrows, scalp hair, and "hating" how she looked, not wanting to go to school. Because she was a bright girl with good verbal skills and an evolving awareness of feelings consistent with her age and emerging adolescence, a conversational hypnosis approach was utilized. When asked if she would *miss* the hair pulling *when* it was *gone*, she said "NO" quite emphatically, and listened carefully. When asked *how* things might be different, she said clearly that she would like the way she looked and would probably be fine to go to school. When asked if she would like to learn a way to *stop* pulling her hair out, she was surprised and readily agreed. Beyond this hypnotic conversation at the first visit, the hair pulling slowed down and she was happy to report as much a week later. A more "formal" self-hypnosis exercise of "hands-helping-hands" (Kohen, 1996) was taught. She agreed to practice this twice a day. By the third visit, visible growth of eyelashes eyebrows and areas of where scalp hair had been pulled were evident. Counseling around her feelings and how she might talk with her girlfriend were concurrent with hypnosis reinforcement at each visit. Full resolution of her hair pulling followed and leads us to conclude this was a habit-problem that began and evolved in association with stress, and not a diagnosis of Trichotillomania. Analogous, but developmentally specific hypnosis approaches have been effective for older adolescents/young adults with the hair pulling of trichotillomania. (Kohen, 1996).

Late Adolescent Development

As young people move into the growing autonomy of late adolescence, they begin to further refine abstract thinking, mature in their awareness and acknowledgment of feelings (their own and others), and are increasingly future-oriented as they contemplate what their life might be or could be following high school. Will they get a job? Will they go to college? What will they become? Awareness and respect for these maturational steps and the challenges thereof will not only facilitate the clinician's rapport with the older adolescent but also serve to guide the determination of hypnosis strategies. While computer games and activity on social media continue from early and mid-adolescence, the older adolescent's world has expanded. They may be by driving a car/riding with friends, playing music and going to concerts, involvement in sports activities as a participant and/or observer, and a myriad of other performance and social engagements. Mutual exploration of these will often provide the ingredients for both hypnosis initiation and active imagery toward the expression of desired outcomes (goals) of hypnosis and the requisite hypnotic suggestions. The creativity of the older adolescent/young adult should be cultivated for their own benefit in determining the process and outcome of therapeutic hypnosis.

For these reasons, it is preferable to help the adolescent patient select most or all of the details of imagery utilized in therapeutic suggestions. For example, the therapist might say "Think of some of the ways you feel comfortable, happy, and safe, like maybe when you're playing that favorite video game with your best friend, or when you're shooting baskets, or when you go mountain biking with your cousins" and then follow their lead instead of suggesting or guessing at a particular plan. If the adolescent is seen over a long period of time, it is important to keep in mind that techniques that were appealing and helpful at one age may have no value or even be aversive at a later age, especially as young adolescents become 18 or 19 years of age and their lives become much different. The normal skepticism many adolescents may have in meeting new adults may manifest in hesitancy about "this hypnosis stuff" and "I don't know if it's real or can really change things ...".

In our experience, many if not most children and teens who learn and utilize hypnosis successfully for one issue or problem in their lives often spontaneously and naturally apply these same skills for other challenges that they encounter as they get older. Awareness of this allows us to implicitly understand how the process of development and maturation naturally influences *how* young people's self-hypnosis strategies, and specifically their imagery, change as they mature. Evidence of this is reflected in a longitudinal study of children and teens who had learned and applied self-hypnosis successfully for migraine and other types of headaches. Kohen (2010) sent surveys to 178 consecutive youths who had previously been referred for treatment of headaches with training in (self)-hypnosis. Of 134 delivered surveys, 52 were returned complete. Strikingly, many years after treatment, 85%

reported continued relief with self-hypnosis, often describing in remarkable detail the ways in which *what* they do and *how* they do their self-hypnosis had changed and evolved since when they first learned, often more than 10–12 years earlier (Kohen, 2010, 2011). Kuttner's videos of children utilizing hypnosis in the treatment of cancer (Kuttner, 1986, 1999) and their discussion of that treatment "13 years later" are also compelling evidence of the ways in which hypnosis learning stays with children as they mature. Beyond being important, exciting, and affirming feedback, this data encourages us to continue to hold fast to our commitment to focus carefully on our rapport in each visit, and to explore with our patients/clients how their lives are evolving and, in turn, how their hypnosis could and should evolve concurrent with and in response to their maturation.

Case example: BG was 17-years-old when referred for hypnosis to help manage "anger outbursts" in response to his perception of his father's "loud chewing noises at the dinner table". This misophonia was very disruptive to family life at mealtimes and even when watching TV together. As rapport developed, anxieties about other issues were revealed, notably the not atypical difficulties with friendships, loss of girlfriend to his previous "best friend", and sense of isolation from his larger peer group. While his pediatrician prescribed anxiolytic and antidepressant medication in the form of an SSRI (selective serotonin reuptake inhibitor), the therapist was asked to help with the misophonia.

He was very skeptical about hypnosis, and preferred to "withdraw" into his video games which include requisite earphones, which had the added benefit of [some] "noise cancellation".

Utilizing his own language and curiosity, he was asked (without any "formal" hypnosis) "Did you know that your brain already knows how to reduce the awareness of all sorts of sounds?" His response was an attentive, quizzical look as though to say, "What do you mean?"

He was invited to "do an experiment" by closing his eyes and turning his attention to the sound of the air flowing in the room and to "let your head nod when you can hear it clearly". An ideomotor head nod followed. He was asked to indicate what number the volume was on a 0–10 scale. He held up 5 fingers. He was invited to turn it up to "7 or 8" and without being asked he nodded that this was done. After a brief pause he was asked to "turn the volume up to maximum, so you're kind of 'blasting' it". He did so, and grimaced. He was asked to then "Turn it way, way, down .... and then CLICK it off and let me know when that's done". He smiled and opened his eyes. He said simply "*That* was very cool!" He was invited to practice this several times a day and especially whenever any loud/disturbing noise started to bother him. He agreed. At the next visit, he complained that "I practiced but it's not working ...". The therapist's response was "not YET ... it's not working the way you want... . YET ... . Continue practicing". He was asked to show the therapist *how* he practiced and did so. By the next visit, he acknowledged he was improving. While struggles with friends continued, he was very proud of having eliminated the misophonia problem, and continued coming to the therapist to talk about ways to manage the relationship struggles (Kohen & Olness, 2023c).

Cross-cultural Variables

Whether overtly demonstrated or not, children and their families bring a cultural framework into each patient–child health professional encounter (Torjesen & Olness, 2018). Child health professionals also bring their own cultural framework. Hence, there may be conflicting ideas about child development, child discipline, parental roles, and treatments. Different cultures have differing ideas about what causes emotional, behavioral, or mental health difficulties. Some immigrant families may be providing their children with traditional herbal treatments. It is important that child health professionals be aware of the possibility of these differing ideas. Before teaching hypnosis, it is important to know what are family perceptions about hypnosis.

Other Developmental Factors to Consider in Teaching Hypnosis

Kohlberg, who developed a theory of moral development, was especially interested in reasoning processes involved in decision-making and how people perceive their rights. As persons move from childhood to adulthood, there are shifts in reasoning about rights and entitlement (Peens & Louw, 2000).

Imagination has a central function in the development of ideas and social function. Most children are skilled in visual imagery. Studies show that these skills wane. A study comparing young adults and elderly indicated that aging might impair the ability to maintain images (Dror & Kosslyn, 1994). It is helpful to ask adult patients about their preferred images, i.e., visual, auditory, kinesthetic, and olfactory.

Factors That Impair Normal Development

Some children experience frustration in school because they have unrecognized subtle learning disabilities or a learning style that does not mesh with the school system. There are many factors that may cause significant injury to the developing brain in utero or early life. These include alcohol and drug use during pregnancy, malnutrition in utero or during the first two years of life, iron deficiency during the first year of life, congenital cardiac defects necessitating surgery, many infectious diseases, and exposure to toxins such as lead or herbicides (Olness, 2003). The outstanding work of Galler and colleagues (Galler et al., 2011; Waber, et al., 2014; Waber, et al., 2018) has demonstrated that brain injury from early malnutrition may not manifest in learning problems until early adolescence and also impacts cognitive abilities in later life. Toxic stress or adverse childhood experiences early in life can lead to psychological problems that impair learning and development (Gilgoff et al., 2020). Childhood, adolescent, and adult head injuries also impact cognitive function. These limitations may be short term or permanent (Petranovich et al., 2020; Watson and Mjaanes, 2019, Narang et al., 2020).

Summary

Changes in human development impact how one learns and responds to hypnosis.

Normal developmental trajectories may be impaired in many ways. It is important that health professionals who teach hypnosis take careful histories about life events that may affect cognition, learning styles, and perceptions about hypnosis.

References

Brown, J. D., King, M. A., & Wissow, L. S. (2017). The central role of relationships with trauma-informed integrated care for children and youth. *Academic Pediatrics*, *17*, S94–S101.

Dror, I. E., & Kosslyn, S. M. (1994). Mental imagery and aging. *Psychology Aging*, *9*, 90–102. doi: 10.1037//0882-7974.9.1.90.

Galler, J. R., Bryce, C. P., Waber, D. P., Medford, G., Eaglesfield, G. D., & Fitzmaurice, G. (2011). Early malnutrition predicts parent reports of externalizing behaviors at ages 9–17. *Nutritional Neuroscience*, *14*, 138–144. Doi: 10.1179/147683011X13009738172521.

Gilgoff, R., Singh, L., Koita, K., Gentile, B., & Marques, S. S. (2020). Adverse childhood experiences, outcomes, and interventions. *Pediatric Clinics of North America*, *67*, 259–273. doi:10.1016/j.pcl.2019.12.001.

Kohen, D. P., & Olness, K. (2023a). Chapter 5 Hypnotic invitations for children: Techniques, strategies and approache. *Hypnosis with children – 5th edition* (pp. 46–71). Routledge Publications, Taylor & Francis. DOI: 10.4324/9781003243687-6

Kohen, D. P., & Olness, K. (2023b). Chapter 7 Facilitating effective interpersonal relationships with hypnosis – Language for clinicians and parents. *Hypnosis with children – 5th edition* (pp. 85–95). Routledge Publications, Taylor & Francis. DOI: 10.4324/9781003243687-9

Kohen, D. P., & Olness, K. (2023c). Chapter 10 Therapeutic hypnosis for habit disorders. *Hypnosis with children – 5th edition* (pp. 140–185). Routledge Publications, Taylor & Francis. DOI: 10.4324/9781003243687-12

Kohen, D. P., & Kaiser, P. (2014). Clinical hypnosis with children and adolescents—What? Why? How? Origins, applications, and efficacy. Children, 1, 74–98. DOI: 10.3390%2Fchildren1020074

Kohen, D. P., & Wynne, E. (1997) Applying hypnosis in a preschool family asthma education program: Uses of storytelling, imagery, and relaxation. *American Journal of Clinical Hypnosis*. *39*, 169–181. 10.1080/00029157.1997.10403382

Kohen, D. P. (1991). Applications of relaxation and mental imagery (self-hypnosis) for habit problems. *Pediatric Annals*, *20*(3), 136–144.

Kohen, D. P. (1996). Management of trichotillomania with relaxation/mental imagery (self-hypnosis): Experience with five children. *Journal of Developmental and Behavioral Pediatrics*, *17*(5), 328–334.

Kohen, D. P. (2010). Long term follow-up of self-hypnosis training for recurrent headaches: What the children say. *The International Journal of Clinical and Experimental Hypnosis*, *58*(4), 417–432.

Kohen, D. P. (2011). Chronic daily headache: Helping adolescents help themselves with self-hypnosis. *American Journal of Clinical Hypnosis*, *54*(1), 32–46.

Kuttner, L. (1986). *No fears, no tears (29 mins)*. DVD available from http://bookstore.cw.bc.ca email: bookstore@cw.bc.ca US or Canada: 1-800-331-1533 x 3 or Crown House Publishing at http://www.chpus.com

Kuttner, L. (1991a). Special considerations for using hypnosis with young children. In W. Wester, & D. O'Grady (Eds.), *Clinical Hypnosis for Children*. (pp. 1336–1444). Brunner/Mazel.

Kuttner, L. (1991b). Helpful strategies in working with preschool children in pediatric practice. *Pediatric Annals*, *20*(3), 120–127.

Kuttner, L. (1999). *No fears, no tears 13 years later: Children coping with pain (46 mins)*. DVD available: http://bookstore.cw.bc.ca email: bookstore@cw.bc.ca; or, Crown House Publishing at http://www.chpus.com

Kuttner, L., & Catchpole, R. E. H. (2013). Development matters: Hypnosis with children. In L. I. Sugarman, & W. C. Wester (Eds.), *Therapeutic hypnosis with children and adolescents, 2nd edition*. (pp. 25–44). Williston, VT: Crown House.

Narang, S. K., Fingarson, A., & Lukefahr, J. (2020) Abusive head trauma in infants and children. *Pediatrics*, *145*(4), e20200203.doi: 10:1542/peds.2020-0203.

Olness, K. (2003). Effects on brain development leading to cognitive impairment: A worldwide epidemic. *Journal of Developmental and Behavioral Pediatrics*, 24, 120–130.

Peens, B. J. , & Louw, D. A. (2000). Kohlberg's theory of moral development: insights into rights reasoning. *Medicine and Law*, *19*, 351–372.

Petranovich, C. L., Smith-Paine, J., Wade, S. L., Yeates, K. W., Taylor, H. G., Stancin, T., & Kurowski, B. G. (2020) From early childhood to adolescence: Lessons about traumatic brain injury from the Ohio head injury outcomes study. *Journal of Head Trauma and Rehabilitation*, *35*, 226–239. doi: 10.1097/HTR.0000000000000555.

Taylor H. G. (2004). Research on outcomes of pediatric traumatic brain injury: Current advances and future directions. *Developmental Neuropsychology*, *25*, 199–225. Doi: 10.1080/87565641.2004.9651928.

Torjesen, K., & Olness, K. (2018). Culturally effective care, in J. Foy (Ed.), *Mental health care of children and adolescents.* (pp. 53–70). Itasca, IL: American Academy of Pediatrics.

Waber, D. P., Bryce, C. P., Girard, J. M., Fischer, L. K., Fitzmaurice, G. M., & Galler, J. R. (2018). Parental history of moderate to severe infantile malnutrition is associated with cognitive deficits in their adult offspring. *Nutritional Neuroscience*, *21*, 195–201. Doi: 10.1080/1028415X.2016.1258379.

Waber, D. P., Bryce, C. P., Girard, J. M., Zichlin, M., Fitzmaurice, G. M., & Galler, J. R. (2014). Impaired IQ and academic skills in adults who experienced moderate to severe infantile malnutrition: A 40-year study. *Nutritional Neuroscience*, *17*, 58–64. Doi: 10.1179/1476830513Y.00000061.

Watson, A., & Mjaanes, J. M. (2019). Soccer injuries in children and adolescents. *Pediatrics*, *144*, 2019–2759. Doi: 10.1542/peds.2019-2759.

14

HYPNOSIS AND INTEGRATIVE ASPECTS OF MUSIC

Anita Jung
JUNG WELLNESS INSTITUTE

Professional Background

As a therapist and trainer, I have been probing the combined intricacies of music and hypnosis in treatment for almost three decades. My interest in the arts eventually guided me to Ericksonian principles after my first impactful encounter with hypnosis in 1995. After years of teaching and training in hypnosis, similarities between musical and hypnotic principles emerged with the conclusion that one does not have to play an instrument to combine musical elements with hypnosis. My commitment to the hypnosis community resulted in serving as the President of the American Society of Clinical Hypnosis and the Central Texas Society of Clinical Hypnosis and as a board member of the International Society of Hypnosis. My passion for music and hypnosis culminated in teaching, creating hypnotherapeutic recordings, and disseminating my acquired knowledge with my professional community globally.

Theoretical Framework

Many definitions of hypnosis have illuminated the horizon, as have many attempts to define music. For me, hypnosis is a powerful tool that elicits ease of entrance into trance, intentionally shifting states and expanding consciousness. I define trance as a state of intense immersion and creative engagement accompanied by a disappearing awareness of time, space, and self in which core beliefs and identity are bypassed, and an expansion of possibilities emerges.

This chapter examines the use of musical elements in hypnosis and describes my theoretical framework by highlighting research similarities between the efficacy of music and hypnosis in treatment. Studies integrating music and hypnosis have increased in the last few years. This chapter unfolds infusing musical elements to enhance therapeutic encounters and accentuate hypnotic techniques in medicine and psychotherapy. Shared elements between music and hypnosis include rhythm, repetition, prosody, and novelty to inform the subject matter.

DOI: 10.4324/9781003449126-19

Review of Research

Applications of Music in Medicine and Psychotherapy

The origins of music and its societal functions, particularly during the Covid-19 pandemic, showed that music might be the food and water of social psychological connectedness, particularly when isolated from people (Greenberg et al., 2021). Music evokes emotions spontaneously, even without external stimuli or associations.

A systematic review and meta-analysis outlined that music can reduce anxiety, fear, depression, and stress (de Witte et al., 2020; Kühlmann et al., 2018). The ability of music to induce intense pleasure, as well as its putative stimulation of endogenous reward systems, suggests a benefit to mental and physical well-being (Blood & Zatorre, 2001) and subsequently, resulted in changes in cerebral blood flow, heart rate, electromyogram, and respiration.

Throughout the years, numerous studies have documented the efficacy of the integration of music in medicine and surgeries (Bernardi et al., 2006; de Witte et al., 2020; Dietrich et al., 2015; Dileo, 2006; Gäbel et al., 2017; Gallagher, 2011; Gutgsell et al., 2013) with promising results in the treatment of pain (Kühlmann et al., 2018; Martin-Saavedra et al., 2018;). In oncology, music has been utilized to manage disease symptoms and treat side effects. Listening to prerecorded music resulted in a beneficial effect on anxiety, pain, mood, and quality of life (Bradt et al., 2011). Music has also positively affected anxiety reduction before breast biopsy and other surgical procedures (Lee et al., 2012).

Hospice patients reported pleasant visualizations accompanied by relaxing and calming sensations of lightness in their body when they participated in receptive music-only therapy in which a custom-built body tambura was played on their body or near their body (Teut et al., 2014). Post-treatment with the body tambura (hospice) in India yielded substantial reduction of pain and reports of pleasant experiences (Dietrich et al., 2015).

Music therapy includes various psychotherapeutic methods using music as a medium for emotional expression and communication through verbal reflections and playing music. After listening to music, studies report a compelling decrease in anxiety (Fachner et al., 2012) and depression (Hanser & Thompson, 1994) and significant improvement in global functioning in everyday life (Erkkilä et al., 2011). Post-treatment results suggest an impact on processing emotions connected to anxiety with lasting electromyography changes in resting electroencephalogram (Fachner et al., 2012).

Applications of Hypnosis in Medicine and Psychotherapy

The focus of hypnosis on the mind–body relationship and its effects on health and disease has proven to be an effective therapeutic tool in medical contexts (Wahbeh et al., 2008). Notable studies depict the efficacy of managing and treating pain with hypnosis (Jensen & Patterson, 2014; Jensen & Turk, 2014). Furthermore, a literature review on the efficacy of hypnotic analgesia in adults shows hypnosis as a viable treatment for chronic and acute pain conditions (Stoelb et al., 2009). Additionally, hypnosis enhances the efficacy of psychodynamic and cognitive-behavioral psychotherapy (Kirsch, 1996).

Integrative Applications of Music and Hypnosis

Few studies on the integrative applications of music and hypnosis exist, but efforts in the last two decades have emerged (e.g., Blankfield et al., 1995; Elkins, 2017; Snodgrass & Lynn, 1989; Wang et al., 2015). Between-group comparisons, music with suggestions (MSG) versus music only (MOG), pre-and post-breast biopsy both showed reduced stress, anxiety, and depression. They increased optimism in the MSG, whereas the MOG yielded reduced stress, anxiety, and pain (Tellez et al., 2016).

Palliative cancer patients listened to rhythmically dominated music with gradually decreasing tempi, similar to a lullaby. The effects showed increased synchronization and coordination of heart rate and musical beat, decreased need for analgesics, and ease of falling asleep. The patients who achieved the highest synchronization occurred in patients with higher relaxation rates (Reinhardt, 1999).

Although hypnosis and music have been widely used in the treatment of mental health problems, self-care, and medicine, no articles describe the use of the elements of music as a tool in hypnosis in particular. Studies combining both pair background music with hypnotic suggestions.

Shared Elements of Music and Hypnosis

Commonalities between music and hypnosis to help individuals shift states are striking, and practitioners of hypnosis can learn from the realm of music. Observing the way music is used in film assists the understanding of creating impact in clinical sessions to benefit the individual's well-being. With this in mind, it has become clear that the neurobiology of music overlaps with the neurobiology of hypnosis (Brown, 1991). The following elements, research-informed, clearly outline how to create impact and inspire change (Table 14.1).

Rhythm

Rhythm is an effective tool to be utilized in hypnosis that can lead to attunement and entrainment, shape brain oscillations, and aid in transforming states and symptoms.

Table 14.1 Musical Elements and Its Use in Hypnosis

Musical Elements	*Techniques*	*Objective*	*Outcome*
1 Rhythm	Pacing and Leading with Rhythm	Brain Oscillations Entrainment	Trance Rapport Attunement
2 Repetition/ Patterns	Threefold Pattern Hypnotic Tihai	Brain Oscillations Conflict Detection ACC Activation	Pattern Interruption Memorable Suggestions
3 Prosody	Vocal Intonations Pauses Pitch Variations	Entrainment Conflict Detection ACC Activation	Memorable Suggestions
4 Novelty	Threefold Pattern Hypnotic Tihai	Conflict Detection ACC Activation	Change of Perspective Transformation of Symptoms

BRAIN OSCILLATIONS

Since the origination of recording the electrical activity of the human brain from the scalp in 1875, activity is usually computed and expressed as amplitude (representing the number of neurons firing) in terms of five frequency bands: delta (1–4 Hz), theta (4–8 Hz), alpha (8–12 Hz), beta (14–30 Hz), and gamma (>30 Hz). Activity in different bandwidths reflects different mental states, such as alert and busy states, that can be observed in the dominance of low-amplitude beta waves. More relaxed and inattentive states, on the other hand, are associated with alpha power. Hypnotic experiences tend to be associated with power in the theta bandwidth and hypnotic responding has been associated with changes in patterns of gamma oscillations which depend on many factors (Jensen et al., 2015). Their role in hypnosis includes recording and recalling declarative memory and emotional limbic circuits, the obvious link between limbic and neocortical circuits in hypnosis (Jensen et al., 2015; see also Jensen, in Section 2).

In music, the 4/4 rhythm shows a tendency toward theta oscillations. The amygdala and hippocampus, for instance, fire in theta rhythm during a trauma state (Seidenbecher et al., 2003). De Benedittis and Sironi (1988) suggested that the amygdala's effects on the arousal at the hypnotic state mediate hypnotic behavior, partially by a dynamic balance of antagonizing effects of discrete limbic structures, the amygdala and the hippocampus, highly significant in the treatment of trauma.

ENTRAINMENT

This scientific process explains how rhythmic repetition of sound influences human experience. Rhythms displayed by two or more phenomena become synchronized, with one of the rhythms often being more dominant, capturing the rhythm of the other. Rather than overlapping, the patterns maintain a consistent relationship with each other (Bluedorn, 2002). Early days of EEG research discovered that alpha and beta waves could be synchronized, entrained, to the frequency of an external, bright strobe light stimulus. Subjects with specific entrained frequencies of an external stimulus entered trance-like states experiencing deep peacefulness, dream-like visions, and other unexpected sensations (Walter, 1953). Communicative rhythms of interacting individuals lead to entrainment (Montagu & Matson, 1979) and may enhance a sense of social belonging (Gerkema, 2002). These rhythms form the basis for rapport and attunement in hypnosis. Music therapists distinguish between three separate modes in the utilization of clinical processes. They range from primary entrainment, matching the music to the physical or cognitive behavior; to secondary entrainment, synchronizing the music with the skill or concept to be learned; to tertiary entrainment, matching the music to cause a change in an unrelated behavior (Rider & Eagle, 1986). The serendipitous variety of music produces internal oscillations that affect sensitivity, emotional availability, and perception. Pulse, tempo, rhythmic patterns, vocal intonations, pre-recorded music, or playing an instrument move us through synchronization processes of entrainment (Levitin et al., 2018) and are elements of an effective hypnosis session.

Prosody

The effects of instinctive vocalizations of lullabies by mothers communicate emotional information that engages and calms the child (Roederer, 1984). Intonations convey emotional states of trust (Trevarthen, 1999–2000). In contrast, we can observe the flat affect, the interrupted flow/rhythm, and the lack of prosody as characteristics observed in trauma survivors. Pursuing prosody instead of monotony, for instance, adding pauses and intonations, can enhance memory beyond its role in comprehension and tends to create tension (Shintel et al., 2014) or make suggestions more memorable. My clinical experience, research-informed, suggests that skillful prosody elicits arousal, creates conflict detection, activates the ACC, heightens the effect of the suggestion, activates self-regulation, and enhances memory.

Repetition

Just as repetition can be an oscillator, *Threefold patterns* (TP) seem deeply rooted in our consciousness. *Omne trium perfectum*, all things that come in three are perfect, a Latin proverb, to be harnessed as a tool to use repetition in hypnosis. The phenomenological effects of TP cultivate the creation of potent, artistic impact. Throughout the ages, TP result in an expected sense of balance, harmony, structure, and satisfaction in creativity, various art forms, and graphic design resonating with our thinking patterns. Composers and performers, at times, also craft elements of unease to artistically evoke a positive psychological effect (Huron, 2006). Hypnotic suggestions enhance, introduce, and add novel perceptual experiences in highly suggestible individuals (Landry et al., 2021). At times, hypnosis must also evoke unease or confusion to work on desensitization, monitor the practice of self-hypnosis skills, or set up the delivery of a posthypnotic suggestion (confusion technique by Milton H. Erickson).

Similarly, the sophisticated tihai, a polyrhythmic technique omnipresent in Indian classical music, sets up a sequence, recognized as a pattern that repeats three times and ends on the one with a dramatic rest, to be followed by a change in pattern or rhythm (Chatterjee, 2005; Ranade, 2006) or marking the ending of a song. The tihai creates tension with a dramatic, unexpected impactful effect, thereby providing catharsis upon its resolution. Our mind finds comfort in the interplay of repetition and its associated expectation. TP phrasings in hypnosis can create conceptually intriguing impact, transform the perception of memories and symptoms, and interrupt the individual's mind from its ordinary thoughts or habits.

The repetitive reorienting of attention by directed saccadic or tracking eye movements are thought to produce specific shifts in regional brain activation and neuromodulation similar to those produced during rapid eye movement (REM) sleep and the potential effectiveness of other stimuli used in the waking state according to eye movement desensitization reprocessing therapy (Stickgold, 2002). Bilateral stimulation such as tapping, clapping, drumming, and binary audio recordings, all rhythmic components, can elicit trance in hypnosis.

Novelty and Change of Perspective

The anterior cingulate cortex (ACC) is involved in conflict monitoring (Raz et al., 2005). During a change in pattern, the incongruency and the element of surprise set up conflict detection, which activates the ACC. The brain notices the prediction error and moves into a state of confusion with heightened arousal. The subsequent hypnotic suggestion is more readily available to the conscious, now receptive, mind. Creating a *Hypnotic Tihai*

(HT) with words and rhythm is one way to increase arousal to evoke involuntary conflict that tends to lead to activation of the ACC, thereby perceiving the posthypnotic suggestion as the resolution that creates novelty. For example, Noe (assumed name), a 38-year-old female who loved the *Beatles*, experienced distress regarding conflict with her sister. While accompanying Noe from the waiting room to my office, I hummed the Beatles song *Let it Be*. The induction started with three breaths to introduce the TP and seed the HT. Once calm and focused, the following HT included: (1) *You can allow yourself to be.* (2) *You can allow yourself to be.* (3) *You can!* (long dramatic pause) *let it be! You can* was dramatically emphasized which tends to heighten the impact of the suggestion. After a brief silence, the recorded song *let it be* played which pleasantly surprised Noe (memorable suggestion). She was instructed to sing along quietly in her mind or out loud. Her homework included singing the song whenever thoughts of conflict arose.

New Research, Perspectives, Applications

This chapter hopes to prompt new studies and research to look deeper into the structure of the arts, particularly music, to combine principles with hypnosis and test its impact. Longitudinal studies on the impact might yield promising results.

Clinical Illustration

This illustration depicts the story of Daniel (assumed name), a middle-aged father and primary caregiver of three sons, who encountered an unwanted divorce and the closing of his business a year prior. A day before the children would leave for their mother's house, Daniel experienced crying spells and spiraled into depressive episodes accompanied by stomach pain that lasted until the children returned from their visit. Referred by his psychiatrist for hypnosis, his current medication regime included antidepressants which kept him fairly stable. Daniel worked from home, and his inability to concentrate had affected his work. No stranger to therapy, he was hopeful that hypnosis might provide relief. It became apparent that his current symptomology mirrored a traumatic event in his childhood (age 6) that centralized into his current situation.

Relevant to this vignette, trauma is defined as the individual experience of an event or enduring conditions in which the individual's ability to integrate his emotional experience is overwhelmed, whereby the individual's experiences constitute a threat to his life, bodily integrity, or that of a caregiver or family (Saakvitne et al., 2000) resulting in lasting adverse effects on the individual's functioning and mental, physical, social, emotional, or spiritual well-being (SAMSHA, 2014).

Daniel was parentified at age 8 when his close Greek family moved across the country, which he describes as traumatizing. His affect and speech, when he spoke of caring for his siblings, afraid that his parents would not return from work, resembled his current symptomatology. Daniel's nervous system had been habitually in a state of high reactivity, as is often the case in trauma states, subsequently lowering his threshold for the perception and the expression of pain. Since music can stimulate brain areas involved in traumatic memory and sensory-emotional processing (Koelsch, 2009) and significantly reduce symptoms, foster resilience, and improve functioning (Landis-Shack et al., 2017), musical elements were woven into the hypnosis sessions. Coupling access to dissociated traumatic memories with positive restructuring of those memories can be placed into a broader perspective in hypnosis (Spiegel & Cardena, 1990).

All hypnosis included the following: Elicitations began with three deep breaths to seed the HT to bypass resistance. The suggestion for listening to a recorded frame drum included feeling grounded, after the rhythm, initially scattered to simulate wandering thoughts, became steady and melodic. A deceleration of the rhythm ratified the trance as a method of deepening. A soothing melody, played by a string instrument called oud, used in Greece, formed the basis for rapport and becoming curious. The musical piece was chosen because of his musical preference and his relation to Greece. The drum, oud, and voice stimulated entrainment. Ideo-motor finger movements were established for unconscious communication.

Session 1

The initial session encompassed discovery, intimation, and set up of positive expectations by harnessing detailed behavioral and internal outcomes. Hypnosis aimed at facilitating entrainment and theta activity in his brain, coupled with suggestions to find ease (TP), anchored an easy return. Daniel was asked to verbalize the rhythm and use his hands to play the rhythm on his body (bilateral stimulation) to set up a somatically based self-hypnosis practice. He imagined a peaceful, green pasture and experienced heightened well-being. His assignments included playing the rhythm several times a day or listening to the recording to evoke a state of well-being.

Session 2

Daniel reported increased hopefulness and motivation. When asked if his stomach felt calmer, he realized that he had not noticed the absence of discomfort but had become aware of a sense of ease. However, he was still tearful as he discussed his children's absence.

Directly, the hypnotic session focused on the primary problem. Indirectly, ambiguous communication included Tolkien's *Lord of the Rings* stories to elicit conceptual realizations and emotions to resolve traumatic memories. A story about the life of hobbits who live in a place with green pastures (utilization) called Shire aimed to activate processing. Particular emphasis focused on the necessity of young hobbits to leave their home to explore and always return safely.

Prosody focused on specific suggestions that were emphasized with a preceding HT. Additionally, the story depicted an elder, wise hobbit who lived peacefully at home, which deeply resonated with Daniel. Active repetitive eye movements and unprompted playing of the rhythm on his body, along with the recorded frame drum, oud, and my spoken voice, were observed during this part of the story. Musical elements included rhythm, prosody, repetition, and novelty embedded in hypnotic techniques such as hypnotic dissociation, pre-suppositions, time distortion, ideomotor signaling, and ambiguous communication (storytelling, metaphors).

Post-hypnotic suggestions included two HPs to create impact and novelty (see Figure 14.1 and 14.2).

Pas ture of Shi re all right Pas ture of Shi re all right Pas ture of Shi re all right
1 2 3 4 1 2 3 4 1 2 3 4 1 2 3 4 1 2 3 4 1 2 3 4
Pas ture of Shi re all right Pas calm now so calm re mem ber the calm
1 2 3 4 1 2 3 4 1 1 2 3 4 1 2 3 4 1 2 3 4 1 2 3 4
now
1 2 3 4

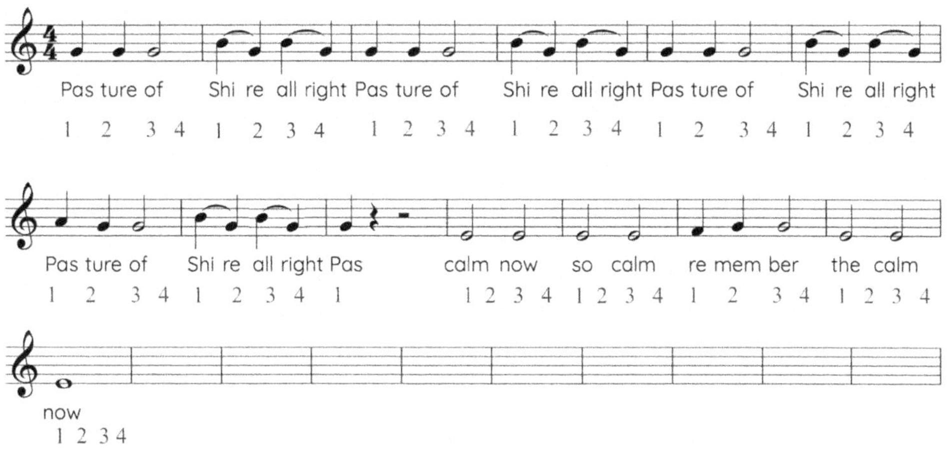

Figure 14.1 Illustration of the first spoken Hypnotic Tihai Notation. The first three measures repeat itself and end on the first note of the first measure followed by a pause which is called a Tihai. The ending of this phrasing is on *Pas* (first note of first measure shown as 1). *Pas* is spoken louder to increase tension. This completes the Tihai. It is followed by a pause with the suggestion of *calm now*. In this example, a word play on *calm* and to remember to be calm follows.

Right here right now Right here right now Right here right now Right
1 2 3 4 1 2 3 4 1 2 3 4 1 2 3 4
in an in - stant calm
1 2 3 4 1 2 3 4 1 2 3 4

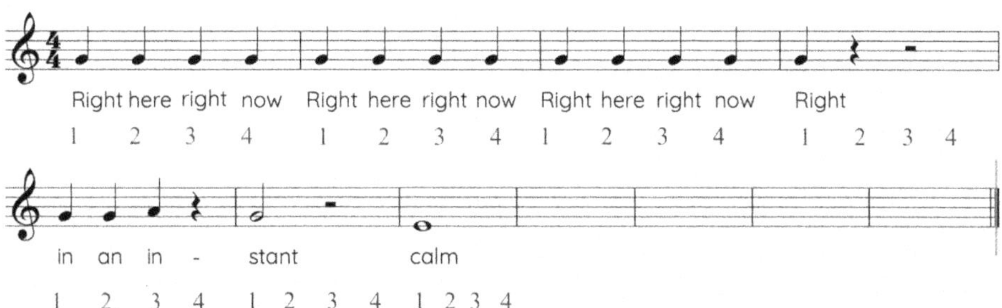

Figure 14.2 Illustration of the second spoken Hypnotic Tihai Notation. The first three measures repeat itself and end on the first note of the first measure followed by a pause which is called a Tihai. The ending of this phrasing is on *Right* (first note of first measure shown as 1). The word *Right* is spoken louder with an abrupt stop which creates tension. This completes the Tihai. It is followed by a pause with the suggestion of *in an instant, calm.*

Session 3

Reporting overall improvement, residues of sadness remained, accompanied by dread a day before his children left. Self-hypnosis skills were monitored (drumming rhythm on body). The intervention included ambiguous indirection addressing the traumatized younger part of Daniel. Since hypnosis optimizes the interaction between the sympathetic and the parasympathetic nervous systems (Boselli et al., 2018), new perspectives on internal or external events might be harnessed, expanded, or created. Therefore, a story about lemba, a bread that the hobbits eat during travels, along with the recorded frame drum and oud, was offered to activate processing including an indirect suggestion (using prosody) that '*lemba sustains*' him to fill any void (utilization: fondness for baking). Musical elements included rhythm, prosody, repetition, and novelty.

Session 4

Continued improvement and transition into an adaptive state resulted in joyful moments and in playing guitar again, even during his children's absence. Daniel continued playing the rhythm on his body (self-hypnosis) to induce calm when needed and had also taught his children to play the rhythm on their body.

Conclusion

Advanced studies regarding music and hypnosis are already in development and the integration of musical elements in hypnosis might yield further research studies in the years to come. Clinical experience, research-informed, supports the inclusion of musical elements to include rhythm, repetition, prosody, and novelty to elicit rapport, strengthen suggestions, interrupt patterns, enhance memory, transform symptoms, and facilitate healing. A hypnosis session can be a defining moment in an individual's life. Hypnosis practitioners can enhance therapeutic encounters by infusing musical elements creatively into their practice. It will take practice to infuse musical elements inside and outside of therapy to become procedural with the guarantee that work might be more creative and enjoyable.

References

Bernardi, L., Porta. C., & Sleight. P. (2006). Cardiovascular, cerebrovascular, and respiratory changes induced by different types of music in musicians and non-musicans: The importance of silence. *Heart*, *92*(4), 445–452.

Blankfield, R. P., Zyzanski, S. J., Flocke, S. A., Alemagno, S., & Scheurman, K. (1995). Taped therapeutic suggestions and taped music as adjuncts in the care of coronary-artery-bypass patients. *American Journal of Clinical Hypnosis*, *37*(3), 32–42. 10.1080/00029157.1995.10403137

Blood, A. J., & Zatorre, R. J. (2001). Intensely pleasurable responses to music correlate with activity in brain regions implicated in reward and emotion. *Proceedings of the National Academy of Sciences of the United States of America*, *98*(20), 11818–11823.

Bluedorn, A. C. (2002). *The human organization of time. Temporal realities and experience.* Stanford, CA: Stanford University Press.

Boselli, E., Musellec, H., Martin, L., Bernard, F., Fusco, N., Guillou, N., Hugot, P., Paqueron, X., Yven, T., & Virot, C. (2018). Effects of hypnosis on the relative parasympathetic tone assessed by ANI (Analgesia/Nociception Index) in healthy volunteers: A prospective observational study. *Journal of Clinical Monitoring and Computing*, *32*(3), 487–492. 10.1007/s10877-017-0056-5

Bradt, J., Dileo, C., Grocke, D., & Magill, L. (2011). Music interventions for improving psychological and physical outcomes in cancer patients. *Cochrane Database Systematic Reviews*, *8*(8), 1–95. Art. No.: CD006911. http://www.ncbi.nlm.nih.gov/pubmed/21833957.

Brown, P. 1991. *The hypnotic brain: Hypnotherapy and social communication.* New Haven: Yale University Press.

Chatterjee, S. (2005). *Tabla: A Study of Tabla.* New York: Chhandayan, Inc.

De Benedittis, G., & Sironi, V. A. (1988). Arousal effects of electrical deep brain stimulation in hypnosis, *International Journal of Clinical and Experimental Hypnosis*, *36*(2), 96–106, 10.1080/00207148808409334 de Witte, M., Pinho, A., Stams, G. J., Moonen, X., Bos, A., & van Hooren, S. (2020). Music therapy for stress reduction: A systematic review and meta-analysis. *Health Psychology Review*, 1–26. Advance online publication. DOI 10.1080/17437199.2020.1846580

Dietrich, C., Teut, M., Samwel, K. L., Narayanasamy, S., Rathapillil, T., & Thathews, G. (2015). Treating palliative care patients with pain with the body tambura: A prospective case study at St. Joseph's Hospice for Dying destitute in Dindigul South India. *Indian Journal of Palliative Care*, *21*(2), 236–241. 10.4103/0973-1075.156509

Dileo, C. (2006). Effects of music and music therapy on medical patients: A meta-analysis of the research and implications for the future. *Journal of the Society for Integrative Oncology*, *4*, 67–70. 10.2310/7200.2006.002

Elkins. G. (2017). Feasibility of music and hypnotic suggestion to manage chronic pain, *International Journal of Clinical and Experimental Hypnosis*, *65*(4), 452–465. 10.1080/00207144.2017.1348858

Erkkilä, J., Punkanen, M., Fachner, J., Ala-Ruona, E., Pöntiö, I., Tervaniemi, M., & Gold, C. (2011). Individual music therapy for depression: Randomised controlled trial. *British Journal of Psychiatry*, *199*(2), 132–139. 10.1192/bjp.bp.110.085431

Fachner, J., Gold, C., & Erkkilä, J. (2012). Music therapy modulates frontol-temporal activity in rest-EEG in depressed clients. *Brain Topography*, *26*(2):338–354. 10.1007/s10548-012-0254-x

Gallagher, L. (2011). The role of music therapy in palliative medicine and supportive care. *Seminars in Oncology*, *38*(3), 403–406. https://doi.org10.1053j.seminoncol.2011.03.010.

Gäbel, C., Garrido, N., Koenig, J., Hillecke, T. K., & Warth, M. (2017). Effects of monochord music on heart rate variability and self-reports of relaxation in healthy adults. *Complementary Medicine Research*, *24*(2), 97–103. German. 10.1159/000455133. Epub 2017 Feb 3. PMID: 28192781.

Gerkema, M. P. (2002). Ultradian rhythms. In V. Kumar (Ed.), *Biological rhythms* (pp. 207–215). Berlin, Germany: Springer-Verlag.

Greenberg, D. M., Decety, J., & Gordon, I. (2021). The social neuroscience of music: Understanding the social brain through human song. *American Psychologist*. Advance online publication. DOI 10.1037/amp0000819

Gutgsell, K., Schluchter, M., Margevicius, S., DeGolia, P., McLaughlin, B., Harris, M., & Wienick, C. (2013). Music therapy reduces pain in palliative care patients: A randomized controlled trial. *Journal of Pain and Symptom Management*, *45*, 822–831. 10.1016/j.jpainsymman.2012.05.008

Hanser, S. B., & Thompson, L. W. (1994). Effects of a music therapy strategy on depressed older adults. *Journal of Gerontology*, *49*(6), P265–P269. 10.1093/geronj/49.6.p265

Huron, D. (2006). *Sweet anticipation: Music and the psychology of expectation*. Cambridge, MA: Massachusetts Institute of Technology Press.

Jensen, M. P., Adachi, T., & Hakimian, S. (2015) Brain oscillations, hypnosis, and hypnotizability. *American Journal of Clinical Hypnosis*, *57*(3), 230–253. 10.1080/00029157.2014.976786

Jensen, M. P., & Patterson, D. R. (2014). Hypnotic approaches for chronic pain management: Clinical implications of recent research findings. *American Psychologist*, *69*(2), 167–177. 10.1037/a0035644

Jensen, M. P., & Turk, D. C. (2014). Contributions of psychology to the understanding and treatment of people with chronic pain: Why it matters to all psychologists. *American Psychologist*, *69*(2), 105–118. doi:10.1037/a0035641

Kirsch, I. (1996). Hypnosis in psychotherapy: Efficacy and mechanisms. *Contemporary Hypnosis*, *13*, 109–114. 10.1002/ch.57

Koelsch S. (2009). A neuroscientific perspective on music therapy. *Annals of the New York Academy of Sciences*, *1169*, 374–384. 10.1111/j.1749-6632.2009.04592.x

Kühlmann, A. Y. R., de Rooij, A., Kroese, L. F., van Dijk, M., Hunink, M. G. M. & Jeekel, J. (2018). Meta-analysis evaluating music interventions for anxiety and pain in surgery. *British Journal of Surgery*, *105*(7), 773–783. 10.1002/bjs.10853

Landis-Shack, N., Heinz, A. J., & Bonn-Miller, M. O. (2017). Music therapy for posttraumatic stress in adults: A theoretical review. *Psychomusicology*, *27*(4), 334–342. 10.1037/pmu0000192

Landry, M., Da Silva Castanheira, J., Sackur, J., & Raz, A. (2021). Difficult turned easy: Suggestion renders a challenging visual task simple. *Psychological Science*, *32*(1), 39–49. 10.1177/095 6797620954856

Lee, K. C., Chao, Y. H., Yiin, J. J., Hsieh, H. Y., Dai, W. J., & Chao, Y. F. (2012). Evidence that music listening reduces preoperative patients' anxiety. *Biological Research for Nursing*, *14*(1), 78–84. 10.1177/1099800410396704

Levitin, D. J., Grahn, J. A., & London, J. (2018). The psychology of music: Rhythm and movement. *Annual Review of Psychology*, *69*, 51–75. doi:10.3389/fnbeh.2014.00037

Martin-Saavedra, J. S., Vergara-Mendez, L. D., Pradilla, I., Vélez-van-Meerbeke, A., & Talero-Gutiérrez, C. (2018). Standardizing music characteristics for the management of pain: A systematic review and meta-analysis of clinical trials. *Complementary Therapies in Medicine*, *41*, 81–89. 10.1016/j.ctim.2018.07.008

Montagu, A., & Matson, F. (1979). *The human connection*. New York: McGraw-Hill.

Ranade, A. D. (2006). Music contexts: A concise dictionary of Hindustani music. p. 167. : Promilla & Co. Publishers.

Raz, A., Fan, J., & Posner, M. I. (2005). Hypnotic suggestion reduces conflict in the human brain. *Proceedings of the National Academy of Sciences of the United States of America*, *102*(28), 9978–9983. 10.1073/pnas.0503064102

Reinhardt, U. (1999). Untersuchungen zur Synchronisation von Herzfrequenz und musikalischem Rhythmus im Rahmen einer Entspannungstherapie bei Patienten mit tumorbedingten Schmerzen. *Forschende Komplementärmedizin*, *6*(3), 135–141.

Rider, M. S., & Eagle, C. T. (1986). Rhythmic entrainment as a mechanism for learning in music therapy. In J. R. Evans, & M. Clynes (Eds.), *Rhythm in psychological, linguistic, and musical processes* (pp. 225–247). Springfield, IL: C.C. Thomas.

Roederer, J. G. (1984). The search for a survival value of music. *Music Perception*, *1*(3), 350–356, Pg. 229. 10.2307/40285265

Saakvitne, K., Gamble, S., Pearlman L., & Tabor Lev, B. (2000). *Risking connection: A training curriculum for working with survivors of childhood abuse*. Baltimore, MD: Sidran Press.

SAMSHA (2014). *HHS Publication No. (SMA) 14-4884*. Rockville, MD: Substance Abuse and Mental Health Services Administration.

Seidenbecher, T., Laxmi, T. R., Stork, O., & Pape, H. C. (2003). Amygdalar and hippocampal theta rhythm synchronization during fear memory retrieval. *Science*, *301*(5634), 846–850. 10.1126/science.1085818

Shintel, H., Anderson, N., & Fenn, K. M. (2014). Talk this way: The effect of prosodically conveyed semantic information on memory for novel words. *Journal of Experimental Psychology. General*, *143*(4), 1437–1442. 10.1037/a0036605

Snodgrass, M., & Lynn, S. J. (1989). Music absorption and hypnotizability. *International Journal of Clinical and Experimental Hypnosis*, *37*(1), 41–54. 10.1080/00207148908410532

Spiegel, D., & Cardena, E. (1990). New uses of hypnosis in the treatment of posttraumatic stress disorder. *The Journal of Clinical Psychiatry*, *51*, (Suppl), 39–46.

Stickgold, R. (2002). EMDR: A putative neurobiological mechanism of action. *Journal of Clinical Psychology*, *58*, 61–75. /10.1002/jclp.1129

Stoelb, B. L., Molton, I. R., Jensen, M. P., & Patterson, D. R. (2009). The efficacy of hypnotic analgesia in adults: A review of the literature. Contemporary hypnosis. *The Journal of the British Society of Experimental and Clinical Hypnosis*, *26*(1), 24–39. 10.1002/ch.370

Tellez, A., Sanchez-Jauregui, T., & Juarez-Garcia, D. M. (2016). Breast biopsy: The effects of hypnosis and music. *International Journal of Clinical and Experimental Hypnosis*, *64*, 456–469. 10.1080/00207144.2016.1209034

Teut, M., Dietrich, C., Deutz, B., Mittring, N., & Witt, C. M. (2014). Perceived outcomes of music therapy with Body Tambura in end of life care: A qualitative pilot study. *British Medical Journal, Palliative Care*, *13*, 18. 10.1186/1472-684x-13-18

Trevarthen, C. (1999-2000). Musicality and the intrinsic motive pulse: Evidence from human psychobiology and infant communication. *Musicae Scientiae, Special Issue*, *3*, 155–215. 10.1177/10298649000030S109

Wahbeh, H., Elsas, S.-M., & Oken, B. S. (2008). Mind–body interventions: Applications in neurology. *Neurology*, *70*, 2321–2328. 10.1212/01.wnl.0000314667.16386.5e

Wang, J. Z., Li, L., Pan, L. L., & Chen, J. H. (2015). Hypnosis and music interventions (HMIs) inactivate HIF-1: A potential curative efficacy for cancers and hypertension. *Medical Hypotheses*, *85*(5), 551–557. 10.1016/j.mehy.2015.07.008

Walter, W. G. (1953). *The living brain*. New York: Norton.

15

UTILIZATION OF METAPHOR AS A THERAPEUTIC TOOL

Consuelo C. Casula

Private Practice, Milan, Italy

Introduction

The main objective of this chapter is to demonstrate how the utilization of metaphor in therapy can help clients and clinicians become more flexible during the hypnotherapeutic process and conversational hypnosis (Short, 2022; Yapko, 2021). A complementary objective is to describe how some metaphors produced by clients can be utilized as a source of information regarding emotions, belief systems, and intentions, and to reframe them.

A final objective is to explore the utilization of metaphor's function of stimulating perceptions, emotions, cognition, behavior, identity, relational and contextual flexibility in accordance with the client's needs. This function is in full agreement with the theory that portrays the brain as a constituent element of the embodied mind, and with the definition of trance as neurobiological plasticity (Siegel, 2017; Sugarman et al., 2020). Neuroplasticity depicts the embodied mind as a problem-solving machine constructed for change where metaphors sow innovative ideas incubating and driving change (Short, 2021).

Background

My passion for metaphors was born during a workshop conducted by Norma and Philip Barretta in 1984, in Milan, Italy. Thanks to them I approached Ericksonian hypnosis and afterwards I attended various congresses organized by the Milton H. Erickson Foundation where I met Robert Dilts, Steve Gilligan, David Gordon, Steve Lankton, Dan Short, Michael Yapko, and Jeff Zeig, among others. Starting from my first book, *Schopenhauer's Porcupines: How to Conduct Training Groups* Casula (1997) better explains some of the phenomena regarding groups in which I used several metaphors and therapeutic stories.

My second book, *Gardeners, Princesses, Porcupines: Metaphors for Personal and Professional Evolution* (Casula, 2002), is entirely dedicated to metaphors, what they are, and how to create them.

Two books have a metaphorical title. The first, *Princess Shoes, Women and the Art of Becoming Themselves,* (Casula, 2009), is born from workshops dedicated to women's empowerment conducted with international colleagues such as Susanna Carolusson, Betty

DOI: 10.4324/9781003449126-20

Alice Erickson, Cecilia Fabre, Julie Linden, and Teresa Robles. The title depicts a princess who loved to walk barefoot; thus her father paved the way for her. One day the princess discovered an unpaved road and wanted to explore it. But her feet hurt. She went to her father to ask him to asphalt it for her. The father answered: "It's time for you to put on your shoes".

Also, *The Golden Bowl: Living the Present, Learning from the Past, Planning the Future in Therapy,* (Casula, 2017), presents itself with a metaphor. It is about a wise monk who was said to be inspired by a golden bowl. One day, a young monk asks the sage if he can see his golden bowl. The wise monk invites him into his home and hands him a wooden bowl. The young man doesn't understand why to call a simple wooden bowl gold. The wise monk replies that that bowl is even more precious than gold because it contains the universal wisdom of the original wood, shares the mysteries of the earth, the sun, the wind, the rain, that it has experienced. It reminds him of natural differences and changes and helps him to remember that everything transforms, passes, and ends.

Metaphors: Transfer of Associations

The word metaphor is rich in meanings and applications. Starting with its etymology, the Greek word *metaphor* is composed of *meta*, "beyond", and *phorà,* from the verb *pherein,* "bringing". Thus, it indicates movement, or transfer. Metaphor transforms a word into a symbol. *Sýmbolon* is a Greek word (symbállō "to join", syn- "with") that combines two different semantic fields: the field of abstract thoughts and that of concrete objects or actions.

In the rhetorical domain, a metaphor means moving a term from one semantic field to another that shares a condensed similarity with the first, but the element of comparison is, however, not stated (Perelman, 1977). This similarity brings together two heterogeneous objects but does not unify them; the metaphor instead creates a closer approach where what is perceived as similar is made identical.

The metaphor is an essential element of language, not just an ornament (Perelman, 1977). It makes up for linguistic deficiency and opens new possibilities to explore innovative reality by following unexplored hypotheses, thus enhancing flexibility. It is a lie that tells a truth, a confusion that brings clarity, a shortcut that gets to a destination first. Metaphor is a game of transformation of an abstract concept into a concrete image or experience that evokes multiple meanings. For instance, when we say, "anger is a volcano", does that mean it is awake and active like Etna? Or is it sleeping like Vesuvius? Similarly, anxiety can be described as a swamp that must be reclaimed. And enthusiasm can be depicted as a choice—the choice of which gods or goddesses at that moment can better inspire the client.

The metaphor, creating wonder and regeneration connected with visual, auditory, tactile, gustatory, and olfactory experiences, suggests the subject explore an innovative reality following unexplored hypotheses, evoking the functions of universal symbols. For instance, when my client Franca said to me, "I see a flame in my heart". I replied, "That flame gives you light and warmth, illuminates you and brings you new ideas while keeping warm the passion for writing the book you want to write".

Both traditional metaphors as well as unexpected but pertinent new metaphors are the fruit of a lively and creative imagination. Several metaphors refer to the human body and establish coordinates that can be traced in the timeless metaphors that have become part of daily language (Lakoff & Johnson, 1980). When clients share metaphors to concretely represent an experience that starts from their own body sensations, the therapist starts a reframing. When the client says they are feeling a swollen heart, having a piece of ice inside, or a weight on the stomach, the therapist makes the listener look in another direction. Thus, a swollen heart needs to be deflated, giving breath to words too long held back; the ice inside needs the process of defrosting to evoke the idea of returning essential warmth. And the weight on the stomach may indicate that something did not go down or that needs to be digested.

When the "burden" metaphor is used by subjects, therapists may use them as marker of change (Levitt et al., 2000). In such a case, I usually propose a contrasting imaginative experience of unloading the burden, getting their backpack off their back, placing it in front of them, opening it, putting their hands inside to remove what has been deposited long time ago (Casula, 2019, 2020, 2021, 2022). This mental action stimulates profound experiential impact, adding a more vivid level of understanding, opening a window that allows both the subject and the hypnotist to highlight what is inside to bring it outside.

Similarly, if the client talks about their depression calling it "a crying of the soul", I might evoke the crying of an athlete who, during a competition, suffers from cramps, muscle sprain, or bone fracture. This switch from the invisible soul to the concrete body evokes the natural biological reparative process of the body. Using this kind of metaphors underlines the idea that the body follows its own ecological automatisms, without the need of conscious oversight.

Other metaphors refer to space (Lakoff & Johnson, 1980). For example, when faced with loss, individuals may say they feel a sense of emptiness or a hollow feeling. In such a case, the searching process allows broader perspective, proposing lateral, horizontal, and vertical views, thus prospecting new shades of meanings. When clients say they have lost their compass, we can remind them that today the compass is always with them, in the GPS of the mobile phone. These kinds of metaphors broaden horizons, enter a border free zone that suggests that there is a new territory to be explored. Most important, these types of metaphors suggest that the resources they are looking for outside of them are already inside.

The therapist can also expand the metaphors the client uses to deepen their experience by creating a metaphoric story to bring novelty, to disturb old patterns, and to suggest how to solve their problems (Peseschkian, 1979; Wallas, 1985, 1991). For example, if the client links therapeutic process to a journey, the therapist might use a typical travel metaphor of climbing a mountain, where the protagonist of the story encounters various obstacles and at the same time elicits internal and external resources to overcome them (Casula, 2020). During the descent, the protagonist can imagine new occasions when the resources elicited in climbing are utilized (Cuadros & Vargas, 2021).

In the metaphoric stories of journeys and explorations of different worlds and places, the protagonist sets off toward the unknown with baggage full of uncertainty and doubts which, during the journey, are dissolved and transformed into awareness of their own resources. There is also an awareness of the objectives to be achieved and of the meaning to give to the experience.

Furthermore, when therapy is represented as a journey, the therapist may be associated either with the notion of a spiritual guide or as an explorer with different maps – depending on the patient's needs. The therapist can also play the role of a private detective or an archeologist who aims at discovering something hidden in ravines, the caves of the embodied mind, or buried under the neglected layers of time. The therapist might be seen as the poet Virgil who accompanied Dante Alighieri to visit hell, purgatory, and paradise in his *Divine Comedy*. No matter the metaphor used in the therapeutic process/journey, the most important aspect of the journey is its destination: reaching individuation, authenticity, and well-being.

Metaphors Used by Clients

For clients, a metaphor is not a poetic embellishment but a form of thought, something to help categorize their experiences (Malcomsen et al., 2021). It is the generative way in which their unconscious mind processes information, showing how they think, weaving a connection between the various threads at their disposal.

Whenever metaphor is used by clients, it is usually attuned to their emotional state (Casula, 2019, 2020, 2021, 2022). It can also reveal an experience or an emotion that can be reconstructed by digging into the hidden parts of their history. The therapist's task is to grasp the patient's emotional experience representing a relational configuration. As a clinical example, Marta told me that since she divorced, she wears high-heeled shoes. I commented that now she is taller than before, and she can distance herself from her ex-husband looking down on what happens to her. As another example, Eugenia told me that when she argued with her husband, she felt like a jellyfish tossed about by the waves. This metaphor connoted Eugenia's perception of herself as passive and inert. It expressed the effect the discussions with her husband had on her and how difficult it was for her to solve the problem and interrupt their pattern of interaction. So, I invited her to explore a contrasting metaphor that could help her to find a solution to the problematic situation. After further analysis of the usual pattern of the discussions between the couple, the metaphor of a surfer seemed able to restore Eugenia's ability to predict the big wave and to ride it with mastery. In this case, the metaphor of the surfer performed the function of a corrective emotional experience, helping to suggest a change of context – from being tossed by the waves, to ride them –, to perceive differently and reframe the problem for the client.

Integrating metaphor into the therapeutic conversation offers an emotional experience rather than conceptual elaboration. It suggests ideas to evoke visual content, convey images, and integrate verbal and imaginative aspects. It can also hold two or more different concepts together, create an abstract bridge and a concrete image, and make itself the bearer of multiple meanings that gradually become salient.

Goal-oriented Metaphors

The use of metaphor in psychotherapy is goal-oriented (Casula, 2019, 2020, 2021, 2022): to focus clients on the feelings embedded in their metaphor and help them to comprehend the meaning in the context of their lives. As a marker of client change, the therapist can develop a core metaphoric theme related to the main therapeutic issues (Levitt et al., 2000).

Metaphor is a linguistic instrument, illustrating by means of an intuitive and fitting image a connection, a configuration, an utterance whose truth exists beyond the language and expressive power of the metaphor. The use of metaphor, in addition to being a linguistic operation, is a way to give meaning to reality, to attribute interpretative schemes to it, and to apply isomorphisms that help to better understand what is going on. Also, metaphor is used as a multiform and ductile tool: multiform because it appears in the guise of a simple word that belongs to another semantic or pragmatic field with respect to the object or concept we are talking about. The chosen metaphoric word evokes a previously unassociated representational world, creates a shift, a disorientation and a logical leap that purposefully creates confusion from which the search for an appropriate and pertinent meaning arises. Metaphor is multiform also in the sense that the therapist creates, or simply tells, metaphoric stories to fit the client's situation creating characters and components that are isomorphic to aspects of the client's circumstances (Hammond, 1990).

The metaphor is also a ductile tool that can be used during both conversational hypnosis and formal trance, which allows the therapist to convey their principles and values without necessarily imposing them on the subject. Thus, as a therapeutic device, metaphor is effective, elegant, and respectful.

The metaphor is a crucial therapeutic tool and a pivot point in the construction of new meanings, sending suggestions at conscious and unconscious levels (Short, 2021). Sometimes it illuminates the dark side of the human soul, with the dim light of a candle, other times with a sharp flashlight, a lighthouse, or a powerful laser.

Using Metaphors and Metaphoric Stories

For Gregory Bateson, interested in syllogism and homology, human beings create stories connected with other narrative and discursive structures (Bateson, 1991; Madonna, 2003; Roffman, 2008). Constructing metaphors and stories means relating different things, using a pattern that connects what is already the product of an elaborate metaphor, so that, metaphor after metaphor, a certain number of variations opens to attain a significant similarity such as to allow for further inferences. No similarity could be grasped if the differences were not embraced at the same time. The metaphor has the power to relate distant realities, creating bridges that unite traits common to the two images and that put them in systemic relation.

Hypnosis as an interpersonal intentional skill, both on the part of the clinician and of the client, influences the psychobiological change process during the trance. Trance is a process of plasticity and flexibility, helping the embodied mind to integrate physical, emotional, and cognitive change (Sugarman et al., 2020; Yapko, 2021). According to Ernest Rossi, the mind is engaged in a continuous and discontinuous chronological dance called the "Novelty Numinosum-Neurogenesis Effect" (Rossi, 2002). Rossi divided this dance into four steps: the first is characterized by the beginning of questioning, doubting, and gathering discomforting information. The second step starts a process of wondering, working out what is happening, thus incubating something new. The third offers a flash of insights, resolution, or revelation through breakthrough and illumination. The fourth and last step happens when the whole experience is quietly reviewed, considered, and verified, and the benefits of the entire process are integrated into everyday life (Sugarman et al., 2020).

These four steps of Rossi's process can be kept in mind in the construction of a metaphoric story in which the protagonist starts by asking them questions, expressing doubts, uncertainties, and goes on in search of information (Cuadros & Vargas, 2021). The exploratory process starts the phase of incubation, during which, often at an unconscious level, the protagonist of the story investigates and deepens what is happening inside and outside them. Incubated cognition may last days or months while the person goes through the imagery process that is not yet ready to be translated into words or actions. Then comes the phase of enlightenment, of insight in which revelation and resolution are glimpsed, ending with the verification of the global experience reviewed and considered through the integration of its benefits into daily life (see also Short, 2020).

Sometimes, metaphors are grouped together to form a narrative, a narrative which is a human method of giving new meanings to the world, including self, identity, personality, others, experience, time, and space (Lakoff & Johnson, 1980; Lankton & Lankton, 1989). Metaphoric stories and their protagonists help clients symbolize their experience, provide a moral compass based on natural laws, general truth, thus evoking universal wisdom and deep understanding (Robles, 2000). The similarities between the structure of our memories and the story as well as the connection to child-like magic thinking and dreams suggest that stories might have a strong relation to the unconscious and carry a dissociative trait in them.

Metaphors are therapeutic tools for healing. By inserting powerful words into a story it helps clients reconstruct their own narrative by deleting faulty elements, adding new positive ones, and externalizing their problems to find better solutions. This use of metaphor creates an interplay between conscious and unconscious intelligence moving from the implicit knowledge of embodied experiences to the explicit awareness and understanding of events (Short, 2022).

A salient metaphor comes from the unconscious intelligence that functions as a unique system of language contained within embodied experience and tacit knowledge. A story takes the listener to another time and place destabilizing critical conscious parameters. A story is meant to stimulate the flexible unconscious intelligence, which is uniquely capable of creative problem-solving and imagination. This empowers subjects to explore a new world of possibilities.

In summary, hypnotic storytelling can be a powerful means of encouraging experiential shifts. By telling a metaphoric story, a clinician focuses the listener's attention, underlines emotionally salient details, structures the perception of events, selects characters, attitudes and values of a protagonist, and seeds solution-oriented behaviors.

Metaphor as Storytelling

Storytelling is perhaps the oldest therapeutic art (Haley, 1986). Almost everyone enjoys listening to coherent and congruent stories as well as telling stories that give meaning to what happens in life. It is a tool that allows clinician to create metaphoric stories embedded with truisms and healing suggestions. Metaphors, stories, narratives, anecdotes, legends, tales of heroes, guided imagery, journeys, and myths are a fulcrum on which healing and growth revolve, not marginal elements of hypnotic techniques (Battino, 2021; Gilligan & Dilts, 2009; Gordon, 1978; Hammond, 1990; Lankton, 2019).

Often, it is the clinician who takes the initiative to tell a therapeutic story that has the same structure as the client's problem situation. This leads the client to an expansion of their model of the world and a vision of change supported by the idea that there is a solution to their problematic situation. The story facilitates a change of context by reframing experience to perceive it differently, offering new interpretations of and meanings to that experience.

Metaphoric communication speaks simultaneously to the conscious mind, that seeks the logic and coherence in the story, and to the unconscious mind, that grasps the affective implications of the characters: it transports the listener into a world in which what happens must be accepted without seeking explanations, justifications, or arbitrary attributions. Several metaphors draw inspiration from nature's character of neutrality, impartiality, and universality to remove the personalism or the touchiness of people who tend to attribute negative intentions to casual acts or occasional circumstances. Some metaphors are also designed to transfer to the listener the lessons offered by nature regarding the acceptance of the differences between individual creatures and species of plants, animals, humans, and all the changes, mysteries, and secrets that nature hides (Casula 2011, 2017; Hadot, 2004).

The therapeutic metaphor makes it easier for the listener to accept the laws of nature, in their impersonal and indifferent manifestations: nature is neutral; it does not favor any living beings by making life easier for them. Every natural creature has its own qualities that help it to live to the best of its possibilities, while also recognizing its own limitations. Skillful adaptation is a matter of differentiating obstacles that can be challenged and overcome from those that must be accepted. The story transports the listeners into a magically realistic world where everything is possible within a realistic framework. The magical thought that is used in metaphors does not feed the protagonist's omnipotence; rather it shows the expression of a full potential that was previously hindered, denied, or neglected.

For instance, Flavio's eight-year-old son made a foam bath for his father to take to the hospital for his second cycle of chemotherapy. I utilized this present, telling Flavio to use the magic ingredients of the bath foam, which are filled with love and tenderness, as healing ingredients to his body and soul.

Therapeutic Metaphors

Therapeutic metaphors propose events that have always happened and will always happen, like myths, heroes, gods, and goddesses, combined with archetype who are universal and therefore credible (Bolen, 1984; Hillman,1980; Jung, 1934; Pearson, 1991; Pesesckian, 1979). The metaphor also proposes unexpected and unpredictable events, which stimulate in the protagonist the ability to grasp an opportunity to change their destiny. The protagonist's ability can simply reside in welcoming those unexpected events with curiosity and trust instead of discarding them as frightening, meaningless, or worthless.

Clinicians can also draw inspiration from ancient myths that deal with the universal themes of the human soul and interpersonal relationships that are still relevant today. In this regard, when I wish to underline a lack of responsibility, I may introduce the Greek heroes described by Homer in the Iliad, Achilles, Ulysses, Aeneas, utilizing Julian Jaynes's theory (Jaynes, 2021). Interestingly, he posits that the minds of the ancients were divided into two parts called *the bicameral mind* (Jaynes, 1976), where one part made decisions and the other part executed them: neither was conscious. The Greek heroes were not responsible for their heroic or vengeful actions: their actions were led by the gods (Jaynes, 2021).

Even anecdotes can be part of the therapeutic narrative repertoire, offering reflections based on personal experience. In this regard, I quote an anecdote from a client married to a man from a different country. One day while the couple was having lunch with my client's parents, and the bottle of wine was emptied, her father said: *the wine is finished*, and my client did not say or do anything. After lunch, her husband asked her why she did not get up to get a bottle of wine, or at least ask her father if he wanted her to do so, out of simple respect. My client replied that she was not brought up to show respect but only to obey explicit orders. Furthermore, growing up, she developed a rebellious attitude against explicit orders and implicit requests. When I share this anecdote of cultural differences to other clients, I stimulate reflection on the indirect style of communication of the father that could be read as form of manipulation, an implicit request or hidden command, and on cultural differences, and different values – respect versus obedience – transmitted by assertive or manipulative parents.

The power of the metaphoric story to change the listener's way of thinking, feeling, and acting lies in mixing up patterns of information and the flow of energy in the embodied mind, and proposing an array of different experiences. The therapeutic metaphor mixes the power of communication with that of the therapeutic alliance, which makes the subject more attentive and receptive to suggestions. Credit should also go to psychobiological plasticity and physical and imaginative agility (Siegel, 2017; Sugarman et al., 2020).

Yapko (2021) states that according to Milton Erickson, subjects' suffering derives from their rigidity; thus, the therapist's primary task is to remove perceptual, emotional, cognitive, behavioral, identity, relational and contextual rigidities. It is as if a tree trunk prevents the flow of the flowing river of life and the therapist's task is to identify where the obstructing trunk is positioned and how to remove it with proper therapeutic tools. The metaphor as a therapeutic tool helps clinicians offer clients the flexibility to continue their lives with the full capacity to utilize internal and external resources, conscious and unconscious mind.

Next, I will propose some examples of metaphors that can be applied to stimulate useful flexibility in the listener – to "remove the trunk" obstructing the flow of the flowing river of life. Let's start with perceptual flexibility.

Metaphors for Stimulating Perceptual Flexibility

Clients who suffer from perceptual rigidity usually concentrate their attention on some pessimistic aspects of their life, on failures, on arbitrary negative meanings and struggle to place them in a wider space-time context. The therapist who intends to soften their rigidity can suggest a perceptive opening that allows a process-oriented malleability previously prevented (Yapko, 2021).

Before using hypnosis to stimulate perceptual flexibility, it is important to locate the client's rigidity. Some tend to perceive details and miss the overall view. Others focus their attention on their internal world, which is made up of perfect ideas whose correspondence they seek in the real world. Because they cannot find perfection, they become lost in frustration. Others are concentrated on the present time, as if what happened in the past is no longer relevant, and what might happen in the future does not depend on them. Then there are those clients who remain nostalgic for the past and would like to replicate a romanticized moment in their present and future. Others are so future-oriented that they miss the opportunities offered by the present.

As a clinical example, Gabriele, a 60-year-old client of mine, met a woman he wanted to live with. He complained that their circadian rhythms were opposite. He liked to go to sleep early, and she preferred stay awake until late. He asked her to respect his needs, while neglecting hers.

With Gabriele, I used a story regarding nocturnal animals, bats, owls, and dormice, who would like to become friends with diurnal animals, songbirds, squirrels, and butterflies. They discovered that they could spend hours together during the transition between day and night and vice versa, respecting their natural characteristics. Thanks to this metaphor, Gabriele recognized that if he really wanted to live with this woman, he must be more empathic and respectful of her circadian rhythm.

To create metaphors to enhance perceptive flexibility, a therapist can insert in the story several sensory instruments: for example, an anosmic needs an auditory cue, a color-blind person needs special glasses to perceive colors; other characters need microscopes or telescopes, binoculars, or magnifying glasses, suitable for evoking different ways of looking at the world around. Mirrors, rearview mirrors, or magic crystal balls might be the tools that help the protagonist of the story to see differences among the present, past, and future.

Metaphors for Stimulating Emotional Flexibility

People who come to therapy sometimes intensify their suffering by reinforcing emotions that they should instead put aside such as envy, jealousy, and resentment. As a clinical example, Giovanna, after failed assisted fertilization procedures due to premature menopause, felt desperate. To restore hope, I invited Giovanna to remember how many times she was surprised to see plants and flowers in apparently sterile soils, like cactuses and oases in the desert; borage, chicory, dandelions in the sand; water lilies in ponds or swamps; orange or fig trees on the sidewalks; capers growing among the rocks or on walls sheltered from the wind.

During conversational hypnosis, it is helpful to remind clients that emotions are inherently fleeting with an average duration of only a few minutes. Emotions last much longer when we combine them with attitudes, thoughts, and behaviors (Casula, 1997, 2009, 2011, 2017; Siegel, 2017; Short, 2018; Yapko, 2019, 2021). Since being able to modulate intensity, duration, and quality is part of emotional intelligence, different stories can be told with protagonists who are good models. Zen masters or Buddhist monks are usually characters capable of responding instead of reacting, of calming down, and of showing loving kindness and compassion, even in moments of tension. Also, animals can be selected to represent a specific emotion. For example, an elephant can be the protagonist of a story that makes meekness win over arrogance.

According to Seligman (1990), optimism is a beneficial attitude that can be taught and learned. I personally like to tell metaphors where emotions such as tenderness, generosity, and gratitude stimulate well-being, where epistemic emotions such as curiosity, trust, and hope are helpful as antidotes to fear, stagnation, anxiety, uncertainty, impotence, and illusion. The appropriate metaphors to stimulate emotional flexibility in patients are those in which the protagonist of the story explores different responses to the same stimulus until they find the one that provides the greatest well-being. An example of a metaphor that promotes self-regulation is that of the orphaned porcupine who had not learned from his parents to manage his quills. Until it met a turtle who taught it not only to contain the quills but also to recognize when to feel confident and trustful or when to defend itself (Casula, 1997, 2020).

Metaphors for Stimulating Cognitive Flexibility

Metaphor is helpful to deal with limited beliefs and to make the subjects aware of their cognitive errors, biases, mental traps, or logical leaps (Yapko, 2019, 2021). Instead of being engaged in a logic or pragmatic competition, metaphors can be used to free subjects from their own mental chains or mind traps, coming out of their custom-built cages. Metaphors that are created for stimulating reflection on one's cognitive patterns are usually stories of confrontation, with dialogues between a protagonist (who has a similar cognitive distortion as the client) and an interlocutor such as a teacher, a spiritual guide.

The interlocutor then shows the fallacy of the distorted way of thinking. The Spanish proverb, "if there is a remedy, why are you worried and if there is no remedy, why are you worried?" may be a suitable metaphor for those who have the illusion to be able to control things that they have no control over (Casula, 2020).

In confrontational stories, a dialogue between two friends can be inserted: one of the protagonists asks questions to the friend who shows rigidity such as: "What advantages have brought you to think what you think so far?" ... Or "How much do you believe in the truthfulness of the statement you have just stated?" ... Or "What evidence have you obtained that these thoughts help you in your personal, relational, and professional life?". Clients react to these types of stories by starting to question their rigidity and becoming open to experiencing the advantages of cognitive flexibility.

As a clinical example, Francesca had perfect ideas of how people should behave, based on how she would behave or would have behaved in a similar situation. For her I created a story of a traveler. The traveler during his first trips was disappointed because the people he met behaved in different ways from what he expected. Only when the traveler began to take a curious stance in the new countries he visited, he transformed from traveler to explorer and later became an anthropologist. Becoming an anthropologist helped him to observe the peculiarity of each villager and recognize that with this new attitude he had much more fun. This story helped Francesca become less judgmental and more open to recognizing the uniqueness of everyone she met.

Metaphors for Stimulating Behavioral Flexibility

In my clinical experience, I have found it is still difficult for some women to assert their rights to be treated fairly, with respect for their social or professional position (Casula, 2009; Linden, 2019).

Here is a clinical example: Paola, during a meeting with colleagues and clients, was sitting next to a colleague a few years older than her. When her colleague asked her to hand him the remote control, she saw it was on the opposite side of the table. She got up, went to get it, and handed it to her colleague, without looking at him to show her discomfort. During our session, Paola realized that she did not like her complacent reaction. With her behavior, she showed her colleague her passive acceptance of a subordinate position in which he put her. Her reflection during our session helped her to understand that it is important for her to act so that similar behavior does not happen again. It is she who must act, assert herself, recognize her empowerment to defend her role and to say a positive NO to inappropriate requests. During our session, I used the metaphor of an actress who had to learn to say a self-defensive NO in different ways: with assertiveness, with indifferent detachment, with a normal or aggressive tone, with grace and dignity, as well as with arrogance and presumption.

Another problem encountered more in women than in men concerns how to respond to unwelcome comments, for example, on choosing a partner or regarding their clothing or their weight. Several subjects have difficulty in responding in kind to those who judge them, give unsolicited advice, or embarrass them even in the presence of other people.

In cases of behavioral rigidity, I find it useful to stimulate subjects' unconscious intelligence and flexibility with a guide imagery in which they identify themselves in different protagonists imagining what they would do if they were a different person from who they are. They are invited to imagine what they would do if they were younger or older; of the opposite sex; of another nation, or continent; of another planet; if they were a spiritual leader, a politician, an entrepreneur, a Nobel winner, an Olympic champion.

Metaphors for Stimulating Identity Flexibility

In addressing identity issues, I created the metaphor of *The Five Petals of Identity* to identify where the difficulty and the resources are located (Casula, 2011, 2017). This metaphor explores (1) body identity – sex/gender, age, body characteristics; (2) social identity, children, parents, partners; (3) professional identity – qualification, profession, occupation; (4) spiritual identity – integrity, honesty, values, and virtues; and (5) secret identity – a secret that the client does not share with others and a secret regarding their identity that the subject did not know. For instance, Anna worked in a homophobic office and did not want to run the risk of being harassed, or even fired revealing her homosexuality. Aldo at the age of 52 discovered that his biological father was a secret lover of his mother, not the man he thought to be his father.

Even today, after years of feminism, some women are not aware of their feminine powers and need others to ratify and legitimize their worth and merit (Casula, 2009; Linden, 2019). As a clinical example, Eugenia reported that her boss told her that she must be the one to ask what job she wanted to do. She was reluctant because she thought that it must be the boss to recognize her potential. But she accepted to obey her boss.

Another clinical example, Stefania is the lover of a married man who for three years has promised her that he will leave his wife for her. In a guided imagery, I suggested Stefania to meet an accountant who multiplies three years by 365 days, 52 weeks and 12 months, and retrospectively helped review her relationship and make a list of give and take, recognizing that the accounts did not add up. This retrospective accounting made Stefania realize that her lover, for 1095 days, 152 weeks and 36 months, has given her crumbs of broken promises, spiced with lies and deceptions. After this retrospective review, I suggested Stefania to look at herself in the mirror to rediscover her integrity. She saw herself in the dark, forced to keep secret her love for that man. She realized that it was time to stop deceiving herself with false illusions. After these interventions, Stefania started a process of detachment and after a few months ended their love affair.

Metaphors for Stimulating Relational Flexibility

We are biologically social animals and live in a network of relationships that define respective and reciprocal roles which support them in formal and informal ways.

As a clinical example, Antonio asked for couples therapy. When the couple arrived, Antonio introduced his wife, Bruna. During the first couples meeting, Antonio complained that Bruna accused him that he has had a lover for four years. When I asked him what he intended to do with this extramarital relationship, he said, "This relationship must evolve". After the first interview with the couple, I had two individual interviews, and a second interview with the couple.

During the individual interviews, Bruna informed me that they were not married and had lived together for 20 years in a house for which she had been paying the mortgage, but Antonio was the only owner. During the second meeting with the couple, I said that they were not married. Antonio explained that for him "marriage is the point of arrival, not the starting point". I asked him if he thought that might be relevant for Bruna who had been living with him for 20 years *more uxorio,* and had paid the mortgage for social, legal, and financial reasons as well as hereditary grounds.

I reminded them of the story of the goddess Juno, who despite her jealousy accepted Jupiter's betrayals in exchange for the prestige of being his wife. I added that in the animal world, there are swans and albatrosses that are monogamous and ants and gorillas that are polygamous. In ancient Greek or Roman times, the most powerful men possessed numerous slaves. I underlined that in Europe bigamy or polygamy is not allowed. Then I asked him what he intended to do with the lover. He gave me the same answer: their relationship must evolve. Bruna replied that she did not want to accept that. At this point I felt blocked, and I asked them: what kind of couple therapy could I do with a couple that was not a couple, but a trio? What couples therapy could I do with two persons in a relationship that showed lack of respect, of reciprocity, of commitment, without clear definition of roles and sharing the same goal?

Metaphors for Stimulating Contextual Flexibility

Contextual flexibility is often used to indicate adequate attention to the explicit and implicit rules of contexts, which are sometimes inextricably linked to the social and professional roles of the people involved.

As a clinical example, Fabio was preparing to spend 21 days isolated in a hospital room for chemotherapy due to a recurrence of his cancer. To be prepared for this ordeal, he said he imagined himself as a warrior ready to start a war against his enemy. I shared with Fabio Lakoff's consideration that it is better not to use *war* as a metaphor when a real war is nearby, like the current between Russia and Ukraine (Lakoff & Johnson, 1980). I proposed to him to find another metaphor, isomorphic with the context of a hospital, a place where the mission of the health personnel is to cure and care, to do everything to help him heal.

Since he played basketball, enjoyed running, and participated in marathons, he told me that he still honored the values coming from those sports. I invited him to focus on the experience in dealing with its deliberate practice, the discipline of preparing for managing the basketball match or the marathon. I also suggested to him to let his unconscious mind remember when he suffered a sprain, a broken ligament, and cramps, and he realized that they were phenomena of practicing sports, just as diseases are part of life. Sportsmen know that accident and illness are temporary and face them with the resilient awareness that they can be cured and healed.

After the first cycle of 21 days in the hospital, Fabio told me that he and his doctors were satisfied with the results of his healing process. He utilized all the metaphors I used with him, such as adopting a bird's eye view to see what was going on in his therapy room, sending his body healing messages to utilize only the positive ingredients of the drugs, encouraging himself with the thought that everything would be fine, and imagining playing basketball with his two kids or running when he felt his weak body longing to stretch a bit. He told me that he discovered he liked being benevolent with himself and respecting that part of himself that was suffering.

Conclusion

This chapter has presented the role of metaphors in human communication and in therapeutic conversation. Metaphor is a linguistic tool essential in evoking implicit meaning, personal memory, and universal experiences, the lock and key to the door of an inner world that would otherwise remain hidden and tacit. This chapter has also presented a metaphor as a metaphoric story that encourages both emotional connection and emotional correction, and that can be told to transform subjects' conscious goals into actions guided by creative imagination, embodied experiences, and unconscious intelligence, free from mind automatisms and body rigidity (Pesesckian, 1979; Wallas, 1985, 1991).

Furthermore, this chapter has shown that the flexibility that the metaphor intends to evoke in subjects must first be experienced by the clinician able to calibrate to a direct or indirect style of communication according to the recipients of the metaphor. This is achieved by combining science and art, contemplation, speculation, theory, research, magical thinking, vivid experiences, and the universal wisdom coming from natural differences, changes, and mysteries, from archetypes, myths, legends, and anecdotes (Casula, 2019, 2020, 2021, 2022; Robles, 2000).

The therapists' aim of enhancing subjects' neurological plasticity is reached also with the careful selection of words based on their semantic and pragmatic implications and on multiple suggestions based on process-oriented hypnosis (Short, 2022; Sugarman et al., 2020; Yapko, 2021).

The use of metaphor has taken on value in hypnosis as it speaks the language of the right hemisphere, whether it is used as an analogy, as an anecdote, or as a story created especially for the client. Its value is appreciated by hypnotists as it allows to send different types of suggestions that stimulate neuroplasticity.

References

Bateson G. (1991). *A sacred unity. Further steps to an ecology of mind.* HarperCollins.

Battino, R. (2021). Brief therapy via guided imagery. In M. Jensen (Ed.), *Handbook of hypnotic techniques: Favorite methods of master clinicians* (Vol 2, pp. 170–195). Kirkland, Washington: Denny Creek Press.

Bolen, J. (1984). *Goddesses in everywoman: A new psychology of women.* New York: Harper & Row.

Casula, C. (1997). *I porcospini di Schopenhauer. Come condurre gruppi di formazione.* Milano, Italy: Franco Angeli.

Casula, C. (2002). *Giardinieri, principesse, porcospini: metafore per l'evoluzione personale e professionale.* Milano, Italy: Franco Angeli.

Casula, C. (2009) (Ed). *Le scarpe della principessa. Donne e l'arte di diventare sé stesse.* Milano, Italy, Franco Angeli.

Casula, C. (2011). *La forza della vulnerabilità: Utilizzare la resilienza per superare le avversità.* Milano, Italy: Franco Angeli.

Casula, C. (2017). *La ciotola d'oro: Vivere il presente, imparare dal passato, progettare il futuro in terapia.* Milano, Italy: Mimesis.

Casula, C. (2019). Utilizing, reframing and expanding patient's metaphors. In M. Jensen (Ed.), *Handbook of hypnotic techniques: Favorite methods of master clinicians.* (Vol. 1, pp. 108–122). Kirkland, Washington: Denny Creek Press.

Casula C. (2020). *Metaphors for personal and professional evolution. Gardeners, princesses, porcupines.* Translated into English by A. Diaz & R. Erickson-Klein. Roxanna Erickson- Klein.

Casula, C. (2021). L'uso delle metafore nella psicoterapia ericksoniana. In G. Debenedittis, C. Loriedo, C. Mammini, & N. Rago, (Eds.), *Trattato di ipnosi. Dai fondamenti teorici alla pratica clinica.* (pp. 138–154). Milano, Italy: Franco Angeli.

Casula, C. (2022). Stimulating unconscious processes with metaphors and narrative. *American Journal of Clinical Hypnosis*, *4*(4). 339–354. 10.1080/00029157.2021.2019670

Cuadros J., & Vargas M. (2021). *Hypnosis y la biologia del bienestar. Metaforas como el lenguage de la mente-cuerpo.* Madrid, Spain: Universo Letras Editorial Planeta.

Gilligan, S., & Dilts, R. (2009). *The heroes journey. A voyage of self discovery.* Crown House Publishing Company.

Gordon, D. (1978). *Therapeutic metaphors. Helping others through the looking glass.* Tucson, AZ: Meta Publication.

Hadot, P. (2004). *Le voile d'Isis. Essai suo l'histoire de l'idée de nature.* Paris, France: Editions Galimard.

Haley, J. (1986). *The power tactics of Jesus Christ and other essays.* New York: W.W. Norton & Co., Inc.

Hammond, C. D. (1990). *Handbook of hypnotic suggestions and metaphors.* New York: Norton & Company.

Hillman, J. (1980). *Facing the gods.* Washington, DC: Spring Publication.

Jaynes, J. (1976). *The origin of consciousness in the break-down of the bicameral mind.* MA: Houghton Mifflin Co.

Jaynes, J. (2021). *Le voci perdute degli dei. Sull'origine della coscienza.* Edizioni Tlon, Pg, Italy, from 2019 the Julian Jaynes Collection, of the Julian Jaynes Society.

Jung, C. G. (1934). Archetypes and the collective unconscious. In H. Read, & M. Fordham (Eds.), *The collected works of C.G. Jung* (pp. 1953–1980). New York: Routledge.

Lakoff, G., & Johnson, M. (1980). *Metaphors we live by.* Chicago, IL: The University of Chicago Press.

Lankton, S. (2019). Use of multiple-embedded metaphors to facilitate change. In M. Jensen (Ed.), *Handbook of hypnotic techniques: Favorite methods of master clinicians* (Vol 1, pp. 82–94). Kirkland, Washington: Denny Creek Press.

Lankton, C., & Lankton, S. (1989). *Tales of enchantment: Goal-oriented metaphors for adults and children in therapy.* New York: Brunner/Mazel.

Levitt, H., Korman, Y., & Angus, L. (2000). A metaphor analysis in treatments of depression: Metaphors as a marker of change, *Counselling Psychology Quarterly*, *13*(1), 23–35. 10.1080/09515070050011042

Linden, J. H. (2019). Ego-strengthening tool for the empowerment of women. In M. Jensen (Ed.), *Handbook of hypnotic techniques: Favorite methods of master clinicians.* (Vol 1, pp. 55–66). Kirkland, Washington: Denny Creek Press.

Madonna G. (2003). *La psicoterapia attraverso Bateson. Verso un'estetica della cura.* Bollati Boringhieri.

Malcomsen, A., Røssberg, J. I., Dammen, T., Willberg, T., Lovgren, A., Ulberg, R., & Evansen, J. (2021). Digging down or scratching the surface: How patients use metaphors to describe their experiences of psychotherapy. *BMC Psychiatry*, 21, 533. doi: 10.1186/s12888-021-03551-1.

Pearson, C. S. (1991). *Awakening the heroes within: Twelve archetypes to help us to find ourselves and transform our world.* New York: Harper Collins.

Perelman, C. (1977). *Il dominio retorico. Retorica e argomentazione.* Torino, Italy: Einaudi.

Peseschkian, N. (1979). *Oriental stories as tools in psychotherapy.* Berlin, Germany: Springer-Verlag.

Robles, T. (2000). *Concierto para cuatro cerebros en psicoterapia, quince años después.* Mexico: Segunda edición, Alom Editores.

Roffman, A. E. (2008). Men are grass. Bateson, Erickson, utilization and metaphor. *The American Journal of Clinical Hypnosis.* *50*(3), 247–257. doi: 10.1080/00029157.2008.10401627.

Rossi, E. L. (2002). *The psychobiology of gene expression: Neuroscience and neurogenesis in therapeutic hypnosis and the healing arts.* W. W. Norton: New York.

Seligman, M. E. P., (1990). *Learned optimism. How to change your mind and your life.* Pocket Book, Simon & Schuster Inc.

Siegel, D. J. (2017). *Mind. A journey to the heart of being human.* Mind Your Brain, Inc.

Short, D. (2018). Conversational hypnosis: Conceptual and technical differences relative to traditional hypnosis. *American Journal of Clinical Hypnosis*, *61*(2), 125–139. doi: 10.1080/00029157.2018.1441802.

Short, D. (2020). *From William James toMilton Erickson: The care of human consciousness*. Archway Publishing.
Short, D. (2021). *Making psychotherapy more effective with unconscious process work*. Routledge.
Short, D. (2022). Beyond words: A conceptual framework for the study and practice of hypnotherapeutic imagery. *American Journal of Clinical Hypnosis*, 64(4), 316–338. doi: 10.1080/00029157.2021.2020709.
Sugarman, L. I., Linden J. H., & Brooks L. W. (2020) *Changing minds with clinical hypnosis*. New York: Routledge.
Wallas L. (1985). *Stories for the third ear*. W. W. Norton: New York.
Wallas L. (1991). *Stories that heal*. W. W. Norton: New York.
Yapko, M. (2019). *Trancework. An introduction to the practice of clinical hypnosis*, (5th ed.). New York: Routledge.
Yapko, M. (2021). *Process-oriented hypnosis: Focusing on the forest, not the trees*. New York: W. W. Norton.

SECTION II

The Neuroscientific Foundations of Hypnosis

Neural Correlates of Hypnosis

16
NEURAL CORRELATES OF HYPNOSIS

Antonio Del Casale[1], *Alessandro Alcibiade*[2], *Clarissa Zocchi*[2], *and Stefano Ferracuti*[3]

[1]Department of Dynamic and Clinical Psychology, and Health Studies, Faculty of Medicine and Psychology, Sapienza University of Rome, Rome, Italy; [2]Department of Neuroscience, Mental Health and Sensory Organs (NESMOS), Faculty of Medicine and Psychology, Sapienza University of Rome, Rome, Italy; [3]Department of Human Neuroscience, Faculty of Medicine and Dentistry, Sapienza University of Rome, Rome, Italy

Background

There is an increasing interest in using hypnosis as a tool in cognitive neuropsychological research (Oakley et al., 2007) and in using brain imaging techniques to investigate hypnosis and related cognitive and behavioral phenomena (Kihlstrom, 2003; Rainville & Price, 2003; Ray & Oathes, 2003; Spiegel, 2003; Woody & Szechtman, 2003). Hypnosis can be used to investigate the nature of suggestibility phenomena more profoundly and as a tool for studying consciousness. Functional neuroimaging studies of hypnotized subjects have highlighted changes in brain activity associated with synchronized behavior changes or responses to a wide range of stimuli. Event-related potentials, functional magnetic resonance imaging (fMRI), magnetoencephalography, positron emission tomography (PET), and single photon emission computed tomography (SPECT) can all measure changes in brain activity. This chapter outlines recent findings on the cognitive and behavioral phenomena associated with hypnosis, focusing on the neurofunctional modifications related to this modified state of consciousness and cognition, evidenced by functional neuroimaging studies.

Resting-State Neural Correlates of Hypnosis

Most neuroimaging studies have focused on studying the functional neural correlates of hypnosis under resting conditions in highly hypnotizable subjects (HHs). The percentage of people considered highly hypnotizable is around 10–15% of the general population (Santarcangelo et al., 2021). Highly hypnotizable individuals are often described as having a strong imagination and a high level of suggestibility, which allows them to enter into a deep state of hypnosis and respond vigorously to suggestions. However, the level of hypnotizability can also vary depending on the situation, the hypnotist, and the individual's mindset and motivations. HHs are readily amenable to hypnosis and capable of exhibiting

DOI: 10.4324/9781003449126-23

the full spectrum of hypnotic phenomena which include altered state of consciousness, heightened suggestibility, analgesia, hallucinations, age regression, increased emotional responses, posthypnotic suggestion, and posthypnotic amnesia (PHA). However, not every HHs experiences all of these phenomena.

The specific techniques the hypnotist uses can also impact the type and severity of the hypnotic phenomena experienced (Santarcangelo et al., 2021). The most recent fMRI studies highlight how hypnosis is associated with a significant modulation of the connectivity and activity of the default mode network (DMN) (Deeley et al., 2012). Other brain areas can be involved depending on the depth of the hypnotic state, the type of mental content, and emotional involvement. HHs during hypnosis showed reduced activity in the anterior part of the DMN and activations of other areas, including the anterior cingulate cortex (ACC), dorsolateral prefrontal cortex (DLPFC), insula, and ventromedial prefrontal cortex, as well as hemispheric asymmetries of frontal lobe connectivity (Lipari et al., 2012). High hypnotizability has been associated with increased functional connectivity between the executive control and the salience networks (Faerman & Spiegel, 2021). During hypnosis, reduced activity in the ACC increased functional connectivity between the DLPFC and insula (salience network), and reduced connectivity between the DLPFC and DMN (posterior cingulate cortex) was reported (Del Casale et al., 2012). These changes in neural activity underlie focused attention, increased somatic and emotional control, and changes in self-awareness that characterize hypnosis (Jiang et al., 2017). Demertzi et al. (2011) analyzed the hypnotic modulation of the default mode and extrinsic network connectivity. Compared to mental imagery, hypnosis-induced modulation of the DMN was associated with reduced connectivity with extrinsic lateral frontoparietal cortical, possibly reflecting decreased sensory awareness. During hypnosis, the DMN showed increased functional connectivity in bilateral angular and middle frontal gyri. In contrast, its posterior midline and parahippocampal structures decreased their connectivity, possibly related to an altered "self" awareness and PHA processing.

McGeown et al. (2009) compared periods of hypnotic and non-hypnotic rest, reporting reductions in activity in the ACC and frontal cortices in HH in the former state compared to the latter. On this basis, brain activity appeared to significantly decrease in the anterior part of the DMN (prefrontal cortex) in HHs when hypnotized. The same region responded to hypnotic suggestions and tasks (McGeown et al., 2009). Deactivating default modality areas in HHs could reflect a state where irrelevant thought processes are inhibited. These people may be able to suspend spontaneous cognition in the absence of simultaneous tasks and may be able to reduce the interference of natural self-directed thoughts. This phenomenon could have to do with preparing for what may be required of upcoming activities or waiting for any instruction that one might receive from another individual (McGeown et al., 2009).

Conflict Monitoring and Attentive Functions

Hypnosis can profoundly change sensory awareness and cognitive processing. Individual differences in hypnotizability should correlate with differences in executive attention control (Egner et al., 2005). Fuster (1997) described how the frontal lobes play a crucial role in attention focus and direction during hypnotic trance by modulating subcortical neural networks. A network constituted by the prefrontal and cingulate cortices, thalamus, and brainstem nuclei is involved in mental absorption and hypnotizability (Santarcangelo et al., 2021).

Together with the ACC, the thalamus is involved in attention, cortical arousal, mood, self-regulation, and awareness (Herrero et al., 2002). Some studies have shown a coactivation in these areas following the induction of hypnosis (Maquet et al., 1999; Rainville et al., 1999). Brainstem nuclei are also critically involved in regulating conscious states, forming part of a neurocircuitry with the thalamus and ACC that regulates sleep-wake rhythm and attention (Aston-Jones et al., 1999; Kinomura et al., 1996). The serial pattern of regional cerebral blood flow changes in the brainstem, thalamus, and ACC may reflect the interrelationships among multiple components of a network (Paus et al., 1997) and may be related to the sense of "mental absorption." Coactivation of the ACC and the ponto-midbrain circuitry may reflect the contribution of the ACC to regulating attention-related activity in the locus coeruleus (Cohen et al., 2000). Rainville et al. (2002) found that mental relaxation correlates with metabolism reductions in the midbrain tegmentum of the brainstem and increased metabolism in the medial ACC and perigenual cortex. In the same study, the authors showed reduced glucose uptake in the brainstem, thalamus, and superior frontal gyrus, extending over the rostral ACC under relaxed states. Although relaxation and mental absorption are both increased during hypnosis, these results indicate that negative correlations in the midbrain stem and thalamus are associated with relaxation, and positive correlations in the upper pons, thalamus, and ACC are associated with absorption (Rainville et al., 2002).

Considerable attention and cognitive control studies have identified a neurocircuit centered on the dorsal ACC, considered a key area for conflict monitoring (Botvinick et al., 2001; Bush et al., 2000; Kerns et al., 2004). A conflict task showing reliable activation of the ACC requires the patient to name the ink color of a displayed word, i.e., the Stroop test (Stroop, 1935). Raz et al. (2005) supported the hypothesis that hypnosis eliminates or reduces conflict, with an early reduction of the activity of the ACC, without diminishing the conflict monitoring processes. Explicit hypnotic suggestion reduces automatic conflict and impairs information processing in HHs. Raz et al. (2005) combined neuroimaging methods to provide high temporal and spatial resolution and to study HHs and low hypnotizable subjects (LHs) with and without hypnotic suggestions to interpret sight words as gibberish. During posthypnotic suggestions, the ACC and visual areas showed reduced activity in HHs compared to the lack of hypnotic suggestions in LHs. ACC activation decreased before response under suggestion but increased upon incorrect responses on incongruent trials, regardless of suggestion (Raz et al., 2005). There is evidence of conflict reductions and uptake changes in the prefrontal cortex (PFC) and ACC under hypnosis, both of which are regions that are known to be involved in attention and cognitive control (Del Casale et al., 2012). These regions also have a relatively high density of dopamine receptors.

Additionally, the nucleus accumbens, a brain area rich in dopamine and involved in reward processing, is activated during hypnotic suggestions for pain relief (Raz, 2004). Because hypnosis can significantly alter HHs' performance on attentional tasks, Raz et al. (2006) hypothesized a potential common mechanism of dopaminergic modulation that affects both attentional task performance and hypnotizability. However, such mechanisms may overlap with different aspects of executive attention, as suggested by an analysis of within-subject correlations of interference in the Attention Network Test and Stroop tasks (Sommer et al., 2004). This approach may emphasize a critical disparity between the cognitive abilities of HHs and LHs and could be a field of future research.

Egner et al. (2005) used event-related fMRI to measure conflict- and control-related ACC and left frontal cortex activation at changing levels of response conflict in a Stroop task in HHs and LHs before and after hypnotic induction. This study supported that differences in executive attention processing mediate the trait of hypnotizability, and executive function is modified in HHs after hypnosis. HHs demonstrated conflict-related ACC hyperactivation during hypnosis, but such hyperactivation was not directly related to increased strategic cognitive control, as expected under normal conditions (Egner et al., 2005). Egner et al. hypothesized that conflict monitoring and cognitive control functions in HHs after hypnotic induction are decoupled, corresponding to a breakdown in the functional integration of two critical components of the frontal attentional control system. Together, these data support that hypnosis in HHs occurs through profound impairment of frontal lobe function and underlying structures (Gruzelier, 1998, 2000).

Mental Imagery

Early SPECT studies showed that the hypnotic state correlated with different metabolic changes in different brain regions such as the right frontal, orbitofrontal, temporal, motor, and somatosensory cortices (Crawford et al., 1993; Diehl et al., 1989; Meyer et al., 1989). This evidence led to the hypothesis that not only areas involved in attentional functions might show functional changes in hypnosis but also brain areas involved in other functions, including visual and motor imagination and learning. In a PET study, Grond et al. (1995) found decreased metabolism of occipital regions and increased sensorimotor areas during the hypnotic state. Existing evidence supports a link between activation of the superior occipital (Rainville et al., 1999) and occipitotemporal (Kosslyn et al., 2000) cortices related to increased visual imagery processes during hypnosis (Kosslyn et al., 2000; Rainville et al., 1999).

In an fMRI study on HHs and LHs performing a task during hypnosis, Raz et al. (2005) reported that decreased signaling in posterior brain activity within an extra-striate visual area in HHs might be related to early occipital modulation or aspects of visual word recognition. Maquet et al. (1999) found that hypnotized subjects who listened to sentences containing pleasant information from their past showed metabolic increases in the bilateral temporal poles (BA 38), superior (BA 42), and middle (BA 21–22) temporal gyri, right ACC (BA 24/32), and basal forebrain. On the left side, significant increases in the entorhinal and premotor cortex were observed (BA 6). These activations were likely related to auditory mental imagery, which is known to activate temporal areas (Zatorre et al., 1996). These studies, therefore, highlight the activity during hypnosis in terms of modifications of the cerebral metabolism of the upper occipital, occipitotemporal, and sensorimotor areas involved in functions such as visual and motor imagination and learning.

Motor Control

Mental imagery processing is crucial in preparing for movement during hypnosis. Some researchers have proposed that hypnosis may induce disconnection or "decoupling" between the prefrontal and posterior regions (Hilgard, 1974; Woody & Farvolden, 1998). Thus, various studies have investigated the functional connection of the motor cortices under hypnosis. In an fMRI study with a Go/No-Go task, Cojan et al. (2009) showed that hypnotic paralysis induces a profound reconfiguration in the functioning of the executive control system, particularly in the anterior prefrontal and parietal cortices. These correlates are distinct from voluntary feigned paralysis and inhibition of motor responses in the normal state. In the same study, the authors reported significant changes in the connectivity of the right motor cortex (M1). During normal alertness, the right M1 was more connected to the right dorsal premotor cortex and the left portion of the cerebellum; during hypnosis, this region was more connected to the right angular gyrus and left precuneus.

Furthermore, both the premotor and precuneus activations are differentially coupled with the right M1 activity across states. The connectivity of the right M1 area in the sham group was similar to that observed in the standard condition for the precuneus, right premotor cortex, and right angular gyrus. By comparing different aspects of motor control (preparation, execution, inhibition), Cojan et al. (2009) argued that hypnotic paralysis did not result from active suppression of motor outputs from the right inferior frontal gyrus, unlike voluntary inhibition (in Go/No-Go trials) or simulated paralysis. Instead, hypnosis forced changes in the prefrontal and parietal areas involved in attentional control and changes in the functional connectivity between M1 and other brain regions. The changes in connectivity resulted in some decoupling with the premotor areas. However, increased coupling with the precuneus is selectively activated during instructions to prepare for left movement during hypnosis (presumably due to imagery-related processes). These data suggest an untangling of motor commands from standard voluntary processes, presumably under the influence of brain systems involved in executive control and autocorrelated imagery (Cojan et al., 2009).

Some studies have reported faster motor reaction time (Braffman & Kirsch, 2001) and higher information processing speed (Ingram et al., 1979) in HHs versus LHs. This evidence is consistent with the finding that HHs can perform differently from LHs even awake.

An fMRI study by Pyka et al. (2011) investigated human brain function during hypnotic paralysis at rest, showing that the precuneus plays a pivotal role during the maintenance of the altered state of consciousness, which correlated with increased connectivity of the precuneus with its dorsal part, and with the right DLPFC and angular gyrus. Furthermore, the increased coupling of selective cortical areas with the precuneus supported the concept that hypnotic paralysis may be mediated by a modified self-representation, which can impact motor abilities (Pyka et al., 2011).

Episodic Memory Suppression in Posthypnotic Amnesia

The impairment of inappropriate selection of memory material has been presented in some memory loss disorders, such as psychogenic or functional amnesia (Markowitsch, 1999), in which the detailed suppression mechanisms may not necessarily be similar to the suppressions that occur in an average recovery. For memory retrieval and the successful subsequent use of this material, both the suppression of some memory representations and the expression of others is required (Bjork, 2007; Gilboa et al., 2006; Hasher & Zacks, 1988; Levy & Anderson, 2002; Racsmány and Conway, 2006; Schnider, 2003). With the aim of better investigating the mechanism of memory suppression in the brain, Mendelsohn et al. (2008) used hypnosis to study the differences between PHA and a model of psychogenic or functional amnesia (Barnier, 2002; Kihlstrom, 1997). During memory performance, this study identified suppression of various neural circuits relative to baseline activity, primarily in the left extra-striatal occipital lobe and left temporal pole. On the other hand, activation was found in the left rostro-lateral prefrontal cortex.

During subsequent suggestion reversal and regular memory performance retrieval, increased activity was observed in several areas, including the occipital, parietal, and dorsolateral frontal regions. Furthermore, the left rostrolateral PFC was preferentially activated during memory performance inhibition (Mendelsohn et al., 2008). Meta-processes and executive functions engaged in episodic memory retrieval are other functions performed in this area (Gilbert et al., 2006; Moscovitch & Winocur, 2002; Nyberg et al., 2000). Burgess et al. (2007) hypothesized that the rostral PFC is a gateway that connects the external and internal worlds, shifting attention between environmental stimuli and self-generated representations. Interestingly, Mendelsohn et al. also proposed that the increased activation of the rostrolateral PFC in PHA can be linked to an early implicit decision about whether or not to activate other recovery processes such as pre-recovery monitoring. They also hypothesized that this activation in memory suppression reflects a more significant retrieval effort. However, the brain substrates involved in the recovery effort have yet to be identified (Rugg & Wilding, 2000). Some evidence led to the hypothesis of the involvement of BA 10 (Schacter et al., 1996) and other PFC regions (Buckner et al., 1998; Heckers et al., 1998; Sohn et al., 2003).

The study of brain activity during memory performance showed that suppression is exerted early in the retrieval process, preventing the activation of regions crucial for effective retrieval. Pre-retrieval monitoring is a top-down process that allows attention to be allocated to relevant stimuli while ignoring irrelevant ones (Gazzaley et al., 2005; Kirsch et al., 1999). This process plays a crucial role in the behavioral manifestations of hypnosis involving the suppression or modulation of sensory input (Raz et al., 2006). Behavioral data showed abolition or reduction of Stroop conflict under posthypnotic suggestion. These findings highlight the role of posthypnotic suggestions in altering cognitive processes and may elucidate the neural correlates of other suggestion-based tasks. They can also help to understand the placebo effect (Wager et al., 2004), which, like hypnosis, is related to suggestion (Hunter, 2007). Therefore, it is essential to compare hypnotic suggestions with other techniques used in the modulation of cognitive control, including placebo and meditation. Only a few studies in the literature compared hypnosis and the meditative state. A mini-review conducted by Penazzi and De Pisapia (2022) pointed out that elements of overlap and difference between the two states can be identified. More specifically, in both cases, focused attention increases. Nevertheless, while hypnosis is mediated by another person capable of suggesting the subject, with the dissociation of executive control and changes of mental imagery processes, meditation is an entirely self-induced way of focusing attention and, with constant training, it can reach progressive depth and differentiation between the individual and the reality.

Conclusions

In the resting condition, brain activity significantly decreases in the anterior part of the DMN (prefrontal cortex) in HHs when hypnotized. This region also responds to hypnotic suggestions and tasks. The cingulate cortex is central to neurocognition under hypnosis and PHA. Furthermore, the activity of the ACC and prefrontal cortices is significantly reduced at rest in a normal state of consciousness in HHs compared to LHs. The right ACC and PCC were also involved in reliving pleasant life experiences under hypnosis.

A common dopaminergic pathway can modulate both attentional task performance and hypnotizability. Hypnosis can eliminate or reduce conflicts through early reduction of ACC activity without reducing conflict monitoring processes. The increase in conflict correlates with increased ACC activation, which is always more significant from the baseline state up to hypnosis in HHs than LHs. This conflict-related activation of the ACC may be related to uncoupling conflict monitoring function and cognitive control or another type of profound impairment of frontal lobe function. Hypnosis can modify the perception of reality by transforming verbal messages into internal images (activation of the occipital areas) and auditory images (activation of the temporal regions). The occipital areas are most activated during encoding or retrieval and never become active in the awake state during the same processes. Hypnosis can increase the activation of some left hemisphere regions, especially the left inferior temporal gyrus. This left-predominant activation may be due to the verbal mediation of hypnotic suggestions, working memory functions, and top-down processes that can reinterpret sensory experience. Hypnosis shifts the control of the action from the voluntary circuits usually involved to the internal representations generated through suggestions and images. This event is mediated by activity in the precuneus and reconfigures executive control of the task performed by the frontal lobes. Motor commands are processed differently during hypnosis; in particular, the precuneus and extrastriate visual areas are active during the preparation of left-hand movements.

Posthypnotic suggestions alter cognitive functions and can elucidate the neural correlates of other suggestion-based tasks. They can also help understand the placebo effect. Memory suppression in PHA correlated with hyperactivation of the rostrolateral PFC, which has shifted attention between external and internal stimuli and pre-retrieval monitoring.

Overall, functional neuroimaging studies confirm Braid's (1843) first central hypothesis of hypnosis as a process of enhancing or depressing neural activity and provide objective evidence that hypnotic phenomena also occur through changes in the functional connectivity between the brain areas.

Neuroimaging studies have provided valuable insights into the neural basis of hypnosis and suggestibility. We still need a complete picture of hypnosis-related phenomena related to individual and personality aspects, hypnosis settings, and personal motivations. Further research is needed to understand better the complex neural mechanisms underlying these phenomena.

References

Aston-Jones, G., Rajkowski, J., & Cohen, J. (1999). Role of locus coeruleus in attention and behavioral flexibility. *Biological Psychiatry*, *46*(9), 1309–1320. 10.1016/s0006-3223(99)00140-7

Barnier A. J. (2002). Posthypnotic amnesia for autobiographical episodes: A laboratory model of functional amnesia? *Psychological Science*, *13*(3), 232–237. 10.1111/1467-9280.00443

Bjork, R. A. (2007). Inhibition: An essential and contentious concept. In H. L. Roediger, Y. Dudai, & S. M. Fitzpatrick (Eds.), *Memory concepts* (pp. 307–313). New York, NY: Oxford University Press.

Botvinick, M. M., Braver, T. S., Barch, D. M., Carter, C. S., & Cohen, J. D. (2001). Conflict monitoring and cognitive control. *Psychological Review*, *108*(3), 624–652. 10.1037/0033-295x.108.3.624

Braid, J. (1843). *Neurohypnology, or the rationale of nervous sleep considered in relation to animal magnetism*. London, United Kingdom: Churchill.

Braffman, W., & Kirsch, I. (2001). Reaction time as a predictor of imaginative suggestibility and hypnotizability. *Contemporary Hypnosis*, *18*, 107–119.

Buckner, R. L., Koutstaal, W., Schacter, D. L., Wagner, A. D., & Rosen, B. R. (1998). Functional-anatomic study of episodic retrieval using fMRI. I. Retrieval effort versus retrieval success. *NeuroImage*, *7*(3), 151–162. 10.1006/nimg.1998.0327

Burgess, P. W., Dumontheil, I., & Gilbert, S. J. (2007). The gateway hypothesis of rostral prefrontal cortex (area 10) function. *Trends in Cognitive Sciences*, *11*(7), 290–298. 10.1016/j.tics.2007.05.004

Burgmer, M., Kugel, H., Pfleiderer, B., Ewert, A., Lenzen, T., Pioch, R., Pyka, M., Sommer, J., Arolt, V., Heuft, G., & Konrad, C. (2013). The mirror neuron system under hypnosis – brain substrates of voluntary and involuntary motor activation in hypnotic paralysis. *Cortex; a journal devoted to the study of the nervous system and behavior*, *49*(2), 437–445. 10.1016/j.cortex.2012.05.023

Bush, G., Luu, P., & Posner, M. I. (2000). Cognitive and emotional influences in anterior cingulate cortex. *Trends in Cognitive Sciences*, *4*(6), 215–222. 10.1016/s1364-6613(00)01483-2

Cohen, J. D., Botvinick, M., & Carter, C. S. (2000). Anterior cingulate and prefrontal cortex: Who's in control? *Nature Neuroscience*, *3*(5), 421–423. 10.1038/74783

Cojan, Y., Waber, L., Schwartz, S., Rossier, L., Forster, A., & Vuilleumier, P. (2009). The brain under self-control: Modulation of inhibitory and monitoring cortical networks during hypnotic paralysis. *Neuron*, *62*(6), 862–875. 10.1016/j.neuron.2009.05.021

Crawford, H. J., Gur, R. C., Skolnick, B., Gur, R. E., & Benson, D. M. (1993). Effects of hypnosis on regional cerebral blood flow during ischemic pain with and without suggested hypnotic analgesia. *International Journal of Psychophysiology: Official Journal of the International Organization of Psychophysiology*, *15*(3), 181–195. 10.1016/0167-8760(93)90002-7

Deeley, Q., Oakley, D. A., Toone, B., Giampietro, V., Brammer, M. J., Williams, S. C., & Halligan, P. W. (2012). Modulating the default mode network using hypnosis. *The International Journal of Clinical and Experimental Hypnosis*, *60*(2), 206–228. 10.1080/00207144.2012.648070

Del Casale, A., Ferracuti, S., Rapinesi, C., Serata, D., Sani, G., Savoja, V., Kotzalidis, G. D., Tatarelli, R., & Girardi, P. (2012). Neurocognition under hypnosis: Findings from recent functional neuroimaging studies. *The International Journal of Clinical and Experimental Hypnosis*, *60*(3), 286–317. 10.1080/00207144.2012.675295

Demertzi, A., Soddu, A., Faymonville, M. E., Bahri, M. A., Gosseries, O., Vanhaudenhuyse, A., Phillips, C., Maquet, P., Noirhomme, Q., Luxen, A., & Laureys, S. (2011). Hypnotic modulation of resting state fMRI default mode and extrinsic network connectivity. *Progress in Brain Research*, *193*, 309–322. 10.1016/B978-0-444-53839-0.00020-X

Diehl, B. J., Meyer, H. K., Ulrich, P., & Meinig, G. (1989). Mean hemispheric blood perfusion during autogenic training and hypnosis. *Psychiatry Research*, *29*(3), 317–318. 10.1016/0165-1781(89)90076-0

Egner, T., Jamieson, G., & Gruzelier, J. (2005). Hypnosis decouples cognitive control from conflict monitoring processes of the frontal lobe. *NeuroImage*, *27*(4), 969–978. 10.1016/j.neuroimage.2005.05.002

Faerman, A., & Spiegel, D. (2021). Shared cognitive mechanisms of hypnotizability with executive functioning and information salience. *Scientific Reports*, *11*(1), 5704. 10.1038/s41598-021-84954-8

Fuster, J. M. (1997). *The prefrontal cortex: Anatomy, physiology, and neuropsychology of the frontal lobe*. Raven.

Gazzaley, A., Cooney, J. W., Rissman, J., & D'Esposito, M. (2005). Top-down suppression deficit underlies working memory impairment in normal aging. *Nature Neuroscience*, *8*(10), 1298–1300. 10.1038/nn1543

Gilbert, S. J., Spengler, S., Simons, J. S., Steele, J. D., Lawrie, S. M., Frith, C. D., & Burgess, P. W. (2006). Functional specialization within rostral prefrontal cortex (area 10): A meta-analysis. *Journal of Cognitive Neuroscience*, *18*(6), 932–948. 10.1162/jocn.2006.18.6.932

Gilboa, A., Alain, C., Stuss, D. T., Melo, B., Miller, S., & Moscovitch, M. (2006). Mechanisms of spontaneous confabulations: A strategic retrieval account. *Brain: A Journal of Neurology*, *129*(Pt 6), 1399–1414. 10.1093/brain/awl093

Grond, M., Pawlik, G., Walter, H., Lesch, O. M., & Heiss, W. D. (1995). Hypnotic catalepsy-induced changes of regional cerebral glucose metabolism. *Psychiatry Research*, *61*(3), 173–179. 10.1016/0925-4927(95)02571-e

Gruzelier, J. H. (1998). A working model of the neurophysiology of hypnosis: A review of the evidence. *Contemporary Hypnosis*, *15*, 3–21.

Gruzelier, J. H. (2000). Redefining hypnosis: Theory, methods and integration. *Contemporary Hypnosis*, *17*, 51–70.

Hasher, L., & Zacks, R. T. (1988). Working memory, comprehension, and aging: A review and a new view. In G. H. Bower (Ed.), *The psychology of learning and motivation* (pp. 193–225). New York, NY: Academic.

Heckers, S., Rauch, S. L., Goff, D., Savage, C. R., Schacter, D. L., Fischman, A. J., & Alpert, N. M. (1998). Impaired recruitment of the hippocampus during conscious recollection in schizophrenia. *Nature Neuroscience*, *1*(4), 318–323. 10.1038/1137

Herrero, M. T., Barcia, C., & Navarro, J. M. (2002). Functional anatomy of thalamus and basal ganglia. *Child's Nervous System: ChNS: Official Journal of the International Society for Pediatric Neurosurgery*, *18*(8), 386–404. 10.1007/s00381-002-0604-1

Hilgard E. R. (1974). Toward a neo-dissociation theory: Multiple cognitive controls in human functioning. *Perspectives in Biology and Medicine*, *17*(3), 301–316. 10.1353/pbm.1974.0061

Hunter P. (2007). A question of faith. Exploiting the placebo effect depends on both the susceptibility of the patient to suggestion and the ability of the doctor to instill trust. *EMBO Reports*, *8*(2), 125–128. 10.1038/sj.embor.7400905

Ingram, R. E., Saccuzzo, D. P., McNeill, B. W., & McDonald, R. (1979). Speed of information processing in high and low susceptible subjects: A preliminary study. *The International Journal of Clinical and Experimental Hypnosis*, *27*(1), 42–47. 10.1080/00207147908407541

Jiang, H., White, M. P., Greicius, M. D., Waelde, L. C., & Spiegel, D. (2017). Brain activity and functional connectivity associated with hypnosis. *Cerebral cortex (New York, N.Y.: 1991)*, *27*(8), 4083–4093. 10.1093/cercor/bhw220

Kerns, J. G., Cohen, J. D., MacDonald, A. W., 3rd, Cho, R. Y., Stenger, V. A., & Carter, C. S. (2004). Anterior cingulate conflict monitoring and adjustments in control. *Science (New York, N.Y.)*, *303*(5660), 1023–1026. 10.1126/science.1089910

Kihlstrom J. F. (1997). Hypnosis, memory and amnesia. *Philosophical Transactions of the Royal Society of London. Series B, Biological sciences*, *352*(1362), 1727–1732. 10.1098/rstb.1997.0155

Kihlstrom J. F. (2003). The fox, the hedgehog, and hypnosis. *The International Journal of Clinical and Experimental Hypnosis*, *51*(2), 166–189. 10.1076/iceh.51.2.166.14611

Kinomura, S., Larsson, J., Gulyás, B., & Roland, P. E. (1996). Activation by attention of the human reticular formation and thalamic intralaminar nuclei. *Science (New York, N.Y.)*, *271*(5248), 512–515. 10.1126/science.271.5248.512

Kirsch, I., Burgess, C. A., & Braffman, W. (1999). Attentional resources in hypnotic responding. *The International Journal of Clinical and Experimental Hypnosis*, *47*(3), 175–191. 10.1080/00207149908410031

Kosslyn, S. M., Thompson, W. L., Costantini-Ferrando, M. F., Alpert, N. M., & Spiegel, D. (2000). Hypnotic visual illusion alters color processing in the brain. *The American Journal of Psychiatry*, *157*(8), 1279–1284. 10.1176/appi.ajp.157.8.1279

Levy, B. J., & Anderson, M. C. (2002). Inhibitory processes and the control of memory retrieval. *Trends in Cognitive Sciences*, *6*(7), 299–305. 10.1016/s1364-6613(02)01923-x

Lipari, S., Baglio, F., Griffanti, L., Mendozzi, L., Garegnani, M., Motta, A., Cecconi, P., & Pugnetti, L. (2012). Altered and asymmetric default mode network activity in a "hypnotic virtuoso": An fMRI and EEG study. *Consciousness and Cognition*, *21*(1), 393–400. 10.1016/j.concog.2011.11.006

Maquet, P., Faymonville, M. E., Degueldre, C., Delfiore, G., Franck, G., Luxen, A., & Lamy, M. (1999). Functional neuroanatomy of hypnotic state. *Biological Psychiatry*, *45*(3), 327–333. 10.1016/s0006-3223(97)00546-5

Markowitsch H. J. (1999). Functional neuroimaging correlates of functional amnesia. *Memory (Hove, England)*, *7*(5-6), 561–583. 10.1080/096582199387751

McGeown, W. J., Mazzoni, G., Venneri, A., & Kirsch, I. (2009). Hypnotic induction decreases anterior default mode activity. *Consciousness and Cognition*, *18*(4), 848–855. 10.1016/j.concog.2009.09.001

Mendelsohn, A., Chalamish, Y., Solomonovich, A., & Dudai, Y. (2008). Mesmerizing memories: Brain substrates of episodic memory suppression in posthypnotic amnesia. *Neuron*, *57*(1), 159–170. 10.1016/j.neuron.2007.11.022

Moscovitch, M., & Winocur, G. (2002). The frontal cortex and working with memory. In D. T. Stuss, & R. T. Knight (Eds.), *The frontal lobes* (pp. 188–209). Oxford, United Kingdom: Oxford University Press.

Nyberg, L., Persson, J., Habib, R., Tulving, E., McIntosh, A. R., Cabeza, R., & Houle, S. (2000). Large scale neurocognitive networks underlying episodic memory. *Journal of Cognitive Neuroscience*, *12*(1), 163–173. 10.1162/089892900561805

Oakley, D. A., Deeley, Q., & Halligan, P. W. (2007). Hypnotic depth and response to suggestion under standardized conditions and during FMRI scanning. *The International Journal of Clinical and Experimental Hypnosis*, *55*(1), 32–58. 10.1080/00207140600995844

Paus, T., Jech, R., Thompson, C. J., Comeau, R., Peters, T., & Evans, A. C. (1997). Transcranial magnetic stimulation during positron emission tomography: A new method for studying connectivity of the human cerebral cortex. *The Journal of Neuroscience: the Official Journal of the Society for Neuroscience*, *17*(9), 3178–3184. 10.1523/JNEUROSCI.17-09-03178.1997

Penazzi, G., & De Pisapia, N. (2022). Direct comparisons between hypnosis and meditation: A mini-review. *Frontiers in Psychology*, *13*, 958185. 10.3389/fpsyg.2022.958185

Pyka, M., Burgmer, M., Lenzen, T., Pioch, R., Dannlowski, U., Pfleiderer, B., Ewert, A. W., Heuft, G., Arolt, V., & Konrad, C. (2011). Brain correlates of hypnotic paralysis: A resting-state fMRI study. *NeuroImage*, *56*(4), 2173–2182. 10.1016/j.neuroimage.2011.03.078

Racsmány, M., & Conway, M. A. (2006). Episodic inhibition. *Journal of Experimental Psychology. Learning, Memory, and Cognition*, *32*(1), 44–57. 10.1037/0278-7393.32.1.44

Rainville, P., & Price, D. D. (2003). Hypnosis phenomenology and the neurobiology of consciousness. *The International Journal of Clinical and Experimental Hypnosis*, *51*(2), 105–129. 10.1076/iceh.51.2.105.14613

Rainville, P., Hofbauer, R. K., Bushnell, M. C., Duncan, G. H., & Price, D. D. (2002). Hypnosis modulates activity in brain structures involved in the regulation of consciousness. *Journal of Cognitive Neuroscience*, *14*(6), 887–901. 10.1162/089892902760191117

Rainville, P., Hofbauer, R. K., Paus, T., Duncan, G. H., Bushnell, M. C., & Price, D. D. (1999). Cerebral mechanisms of hypnotic induction and suggestion. *Journal of Cognitive Neuroscience*, *11*(1), 110–125. 10.1162/089892999563175

Ray, W. J., & Oathes, D. (2003). Brain imaging techniques. *The International Journal of Clinical and Experimental Hypnosis*, *51*(2), 97–104. 10.1076/iceh.51.2.97.14616

Raz, A. (2004). Atypical attention: Hypnosis and conflict reduction. In M. I., Posner (Ed.), *Cognitive neuroscience of attention* (pp. 420–429). Guilford.

Raz, A., Fan, J., & Posner, M. I. (2005). Hypnotic suggestion reduces conflict in the human brain. *Proceedings of the National Academy of Sciences of the United States of America*, *102*(28), 9978–9983. 10.1073/pnas.0503064102

Raz, A., Fan, J., & Posner, M. I. (2006). Neuroimaging and genetic associations of attentional and hypnotic processes. *Journal of Physiology, Paris*, *99*(4–6), 483–491. 10.1016/j.jphysparis.2006.03.003

Raz, A., Shapiro, T., Fan, J., & Posner, M. I. (2002). Hypnotic suggestion and the modulation of Stroop interference. *Archives of general psychiatryGeneral Psychiatry*, *59*(12), 1155–1161. 10.1001/archpsyc.59.12.1155

Rugg, M. D., & Wilding, E. L. (2000). Retrieval processing and episodic memory. *Trends in Cognitive Sciences*, *4*(3), 108–115. 10.1016/s1364-6613(00)01445-5

Santarcangelo, E. L., Carli, G., & Sebastiani, L. (2021). An evolutionary approach to hypnotizability. *The American Journal of Clinical Hypnosis*, *63*(4), 294–301. 10.1080/00029157.2020.1860893

Schacter, D. L., Alpert, N. M., Savage, C. R., Rauch, S. L., & Albert, M. S. (1996). Conscious recollection and the human hippocampal formation: Evidence from positron emission tomography. *Proceedings of the National Academy of Sciences of the United States of America*, *93*(1), 321–325. 10.1073/pnas.93.1.321

Schnider A. (2003). Spontaneous confabulation and the adaptation of thought to ongoing reality. *Nature Reviews. Neuroscience*, *4*(8), 662–671. 10.1038/nrn1179

Sohn, M. H., Goode, A., Stenger, V. A., Carter, C. S., & Anderson, J. R. (2003). Competition and representation during memory retrieval: Roles of the prefrontal cortex and the posterior parietal cortex. *Proceedings of the National Academy of Sciences of the United States of America*, *100*(12), 7412–7417. 10.1073/pnas.0832374100

Sommer, T., Fossella, J. A., Fan, J., & Posner, M. I. (2004). Inhibitory control: Cognitive subfunctions, individual differences and variation in dopaminergic genes. In: J. Reinvang, M. W. Greenlee, & M. Herrmann (Eds.), *The cognitive neuroscience of individual differences: New perspectives* (pp. 28–44). Oldenburg, Germany: Bibliotheks-und Informationssystem der Universität.

Spiegel D. (2003). Negative and positive visual hypnotic hallucinations: Attending inside and out. *The International Journal of Clinical and Experimental Hypnosis*, *51*(2), 130–146. 10.1076/iceh.51.2.130.14612

Stroop, J. R. (1935). Studies of interference in serial verbal reactions. *Journal of Experimental Psychology*, *18*, 643–661.

Wager, T. D., Rilling, J. K., Smith, E. E., Sokolik, A., Casey, K. L., Davidson, R. J., Kosslyn, S. M., Rose, R. M., & Cohen, J. D. (2004). Placebo-induced changes in FMRI in the anticipation and experience of pain. *Science (New York, N.Y.)*, *303*(5661), 1162–1167. 10.1126/science.1093065

Woody, E. Z., & Szechtman, H. (2003). How can brain activity and hypnosis inform each other?. *The International Journal of Clinical and Experimental Hypnosis*, *51*(3), 232–255. 10.1076/iceh.51.3.232.15521

Woody, E., & Farvolden, P. (1998). Dissociation in hypnosis and frontal executive function. *The American Journal of Clinical Hypnosis*, *40*(3), 206–216. 10.1080/00029157.1998.10403427

Zatorre, R. J., Halpern, A. R., Perry, D. W., Meyer, E., & Evans, A. C. (1996). Hearing in the mind's ear: A PET investigation of musical imagery and perception. *Journal of Cognitive Neuroscience*, *8*(1), 29–46. 10.1162/jocn.1996.8.1.29

17

EEG OSCILLATORY ACTIVITY CONCOMITANT WITH HYPNOSIS AND HYPNOTIZABILITY

Vilfredo De Pascalis

Department of Psychology, Sapienza University of Rome, Italy; University of New England, Armidale, NSW, Australia

Introduction

In recent years, hypnosis has been used in clinics and education (De Benedittis, 2020). However, the neural mechanisms of hypnosis and cognitive processes underlying responsiveness to hypnotic suggestions are not well explored and remain poorly understood (Halsband & Wolf, 2019; Terhune et al., 2017). According to Jensen and Patterson (2014), the lack of a widely accepted definition of hypnosis (Barnier & Nash, 2008) is one cause of the limited research and the consequent insufficient knowledge of mechanisms characterizing hypnosis. Hypnosis is a complex phenomenon embodying several elements such as interpersonal interaction, suggestion, relaxation, focused attention, concentration, imagination, altered perception of the environment, amnesia, analgesia, and letting go of thoughts, along with the disengagement of discursive and critical analytical reasoning. Given this complexity, researchers and clinicians need to specify the definition or reference model of hypnosis they use in their work. The improved understanding of neurophysiological mechanisms underlying hypnosis responding could strengthen our knowledge of essential brain functions underpinning mental processes.

The present review aims to provide a focused overview of the link between brain oscillation patterns measured by electroencephalogram (EEG) and hypnosis and individual differences in hypnotizability. Most of the research in this area focuses on three related questions: (1) changes in conventional oscillatory EEG-band activity before and following the induction of hypnosis, especially in highly hypnotizables (HHs) relative to low hypnotizables (LHs); (2) EEG functional connectivity changes to hypnotic responding, and hypnotizability; (3) differences in resting functional connectivity at baseline and following hypnosis induction.

We first report a concise classification of conventional EEG signals to facilitate understanding of the reported findings (for more information, see reviews by Barabasz & Barabasz, 2008; Jensen et al., 2015a,b; Terhune et al., 2017).

 DOI: 10.4324/9781003449126-24

EEG Frequency Oscillations

The oscillatory nature of the EEG is conventionally classified as bandwidths of oscillations that occur between specific frequency ranges and are labeled as delta (0.5–4 Hz), theta (4–8 Hz), alpha (8–13 Hz), beta (13–30 Hz), gamma (> 30 Hz). It is widely assumed that EEG oscillations provide essential links to brain functions, especially for communication between brain regions and associative processes. The delta, theta, alpha, beta, and gamma frequency oscillations are selectively distributed into oscillatory systems controlling the integrative brain functions of sensory registration, perception, movement, and cognitive processes related to attention, learning, memory, and emotions and represent a sort of alphabet of brain function (see, e.g., Başar, 2011; Buzsáki, 2006). For more details on the description of EEG rhythms, the reader is invited to read the review by Jensen et al. (2015a).

Hypnotizability, Hypnosis, and EEG oscillations

The study of electrical brain oscillations as potential indices of hypnosis began about 50 years ago (e.g., Galbraith et al., 1970; Nowlis & Rhead, 1968).

Until today, the research using EEG-band oscillations for neural bases of hypnotic susceptibility, hypnosis, and hypnotic responding has been of great interest to the neuroscience of hypnosis (Halsband & Wolf, 2019; Jensen et al., 2015a). Early EEG research initially highlighted changes in cortical electrical activity during hypnosis, indicating a higher occurrence of occipital alpha waves in HHs than LHs (Bakan & Svorad, 1969; Edmonston & Grotevant, 1975; Engstrom et al., 1970; London et al., 1968; Morgan et al., 1974; Ulett et al., 1972). However, this early finding was not replicated in subsequent studies (e.g., Barabasz, 1983; Perlini & Spanos, 1991). Other findings show a higher alpha activity among HHs relative to LHs out of hypnosis (De Pascalis & Palumbo, 1986) and increases in alpha following hypnotic procedures (Graffin et al., 1995; MacLeod-Morgan, 1979; Williams & Gruzelier, 2001). However, several reports did not favor an increase in alpha power with hypnosis, even when the significant effects of hypnosis did not show a decrease in alpha power (Kihlstrom, 2013; Ray, 1997; Sabourin et al., 1990).

The most consistent relationship between EEG activity and hypnosis has been reported in the 4–8 Hz theta band (see Crawford & Gruzelier, 1992; Jensen et al., 2015a). Several authors have reported increased spectral power in the EEG-theta band during hypnosis (Crawford, 1990; De Pascalis et al., 1998; Graffin et al., 1995; Sabourin et al., 1990; Tebecis et al., 1975). Crawford and colleagues (Crawford et al., 1996) reported a greater spectral power for high alpha (11.5–13.45 Hz), beta (16.5–25.45 Hz), and high theta (5.5–7.45 Hz) band in the right parietal cortex of HHs. There are also findings of increases in theta activity, mainly in HHs, during hypnotic inductions and suggestions (e.g., Jensen et al., 2013; Sabourin et al., 1990). However, De Pascalis and Perrone (1996), in HHs, observed an amplitude reduction in the low-theta band (4–5.75 Hz) in the left hemisphere during hypnosis/analgesia and hypnosis/no-analgesia conditions relative to a waking condition. In a subsequent experiment by De Pascalis et al. (1998), HHs, compared to LHs, in both waking- and hypnosis resting conditions, produced (1) increases in low theta amplitude (4–6 Hz) in bilateral frontal and right posterior areas and (2) decreases in alpha1 (8.25–10 Hz) amplitude bilaterally in the frontal cortex.

Additionally, in several reports, HHs tend to evidence more baseline theta activity than LHs during hypnosis and waking conditions (Freeman et al., 2000; Galbraith et al., 1970;

Sabourin et al., 1990; Tebecis et al., 1975), although there are studies where these differences have not been found (see, e.g., Rho et al., 2021). Jensen and collaborators (Jensen et al., 2008), in their seminal review on cortical neuromodulation of pain by self-hypnosis training, neurofeedback, and other behavioral treatments, hypothesized that greater theta oscillatory power prior to hypnosis might predict variability in hypnotic analgesia (see Jensen, EEG-Assessed Bandwidth Power and Hypnosis, in this volume).

The most pronounced and consistent differences for hypnotizability in hypnosis conditions have been reported in the theta spectrum, although these differences were obtained mainly considering HH and LH participants and excluding MH ones. Except for theta activity, findings regarding EEG measures in most of the other frequency bands show both increases and decreases with hypnosis (see review by Wolf et al., 2022).

Crawford (1994) proposed a dynamic neuropsychophysiological model of hypnosis (Crawford, 1989; Crawford & Gruzelier, 1992), suggesting that hypnosis is a state of enhanced attention that activates a fronto-limbic attentional dynamic system during hypnotic phenomena such as hypnotic analgesia. This model identifies low-frequency theta (3–6 Hz) and high theta (6–8 Hz) rhythms as candidates for frequency bandwidths that underlie the attentional and disattentional processes characteristic of hypnosis and hypnotic responses to suggestions. In one study, HHs presented higher attentional filtering abilities than LHs, and these differences were found to be reflected in the underlying brain dynamics. For example, Sabourin et al. (1990) observed an enhanced theta power (4–7.75 Hz) during hypnosis in both LHs and HHs, suggesting an intensification of attentional processes and imagery in hypnosis. Further research has provided consistent findings indicating that HHs show greater power in the lower theta bandwidth than LHs at resting baseline before hypnotic inductions and during hypnosis, whereas HHs, and to a less extent LHs, show an increase in slow wave activity after hypnotic induction (Crawford, 1990; Williams & Gruzelier, 2001).

However, some later findings did not support hypnosis-related power changes in the theta band and any other of the EEG frequency bands (Jamieson & Burgess, 2014; White et al., 2008). In addition, Terhune et al. (2011b) found a power increase in the alpha2 (10.5–12 Hz) frequency band during hypnosis, while no significant differences for any other EEG band were reported. Concerning resting state bandwidth power, the majority of the studies comparing HHs to LHs have shown a relatively higher theta power in HHs (Graffin et al., 1995; Kirenskaya et al., 2011; Vanhaudenhuyse et al., 2014), although findings with no significant differences in theta amplitude between hypnotizability groups have also been reported (De Pascalis, 1999).

In terms of gamma EEG activity, a pioneering study by Ulett et al. (1972) reported increased alpha, beta, and gamma (40 Hz) activities in the right occipital cortex during hypnotic induction. Later, De Pascalis and colleagues reported that in both nonhypnotic (De Pascalis et al., 1987) and hypnotic (De Pascalis et al., 1989) conditions, HHs (but not LHs) evidenced a greater 40 Hz EEG amplitude density at left and right temporo-parieto-occipital scalp regions during emotional experience compared to a resting condition. Later, these emotional findings were not confirmed by Crawford et al. (1996). Further, Schnyer and Allen (1995) observed a greater gamma density in the 36–44 Hz frequency band in HHs; participants responding with recognition amnesia to posthypnotic amnesia suggestion (but not those HHs without recognition amnesia) showed significantly greater 40 Hz activity over the LHs in the waking rest condition. De Pascalis et al. (1998) reported higher 40 Hz EEG amplitudes and heart-rate activity in HHs relative to LHs during a resting-hypnosis condition. Croft and colleagues (Croft et al., 2002), using painful electric stimuli, found that prefrontal gamma power (32–100 Hz), measured during the 40–540 ms period following phasic electrical stimulations to the right hand, predicted subjective pain ratings in a control condition out of hypnosis. This association was unchanged by hypnosis in LHs, while it was lacking during hypnosis and hypnotic analgesia in HHs, suggesting that hypnosis interferes with this pain-gamma relationship. De Pascalis and coworkers (De Pascalis et al., 2004) replicated and extended these findings to medium hypnotizables (MHs) by using a measure of phase-ordered gamma response (38–42 Hz) to painful electric stimuli in waking and hypnosis.

In sum, the extant findings show that enhanced theta power is the most frequent significant bandwidth associated with response to hypnosis. Changes in alpha power are relatively less frequently found. However, when significant effects for alpha are found, the evidence indicates that more alpha power is associated with more response to hypnosis. On the other hand, when significant effects are found for gamma power during hypnosis, those effects are found in both directions. This variability may depend not only on contextual differences and delivered hypnotic suggestions but also on the fact that theta-gamma coupling may be at work (see Jensen et al., 2015b). An increase or decrease in gamma activity may depend upon phases of theta oscillations.

Based on the present review, theta activity appears to be the most robust and reliable EEG measure sensitive to hypnosis responding and individual differences in hypnotizability. The current suggestion is in line with Jensen et al. (2015a) conceptualization of a preliminary theta/gamma oscillation model of hypnosis. These authors, starting from the assumption that theta-wave oscillations play a leading role in declarative memory processes and that these processes are central to many hypnotic suggestions, hypothesized that theta oscillations are linked to individual differences in hypnotizability and hypnotic responding. This model proposes that responses to hypnosis and hypnotic suggestions should be associated with an increase in theta oscillations and an increase or decrease, depending on the conveyed suggestion and contextual experience, in gamma oscillations. Notably, several hypotheses can be derived from the model that need to be tested for predicting and understanding hypnotic responding and improving hypnosis treatments.

EEG Connectivity Studies of Hypnosis and Hypnotizability

The extant EEG and fMRI research has provided convergent findings indicating that peculiar neural network connectivities characterize high hypnotic suggestibility and hypnotic responding. It is generally known that the electrical activity in the brain is the product of the dynamic interactions between and among distributed neural networks that exhibit transient and quasi-stationary activity. Statistical interdependencies between physiological time series recorded from different brain areas are labeled as *functional connectivity* (Lee et al., 2003) and include synchronous oscillatory activity essential for neural assemblies and coordination between different cell assemblies involved in multiple systems.

One possible assumption in the study of hypnotic suggestions is that suggestion-induced alterations in the experiential content are peculiarly associated with distinct changes in functional connectivity. The EEG coherence between two cortical regions or scalp sites is a classic putative measure of functional connectivity, and the degree of this measure is believed to reflect the strength of the interconnections between different cortical areas (Bullock et al., 2003). However, the poor temporal resolution, linearity, and the critical disadvantage of volume conduction limit the functional meaning of coherence measurements between electrode sites in EEG research (Burgess, 2007).

Several connectivity measures have been developed to account for volume conduction, even if only partially (e.g., Stam et al., 2007). The most frequently used functional connectivity measures between two electrodes are those that control for volume conduction artifacts and include: (1) imaginary component of coherency (iCOH; Nolte et al., 2004); (2) phase lag index (PLI; Stam et al., 2007); and (3) source space analysis. The first two measures are derived from computations of coherence between electrodes. The third measure requires applying source localization methods to the EEG signal (e.g., standardized or exact low-resolution brain electromagnetic tomography sLORETA or eLORETA) to identify the specific brain regions generating an EEG signal prior to calculating a measure of coherence controlled for volume conduction. Although the accuracy in localizing sources using the EEG is known to be very limited, the source connectivity findings that a specific brain area is selectively and specifically connected (or disconnected) with another area could provide good evidence that hypnosis is an exceptional mental condition (i.e., "state").

Studies using functional magnetic resonance imaging (fMRI) and EEG neuroimaging have provided new findings on the neurophysiological concomitant of hypnosis, hypnotic suggestions, and hypnotizability (see Halsband & Wolf, 2021; Oakley & Halligan, 2013; Terhune et al., 2017). These studies have demonstrated that the effects of suggestion are distinct from those of imagination and that there are similar cortical activation patterns between suggested experiences and the corresponding perceptual states.

In terms of EEG coherence, an unpublished EEG study by Kaiser (cited in Gruzelier, 1998) reported a relative reduction in upper-alpha band coherence at a bipolar left frontal, lateral electrode pair, and medial pair in HHs during hypnosis. In contrast, the LHs showed increased alpha coherence between these electrode pairs. The decreased coherence in HHs reflected a reduced synchronization of left frontal functional processes in hypnosis. Following a virtual reality hypnosis induction, White et al. (2008) reported decreased EEG coherence between medial frontal and lateral left prefrontal sites within the beta frequency band (13–30 Hz) in HHs but found increasing coherence in this frequency band in LHs. This finding is consistent with Egner et al. (2005) and suggests a functional dissociation between medial and lateral frontal regions in hypnosis.

Functional connectivity has also been assessed in a case study of a HH individual after a "neutral" hypnotic induction (Fingelkurts et al., 2007). Consistent with impaired functional connectivity, these investigators found that synchrony between anterior sites was significantly lower across multiple frequency bands (delta, theta, alpha, beta, and gamma). These authors reported local disruption in the left frontal and long-range functional cortical connectivity. They regarded their observed hypofrontality finding as a neuronal correlate of hypnosis in which separate cognitive modules of the brain may be temporarily unable to communicate normally. This observation is consistent with Gruzelier's results of left-hemisphere inhibition in hypnosis (Gruzelier, 2000). Miltner and Weiss (2007) reported a decrease in EEG coherence within the gamma band between somatosensory and frontal cortical regions during hypnotic analgesia in hypnosis compared to a control condition. According to Miltner and Weiss, the loss of gamma coherence between somatosensory and frontal brain areas during hypnotic analgesia reflects a breakdown of functional connectivity between the brain areas involved in the analysis of the somatosensory aspects of the noxious input (S2/insula) and areas organizing the emotional and behavioral responses to pain. They argued that hypnosis is characterized by a breakdown of coherent large-scale cortical oscillations organized and controlled by regions within the frontal cortex.

More recently, Jamieson and coworkers (Jamieson et al., 2017) conducted an excellent EEG connectivity study (using eLORETA procedures) testing the hypothesis that hypnotic amnesia reflects a functional dissociation from awareness. Using an old-new paradigm, they found that changes in regional cortical oscillations within the upper-alpha (10–12 Hz) band selectively inhibited the recall of memories of previously presented faces during hypnotic amnesia. During hypnotic amnesia, they observed that spatial and temporal coordination of upper alpha appears to suppress lagged nonlinear connectivity between right BA34 (parahippocampal gyrus) and right parietal (BA7), inferior temporal (BA20), and superior temporal (BA22) regions. In contrast, these patterns were absent after the reversal of the amnesia suggestion.

Resting Functional Connectivity in Control and Hypnosis Conditions

Terhune et al. (2011a) recorded EEG during resting in control and hypnosis conditions and computed the PLI. The PLI measures the extent to which a distribution of phase angle differences between two EEG time series is asymmetrically distributed (Stam et al., 2007). The concept is that if spurious connectivity is due to volume conduction, the between-signal phase angle differences will be distributed around 0 and should be avoided. The PLI only includes non-zero phase differences in which one signal is leading or lagging behind another. PLI values range from 0 to 1, and increased values indicate enhanced synchronization. In this study, HHs, as compared to the LHs, reliably experienced a relatively higher dissociation paralleled by relatively lower frontal-parietal phase synchrony in the upper-alpha band (10.5–12 Hz) during hypnosis. This finding appears consistent with the original findings of greater posterior upper alpha power in HHs (Williams & Gruzelier, 2001). Later, Jamieson and Burgess (2014), using both coherence and iCOH as measures of functional connectivity, compared resting pre-hypnosis with hypnosis condition in HHs and reported increased posterior connectivity (iCOH) in the theta band (4–7.9 Hz) and decreased anterior iCOH in the beta1 band (13–19.9Hz) during hypnosis. The authors interpreted their results as indicating that the hypnotic induction, in HHs more than LHs, elicited a qualitative change in the functional organization of specific brain systems. These findings are consistent with previous resting state EEG findings reported by Egner et al. (2005) of decreased functional connectivity, as measured with EEG gamma coherence, between frontal midline and left lateral scalp sites in highly susceptible subjects after hypnosis.

Additional preliminary resting state findings have been reported by Cardeña and colleagues (Cardeña et al., 2013). They adopted a neurophenomenological approach to investigate neutral hypnosis—which involves no specific suggestion other than to go into hypnosis—using the EEG power measures within conventional frequency bands and an EEG measure of global functional connectivity. Hypnotizability was marginally associated with lower global functional connectivity during hypnosis. They also found that experienced hypnotic depth and spontaneous phenomena following a neutral hypnotic induction vary as a function of hypnotizability and are related to global functional connectivity and EEG band oscillation activity. Finally, Li et al. (2017) investigated changes in resting state EEG coherence induced by hypnosis treatment for nicotine addiction in male smokers.

They found a significant increase in EEG coherence in delta and theta frequency and a significant decrease in alpha and beta frequency between a resting state in baseline and hypnosis, indicating alterations in consciousness after hypnotic induction.

Overall, the findings from EEG studies examining functional connectivity indicate that highly suggestible individuals exhibit reduced frontal connectivity across a number of frequency bands. Further research is needed to clarify the oscillatory specificity of these effects.

Research using resting-state fMRI and structural MRI have found that, following a hypnotic induction, HHs have more significant activity reductions in anterior default mode network (DMN) regions (anterior cingulate, medial and superior frontal gyri bilaterally) or medial prefrontal cortex than LHs (Jiang et al., 2017; McGeown et al., 2009). Original neuroimaging studies conceptualized the DMN of brain function as a distinct network of brain regions more active at rest or in low-demanding conditions than during goal-directed cognitive tasks (Gusnard & Raichle, 2001; Mazoyer et al., 2001). More recent research has established that various networks are involved in resting conditions other than the DMN such as the sensorimotor and dorsal attention networks (Zhang & Raichle, 2010). Additionally, the state of attentional absorption, following a hypnotic induction under invariant conditions of spontaneous changes in cognitive and perceptual states, has been associated with reduced activity in the DMN and increased activity in prefrontal attentional systems (Deeley et al., 2012). In a more recent and well-conducted fMRI study, Jiang et al. (2017) found that HH individuals, following hypnotic induction, exhibit an increased functional coupling between bilateral dorsolateral prefrontal and insular cortices. The study has also highlighted that a reduced coupling between the dorsolateral prefrontal cortex and posterior regions of the DMN (e.g., posterior cingulate cortex) enhances self-consciousness of being hypnotized, i.e., reduces the sense of agency that identifies hypnosis.

In conclusion, the resting fMRI studies cited above have provided promising results indicating that high hypnotic suggestibility is characterized by a peculiar pattern of functional connectivity of the prefrontal lobe with posterior regions known to engage in cognitive and self-related processing in self-monitoring and mind-wandering, which suggests the involvement of these functions in hypnosis.

Concluding Remarks

Original and current research has provided evidence that different brain oscillations can be modulated in response to hypnotic inductions and suggestions. In particular, hypnosis has been demonstrated to be associated with increased theta oscillations. Although significant effects associated with the alpha bandwidth are not always found, when significant effects do emerge, higher alpha power tends to be associated with a more significant response to hypnosis. Research reports on gamma power changes with hypnosis have highlighted variations in both directions, i.e., increases or decreases, depending on task requirements and delivered suggestions. Thus, preliminary evidence suggests the possibility that the magnitude of theta band oscillations is the most reliable concomitant and sensitive to hypnosis responding and hypnotizability. Further support for this hypothesis would have important implications for understanding the mechanisms underlying hypnosis that are necessary for developing new innovative clinical hypnosis treatments.

Hypnosis studies using EEG functional connectivity have found that hypnosis can affect connectivity across the spectrum of EEG oscillations, from delta to gamma. Thus, these studies suggest that the frequency of the connectivity of EEG oscillations is not central to hypnosis responding and hypnotic susceptibility. Common to EEG functional connectivity and fMRI studies are the findings that hypnosis reduces activity in the dorsal anterior cingulate cortex (focused attention), increases functional connectivity between the dorsolateral prefrontal cortex and the insula in the salience network (enhanced somatic and emotional control), and decreases connectivity with posterior cingulate activity in the DMN (lack of self-consciousness) (Jiang et al., 2017). The reduced interdependence of brain processes reflects the experience of involuntariness in hypnotic responding and amnesia. This pattern of results is consistent with increasing reduced conflict-related activity in the anterior cingulate cortex as hypnotizable subjects become hypnotized (Egner et al., 2005; Gruzelier, 1998). Recent upper-alpha (10–12 Hz) functional connectivity findings are also consistent with the dissociated control model of hypnosis (Woody & Bowers, 1994) and with a more recent model proposed by Jamieson and Woody (2007) in which breakdowns in the functional integration between different components of executive control networks account for core features in the phenomenology of the hypnotic condition.

However, based on the reviewed findings, it is not easy to generalize and highlight the resulting EEG oscillatory activity as a distinctive neurophysiological marker of hypnosis and hypnotizability. The above weak conclusion is mainly due to the heterogeneity of the studies and the different techniques employed in various application areas of hypnosis, making comparability among studies impossible. There are good reasons for thinking that EEG investigations using sophisticated measures of functional connectivity within the EEG frequency spectrum will improve our understanding of the role played by the frontal lobes in hypnosis and its functional relation with other cortical structures (see review by Kihlstrom, 2013). Future hypnosis research will need to develop sophisticated experimental designs and signal processing methods geared to increase our understanding of the neural mechanisms underlying experiential and behavioral aspects of hypnotic phenomena such as the divisions of awareness and the experience of involuntariness. Mainly researchers should include MH participants in their studies, given that these individuals may differ in important aspects of hypnotic responding from both HH and LH, making experimental findings more reliable (see Jensen et al., 2017).

Additionally, a more uniform and extended design is recommended in future EEG-hypnosis research, making a proper distinction between inductions, neutral hypnosis (Cardeña et al., 2013), and experimentally designed hypnotic suggestions. The success of experimental hypnosis research strictly depends on the robustness of hypnotic susceptibility scales since individual hypnotizability is essential for relating this measure to cognitive and neurophysiological variables (e.g., Terhune et al., 2017).

In conclusion, searching for neurophysiological signatures of hypnosis should be seen from a perspective of a productive talk between the laboratory and clinical practice. Making laboratory findings more easily translated into clinical practice and clinical observations communicated to science should lead to new knowledge on the neurophysiology of hypnosis phenomena and extend the range of possible clinical applications, and vice versa.

References

Bakan, P., & Svorad, D. (1969). Resting EEG alpha and asymmetry of reflective lateral eye movements. *Nature*, *223*(5209), 975–976. doi:10.1038/223975a0.

Barabasz, A. F. (1983). EEG alpha-hypnotizability correlations are not simple covariates of subject self-selection. *Biological Psychology*, *17*(2), 169–172. doi:10.1016/0301-0511(83)90017-0.

Barabasz, A. F., & Barabasz, M. (2008). Hypnosis and the brain. In R. M., Nash , & A. J., Barnier (Eds), *The Oxford handbook of hypnosis: Theory, research, and practice*, pp. 337–364.
Barnier, A. J., & Nash, M. R. (2008). 1 Introduction: A roadmap for explanation, a working definition. In A. J. Barnier & M. R. Nash (Eds.), *The Oxford handbook of hypnosis: Theory, research, and practice* (pp. 1–18). Oxford University Press.
Başar, E. (2011). *Brain-body-mind in the nebulous Cartesian system: A holistic approach by oscillations*. Springer.
Bullock, T. H., McClune, M. C., & Enright, J. T. (2003). Are the electroencephalograms mainly rhythmic? Assessment of periodicity in wide-band time series. *Neuroscience*, *121*(1), 233–252. doi:10.1016/S0306-4522(03)00208-2.
Burgess, A. (2007). On the contribution of neurophysiology to hypnosis research: Current state and future directions. In G. Jamieson (Ed.), *Hypnosis and conscious states: The cognitive neuroscience perspective* (pp. 195–219). Oxford University Press.
Buzsáki, G. (2006). *Rhythms of the brain*. Oxford University Press.
Cardeña, E., Jönsson, P., Terhune, D. B., & Marcusson-Clavertz, D. (2013). The neurophenomenology of neutral hypnosis. *Cortex*, *49*(2), 375–385. doi:10.1016/j.cortex.2012.04.001.
Crawford, H. J. (1989). Cognitive and physiological flexibility: Multiple pathways to hypnotic responsiveness. In: V. A. Gheorghiu, P. Netter, H. J. Eysenck, & R. Rosenthal (Eds.), *Suggestion and suggestibility: Theory and research* (pp. 165–167). Berlin, Heidelberg: Springer. 10.1007/978-3-642-73875-3_11
Crawford, H. J. (1990). Cognitive and psychophysiological correlates of hypnotic responsiveness and hypnosis. In M. L. Fass, & D. Brown (Eds.), *Creative mastery in hypnosis and hypnoanalysis: A festschrift for Erika Fromm* (pp. 155–168). Hillsdale, NJ: Lawrence Erlbaum.
Crawford, H. J. (1994). Brain dynamics and hypnosis: Attentional and disattentional processes. *International Journal of Clinical and Experimental Hypnosis*, *42*(3), 204–232. doi:10.1080/00207149408409352.
Crawford, H. J., Clarke, S. W., & Kitner-Triolo, M. (1996). Self-generated happy and sad emotions in low and highly hypnotizable persons during waking and hypnosis: Laterality and regional EEG activity differences. *International Journal of Psychophysiology*, *24*(3), 239–266. doi:10.1016/S0167-8760(96)00067-0.
Crawford, H. J., & Gruzelier, J. H. (1992). A midstream view of the neuropsychophysiology of hypnosis: Recent research and future directions. In E. Fromm, & M. R. Nash (Eds.), *Contemporary hypnosis research* (pp. 227–266). New York: Guilford Press.
Croft, R. J., Williams, J. D., Haenschel, C., & Gruzelier, J. H. (2002). Pain perception, hypnosis and 40 Hz oscillations. *International Journal of Psychophysiology*, *46*(2), 101–108. doi:10.1016/S0167-8760(02)00118-6.
De Benedittis, G. (2020). Neural mechanisms of hypnotic analgesia. *OBM Integrative and Complementary Medicine*, *5*(2), 023. doi:10.21926/obm.icm.2002023.
De Pascalis, V. (1999). Psychophysiological correlates of hypnosis and hypnotic susceptibility. *International Journal of Clinical and Experimental Hypnosis*, *47*(2), 117–143. doi:10.1080/00207149908410026.
De Pascalis, V., Cacace, I., & Massicolle, F. (2004). Perception and modulation of pain in waking and hypnosis: Functional significance of phase-ordered gamma oscillations. *Pain*, *112*(1), 27–36. doi:10.1016/j.pain.2004.07.003.
De Pascalis, V., Marucci, F. S., & Penna, P. M. (1989). 40-Hz EEG asymmetry during recall of emotional events in waking and hypnosis: Differences between low and high hypnotizables. *International Journal of Psychophysiology*, *7*(1), 85–96. doi:10.1016/0167-8760(89)90034-2.
De Pascalis, V., Marucci, F. S., Penna, P. M., & Pessa, E. (1987). Hemispheric activity of 40 Hz EEG during recall of emotional events: Differences between low and high hypnotizables. *International Journal of Psychophysiology*, *5*(3), 167–180. doi:10.1016/0167-8760(87)90003-1.
De Pascalis, V., & Palumbo, G. (1986). EEG alpha asymmetry: Task difficulty and hypnotizability. *Perceptual and Motor Skills*, *62*(1), 139–150. doi:10.2466/pms.1986.62.1.139.
De Pascalis, V., & Perrone, M. (1996). EEG asymmetry and heart rate during experience of hypnotic analgesia in high and low hypnotizables. *International Journal of Psychophysiology*, *21*(2), 163–175. doi:10.1016/0167-8760(95)00050-X.

De Pascalis, V., Ray, W. J., Tranquillo, I., & D'Amico, D. (1998). EEG activity and heart rate during recall of emotional events in hypnosis: Relationships with hypnotizability and suggestibility. *International Journal of Psychophysiology*, *29*(3), 255–275. doi:10.1016/S0167-8760(98)00009-9.

Deeley, Q., Oakley, D. A., Toone, B., Giampietro, V., Brammer, M. J., Williams, S. C. R., & Halligan, P. W. (2012). Modulating the default mode network using hypnosis. *International Journal of Clinical and Experimental Hypnosis*, *60*(2), 206–228. doi:10.1080/00207144.2012.648070.

Edmonston, W. E., & Grotevant, W. R. (1975). Hypnosis and alpha density. *American Journal of Clinical Hypnosis*, *17*(4), 221–232. doi:10.1080/00029157.1975.10403748.

Egner, T., Jamieson, G., & Gruzelier, J. H. (2005). Hypnosis decouples cognitive control from conflict monitoring processes of the frontal lobe. *Neuroimage*, *27*(4), 969–978. doi:10.1016/j.neuroimage.2005.05.002.

Engstrom, D. R., London, P., & Hart, J. T. (1970). Hypnotic susceptibility increased by EEG alpha training. *Nature*, *227*(5264), 1261–1262. doi:10.1038/2271261a0.

Fingelkurts, A. A., Fingelkurts, A. A., Kallio, S., & Revonsuo, A. (2007). Hypnosis induces a changed composition of brain oscillations in EEG: A case study. *Contemporary Hypnosis*, *24*(1), 3–18. doi:10.1002/ch.327.

Freeman, R., Barabasz, A., Barabasz, M., & Warner, D. (2000). Hypnosis and distraction differ in their effects on cold pressor pain. *American Journal of Clinical Hypnosis*, *43*(2), 137–148. doi:10.1080/00029157.2000.10404266.

Galbraith, G. C., London, P., Leibovitz, M. P., Cooper, L. M., & Hart, J. T. (1970). EEG and hypnotic susceptibility. *Journal of Comparative and Physiological Psychology*, *72*, 125–131. doi:10.1037/h0029278.

Graffin, N. F., Ray, W. J., & Lundy, R. (1995). EEG concomitants of hypnosis and hypnotic susceptibility. *Journal of Abnormal Psychology*, *104*(1), 123–131. doi:10.1037/0021-843X.104.1.123.

Gruzelier, J. H. (1998). A working model of the neurophysiology of hypnosis: A review of evidence. *Contemporary Hypnosis*, *15*(1), 3–21. doi:10.1002/ch.112.

Gruzelier, J. H. (2000). Redefining hypnosis: Theory, methods and integration. *Contemporary Hypnosis*, *17*(2), 51–70.

Gusnard, D. A., & Raichle, M. E. (2001). Searching for a baseline: Functional imaging and the resting human brain. *Nature Reviews Neuroscience*, *2*(10), 685–694. doi:10.1038/35094500.

Halsband, U., & Wolf, T. G. (2019). Functional changes in brain activity after hypnosis: Neurobiological mechanisms and application to patients with a specific phobia—limitations and future directions. *International Journal of Clinical and Experimental Hypnosis*, *67*(4), 449–474. doi:10.1080/00207144.2019.1650551.

Halsband, U., & Wolf, T. G. (2021). Current neuroscientific research database findings of brain activity changes after hypnosis. *American Journal of Clinical Hypnosis*, *63*(4), 372–388. doi:10.1080/00029157.2020.1863185.

Jamieson, G. A., & Burgess, A. P. (2014). Hypnotic induction is followed by state-like changes in the organization of EEG functional connectivity in the theta and beta frequency bands in high-hypnotically susceptible individuals. *Frontiers in Human Neuroscience*, *8*. doi:10.3389/fnhum.2014.00528.

Jamieson, G. A., Kittenis, M. D., Tivadar, R. I., & Evans, I. D. (2017). Inhibition of retrieval in hypnotic amnesia: Dissociation by upper-alpha gating. *Neuroscience of Consciousness*, *2017*(1), nix005. doi:10.1093/nc/nix005.

Jamieson, G. A., & Woody, E. (2007). Dissociated control as a paradigm for cognitive neuroscience research and theorizing in hypnosis. In G. A. Jamieson (Ed.), *Hypnosis and conscious states: The cognitive neuroscience perspective* (pp. 111–132). Oxford University Press.

Jensen, M. P., Adachi, T., & Hakimian, S. (2015a). Brain oscillations, hypnosis, and hypnotizability. *American Journal of Clinical Hypnosis*, *57*(3), 230–253. doi:10.1080/00029157.2014.976786.

Jensen, M. P., Adachi, T., Tomé-Pires, C., Lee, J., Osman, Z. J., & Miró, J. (2015b). Mechanisms of hypnosis: Toward the development of a biopsychosocial model. *International Journal of Clinical and Experimental Hypnosis*, *63*(1), 34–75. doi:10.1080/00207144.2014.961875.

Jensen, M. P., Hakimian, S., Sherlin, L. H., & Fregni, F. (2008). New insights into neuromodulatory approaches for the treatment of pain. *The Journal of Pain*, *9*(3), 193–199. doi:10.1016/j.jpain.2007.11.003.

Jensen, M. P., Jamieson, G. A., Lutz, A., Mazzoni, G., McGeown, W. J., Santarcangelo, E. L., ... Terhune, D. B. (2017). New directions in hypnosis research: Strategies for advancing the cognitive and clinical neuroscience of hypnosis. *Neuroscience of Consciousness*, *2017*(1). doi:10.1093/nc/nix004.

Jensen, M. P., & Patterson, D. R. (2014). Hypnotic approaches for chronic pain management: Clinical implications of recent research findings. *American Psychologist*, *69*, 167–177. doi:10.1037/a0035644.

Jensen, M. P., Sherlin, L. H., Askew, R. L., Fregni, F., Witkop, G., Gianas, A., ... Hakimian, S. (2013). Effects of non-pharmacological pain treatments on brain states. *Clinical Neurophysiology*, *124*(10), 2016–2024. doi:10.1016/j.clinph.2013.04.009.

Jiang, H., White, M. P., Greicius, M. D., Waelde, L. C., & Spiegel, D. (2017). Brain Activity and functional connectivity associated with hypnosis. *Cerebral Cortex*, *27*(8), 4083–4093. doi:10.1093/cercor/bhw220.

Kihlstrom, J. F. (2013). Neuro-hypnotism: Prospects for hypnosis and neuroscience. *Cortex*, *49*(2), 365–374. doi:10.1016/j.cortex.2012.05.016.

Kirenskaya, A. V., Novototsky-Vlasov, V. Y., Chistyakov, A. N., & Zvonikov, V. M. (2011). The Relationship between hypnotizability, internal imagery, and efficiency of neurolinguistic programming. *International Journal of Clinical and Experimental Hypnosis*, *59*(2), 225–241. doi:10.1080/00207144.2011.546223.

Lee, L., Harrison, L. M., & Mechelli, A. (2003). A report of the functional connectivity workshop, Dusseldorf 2002. *Neuroimage*, *19*(2), 457–465. doi:10.1016/S1053-8119(03)00062-4.

Li, X., Ma, R., Pang, L., Lv, W., Xie, Y., Chen, Y., ... Zhang, X. (2017). Delta coherence in resting-state EEG predicts the reduction in cigarette craving after hypnotic aversion suggestions. *Scientific Reports*, *7*(1), 2430. doi:10.1038/s41598-017-01373-4.

London, P., Hart, J. T., & Leibovitz, M. P. (1968). EEG alpha rhythms and susceptibility to hypnosis. *Nature*, *219*(5149), 71–72. doi:10.1038/219071a0.

MacLeod-Morgan, C. (1979). Hypnotic susceptibility, EEG theta and alpha waves, and hemispheric specificity. In D. R. C. G. D. Burrows, & L. Dennerstein (Eds.), *Hypnosis 1979: Proceedings of the 8th International Congress of Hypnosis and Psychosomatic Medicine, Melbourne, Australia, August 19–24, 1979* (pp. 181–188). Amsterdam: Elsevier.

Mazoyer, B., Zago, L., Mellet, E., Bricogne, S., Etard, O., Houdé, O., ... Tzourio-Mazoyer, N. (2001). Cortical networks for working memory and executive functions sustain the conscious resting state in man. *Brain Research Bulletin*, *54*(3), 287–298. doi:10.1016/S0361-9230(00)00437-8.

McGeown, W. J., Mazzoni, G., Venneri, A., & Kirsch, I. (2009). Hypnotic induction decreases anterior default mode activity. *Consciousness and Cognition*, *18*(4), 848–855. doi:10.1016/j.concog.2009.09.001.

Miltner, W. H. R., & Weiss, T. (2007). Cortical mechanisms of hypnotic pain control. In G. A., Jamieson (Ed.), *Hypnosis and conscious states: The cognitive neuroscience perspective*. (pp. 51–66). New York: Oxford University Press.

Morgan, A. H., Macdonald, H., & Hilgard, E. R. (1974). EEG alpha: Lateral asymmetry related to task, and hypnotizability. *Psychophysiology*, *11*(3), 275–282. doi:10.1111/j.1469-8986.1974.tb00544.x.

Nolte, G., Bai, O., Wheaton, L., Mari, Z., Vorbach, S., & Hallett, M. (2004). Identifying true brain interaction from EEG data using the imaginary part of coherency. *Clinical Neurophysiology*, *115*(10), 2292–2307. doi:10.1016/j.clinph.2004.04.029.

Nowlis, D. P., & Rhead, J. C. (1968). Relation of eyes-closed resting EEG alpha activity to hypnotic susceptibility. *Perceptual and Motor Skills*, 27(3_suppl), 1047–1050. doi:10.2466/pms.1968.27.3f.1047.

Oakley, D. A., & Halligan, P. W. (2013). Hypnotic suggestion: Opportunities for cognitive neuroscience. *Nature Reviews Neuroscience*, *14*(8), 565–576. doi:10.1038/nrn3538.

Perlini, A. H., & Spanos, N. P. (1991). EEG alpha methodologies and hypnotizability: A critical review. *Psychophysiology*, *28*(5), 511–530. doi:10.1111/j.1469-8986.1991.tb01989.x.

Ray, W. J. (1997). Eeg concomitants of hypnotic susceptibility. *International Journal of Clinical and Experimental Hypnosis*, *45*(3), 301–313. doi:10.1080/00207149708416131.

Rho, G., Callara, A. L., Petri, G., Nardelli, M., Scilingo, E. P., Greco, A., & De Pascalis, V. (2021). Linear and nonlinear quantitative EEG analysis during neutral hypnosis following an opened/closed eye paradigm. *Symmetry*, *13*(8), 1423.

Sabourin, M. E., Cutcomb, S. D., Crawford, H. J., & Pribram, K. (1990). EEG correlates of hypnotic susceptibility and hypnotic trance: Spectral analysis and coherence. *International Journal of Psychophysiology*, *10*(2), 125–142. doi:10.1016/0167-8760(90)90027-B.

Schnyer, D. M., & Allen, J. J. (1995). Attention-related electroencephalographic and event-related potential predictors of responsiveness to suggested posthypnotic amnesia. *International Journal of Clinical and Experimental Hypnosis*, *43*(3), 295–315. doi:10.1080/00207149508409972.

Stam, C. J., Nolte, G., & Daffertshofer, A. (2007). Phase lag index: Assessment of functional connectivity from multi channel EEG and MEG with diminished bias from common sources. *Human Brain Mapping*, *28*(11), 1178–1193. doi:10.1002/hbm.20346.

Tebecis, A. K., Provins, K. A., Farnbach, R. W., & Pentony, P. (1975). Hypnosis and the EEG: A quantitative investigation. *Journal of Nervous and Mental Disease*, *161*, 1–17. doi:10.1097/00005053-197507000-00001.

Terhune, D. B., Cardeña, E., & Lindgren, M. (2011a). Differential frontal-parietal phase synchrony during hypnosis as a function of hypnotic suggestibility. *Psychophysiology*, *48*(10), 1444–1447. doi:10.1111/j.1469-8986.2011.01211.x.

Terhune, D. B., Cardeña, E., & Lindgren, M. (2011b). Dissociative tendencies and individual differences in high hypnotic suggestibility. *Cognitive Neuropsychiatry*, *16*(2), 113–135. doi:10.1080/13546805.2010.503048.

Terhune, D. B., Cleeremans, A., Raz, A., & Lynn, S. J. (2017). Hypnosis and top-down regulation of consciousness. *Neuroscience & Biobehavioral Reviews*, *81*, 59–74. doi:10.1016/j.neubiorev.2017.02.002.

Ulett, G. A., Akpinar, S., & Itil, T. M. (1972). Quantitative EEG analysis during hypnosis. *Electroencephalography and Clinical Neurophysiology*, *33*(4), 361–368. doi:10.1016/0013-4694(72)90116-2.

Vanhaudenhuyse, A., Laureys, S., & Faymonville, M. E. (2014). Neurophysiology of hypnosis. *Neurophysiologie Clinique/Clinical Neurophysiology*, *44*(4), 343–353. doi:10.1016/j.neucli.2013.09.006.

White, D., Ciorciari, J., Carbis, C., & Liley, D. (2008). EEG correlates of virtual reality hypnosis. *International Journal of Clinical and Experimental Hypnosis*, *57*(1), 94–116. doi:10.1080/00207140802463690.

Williams, J. D., & Gruzelier, J. H. (2001). Differentiation of hypnosis and relaxation by analysis of narrow band theta and alpha frequencies. *International Journal of Clinical and Experimental Hypnosis*, *49*(3), 185–206. doi:10.1080/00207140108410070.

Wolf, T. G., Faerber, K. A., Rummel, C., Halsband, U., & Campus, G. (2022). Functional changes in brain activity using hypnosis: A systematic review. *Brain Sciences*, *12*(1), 108.

Woody, E. Z., & Bowers, K. S. (1994). A frontal assault on dissociated control. In S.J., Lynn, & J.W., Rhue (Eds.), *Dissociation: Clinical and theoretical perspectives* (pp. 52–79). New York: The Guilford Press.

Zhang, D., & Raichle, M. E. (2010). Disease and the brain's dark energy. *Nature Reviews Neurology*, 6(1), 15–28. doi:10.1038/nrneurol.2009.198.

18

BEYOND THE NEURAL SIGNATURE OF HYPNOSIS

Neuroimaging Studies Support a Multifaceted View of Hypnotic Phenomena

Mathieu Landry and Pierre Rainville

Université de Montréal, Canada

The Quest to Uncover the Neural Signature of Hypnosis

Hypnosis engulfs a wide variety of mental phenomena marked by inter-individual differences, spontaneous changes in subjective experiences, and the ability to respond to assorted suggestions for individuals to change their perception, cognitions, emotions, or ideomotor actions (Elkins et al., 2015; Terhune et al., 2017). Thus, hypnotic phenomena hardly reduce to a single component and involve several facets of the mind and brain. Some of these facets relate to variability in the capacity to respond to hypnotic suggestions (McConkey & Barnier, 2004). Others, the fact that individuals undergoing hypnosis often experience changes in their phenomenology such as intense feelings of absorption, temporal distortions, a sense of responding to suggestions in an automatic and involuntary manner, or deep feelings of relaxation and appeasement (Rainville & Price, 2003). At the same time, hypnosis also changes how information is processed in a manner that is consistent with the content of hypnotic suggestions, which means that different suggestions will elicit different neural responses (Landry & Raz, 2015). For example, a suggestion that targets pain perception will change the perception and interpretation of nociceptive inputs (Rainville et al., 1999). The inherent complexity of hypnotic phenomena has challenged attempts to discover the underlying mechanisms of hypnotic phenomena – a difficulty that has permeated the field in various ways. For example, it remains unclear which aspects should be prioritized when trying to characterize hypnotic phenomena, especially considering that the relationship between the phenomenological dimensions of hypnosis and hypnotic responses remains ambiguous (Pekala, 2015; Terhune, 2014). Attempts to uncover mechanisms have also been challenged by evidence showing that inter-individual differences in the ability to generate efficient hypnotic responses are likewise multifaceted (Barnier et al., 2022). Obviously, these challenges similarly impact ongoing efforts to discover the neural basis of hypnosis. While neuroimaging has become a prominent methodological approach to investigate hypnotic phenomena, the current body of work is largely characterized by heterogeneity in the findings (Landry et al., 2017). The lack of commonalities among neuroimaging results is consistent with the notion that hypnosis

 DOI: 10.4324/9781003449126-25

relates to multiple neural patterns, rather than one. In this chapter, we review different factors that play an important role in shaping the emergence of hypnotic phenomena and then relate these factors to modulations of various brain networks. Ultimately, we show how it remains difficult to pinpoint a single neural process that seems critical for hypnosis, and instead argue for a multifaceted view regarding the evidence from neuroimaging studies.

The lack of commonalities across neuroimaging findings contrasts with claims that hypnosis involves a particular brain state – a neurobiological signature that would reflect a critical process for the emergence of hypnotic phenomena. The notion that hypnotic phenomena involve one such specific cerebral state or neural pattern has often been presented alongside theoretical frameworks. For example, the research group of David Spiegel, a leading researcher in the field, emphasizes mental absorption as a critical component of hypnosis that relates to activity in the anterior cingulate cortex (ACC; e.g., DeSouza et al., 2020). This cortical region is a key node of thalamo-cortical attentional networks where activity has been previously associated with self-reports of mental absorption following hypnotic induction (Rainville et al., 2002). Unraveling the functional role of this cortical region in the context of hypnosis may be critical to understanding the neural basis of hypnotic phenomena. In the same way, proponents of the cold control theory of hypnosis, a theoretical framework predicated upon metacognition of intentions, link the emergence of hypnotic phenomena to the dorsolateral prefrontal cortex (DLPFC; Dienes & Hutton, 2013), a brain region strongly related to metacognitive abilities (Shekhar & Rahnev, 2018). Hypnotic phenomena have also been related to modulations of theta oscillations – a brain rhythm that putatively relates to various cognitive processes involved in the production of hypnotic responses (Jensen et al., 2015). These examples present theoretical proposals that argue for a neural signature of hypnotic phenomena. In contrast to such a proposal, the multifaceted view of hypnosis contends that hypnotic responsiveness reflects multiple underlying components (Woody et al., 2005). In this way, rather than reduce hypnotic phenomena to a single mechanism, this proposal argues for the decomposition of hypnosis into sub-components, much like other complex cognitive abilities. This componential view entails that hypnotic responsiveness comprises multiple neural processes, which aligns with the heterogeneity we observe in the neuroimaging literature. Barnier and colleagues (2022) recently submitted a list of potential such sub-components. Our proposal aligns with this idea and proposes to explore potential neural processes linked to various components of hypnosis. In our view, the goal of developing a mechanistic account of hypnotic phenomena encompasses a variety of brain dynamics.

We previously mentioned how the heterogeneity of neuroimaging findings weakens overarching conclusions about the neural basis of hypnosis. A useful taxonomy to understand the current body of results in the field proposes to organize them according to variables of interests: susceptibility to hypnotic suggestions, hypnotic induction, and the effects of suggestions (Landry & Raz, 2015; Landry et al., 2017; Mazzoni et al., 2013). While this approach fails to deliver a reliable theoretical framework for explaining hypnotic phenomena, it nevertheless groups the various findings according to some of the key variables in the field, which ultimately allows us to evaluate and uncover the latent components of hypnotic responding (Figure 18.1). More specifically, the logic of this taxonomy is that most experimental protocols can be separated into observations related to hypnotic susceptibility, hypnotic induction, and hypnotic suggestions because these key variables can inform our hypotheses about the causal relationship between latent components that

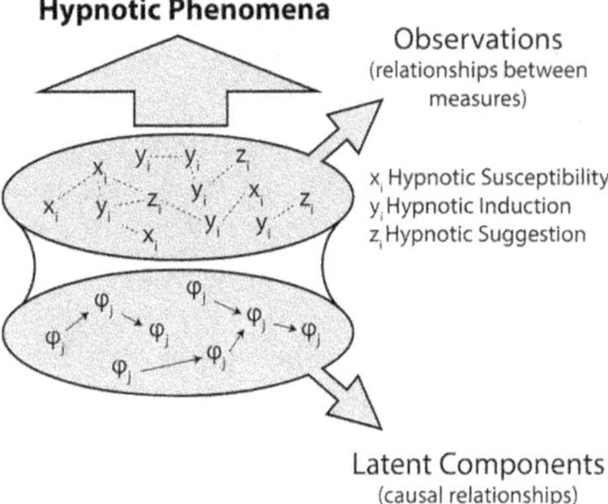

Figure 18.1 The emergence of hypnotic phenomena. Hypnotic phenomena result from the causal relationship of several latent components (phi variables). However, latent components are not directly observable. To infer the presence of these latent components and their causal relationships, researchers rely on observations (i.e., variables that can be measured). Observations can be separated based on the following taxonomy: hypnotic susceptibility (variable x), hypnotic induction (variable y), hypnotic suggestion (variable z). Inference of causal relationships is based on these observations.

yield hypnotic phenomena. For example, induction procedures typically yield spontaneous changes in phenomenology (Pekala & Kumar, 2007). Therefore, neuroimaging protocols that evaluates neural activity as a function of induction will be relevant to understand the neurophenomenology of hypnosis and the relevancy of these changes in phenomenology for explaining the neural mechanisms of hypnotic phenomena. Note that observations are not limited to neural activity and include all observations for assessing hypotheses such as subjective reports or task performance. Applying this approach in light of the componential view of hypnosis, we anticipate that several causal relationships lead to the emergence of hypnotic phenomena. This basic and overarching framework can help us to infer these causal relationships.

Decomposing Hypnosis into Components

Divide findings according to variables of interest provided, we see that neuroimaging of hypnotic susceptibility applies to a variety of experimental protocols that are mainly divided into three streams: studies aiming to investigate structural differences (e.g., Horton et al., 2004), those investigating functional differences at rest (e.g., Hoeft et al., 2012), and others investigating functional differences during cognitive tasks (e.g., Lifshitz & Raz, 2015). This work often contrasts low hypnotic susceptible individual (LHSI) and high hypnotic susceptible individual (HHSI). From a functional point of view, one study that links hypnotic susceptibility relates to variations in baseline attention capacities, while these effects relate to modulations of cortical associated with attention processing and executive functions (Cojan et al., 2015). These findings align with the prevailing view that attention capacities play a central role in shaping how individuals respond to the process of hypnosis (Gruzelier, 1998). Here, we can appreciate how various functional aspects of voluntary attention, such as the selection of specific information, the maintenance of their focus, and the suppression of task-irrelevant distractions, relate to core aspects of mental absorption, executive control, and hypnosis (Egner & Raz, 2007; Lifshitz et al., 2019; Raz, 2004, 2005). Brain networks underlying these attention processes involve thalamocortical and cortico-cortical interactions that may explain the gating of bottom-up sensory-perceptual responses in a variety of contexts including hypnotic analgesia (Del Casale et al., 2015; Kiernan et al., 1995). In short, attention processes facilitate goal-driven behaviors through the selection of task relevant and suppression of task-irrelevant information to facilitate the production of an efficient hypnotic response.

Despite the putative prominence of attention processes in hypnosis, it is important to note that HHSIs do not represent a homogenous group (Terhune, 2015; Terhune & Cardeña, 2010), which means that attention capabilities may only facilitate the production of efficient responses for some of them (Terhune et al., 2011). Hence, while some individuals efficiently respond to hypnotic suggestions due to their attention capacities, others may rely on different capacities such as the capacity to experience dissociation, i.e., disruption in the integration of consciousness (Barnier et al., 2022). Specifically, evidence indicates that only a subset of HHSIs exhibit dissociative tendencies in the context of executive control and hypnosis (Terhune et al., 2011). Consistent with this hypothesis, one neuroimaging study observed that, following a hypnotic induction, HHSIs showed altered patterns of activity in the ACC, a brain region related to executive control and conflict monitoring, when they completed the Stroop task – a cognitive task that engages cognitive control by generating cognitive conflict (Egner et al., 2005). In line with the dissociation account of hypnosis, the authors interpreted this outcome as a disconnection between monitoring and executive control. In this regard, dissociation is also viewed as a core component of hypnosis (Wieder et al., 2022). A disruption in the feeling of authorship represents another way by which dissociation seemingly occurs during hypnotic responding (Polito et al., 2014). Specifically, HHSIs tend to experience feelings of automaticity and involuntariness when responding to hypnotic suggestions, while neuroimaging studies relate these phenomenological facets to the parietal region (Blakemore et al., 2003), including connectivity patterns between the parietal operculum and the middle ACC regions (Figure 18.2A; Rainville et al., 2019). In sum, various neural patterns are related to hypnotic susceptibility with some of them pertaining to attention processes and others to dissociation tendencies.

The induction procedure impacts HHSIs and LHSIs differently, both at subjective (Cardeña et al., 2013; Jiang et al., 2016; Kumar & Pekala, 1988) and neural levels (Rainville et al., 2002). Individuals undergoing hypnosis are often guided toward experiencing a strong sense of mental absorption, which leads them to disconnect from their immediate environment and extraneous concerns. This state of intense focus seemingly prepares them to respond to upcoming suggestions by directing mental resources toward maintaining focus and producing an efficient response, rather than engaging task-irrelevant thoughts (Terhune & Cardeña, 2016). At the neural level, the effects of induction relate to several brain networks, including the dorsal attention, the central executive, the salience, and the default networks (Figure 18.2B). Research relates ongoing dynamics of these networks to higher-order cognitive abilities (Bressler & Menon, 2010). Most notably, in the absence of hypnosis, the dorsal attention and the default networks exhibit anti-correlated patterns – i.e., when one network is more active, the other is less active, and vice versa (Fox et al., 2005). Interestingly, changes in these anti-correlated patterns relate to the flow of attention processes (Turnbull et al., 2019). Dynamics between the dorsal attention

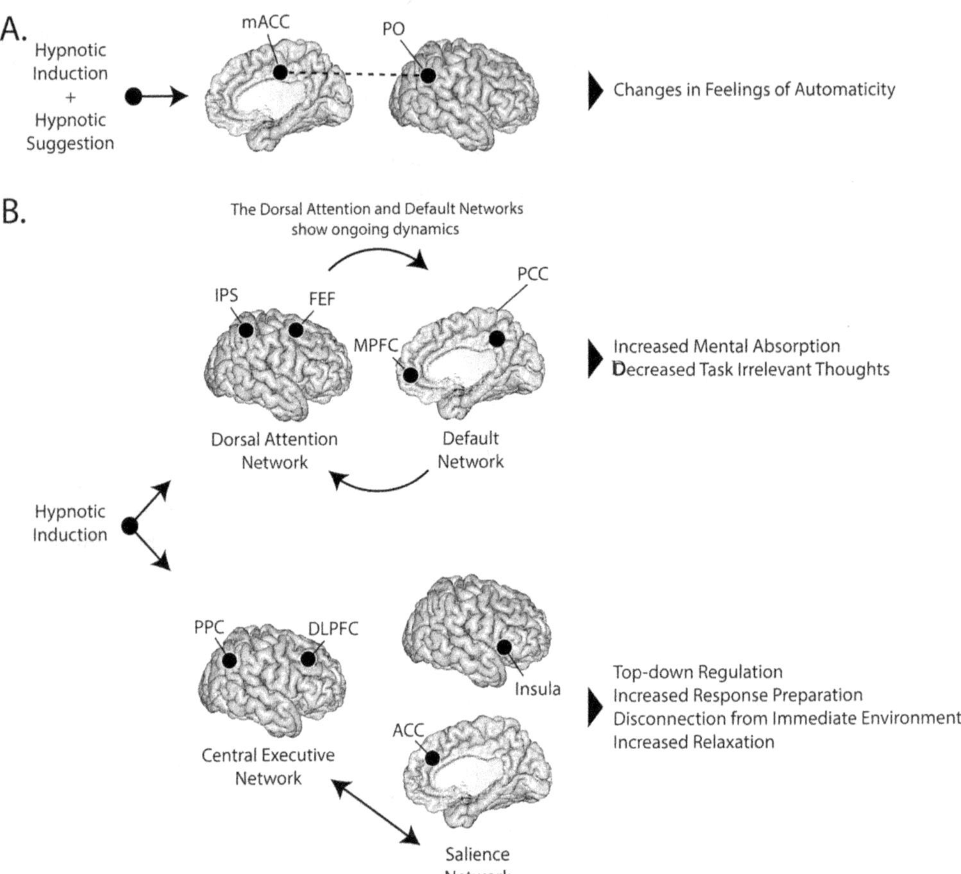

Figure 18.2 Brain dynamics related to hypnotic induction. A. Hypnotic responding relates to altered feelings of authorship, whereby responding to suggestions feels automatic and involuntary. Neuroimaging findings relate this phenomenological aspect of hypnosis to modulations of the parietal operculum (PO), as well as changes in connectivity between the PO and the middle anterior cingulate cortex (mACC). Dotted lines represent functional connectivity pattern. B. The dorsal attention and default networks show anti-correlated patterns. The hypnotic induction alters these dynamics. These effects relate to increased feelings of absorption and decreased task irrelevant thoughts. Moreover, the induction procedure also involves changes in the central executive and salience networks. These effects relate to top-down regulation, increased response preparation, disconnection from immediate environment, and increased relaxation. Intraparietal sulcus (IPS); frontal eye field (FEF); medial prefrontal cortex (MPFC); posterior cingulate cortex (PCC); posterior parietal cortex (PPC); dorsolateral prefrontal cortex (DLPFC); anterior cingulate cortex (ACC).

and default networks therefore reflect the engagement of attention resources toward certain events for extended periods of time. Hence, it seems hardly surprising to observe that the hypnotic induction alters activity in both the dorsal attention and the default networks as individuals become increasingly absorbed (Figure 18.2B; McGeown et al., 2009; Rainville et al., 2002). This neural pattern therefore reflects that individuals are focused on a specific mental object during the induction (i.e., a sensory stimulus, an imaginary representation, or a memory), while also suppressing task-irrelevant thoughts. In parallel to these effects, this procedure also involves changes in the central executive and the salience networks, as evidenced by a systematic review of neuroimaging studies of hypnosis (Landry et al., 2017). One can speculate that these additional patterns of neural activity further reflect the recruitment of executive resources while individuals maintain their focus and prepare their responses, as well as a disconnection from the immediate environment (Figure 18.2B). These speculations follow from research relating the central executive network to the coordination of mental strategies and top-down regulation, whereas the salience network is implicated in the processing and detection of salient events (Seeley et al., 2007). Moreover, changes in the salience network also relate to increased relaxation, as most induction procedures comprise instructions and directives to elicit a calming effect in individuals undergoing hypnosis. Altogether, neuroimaging investigations of the induction procedure indicate that hypnosis is hardly limited to a particular brain region, but instead involves changes across several large-scale brain networks. In turn, these changes seemingly relate to various phenomenological facets of hypnosis, including increased feelings of absorption and disengagement from task-irrelevant thoughts, increased feelings of relaxation, or increased feelings of involuntariness. These neural patterns could also indicate that individuals are mentally preparing to respond to hypnotic suggestion or their disconnection from the immediate environment.

Evidence further highlights the centrality of top-down regulation and response preparation in the generation of an efficient hypnotic response. These effects can be observed using the Stroop task – a well-established protocol in cognitive psychology to examine executive control resources. In this experimental task, participants must recruit executive control to resolve a conflict between automatic and controlled processes (MacLeod, 1991). Raz and colleagues (as well as other research groups) have used this experimental approach to demonstrate that hypnotic suggestions can bolster top-down executive control in HHSIs to the point where both the behavioral and neural markers of cognitive conflict in the Stroop task are largely eliminated (Raz et al., 2005). These findings underline the capacity of HHSIs to exert greater control over automatic processes – i.e., automatic processes are notoriously difficult to control because they fall beyond the purview of volition. This outcome highlights the potency of hypnosis as a clinical tool for enabling individuals to exert greater control over otherwise difficult-to-control mental processes. It also emphasizes the centrality of top-down control for shaping one's mental state during hypnotic phenomena (Terhune et al., 2017).

The dual mechanisms framework of cognitive control proposes that the engagement of executive control resources occurs in two ways: proactively, where resources are recruited in anticipation of upcoming cognitive conflict, or retroactively in response to the emergence of a cognitive conflict (Braver, 2012). A recent study tested whether the elimination of the Stroop effect in the context of hypnosis reflects proactive or retroactive executive control (Landry et al., 2021). Evidence supported the proactive view, thereby implying that individuals capable of suppressing the Stroop effect primarily rely on response preparation to produce an efficient hypnotic response. This finding stresses the importance of response preparation in hypnosis and aligns with neurophysiological evidence showing that HHSIs exhibit greater motor preparation during a simple response-time task following a hypnotic induction (Srzich et al., 2019). Neuroimaging findings further support the idea that response preparation is central to hypnotic responding. Here, we observed that neural

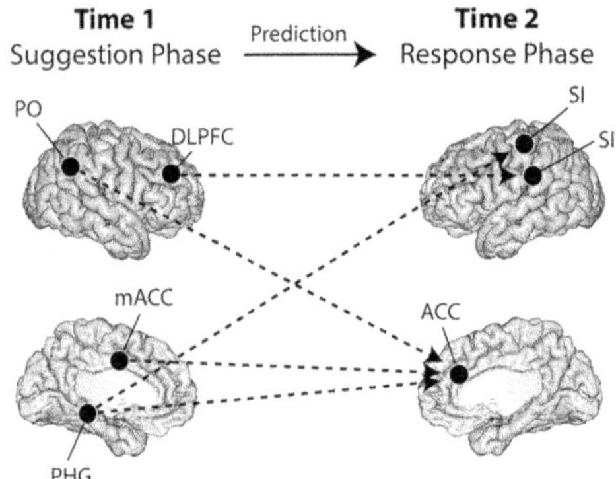

Figure 18.3 Time course of neural responses to hypnotic suggestions. Neural responses during the suggestion phase (Time 1) predict neural activity that occurs later during hypnotic responding in the context of hypnotic analgesia and hyperalgesia (Time 2). Activity in the parietal operculum (OP) during Time 1 predicts activity in the anterior cingulate cortex (ACC) at Time 2 (Desmarteaux et al., 2021). Activity in the dorsolateral prefrontal cortex (DLPFC) during Time 1 predicts activity in the secondary somatosensory cortex (SII) at Time 2 (Raij et al. 2009). Activity in the middle anterior cingulate cortex (mACC) during Time 1 predicts activity in the ACC at Time 2 (Desmarteaux et al., 2021). Activity in the parahippocampal gyrus (PHG) during Time 1 predicts activity in the ACC and the primary somatosensory cortex (SI) at Time 2 (Desmarteaux et al., 2021). Dotted lines represent temporal predictions.

activity in several brain regions while participants are hearing suggestions can successfully predict the neural activity when they are producing the hypnotic response (see Figure 18.3; Desmarteaux et al., 2021; Raij et al., 2009). In short, the suggestion phase predicts the response phase. A recent study underlines the centrality of the parietal operculum, mid-cingulate cortex, and left parahippocampal gyrus in predicting these effects (Desmarteaux et al., 2021), whereas a previous one shows that DLPFC activity during the encoding of the suggestion relates to the upcoming response. Altogether, these results imply that hypnosis reflects a build-up toward producing an efficient response that comprises both the interpretation of verbal suggestions and the implementation of corresponding mental strategies. The recruitment of the DLPFC and mid-cingulate cortex, two regions associated with the central executive network, during preparation aligns with the idea that hypnosis involves proactive executive control.

Greater top-down cognitive control and response preparation therefore represent additional components of hypnosis that recruit different neural patterns. The idea that response preparation shapes hypnotic responses dovetails theoretical frameworks that emphasize the importance of expectations in hypnotic phenomena (Lynn et al., 2008; Martin & Pacherie, 2019). According to this viewpoint, expectations about one's own responsiveness to suggestions, including the behavioral and subjective changes that will occur, are central to generating an efficient response. Empirical evidence underlines the connection between expectancies and subsequent responses to hypnosis (e.g., Green & Lynn, 2010; however, see Ludeña et al., 2016). For example, merely using the term "hypnosis" in the context of an induction, as opposed to an alternative terminology, enhances the hypnotic response thereafter, which highlights the potency of expectations and beliefs relative to hypnotic phenomena (Gandhi & Oakley, 2005). Hypnotic phenomena therefore partly result from response-expectancies that can yield greater preparation toward producing a response. This is why clinicians should adapt their interventions to maximize positive expectations of their patient, which ultimately boosts preparation and the efficiency of the response (Yapko, 2015).

Mental imagery represents another component typically considered relevant to the emergence of hypnotic phenomena (Kunzendord et al., 1996). The notion of imagery refers to the endogenous production of mental representations that share key properties with perceptual representations (Pearson et al., 2015). Imagery therefore corresponds to internal representations capable of inducing potent subjective experiences that feels like perception in the absence of sensory inputs. In the context of clinical hypnosis, health professionals often rely on imagery to guide the response of their patients (Yapko, 2015). During the induction procedure, they may lead their patients into evoking images that deepen their feelings of absorption and relaxation. Likewise, they can also use imagery as a strategy to guide responses to hypnotic suggestions. For example, they may encourage their patients to imagine the process of healing for producing an analgesic response. In this regard, combining hypnosis with technological development in virtual reality seemingly uses the same mechanisms to bolster the hypnotic response in clinical context (Patterson et al., 2010; Rousseaux et al., 2020).

However, the specific role of imagery in the context of hypnosis remains uncertain, as evidenced by mixed findings on this topic (Terhune & Oakley, 2020). In this regard, neuroimaging shows that hypnosis and imagination yield different effects at the brain level, thereby corroborating the idea that, despite overlap between them, hypnotic phenomena hardly reduce to imagination (Derbyshire et al., 2004; Szechtman et al., 1998). Nevertheless, different lines of research promote the idea that imagery plays an important role in hypnotic phenomena. First, several reports highlight a relationship between hypnotic susceptibility and the propensity for spontaneous imaginative experience in daily life (Cardeña & Terhune, 2014). Second, as we noted in the previous paragraph, technology designed to boost imagery enhances the hypnotic response. Therefore, directly targeting imagery can improve hypnotic responding. Third, the simple use of visual imagery to alter nociception outside of hypnosis can have similar effects to hypnotic analgesia, which implies possible overlapping mechanisms between the visual imagery and hypnotic phenomena (Fardo et al., 2015). Fourth, at least for some individuals, hypnosis can generate vivid perceptual experiences – analogous to perceptual hallucinations (Woody & Szechtman, 2000). A recent study assessed whether these effects reflect genuine perceptual experiences using a difficult perceptual task where missing visual information on the screen makes it nearly impossible to perform above chance level (Landry et al., 2021). Evidence confirmed that hypnotic suggestions to imagine this missing perceptual information allowed HHSIs to dramatically improve performance on this difficult task. This outcome is consistent with the idea that hypnosis can elicit genuine perceptual experiences. In the same vein, neuroimaging reveals that suggestions for experiencing altered color perception modulate visual areas in the absence of an induction procedure for HHSIs (Kosslyn et al., 2000; McGeown et al., 2012). These findings emphasize the potency of suggestions for dramatically altering how information is being processed, while we observe corresponding changes in the sensory areas. Lastly, evidence in electrophysiology indicates that HHSIs exhibit greater equivalence in neural activity between imagery and perception compared to LHSIs (Ibáñez-Marcelo et al., 2019; Santarcangelo, Current Volume). Overall, evidence indicates that imagery likely represents an efficient strategy for bolstering responsiveness to hypnosis, while this component rests on neural patterns related to perception rather than the ones we previously indicated.

Conclusion

Altogether, mounting evidence indicates that hypnosis is multifaceted and hardly reduces to a single process. Insofar as each facet reflects a different brain dynamic, hypnosis therefore involves several neural patterns, rather than a single one. In this chapter, we underlined several of these patterns and explained how each correspond to various facets of hypnotic phenomena, including those pertaining to hypnotic susceptibility, induction, and suggestion. However, it remains uncertain which ones play a causal role in the emergence of hypnotic phenomena, and which ones reflect epiphenomena. An important consequence that follows from the componential view of hypnosis is that individuals can efficiently respond to suggestions in various ways, i.e., the equifinality principle. This theoretical proposal entails that uncovering a single neural signature represents an unattainable goal. In support of this hypothesis, a neuroimaging compared hypnotic responses for modulating clinical pain and nociceptive pain to determine whether the same neural networks are recruited in both hypno-analgesic conditions (Derbyshire et al., 2016). Critically, while hypnosis yielded similar effects at the subjective level, both groups showed significantly different patterns at the neural level. In other words, the same outcome can be achieved via distinct neural circuits. The idea of a specific neural signature is therefore difficult to reconcile with the heterogeneity of findings in the field.

This chapter highlights the challenges of uncovering the neural mechanisms of hypnosis. To address these challenges, we have presented evidence that supports a componential view of hypnosis, whereby hypnotic phenomena are viewed through a multifaceted lens – which means that they occur via a variety of strategies. This viewpoint accounts for the diversity of findings in the field. Here, we have briefly described neural dynamics related to some of these components such as mental absorption, relaxation, reduced awareness of the environment, greater cognitive control, altered feelings of agency and automaticity, the interpretation of suggestion and response preparation, and visual imagery. One possible conclusion that follows from the work we presented is that hypnotic phenomena emerge from combining these various components. From a theoretical perspective, this conclusion brings about the need to carefully take into consideration inter-individual differences beyond hypnotic susceptibility. From a clinical perspective, it further highlights the need to mold clinical protocols to the strengths of patients to maximize their responses.

References

Barnier, A. J., Terhune, D. B., Polito, V., & Woody, E. Z. (2022). A componential approach to individual differences in hypnotizability. *Psychology of Consciousness: Theory, Research, and Practice*, *9*(2), 130. 10.1037/cns0000267

Blakemore, S. J., Oakley, D. A., & Frith, C. D. (2003). Delusions of alien control in the normal brain. *Neuropsychologia*, *41*(8), 1058–1067. 10.1016/S0028-3932(02)00313-5

Braver, T. S. (2012). The variable nature of cognitive control: A dual mechanisms framework. *Trends in Cognitive Sciences*, *16*(2). 10.1016/j.tics.2011.12.010

Bressler, S. L., & Menon, V. (2010). Large-scale brain networks in cognition: Emerging methods and principles. *Trends in Cognitive Sciences*, *14*(6), 277–290. 10.1016/j.tics.2010.04.004

Cardeña, E., Jönsson, P., Terhune, D. B., & Marcusson-Clavertz, D. (2013). The neurophenomenology of neutral hypnosis. *Cortex*, *49*(2), 375–385. 10.1016/j.cortex.2012.04.001

Cardeña, E., & Terhune, D. B. (2014). Hypnotizability, personality traits, and the propensity to experience alterations of consciousness. *Psychology of Consciousness: Theory, Research, and Practice*, *1*(3), 292. 10.1037/cns0000026

Cojan, Y., Piguet, C., & Vuilleumier, P. (2015). What makes your brain suggestible? Hypnotizability is associated with differential brain activity during attention outside hypnosis. *NeuroImage*, *117*, 367–374. 10.1016/j.neuroimage.2015.05.076

Del Casale, A., Ferracuti, S., Rapinesi, C., De Rossi, P., Angeletti, G., Sani, G.,... Girardi, P. (2015). Hypnosis and pain perception: An activation likelihood estimation (ALE) meta-analysis of functional neuroimaging studies. *Journal of Physiology-Paris*, *109*(4–6), 165–172. 10.1016/j.jphysparis.2016.01.001

Derbyshire, S. W. G., Whalley, M. G., Seah, S. T. H., & Oakley, D. A. (2016). Suggestions to reduce clinical fibromyalgia pain and experimentally induced pain produce parallel effects on perceived pain but divergent functional MRI-based brain activity. *Psychosomatic Medicine*, *79*(2), 189. DOI: 10.1097/PSY.0000000000000370

Derbyshire, S. W. G., Whalley, M. G., Stenger, V. A., & Oakley, D. A. (2004). Cerebral activation during hypnotically induced and imagined pain. *NeuroImage*, *23*(1), 392–401. 10.1016/j.neuroimage.2004.04.033

Desmarteaux, C., Streff, A., Chen, J.-I., Houzé, B., Piché, M., & Rainville, P. (2021). Brain responses to hypnotic verbal suggestions predict pain modulation. *Frontiers in Pain Research*, *2*, 757384. 10.3389/fpain.2021.757384

DeSouza, D. D., Stimpson, K. H., Baltusis, L., Sacchet, M. D., Gu, M., Hurd, R.,... Spiegel, D. (2020). Association between anterior cingulate neurochemical concentration and individual differences in hypnotizability. *Cerebral Cortex*, *30*(6), 3644–3654. 10.1093/cercor/bhz332

Dienes, Z., & Hutton, S. (2013). Understanding hypnosis metacognitively: rTMS applied to left DLPFC increases hypnotic suggestibility. *Cortex*, *49*(2), 386–392. 10.1016/j.cortex.2012.07.009

Egner, T., Jamieson, G. A., & Gruzelier, J. H. (2005). Hypnosis decouples cognitive control from conflict monitoring processes of the frontal lobe. *NeuroImage*, *27*(4), 969–978. 10.1016/j.neuroimage.2005.05.002

Egner, T., & Raz, A. (2007). Cognitive control processes and hypnosis. In G. A. Jamieson (Ed.), *Hypnosis and conscious states: The cognitive neuroscience perspective* (pp. 29–50). New York: Oxford University Press.

Elkins, G. R., Barabasz, A. F., Council, J. R., & Spiegel, D. (2015). Advancing research and practice: The revised APA Division 30 definition of hypnosis. *American Journal of Clinical Hypnosis*, *57*(4), 378–385. 10.1080/00207144.2014.961870

Fardo, F., Allen, M., Jegindø, E.-M. E., Angrilli, A., & Roepstorff, A. (2015). Neurocognitive evidence for mental imagery-driven hypoalgesic and hyperalgesic pain regulation. *NeuroImage*, *120*, 350–361. 10.1016/j.neuroimage.2015.07.008

Fox, M. D., Snyder, A. Z., Vincent, J. L., Corbetta, M., Van Essen, D. C., & Raichle, M. E. (2005). The human brain is intrinsically organized into dynamic, anticorrelated functional networks. *Proceedings of the National Academy of Sciences of the United States of America*, *102*(27), 9673–9678. 10.1073/pnas.050413610

Gandhi, B., & Oakley, D. A. (2005). Does 'hypnosis' by any other name smell as sweet? The efficacy of 'hypnotic' inductions depends on the label 'hypnosis'. *Consciousness and Cognition*, *14*(2), 304–315. 10.1016/j.concog.2004.12.004

Green, J. P., & Lynn, S. J. (2010). Hypnotic responsiveness: Expectancy, attitudes, fantasy proneness, absorption, and gender. *International Journal of Clinical and Experimental Hypnosis*, *59*(1), 103–121. 10.1080/00207144.2011.522914

Gruzelier, J. H. (1998). A working model of the neurophysiology of hypnosis: A review of evidence. *Contemporary Hypnosis*, *15*(1), 3–21. 10.1002/ch.112

Hoeft, F., Gabrieli, J. D., Whitfield-Gabrieli, S., Haas, B. W., Bammer, R., Menon, V., & Spiegel, D. (2012). Functional brain basis of hypnotizability. *Archives of General Psychiatry*, *69*(10), 1064–1072. doi:10.1001/archgenpsychiatry.2011.2190

Horton, J. E., Crawford, H. J., Harrington, G., & Downs, J. H. (2004). Increased anterior corpus callosum size associated positively with hypnotizability and the ability to control pain. *Brain, 127*(8), 1741–1747. 10.1093/brain/awh196

Ibáñez-Marcelo, E., Campioni, L., Phinyomark, A., Petri, G., & Santarcangelo, E. L. (2019). Topology highlights mesoscopic functional equivalence between imagery and perception: The case of hypnotizability. *NeuroImage, 200*, 437–449. 10.1016/j.neuroimage.2019.06.044

Jensen, M. P., Adachi, T., & Hakimian, S. (2015). Brain oscillations, hypnosis, and hypnotizability. *American Journal of Clinical Hypnosis, 57*(3), 230–253. 10.1080/00029157.2014.976786

Jiang, H., White, M. P., Greicius, M. D., Waelde, L. C., & Spiegel, D. (2016). Brain activity and functional connectivity associated with hypnosis. *Cerebral Cortex, 27*(8), 4083–4093. 10.1093/cercor/bhw220

Kiernan, B. D., Dane, J. R., Phillips, L. H., & Price, D. D. (1995). Hypnotic analgesia reduces R-III nociceptive reflex: Further evidence concerning the multifactorial nature of hypnotic analgesia. *Pain, 60*(1), 39–47. 10.1016/0304-3959(94)00134-Z

Kosslyn, S. M., Thompson, W. L., Costantini-Ferrando, M. F., Alpert, N. M., & Spiegel, D. (2000). Hypnotic visual illusion alters color processing in the brain. *The American Journal of Psychiatry, 157*(8), 1279–1284. 10.1176/appi.ajp.157.8.1279

Kumar, V. K., & Pekala, R. J. (1988). Hypnotizability, absorption, and individual differences in phenomenological experience. *International Journal of Clinical and Experimental Hypnosis, 36*(2), 80–88. 10.1080/00207148808409332

Kunzendord, R. G., Spanos, N. P., & Wallace, B. (Eds.). (1996). *Hypnosis and imagination.* Amityville, NY: Baywood publishing.

Landry, M., Da Silva Castanheira, J., Milton, D., & Raz, A. (2021). Suggestion alters Stroop automaticity: Hypnotic alexia through a proactive lens. *Psychology of Consciousness: Theory, Research, and Practice, 9*(2), 159. 10.1037/cns0000268

Landry, M., Da Silva Castanheira, J., Sackur, J., & Raz, A. (2021). Difficult turned easy: Suggestion renders a challenging visual task simple. *Psychological Science, 20*(2), 258–265. 10.1177/0956797620954856

Landry, M., Lifshitz, M., & Raz, A. (2017). Brain correlates of hypnosis: A systematic review and meta-analytic exploration. *Neuroscience & Biobehavioral Reviews, 81*, 75–98. 10.1016/j.neubiorev.2017.02.020

Landry, M., & Raz, A. (2015). Hypnosis and imaging of the living brain. *American Journal of Clinical Hypnosis, 57*(3), 285–313. 10.1080/00029157.2014.978496

Lifshitz, M., & Raz, A. (2015). Hypnotic ability and baseline attention: fMRI findings from Stroop interference. *Psychology of Consciousness: Theory, Research, and Practice, 2*(2), 134. 10.1037/cns0000050

Lifshitz, M., van Elk, M., & Luhrmann, T. M. (2019). Absorption and spiritual experience: A review of evidence and potential mechanisms. *Consciousness and Cognition, 73*, 102760. 10.1016/j.concog.2019.05.008

Ludeña, M., Pires, C., & Pires, C. (2016). Are expectancies about hypnosis predictive of responsiveness and phenomenology? *International Journal of Psychology and Neuroscience, 2*, 22–43.

Lynn, S. J., Kirsch, I., & Hallquist, M. N. (2008). Social cognitive theories of hypnosis. In M. R. Nash, & A. J. Barnier (Eds.), *The Oxford handbook of hypnosis: Theory, research and practice* (pp. 111–139). Oxford: Oxford University Press Oxford.

MacLeod, C. M. (1991). Half a century of research on the Stroop effect: An integrative review. *Psychological Bulletin, 109*(2), 163. 10.1037/0033-2909.109.2.163

Martin, J.-R., & Pacherie, E. (2019). Alterations of agency in hypnosis: A new predictive coding model *Psychological Review, 126*, 133–152. 10.1037/rev0000134

Mazzoni, G., Venneri, A., McGeown, W. J., & Kirsch, I. (2013). Neuroimaging resolution of the altered state hypothesis. *Cortex, 49*(2), 400–410. 10.1016/j.cortex.2012.08.005

McConkey, K. M., & Barnier, A. J. (2004). High hypnotisability: Unity and diversity in behaviour and experience. In M. Heap, R. J. Brown, & D. A. Oakley (Eds.), *The highly hypnotizable person: Theoretical, experimental and clinical issues* (pp. 61–84). New York: Routledge.

McGeown, W. J., Mazzoni, G., Venneri, A., & Kirsch, I. (2009). Hypnotic induction decreases anterior default mode activity. *Consciousness and Cognition, 18*(4), 848–855. 10.1016/j.concog.2009.09.001

McGeown, W. J., Venneri, A., Kirsch, I., Nocetti, L., Roberts, K., Foan, L., & Mazzoni, G. (2012). Suggested visual hallucination without hypnosis enhances activity in visual areas of the brain. *Consciousness and Cognition*, *21*(1), 100–116. 10.1016/j.concog.2011.10.015

Patterson, D. R., Jensen, M. P., Wiechman, S. A., & Sharar, S. R. (2010). Virtual reality hypnosis for pain associated with recovery from physical trauma. *International Journal of Clinical and Experimental Hypnosis*, *58*(3), 288–300. 10.1080/00207141003760595

Pearson, J., Naselaris, T., Holmes, E. A., & Kosslyn, S. M. (2015). Mental imagery: Functional mechanisms and clinical applications. *Trends in Cognitive Sciences*, *19*(10), 590–602.m 10.1016/j.tics.2015.08.003

Pekala, R. J. (2015). Hypnosis as a "state of consciousness": How quantifying the mind can help us better understand hypnosis. *American Journal of Clinical Hypnosis*, *57*(4), 402–424. 10.1080/00029157.2015.1011480

Pekala, R. J., & Kumar, V. K. (2007). An empirical-phenomenological approach to quantifying consciousness. In G. Jamieson (Ed.), *Hypnosis and conscious states: The cognitive neuroscience perspective* (pp. 167–194). New York: Oxford University Press.

Polito, V., Barnier, A. J., Woody, E. Z., & Connors, M. H. (2014). Measuring agency change across the domain of hypnosis. *Psychology of Consciousness: Theory, Research, and Practice*, *1*(1), 3. 10.1037/cns0000010

Raij, T. T., Numminen, J., Närvänen, S., Hiltunen, J., & Hari, R. (2009). Strength of prefrontal activation predicts intensity of suggestion-induced pain. *Human Brain Mapping*, *30*(9), 2890–2897. 10.1002/hbm.20716

Rainville, P., Carrier, B., Hofbauer, R. K., Bushnell, M. C., & Duncan, G. H. (1999). Dissociation of sensory and affective dimensions of pain using hypnotic modulation. *Pain*, *82*(2), 159–171. 10.1016/S0304-3959(99)00048-2

Rainville, P., Hofbauer, R. K., Bushnell, M. C., Duncan, G. H., & Price, D. D. (2002). Hypnosis modulates activity in brain structures involved in the regulation of consciousness. *Journal of Cognitive Neuroscience*, *14*(6), 887–901. 10.1162/089892902760191117

Rainville, P., & Price, D. D. (2003). Hypnosis phenomenology and the neurobiology of consciousness. *International Journal of Clinical and Experimental Hypnosis*, *51*(2), 105–129. 10.1076/iceh.51.2.105.14613

Rainville, P., Streff, A., Chen, J.-I., Houzé, B., Desmarteaux, C., & Piché, M. (2019). Hypnotic automaticity in the brain at rest: An arterial spin labelling study. *International Journal of Clinical and Experimental Hypnosis*, *67*(4), 512–542. 10.1080/00207144.2019.1650578

Raz, A. (2004). Atypical attention: Hypnosis and conflict reduction. In M. I. Posner (Ed.), *Cognitive Neuroscience of Attention*. New York: Guilford Press.

Raz, A. (2005). Attention and hypnosis: Neural substrates and genetic associations of two converging processes. *International Journal of Clinical and Experimental Hypnosis*, *53*(3), 237–258. 10.1080/00207140590961295

Raz, A., Fan, J., & Posner, M. I. (2005). Hypnotic suggestion reduces conflict in the human brain. *Proceedings of the National Academy of Sciences of the United States of America*, *102*(28), 9978–9983. 10.1073/pnas.050306410

Rousseaux, F., Bicego, A., Ledoux, D., Massion, P., Nyssen, A.-S., Faymonville, M.-E., ... Vanhaudenhuyse, A. (2020). Hypnosis associated with 3D immersive virtual reality technology in the management of pain: a review of the literature. *Journal of Pain Research*, *13*, 1129. 10.2147/JPR.S231737

Santarcangelo, E. L. (Current Volume). Hypnotizability and experimental hypnosis. In J. Linden, L. Sugarman, G. de Benedittis, & K. Varga (Eds.), *Routledge international handbook of clinical hypnosis*. London: Taylor & Francis.

Seeley, W. W., Menon, V., Schatzberg, A. F., Keller, J., Glover, G. H., Kenna, H., ...Greicius, M. D. (2007). Dissociable intrinsic connectivity networks for salience processing and executive control. *Journal of Neuroscience*, *27*(9), 2349–2356. 10.1523/JNEUROSCI.5587-06.2007

Shekhar, M., & Rahnev, D. (2018). Distinguishing the roles of dorsolateral and anterior PFC in visual metacognition. *Journal of Neuroscience*, *38*(22), 5078–5087. 10.1523/JNEUROSCI.3484-17.2018

Srzich, A. J., Cirillo, J., Stinear, J. W., Coxon, J. P., McMorland, A. J. C., & Anson, J. G. (2019). Does hypnotic susceptibility influence information processing speed and motor cortical preparatory activity? *Neuropsychologia*, *129*, 179–190. 10.1016/j.neuropsychologia.2019.03.014

Szechtman, H., Woody, E. Z., Bowers, K. S., & Nahmias, C. (1998). Where the imaginal appears real: A positron emission tomography study of auditory hallucinations. *The Proceedings of the National Academy of Sciences of the United States of America*, *95*(4), 1956–1960. 10.1073/pnas.95.4.195

Terhune, D. B. (2014). Defining hypnosis: The pitfalls of prioritizing spontaneous experience over response to suggestion. *The Journal of Mind–Body Regulation*, *2*(2), 115–117.

Terhune, D. B. (2015). Discrete response patterns in the upper range of hypnotic suggestibility: A latent profile analysis. *Consciousness and Cognition*, *33*, 334–341. 10.1016/j.concog.2015.01.018

Terhune, D. B., & Cardeña, E. (2010). Differential patterns of spontaneous experiential response to a hypnotic induction: A latent profile analysis. *Consciousness and Cognition*, *19*(4), 1140–1150. 10.1016/j.concog.2010.03.006

Terhune, D. B., & Cardeña, E. (2016). Nuances and uncertainties regarding hypnotic inductions: Toward a theoretically informed praxis. *American Journal of Clinical Hypnosis*, *59*(2), 155–174. 10.1080/00029157.2016.1201454

Terhune, D. B., Cardeña, E., & Lindgren, M. (2011). Dissociated control as a signature of typological variability in high hypnotic suggestibility. *Consciousness and Cognition*, *20*(3), 727–736. 10.1016/j.concog.2010.11.005

Terhune, D. B., Cleeremans, A., Raz, A., & Lynn, S. J. (2017). Hypnosis and top-down regulation of consciousness. *Neuroscience & Biobehavioral Reviews*. 10.1016/j.neubiorev.2017.02.002

Terhune, D. B., & Oakley, D. A. (2020). Hypnosis and imagination. In A. Abraham (Ed.), *Cambridge handbook of imagination* (pp. 711–727). Cambridge University Press.

Turnbull, A., Wang, H.-T., Schooler, J. W., Jefferies, E., Margulies, D. S., & Smallwood, J. (2019). The ebb and flow of attention: Between-subject variation in intrinsic connectivity and cognition associated with the dynamics of ongoing experience. *NeuroImage*, *185*, 286–299. 10.1016/j.neuroimage.2018.09.069

Wieder, L., Brown, R. J., Thompson, T., & Terhune, D. B. (2022). Hypnotic suggestibility in dissociative and related disorders: A meta-analysis. *Neuroscience & Biobehavioral Reviews*, 104751. 10.1016/j.neubiorev.2022.104751

Woody, E. Z., Barnier, A. J., & McConkey, K. M. (2005). Multiple hypnotizabilities: Differentiating the building blocks of hypnotic response. *Psychological Assessment*, *17*(2), 200. 10.1037/1040-3590.17.2.200

Woody, E. Z., & Szechtman, H. (2000). Hypnotic hallucinations: Towards a biology of epistemology. *Contemporary Hypnosis*, *17*(1), 4–14. 10.1002/ch.186

Yapko, M. D. (2015). *Essentials of hypnosis* (2nd ed.). New York: Routledge.

19

THE NEUROCHEMICAL BASES OF VERBAL SUGGESTION AND HYPNOSIS

Derek M. Smith[1], *David J. Acunzo*[2], *Peter Q. Deeley*[3], *Mitul A. Mehta*[3], *and Devin B. Terhune*[3]

[1]Department of Neurology, Johns Hopkins University School of Medicine, Baltimore, MD; [2]Department of Psychology, University of Birmingham, Birmingham, UK; [3]Institute of Psychiatry, Psychology & Neuroscience, King's College London, London, UK

Introduction

The most robust finding in both experimental and clinical research on hypnosis is that hypnotic effects and treatment outcomes are constrained by trait verbal suggestibility (Laurence et al., 2008; Montgomery et al., 2011; Terhune et al., 2017). Owing to its clinical and theoretical impact, attempts have been made to modulate direct verbal suggestibility, with varying success (Gorassini, 2004). Pharmacological agents are one promising modulator of direct verbal suggestibility (Acunzo et al., 2021). Determining the neurochemical contributors to hypnosis is of great importance as it offers the possibility to understand and modulate the neurocognitive mechanisms associated with suggestion and devise methods by which treatment outcomes can be strengthened.

Our current understanding of the potential role of neurochemical systems in direct verbal suggestibility remains in its infancy (Acunzo et al., 2021), but multiple potentially converging lines of research provisionally implicate different neurochemical systems. Here we aim to build upon our recent synthesis of this research domain (Acunzo et al., 2021). We first briefly review links between four neurochemicals and suggestibility, focusing on more recent research (for historical reviews, see Moll, 1911; Pettey, 1913; and Vingoe, 1973). We next consider the implications of this research for theories of hypnosis and clinical applications of suggestion. Finally, we highlight salient limitations in this research domain and describe challenges and potentially fruitful lines of research in this understudied area.

The Neurochemistry and Psychopharmacology of Hypnosis and Suggestion

Dopamine

Dopamine is a monoamine neurotransmitter belonging to catecholamines, which also include epinephrine and norepinephrine. Dopamine is involved in the neuromodulation of

DOI: 10.4324/9781003449126-26

a variety of systems and functions including motivation, reward, reinforcement (Gershman & Uchida, 2019; Wise & Robble, 2020) working memory, cognitive control (Cools, 2019; Ott & Nieder, 2019), and motor control (Joshua et al., 2009). Dopamine modulation also appears to be key in default mode network integration, suggesting a central role in consciousness maintenance (Spindler et al., 2021).

Preliminary research suggests that dopamine concentration is positively associated with response to suggestion, but some findings are mixed or contradictory (see Acunzo et al. (2021) for a review). Sensory gating, as measured by the prepulse inhibition of the startle reflex, which is attenuated with dopamine agonist administration, appears to be reduced in highly suggestible individuals (Levin et al., 2011; Lichtenberg et al., 2008; Storozheva et al., 2018). This result has been interpreted to reflect elevated dopamine in these individuals (but see De Pascalis & Russo, 2013). Cerebrospinal fluid concentrations of dopamine metabolite homovanillic acid have been positively linked with trait hypnotic suggestibility (Spiegel & King, 1992). More direct and causal evidence for the role of dopamine in increasing suggestibility comes from pharmacological studies: dopamine reuptake inhibitor methylphenidate treatment was found to increase hypnotic suggestibility in individuals with attention-deficit/hyperactivity disorder (ADHD) (Lotan et al., 2015) and dextroamphetamine administration, which increases extracellular levels of dopamine, seems to increase response to suggestion compared to a placebo in healthy volunteers (Ulett et al., 1972). Although speculative, one interpretation is that potentiation of dopamine transmission augments suggestibility by promoting focused attention toward verbal suggestions. Proxy measures for dopaminergic function and their association with hypnotic suggestibility have yielded contradictory results (see Acunzo et al., 2021; Cardeña et al., 2017), although recent analyses have begun to question the sensitivity of these proxies (Sescousse et al., 2018; van den Bosch et al., 2022); similar inconsistencies have been observed with research on the genetic polymorphisms (some implicated in dopamine transmission) related to suggestibility (Lichtenberg et al., 2000; Presciuttini et al., 2014; Rominger et al., 2014; Storozheva et al., 2018; Szekely et al., 2010). Given dopamine's inverted U-shaped relationship with cognitive performance, it would not be surprising if dopamine exhibited such a relationship with hypnotic suggestibility (Cools & D'Esposito, 2011).

Serotonin

Serotonin (5-HT) plays a broad role in cognition, affect regulation, and social influence (Duerler et al., 2022; Štrac et al., 2016). Additionally, serotonin has a role in the formation of social hierarchy with dominance in primates being associated with higher serotonin levels (Moskowitz et al., 2001; Raleigh et al., 1991; Raleigh et al., 1984).

Multiple studies have reported that classic psychedelics, such as lysergic acid diethylamide (LSD), produce an increase in suggestibility (for a review, see (Acunzo et al., 2021). The psychoactive effects of classic psychedelics seem to be mostly mediated through 5-HT$_{2A}$ receptor (Carhart-Harris & Nutt, 2017). Insofar as these drugs primarily act as partial serotonin agonists (Nichols, 2016), this research arguably implicates the serotonin system in responsiveness to suggestion. In particular, suggestibility has been shown to be enhanced by LSD, mescaline, and a combination of LSD, mescaline, and psilocybin (Sjoberg & Hollister, 1965); for similar effects, see Middlefell (1967) and Ulett et al. (1972). More recently, it was reported that suggestibility, as indexed by the *Creative*

Imagination Scale, was greater following LSD administration than placebo in a within-subjects single-blind study (Carhart-Harris et al., 2015), a result that was subsequently independently replicated (Wießner et al., 2021). A potentially convergent finding is that a variant of the T102C polymorphism that results in stronger binding potential for the 5-HT_{2A} receptor is associated with higher absorption, a well-established correlate of hypnotic suggestibility (Ott et al., 2005). However, independent research failed to observe an association between the serotonin transporter polymorphism 5-HTTLPR and hypnotic suggestibility (Katonai et al., 2017; Rominger et al., 2014). However, it should be noted that Katonai and colleagues did find an association between 5-HTTLPR and a self-report measure capturing the perceived intimacy of the hypnotic interaction. Limited suggestibility research has been conducted on serotonergic drugs other than psychedelics.

In summary, these results imply that suggestibility is potentially associated with the 5-HT_{2A} receptor but its relationship to the serotonin system more broadly is less clear. The cognitive-perceptual mechanisms that mediate this link are similarly unclear given the broad psychological effects of psychedelic drugs.

GABA

GABA is the primary inhibitory neurochemical in the brain. In addition to a central role in governing neuronal inhibition, it is prominently involved in neuronal plasticity and modulation of cortical network dynamics (Ende, 2015). At the psychological level, GABA is involved in a diverse array of cognitive functions including memory and learning and is aberrant in multiple disorders (Reddy-Thootkur et al., 2022).

Multiple lines of research provide preliminary evidence that elevated GABA is associated with greater (hypnotic) suggestibility (Spiegel, 1980). The most robust evidence for this link comes from a recent magnetic resonance spectroscopy study, which found that hypnotic suggestibility was positively associated with GABA concentrations in anterior cingulate cortex (DeSouza et al., 2020), although the lack of a control voxel renders the anatomical specificity of this result ambiguous. To our knowledge, there have been few controlled studies of the impact of GABAergic agents on suggestibility. One placebo-controlled study found that alcohol, a GABA agonist, enhances hypnotic suggestibility (Semmens-Wheeler et al., 2013; see also Hull, 1933). By contrast, a well-powered study reported that another GABA agonist, diazepam, did not significantly enhance hypnotic suggestibility relative to nicotinic acid, although this was potentially attributed to sample heterogeneity (Gibson et al., 1977; see also Halpern & Merlis, 1961). Multiple anecdotal findings have also suggested that GABA agonists, such as benzodiazepines, enhance responsiveness to suggestion (for a review, see Acunzo et al., 2021). Similarly, an uncontrolled study of hypnotic suggestibility in different medicated patient groups suggested that those receiving anti-anxiety medication (typically GABA agonists) tended to display higher hypnotic suggestibility (Spiegel, 1980).

Glutamate

Glutamate is the brain's primary excitatory neurotransmitter and is involved in a wide range of cognitive functions including learning and memory (Olney & Farber, 1995; Riedel et al., 2003). The N-methyl-D-aspartate (NMDA) receptor antagonists ketamine and nitrous oxide are known to induce pronounced dissociative states, such as depersonalization and derealization, as well as a range of psychotomimetic effects, including hallucinations and delusions (Piazza et al., 2022).

Research showing that glutamate concentrations in anterior cingulate cortex are negatively correlated with dissociative absorption provides an indirect association between glutamate and suggestibility (DeSouza et al., 2020). Research has shown that 20–40% nitrous oxide inhalation was associated with greater nonhypnotic (Whalley & Brooks, 2009) and hypnotic (Barber et al., 1979) suggestibility than placebo (medical air or oxygen) inhalation (this is further supported by earlier preliminary research, e.g., Eysenck & Rees, 1945). Importantly, in Whalley and Brooks' study, expectations did not predict suggestibility change although increases in imagination vividness correlated with suggestibility increases. Moreover, participants were unable to reliably identify which condition they were in (Whalley & Brooks, 2009), which suggests that the effects were not attributable to inadequate participant blinding, which is a salient confound in most psychedelic research (Burke & Blumberger, 2021). Preliminary research suggests that ketamine also increases hypnotic suggestibility but possibly only in low suggestible participants (Patterson et al., 2018; Sklar et al., 1981). The dissociative effects of NMDA receptor antagonists parallel the elevation in state dissociation (e.g., depersonalization) that accompanies hypnotic inductions (Cleveland et al., 2015). Taken together, these studies provide preliminary evidence for the role of glutamatergic function in suggestibility.

Other Substances

Unfortunately, little attention has been allocated to understanding the influence of other neurochemical systems on suggestibility. Acetylcholine and opioids are prime examples of substances that are understudied (Goldstein & Hilgard, 1975; Spiegel & Albert, 1983; Sternbach, 1982). Research suggests that highly suggestible participants might have lower responsiveness to opioids (Goldstein & Hilgard, 1975; Presciuttini et al., 2018; Spiegel & Albert, 1983). In particular, several research groups have failed to attenuate hypnotic analgesia with the opioid antagonist naloxone (Goldstein & Hilgard, 1975; Spiegel & Albert, 1983) or observe significant changes in beta-endorphin plasma levels during hypnotic suggestions of analgesia (Debenedittis et al., 1989; Moret et al., 1991), suggesting that hypnotic analgesia is not dependent on opioid-based mechanisms. Early research similarly implied that cannabis, which targets the cannabinoid system, enhances hypnotic suggestibility (Beahrs et al., 1974). There is also growing interest in the impact of oxytocin, a neuropeptide involved in social cognition and attachment (Shamay-Tsoory & Abu-Akel, 2016) on hypnotic suggestibility (Bryant & Hung, 2013; Bryant et al., 2012; Kasos et al., 2018; Varga & Kekecs, 2014), although the data are inconclusive to date and marked by contradictory findings and caveats (Acunzo et al., 2021).

Implications for Theories of Hypnosis

To our knowledge, no contemporary theories of hypnosis make explicit reference to the neurochemical systems subserving responsiveness to verbal suggestions. In turn, most pharmacological research on verbal suggestion effects has not been theory-driven and thus it is difficult to leverage the foregoing body of research to provide support for, or falsification of, these theories. Nevertheless, in this section, we bring these data to bear on contemporary theories and highlight congruencies and inconsistencies (Table 19.1) with a

Table 19.1 Features of Prominent Hypnosis Theories and Relevance to Neurochemical Systems Implicated in Hypnosis and Suggestion

	Mechanisms Underlying Response to Hypnotic Suggestion			
Theory	*Primary Cognitive Mechanisms*	*Primary Neurophysiological Mechanisms*	*Primary Neurochemical Mechanisms*	*Relevant Neurochemical Evidence*
Cold control	Diminished awareness of intentions	Atypical prefrontal functioning	Not specified	**Consistent**: Suggestibility enhancing agents also disrupt prefrontal connectivity (Driesen et al., 2013; Kummerfeld et al., 2020; Pallavicini et al., 2019; Ryu et al., 2017); Ketamine impairs metacognition (Lehmann et al., 2021) **Inconsistent**: Suggestibility enhancing substances impair cognitive control (Blackman et al., 2013; Kummerfeld et al., 2020; Pokorny et al., 2020; Umbricht et al., 2003)
Dissociated experience	Diminished executive monitoring	Not specified	Not specified	**Consistent/inconsistent**: Same as evidence for/against cold control theory
Dissociated control	Diminished executive control	Diminished lateral prefrontal cortex functioning	Not specified	**Consistent**: NMDAR antagonism impairs post-error performance adjustments (Skoblenick & Everling, 2014); Suggestibility enhancing agents disrupt prefrontal connectivity (Driesen et al., 2013; Kummerfeld et al., 2020; Pallavicini et al., 2019; Ryu et al., 2017); Suggestibility enhancing agents impair cognitive control (Blackman et al., 2013; Kummerfeld et al., 2020; Pokorny et al., 2020; Umbricht et al., 2003) **Inconsistent**: None
Second-order dissociated control	Diminished communication between executive monitoring and control	Reduced connectivity between anterior cingulate and lateral prefrontal cortices	Not specified	**Consistent**: Same as evidence for dissociated control theory **Inconsistent**: None
Interoceptive predictive coding	Diminished interoceptive prediction mismatch fosters a sense of reality/feeling of knowing	Aberrant interoceptive predictive processing in the insula leads to reduced responsiveness in the salience network	Not specified	**Consistent**: (Barber et al., 1979; Patterson et al., 2018; Whalley & Brooks, 2009) and may regulate precision (Adams et al., 2013) **Inconsistent**: None

(*Continued*)

Table 19.1 (Continued)

	Mechanisms Underlying Response to Hypnotic Suggestion			
Theory	*Primary Cognitive Mechanisms*	*Primary Neurophysiological Mechanisms*	*Primary Neurochemical Mechanisms*	*Relevant Neurochemical Evidence*
Predictive coding	Motor suggestions via attention modulate the strength of sensory evidence, proprioceptive predictions, and prediction errors	Not specified	Not specified	**Consistent:** same as evidence for interoceptive predictive coding **Consistent/Inconsistent:** Data on the impact of suggestibility enhancing substances on attention are mixed (Bălăeţ, 2022; Fried et al., 1995; Oranje et al., 2000)
Response expectancy	Response expectancies produce subjective experiences	Not specified	Not specified	**Consistent:** None **Inconsistent:** None

view toward future interrogation of these models on the basis of systems neuroscience research into these neurochemical systems.

Dissociation and Cold Control Theories

Hypnosis has long been conceptually linked to dissociation (Bell et al., 2011; Ellenberger, 1970), which includes various disruptions of normally integrated cognitive systems such as those governing awareness, identity, and memory (Kihlstrom et al., 1994). Dissociation theories of hypnosis coalesce around the proposal that responding to hypnotic suggestion involves a disruption or reduction in the coordination of cognitive modules that are normally coupled in the execution of complex behaviors (for a review, see Woody & Sadler, 2008). These theories have alternatively proposed that hypnotic responding is supported by a breakdown in the coordination of executive control and monitoring (*Neo-dissociation* or *Dissociated Experience Theory*), executive control and lower-level systems supporting automatic behaviors (contention scheduling; *Dissociated Control Theory*), or an asymmetrical disruption whereby control cannot be updated from executive monitoring (*Second-order Dissociated Control Theory*). A similar model, *Cold Control Theory*, proposes that responsiveness to suggestion is facilitated by reduced awareness of intentions supporting goal-directed responses (Dienes & Perner, 2007). Although this account does not mechanistically invoke dissociation, and more parsimoniously focuses on metacognition, cold control theory is indistinguishable from dissociation theories at the neurophysiological level (Terhune, 2012).

Congruence with Pharmacological Findings

The pharmacological research reviewed above is broadly consistent with dissociation (and cold control) theories of hypnosis and suggestion but for the most part does not provide preferential support for specific predictions from these accounts. The dissociation theories postulate that there is a critical link between dissociation and suggestibility. At the phenomenological level, it is notable that different pharmacological agents that appear to enhance suggestibility including LSD and nitrous oxide produce dissociative states such as depersonalization (Liechti, 2017; Piazza et al., 2022). Further work should clarify this apparent association by examining whether suggestibility enhancement depends on the experience of dissociative states in response to these drugs, such as by pharmacological reduction of dissociative states through concurrent administration of GABA agonists (Gitlin et al., 2020). Moreover, suggestion effects have been theorized to share greater mechanistic overlap with compartmentalization states (e.g., functional symptoms) (Brown, 2006) rather than detachment states (e.g., depersonalization) and it will be important to probe this in future research. Conversely, both *Dissociated Control* and *Cold Control*, but not *Neo-Dissociation*, theories predict that prefrontal dysfunction is conducive to hypnotic responding (Coltheart et al., 2018; Dienes & Hutton, 2013). A decoupling between anterior and posterior regions seems to be associated both with high hypnotic suggestibility (Jamieson & Burgess, 2014; Terhune et al., 2011) as well as the impact of NMDA receptor antagonists and classic psychedelics (Pallavicini et al., 2019) and provides a potential neurophysiological mechanism underlying suggestibility enhancement (see also Reiser et al., 2012). Congruent with these findings, NMDA receptor antagonism reduces the ability to use contextual information held in working memory to determine the correct response to subsequent stimuli (Blackman et al., 2013; Kummerfeld et al., 2020; Umbricht et al., 2000) an effect which is likely mediated by disruptions in prefrontal connectivity (Driesen et al., 2013; Kummerfeld et al., 2020; Ryu et al., 2017) and broadly aligns with the proposal that prefrontal hypofunction is conducive to enhanced suggestibility. NMDA receptor antagonism has also been shown to induce a shift from a cortically centered to a subcortically centered connectivity profile; this might imply a greater dependence on basal ganglia and cerebellar mechanisms in action selection and execution, which indirectly aligns with dissociated control theory (Joules et al., 2015; Santarcangelo, 2014).

Dissociation, particularly dissociated control theories, which emphasize compromised executive functioning, and cold control theories, which emphasize compromised metacognition, part ways when it comes to their cognitive predictions. In turn, considering the broader cognitive effects of the drugs considered above may help to clarify the cognitive bases of their suggestibility enhancement. Ketamine has been shown to impair metacognition of episodic memory (Lehmann et al., 2021) – this aligns with cold control and neo-dissociation theories although it does not explicitly contradict dissociated control theory. By contrast, Dissociated Control Theory predicts some sort of disruption of cognitive control should accompany suggestibility enhancement and this prediction sits well with the cognitive control disruptions induced by NMDA receptor antagonism (Blackman et al., 2013; Kummerfeld et al., 2020; Umbricht et al., 2000) as well as serotonergic psychedelics (Heekeren et al., 2008; Umbricht et al., 2003). Along similar lines, one finding that is especially congruent with the predictions of Second-Order Dissociated Control Theory is that ketamine impairs post-error adjustments in non-human primates implying a breakdown of the normal integration of executive monitoring and control (Skoblenick & Everling, 2014). Importantly, cold control and neo-dissociation theories assume that hypnotic suggestions are implemented via executive control without accompanying higher order thoughts and thus pharmacological impairments in cognitive control should reduce hypnotic responding. This has not been observed and thus the available evidence *slightly* favors dissociated control theory. Nevertheless, to our knowledge, the dissociative, decoupling, and control effects of these drugs (Kummerfeld et al., 2020; Pallavicini et al., 2019) have not yet been related to suggestibility enhancement.

Response Expectancy and Predictive Coding Theories

Suggestions can be construed as communications that allow an individual to form specific predictions regarding subsequent experiences. The proposal that one's response expectancies drive, or at least partly shape, responses to hypnotic suggestions is a central tenet within social cognitive theories of hypnosis, including response expectancy theory (Kirsch, 1985) and response set theory (Kirsch & Lynn, 1999). Although a wealth of evidence indicates that response expectancies are a reliable predictor of responsiveness to (hypnotic) suggestions, there are ongoing questions regarding the magnitude of these effects as well as the underlying mechanisms (for reviews see Lynn et al., 2022; Lynn et al., 2008; Terhune et al., 2017). Similar ideas are present in more recent theories of hypnotic suggestion (Jamieson, 2018, 2022; Martin & Pacherie, 2019) embedded within the predictive coding framework (Clark, 2013; Friston, 2010). This framework views the brain as a hierarchical Bayesian inference machine that works to minimize the discrepancy between predictions and sensory evidence while weighting these factors based on their respective confidence levels (precision). Although these accounts differ, they maintain that behavioral and phenomenological responses to suggestions are routed in abnormalities in the precision assigned to priors (predictions) and/or prediction errors (mismatch between priors and sensory evidence), such that behavior and experience are more strongly shaped by priors engendered by suggestions.

Congruence with Pharmacological Findings

As with other theories, response expectancy and predictive coding theories of hypnosis do not stipulate specific neurochemical processes. How drugs and/or hypnosis modulate precision may depend on the cortical level of a predictive hierarchy, thus complicating the interpretation of results. For example, it has been argued that psychedelics exert their effects by dampening the precision of high-level priors, leading ascending prediction errors to better update beliefs (Carhart-Harris & Friston, 2019). At first glance, this would seem to be incompatible with predictive coding models of hypnosis, which plausibly would attribute suggestibility enhancement under psychedelics to increased prior precision. However, the latter priors arguably manifest at a lower level in the cortical hierarchy, which would mean that more precise lower level sensorimotor priors would tend to override mismatches in sensory feedback. In keeping with this hypothesis, the mismatch negativity amplitude (MMN), an electrophysiological response (difference between deviant and standard events), which is believed to be a manifestation of low-level prediction errors, is attenuated by ketamine and some psychedelic drugs (Heekeren et al., 2008; Timmermann et al., 2018). However, the MMN does not exhibit a consistent relationship with hypnosis and hypnotic suggestibility (Hiltunen et al., 2019; Jamieson et al., 2005). Also, in the framework of predictive coding, precision is typically conceived of at a psychological level as attention (Adams et al., 2013; Feldman & Friston, 2010) but the impact of suggestibility enhancing substances on attention is mixed (Bălăeţ, 2022; Fried et al., 1995; Oranje et al., 2000). Changes in insula connectivity associated with hypnosis (Jiang et al., 2017) hint at the possibility of a change in interoceptive predictive coding, as suggested by Jamieson (2022), but these findings should be interpreted with caution. Over-weighting of priors in perception has also been shown to relate to lower glutamate concentrations in insula in psychosis (Leptourgos et al., 2022), which arguably provides preliminary support for the possibility that NMDAR antagonists enhance suggestibility by increasing prior precision. However, more research is required before firmer conclusions can be made regarding how to best explain hypnosis and pharmacologically facilitated suggestibility within a predictive coding framework.

Therapeutic Implications and Applications

Enhanced Suggestibility

There is increasing evidence for the use of targeted suggestions to augment the effectiveness of established psychological treatments for a range of mental health and functional disorders – for example, anxiety disorders, depression, and functional neurological symptoms (Deeley, 2016; Elkins, 2016; Valentine et al., 2019). Improved understanding of the neuropharmacology of suggestive and dissociative processes could potentially lead to additional augmentation of psychological treatments with pharmacotherapy. However, several provisos should be borne in mind. Ideally, any pharmacotherapy would need to be evaluated in the context of an existing protocolized psychological treatment using suggestion for which a robust evidence base exists. Although psychological treatments augmented with suggestion have been described in case reports and case series (Lemercier & Terhune, 2018), at present there continues to be a lack of large-scale randomized controlled trials demonstrating the safety and effectiveness of specific treatments augmented with suggestion. This limits the justification for the addition of pharmacotherapy to enhance the effectiveness of suggestion to psychological treatments that employ them. However, an alternative approach could be to take conditions for which the safety and effectiveness of pharmacotherapy have been established (e.g., selective serotonin reuptake inhibitors for depression and anxiety disorders), or those for which there is emerging evidence (e.g., research demonstrating the effectiveness of psilocybin for the treatment of depression with appropriate therapeutic support, Carhart-Harris et al., 2016) and to evaluate the addition of suggestion to augment treatment (i.e., what was once referred to as the hypnodelic approach, Lemercier & Terhune, 2018). With appropriate control conditions, this would also allow assessment of drug x condition x suggestion interactions to determine the extent to which the effects of suggestions are modulated by psychoactive agents and neuropsychiatric conditions. In addition to investigating therapeutic efficacy, this may provide insights into the neuropharmacology of suggestive processes.

Challenges and Future Directions

Limitations of the Literature

Despite some intriguing convergences across studies, this literature possesses multiple methodological limitations that need to be considered when interpreting their theoretical and therapeutic implications (Acunzo et al., 2021). Perhaps most importantly, most of these studies concerned psychoactive drugs and thus did not adhere to conventional double-blind designs (for a counterexample, see Whalley & Brooks, 2009) and opens up the possibility that the observed effects are driven, or exacerbated, by expectancy and placebo effects (Burke & Blumberger, 2021). Relatedly, nearly all previous pharmacological studies involved live administration, and experimenter scoring, of suggestibility scales by an experimenter who was not blinded, which can further exacerbate the impact of participant unblinding. To improve the rigor and generalizability of empirical results, future research will benefit from the use of active control agents, double-blind designs, comparisons across psychoactive agents, and standardized recorded scales (for a review, see Acunzo et al., 2021). The majority of research on the neurochemistry of suggestion has focused on overt responsiveness to suggestion and future research would benefit from more attention being paid to subjective reports, which can provide valuable information regarding the experience of avolition accompanying responses to suggestion, i.e., the *classic suggestion effect* (Weitzenhoffer, 1974). Another limitation of the literature is that some of the non-pharmacological studies of the neurochemical basis of hypnosis made use of peripheral neurochemical measurements (Kasos et al., 2018; Varga & Kekecs, 2014). Finally, as noted above, relatively few studies have considered the variables that mediate or correlate with suggestibility enhancement, such as dissociative states, aberrant functional decoupling, or other neurocognitive changes, and this limits the mechanistic insights that can be gained from these studies.

Determining Causal Pathways

Targeting specific neurochemical systems with pharmacological agents affords the promise of establishing their causal role in suggestibility enhancement. However, causal inferences are severely limited due to the neurochemical complexity and psychoactive nature of these drugs. Pharmacological agents implicated in suggestibility enhancement rarely target a specific neurochemical system and often have complex neurochemical interactions and downstream effects. For example, both serotonergic psychedelics and glutamatergic dissociatives seem to modulate dopamine release (De Gregorio et al., 2016; Gupta et al., 2019). Perhaps more problematically, rather than suggestibility enhancement being attributable to specific neurochemicals, one possibility is that drugs with psychoactive effects might enhance suggestibility (Spiegel, 1980). That is, suggestibility enhancement might be a product of phenomenological changes shared across these drugs. This proposal can arguably explain why such a diverse set of drugs with markedly different neurochemical profiles from LSD to cannabis (Beahrs et al., 1974) to nitrous oxide seem to enhance suggestibility. A further consideration is phenomenological heterogeneity in response to these agents and how this might differentially impact suggestibility alteration (Acunzo et al., 2021). For example, alcohol, nitrous oxide, and ketamine have stimulant effects in some individuals and sedative effects in others (e.g., Walsh et al., 2017). Anecdotal research suggests that sedatives might attenuate hypnotic suggestibility (Spiegel, 1980). Greater consideration of these issues is warranted in future research such as with active control agents, investigation of mediation and moderating phenomenological and cognitive variables, and investigation of pharmacological agents that attenuate, rather than enhance, suggestibility.

Apples and Oranges

A salient methodological issue for future research is determining whether (high) suggestibility in the absence of pharmacological facilitation and pharmacologically modulated (high) suggestibility depend on overlapping mechanisms. That is, it is not yet clear if the dissociative states and increases in suggestibility associated with the substances covered here share neurocognitive features with those observed in clinical populations or in highly suggestible individuals. Parallels between pharmacological dissociative states and suggestibility enhancement and elevated suggestibility in dissociative psychopathology (Bell et al., 2011; Wieder et al., 2022) are intriguing and warrant greater attention. By contrast, if many or all cases of pharmacologically elevated suggestibility are dissimilar to non-modulated high hypnotic suggestibility, pharmacological research is less likely to yield insights into the nature of suggestion.

Orexin: A New Frontier?

A potentially fruitful pathway for future research is the modulatory influence of orexin on suggestibility. Orexin is a neuropeptide that helps regulate arousal and appetite and influences multiple neuromodulatory systems and attentional processing (Brown et al., 2001; Tsujino & Sakurai, 2009). Plasma and cerebrospinal fluid levels of orexin-A have been shown to be lower in PTSD (Higuchi et al., 2002), a condition associated with elevated hypnotic suggestibility (Spiegel et al., 1988) and narcolepsy, which is characterized by the loss of orexin neurons in lateral hypothalamus and elevated dissociative symptoms (Quaedackers et al., 2022). It has been recently proposed that orexin antagonists might facilitate dissociative experiences and enhance responsiveness to suggestion (Smith & Terhune, 2023); however, to our knowledge, this remains to be demonstrated.

Non-Linear Effects

A further challenge is posed by the non-linear effects of neurochemical systems on cognition and perception. Both norepinephrine and dopamine exhibit quadratic relationships with behavioral performance (Aston-Jones et al., 1999; Cools & D'Esposito, 2011) and it is plausible that hypnotic suggestibility might exhibit non-linear relationships with the neurochemical systems considered here, resulting in a sensitivity to drug dose and a "baseline" dependency (Cools & D'Esposito, 2011). Clearly, the relationships between suggestibility and substances capable of inducing a loss of consciousness (e.g., GABAergic drugs) are non-linear. Accordingly, closer attention should be allocated to more subtle effects by examining multiple doses in future pharmacological studies.

Conclusion

In summary, preliminary research suggests that NMDAR hypofunction, elevated concentrations of dopamine and GABA, a greater serotonin receptor binding affinity, are conducive to responding to (hypnotic) suggestions. Despite multiple converging findings, a clear interpretation of these results is limited by methodological considerations and limitations. The results align with several theoretical orientations, signaling the need for greater stipulation of neurochemical mechanisms within theories of hypnosis and greater interrogation of mediating and moderating cognitive factors. We have outlined fruitful avenues for future lines of research. The limited amount of research conducted in this area means that future researchers have an abundance of low hanging fruit to pick from, although there are many caveats and complications to take into consideration. Despite these challenges, a better understanding of the neurochemistry of suggestion will allow us to test theories of hypnosis and potentially develop novel pharmacological approaches to enhancing the efficacy of hypnotic suggestion in therapeutic and clinical contexts (Lemercier & Terhune, 2018).

References

Acunzo, D. J., Oakley, D. A., & Terhune, D. B. (2021). The neurochemistry of hypnotic suggestion. *American Journal of Clinical Hypnosis*, *63*(4), 355–371. 10.1080/00029157.2020.1865869

Adams, R. A., Stephan, K. E., Brown, H. R., Frith, C. D., & Friston, K. J. (2013). The computational anatomy of psychosis. *Frontiers in Psychiatry*, *4*, 47. 10.3389/fpsyt.2013.00047

Aston-Jones, G., Rajkowski, J., & Cohen, J. (1999). Role of locus coeruleus in attention and behavioral flexibility. *Biological Psychiatry*, *46*(9), 1309–1320. 10.1016/s0006-3223(99)00140-7

Bălăeţ, M. (2022). Psychedelic cognition: The unreached frontier of psychedelic science. *Frontiers in Neuroscience*, *16*, 1–12. 10.3389/fnins.2022.832375

Barber, J., Donaldson, D., Ramras, S., & Allen, G. D. (1979). The relationship between nitrous oxide conscious sedation and the hypnotic state. *Journal of the American Dental Association (1939)*, *99*(4), 624–626. 10.14219/jada.archive.1979.0353

Beahrs, J. O., Carlin, A. S., & Shehorn, J. (1974). Impact of psychoactive drugs on hypnotizability. *American Journal of Clinical Hypnosis*, *16*(4), 267–269. 10.1080/00029157.1974.10403692

Bell, V., Oakley, D. A., Halligan, P. W., & Deeley, Q. (2011). Dissociation in hysteria and hypnosis: Evidence from cognitive neuroscience. *Journal of Neurology, Neurosurgery & Psychiatry*, *82*(3), 332–339. 10.1136/jnnp.2009.199158

Blackman, R. K., MacDonald, A. W., & Chafee, M. V. (2013). Effects of ketamine on context-processing performance in monkeys: A new animal model of cognitive deficits in schizophrenia. *Neuropsychopharmacology*, *38*(11), 2090–2100. 10.1038/npp.2013.118

Brown, R. E., Sergeeva, O., Eriksson, K. S., & Haas, H. L. (2001). Orexin A excites serotonergic neurons in the dorsal raphe nucleus of the rat. *Neuropharmacology*, *40*(3), 457–459. 10.1016/s0028-3908(00)00178-7

Brown, R. J. (2006). Different types of "dissociation" have different psychological mechanisms. *Journal of Trauma & Dissociation*, *7*(4), 7–28. 10.1300/J229v07n04_02

Bryant, R. A., & Hung, L. (2013). Oxytocin enhances social persuasion during hypnosis. *PloS One*, *8*(4), e60711. 10.1371/journal.pone.0060711

Bryant, R. A., Hung, L., Guastella, A. J., & Mitchell, P. B. (2012). Oxytocin as a moderator of hypnotizability. *Psychoneuroendocrinology*, *37*(1), 162–166. 10.1016/j.psyneuen.2011.05.010

Burke, M. J., & Blumberger, D. M. (2021). Caution at psychiatry's psychedelic frontier. *Nature Medicine*, *27*(10), 1687–1688. 10.1038/s41591-021-01524-1

Cardeña, E., Nordhjem, B., Marcusson-Clavertz, D., & Holmqvist, K. (2017). The "hypnotic state" and eye movements: Less there than meets the eye? *PloS One*, *12*(8), e0182546. 10.1371/journal.pone.0182546

Carhart-Harris, R., & Nutt, D. (2017). Serotonin and brain function: A tale of two receptors. *Journal of Psychopharmacology*, *31*(9), 1091–1120. 10.1177/0269881117725915

Carhart-Harris, R. L., Bolstridge, M., Rucker, J., Day, C. M., Erritzoe, D., Kaelen, M., Bloomfield, M., Rickard, J. A., Forbes, B., & Feilding, A. (2016). Psilocybin with psychological support for treatment-resistant depression: An open-label feasibility study. *The Lancet Psychiatry*, *3*(7), 619–627. 10.1016/S2215-0366(16)30065-7

Carhart-Harris, R. L., & Friston, K. (2019). REBUS and the anarchic brain: Toward a unified model of the brain action of psychedelics. *Pharmacological Reviews*, *71*(3), 316–344. 10.1124/pr.118.017160

Carhart-Harris, R. L., Kaelen, M., Whalley, M., Bolstridge, M., Feilding, A., & Nutt, D. J. (2015). LSD enhances suggestibility in healthy volunteers. *Psychopharmacology*, *232*(4), 785–794. 10.1007/s00213-014-3714-z

Clark, A. (2013). Are we predictive engines? Perils, prospects, and the puzzle of the porous perceiver. *Behavioral and Brain Sciences*, *36*(3), 233. 10.1017/s0140525x12002440

Cleveland, J. M., Korman, B. M., & Gold, S. N. (2015). Are hypnosis and dissociation related? New evidence for a connection. *International Journal of Clinical and Experimental Hypnosis*, *63*(2), 198–214. 10.1080/00207144.2015.1002691

Coltheart, M., Cox, R., Sowman, P., Morgan, H., Barnier, A., Langdon, R., Connaughton, E., Teichmann, L., Williams, N., & Polito, V. (2018). Belief, delusion, hypnosis, and the right dorsolateral prefrontal cortex: A transcranial magnetic stimulation study. *Cortex*, *101*, 234–248. 10.1016/j.cortex.2018.01.001

Cools, R. (2019). Chemistry of the adaptive mind: Lessons from dopamine. *Neuron*, *104*(1), 113–131. 10.1016/j.neuron.2019.09.035

Cools, R., & D'Esposito, M. (2011). Inverted-U-shaped dopamine actions on human working memory and cognitive control. *Biological Psychiatry*, *69*(12), e113–e125. 10.1016/j.biopsych.2011.03.028

De Gregorio, D., Comai, S., Posa, L., & Gobbi, G. (2016). d-Lysergic acid diethylamide (LSD) as a model of psychosis: Mechanism of action and pharmacology. *International Journal of Molecular Sciences*, *17*(11), 1953. 10.3390/ijms17111953

De Pascalis, V., & Russo, E. (2013). Hypnotizability, hypnosis and prepulse inhibition of the startle reflex in healthy women: An ERP analysis. *PloS One*, *8*(11), e79605. 10.1371/journal.pone.0079605

Debenedittis, G., Panerai, A. A., & Villamira, M. A. (1989). Effects of hypnotic analgesia and hypnotizability on experimental ischemic pain. *International Journal of Clinical and Experimental Hypnosis*, *37*(1), 55–69. 10.1080/00207148908410533

Deeley, Q. (2016). Hypnosis as therapy for functional neurologic disorders. *Handbook of Clinical Neurology*, *139*, 585–595. 10.1016/B978-0-12-801772-2.00047-3

DeSouza, D. D., Stimpson, K. H., Baltusis, L., Sacchet, M. D., Gu, M., Hurd, R., Wu, H., Yeomans, D. C., Willliams, N., & Spiegel, D. (2020). Association between anterior cingulate neurochemical concentration and individual differences in hypnotizability. *Cerebral Cortex*, *30*(6), 3644–3654. 10.1093/cercor/bhz332

Dienes, Z., & Hutton, S. (2013). Understanding hypnosis metacognitively: rTMS applied to left DLPFC increases hypnotic suggestibility. *Cortex*, *49*(2), 386–392. 10.1016/j.cortex.2012.07.009

Dienes, Z., & Perner, J. (2007). Executive control without conscious awareness: The cold control theory of hypnosis. In G. A., Jamieson (Ed.), *Hypnosis and conscious states: The cognitive neuroscience perspective*, pp. 293–314.

Driesen, N. R., McCarthy, G., Bhagwagar, Z., Bloch, M. H., Calhoun, V. D., D'souza, D. C., Gueorguieva, R., He, G., Leung, H.-C., & Ramani, R. (2013). The impact of NMDA receptor blockade on human working memory-related prefrontal function and connectivity. *Neuropsychopharmacology*, *38*(13), 2613–2622. 10.1038/npp.2013.170

Duerler, P., Vollenweider, F. X., & Preller, K. H. (2022). A neurobiological perspective on social influence: Serotonin and social adaptation. *Journal of Neurochemistry*, *162*(1), 60–79. 10.1111/jnc.15607

Elkins, G. R. (2016). *Handbook of medical and psychological hypnosis: Foundations, applications, and professional issues*. Springer Publishing Company. 10.1891/9780826124876

Ellenberger, H. F. (1970). *The discovery of the unconscious: The history and evolution of dynamic psychiatry* (Vol. 1). Basic books.

Ende, G. (2015). Proton magnetic resonance spectroscopy: Relevance of glutamate and GABA to neuropsychology. *Neuropsychology Review*, *25*(3), 315–325. 10.1007/s11065-015-9295-8

Eysenck, H. J., & Rees, W. L. (1945). States of heightened suggestibility: Narcosis. *Journal of Mental Science*, *91*, 301–310. 10.1192/bjp.91.384.301

Feldman, H., & Friston, K. J. (2010). Attention, uncertainty, and free-energy. *Frontiers in Human Neuroscience*, *4*, 215. 10.3389/fnhum.2010.00215

Fried, M., Garrioch, M., Tiplady, B., & Wildsmith, J. (1995). The effects of inhaled nitrous oxide on some measures of attention. *Journal of Psychopharmacology*, *9*(2), 123–126. 10.1177/026988119500900206

Friston, K. (2010). The free-energy principle: A unified brain theory? *Nature Reviews Neuroscience*, *11*(2), 127–138. 10.1038/nrn2787

Gershman, S. J., & Uchida, N. (2019). Believing in dopamine. *Nature Reviews Neuroscience*, *20*(11), 703–714. 10.1038/s41583-019-0220-7

Gibson, H., Corcoran, M., & Curran, J. (1977). Hypnotic susceptibility and personality: The consequences of diazepam and the sex of the subjects. *British Journal of Psychology*, *68*(1), 51–59. 10.1111/j.2044-8295.1977.tb01558.x

Gitlin, J., Chamadia, S., Locascio, J. J., Ethridge, B. R., Pedemonte, J. C., Hahm, E. Y., Ibala, R., Mekonnen, J., Colon, K. M., & Qu, J. (2020). Dissociative and analgesic properties of ketamine are independent. *Anesthesiology*, *133*(5), 1021–1028. 10.1097/ALN.0000000000003529

Goldstein, A., & Hilgard, E. R. (1975). Failure of the opiate antagonist naloxone to modify hypnotic analgesia. *Proceedings of the National Academy of Sciences*, 72(6), 2041–2043. 10.1073/pnas.72.6.2041

Gorassini, D. R. (2004). Enhancing hypnotizability. In M. Heap, R. Brown, & D. Oakley (Eds.), *The highly hypnotizable person: Theoretical, experimental and clinical issues* (pp. 213–239). Routledge. 10.4324/9780203487822

Gupta, K., Emmanouil, D., & Sethi, A. (2019). *Nitrous oxide in pediatric dentistry: A clinical handbook*. Springer. 10.1007/978-3-030-29618-6

Halpern, S., & Merlis, S. (1961). Hypnosis and psychotropic agents: Their interactions in mental patients. *Neuro-Psychopharmacology*, 2, 258–262.

Heekeren, K., Daumann, J., Neukirch, A., Stock, C., Kawohl, W., Norra, C., Waberski, T. D., & Gouzoulis-Mayfrank, E. (2008). Mismatch negativity generation in the human 5HT2A agonist and NMDA antagonist model of psychosis. *Psychopharmacology*, *199*(1), 77–88. 10.1007/s00213-008-1129-4

Higuchi, S., Usui, A., Murasaki, M., Matsushita, S., Nishioka, N., Yoshino, A., Matsui, T., Muraoka, H., Ishizuka, Y., & Kanba, S. (2002). Plasma orexin-A is lower in patients with narcolepsy. *Neuroscience Letters*, *318*(2), 61–64. 10.1016/s0304-3940(01)02476-4

Hiltunen, S., Virta, M., Kallio, S., & Paavilainen, P. (2019). The effects of hypnosis and hypnotic suggestions on the mismatch negativity in highly hypnotizable subjects. *International Journal of Clinical and Experimental Hypnosis*, *67*(2), 192–216. 10.1080/00207144.2019.1580966

Hull, C. L. (1993). *Hypnosis and suggestibility*. Appleton-Century.

Jamieson, G. A. (2018). Expectancies of the future in hypnotic suggestions. *Psychology of Consciousness: Theory, Research, and Practice*, *5*(3), 258. 10.1037/cns0000170

Jamieson, G. A. (2022). An insula view of predictive processing in hypnotic responses. *Psychology of Consciousness: Theory, Research, and Practice*, *9*(2), 117. 10.1037/cns0000266

Jamieson, G. A., & Burgess, A. P. (2014). Hypnotic induction is followed by state-like changes in the organization of EEG functional connectivity in the theta and beta frequency bands in high-hypnotically susceptible individuals. *Frontiers in Human Neuroscience*, *8*, 528. 10.3389/fnhum.2014.00528

Jamieson, G. A., Dwivedi, P., & Gruzelier, J. H. (2005). Changes in mismatch negativity across pre-hypnosis, hypnosis and post-hypnosis conditions distinguish high from low hypnotic susceptibility groups. *Brain Research Bulletin*, *67*(4), 298–303. 10.1016/j.brainresbull.2005.06.033

Jiang, H., White, M. P., Greicius, M. D., Waelde, L. C., & Spiegel, D. (2017). Brain activity and functional connectivity associated with hypnosis. *Cerebral Cortex*, *27*(8), 4083–4093. 10.1093/cercor/bhw220

Joshua, M., Adler, A., & Bergman, H. (2009). The dynamics of dopamine in control of motor behavior. *Current Opinion in Neurobiology*, *19*(6), 615–620. 10.1016/j.conb.2009.10.001

Joules, R., Doyle, O., Schwarz, A., O'daly, O., Brammer, M., Williams, S., & Mehta, M. (2015). Ketamine induces a robust whole-brain connectivity pattern that can be differentially modulated by drugs of different mechanism and clinical profile. *Psychopharmacology*, *232*(21), 4205–4218. 10.1007/s00213-015-3951-9

Kasos, E., Kasos, K., Pusztai, F., Polyák, Á., Kovács, K. J., & Varga, K. (2018). Changes in oxytocin and cortisol in active-alert hypnosis: Hormonal changes benefiting low hypnotizable participants. *International Journal of Clinical and Experimental Hypnosis*, *66*(4), 404–427. 10.1080/00207144.2018.1495009

Katonai, E. R., Szekely, A., Vereczkei, A., Sasvari-Szekely, M., Bányai, É. I., & Varga, K. (2017). Dopaminergic and serotonergic genotypes and the subjective experiences of hypnosis. *International Journal of Clinical and Experimental Hypnosis*, *65*(4), 379–397. 10.1080/00207144.2017.1348848

Kihlstrom, J. F., Glisky, M. L., & Angiulo, M. J. (1994). Dissociative tendencies and dissociative disorders. *Journal of Abnormal Psychology*, *103*(1), 117. 10.1037//0021-843x.103.1.117

Kirsch, I. (1985). Response expectancy as a determinant of experience and behavior. *American Psychologist*, *40*(11), 1189. 10.1037/0003-066X.40.11.1189

Kirsch, I., & Lynn, S. J. (1999). Automaticity in clinical psychology. *American Psychologist*, *54*(7), 504. 10.1037//0003-066x.54.7.504

Kummerfeld, E., Ma, S., Blackman, R. K., DeNicola, A. L., Redish, A. D., Vinogradov, S., Crowe, D. A., & Chafee, M. V. (2020). Cognitive control errors in nonhuman primates resembling those in schizophrenia reflect opposing effects of NMDA receptor blockade on causal interactions between cells and circuits in prefrontal and parietal cortices. *Biological Psychiatry: Cognitive Neuroscience and Neuroimaging*, *5*(7), 705–714. 10.1016/j.bpsc.2020.02.013

Laurence, J.-R., Beaulieu-Prevost, D., & Chéné, T. d. (2008). Measuring and understanding individual differences in hypnotizability. In M. R. Nash, & A. J. Barnier (Eds.), *The Oxford handbook of hypnosis: Theory, research, and practice* (pp. 225–253). Oxford University Press. 10.1093/oxfordhb/9780198570097.013.0009

Lehmann, M., Neumann, C., Wasserthal, S., Schultz, J., Delis, A., Trautner, P., Hurlemann, R., & Ettinger, U. (2021). Effects of ketamine on brain function during metacognition of episodic memory. *Neuroscience of Consciousness*, *2021*(1), niaa028. 10.1093/nc/niaa028

Lemercier, C. E., & Terhune, D. B. (2018). Psychedelics and hypnosis: Commonalities and therapeutic implications. *Journal of Psychopharmacology*, *32*(7), 732–740. 10.1177/0269881118780714

Leptourgos, P., Bansal, S., Dutterer, J., Culbreth, A., Powers III, A., Suthaharan, P., Kenney, J., Erickson, M., Waltz, J., & Wijtenburg, S. A. (2022). Relating glutamate, conditioned, and clinical hallucinations via 1H-MR spectroscopy. *Schizophrenia Bulletin*, *48*(4), 912–920. 10.1093/schbul/sbac006

Levin, R., Heresco-Levy, U., Edelman, S., Shapira, H., Ebstein, R. P., & Lichtenberg, P. (2011). Hypnotizability and sensorimotor gating: A dopaminergic mechanism of hypnosis. *International Journal of Clinical and Experimental Hypnosis*, *59*(4), 399–405. 10.1080/00207144.2011.594678

Lichtenberg, P., Bachner-Melman, R., Gritsenko, I., & Ebstein, R. P. (2000). Exploratory association study between catechol-O-methyltransferase (COMT) high/low enzyme activity polymorphism and hypnotizability. *American Journal of Medical Genetics*, *96*(6), 771–774. 10.1002/1096-8628(20001204)96:6<771::aid-ajmg14>3.0.co;2-t

Lichtenberg, P., Even-Or, E., Bar, G., Levin, R., Brin, A., & Heresco-Levy, U. (2008). Reduced prepulse inhibition is associated with increased hypnotizability. *International Journal of Neuropsychopharmacology*, *11*(4), 541–545. 10.1017/S1461145707008231

Liechti, M. E. (2017). Modern clinical research on LSD. *Neuropsychopharmacology*, *42*(11), 2114–2127. 10.1038/npp.2017.86

Lotan, A., Bonne, O., & Abramowitz, E. G. (2015). Methylphenidate facilitates hypnotizability in adults with ADHD: A naturalistic cohort study. *International Journal of Clinical and Experimental Hypnosis*, *63*(3), 294–308. 10.1080/00207144.2015.1031547

Lynn, S. J., Green, J. P., Zahedi, A., & Apelian, C. (2022). The response set theory of hypnosis reconsidered: Toward an integrative model. *American Journal of Clinical Hypnosis*, *65*, 1–25. 10.1080/00029157.2022.2117680

Lynn, S. J., Kirsch, I., & Hallquist, M. N. (2008). Social cognitive theories of hypnosis. In M. R. Nash, & A. J. Barnier (Eds.), *The Oxford handbook of hypnosis: Theory, research, and practice* (pp. 111–139). Oxford University Press. 10.1080/00029157.2022.2117680

Martin, J.-R., & Pacherie, E. (2019). Alterations of agency in hypnosis: A new predictive coding model. *Psychological Review*, *126*(1), 133. 10.1037/rev0000134

Middlefell, R. (1967). The effects of LSD on body sway suggestibility in a group of hospital patients. *British Journal of Psychiatry*, *113*, 277–280. 10.1192/bjp.113.496.277

Moll, A. (1911). *Hypnotism*. Walter Scott.

Montgomery, G. H., Schnur, J. B., & David, D. (2011). The impact of hypnotic suggestibility in clinical care settings. *International Journal of Clinical and Experimental Hypnosis*, *59*(3), 294–309. 10.1080/00207144.2011.570656

Moret, V., Forster, A., Laverrière, M.-C., Lambert, H., Gaillard, R., Bourgeois, P., Haynal, A., Gemperle, M., & Buchser, E. (1991). Mechanism of analgesia induced by hypnosis and acupuncture: Is there a difference? *Pain*, *45*(2), 135–140. 10.1016/0304-3959(91)90178-Z

Moskowitz, D., Pinard, G., Zuroff, D. C., Annable, L., & Young, S. N. (2001). The effect of tryptophan on social interaction in everyday life: A placebo-controlled study. *Neuropsychopharmacology*, *25*(2), 277–289. 10.1016/S0893-133X(01)00219-6

Nichols, D. E. (2016). Psychedelics. *Pharmacological Reviews*, *68*(2), 264–355. 10.1124/pr.115.011478

Olney, J. W., & Farber, N. B. (1995). Glutamate receptor dysfunction and schizophrenia. *Archives of General Psychiatry*, *52*(12), 998–1007. 10.1001/archpsyc.1995.03950240016004

Oranje, B., Van Berckel, B., Kemner, C., Van Ree, J., Kahn, R., & Verbaten, M. (2000). The effects of a sub-anaesthetic dose of ketamine on human selective attention. *Neuropsychopharmacology*, *22*(3), 293–302. 10.1016/S0893-133X(99)00118-9

Ott, T., & Nieder, A. (2019). Dopamine and cognitive control in prefrontal cortex. *Trends in Cognitive Sciences*, *23*(3), 213–234. 10.1016/j.tics.2018.12.006

Ott, U., Reuter, M., Hennig, J., & Vaitl, D. (2005). Evidence for a common biological basis of the absorption trait, hallucinogen effects, and positive symptoms: Epistasis between 5-HT2a and COMT polymorphisms. *American Journal of Medical Genetics Part B: Neuropsychiatric Genetics*, *137*(1), 29–32. 10.1002/ajmg.b.30197

Pallavicini, C., Vilas, M. G., Villarreal, M., Zamberlan, F., Muthukumaraswamy, S., Nutt, D., Carhart-Harris, R., & Tagliazucchi, E. (2019). Spectral signatures of serotonergic psychedelics and glutamatergic dissociatives. *Neuroimage*, *200*, 281–291. 10.1016/j.neuroimage.2019.06.053

Patterson, D. R., Hoffer, C., Jensen, M. P., Wiechman, S. A., & Sharar, S. R. (2018). Ketamine as a possible moderator of hypnotizability: A feasibility study. *International Journal of Clinical and Experimental Hypnosis*, *66*(3), 298–307. 10.1080/00207144.2018.1460559

Pettey, G. E. (1913). *The narcotic drug diseases and allied ailments: Pathology, pathogenesis, and treatment*. Davis.

Piazza, G. G., Iskandar, G., Hennessy, V., Zhao, H., Walsh, K., McDonnell, J., Terhune, D. B., Das, R. K., & Kamboj, S. K. (2022). Pharmacological modelling of dissociation and psychosis: An evaluation of the Clinician Administered Dissociative States Scale and Psychotomimetic States Inventory during nitrous oxide ('laughing gas')-induced anomalous states. *Psychopharmacology*, *239*(7), 2317–2329. 10.1007/s00213-022-06121-9

Pokorny, T., Duerler, P., Seifritz, E., Vollenweider, F. X., & Preller, K. H. (2020). LSD acutely impairs working memory, executive functions, and cognitive flexibility, but not risk-based decision-making. *Psychological Medicine*, *50*(13), 2255–2264. 10.1017/S0033291719002393

Presciuttini, S., Curcio, M., Sciarrino, R., Scatena, F., Jensen, M. P., & Santarcangelo, E. L. (2018). Polymorphism of opioid receptors µ1 in highly hypnotizable subjects. *International Journal of Clinical and Experimental Hypnosis*, *66*(1), 106–118. 10.1080/00207144.2018.1396128

Presciuttini, S., Gialluisi, A., Barbuti, S., Curcio, M., Scatena, F., Carli, G., & Santarcangelo, E. L. (2014). Hypnotizability and catechol-o-methyltransferase (COMT) polymorphysms in Italians. *Frontiers in Human Neuroscience*, *7*, 929. 10.3389/fnhum.2013.00929

Quaedackers, L., Droogleever Fortuyn, H., Van Gilst, M., Lappenschaar, M., & Overeem, S. (2022). Dissociative symptoms are highly prevalent in adults with narcolepsy type 1. *Behavioral Sleep Medicine*, *20*(1), 63–73. 10.1080/15402002.2021.1888729

Raleigh, M. J., McGuire, M. T., Brammer, G. L., Pollack, D. B., & Yuwiler, A. (1991). Serotonergic mechanisms promote dominance acquisition in adult male vervet monkeys. *Brain Research*, *559*(2), 181–190. 10.1016/0006-8993(91)90001-c

Raleigh, M. J., McGuire, M. T., Brammer, G. L., & Yuwiler, A. (1984). Social and environmental influences on blood serotonin concentrations in monkeys. *Archives of General Psychiatry*, *41*(4), 405–410. 10.1001/archpsyc.1984.01790150095013

Reddy-Thootkur, M., Kraguljac, N. V., & Lahti, A. C. (2022). The role of glutamate and GABA in cognitive dysfunction in schizophrenia and mood disorders: A systematic review of magnetic resonance spectroscopy studies. *Schizophrenia Research*, *249*, 74–84. 10.1016/j.schres.2020.02.001

Reiser, E. M., Schulter, G., Weiss, E. M., Fink, A., Rominger, C., & Papousek, I. (2012). Decrease of prefrontal-posterior EEG coherence: Loose control during social-emotional stimulation. *Brain and Cognition*, *80*(1), 144–154. 10.1016/j.bandc.2012.06.001

Riedel, G., Platt, B., & Micheau, J. (2003). Glutamate receptor function in learning and memory. *Behavioural Brain Research*, *140*(1–2), 1–47. 10.1016/s0166-4328(02)00272-3

Rominger, C., Weiss, E. M., Nagl, S., Niederstätter, H., Parson, W., & Papousek, I. (2014). Carriers of the COMT Met/Met allele have higher degrees of hypnotizability, provided that they have good attentional control: A case of gene–trait interaction. *International Journal of Clinical and Experimental Hypnosis*, *62*(4), 455–482. 10.1080/00207144.2014.931177

Ryu, J.-H., Kim, P.-J., Kim, H.-G., Koo, Y.-S., & Shin, T. J. (2017). Investigating the effects of nitrous oxide sedation on frontal-parietal interactions. *Neuroscience Letters*, *651*, 9–15. 10.1016/j.neulet.2017.04.036

Santarcangelo, E. L. (2014). New views of hypnotizability. *Frontiers in Behavioral Neuroscience*, *8*, 224. 10.3389/fnbeh.2014.00224

Semmens-Wheeler, R., Dienes, Z., & Duka, T. (2013). Alcohol increases hypnotic susceptibility. *Consciousness and Cognition*, *22*, 1082–1091. 10.1016/j.concog.2013.07.001

Sescousse, G., Ligneul, R., van Holst, R. J., Janssen, L. K., de Boer, F., Janssen, M., Berry, A. S., Jagust, W. J., & Cools, R. (2018). Spontaneous eye blink rate and dopamine synthesis capacity: Preliminary evidence for an absence of positive correlation. *European Journal of Neuroscience*, *47*(9), 1081–1086. 10.1111/ejn.13895

Shamay-Tsoory, S. G., & Abu-Akel, A. (2016). The social salience hypothesis of oxytocin. *Biological Psychiatry*, *79*(3), 194–202. 10.1016/j.biopsych.2015.07.020

Sjoberg, B., & Hollister, L. E. (1965). The effects of psychotomimetic drugs on primary suggestibility. *Psychopharmacologia*, *8*(4), 251–262. 10.1007/BF00407857

Sklar, G. S., Zukin, S. R., & Reilly, T. A. (1981). Adverse reactions to ketamine anaesthesia *Anaesthesia*, *36*, 183–187. 10.1111/j.1365-2044.1981.tb08721.x

Skoblenick, K., & Everling, S. (2014). N-methyl-d-aspartate receptor antagonist ketamine impairs action-monitoring activity in the prefrontal cortex. *Journal of Cognitive Neuroscience*, *26*(3), 577–592. 10.1162/jocn_a_00519

Smith, D. M., & Terhune, D. B. (2023). Pedunculopontine-induced cortical decoupling as the neurophysiological locus of dissociation. *Psychological Review 130*, 183–210. 10.1037/rev0000353
Spiegel, D. (1980). Hypnotizability and psychoactive medication. *American Journal of Clinical Hypnosis*, *22*(4), 217–222. 10.1080/00029157.1980.10403231
Spiegel, D., & Albert, L. H. (1983). Naloxone fails to reverse hypnotic alleviation of chronic pain. *Psychopharmacology*, *81*(2), 140–143. 10.1007/BF00429008
Spiegel, D., Hunt, T., & Dondershine, H. E. (1988). Dissociation and hypnotizability in posttraumatic stress disorder. *The American Journal of Psychiatry*, *145*(3), 301–305. 10.1176/ajp.145.3.301
Spiegel, D., & King, R. (1992). Hypnotizability and CSF HVA levels among psychiatric patients. *Biological Psychiatry*, *31*(1), 95–98. 10.1016/0006-3223(92)90009-o
Spindler, L. R., Luppi, A. I., Adapa, R. M., Craig, M. M., Coppola, P., Peattie, A. R., Manktelow, A. E., Finoia, P., Sahakian, B. J., & Williams, G. B. (2021). Dopaminergic brainstem disconnection is common to pharmacological and pathological consciousness perturbation. *Proceedings of the National Academy of Sciences*, *118*(30), e2026289118. 10.1073/pnas.2026289118
Sternbach, R. A. (1982). On strategies for identifying neurochemical correlates of hypnotic analgesia: A brief communication. *International Journal of Clinical and Experimental Hypnosis*, *30*(3), 251–256. 10.1080/00207148208407262
Storozheva, Z. I., Kirenskaya, A. V., Gordeev, M. N., Kovaleva, M. E., & Novototsky-Vlasov, V. Y. (2018). COMT genotype and sensory and sensorimotor gating in high and low hypnotizable subjects. *International Journal of Clinical and Experimental Hypnosis*, *66*(1), 83–105. 10.1080/00207144.2018.1396120
Štrac, D. Š., Pivac, N., & Mück-Šeler, D. (2016). The serotonergic system and cognitive function. *Translational Neuroscience*, *7*(1), 35–49. 10.1515/tnsci-2016-0007
Szekely, A., Kovacs-Nagy, R., Bányai, É. I., Gősi-Greguss, A. C., Varga, K., Halmai, Z., Ronai, Z., & Sasvari-Szekely, M. (2010). Association between hypnotizability and the catechol-O-methyltransferase (COMT) polymorphism. *International Journal of Clinical and Experimental Hypnosis*, *58*(3), 301–315. 10.1080/00207141003760827
Terhune, D. B. (2012). Metacognition, cold control and hypnosis. *Journal of Mind-Body Regulation*, *2*(1), 75–79. https://journalhosting.ucalgary.ca/index.php/mbr/article/view/16009
Terhune, D. B., Cardeña, E., & Lindgren, M. (2011). Differential frontal-parietal phase synchrony during hypnosis as a function of hypnotic suggestibility. *Psychophysiology*, *48*(10), 1444–1447. 10.1111/j.1469-8986.2011.01211.x
Terhune, D. B., Cleeremans, A., Raz, A., & Lynn, S. J. (2017). Hypnosis and top-down regulation of consciousness. *Neuroscience & Biobehavioral Reviews*, *81*, 59–74. 10.1016/j.neubiorev.2017.02.002
Timmermann, C., Spriggs, M. J., Kaelen, M., Leech, R., Nutt, D. J., Moran, R. J., Carhart-Harris, R. L., & Muthukumaraswamy, S. D. (2018). LSD modulates effective connectivity and neural adaptation mechanisms in an auditory oddball paradigm. *Neuropharmacology*, *142*, 251–262. 10.1016/j.neuropharm.2017.10.039
Tsujino, N., & Sakurai, T. (2009). Orexin/hypocretin: A neuropeptide at the interface of sleep, energy homeostasis, and reward system. *Pharmacological Reviews*, *61*(2), 162–176. 10.1124/pr.109.001321
Ulett, G. A., Akpinar, S., & Itil, T. M. (1972). Hypnosis: Physiological, pharmacological reality. *American Journal of Psychiatry*, *128*(7), 799–805. 10.1176/ajp.128.7.799
Umbricht, D., Schmid, L., Koller, R., Vollenweider, F. X., Hell, D., & Javitt, D. C. (2000). Ketamine-induced deficits in auditory and visual context-dependent processing in healthy volunteers: Implications for models of cognitive deficits in schizophrenia. *Archives of General Psychiatry*, *57*(12), 1139–1147. 10.1001/archpsyc.57.12.1139
Umbricht, D., Vollenweider, F. X., Schmid, L., Grübel, C., Skrabo, A., Huber, T., & Koller, R. (2003). Effects of the 5-HT2A agonist psilocybin on mismatch negativity generation and AX-continuous performance task: Implications for the neuropharmacology of cognitive deficits in schizophrenia. *Neuropsychopharmacology*, *28*(1), 170–181. 10.1038/sj.npp.1300005
Valentine, K. E., Milling, L. S., Clark, L. J., & Moriarty, C. L. (2019). The efficacy of hypnosis as a treatment for anxiety: A meta-analysis. *International Journal of Clinical and Experimental Hypnosis*, *67*(3), 336–363. 10.1080/00207144.2019.1613863

van den Bosch, R., Hezemans, F. H., Määttä, J. I., Hofmans, L., Papadopetraki, D., Verkes, R.-J., Marquand, A. F., Booij, J., & Cools, R. (2022). Evidence for absence of links between striatal dopamine synthesis capacity and working memory capacity, spontaneous eye-blink rate, and trait impulsivity. *bioRxiv*. 10.1101/2022.07.11.499570

Varga, K., & Kekecs, Z. (2014). Oxytocin and cortisol in the hypnotic interaction1. *International Journal of Clinical and Experimental Hypnosis*, *62*(1), 111–128. 10.1080/00207144.2013.841494

Vingoe, F. J. (1973). More on drugs, hypnotic susceptibility and experimentally controlled conditions. *Bulletin of the British Psychological Society*, *26*(91), 95–103.

Walsh, K., Das, R. K., & Kamboj, S. K. (2017). The subjective response to nitrous oxide is a potential pharmaco-endophenotype for alcohol use disorder: A preliminary study with heavy drinkers. *International Journal of Neuropsychopharmacology*, *20*(4), 346–350. 10.1093/ijnp/pyw063

Weitzenhoffer, A. M. (1974). When is an "instruction" an "instruction"? *International Journal of Clinical and Experimental Hypnosis*, *22*(3), 258–269. 10.1080/00207147408413005

Whalley, M., & Brooks, G. (2009). Enhancement of suggestibility and imaginative ability with nitrous oxide. *Psychopharmacology*, *203*(4), 745–752. 10.1007/s00213-008-1424-0

Wieder, L., Brown, R. J., Thompson, T., & Terhune, D. B. (2022). Hypnotic suggestibility in dissociative and related disorders: A meta-analysis. *Neuroscience and Biobehavioral Reviews*, *139*, 104751. 10.1016/j.neubiorev.2022.104751

Wießner, I., Falchi, M., Palhano-Fontes, F., Feilding, A., Ribeiro, S., & Tófoli, L. F. (2021). LSD, madness and healing: Mystical experiences as possible link between psychosis model and therapy model. *Psychological Medicine*, *53*, 1–15. 10.1016/j.neubiorev.2022.104751

Wise, R. A., & Robble, M. A. (2020). Dopamine and addiction. *Annual Review of Psychology*, *71*, 79–106. 10.1146/annurev-psych-010418-103337

Woody, E. Z., & Sadler, P. (2008). Dissociation theories of hypnosis. In M. R. Nash, & A. J. Barnier (Eds.), *The Oxford handbook of hypnosis: Theory, research, and practice* (pp. 81–110). Oxford University Press. 10.1093/oxfordhb/9780198570097.013.0004

Hypnotizability

20
THE NEUROPSYCHOLOGY OF HYPNOTIZABILITY

Afik Faerman and David Spiegel
Stanford University, Stanford, CA, USA

Introduction

People react differently to hypnosis. This fact was realized at least as early as the 18th century by Franz Mesmer (Laurence et al., 2008), noting that "*I have noticed also that not all men can be equally magnetized: of ten persons that were present, there was one who could not be magnetized, who stopped the communication of magnetism. On the other hand, there was one of these ten persons who was so susceptible to magnetization that he could not approach a patient within ten feet without causing him tremendous pain*" (Mesmer, 1775; as cited in Laurence & Perry, 1988, p. 59, our italics). The search for factors explaining the differential interindividual effects of hypnosis has led to the formation of a latent concept encompassing a person's responsiveness to various types of suggestions given in the context of hypnosis. While no clear consensus about the terminology and exact definition of this latent concept has been achieved, it has largely been perceived as a dimension spanning from low to high. As such, several measurements have been developed to capture hypnotizability, some individually administered while others group based.

Tellegen's (1978) "Minimal" definition described *hypnotizability* as "the ability to represent suggested events and states imaginatively and enactively in such a manner that they are experienced as real." Since Tellegen's definition, this ability and its determinants have been the center of research in an effort to understand what makes some people respond more to hypnosis than others. Kirsch and Braffman (2001) classify responsiveness to suggestions that follow a formal induction as h*ypnotic suggestibility*, and referred to hypnotizability as the degree of responding to hypnotic suggestions that is unexplained by other factors that might impact responsiveness to suggestions such as the ability to have experiences using imagination instructions without hypnotic inductions (i.e., *imaginative suggestibility*), expectancy, and motivation. They argue that the amount of variance accounted for by imaginative suggestibility and contextual factors is as great as the reliability of hypnotic suggestibility scales and, therefore, no additional variables (e.g., hypnotizability) are necessary to explain responsiveness to suggestions, even when a hypnotic induction is present (Braffman & Kirsch, 1999; Kirsch & Braffman, 2001). At the heart of

DOI: 10.4324/9781003449126-28

this model lies the astute observation that expectancies contextualize our experiences, and that they play a notable role in responsiveness to hypnosis. This perspective has been supported by some (e.g., Meyer & Lynn, 2011; Milling et al., 2005; Poulsen & Matthews, 2003) and challenged by others. For example, Benham et al. (2006) used structural equation modeling and found substantial residual variability in hypnotic responsiveness that was not explained by either direct or indirect expectancies. Furthermore, several studies suggested that, particularly for highly hypnotizable individuals, hypnotic suggestions are significantly more effective in facilitating experiential change than placebo expectations (e.g., Knox et al., 1981; McGlashan et al., 1969; Miller & Bowers, 1986; Sharav et al., 2023; Sliwinski & Elkins, 2017; Spanos et al., 1989), and that hypnosis and placebo are facilitated by largely different brain regions (Parris, 2016). Beyond expectancy, whether there is a conceptual difference between hypnotic and imaginative suggestions (i.e., does hypnosis require a formal induction or a mentioning of the term 'hypnosis') is not yet clear. Nevertheless, the findings of Kirsch and Braffman across multiple studies (e.g., Braffman & Kirsch, 1999; Kirsch, 2001; Kirsch & Braffman, 2001) emphasize that hypnotizability has implications outside the context of hypnosis such as the general ability to experience phenomena independent from sensory stimuli (also termed *phenomenological control*; Dienes et al., 2022) in response to verbal suggestions (e.g., imaginative suggestibility).

Another contextual factor, originally stemming from psychological research, that has been shown relevant to people's responsiveness to hypnosis is demand characteristics (i.e., changes in people's behaviors, often unknowingly, in response to their interpretation of what is expected of them; Orne, 1962). As responding to the hypnotic process involves following instructions and accepting suggestions, factors that implicitly increase cooperation could reduce resistance to experiencing changes in the context of hypnosis. As such, familiarity with hypnosis, beliefs about hypnosis, and previous experience with hypnosis could shape implicit and explicit expectations from a hypnosis session (Apelian et al., 2022; Molina-Peral et al., 2020), thereby influencing both expectancy and demand characteristics. In turn, these factors could explain some of the variance in responding to suggestions in hypnosis (e.g., Green, 2012).

Aside from the important yet relatively understudied element of how to most effectively facilitate hypnosis (i.e., factors intrinsic and/or extrinsic to the *facilitator* or the hypnosis session itself that contribute to clinical outcome and/or subjective experience of the client), it appears that intrinsic and extrinsic factors in the person receiving the suggestions play a role in their reported and observed responsiveness to hypnosis. Alongside extrinsic factors (e.g., social context, demand characteristics, emotional cues), hypnotizability has also been studied as a neurobehavioral trait representing an inherent capability to experience cognitive, perceptual, emotional, physiological, and behavioral phenomena in response to suggestions in the context of hypnosis (e.g., Elkins et al., 2015). Conceptualized as a trait, hypnotizability shows minimal increases with aging (Page & Green, 2007), with a test-retest of $r = .71$ across 25 years during adulthood (Piccione et al., 1989). More than two-thirds of adults score are at least medium hypnotizable, with about 15% having high hypnotizability (Lynn et al., 2004). However, low scores on hypnotizability measures do not exclude benefitting from hypnosis-based treatments, and low hypnotizables might respond better when the same intervention is not labeled as "hypnosis" (Lynn & Shindler, 2002; Scacchia & De Pascalis, 2020).

A Neuropsychological Approach for Hypnotizability

Neuropsychology is a specialty field within psychology dedicated to understanding the relationships between the brain and behavior, particularly as these relationships can be applied to the diagnosis of neurological or psychiatric disorders, assessment of cognitive and behavioral functioning, and the design of effective treatment (Bellone & Van Patten, 2021). The neuropsychological evaluation includes gathering relevant historical context, testing and interpretation of cognitive functioning, assessing psychological factors (e.g., mood, processing styles, behavior, and personality), and analyzing and integrating neuroimaging data and findings. Applying the neuropsychological approach to the study of hypnotizability could, in theory, help portray its neurocognitive correlates in an integrative manner and identify distinct biopsychosocial profiles of responsiveness to suggestions in hypnosis. The idea is not to argue for or against one view or the other (e.g., neurobehavioral trait versus expectancy effects versus social responding) but to provide a framework through which those different explanations could be integrated into a unified neurocognitive cascade. Rather than being a "theory" of its own, this unifying approach is an effort to weave an operational thread between different theories, previous and recent findings, and future questions. Such exploration could, in turn, pave the way toward using hypnotizability scores as a marker for other forms of functioning as well as understanding hypnotizability as a modifiable factor via its neurocognitive mechanisms.

It is prudent to keep in mind that, aside from providing insights for neuroscience and cognitive psychology, studying hypnotizability has clinical significance. There is supportive evidence that hypnotizability moderates the effectiveness of hypnosis-based interventions (Lynn & Shindler, 2002). The most robust evidence applies to hypnotic analgesia used for both clinical (Milling et al., 2021) and experimental (Thompson et al., 2019) pain management. Further, yet inconsistent findings suggest that hypnotizability may be of importance in hypnosis-based interventions for weight management (e.g., Barabasz & Spiegel, 1989), smoking (e.g., Spiegel et al., 1993), and anxiety (Lynn et al., 2003). In recent years, hypnotizability measurement has also become more feasible in both clinical and research settings, with demonstrations of valid and reliable remote and computerized measurement approaches (e.g., Kittle et al., 2021; Lush et al., 2021).

Theoretical Conceptualization of Hypnotizability

Several theories attempted to explain hypnotizability from a neurocognitive perspective. In their *midstream neuropsychophysiology of hypnosis* theory, Crawford and Gruzelier (1992) proposed that hypnotizability is derived from the ability of frontal executive processes to inhibit attention and information processing during hypnosis. Furthermore, they emphasize evidence demonstrating that highly hypnotizable individuals are better at shifting between cognitive strategies, suggesting that high hypnotizability is a manifestation of stronger baseline cognitive flexibility (Crawford & Gruzelier, 1992) and executive control (Crawford, 1994).

Similarly, the *dissociated control theory*[1] (DCT; Jamieson & Woody, 2007) argued that, during hypnosis, the executive control network (ECN; central to maintenance, manipulation, and expansion of information; Menon, 2021) dissociates from the salience network (SN; involved in identifying and processing salient stimuli and moderating involvement of other brain systems in attended information; Menon, 2021), and hinted that hypnotizability is the brain's ability to facilitate such decoupling in the context of hypnosis. The DCT equates the hypnosis-related ECN-SN dissociation to frontal lobe damage (Jamieson & Woody, 2007). Following studies provided both behavioral and neuroimaging evidence that challenged the DCT assumptions. For example, Kihlstrom et al. (2013) found no differences in hypnotizability between patients with unilateral stroke in either right or left hemisphere (including frontal-temporal-parietal strokes) and healthy college students. Hoeft et al. (2012) showed that high hypnotizability was associated with greater ECN-SN resting-state connectivity (outside the context of hypnosis) than low hypnotizability. Furthermore, Jiang et al. (2017) expanded on these findings and reported increased ECN-SN connectivity via the insula, and inhibition of the SN (as seen in previous studies as well; Landry et al., 2017). Taken together, it is possible that, in hypnosis, the ECN asserts control over the SN, thereby facilitating top down modulation of conscious experiences (Terhune et al., 2017). Jiang et al. (2017) also noted uncoupling of the ECN and the default mode network (DMN; often referred to as involved in self-referential thinking; Menon, 2021) during hypnosis associated with greater subjective "depth" of hypnosis and hypnotizability. This ECN-DMN uncoupling was interpreted as a potential marker for the dissociation of information processing during hypnosis from self-referential processes such as self-reflection and mind wandering (Jiang et al., 2017).

The COLD control theory (CCT) of hypnosis (Dienes & Perner, 2007) argues that successfully following suggestions in hypnosis is done intentionally but with limited higher-order thinking (e.g., metacognition) about such intentions and, thus, is experienced as involuntary. A similar hypothesis was previously proposed in the *neo-dissociation theory* (e.g., misattribution of the intention behind responses in hypnosis to external suggestions; Hilgard, 1973, 1991), and subsequently by Kirsch and Lynn (1998) in their socio-cognitive explanation of hypnotic involuntariness (e.g., prior beliefs and expectancies influence subjective experiences and attentional processes that provide cues coherent with the suggested phenomena, which then lead to the interpretation of the intentionally allowed response as nonvolitional). In that context, hypnotizability is a manifestation of the extent of executive control in the form of higher-order thought suppression (Dienes et al., 2022). Originally, the CCT predicted that a compromise of ECN would lead to lower hypnotizability given the involvement of executive functions in responding to suggestions (Dienes & Perner, 2007). In later accounts of the CCT, this prediction was adapted and ECN inhibition was hypothesized to reduce metacognitive awareness of intentions in high hypnotizables, which is not limited to hypnosis and may happen in other contexts (Dienes et al., 2022; Dienes & Hutton, 2013).

Recent applications of predictive processing portray hypnotizability as the ability to prioritize prior expectations over perceptual evidence when forming perceptual inferences during hypnosis (Martin & Pacherie, 2019). From a neurocognitive perspective, in hypnosis, counterfactual suggested logical rules and active inference-like experiences are accepted when interoceptive inference (modulated by the SN) suppresses interoceptive prediction errors (managed by the ECN; Jamieson, 2022). This view may present an updated conceptualization of ECN involvement in hypnosis and is also in line with the increase in SN-ECN connectivity observed in hypnosis. Furthermore, this might explain why baseline SN-ECN connectivity is greater in high versus low hypnotizability, as a greater propensity to facilitate an SN-modulated suppression of the ECN following suggestions in hypnosis.

Biological Bases of Hypnotizability

Growing genetic evidence further substantiates the likelihood that hypnotizability has intrinsic biological elements. Initial results of twin studies indicated that hypnotizability is estimated to be 44–64% heritable (Bauman & Bul, 1981; Morgan, 1973). Several studies found associations of hypnotizability with polymorphisms in the catechol-O-methyltransferase (COMT) gene, responsible for the COMT enzyme that affects neuro-transmitters such as dopamine, adrenaline, and noradrenaline (Katonai et al., 2017; Rominger et al., 2014; Szekely et al., 2010). This finding, although inconsistent across studies, is often interpreted by linking hypnotizability to dopaminergic pathways. These associations were observed with the Stanford Hypnotic Susceptibility Scale, Form C (SHSS:C; Lichtenberg et al., 2000, 2004; Raz, 2005; Raz et al., 2006; Rominger et al., 2014) and the Waterloo-Stanford Group Scale, Form C (WSGC; Szekely et al., 2010), but not with the SHSS Form A (Presciuttini et al., 2014) or a ten-item adaptation of the Harvard Group Scale of Hypnotic Susceptibility, Form A (HGSHS:A; Bryant et al., 2013). In particular, these relationships were stronger with the val/met polymorphism of the COMT gene, as compared with those who were homozygous for either valine or methionine. In a murine model, the *val* allele of COMT increases metabolic activity by increasing its thermostability, thereby reducing dopamine activity in the synapse, while *met* decreases metabolic activity (Simpson et al., 2014). Consistently, levels of homovanillic acid, a metabolite of dopamine in cerebrospinal fluid, have been found to be significantly correlated with hypnotizability in a population of psychiatric patients and controls (Spiegel & King, 1992). Rominger et al. (2014) found that homozygosity for the COMT Met allele, theoretically linked to dissociative abilities, links to high hypnotizability only in the presence of high working memory abilities. The authors argued that investigations of genetic effects on behavior need to consider the context of relevant neuropsychological factors. Since the prefrontal cortex is particularly rich in dopaminergic neurons, modulation of the rate of dopamine turnover would putatively affect ECN activity, and it may be that a moderate metabolic rate allows for optimal dopaminergic activity in the ECN. A point-of-care test for this polymorphism that has just become available as a potential diagnostic screen for hypnotizability used proposed optimal COMT diplotypes and identified 89.5% of people with pain who are highly hypnotizable according to the hypnotic induction profile (HIP; Cortade et al., 2023).

Other associations were observed between SHSS:A scores and a polymorphism in the opioid receptor μ1 (OPRM1), the gene responsible for a key opioid receptor in nociception (Presciuttini et al., 2018). As the observed polymorphism is associated with decreased effectiveness of opioids in reducing pain, the authors suggest that hypnotic analgesia is unlikely to utilize the opioid system for pain reduction, which has been previously demonstrated by Spiegel and Albert (1983). In a later study, the same group found that hypnosis possibly modulates pain experience via the endocannabinoid system, as hypnotizability was associated with a polymorphism that weakens a gene responsible for fatty acid amide hydrolase (FAAH), an enzyme that deconstructs anandamide, one of the main neurotransmitters in the endocannabinoid system (Presciuttini et al., 2020). Hypnotizability was also related to polymorphisms in other genes such as the oxytocin receptor (OXTR; Bryant et al., 2013) and the nitric oxide synthase 3 (NOS3; Presciuttini et al., 2009) genes. Additional potential hormonal effects are suggested by the significant and meaningful increase in hypnotizability during pregnancy (Alexander et al., 2009).

Neurocognitive Factors in Hypnotizability

A central pillar of neuropsychological evaluations is to assess cognitive functions and identify profiles of individual and relative strengths and weaknesses. Based on the theoretical approaches to hypnotizability, it is possible that ECN and SN activation and connectivity are altered during hypnosis in highs more so than in lows. Several reviews provided summaries of the modulation of cognitive performance during hypnosis, primarily frontal and attentional functions (e.g., Parris, 2017; Terhune et al., 2017). However, to explore inherent cognitive differences as correlates of hypnotizability, here we focus mainly on performance on cognitive tests outside the context of hypnosis.

From a procedural standpoint, most hypnosis sessions include a form of induction including or followed by a set of suggestions. Although the exact role of induction in contributing to a person's benefit from hypnosis is still debated (Martin, 2019; Terhune & Cardeña, 2016), at the least, induction provides the psychosocial context in which a person's expectancy might increase, at the least indirectly impacting their responsiveness to the suggestions given in hypnosis. Furthermore, in the vast majority of cases, the induction and suggestions are provided verbally (i.e., auditorily). This paves the way for a narrative (at the cost of oversimplifying) of a stepwise investigation into the cognitive processes that participate in responding to hypnosis. First, auditory information is processed in the temporoparietal regions.[2] Then, this sensory information needs to be attended, followed by higher-order processing, which leads to responsiveness (i.e., following suggestions), evaluation of agency and allocation of cognitive and emotional resources (i.e., involuntariness and effortlessness), and consequent reorganization of planned behaviors (i.e., posthypnotic phenomena). In individuals with intact auditory processing, these highlight attention, working memory, executive functions, and memory. Moreover, recent literature suggests that hypnotizability plays a role in multisensory integration (Mioli et al., 2021) and is associated with greater interoceptive accuracy in perceiving sleep depth (Cordi & Rasch, 2022) but potentially poorer in perceiving heartbeats (Rosati et al., 2021). Additionally, the baseline amplitude of the heartbeat evoked cortical potential (HEP) may be reduced in highs in the parietal cortex but increases in highs and decreases in lows during hypnosis, interpreted as the highs' enhancement of attentional focus (mainly internally) and low's difficulty with engaging with the hypnotic suggestions (Callara et al., 2023). Phenomenological control may also be supported by similarities in neural activations between actual and imagined perception or action (i.e., functional equivalence; Kosslyn et al., 2006), which has recently been found to be greater in high compared to low hypnotizables (Ibáñez-Marcelo et al., 2019). These paint a complex picture with multiple parts, and, as such, it is unlikely that any single cognitive task would be a dominant indicator of hypnotizability. Importantly, despite an intent on converging findings from different studies to create coherent, evidence-based cognitive profiles of hypnotizability, there is notable variety in cognitive tasks and hypnotizability measures across studies and relatively consistent small samples, a concern previously raised by Wagstaff (2004). This makes drawing clear lines between different studies challenging and presents a lack of clarity in identifying consistent findings across cognitive domains.

Attention and Working Memory

Simple attention has been found to be greater in high versus low hypnotizability across different tasks and designs. Braffman and Kirsch (2001) found a significant negative correlation between hypnotizability and both reaction time and error rates on a task with simple attentional demands. Srzich et al. (2019) observed similar effects with faster simple and choice reaction times in highs compared to lows on a task that better utilizes stimulus-response compatibility, to better capture attentional abilities and reduce demands of visual discrimination. Furthermore, they found that highs had faster premotor times (i.e., time from presentation of the target stimulus to the increased in muscle firing as measured by electromyography) compared to lows, which were associated with larger mean C3/C4 contingent negative variation amplitude, a marker of preparation toward a rapid precued movement. They interpreted these findings as a likely role of greater focused attention (i.e., an ability to prepare for a precued response and detect the onset of a target stimulus), leading to a faster response and motor preparatory cortical activity in hypnotizability. Similarly, using a modified version of the Attentional Network Task, Castellani et al. (2007) showed that high hypnotizables were faster than lows in two conditions with no inhibitory demands. Additionally, Schmidt et al. (2017) observed significantly better accuracy (correct counting) on the Oddball test in high compared to medium and low hypnotizables. In contrast, Khodaverdi-Khani and Laurence (2016) found no differences between high and low hypnotizables on the Digit Span Forward, a task of simple auditory attention span (without the manipulation of content which relies more heavily on working memory abilities such as in Digit Span Backward; Sattler & Ryan, 2009; Wechsler, 2008).

On tasks of sustained attention, highly hypnotizables were significantly slower yet more accurate than medium or low hypnotizables (Varga et al., 2011). Similarly, Priebe and Wallace (1986) reported that high hypnotizables were more accurate on a timed visual tracking task (made fewer errors) than low hypnotizables, with no significant difference in the number of target stimuli correctly identified. Some studies argued that high hypnotizability involves the ability to focus attention on specific stimuli while rendering non-target stimuli irrelevant (Crawford, 1994; Mitchell, 1970). This claim is not clearly substantiated by neuropsychological studies, and further evidence is warranted. However, it can be supported by neuroimaging evidence of greater connectivity of the ECN with the SN (i.e., greater potential for frontal modulation of attentional processes; Hoeft et al., 2012) and a positive correlation between extracellular gamma-aminobutyric acid concentration in the anterior cingulate cortex (ACC) and HIP scores (interpreted as a greater baseline capacity to inhibit ACC functions as hypnotizability increases; DeSouza et al., 2020).

With regard to working memory, Khodaverdi-Khani and Laurence (2016) found performance on the Digit Span Backwards, a measure of auditory working memory, to correlate negatively with hypnotizability. High hypnotizability was also associated with significant improvements in visual working memory performance over time (on the N-back test), while the performance of those with low hypnotizability worsened (Khodaverdi-Khani & Laurence, 2016). Echoing previous similar arguments (e.g., Dixon et al., 1990; Dixon & Laurence, 1992), the authors suggested that high hypnotizability might favor automatizing task performance, which reduces working memory load (Khodaverdi-Khani & Laurence, 2016). Terhune et al. (2011) found that high hypnotizables that are also high in dissociative phenomenology show poorer performance on the counting span task, a measure of visual working memory, than both highs with low dissociative tendencies and lows. They posed the question of whether poor working memory is, therefore, a feature of dissociative tendencies and not of hypnotizability (Terhune et al., 2011).

Executive Functions

Previous approaches to the cognitive bases of hypnosis hypothesized that hypnosis involves suppression of controlled cognitive processes (e.g., critical judgment), and high hypnotizability was theorized to be associated with a better ability to abandon logical rules that lead to the implementation of cognitive strategies (Dixon et al., 1990). This notion was partially supported by our recent finding that high hypnotizability was associated with less perseveration on inapplicable logical rules in the Wisconsin Card Sorting Test (WCST; Faerman & Spiegel, 2021), as well as by Aikins and Ray (2001) who, using a rather small sample, found significantly better overall performance on the WCST (fewer trials to completion) in high versus low hypnotizable individuals. Although some interpreted these results as evidence of better set-shifting abilities, it is quite an underestimation of the complex set of executive functions required for such performance. In the WCST, examinees need to use non-directive feedback to understand the presence of a logical rule (which is not disclosed to them by the examiner), abandon a previously tested and successfully applied logical rule, and switch response sets as the logical rules update according to task progression (Folden, 2014). This is also supported by evidence that high hypnotizables are more sensitive to incoming contextualizing information, which likely influences information processing strategies (Martin et al., 2018). Therefore, it indeed involves set-shifting but also aspects of problem-solving and distractibility management and might be more accurately encompassed under the more broad term of cognitive flexibility (Miles et al., 2021).

Despite these strengths, the disadvantage of highs in timed tasks previously described for attention performance appears to apply to set-shifting as well. Using a computerized set-shifting task, in which performance was conceptualized as the delay in response time as a result of switching, Varga et al. (2011) found that response time was significantly slower in high versus low hypnotizable individuals, with no significant difference between high and medium or low and medium hypnotizability. However, they noted that highly hypnotizable participants were significantly more accurate than both low and medium hypnotizables, meaning they performed set-shifting with fewer errors but at a potential cost of response time (Varga et al., 2011). Similarly, Cojan et al. (2015) compared performance and neural activation during the flanker task between high and low hypnotizables and found slower reaction time and greater accuracy in high versus low hypnotizable individuals, which they interpreted as evidence for superior attentional flexibility. Dixon and Laurence (1992) found significantly slower reaction times on incongruent than congruent trials at the shortest interstimulus intervals of a Stroop color naming task in high but not in low hypnotizables. However, at the longest interstimulus interval, both high and low hypnotizables showed similar reaction time profiles. These findings indicate that highly hypnotizable individuals largely perform better when given enough time, which might go hand in hand with previous statements about a differential benefit from practice and the tendency to automatize performance and reduce cognitive demands over time.

In an attempt to test the assumptions of the DCT, Farvolden and Woody (2004) administered to 30 highs and 30 lows a series of tasks and tests that were previously found to show significant performance differences between patients with frontal lobe injuries and healthy controls. Consistent with previous studies (see Parris, 2017), they found no significant differences in verbal fluency performance or perseveration between highs and lows outside the context of hypnosis. However, they did find that high hypnotizables made significantly more errors across different tasks, including free-recall, proactive interference, and source amnesia

(Farvolden & Woody, 2004). These results highlight that executive functioning in highs is not clear-cut across different tasks and that it is unlikely that we can make an umbrella statement about overall executive functioning and hypnotizability (Parris, 2017).

With regard to cognitive inhibition, the evidence is grossly inconsistent. Some groups found high hypnotizability to be associated with better baseline performance on the Stroop test (Egner et al., 2005; Kaiser et al., 1997; Nordby et al., 1999; Raz et al., 2005; Rubichi et al., 2005). These findings were complemented by evidence of greater P300 (an EEG event-related potential associated with decision-making; Kaiser et al., 1997) and ACC recruitment (a central brain region part of the SN; Egner et al., 2005) in high compared to low hypnotizables. In contrast, Dixon et al. (1990, 1992) demonstrated that when task design allows minimizing the impact of strategy (mainly via shorter interstimulus intervals), highly hypnotizables had a greater Stroop effect. Consistently, Braffman and Kirsch (2001) reported a positive correlation between hypnotizability and go/no-go reaction time, indicating that inhibition likely requires greater cognitive demands in high than in low hypnotizables. Interestingly, when not provided with specific instructions targeted to modulate the Stroop interference, high hypnotizables appear to have a significant increase in the Stroop effects during hypnosis as compared to outside the context of hypnosis (Blum & Graef, 1971; Egner et al., 2005; Kaiser et al., 1997; Sheehan et al., 1988). However, Terhune et al. (2011) clarified that only dissociative highs display poorer cognitive control (via the sequential congruency effect on the Stroop) and that most highs actually displayed superior cognitive control following a hypnotic induction (also supported by previous results; Nordby et al., 1999). David and Brown (2002) also demonstrated positive correlations between inhibition (on a semantic negative priming task) and scores on both the HGSHS:A and SHSS:C (both objective and subjective). Contrary to the findings cited above, Dienes et al. (2009) found no evidence of a relationship between hypnotizability (via the WGSC) and three tasks of cognitive inhibition in a large sample of 180 participants. This, again, emphasizes the inconsistencies when it comes to linking executive functioning and hypnotizability.

Unfortunately, while reductions in frontal processes have been associated with hypnosis, both observed (Landry et al., 2017) and experimentally induced (Coltheart et al., 2018; Dienes & Hutton, 2013) neuroimaging data provided relatively little clarity on executive functions as studies report contradictory findings of both increase and decrease in frontal activation during hypnosis (Landry et al., 2017; Parris, 2017). Cojan et al. (2015) observed greater right inferior frontal gyrus recruitment and less ACC and intraparietal sulcus recruitment in highs during performance on the flanker task. Lifshitz and Raz (2015) showed that, compared to low hypnotizable individuals, highs had increased activity in the thalamus (specifically, the pulvinar nucleus) and fusiform gyrus during the Stroop task. Egner et al. (2005) saw no difference between high and low hypnotizables at baseline on either behavioral or neural activation during the Stroop task. Parris (2017) points out that it is yet unclear whether frontal inhibition is truly a unique feature of hypnosis or whether it represents the neurocognitive correlates of demand characteristics, which he identifies as a "dual-task-like state."

Memory

Some evidence indicates that hypnotizability might be associated with poorer learning of verbal information. On a verbal paired association task, Farvolden and Woody (2004) observed no significant difference in performance on initial pair learning. However, on a second trial using the same cue words to learn new associations, high hypnotizables demonstrated greater sensitivity to proactive interference (more errors). Furthermore, using a modified timed version of the Rey Auditory Verbal Learning Task (RAVLT), Farvolden and Woody (2004) also showed that highly hypnotizable individuals demonstrated less efficient learning (fewer words recalled on the last learning trial) and made more repetition errors than low hypnotizables. Terhune et al. (2011) expanded this finding and clarified that this performance difference is only significant for highly dissociative high hypnotizables. Low-dissociative high hypnotizables performed significantly better than high-dissociative high hypnotizables and showed no significant performance difference from low hypnotizables (Terhune et al., 2011). This finding appears logical, particularly if the dissociative tendencies are applicable during the learning or performing phase of the test.

Interestingly, delayed recall of verbal information seems to be stronger in high hypnotizables. Farvolden and Woody (2004) found that highly hypnotizable individuals performed significantly better on a task of word sequence memory than low hypnotizables. Similarly, Dasse et al. (2015) found that high hypnotizables were more accurate in both recall and recognition of previously learned words.

Furthermore, there is evidence to suggest that highly hypnotizable individuals have more malleable memory and are more susceptible to pseudomemory than low hypnotizables (Malinoski & Lynn, 1999). This, in turn, translates to an ability to develop false memories in response to suggestions in hypnosis, which was observed in high but not low hypnotizables (Barnier & McConkey, 1992; Dasse et al., 2015). This might also explain high hypnotizables' sensitivity to proactive interference on memory tasks (Farvolden & Woody, 2004). This malleability, however, goes both ways, as hypnosis could also be used as a tool to remediate the effects of false memory formation (Wagstaff et al., 2008).

Integration and Future Directions

Previous literature elaborated on psychological, social, and contextual factors that may play into responsiveness to suggestions in the context of hypnosis. Recent evidence contributed to a deeper understanding of the neurocognitive, genetic, and physiological factors in hypnotizability. During and following hypnosis, individuals can experience internally initiated cognitive, perceptual, emotional, physiological, and behavioral phenomena.

Based on the reviewed evidence, hypnotizability is best conceptualized as a neurobehavioral ability of the brain (as suggested by others; e.g., Benham et al., 2006; Elkins et al., 2015), influenced by both genetic and biopsychosocial factors (as highlighted by Braffman and Kirsch and following studies). In essence, hypnotizability reflects a brain's ability to construct veridical experiences independent from or only partially dependent on external sensorimotor, interoceptive, and proprioceptive information in the context of hypnosis. Given the instructive and even directive nature of suggestions in hypnosis, engaging the systems that allow for such top-down formation of conscious experiences in hypnosis can be involuntary (e.g., DCT) or intentional but with no awareness of such intentions so that it feels involuntary (e.g., CCT). There is a general agreement across theories and supportive evidence that hypnosis is likely facilitated by higher-order processes. Thus, it is probable that hypnosis-related cognitive processes could be impacted by factors that universally modify psychosocial functioning (e.g., expectancy, demand characteristics, emotional cues). In other words, hypnotizability appears to be an inherent ability to facilitate phenomenological control (Dienes et al., 2022) during hypnosis (at least), which builds on neurocognitive processes and could be moderated, in some cases and to some extent, by psychosocial factors.

Overall, but not across the board, highly hypnotizable people appear to perform better than low hypnotizables on tasks of simple attention. However, as task complexity increases, highly hypnotizables experience greater cognitive load, likely in an attempt to automatize responses and lower processing demands. Behaviorally, this translates to slower reaction times yet greater accuracy on tasks of sustained and complex attention, particularly when performance is measured over time. This highlights a potential disadvantage of high hypnotizables on timed tasks, but more efficient learning of task demands and performance management over time. This may also explain some of the results observed in the learning of verbal information; during a timed learning task with a timed response window, high hypnotizables show less efficient verbal learning than low hypnotizables (although this might only apply for the dissociative subtype of highs). However, highs appear to benefit more than low hypnotizables from time for information consolidation and outperform lows on delayed recall tests. After accounting for their disadvantages on timed measures of performance, highly hypnotizables demonstrate greater accuracy on tasks of cognitive flexibility. Additionally, although inhibition might pose higher cognitive demands on high hypnotizables (in some but not all studies), they largely seem to be better at implementing strategies to more efficiently manage these demands (e.g., when provided to them in the form of suggestions within or outside the context of hypnosis). Lastly, effective cognitive flexibility but limited inhibition might be a double-edged sword, as it may favor strategies that are more prone to distortion. Although this could support previous notions of reduced critical evaluation in high hypnotizables (e.g., Dixon et al., 1990), correlations between hypnotizability and interrogative suggestibility are weak at best (Stein et al., 2022). Nevertheless, the evidence grossly supports the possibility that the reliance of several cognitive processes on previously learned information might be less rigid in high hypnotizables, leading to increased proneness to proactive interference, memory inaccuracies when given false leading information, and greater phenomenological control. These could also help explain other observations made across the literature, such as that highs are likely better in managing their pain (not necessarily through hypnosis; Faerman et al., 2021), report overall greater well-being (Biscuola et al., 2022), are more accepting of paranormal or spiritual beliefs, and tend toward external locus of control (Green & Hina, 2022).

The many parts of the relationships between hypnotizability and cognitive processes also highlight a key limitation of current and previous theories of hypnosis. As these theories make predictions on such relationships, they tend toward generalized, broad statements about cognition. For example, several theories refer to frontal, executive, or attentional functions, all of which represent an umbrella of specific cognitive abilities that vary among people, situations, and neurocognitive conditions. A more comprehensive approach to conceptualizing the cognitive underpinnings of hypnotizability, evidently, should address the building blocks rather than the overall structure. While this approach risks constructivist bias and might miss the mark when it comes to drawing practical predictions, it would allow the field to develop a precision medicine framework to hypnotizability and, hopefully, prove impactful on future clinical translations.

Hypnosis is one context, Western in its medically oriented approach, in which the neurocognitive systems that facilitate hypnotizability can be effectively engaged to lead to clinically meaningful change. It is highly likely that hypnosis is *not* the only context in which similar top-down modulations of conscious experiences can be evoked. For example, similarities have been drawn between hypnosis and various ritualistic healing traditions (Cardeña & Krippner, 2010). Although hypnotizability might not overlap perfectly with the extent and richness of veridical experiences in such contexts, some overlap is likely in neurocognitive mechanisms that facilitate these functions. That is not to say that hypnotizability is akin to a rich imagination. In their review of the link between hypnosis and imagination, Terhune and Oakley (2020) concluded that, while hypnotizability may associate with specific aspects of imagination, the evidence that imaginative abilities translate into hypnotic responsiveness is weak at best and that hypnosis and voluntary imaginative actions differ in their underlying neurocognitive mechanisms.

Limitations

As noted previously, there is very little overlap between studies on the neurocognitive tasks and measures used to conceptualize specific cognitive abilities. Furthermore, there seems to be a lack of consensus across different cognitive fields as to the boundaries of specific cognitive domains and, subsequently, their operational definitions (e.g., Baddeley, 2021). While here we assumed the conceptualization of clinical neuropsychology, disagreement on the cognitive ability primarily isolated by a given task could lead to different conclusions.

Additionally, the vast majority of studies into the neurocognitive correlates of hypnotizability utilize group comparisons between high, low, and rarely medium hypnotizables (Perri, 2021). While these designs allow for greater power in identifying effects, they pose obstacles on the path to understanding hypnotizability as a spectrum (e.g., by introducing extreme-groups effects; Jensen et al., 2017), despite evidence that hypnotizability is better conceptualized as a dimension rather than through taxonomic grouping (Reshetnikov & Terhune, 2022). Furthermore, a recent analysis of 66 normalization studies of hypnotizability measures (Peter & Roberts, 2022) found that almost 60% of the participants on whom the norms were created were college and university students (mostly psychology students), almost 30% were patients already treated with hypnosis, and more than 80% were told that they were about to participate in a hypnosis study. These findings highlight a clear risk of bias that serves as a hindrance in generalizing the norms to the general population. Therefore, it is possible that our categorization of high versus low hypnotizables is skewed, might mask observed effects, and could lead to conflicting evidence.

However, the major limitation in formalizing a clear understanding of the neuropsychological profiles of hypnotizability lies in the different ways the field has been conceptualizing and measuring hypnotizability. There is great variability in the domains and types of suggestions and, likely, their corresponding cognitive processes across commonly used hypnotizability measures (see Table 20.1 for a summary). Most, if not all hypnotizability measures attempt to capture a unitary global score representing an individual's ability to experience suggestions in hypnosis by testing responsiveness to a variety of suggestion domains and contents. Neuropsychological investigations acknowledge that global scores (e.g., general intelligence or g-factor) are less informative than considering cognitive domain subscores which are often required to identify individualized patterns (i.e., "profiles") in cognitive functioning. In the context of hypnotizability, this includes the finding that responsiveness to different domains of suggestions in hypnosis involves different brain networks or regions, even after controlling for demand characteristics (Landry et al., 2017; Perri et al., 2021). For example, hypnotic analgesia suggestions directed at the nociceptive aspects of pain are associated with involvement of the somatosensory cortex,

Table 20.1 Summary of Suggestion Domains Across Commonly Used Hypnotizability Measures

Suggestion Domain		*Suggestion Content*	*HGSHS:A*	*SHSS:A*	*SHSS:C*	*RSPS*	*HIP*	*BSS*	*SHCS*	*WSGC*	*EHS*	*SWASH*
Motor	**Facilitative**	Head falling	✓									
		Eye closure	✓	✓								
		Hand lowering	✓	✓	✓			✓	✓	✓		✓
		Moving hands together	✓	✓	✓				✓	✓		✓
		Arm levitation					✓	✓			✓	
		Postural sway		✓								
	Inhibitory	Immobilization	✓	✓	✓			✓		✓	✓	✓
		Finger lock	✓	✓				✓				
		Arm rigidity	✓	✓	✓					✓		✓
		Communication inhibition	✓	✓				✓				
		Eye catalepsy	✓									
Perceptual	**Facilitative**	Fly hallucination	✓		✓					✓		✓
		Visual hallucination		✓		✓					✓	
		Thirst hallucination						✓				
		Taste/olfactory hallucination			✓					✓		✓
		Auditory hallucination			✓	✓				✓		✓
		Kinesthetic hallucination					✓					
	Inhibitory	Anosmia			✓	✓						
		Negative visual hallucination			✓					✓		✓
		Analgesia				✓						
Cognitive	**Facilitative**	Posthypnotic suggestion	✓	✓	✓	✓		✓	✓	✓	✓	✓
		Dream			✓	✓			✓	✓		
		Age regression			✓	✓			✓	✓		
	Inhibitory	Amnesia	✓	✓	✓		✓	✓	✓	✓		✓
		Agency alteration					✓				✓	
		Agnosia				✓						
		Arithmetic impairment				✓						

Note. BSS = Barber Suggestibility Scale; EHS = Elkins Hypnotizability Scale; HGSHS:A = Harvard Group Scale of Hypnotic Susceptibility; HIP = Hypnotic Induction Profile; SHSS:A= Stanford Hypnotic Susceptibility Scale (Form A); SHSS:C = Stanford Hypnotic Susceptibility Scale (Form C); SHCS = Stanford Hypnotic Clinical Scales; RSPS = Revised Stanford Profile Scales (previously Stanford Profile Scales for Hypnotic Susceptibility); SWASH = Sussex-Waterloo Scale of Hypnotizability; WSGC = Waterloo-Stanford Group Scale of Hypnotic Susceptibility (Form C).

while targeting the affective or attentional components of experiencing pain shows greater ACC involvement (Landry et al., 2017). Likewise, among highly hypnotizable individuals, hypnotic suggestions to add color to a black and white grid resulted in both phenomenological increase in color perception and increased activation of the lingual and fusiform gyri of the visual system, while hypnotic suggestions to drain color from a color grid resulted in the opposite effect – decreased color perception and activity in those regions (Kosslyn et al., 2000). Similar neural representations can be seen in studies of hypnotic alexia. When suggestions state that the letters appear as "meaningless symbols ... and *you will not attempt to attribute any meaning* to them" (Raz et al., 2005, p. 9979), the ACC (a central note of the SN) shows reduced activation. However, when suggestions claim that "you know how difficult ... how *impossible it is to comprehend* the meaning of entirely foreign symbols" (Ulrich et al., 2015, p. 4), the reductions in neural activation are seen in temporal and supplementary motor areas, and pre- and post-central gyri, regions associated with semantic processing. As such, based on individual differences in the structures and functions of our neurocognitive real estate, people may differ in their responsiveness to different suggestion domains. This can lead to scenarios where individuals receive a similar hypnotizability score despite responding to different suggestion domains. Indeed, differential responsiveness to different suggestions has been evident since the early standardization of hypnotizability measurement (Hilgard et al., 1961; Shor & Orne, 1963).

Furthermore, all measures have "floors" and "ceilings," or limits to their ability to identify differences at the low and high ends of the hypnotizability spectrum. This is an important limitation of hypnotizability measurement, as highly hypnotizable individuals still show differential responsiveness (Barnier et al., 2014). Moreover, individuals at the ceiling of hypnotizability show discrete response patterns, indicating different subtypes of high hypnotizability (Terhune, 2015). Unfortunately, only a few studies addressed cognitive performance across the different subgroups of high hypnotizability (e.g., Terhune et al., 2011) and, therefore, could not be easily integrated into the current framework. Following these lines of evidence and seminal work by Woody (e.g., Woody & McConkey, 2003), Barnier et al. (2022) recently called for adopting a componential approach in hypnotizability research and practice, disengaging from the unitary construct of hypnotizability, and proposed a componential model to advance.

Conclusion

Hypnotizability is a complex cognitive ability that represents a person's capacity for a variety of experiences and ability to generate an array of behaviors in response to suggestions given in the context of hypnosis. The effects of hypnotizability appear to be greater in the context of hypnosis than outside of it. However, the evidence against a unique contribution of hypnotic inductions, alongside evidence of neurocognitive differences between high and low hypnotizables and reports of highly hypnotizable individuals' phenomenological control outside the context of hypnosis, indicates that the capacity captured by hypnotizability is unlikely to be exclusively applicable in the context of hypnosis.

The neuropsychological profiles of hypnotizability are difficult to pinpoint due to several limitations in the literature and inconsistent (and, at times, contradictory) findings. However, several potential differences between high and low hypnotizables are established, including better performance on simple attention tasks, a greater burden from increasing task complexity and time constraints, efficient cognitive flexibility, and potentially limited performance on some forms of inhibition. Taken together, hypnotizability is more likely an ability than a liability.

Disclosures

D.S. is co-founder of Reveri Health Inc., which offers an AI-based application providing self-hypnosis. A.F. is a consultant for Reveri Health Inc.

Notes

1 We discuss here the second-order DCT (Jamieson & Woody, 2007) rather than DCT as originally formulated (Woody & Bowers, 1994), which make slightly different predictions.
2 The vast majority of research on hypnosis and its use in clinical practice has utilized hypnosis almost exclusively in the form of verbal suggestions (mostly via speech and, to a lesser extent using printed text). Although it is possible the processes participating in the phenomenological and behavioral phenomena observed and reported in hypnosis could be engaged by other means (e.g., non-verbal visual stimuli, tactile stimuli, etc.), no clear evidence currently exists to our knowledge.

References

Aikins, D., & Ray, W. J. (2001). Frontal lobe contributions to hypnotic susceptibility: A neuropsychological screening of executive functioning. *International Journal of Clinical and Experimental Hypnosis*, *49*(4), 320–329.

Alexander, B., Turnbull, D., & Cyna, A. (2009). The effect of pregnancy on hypnotizability. *American Journal of Clinical Hypnosis*, *52*(1), 13–22. 10.1080/00029157.2009.10401688

Apelian, C., De Vignemont, F., & Terhune, D. B. (2023). Comparative effects of hypnotic suggestion and imagery instruction on bodily awareness. *Consciousness and Cognition*, *108*, 103473.

Baddeley, A. D. (2021). Developing the concept of working memory: The role of neuropsychology1. *Archives of Clinical Neuropsychology*, *36*(6), 861–873. 10.1093/arclin/acab060

Barabasz, M., & Spiegel, D. (1989). Hypnotizability and weight loss in obese subjects. *International Journal of Eating Disorders*, *8*(3), 335–341. 10.1002/1098-108X(198905)8:3<335::AID-EAT2260080309>3.0.CO;2-O

Barnier, A. J., Cox, R. E., & McConkey, K. M. (2014). The province of "highs": The high hypnotizable person in the science of hypnosis and in psychological science. *Psychology of Consciousness: Theory, Research, and Practice*, *1*(2), 168–183. 10.1037/cns0000018

Barnier, A. J., & McConkey, K. M. (1992). Reports of real and false memories: The relevance of hypnosis, hypnotizability, and context of memory test. *J Abnorm Psychol*, *101*(3), 521–527.

Barnier, A. J., Terhune, D. B., Polito, V., & Woody, E. Z. (2022). A componential approach to individual differences in hypnotizability. *Psychology of Consciousness: Theory, Research, and Practice*, *9*(2), 130–140. 10.1037/cns0000267

Bauman, D. E., & Bul, P. I. (1981). Human inheritability of hypnotizability. *Genetika*, *17*(2), 352–356.

Bellone, J., & Van Patten, R. (2021). What Is neuropsychology? In J. A. Bellone, & R. Van Patten (Eds.), *Becoming a neuropsychologist: Advice and guidance for students and trainees* (pp. 3–28). Springer International Publishing. 10.1007/978-3-030-63174-1_1

Benham, G., Woody, E. Z., Wilson, K. S., & Nash, M. R. (2006). Expect the unexpected: Ability, attitude, and responsiveness to hypnosis. *Journal of Personality and Social Psychology*, *91*(2), 342–350. 10.1037/0022-3514.91.2.342

Biscuola, E., Bongini, M., Belcari, I., Santarcangelo, E. L., & Sebastiani, L. (2022). Well-being in highly hypnotizable persons. *International Journal of Clinical and Experimental Hypnosis*, *70*(2), 123–135. 10.1080/00207144.2022.2049972

Blum, G. S., & Graef, J. R. (1971). The detection over time of subjects simulating hypnosis. *International Journal of Clinical and Experimental Hypnosis*, *19*(4), 211–224. 10.1080/00207147108407168

Braffman, W., & Kirsch, I. (1999). Imaginative suggestibility and hypnotizability: An empirical analysis. *Journal of Personality and Social Psychology*, *77*(3), 578–587. 10.1037/0022-3514.77.3.578
Braffman, W., & Kirsch, I. (2001). Reaction time as a predictor of imaginative suggestibility and hypnotizability. *Contemporary Hypnosis*, *18*(3), 107–107.
Bryant, R. A., Hung, L., Dobson-Stone, C., & Schofield, P. R. (2013). The association between the oxytocin receptor gene (OXTR) and hypnotizability. *Psychoneuroendocrinology*, *38*(10), 1979–1984. 10.1016/j.psyneuen.2013.03.002
Callara, A., Fontanelli, L., Belcari, I., Rho, G., Greco, A., Zelič, Ž., Sebastiani, L., & Santarcangelo, E. (2023). Modulation of the heartbeat evoked cortical potential by hypnotizability and hypnosis. *Psychophysiology*. e14309. 10.22541/au.167407911.13110099/v1
Cardeña, E., & Krippner, S. (2010). The cultural context of hypnosis. In S. J. Lynn , J. W. Rhue , & I. Kirsch (Eds.), *Handbook of clinical hypnosis, 2nd ed.* (pp. 743–771). American Psychological Association. 10.2307/j.ctv1chs5qj.34
Castellani, E., Alessandro, L. D., & Sebastiani Laura, L. (2007). Hypnotizability and spatial attentional functions. *Archives Italiennes de Biologie*, *145*(1), 23–3710.4449/aib.v145i1.864
Cojan, Y., Piguet, C., & Vuilleumier, P. (2015). What makes your brain suggestible? Hypnotizability is associated with differential brain activity during attention outside hypnosis. *NeuroImage*, *117*, 367–374. 10.1016/j.neuroimage.2015.05.076
Coltheart, M., Cox, R., Sowman, P., Morgan, H., Barnier, A., Langdon, R., Connaughton, E., Teichmann, L., Williams, N., & Polito, V. (2018). Belief, delusion, hypnosis, and the right dorsolateral prefrontal cortex: A transcranial magnetic stimulation study. *Cortex*, *101*, 234–248. 10.1016/j.cortex.2018.01.001
Cordi, M. J., & Rasch, B. (2022). Hypnotizability may relate to interoceptive ability to accurately perceive sleep depth: An exploratory study. *International Journal of Clinical and Experimental Hypnosis*, *70*(4), 385–402. 10.1080/00207144.2022.2130068
Cortade, D. L., Markovits, J., Spiegel, D., & Wang, S. X. (2023). Point-of-care testing of enzyme polymorphisms for predicting hypnotizability and postoperative pain. *The Journal of Molecular Diagnostics*, *25*(4), 197–210. 10.1016/j.jmoldx.2023.01.002
Crawford, H. J. (1994). Brain dynamics and hypnosis: Attentional and disattentional processes. *International Journal of Clinical and Experimental Hypnosis*, *42*(3), 204–232. 10.1080/0020714 9408409352
Crawford, H. J., & Gruzelier, J. H. (1992). A midstream view of the neuropsychophysiology of hypnosis: Recent research and future directions. In E. Fromm, & M. R. Nash (Eds.), *Contemporary hypnosis research* (pp. 227–266). Guilford Press.
Dasse, M. N., Elkins, G. R., & Weaver, C. A. (2015). Hypnotizability, not suggestion, influences false memory development. *International Journal of Clinical and Experimental Hypnosis*, *63*(1), 110–128. 10.1080/00207144.2014.961880
David, D., & Brown, R. J. (2002). Suggestibility and negative priming: Two replication studies. *International Journal of Clinical and Experimental Hypnosis*, *50*(3), 215–228. 10.1080/0020714 0208410100
DeSouza, D. D., Stimpson, K. H., Baltusis, L., Sacchet, M. D., Gu, M., Hurd, R., Wu, H., Yeomans, D. C., Willliams, N., & Spiegel, D. (2020). Association between anterior cingulate neurochemical concentration and individual differences in hypnotizability. *Cerebral Cortex*, *30*(6), 3644–3654. 10.1093/cercor/bhz332
Dienes, Z., Brown, E., Hutton, S., Kirsch, I., Mazzoni, G., & Wright, D. B. (2009). Hypnotic suggestibility, cognitive inhibition, and dissociation. *Consciousness and Cognition*, *18*(4), 837–847. 10.1016/j.concog.2009.07.009
Dienes, Z., & Hutton, S. (2013). Understanding hypnosis metacognitively: RTMS applied to left DLPFC increases hypnotic suggestibility. *Cortex*, *49*(2), 386–392. 10.1016/j.cortex.2012.07.009
Dienes, Z., Lush, P., Palfi, B., Roseboom, W., Scott, R., Parris, B., Seth, A., & Lovell, M. (2022). Phenomenological control as cold control. *Psychology of Consciousness: Theory, Research, and Practice*, *9*(2), 101–116. 10.1037/cns0000230
Dienes, Z., & Perner, J. (2007). Executive control without conscious awareness: The cold control theory of hypnosis. In G. A. Jamieson (Ed.), *Hypnosis and conscious states: The cognitive neuroscience perspective* (pp. 293–314).

Dixon, M., Brunet, A., & Laurence, J. R. (1990). Hypnotizability and automaticity: Toward a parallel distributed processing model of hypnotic responding. *Journal of Abnormal Psychology*, *99*(4), 336–343.

Dixon, M., & Laurence, J.-R. (1992). Hypnotic susceptibility and verbal automaticity: Automatic and strategic processing differences in the Stroop color-naming task. *Journal of Abnormal Psychology*, *101*(2), 344. 10.1037/0021-843X.101.2.344

Egner, T., Jamieson, G., & Gruzelier, J. (2005). Hypnosis decouples cognitive control from conflict monitoring processes of the frontal lobe. *NeuroImage*, *27*(4), 969–978. 10.1016/j.neuroimage.2005.05.002

Elkins, G. R., Barabasz, A. F., Council, J. R., & Spiegel, D. (2015). Advancing research and practice: The revised APA Division 30 definition of hypnosis. *International Journal of Clinical and Experimental Hypnosis*, *63*(1), 1–9. 10.1080/00207144.2014.961870

Faerman, A., & Spiegel, D. (2021). Shared cognitive mechanisms of hypnotizability with executive functioning and information salience. *Scientific Reports*, *11*(1), Article 1. 10.1038/s41598-021-84954-8

Faerman, A., Stimpson, K. H., Bishop, J. H., Neri, E., Phillips, A., Gülser, M., Amin, H., Nejad, R., Fotros, A., Williams, N. R., & Spiegel, D. (2021). Hypnotic predictors of agency: Responsiveness to specific suggestions in hypnosis is associated with involuntariness in fibromyalgia. *Consciousness and Cognition*, *96*, 103221. 10.1016/j.concog.2021.103221

Farvolden, P., & Woody, E. Z. (2004). Hypnosis, memory, and frontal executive functioning. *International Journal of Clinical and Experimental Hypnosis*, *52*(1), 3–26. 10.1076/iceh.52.1.3.23926

Folden, D. (2014). Frontal lobe function. In M. W. Parsons, T. A. Hammeke, & P. J. Snyder (Eds.), *Clinical neuropsychology: A pocket handbook for assessment* (pp. 498–524). American Psychological Association. https://www.jstor.org/stable/j.ctv1chs48b

Green, J. P. (2012). The Valencia Scale of Attitudes and Beliefs Toward Hypnosis–Client version and hypnotizability. *International Journal of Clinical and Experimental Hypnosis*, *60*(2), 229–240. 10.1080/00207144.2012.648073

Green, J. P., & Hina, S. R. (2022). God locus of health control, paranormal beliefs, and hypnotizability. *International Journal of Clinical and Experimental Hypnosis*, *70*(2), 174–195. 10.1080/00207144.2022.2049445

Hilgard, E. R. (1973). A neodissociation interpretation of pain reduction in hypnosis. *Psychological Review*, *80*(5), 396. 10.1037/h0020073

Hilgard, E. R. (1991). A neodissociation interpretation of hypnosis. In S. J. Lynn & J. W. Rhue (Eds.), *Theories of hypnosis: Current models and perspectives* (pp. 83–104). Guilford Press.

Hilgard, E. R., Weitzenhoffer, A. M., Landes, J., & Moore, R. K. (1961). The distribution of susceptibility to hypnosis in a student population: A study using the Stanford Hypnotic Susceptibility Scale. *Psychological Monographs: General and Applied*, *75*(8), 1–22. 10.1037/h0093802

Hoeft, F., Gabrieli, J. D. E., Whitfield-Gabrieli, S., Haas, B. W., Bammer, R., Menon, V., & Spiegel, D. (2012). Functional brain basis of hypnotizability. *Archives of General Psychiatry*, *69*(10), 1064–1072. 10.1001/archgenpsychiatry.2011.2190

Ibáñez-Marcelo, E., Campioni, L., Phinyomark, A., Petri, G., & Santarcangelo, E. L. (2019). Topology highlights mesoscopic functional equivalence between imagery and perception: The case of hypnotizability. *NeuroImage*, *200*, 437–449. 10.1016/j.neuroimage.2019.06.044

Jamieson, G. A. (2022). An insula view of predictive processing in hypnotic responses. *Psychology of Consciousness: Theory, Research, and Practice*, *9*(2), 117–129. 10.1037/cns0000266

Jamieson, G. A., & Woody, E. (2007). Dissociated control as a paradigm for cognitive neuroscience research and theorizing in hypnosis. In G. A. Jamieson (Ed.), *Hypnosis and conscious states: The cognitive neuroscience perspective* (pp. 111–129). Oxford University Press.

Jensen, M. P., Jamieson, G. A., Lutz, A., Mazzoni, G., McGeown, W. J., Santarcangelo, E. L., Demertzi, A., De Pascalis, V., Banyai, E. I., Rominger, C., Vuilleumier, P., Faymonville, M. E., & Terhune, D. B. (2017). New directions in hypnosis research: Strategies for advancing the cognitive and clinical neuroscience of hypnosis. *Neuroscience of Consciousness*, *3*(1), 1–14.

Jiang, H., White, M. P., Greicius, M. D., Waelde, L. C., & Spiegel, D. (2017). Brain activity and functional connectivity associated with hypnosis. *Cerebral Cortex*, *27*(8), 4083–4093. 10.1093/cercor/bhw220

Kaiser, J., Barker, R., Haenschel, C., Baldeweg, T., & Gruzelier, J. H. (1997). Hypnosis and event-related potential correlates of error processing in a stroop-type paradigm: A test of the frontal hypothesis. *International Journal of Psychophysiology*, *27*(3), 215–222. 10.1016/S0167-8760(97)00055-X

Katonai, E. R., Szekely, A., Vereczkei, A., Sasvari-Szekely, M., Bányai, É. I., & Varga, K. (2017). Dopaminergic and serotonergic genotypes and the subjective experiences of hypnosis. *International Journal of Clinical and Experimental Hypnosis*, *65*(4), 379–397. 10.1080/00207144.2017.1348848

Khodaverdi-Khani, M., & Laurence, J.-R. (2016). Working memory and hypnotizability. *Psychology of Consciousness: Theory, Research, and Practice*, *3*(1), 80–92. 10.1037/cns0000058

Kihlstrom, J. F., Glisky, M. L., McGovern, S., Rapcsak, S. Z., & Mennemeier, M. S. (2013). Hypnosis in the right hemisphere. *Cortex*, *49*(2), 393–399. 10.1016/j.cortex.2012.04.018

Kirsch, I. (2001). The response set theory of hypnosis: Expectancy and physiology. *American Journal of Clinical Hypnosis*, *44*(1), 69–73. 10.1080/00029157.2001.10403458

Kirsch, I., & Braffman, W. (2001). Imaginative suggestibility and hypnotizability. *Current Directions in Psychological Science*, *10*(2), 57–61. 10.1111/1467-8721.00115

Kirsch, I., & Lynn, S. J. (1998). Social–cognitive alternatives to dissociation theories of hypnotic involuntariness. *Review of General Psychology*, *2*(1), 66–80. 10.1037/1089-2680.2.1.66

Kittle, J., Zhao, E., Stimpson, K., Weng, Y., & Spiegel, D. (2021). Testing hypnotizability by phone: Development and validation of the remote hypnotic induction profile (rHIP). *International Journal of Clinical and Experimental Hypnosis*, *69*(1), 94–111. 10.1080/00207144.2021.1827937

Knox, V. J., Gekoski, W. L., Shum, K., & Mclaughlin, D. M. (1981). Analgesia for experimentally induced pain: Multiple sessions of acupuncture compared to hypnosis in high- and low-susceptible subjects. *Journal of Abnormal Psychology*, *90*, 28–34.

Kosslyn, S. M., Thompson, W. L., Costantini-Ferrando, M. F., Alpert, N. M., & Spiegel, D. (2000). Hypnotic visual illusion alters color processing in the brain. *American Journal of Psychiatry*, *157*(8), 1279–1284. 10.1176/appi.ajp.157.8.1279

Kosslyn, S. M., Thompson, W. L., & Ganis, G. (2006). *The case for mental imagery*. Oxford University Press.

Laurence, J.-R., Beaulieu-Prévost, D., & Chéné, T. du. (2008). Measuring and understanding individual differences in hypnotizability. In M. Nash , & A. Barnier (Eds.), *The Oxford handbook of hypnosis: Theory, research, and practice* (pp. 225–253). Oxford University Press.

Landry, M., Lifshitz, M., & Raz, A. (2017). Brain correlates of hypnosis: A systematic review and meta-analytic exploration. *Neuroscience & Biobehavioral Reviews*, *81*, 75–98. 10.1016/j.neubiorev.2017.02.020

Laurence, J.-R., & Perry, C. (1988). *Hypnosis, will, and memory: A psycho-legal history* (p. xxi, 432). Guilford Press.

Lichtenberg, P., Bachner-Melman, R., Ebstein, R. P., & Crawford, H. J. (2004). Hypnotic susceptibility: Multidimensional relationships with Cloninger's tridimensional personality questionnaire, COMT polymorphisms, absorption, and attentional characteristics. *International Journal of Clinical and Experimental Hypnosis*, *52*(1), 47–72. 10.1076/iceh.52.1.47.23922

Lichtenberg, P., Bachner-Melman, R., Gritsenko, I., & Ebstein, R. P. (2000). Exploratory association study between catechol-O-methyltransferase (COMT) high/low enzyme activity polymorphism and hypnotizability. *American Journal of Medical Genetics*, *96*(6), 771–774. 10.1002/1096-8628(20001204)96:6<771::AID-AJMG14>3.0.CO;2-T

Lifshitz, M., & Raz, A. (2015). Hypnotic ability and baseline attention: FMRI findings from Stroop interference. *Psychology of Consciousness: Theory, Research, and Practice*, *2*(2), 134–143. 10.1037/cns0000050

Lush, P., Scott, R. B., Moga, G., & Dienes, Z. (2021). Computer versus live delivery of the Sussex Waterloo Scale of Hypnotizability (SWASH). *Psychology of Consciousness: Theory, Research, and Practice*. 10.1037/cns0000292

Lynn, S. J., Meyer, E., & Shindler, K. (2004). Clinical correlates of high hypnotizability. In M. Heap, R. J. Brown, & D. A. Oakley (Eds.), *The highly hypnotizable person: Theoretical, experimental and clinical issues* (pp. 187–212). Routledge.

Lynn, S. J., & Shindler, K. (2002). The role of hypnotizability assessment in treatment. *American Journal of Clinical Hypnosis*, *44*(3–4), 185–197. 10.1080/00029157.2002.10403479

Lynn, S. J., Shindler, K., & Meyer, E. (2003). Hypnotic suggestibility, psychopathology, and treatment outcome. *Sleep and Hypnosis*, *5*(1), 17–25.
Malinoski, P. T., & Lynn, S. J. (1999). The plasticity of early memory reports: Social pressure, hypnotizability, compliance and interrogative suggestibility. *International Journal of Clinical and Experimental Hypnosis*, *47*(4), 320–345. 10.1080/00207149908410040
Martin, J.-R. (2019). Bayes to the rescue: Does the type of hypnotic induction matter? *Psychology of Consciousness: Theory, Research, and Practice*, *6*(4), 359. 10.1037/cns0000189
Martin, J.-R., & Pacherie, E. (2019). Alterations of agency in hypnosis: A new predictive coding model. *Psychological Review*, *126*(1), 133–152. 10.1037/rev0000134
Martin, J.-R., Sackur, J., & Dienes, Z. (2018). Attention or instruction: Do sustained attentional abilities really differ between high and low hypnotisable persons? *Psychological Research*, *82*(4), 700–707. 10.1007/s00426-017-0850-1
McGlashan, T. H., Evans, F. J., Orne, M. T., Neisser, U., O'connell, D. N., Orne, E. C., Paskewitz, D. A., & Perry, C. W. (1969). The nature of hypnotic analgesia and placebo response to experimental pain. *Psychosomatic Medicine*, *31*(3), 227–246.
Menon, V. (2021). Dissociation by network integration. *American Journal of Psychiatry*, *178*(2), 110–112. 10.1176/appi.ajp.2020.20121728
Meyer, E. C., & Lynn, S. J. (2011). Responding to hypnotic and nonhypnotic suggestions: *Performance standards, imaginative suggestibility, and response expectancies. International Journal of Clinical and Experimental Hypnosis*, *59*(3), 327–349. 10.1080/00207144.2011.570660
Miles, S., Howlett, C. A., Berryman, C., Nedeljkovic, M., Moseley, G. L., & Phillipou, A. (2021). Considerations for using the Wisconsin Card Sorting Test to assess cognitive flexibility. *Behavior Research Methods*, *53*(5), 2083–2091. 10.3758/s13428-021-01551-3
Miller, M. E., & Bowers, K. S. (1986). Hypnotic analgesia and stress inoculation in the reduction of pain. *Journal of Abnormal Psychology*, *95*(1), 6. 10.1037/0021-843X.95.1.6
Milling, L. S., Kirsch, I., Allen, G. J., & Reutenauer, E. L. (2005). The effects of hypnotic and nonhypnotic imaginative suggestion on pain. *Annals of Behavioral Medicine*, *29*(2), 116–127. 10.1207/s15324796abm2902_6
Milling, L. S., Valentine, K. E., LoStimolo, L. M., Nett, A. M., & McCarley, H. S. (2021). Hypnosis and the alleviation of clinical pain: A comprehensive meta-analysis. *International Journal of Clinical and Experimental Hypnosis*, *69*(3), 297–322. 10.1080/00207144.2021.1920330
Mioli, A., Diolaiuti, F., Zangrandi, A., Orsini, P., Sebastiani, L., & Santarcangelo, E. L. (2021). Multisensory integration is modulated by hypnotizability. *International Journal of Clinical and Experimental Hypnosis*, *69*(2), 215–224. 10.1080/00207144.2021.1877089
Mitchell, M. B. (1970). Hypnotizability and distractibility. *American Journal of Clinical Hypnosis*, *13*(1), 35–45. 10.1080/00029157.1970.10402076
Molina-Peral, J. A., Rodríguez, J. S.-, Capafons, A., & Mendoza, M. E. (2020). Attitudes toward hypnosis based on source of information and experience with hypnosis. *American Journal of Clinical Hypnosis*, *62*(3), 282–297. 10.1080/00029157.2019.1584741
Morgan, A. H. (1973). The heritability of hypnotic susceptibility in twins. *Journal of Abnormal Psychology*, *82*(1), 55–61. 10.1037/h0034854
Nordby, H., Hugdahl, K., Jasiukaitis, P., & Spiegel, D. (1999). Effects of hypnotizability on performance of a Stroop task and event-related potentials. *Perceptual and Motor Skills*, *88*(3), 819–830. 10.2466/pms.1999.88.3.819
Orne, M. T. (1962). On the social psychology of the psychological experiment: With particular reference to demand characteristics and their implications. *American Psychologist*, *17*(11), 776–783. 10.1037/h0043424
Page, R. A., & Green, J. P. (2007). An update on age, hypnotic suggestibility, and gender: A brief report. *American Journal of Clinical Hypnosis*, *49*(4), 283–287. 10.1080/00029157.2007.10524505
Parris, B. A. (2016). The prefrontal cortex and suggestion: Hypnosis vs. placebo effects. *Frontiers in Psychology*, *7*, 211–229. 10.3389/fpsyg.2016.00415
Parris, B. A. (2017). The role of frontal executive functions in hypnosis and hypnotic suggestibility. *Psychology of Consciousness: Theory, Research, and Practice*, *4*(2), 211–229. 10.1037/cns0000106
Perri, R. L. (2021). In medio stat virtus: The importance of studying mediums in hypnosis research. *American Journal of Clinical Hypnosis*, *64*(1), 4–11. 10.1080/00029157.2020.1859980

Perri, R. L., Bianco, V., Facco, E., & Di Russo, F. (2021). Now you see one letter, now you see meaningless symbols: Perceptual and semantic hypnotic suggestions reduce Stroop errors through different neurocognitive mechanisms. *Frontiers in Neuroscience, 14*. https://www.frontiersin.org/articles/10.3389/fnins.2020.600083

Peter, B., & Roberts, R. L. (2022). Hypnotizability norms may not be representative of the general population: Potential sample and self-selection bias considerations. *International Journal of Clinical and Experimental Hypnosis, 70*(1), 49–67. 10.1080/00207144.2021.2003694

Piccione, C., Hilgard, E. R., & Zimbardo, P. G. (1989). On the degree of stability of measured hypnotizability over a 25-year period. *Journal of Personality and Social Psychology, 56*(2), 289–295. 10.1037/0022-3514.56.2.289

Poulsen, B. C., & Matthews Jr, W. J. (2003). Correlates of imaginative and hypnotic suggestibility in children. *Contemporary Hypnosis, 20*(4), 198–208. 10.1002/ch.278

Presciuttini, S., Carli, G., & Santarcangelo, E. L. (2020). Hypnotizability-related FAAH C385A polymorphism: Possible endocannabinoid contribution to suggestion-induced analgesia. *International Journal of Clinical and Experimental Hypnosis, 68*(1), 29–37. 10.1080/00207144.2020.1682254

Presciuttini, S., Curcio, M., Chillemi, R., Barbuti, S., Scatena, F., Carli, G., Ghelarducci, B., & Santarcangelo, E. L. (2009). Promoter polymorphisms of the NOS3 gene are associated with hypnotizability-dependent vascular response to nociceptive stimulation. *Neuroscience Letters, 467*(3), 252–255. 10.1016/j.neulet.2009.10.056

Presciuttini, S., Curcio, M., Sciarrino, R., Scatena, F., Jensen, M. P., & Santarcangelo, E. L. (2018). Polymorphism of opioid receptors µ1 in highly hypnotizable subjects. *International Journal of Clinical and Experimental Hypnosis, 66*(1), 106–118. 10.1080/00207144.2018.1396128

Presciuttini, S., Gialluisi, A., Barbuti, S., Curcio, M., Scatena, F., Carli, G., & Santarcangelo, E. L. (2014). Hypnotizability and catechol-O-methyltransferase (COMT) polymorphysms in Italians. *Frontiers in Human Neuroscience, 7*. 10.3389/fnhum.2013.00929

Priebe, F. A., & Wallace, B. (1986). Hypnotizability, imaging ability, and the detection of embedded objects. *International Journal of Clinical and Experimental Hypnosis, 34*(4), 320–329. 10.1080/00207148608406997

Raz, A. (2005). Attention and hypnosis: Neural substrates and genetic associations of two converging processes. *International Journal of Clinical and Experimental Hypnosis, 53*(3), 237–258. 10.1080/00207140590961295

Raz, A., Fan, J., & Posner, M. I. (2005). Hypnotic suggestion reduces conflict in the human brain. *Proceedings of the National Academy of Sciences of the United States of America, 102*(28), 9978–9983. 10.1073/pnas.0503064102

Raz, A., Fan, J., & Posner, M. I. (2006). Neuroimaging and genetic associations of attentional and hypnotic processes. *Journal of Physiology-Paris, 99*(4–6), 483–491. 10.1016/j.jphysparis.2006.03.003

Reshetnikov, M., & Terhune, D. B. (2022). Taxometric evidence for a dimensional latent structure of hypnotic suggestibility. *Consciousness and Cognition, 98*, 103269. 10.1016/j.concog.2022.103269

Rominger, C., Weiss, E. M., Nagl, S., Niederstätter, H., Parson, W., & Papousek, I. (2014). Carriers of the COMT Met/Met allele have higher degrees of hypnotizability, provided that they have good attentional control: A case of gene–trait interaction. *International Journal of Clinical and Experimental Hypnosis, 62*(4), 455–482. 10.1080/00207144.2014.931177

Rosati, A., Belcari, I., Santarcangelo, E. L., & Sebastiani, L. (2021). Interoceptive accuracy as a function of hypnotizability. *International Journal of Clinical and Experimental Hypnosis, 64*(4), 1–12. 10.1080/00207144.2021.1954859

Rubichi, S., Ricci, F., Padovani, R., & Scaglietti, L. (2005). Hypnotic susceptibility, baseline attentional functioning, and the Stroop task. *Consciousness and Cognition, 14*(2), 296–303. 10.1016/j.concog.2004.08.003

Sattler, J. M., & Ryan, J. J. (2009). *Assessment with the WAIS-IV*. Jerome M Sattler Publisher.

Scacchia, P., & De Pascalis, V. (2020). Effects of prehypnotic instructions on hypnotizability and relationships between hypnotizability, absorption, and empathy. *American Journal of Clinical Hypnosis, 62*(3), 231–266. 10.1080/00029157.2019.1586639

Schmidt, B., Hecht, H., Naumann, E., & Miltner, W. H. R. (2017). The power of mind: Blocking visual perception by hypnosis. *Scientific Reports*, *7*(1), Article 1. 10.1038/s41598-017-05195-2
Sharav, Y., Haviv, Y., & Tal, M. (2023). Placebo or nocebo interventions as affected by hypnotic susceptibility. *Applied Sciences*, *13*(2), Article 2. 10.3390/app13020931
Sheehan, P. W., Donovan, P., & MacLeod, C. M. (1988). Strategy manipulation and the Stroop effect in hypnosis. *Journal of Abnormal Psychology*, *97*, 455–460.
Shor, R. E., & Orne, E. C. (1963). Norms on the Harvard Group Scale of Hypnotic Susceptibility, Form A. *International Journal of Clinical and Experimental Hypnosis*, *11*(1), 39–47. 10.1080/00207146308409226
Simpson, E. H., Morud, J., Winiger, V., Biezonski, D., Zhu, J. P., Bach, M. E., Malleret, G., Polan, H. J., Ng-Evans, S., Phillips, P. E. M., Kellendonk, C., & Kandel, E. R. (2014). Genetic variation in COMT activity impacts learning and dopamine release capacity in the striatum. *Learning & Memory*, *21*(4), 205–214. 10.1101/lm.032094.113
Sliwinski, J. R., & Elkins, G. R. (2017). Hypnotherapy to reduce hot flashes: Examination of response expectancies as a mediator of outcomes. *Journal of Evidence-Based Complementary & Alternative Medicine*, *22*(4), 652–659. 10.1177/2156587217708523
Spanos, N. P., Perlini, A. H., & Robertson, L. A. (1989). Hypnosis, suggestion, and placebo in the reduction of experimental pain. *Journal of Abnormal Psychology*, *98*(3), 285–293.
Spiegel, D., & Albert, L. H. (1983). Naloxone fails to reverse hypnotic alleviation of chronic pain. *Psychopharmacology*, *81*(2), 140–143. 10.1007/BF00429008
Spiegel, D., Frischholz, E. J. D. P., Fleiss, J. L. D. P., & Spiegel, H. (1993). Predictors of smoking abstinence following a single-session restructuring intervention with self-hypnosis. *American Journal of Psychiatry*, *150*, 1090–1097.
Spiegel, D., & King, R. (1992). Hypnotizability and CSF HVA levels among psychiatric patients. *Biological Psychiatry*, *31*(1), 95–98. 10.1016/0006-3223(92)90009-O
Srzich, A. J., Cirillo, J., Stinear, J. W., Coxon, J. P., McMorland, A. J. C., & Anson, J. G. (2019). Does hypnotic susceptibility influence information processing speed and motor cortical preparatory activity? *Neuropsychologia*, *129*, 179–190. 10.1016/j.neuropsychologia.2019.03.014
Stein, M. V., Faerman, A., Thompson, T., Kirsch, I., Lynn, S. J., & Terhune, D. B. (2022). *Revisiting the domain of suggestion: A meta-analysis of suggestibility across different contexts*. Association of the Scientific Study of Consciousness.
Szekely, A., Kovacs-Nagy, R., Bányai, É. I., Gősi-Greguss, A. C., Varga, K., Halmai, Z., Ronai, Z., & Sasvari-Szekely, M. (2010). Association between hypnotizability and the catechol-O-methyltransferase (COMT) polymorphism. *International Journal of Clinical and Experimental Hypnosis*, *58*(3), 301–315. 10.1080/00207141003760827
Tellegen, A. (1978). On measures and conceptions of hypnosis. *American Journal of Clinical Hypnosis*, *21*(2–3), 219–237. 10.1080/00029157.1978.10403973
Terhune, D. B. (2015). Discrete response patterns in the upper range of hypnotic suggestibility: A latent profile analysis. *Consciousness and Cognition*, *33*, 334–341. 10.1016/j.concog.2015.01.018
Terhune, D. B., & Cardeña, E. (2016). Nuances and uncertainties regarding hypnotic inductions: Toward a theoretically informed praxis. *American Journal of Clinical Hypnosis*, *59*(2), 155–174. 10.1080/00029157.2016.1201454
Terhune, D. B., Cardeña, E., & Lindgren, M. (2011). Dissociative tendencies and individual differences in high hypnotic suggestibility. *Cognitive Neuropsychiatry*, *16*(2), 113–135. 10.1080/13546805.2010.503048
Terhune, D. B., Cleeremans, A., Raz, A., & Lynn, S. J. (2017). Hypnosis and top-down regulation of consciousness. *Neuroscience & Biobehavioral Reviews*, *81*, 59–74. 10.1016/j.neubiorev.2017.02.002
Terhune, D. B., & Oakley, D. A. (2020). Hypnosis and imagination. In A. Abraham, (Ed), *The Cambridge Handbook of the Imagination* (pp. 711–727). Cambridge University Press. https://www.cambridge.org/core/books/cambridge-handbook-of-the-imagination/B4080A5A7D13689D97D73E916A8DDDA5
Thompson, T., Terhune, D. B., Oram, C., Sharangparni, J., Rouf, R., Solmi, M., Veronese, N., & Stubbs, B. (2019). The effectiveness of hypnosis for pain relief: A systematic review and meta-analysis of 85 controlled experimental trials. *Neuroscience & Biobehavioral Reviews*, *99*, 298–310. 10.1016/j.neubiorev.2019.02.013

Ulrich, M., Kiefer, M., Bongartz, W., Grön, G., & Hoenig, K. (2015). Suggestion-induced modulation of semantic priming during functional magnetic resonance imaging. *PLoS ONE*, *10*(4). 10.1371/journal.pone.0123686

Varga, K., Németh, Z., & Szekely, A. (2011). Lack of correlation between hypnotic susceptibility and various components of attention. *Consciousness and Cognition*, *20*(4), 1872–1881. 10.1016/j.concog.2011.09.008

Wagstaff, G. F. (2004). High hypnotizability in a sociocognitive framework. In M. Heap, R. Brown, & D. Oakley (Eds.), *The Highly Hypnotizable Person* (pp. 85–14). Routledge.

Wagstaff, G. F., Cole, J., Wheatcroft, J., Anderton, A., & Madden, H. (2008). Reducing and reversing pseudomemories with hypnosis. *Contemporary Hypnosis*, *25*(3–4), 178–191. 10.1002/ch.366

Wechsler, D. (2008). *Wechsler Adult Intelligence Scale, Fourth Edition: Technical and interpretive manual* (4th ed.). Psychological Corporation.

Woody, E. Z., & McConkey, K. M. (2003). What we don't know about the brain and hypnosis, but need to: A view from the Buckhorn Inn. *International Journal of Clinical and Experimental Hypnosis*, *51*(3), 309–338. 10.1076/iceh.51.3.309.15523

21
PHYSIOLOGICAL CORRELATES OF HYPNOTIZABILITY

Enrica L. Santarcangelo

Department of Translational Research, University of Pisa, Pisa, Italy

The latest report of the American Psychological Association (Elkins et al., 2015) defined hypnotizability as "an individual's ability to experience suggested alterations in physiology, sensations, emotions, thoughts, or behavior during hypnosis". The suggested alterations consist of the request to imagine and experience cognitive-emotional and sensorimotor contexts different from the real ones. Nonetheless, hypnotizability modulates the effects of suggestions also in the ordinary state of consciousness, although sometimes less than during hypnosis (DeBenedittis et al., 1989; Derbyshire et al., 2009). Moreover, experimental evidence shows that it is associated with physiological correlates in the absence of suggestions (Santarcangelo & Scattina, 2016). This chapter reports such evidence and shows that hypnotizability is a very pervasive trait influencing everyday life in several domains.

Genetic Markers

Catechol-O-Methyltransferase

Attention is more efficiently controlled in subjects with the Met/Met or Val/Met variant of the single nucleotide polymorphism rs4680 of the catechol-O-methyltransferase (COMT) gene than in the homozygous Val/Val individuals. This depends on the Met-carriers less efficient enzymatic activity resulting in higher dopamine content in the prefrontal and anterior cingulate cortices. Met carriers have more pronounced attentional stability, whereas Val/Val homozygous individuals exhibit greater proneness to shift attention from one object to another one (Colzato et al., 2010). Nonetheless, a few authors failed to demonstrate any correlation between COMT polymorphism and executive attention (Fossella et al., 2002).

Most research reported higher frequency of Val/Met polymorphism in highs than in low hypnotizable individuals (lows) (Storozheva et al., 2018). In contrast, one study found that the association between Val/Met polymorphism and high hypnotizability was significant in females only (Lichtenberg et al., 2000), another reported that it was significant only if hypnotizability was paired with high attentional abilities (Rominger et al., 2014) and other authors did not find any difference between highs and lows

DOI: 10.4324/9781003449126-29

(Bryant et al., 2013; Presciuttini et al., 2014). Moreover, the highs' greater proneness to "absorption" – i.e., attention deeply focused on mental images, implying attentional stability – which was suggested for highs in the 1970s (Tellegen & Atkinson, 1974) at least in specific conditions (Tellegen, 1981) – has not been unanimously confirmed (Vanhaudenhuyse et al., 2019). Finally, hypnotizability-related differences in sustained/selective/divided attention and task switching have not been supported by experimental evidence (Varga et al., 2011). Thus, the debate on the relation between hypnotizability, attentional characteristics, and COMT must be considered still open.

Oxytocin (OXT) Receptors

OXT has complex effects on experience and behavior. It makes us more sensitive to the social cues, as in a positive atmosphere its administration enhances trust, attention to social stimuli (Bakermans-Kranenburg & van Jizendoorn, 2018), whereas avoidance or aggressive motivational systems are stimulated if the context is untrustful. Moreover, a post-hypnotic suggestion for word blindness has been found more effective in a placebo group than in a group receiving OXT (possibly due to memory impairment), and OXT administration did not modulate pain perception in placebo and nocebo conditions (Acunzo et al., 2021).

Intranasally administered OXT increases the subjects' susceptibility to suggestion (Bryant, et al., 2012). The individuals with the GG genotype at rs53576 of the oxytocin receptor exhibit lower hypnotizability and absorption than those with the A allele (Bryant et al., 2013), who are more prone to accept suggestions. On the other hand, during hypnotic sessions, the lows' oxytocin release is larger than the highs' one (Varga & Kekecs, 2014; Kasos et al., 2018). Thus, although the OXT receptor polymorphism make highs more prone to accept suggestions, lows could accept them owing to larger OXT release (Santarcangelo & Carli, 2021). On these bases, the assumptions of experimental and clinical hypnosis – selected persons or all people can respond to suggestions – can reconcile by assuming that most individuals accept suggestions, although through different physiological mechanisms.

Opioids μ1 Receptors

The OPRM1 gene encodes the μ1 opioid receptor, which is the main site of action for opioids. Its A118G (rs1799971) polymorphism is associated with lower levels of OPRM1 mRNA and protein, so G carriers require higher dosages of opiates for post-surgery and cancer pain. The frequency of the G allele is significantly higher in highs compared to lows and controls (umbilical cords). Thus, highs display a less efficient opioid system than lows (Santarcangelo & Carli, 2021), which accounts for the observation that "for subjects highly susceptible to hypnosis ... the average placebo response is negligible or even negative" (Hilgard & Hilgard, 1975).

Unfortunately, suggestion-induced analgesia has been studied almost exclusively during hypnosis. It is not associated with opioids release (Goldstein & Hilgard, 1975; Spiegel & Albert, 1983; Moret et al., 1991), unless nociceptive stimulation had very high intensity (Zachariae, et al., 1998) or was administered in stressful conditions (Frid & Singer, 1979). The findings of endogenous opioids release and μ1 receptors sensitivity as a function of hypnotizability could assist in the setup of personalized pharmacological treatments of pain.

Fatty Acid Amide Hydrolase

The activity of endocannabinoids (eCBs) is mostly regulated by their degradation by the fatty acid amide hydrolase (FAAH). In particular, the A allele of the FAAH C385A polymorphism (rs324420) has been associated with lower pain sensitivity due to lower FAAH activity. Although no significant difference was observed between highs, lows, and controls (umbilical cords), the trend of A frequency to increase from lows to controls to highs suggests a possible indirect contribution of the FAAH polymorphism to the highs' analgesia. The production of CB1 receptors, in fact, is influenced by OXT, and their activity influences noradrenergic and dopaminergic pathways (Santarcangelo & Carli, 2021). A contribution of eCBs to placebo analgesia has already been shown, in fact, in individuals whose placebo-induced analgesia was not influenced by naloxone (Vase et al., 2005), as occurs in highs unless the nociceptive stimulation is very intense (Zachariae et al., 1998).

Sensorimotor Integration and Imagery

Spinal and Trigeminal Reflexes

The earliest report of hypnotizability-related excitability of spinal motoneurons was the observation of the decreasing amplitude of the soleus monosynaptic Hoffmann reflex (H) during long-lasting relaxation in highs receiving low intensity, low frequency stimulation of the proprioceptive fibers Ia elicited at approximately similar time intervals (Santarcangelo et al., 1989). The stimulation characteristics suggested that the H reflex decrease was due to habituation. In fact, when H reflexes were evoked randomly, at shorter and variable intervals (Busse, 1991), or intermingled with different spinal stimulations (Kiernan et al., 1995), their amplitude did not decrease. Moreover, the H amplitudes time series revealed a correlation of H reflex amplitudes with the preceding time interval duration in highs and with the amplitude of the preceding H reflex in lows, suggesting subtle differences between highs and lows in the control of their spinal cord excitability (Busse, 1991).

The F wave is a motor neuron response occurring after supramaximal, antidromic stimulation of peripheral nerves and indicates the motoneurons post-synaptic excitability. It involves about 2% of the antidromically stimulated pool of motoneurons and shows, in the same flexor muscle, a large variability in frequency of occurrence, latency, duration, amplitude and shape. During both long-lasting relaxation and neutral hypnosis, its frequency of occurrence decreased in the highs' right, but not left *abductor digiti minimi,* and did not change in lows (Santarcangelo et al., 2003). This fits with the theory of a progressive shift from left to right cerebral activation during hypnotic induction in highs (Gruzelier, 2006; Naish, 2010), who may have changed their state independently from hypnotic induction (Kirsch, 2000). In lower limbs, there was no change in the F frequency of occurrence (Santarcangelo et al., 2003), but its amplitude and latency decreased and increased, respectively. Such changes indicated a shift of the antidromic response from large to small motoneurons (unpublished observation), which could be accounted for by relaxation-related reduction of the activity of the coeruleo-spinal pathway, with consequently increased activity of the Renshaw cells (Fung et al., 1991). These cells inhibit the motoneurons which excite them, and their action may be more effective on large than small motoneurons. In fact, the former provides stronger excitatory input to their Renshaw cells which, in turn, exert stronger inhibition of the same motoneurons (Hultborn et al., 1988).

The withdrawal, spinal flexor reflex (FR) consists of an earlier, spinal response and of later, trans-bulbar/cortical responses to nociceptive stimulation. It has been widely studied during hypnosis, whereas only one study dealt with hypnotizability-related differences in FR in the absence of suggestions. It did not report any difference between highs and lows (Sandrini et al., 2000), while a reduction of the FR amplitude has been reported during wakeful suggestions of hypoalgesia (Houzé et al., 2021).

The spontaneous eye blink rate (sBR), of trigeminal origin, protects the eyes from external agents, has been positively associated with the cortico-striatal dopaminergic tone, and varies according to attentional levels and cognitive load. It has been reported both lower or higher in highs with respect to lows and medium hypnotizables (mediums) (Lindsay et al., 1993; Lichtenberg et al., 2008), possibly depending on experimental conditions, i.e., the time of the day (Barbato et al., 2000), large intersubjects variability, and attentional conditions (Bonfiglio et al., 2005). sBR was also found higher in highs than in lows during the earliest minutes of long-lasting relaxation and progressively decreasing throughout the session (Di Gruttola et al., 2014). The initial higher sBR could be sustained by higher cortico-striatal dopaminergic tone, and its progressive decrease could be due to attentional engagement in the "relaxation task". This interpretation fits with the idea that relaxation is achieved by highs and lows differentially, being associated with increasing EEG gamma activity (Sebastiani et al., 2005) and decreasing determinism (Marwan et al., 2007) of the EEG recurrence plot (RP) in highs (Madeo et al., 2013) and with decreasing gamma power and unchanged RP determinism in lows.

The nociceptive nBR is a trigeminal reflex elicited by nociceptive stimulation of the trigeminal receptive field or of other body parts in the peripersonal space (Sambo et al., 2012). It can be induced by stimulation of the supraorbital nerve and consists of an ipsilateral, spinal short latency component and of bilateral, later components controlled by pontine and medullary circuits. In the absence of suggestions, nBR does not differ between highs and lows, like the spinal withdrawal reflex (Sandrini et al., 2000), and no hypnotizability-related difference appears when it is cued by visual stimuli (Santarcangelo et al., 2016). Nonetheless, similar amplitudes are associated with different cortical mechanisms in highs and lows, as nociceptive stimulation changes global and local features of pain-related cortical networks almost exclusively in lows (Zarei et al., 2020), in line with the observation of cortical correlates of actual and imaginative sensorimotor tasks (Ibáñez-Marcelo et al., 2019a; Ruggirello et al., 2019).

Postural and Visuomotor Control

Postural control is influenced by sensori-motor, cognitive and emotional information. It is impaired by concomitant tasks and in patients with cognitive decline (Monaghan et al., 2022; Salihu et al., 2022). The different attentional characteristics of highs and lows suggested that the highs' postural control may be less impaired than the lows' one by cognitive load and sensorimotor alteration. The first hypothesis – cognitive load – was not supported by measures of the area and velocity of body sway. In contrast, during visual and/or leg proprioceptive alteration (closed/open eyes, stable/unstable support) highs exhibited a less close postural control indicated by larger and faster body sway with respect to lows, despite the same perception of sway. This can be accounted for by a different "critical point" for postural control (Collins & De Luca, 1993), that is the distance from the origin of the movement at which the peripheral information due to movement is integrated with

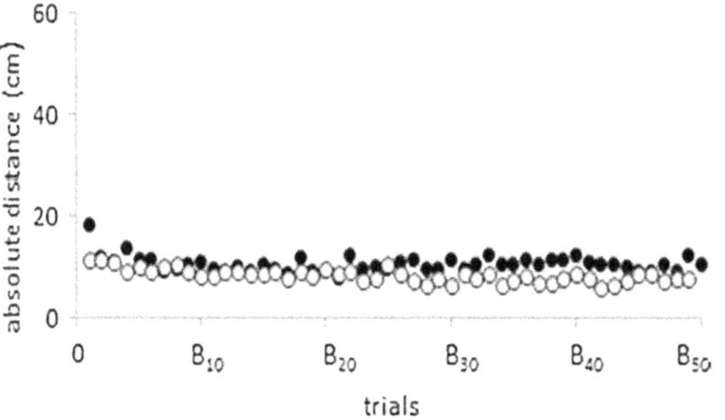

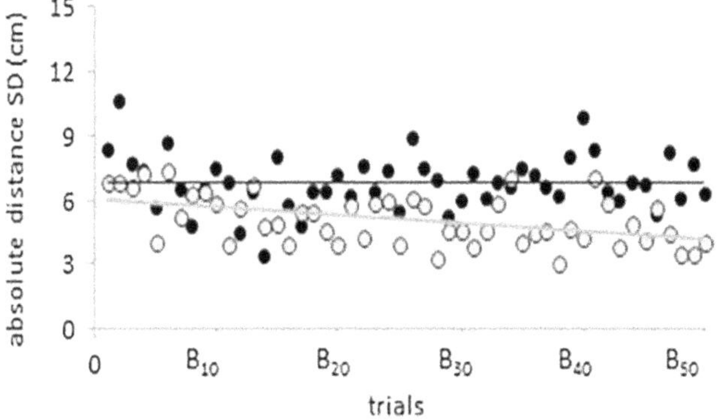

Figure 21.1 Launches absolute error. Launches absolute error (upper panel) and standard deviation (lower panel) in baseline conditions. Black and gray dots: highs and lows, respectively. Larger error and variability and no learning across trials in highs. Modified from Menzocch et al., 2014).

central commands (Santarcangelo et al., 2008a). The highs' posture is also less sensitive than lows' to changes in the neck tonic proprioceptive input due to the rotated posture of the head, which modulates the neck proprioceptive input to high brain centers in the general population (Santarcangelo et al., 2008b). Nonetheless, highly demanding postural tasks similarly engage highs and lows, suggesting that the former can compensate for their less close postural control by attention (Santarcangelo & Scattina, 2016).

Postural studies indicated a different cerebellar function in highs and lows (Koziol et al., 2014). Thus, a classical cerebellar task consisting of launching small balls against a target before (Figure 21.1), during, and after the application of ocular prisms was proposed to the two groups. It revealed that the highs' cerebellum allows them to appropriately change the direction of launches according to the gaze direction when prisms were applied or removed, but the variability of the error (distance from the target) is larger in highs than in lows in all prism conditions (Menzocchi et al., 2015). Importantly, learning due to task repetition (ball launches, sensory alteration in standing subjects) does not occur in highs (Santarcangelo & Scattina, 2016). Overall, these findings support the view that the highs' cerebellum may be "less smart" than the lows' one (Koziol et al., 2014; Tzvi et al., 2022).

Motor Cortex Excitability and Functional Equivalence between Imagery and Perception/Action

The highs' right motor cortex is more excitable than lows', with mediums showing intermediate amplitudes of the motor evoked potentials at threshold (Figure 21.2) and suprathreshold levels of transcranial magnetic stimulation (TMS) (Spina et al., 2020). In contrast, the left motor cortex excitability is similar in highs and lows (Cesari et al., 2020). In both cases, motor imagery increases the motor cortex excitability only in highs. The greater excitability of their right motor cortex cannot be sustained by larger prefrontal and cingulate dopamine content, unable to explain the laterality of the observation, whereas reduced inhibition of the right motor cortex by the left cerebellum could be involved (see Section 2.4).

The highs' further enhancement of the cortical excitability during motor imagery must be attributed to greater functional equivalence (FE) between imagery and perception/action (Ibáñez-Marcelo et al., 2019a, b).

FE indicates the degree of similarity between actual and imagined perception/action sustained by the same brain activations and activation profiles (Jeannerod, 1995; Kosslyn et al., 2006). Topological data analysis of EEG, which detects brain activities configurations, revealed that FE is stronger in highs than in lows (Ibáñez-Marcelo et al., 2019a), as earlier suggested by behavioral studies (Santarcangelo et al., 2010). Such stronger FE may promote ideomotor behaviors and account for the highs' report of involuntariness.

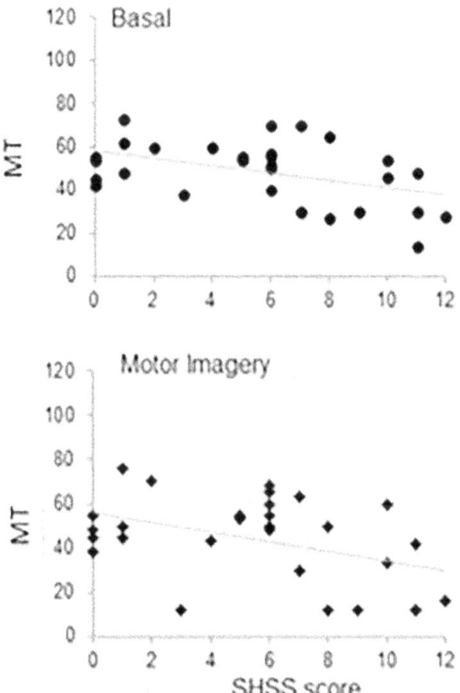

Figure 21.2 Right motor cortex excitability. Left motor threshold (MT) after transcranial magnetic stimulation of the right primary motor cortex as a function of hypnotizability. Upper panel, baseline conditions; lower panel; sensorimotor imagery. Negative correlation between hypnotizability scores and MT. Modified from Spina et al., 2020.

FE could contribute to the construction of the individual sensorimotor self together with physical experiences, thus being relevant to neurodevelopment.

EEG topology suggested also different modes of information processing – small, although significant, widely distributed EEG changes with respect to baseline in highs, and focal changes in lows (Ibáñez-Marcelo et al., 2019b) which may be relevant to clinical conditions. Moreover, owing to the highs' stronger FE, hypnotic assessment could efficaciously predict the outcome of mental imagery training and brain computer interface interventions (Fontanelli et al., 2022). Studies aimed at the enhancement of FE in medium/lows – by imagery training and/or TMS/tDCS of motor areas – could extend the efficacy of imagery training and brain computer interface interventions to mediums/lows themselves (Fontanelli et al., 2022).

The Cerebellum

The hypnotizability-related differences in attentional stability, sensorimotor integration, and right motor cortex excitability suggested differences in cerebellar functional characteristics. The cerebellum, in fact, controls motor and non-motor functions (Buckner, 2013; Koziol et al., 2014) through its functional connections to sensorimotor and associative cortical areas (De Benedictis et al., 2022).

Reduced gray matter volume was observed in the highs' left cerebellar lobules IV–VI. The variation of lobules IV–V is compatible with the differences observed in sensori-motor integration and excitability of the right motor cortex, while lobule VI variation can account for the highs' low proneness to attentional shifts and higher emotional intensity (Picerni et al., 2019). The reduced gray matter volume of cerebellar lobules could also be involved in the paradoxical control of pain (Figure 21.3) observed in healthy highs receiving nociceptive laser stimulation of the left hand after bilateral anodal stimulation (tDCS) of the cerebellum at low frequency (3–5 interstimulus intervals). In contrast to the general population, who decreases the amplitude of nociceptive cortical potentials, in fact, in highs the cerebellar anodal tDCS increases the amplitude of nociceptive cortical potentials (Bocci et al., 2017). The cerebellar mechanisms of pain modulation engage both somatosensory, cingulate, and motor cortex (Li et al., 2022). Thus, the paradoxical effects of anodal stimulation could be due to a complex modulation of the highs' pain matrix, possibly mediated by variations of

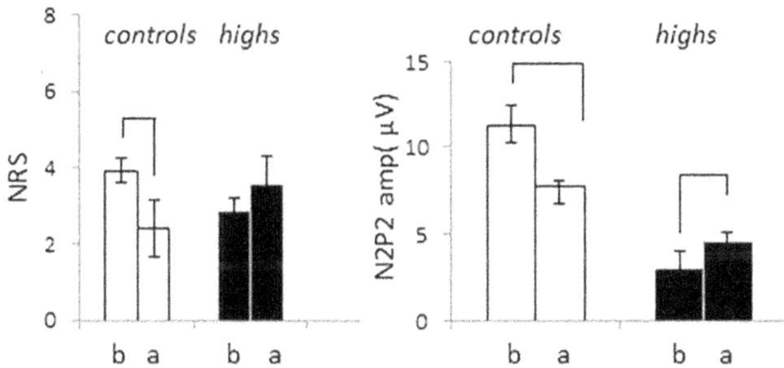

Figure 21.3 Cerebellar modulation of subjective experience and nociceptive potentials. Subjective experience and nociceptive potentials before and after bilateral anodal tDCS of the cerebellum. No reduction in pain perception (NRS) and increase in the cortical potentials amplitude in highs. Controls include lows and mediums. Modified from Bocci et al., 2017.

the insula and of its connections to cingulate and prefrontal regions (Landry et al., 2017). The inhibitory role of the motor cortex on pain (Yao et al., 2021) is not a good candidate to account for the highs' experience and cortically evoked potentials after cerebellar tDCS, as their right motor cortex is more excitable than lows/mediums' (Spina et al., 2020) and the left motor cortex' excitability is like lows' (Cesari et al., 2020).

Cardiovascular Control

Heart Rate and Variability, Blood Pressure, Skin Blood Flow, Electrodermal Activity

Heart rate (HR) and heart rate variability (HRV) are largely used as correlates of the experience of relaxation and emotion. HRV is usually indicated by the high frequency (HF), vagal and low frequency (LF), sympathetic components of the power spectrum of the tachogram (the series of the time differences between the ECG consecutive R waves), despite these components represent only 5% of the total HRV (largely due to Very Low Frequency (VLF) components related to thermoregulation and renin-angiotensin activity). Most studies of hypnotizability-related differences in cardiovascular control have been based, in fact, on LF and HF. A weakness in this approach is the inconsistent use of their absolute (Santarcangelo et al., 1992) or normalized values (De Benedittis et al., 1994), which may lead to different conclusions about the underlying mechanisms. Overall, however, different hypnotizability levels can be associated with different modes of autonomic control.

During long lasting relaxation, both highs and lows reduce their HR, but highs display stronger vagal and lower sympathetic contribution to HRV than lows (Santarcangelo et al., 2012). In the same study, no change in blood pressure occurred in both groups, but highs increased their peripheral blood flow, indicating consistent sympathetic activity at cardiac and vascular levels. In contrast, other studies showed higher skin conductance in highs than in mediums and lows suggesting higher sympathetic tone (Jørgensen & Zachariae, 2002), despite the absence of differences in HR and HRV. Theoretically, highs can exhibit higher sympathetic tone during relaxation owing to attentional engagement in the "relaxation task" (Sebastiani et al., 2005; Madeo et al., 2013), in contrast to the lows' mere disengagement from environmental information (Sebastiani et al., 2005).

Upright stance induces similar HR increases in highs and lows and decreases in total HRV and vagal control only in lows. Highs, in contrast, exhibit non-significant decreases in absolute HF and non-significant increases in LF and VLF, as occurs in the general population during the 0 G phase of parabolic flights, when baroreceptive responses cannot be elicited (Santarcangelo et al., 2008). During tonic pressure pain (Paoletti et al., 2010) and cold pressure test (Santarcangelo et al., 2013), similar cardiovascular changes occur in highs and lows. The suggestions of analgesia, subjectively effective only in highs, are associated with similar autonomic activity in the two groups, in contrast to cortical activity (De Pascalis et al., 2015) and somatic reflexes (Sandrini et al., 2000), which can be accounted for by separate descending controls (Piché et al., 2010). Other authors, however, reported decreased skin conductance during nociceptive stimulation in highs receiving suggestions of hypoalgesia (Houzé et al., 2021). Unpleasant imagery increases skin conductance in both groups, whereas HR increases in lows and decreases in highs, suggesting a possible defensive mechanism making highs able to partially buffer negative emotion (Sebastiani et al., 2003). During phase completion (Jørgensen & Zachariae, 2002), mediums show greater reduction in the parasympathetic activity than both lows and highs, whereas highs exhibit larger increase in sympathetic activity than mediums/lows. Finally, mental computation (MC) induces similar increases in HR/blood pressure and decreases in the skin blood flow in highs and lows (Paoletti et al., 2010).

Electrodermal levels and responses have been widely studied as a function of hypnotizability, although almost exclusively during and after hypnotic induction. Generally, no baseline differences between highs and lows were observed, with the exception of higher left than right side responses to tones, and of faster habituation in highs with respect to lows (Kasos et al., 2020). The latter findings accord with the reduction in the H reflex amplitude and in the F wave frequency of occurrence observed in highs during simple relaxation (Santarcangelo et al., 1989, 2003).

Interoceptive Accuracy and Sensitivity

Interoception is the sense of the physiological condition of the body (Craig, 2002). It includes interoceptive accuracy (IA) – the ability to appropriately detect bodily signals – and the interoceptive awareness/sensitivity (IS), that is the mode of their interpretation. Both aspects contribute to body image, social behavior, and physical and mental health (Nord & Garfinkel, 2022). They are associated with specific activities and connectivity of a few brain regions (Quadt et al., 2022), including some structures also displaying hypnotizability-related morpho-functional characteristics, i.e., the insular, cingulate, temporal cortices (Landry et al., 2017), and the cerebellum (Picerni et al., 2019). IA is measured by behavioral tests, mainly the heartbeats count, which allows to compare the counted and ECG recorded heartbeats. This measure, however, is not highly reliable, as it is influenced by experimental conditions (Ring et al., 2015), previous experience (Ferentzi et al., 2022), and measurement devices (Murphy et al., 2019). Moreover, it is modulated by heart rate variability (Lischke et al., 2021).

During relaxation, hypnotizability and IA (Figure 21.4) are negatively correlated with each other (Rosati et al., 2021). Theoretically, the low IA may contribute to the highs' greater proneness to perceive body conditions as different from the real ones after suggestions.

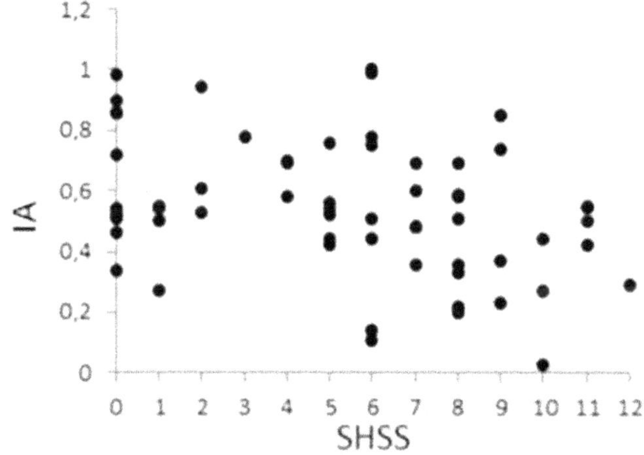

Figure 21.4 Interoceptive accuracy (IA) as a function of hypnotizability. Negative correlation between hypnotizability scores and IA. Modified from Rosati et al., 2021.

On the other hand, during a cold pressure test, there was a positive correlation between the pain threshold and the RR duration (time distance (ms) between consecutive R waves of the ECG) observed before the occurrence of the pain threshold itself (Varanini et al., 2018)). Thus, interoceptive signals seem to be better integrated into the subjective unconscious experience of highs with respect to lows, likely based on different processing of interoceptive signals by structures, i.e., the insula and the cerebellum (Forstenpointner et al., 2022), which show hypnotizability-related structural variations and functional connectivity (Landry et al., 2017; Picerni et al., 2019). In contrast to IA, highs display greater interoceptive sensitivity/awareness than mediums and lows. The Multidimensional Assessment of Interoceptive Awareness (MAIA) (Mehling et al., 2012) reveals, in fact, higher scores of the proneness to take into consideration bodily signals independently from their emotional content (*noticing*), to realize that certain body sensations are the sensory aspects of emotional states (*emotional awareness*), to control emotional distress by attention to body sensations (*self-regulation*), and, in general, to actively listen to the body (*body listening*) and consider its experience as trustworthy (*trusting*). Overall, these differences indicate a more adaptive body-mind interaction in highs than in mediums/lows (Diolaiuti et al., 2019).

Peripheral Arteries Flow Mediated Dilation, Cerebrovascular Reactivity

The brachial artery post-occlusion, flow mediated dilation (FMD) is a measure of the artery reaction to occlusion. It is largely due to the release of nitric oxide (NO) from endothelial cells induced by shear stress. Stress (Xue et al., 2015; Sara et al., 2022) and pain (Coyle et al., 2021) impair FMD and the cardiovascular function. Larger FMD predicts better cardiovascular health (Matsuzawa et al., 2015).

MC reduces FMD in lows, but not in highs (Jambrik et al.,2004), and nociceptive stimulation reduces it much more in lows than in highs (Jambrik et al., 2005) (Figure 21.5). Thus, highs seem to be protected against cardiovascular events and, possibly, against the cardiovascular consequences of chronic pain. Clinical trials are required to support this thesis.

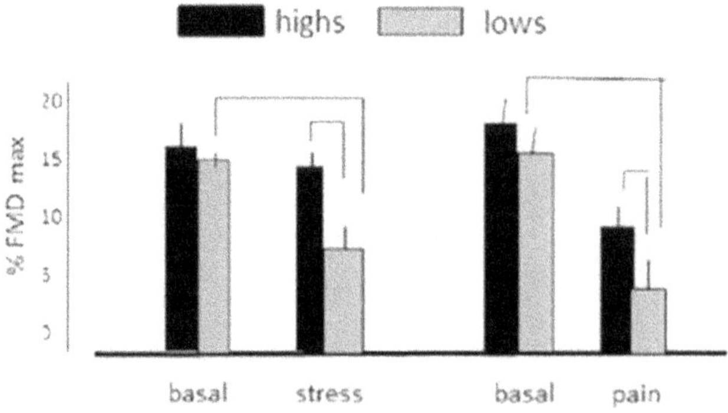

Figure 21.5 Post occlusion FMD during mental computation and nociceptive pain. Post occlusion flow-mediated dilation (FMD) of the brachial artery during mental computation (stress) and nociceptive stimulation (pain). Lines indicate significant differences between highs and low as well as between conditions. Modified from Jambrik et al., 2004, 2005.

Near infrared spectroscopy (NIRS) shows that during MC and a Trail Making Task (TMT), the tissue hemoglobin index (THI) and the tissue oxygenation index (TOI) increase only in the participants with medium-to-high hypnotizability scores (med-highs). In this group, TOI is larger during MC (requiring internally directed attention) than during TMT (requiring externally directed attention), although the performance is like med-lows'. Thus, during cognitive tasks, the med-highs' tissue oxygenation is more finely adjusted to metabolic demands than med-lows' in the presence of similar increases in systemic blood pressure (Rashid et al., 2022a). The internally directed attention during MC, in fact, is cognitively more costly than the externally directed attention during TMT (Ceh et al., 2021). NO may play a role in these hypnotizability-related differences, as suggested for the cerebrovascular reactivity to hyperventilation (Rashid et al., 2022b). In this condition, the cerebrovascular reactivity is controlled by the systemic blood pressure only in the participants with medium-to-high hypnotizability scores, likely owing to NO-related mechanisms. The role of NO in the cerebrovascular reactivity during tasks associated with changes in the systemic blood pressure fits with the observation that the conditions not associated with such changes like visual stimulation (Rashid et al., 2022c), hypnotizability-related differences in cerebrovascular reactivity do not occur.

Limitations and Conclusions

Most of the described studies have limitations due to small sample size and/or the absence of medium hypnotizable participants (Jensen et al., 2017). Nonetheless, they indicate that hypnotizability-related differences can influence several aspects of everyday life even in the absence of suggestions. Unfortunately, despite the several correlates of hypnotizability described till now, a discriminant index of hypnotizability has not been proposed. The determinism extracted from the EEG Recurrence Plot (Marwan et al., 2007) allows to discriminate highs from lows with good, but not absolute precision (Madeo et al., 2013; Chiarucci et al., 2014), while other studies aimed at classifying highs, mediums, and lows have been conducted after hypnotic induction (Yargholi & Nasrabadi, 2015). Further efforts are required to be able to classify highs, mediums, and lows in the ordinary state of consciousness instrumentally.

In conclusion, current evidence indicates a relevant contribution of neuroscience to the bio-psycho-social model of hypnosis (Jensen et al., 2015). The physiological correlates of hypnotizability account for the construction of different individual selves and for the variability of the general population in the sensorimotor, autonomic, and cognitive-emotional domains.

In a medical perspective, hypnotic assessment may assist in the setup of personalized pharmacological and non-pharmacological pain treatments, in the choice of rehabilitation strategies for brain injured patients, and in the prognosis of cardiovascular patients. The highs' high well-being (Biscuola et al., 2022), which in the general population is associated with high serotoninergic tone, low cortisol, and inflammation markers levels (de Vries et al., 2022), could contribute to better physical health. One of the next challenges, for clinicians, is to assess whether imagery/relaxation training which controls immune activity during hypnotic treatments (Carlson et al., 2017; Derbyshire et al., 2009; Gruzelier, 2002; Kovács, et al., 2008; Minowa & Koitabashi, 2014; Moser, 2014; Ruzyla-Smith et al., 1995; Zachariae et al., 1994) is effective out of hypnosis, as expected (Derbyshire et al., 2009; Lynn & Green, 2011).

Although the highs' favorable cardiovascular characteristics observed in healthy participants (Jambrik et al., 2004, 2005; Santarcangelo et al., 2012) should be tested in clinical trials, they may have contributed to the highs' survival to natural selection together with their imagery abilities possibly facilitating the recovery from brain injuries (Ibáñez-Marcelo et al., 2019). In contrast, the lows' survival might be due to better visuomotor control (Menzocchi et al., 2015) allowing them greater success in hunting, and to higher proneness to avoid unpleasant situations (Diolaiuti et al., 2019). One may also wonder whether, among our ancestors possibly displaying inefficient opioid systems (not allowing them to efficiently cope with pain), only those who developed an efficient non-opioid system to adaptively control pain and pain-related behavior may have survived (Santarcangelo et al., 2021).

References

Acunzo, D. J., Oakley, D. A., & Terhune, D. B. (2021). The neurochemistry of hypnosis. *American Journal of Clinical Hypnosis*, *63*, 355–371 10.1080/00029157.2020.

Bakermans-Kranenburg, M. J., & van Jizendoorn, M. H. (2018). Oxytocin and human sensitive and protective parenting. *Current Topics in Behavioral Neuro*science, *35*, 421–448. doi:10.1007/7854_2017_23.

Barbato, G., Ficca, G., Muscettola, G. Fichele, M., Beatrice, M., & Rinaldi, F. (2000). Diurnal variation in spontaneous eye-blink rate. *Psychiatry Research*, *93*, 145–151.

Biscuola, E., Bongini, M., Belcari, I., Santarcangelo, E. L., & Sebastiani L. (2022). Well-being in highly hypnotizable persons. *International Journal of Clinical and Experimental Hypnosis*, *70*(2), 123–135. doi: 10.1080/00207144.2022.2049972.

Bocci, T., Barloscio, D., Parenti, L., Sartucci, F., Carli G., & Santarcangelo, E. L. (2017). High hypnotizability impairs the cerebellar control of pain. *Cerebellum*, *16*(1), 55–61. doi: 10.1007/s12311-016-0764-2.

Bonfiglio, L., Carboncini, M. C., Bongioanni, P., Andre, P., Minichilli, F., Forni, M., & Rossi, B. (2005). Spontaneous blinking behaviour in persistent vegetative and minimally conscious states: Relationships with evolution and outcome. *Brain Research Bulletin*, *68*, 163–170.

Bryant, R. A., Hung, L., Dobson-Stone, C., & Schofield, P. R. (2013). The association between the oxytocin receptor gene (OXTR) and hypnotizability. *Psychoneuroendocrinology*, *38*(10), 1979–1984. doi: 10.1016/j.psyneuen.2013.03.002.

Bryant, R. A., Hung, L., Guastella, A. J., & Mitchell, P. B. (2012). Oxytocin as a moderator of hypnotizability. *Psychoneuroendocrinology*, *37*(1), 162–166. doi:10.1016/j.psyneuen.2011.05.010.

Buckner, R. L. (2013). The cerebellum and cognitive function: 25 years of insight from anatomy and neuroimaging. *Neuron*, *80*(3), 807–815.

Busse, K. (1991). Modulazione del riflesso monosinaptico in funzione della frequenza di stimolazione in soggetti di diversa suscettibilità ipnotica. Master's degree. University of Siena.

Carlson, L. E., Zelinski, E., Toivonen, K., Flynn, M., Qureshi, M., Piedalue, K. A., & Grant, R. (2017). Mind-body therapies in cancer: What is the latest evidence? *Current Oncology Reports*, *19*(10), 67. doi: 10.1007/s11912-017-0626-1.

Ceh, S. M., Annerer-Walcher, S., Koschutnig, K., Körner, C., Fink, A., & Benedek, M. (2021). Neurophysiological indicators of internal attention: An fMRI-eye-tracking coregistration study. *Cortex*, *143*, 29–46. 10.1016/j.cortex.2021.07.005

Cesari, P., Modenese, M., Benedetti, S., Emadi Andani, M., & Fiorio, M. (2020). Hypnosis-induced modulation of corticospinal excitability during motor imagery. *Scientific Reports*, *10*(1),16882. doi: 10.1038/s41598-020-74020-0.

Chiarucci, R., Madeo, D., Loffredo, M. I., Castellani, E., Santarcangelo, E. L., & Mocenni, C. (2014). Cross-evidence for hypnotic susceptibility through nonlinear measures on EEGs of non-hypnotized subjects. *Scientific Reports*, *8*(4), 5610. doi: 10.1038/srep05610.

Collins, J. J., & De Luca, C. J. (1993). Open-loop and closed-loop control of posture: A random-walk analysis of center-of-pressure trajectories. *Experimental Brain Research*, *95*(2), 308–318. doi: 10.1007/BF00229788.

Colzato, L. S., Waszak, F., Nieuwenhuis S., Posthuma D., & Hommel B. (2010). The flexible mind is associated with the catechol-O-methyltransferase (COMT) Val158Met polymorphism: Evidence for a role of dopamine in the control of task-switching. Neuropsychologia, *48*, 2764–2768. 10.1016/j.neuropsychologia.2010.04.023

Coyle, P. C., O'Brien, V. A., Edwards, D. G., Pohlig, R. T., & Hicks, G. E. (2021). Markers of cardiovascular health in older adults with and without chronic low back and radicular leg pain: A comparative analysis. *Pain Medicine*, *22*(6),1353–1359. doi: 10.1093/pm/pnaa426.

Craig, A. (2002). How do you feel? Interoception: The sense of the physiological condition of the body. *Nature Reviews Neuroscience*, *3*, 655–666. 10.1038/nrn894

De Benedictis, A., Rossi-Espagnet, M. C., de Palma, L., Carai, A., & Marras, C. E. (2022). Networking of the human cerebellum: From anatomo-functional development to neurosurgical implications. *Frontiers in Neurology*, *13*, 806298. doi: 10.3389/fneur.2022.806298.

De Benedittis, G., Cigada, M., Bianchi, A., Signorini, M., & Cerutti, S. (1994). Autonomic changes duringhypnosis: A heart rate variability power spectrum analysis as a marker of sympatho-vagal balance. *International Journal of Clinical and Experimental Hypnosis*, *42*(2), 140–152. doi: 10.1080/00207149408409347.

DeBenedittis, G., Panerai, A. A., & Villamira, M. A. (1989). Effects of hypnotic analgesia and hypnotizability on experimental ischemic pain. *International Journal of Clinical and Experimental Hypnosis*, *37*(1), 55–69. doi: 10.1080/00207148908410533.

De Pascalis, V., Varriale, V., & Cacace, I. (2015). Pain modulation in waking and hypnosis in women: Event-related potentials and sources of cortical activity. *PLoS One*, *10*(6), e0128474. doi: 10.1371/journal.pone.0128474.

de Vries, L. P., van de Weijer, M. P., & Bartels, M. (2022). The human physiology of well-being: A systematic review on the association between neurotransmitters, hormones, inflammatory markers, the microbiome and well-being. *Neuroscience and Biobehavioral Reviews*, *104733*. doi: 10.1016/j.neubiorev.2022.104733.

Derbyshire, S. W., Whalley, M. G., & Oakley, D. A. (2009). Fibromyalgia pain and its modulation by hypnotic and non-hypnotic suggestion: An fMRI analysis. *European Journal of Pain*, *13*(5), 542–550. doi: 10.1016/j.ejpain.2008.06.010.

Di Gruttola, F., Orsini, P., Carboncini, M. C., Rossi, B., & Santarcangelo, E. L. (2014). Revisiting the association between hypnotizability and blink rate. *Experimental Brain Research*, *232*(12), 3763–3769. doi: 10.1007/s00221-014-4073-z.

Diolaiuti, F., Huber, A., Ciaramella, A., Santarcangelo, E. L., & Sebastiani, L. (2019). Hypnotizability-related interoceptive awareness and inhibitory/activating emotional traits. *Archives Italiennes de Biologie*, 157(4), 111–119. doi: 10.12871/00039829202042.

Elkins, G. R., Barabasz, A. F., Council, J. R., & Spiegel, D. (2015). Advancing research and practice: The revised APA Division 30 definition of hypnosis. *International Journal of Clinical and Experimental Hypnosis*, *63*(1),1–9. doi: 10.1080/00207144.2014.961870.

Ferentzi, E., Wilhelm, O., & Köteles, F. (2022). What counts when heartbeats are counted. *Trends in Cognitive Science*, *S1364-6613*(22), 00166–00168. doi:10.1016/j.tics.2022.07.009.

Fontanelli, L., Spina, V., Chisari, C., Siciliano, G., & Santarcangelo, E. L. (2022). Is hypnotic assessment relevant to neurology? *Neurological Sciences*, *43*, 4655-4661, doi: 10.1007/s10072-022-06122-8.

Forstenpointner, J., Maallo, A. M. S., Elman, I., Holmes, S., Freeman, R., Baron, R., & Borsook, D. (2022). The solitary nucleus connectivity to key autonomic regions in humans. *European Journal of Neuroscience*, *56*(2), 3938–3966. doi: 10.1111/ejn.15691.

Fossella, J., Sommer, T., Fan J., Wu Y., Swanson J. M., Pfaff D. W., Pfaff, D. W., & Posner, M. I. (2002). Assessing the molecular genetics of attention networks. *BMC Neuroscience*, *3*, 14. doi: 10.1186/1471-2202-3-14.

Frid, M., & Singer, G. (1979). Hypnotic analgesia in conditions of stress is partially reversed by naloxone. *Psychopharmacology (Berl)*, *63*(3), 211–215. doi: 10.1007/BF00433552.

Fung, S. J., Manzoni, D., Chan, J. Y., Pompeiano, O., & Barnes, C. D. (1991). Locus coeruleus control of spinal motor output. *Progress in Brain Research*, *88*, 395–409. doi:10.1016/s0079-6123(08)63825-x.

Goldstein, A., & Hilgard, E. R. (1975) Failure of opiate antagonist naloxone to modify hypnotic analgesia. *Proceedings of the National Academy of Sciences*, *72*, 2041–2043.

Gruzelier, J. H. (2002) A review of the impact of hypnosis, relaxation, guided imagery and individual differences on aspects of immunity and health. *Stress*, *5*(2), 147–163. 10.1080/1025389029002 7877

Gruzelier, J. H. (2006). Frontal functions, connectivity and neural efficiency underpinning hypnosis and hypnotic susceptibility (2006). *Contemporary Hypnosis*, *23*(1), 15–32. DOI: 10.1002/ch.35

Hilgard, E. R., & Hilgard, J. R. (1975). *Hypnosis in the relief of pain*. Los Altos, CA: William Kaufmann.

Houzé, B. A., Piché M., & Rainville, P. (2021). Spinal and supraspinal modulation of pain responses by hypnosis, suggestions, and distraction. *American Journal of Clinical Hypnosis*, *3*(4), 329–354. doi: 10.1080/00029157.2020.1863184.

Hultborn, H., Lipski, J., Mackel, R., & Wigström, H. (1988). Distribution of recurrent inhibition within a motor nucleus. I. Contribution from slow and fast motor units to the excitation of Renshaw cells. *Acta Physiologica Scandinavica*, *134*(3), 347–361. doi: 10.1111/j.1748-1716. 1988.tb08503.x.

Ibáñez-Marcelo, E., Campioni, L., Phinyomark, A., Petri, G., & Santarcangelo, E. L. (2019a). Topology highlights mesoscopic functional equivalence between imagery and perception: The case of hypnotizability. *Neuroimage*, *200*, 437–449. doi: 10.1016/j.neuroimage.2019.06.044.

Ibáñez-Marcelo, E., Campioni, L., Manzoni, D., Santarcangelo, E. L., & Petri, G. (2019b). Spectral and topological analyses of the cortical representation of the head position: Does hypnotizability matter? *Brain & Behavior*, *9*(6), e01277. doi: 10.1002/brb3.1277.

Jambrik, Z., Santarcangelo, E. L., Ghelarducci, B., Picano, E., & Sebastiani, L. (2004). Does hypnotizability modulate the stress-related endothelial dysfunction? *Brain Research Bulletin*, *63*(3), 213–216. doi: 10.1016/j.brainresbull.2004.01.011.

Jambrik, Z., Santarcangelo, E. L., Rudisch, T., Varga, A., Forster, T., & Carli, G. (2005). Modulation of pain-induced endothelial dysfunction by hypnotisability. *Pain*, *116*(3), 181–186. doi: 10.1016/j.pain.2005.03.041.

Jeannerod, M. (1995). Mental imagery in motor context. *Neuropsychologia*, *33*(11), 1419–1432.

Jensen, M. P., Adachi, T., Tomé-Pires, C., Lee, J., Osman, Z. J., & Miró, J. (2015). Mechanisms of hypnosis: Toward the development of a biopsychosocial model. *International Journal of Clinical and Experimental Hypn*osis, *63*(1),34–75. doi: 10.1080/00207144.2014.961875.

Jensen, M. P., Jamieson, G. A., Lutz, A., Mazzoni, G., McGeown, W. J., Santarcangelo, E. L., Demertzi, A., De Pascalis, V., Bányai, É.I., Rominger, C., Vuilleumier, P., Faymonville, M. E., & Terhune, D. B. (2017). New directions in hypnosis research: Strategies for advancing the cognitive and clinical neuroscience of hypnosis. *Neuroscience of Consciousness*, *3*(1), nix004. doi: 10.1093/ nc/nix004.

Jørgensen, M. M., & Zachariae, R. (2002). Autonomic reactivity to cognitive and emotional stress of low, medium, and high hypnotizable healthy subjects: Testing predictions from the high-risk model of threat perception. *International Journal of Clinical and Experimental Hypn*osis, *50*(3), 248–275. doi: 10.1080/00207140208410102.

Kasos, E., Kasos, K., Pusztai, F., Polyák, Á., Kovács, K. J., & Varga, K. (2018). Changes in oxytocin and cortisol in active-alert hypnosis: Hormonal changes benefiting low hypnotizable participants. *International Journal of Clinical and Experimental Hypn*osis, 66(4), 404–427. doi: 10.1080/002 07144.2018.1495009.

Kasos, K., Csirmaz, L., Vikor, F., Zimonyi, S., Varga, K., & Székely, A. (2020). Electrodermal correlates of hypnosis: Current developments. *OBM Integrative and Complementary Medicine 2020*, *5*(2), 017.

Kiernan, B. D., Dane, J. R., Phillips, L. H., & Price, D. D. (1995). Hypnotic analgesia reduces R-III nociceptive reflex: Further evidence concerning the multifactorial nature of hypnotic analgesia. *Pain*, *60*, 39–47. doi: 10.1016/0304-3959(94)00134-Z

Kirsch, I. (2000). The response set theory of hypnosis. *Americn Journal of Clinical Hypnosis*, *42*(3-4), 274–292. doi: 10.1080/00029157.2000.10734362.

Kosslyn, S. M., Thompson, W. L., & Ganis, G. (2006). *The case for mental imagery*. Oxford, UK: Oxford University Press.

Kovács, Z. A., Puskás, L. G., Juhász, A., Rimanócz, y. A., Hackler, L. Jr, Kátay, L., Gali, Z., Vetró, A., Janka, Z., & Kálmán, J. (2008). Hypnosis upregulates the expression of immune-related genes in lymphocytes. *Psychotherapy & Psychosomatics*, *77*(4), 257–259. 10.1159/000128165

Koziol, L. F., Budding, D., Andreasen, N., D'Arrigo, S., Bulgheroni, S., Imamizu, H., Ito, M., Manto, M., Marvel, C., Parker, K., Pezzulo, G., Ramnani, N., Riva, D., Schmahman, n J., Vandervert, L., & Yamazaki, T. (2014). Consensus paper: The cerebellum's role in movement and cognition. *Cerebellum*, *13*(1), 151–177. doi: 10.1007/s12311-013-0511-x.

Landry, M., Lifshitz, M., & Raz, A. (2017). Brain correlates of hypnosis: A systematic review and meta-analytic exploration. *Neuroscience & Biobehavioral Reviews*, *81*(Pt A), 75–98. doi: 10.1016/j.neubiorev.2017.02.020.

Li, X., Lin, X., Yao, J., Chen, S., Hu, Y., Liu, J., & Jin, R. (2022). Effects of high-definition transcranial direct current stimulation over the primary motor cortex on cold pain sensitivity among healthy adults. *Frontiers in Molecular Neuroscience*, *15*, 853509. doi: 10.3389/fnmol.2022.853509.

Lichtenberg, P., Bachner-Melman, R., Gritsenko, I., & Ebstein, R. P. (2000). Exploratory association study between catechol-O-methyltransferase (COMT) high/low enzyme activity polymorphism and hypnotizability. *American Journal of Medical Genetics*, *96*(6), 771–774. doi: 10.1002/1096-8628(20001204)96::6<771:aid-ajmg14>3.0.co;2-t.

Lichtenberg, P., Even-Or, E., Bachner-Melman, R., Levin, R., Brin, A., & Heresco-Levy, U. (2008). Hypnotizability and blink rate: A test of the dopamine hypothesis. *International Journal of Clinical and Experimental Hypnosis*, *56*(3), 243–254. doi: 10.1080/00207140802039474.

Lindsay, S., Kurtz, R. M., & Stern, J. A. (1993) Hypnotic susceptibility and the endogenous eye-blink: A brief communication. *International Journal of Clinical and Experimental Hypnosis*, *41*, 92.

Lischke A., Pahnke, R., Mau-Moeller, A., & Weippert, M. (2021). Heart rate variability modulates interoceptive accuracy. *Frontiers in Neuroscience*, *14*, 612445. doi: 10.3389/fnins.2020.612445.

Lynn, S. J., & Green, J. P. (2011). The sociocognitive and dissociation theories of hypnosis: Toward a rapprochement. *International Journal of Clinical and Experimental Hypnosis*, *59*(3), 277–293. doi: 10.1080/00207144.2011.570652.

Madeo, D., Castellani, E., Santarcangelo, E. L., & Mocenni, C. (2013). Hypnotic assessment based on the recurrence quantification analysis of EEG recorded in the ordinary state of consciousness. *Brain & Cognition*, *83*(2), 227–233. doi: 10.1016/j.bandc.2013.08.002.

Marwan, N. C., Thiel, M., & Kurths, J. (2007). Recurrence plots for the analysis of complex systems. *Physics Reports*, *438*, 237–329.

Matsuzawa, Y., Kwon, T. G., Lennon, R. J., Lerman, L. O., & Lerman, A. (2015). A. prognostic value of flow-mediated vasodilation in brachial artery and fingertip artery for cardiovascular events: A systematic review and meta-analysis. *Journal of American Heart Association*, *4*(11), e002270. doi: 10.1161/JAHA.115.002270.

Mehling, W. E., Acree, M., Stewart, A., Silas, J., & Jones, A. (2012). The multidimensional assessment of interoceptive awareness, Version 2 (MAIA-2). *PLoS One*, *13*(12), e0208034. doi: 10.1371/journal.pone.0208034.

Menzocchi, M., Mecacci, G., Zeppi, A., Carli, G., & Santarcangelo, E. L. (2014). Hypnotizability and performance on a prism adaptation test. *Cerebellum*, *4*(6),699–706. doi: 10.1007/s12311-015-0671-y.

Minowa, C., & Koitabashi, K. (2014). The effect of autogenic training on salivary immunoglobulin A in surgical patients with breast cancer: A randomized pilot trial. *Complementary Therapy in Clinical Practice*, *20*(4), 193–196. 10.1016/j.ctcp.2014.07.001

Monaghan, A. S., Johansson, H., Torres, A., Brewer, G. A., & Peterson, D. S. (2022). The impact of divided attention on automatic postural responses: A systematic review and meta-analysis. *Experimental Gerontology*, *162*, 111759. doi: 10.1016/j.exger.2022.111759.

Moret, V., Forster, A., Laverrière, M.-C., Lambert, H., Gaillard, R. C., Bourgeois, P., Haynal, A., Gemperle, M., & Buchser, E. (1991). Mechanism of analgesia induced by hypnosis and acupuncture: Is there a difference? *Pain*, *45*(2), 135–140. 10.1016/0304-3959(91)90178-Z.

Moser, G. (2014). The role of hypnotherapy for the treatment of inflammatory bowel diseases. *Expert Reviews in Gastroenterology & Hepatology*, *8*(6):601–606. doi: 10.1586/17474124.2014.917955.

Murphy, J., Brewer, R., Coll, M. P., Plans, D., Hall, M., Shiu, S. S., Catmur,.C., & Bird, G. (2019). I feel it in my finger: Measurement device affects cardiac interoceptive accuracy. *Biological Psychology*, *148*, 107765. doi: 10.1016/j.biopsycho.2019.107765.

Naish, P. L. (2010). Hypnosis and hemispheric asymmetry. *Consciousness & Cognition*, *19*(1), 230–234. doi: 10.1016/j.concog.2009.10.003.

Nord, C. L., & Garfinkel, S. N. (2022). Interoceptive pathways to understand and treat mental health conditions. *Trends in Cognitive Science*, *26*(6), 499–513. doi: 10.1016/j.tics.2022.03.004.

Paoletti, G., Varanini, M., Balocchi, R., Morizzo, C., Palombo, C., & Santarcangelo, E. L. (2010). Cardiovascular and respiratory correlates of deep nociceptive stimulation, suggestions for analgesia, pain imagery and cognitive load as a function of hypnotizability. *Brain Research Bulletin*, *82*(1-2),5–73. doi: 10.1016/j.brainresbull.2010.03.003.

Picerni E., Santarcangelo E. L., Laricchiuta D., Cutuli D., Petrosini L., Spalletta G., Piras F. (2019). Cerebellar structural variations in subjects with different hypnotizability. *Cerebellum*, *18*(1),109–118. doi: 10.1007/s12311-018-0965-y.

Piché, M., Arsenault, M., & Rainville, P. (2010). Dissection of perceptual, motor and autonomic components of motor of brain activity evoked by noxious stimulation. *Pain*, *149*(3), 453–462. doi: 10.1016/j.pain.2010.01.005.

Presciuttini, S., Gialluisi, A., Barbuti, S., Curcio, M., Scatena, F., Carli, G., & Santarcangelo, E. L. (2014). Hypnotizability and catechol-O-methyltransferase (COMT) polymorphysms in Italians. *Frontiers in Human Neuroscience*, 7, 929. doi: 10.3389/fnhum.2013.00929.

Quadt, L., Critchley, H., & Nagai, Y. (2022). Cognition, emotion, and the central autonomic network. *Autonomic Neuroscience*, *238*, 102948. doi: 10.1016/j.autneu.2022.102948.

Rashid, A., Santarcangelo, E. L., & Roatta, S. (2022a). Does hypnotizability affect neurovascular coupling during cognitive tasks? *Physiology & Behavior*, *113915*. doi: 10.1016/j.physbeh.2022.113915.

Rashid, A., Santarcangelo, E. L., & Roatta, S. (2022b). Cerebral blood flow in healthy subjects with different hypnotizability scores. *Brain Sciences*, *12*(5), 558. doi: 10.3390/brainsci12050558.

Rashid, A., Santarcangelo, E. L., & Roatta, S. (2022c). Cerebrovascular reactivity during visual stimulation: Does hypnotizability matter? *Brain Research*, *1794*, 148059. doi: 10.1016/j.brainres.2022.148059.

Ring, C., Brener, J., Knapp, K., & Mailloux, J. (2015). Effects of heartbeat feedback on beliefs about heart rate and heartbeat counting: A cautionary tale about interoceptive awareness. *Biological Psychology*, *104*, 193–198. 10.1016/i.biopsycho.2014.12.010.

Rominger, C., Weiss, E. M., Nagl, S., Niederstätter, H., Parson, W., & Papousek, I. 8(2014). Carriers of the COMT Met/Met allele have higher degrees of hypnotizability, provided that they have good attentional control: A case of gene-trait interaction. *International Journal of Clinical and Experimental Hypnosis*, *62*(4), 55–82. doi: 0.1080/00207144.2014.931177.

Rosati, A., Belcari, I., Santarcangelo, E. L., & Sebastiani, L. (2021). Interoceptive accuracy as a function of hypnotizability. *International Journal of Clinical and Experimental Hypnosis*, *69*(4), 441–452. doi: 10.1080/00207144.2021.1954859.

Ruggirello, S., Campioni, L., Piermanni, S., Sebastiani, &, Santarcangelo, E. L. (2019). Does hypnotic assessment predict the functional equivalence between motor imagery and action? *Brain & Cognition*, *136*, 103598. doi: 10.1016/j.bandc.2019.103598.

Ruzyla-Smith, P., Barabasz, A., Barabasz, M., & Warner, D. (1995). Effects of hypnosis on the immune response: B-cells, T-cells, helper and suppressor cells. *American Journal of Clinical Hypnosis*, *38*(2), 71–79. 10.1080/00029157.1995.10403185

Salihu, A. T., Hill, K. D., & Jaberzadeh, S. (2022). Effect of cognitive task complexity on dual task postural stability: A systematic review and meta-analysis. *Experimental Brain Research*, *240*(3), 703–731. doi: 10.1007/s00221-021-06299-y.

Sambo, C. F., Liang, M., Cruccu, G., & Iannetti, G. D. (2012). Defensive peripersonal space: The blink reflex evoked by hand stimulation is increased when the hand is near the face. *Journal of Neurophysiology*, *107*(3), 880–889. doi: 10.1152/jn.00731.2011.

Sandrini, G., Milanov, I., Malaguti, S., Nigrelli, M. P., Moglia, A., & Nappi, G. (2000). Effects of hypnosis on diffuse noxious inhibitory controls. *Physiology & Behavior*, *69*(3), 295–300. doi: 10.1016/s0031-9384(00)00210-9.

Santarcangelo, E. L., Balocchi, R., Scattina, E., Manzoni, D., Bruschini, L., Ghelarducci, B., & Varanini, M. (2008). Hypnotizability-dependent modulation of the changes in heart rate control induced by upright stance. *Brain Research Bulletin*, *75*(5), 692–697. doi: 10.1016/j.brainresbull.2007.11.012.

Santarcangelo, E. L., Briscese, L., Capitani, S., Orsini, P., Varanini, M., Rossi, B., & Carboncini, M. C. (2016). Blink reflex in subjects with different hypnotizability: New findings for an old debate. *Physiology & Behavior*, *163*, 288–293. doi: 10.1016/j.physbeh.2016.05.021.
Santarcangelo, E. L., Busse, K., & Carli, G. (1989). Changes in electromyographically recorded human monosynaptic reflex in relation to hypnotic susceptibility and hypnosis. *Neuroscience Letters*, *104*, 157–160. doi: 10.1016/0304-3940(89)90347-9.
Santarcangelo, E. L., Busse, K., & Carli, G.(2003). Frequency of occurrence of the F wave in distal flexor muscles as a function of hypnotic susceptibility and hypnosis. *Cognitive Brain Research*, *16*(1), 99–103. doi: 10.1016/s0926-6410(02)00224-0.
Santarcangelo, E. L., & Carli, G. (2021). Individual traits and pain treatment: The case of hypnotizability. *Frontiers in Neuroscience*, *15*, 683045. doi: 10.3389/fnins.2021.683045. PMID: 34149351
Santarcangelo, E. L., Carli, G., & Sebastiani, L. (2021). An evolutionary approach to hypnotizability. *American Journal of Clinical Hypnosis*, *63*(4), 294–301. doi: 10.1080/00029157.2020.1860893.
Santarcangelo, E. L., Emdin, M., Picano, E., Raciti, M., Macerata, A., Michelassi, C., Ktaft, G., Riva, A., & L'Abbate, A. (1992). Can hypnosis modify the sympathetic-parasympathetic balance at heart level?: Methodological aspects and pathophysiological relevance. Workshop on continuous monitoring of respiration. *Journal of Ambulatory Monitoring*, *5*, 191–196.
Santarcangelo, E. L., Paoletti, G., Balocchi, R., Carli, G., Morizzo, C., Palombo, C., & Varanini, M. (2012). Hypnotizability modulates the cardiovascular correlates of subjective relaxation. *International Journal of Clinical and Experimental Hypnosis*, *60*(4), 383–396. doi: 10.1080/00207144.2012.700609.
Santarcangelo, E. L., Paoletti, G., Chiavacci, I., Palombo, C., Carli, G., & Varanini, M.(2013). Cognitive modulation of psychophysical, respiratory and autonomic responses to cold pressor test. *PLoS One*, *8*(10), 75023. doi: 10.1371/journal.pone.0075023.
Santarcangelo, E. L., & Scattina, E. (2016). Complementing the latest APA Definition of hypnosis: Sensory-motor and vascular peculiarities involved in hypnotizability. *International Journal of Clinical and Experimental Hypnosis*, *64*(3), 318–330. doi: 10.1080/00207144.2016.1171093.
Santarcangelo, E. L., Scattina, E., Carli, G., Macerata, A., & Manzoni, D. (2008a). Hypnotizability-dependent modulation of postural control: Effects of alteration of the visual and leg proprioceptive inputs. *Experimental Brain Research*, *191*(3), 331–340. doi: 10.1007/s00221-008-1526-2.
Santarcangelo, E. L., Scattina, E., Orsini, P., Bruschini, L., Ghelarducci, B., &Manzoni, D. (2008b). Effects of vestibular and neck proprioceptive stimulation on posture as a function of hypnotizability. *International Journal of Clinical and Experimental Hypnosis*, *56*(2), 170–184. doi: 10.1080/00207140701849510.
Santarcangelo, E. L., Scattina, E., Carli, G., Ghelarducci, B., Orsini, P., & Manzoni, D. (2010). Can imagery become reality? *Experimental Brain Research*, *206*(3), 329–335. doi: 10.1007/s00221-010-2412-2.
Sara, J. D. S., Toya, T., Ahmad, A., Clark, M. M., Gilliam, W. P., Lerman, L. O., & Lerman, A. (2022). Mental stress and its effects on vascular health. *Mayo Clinic Proceedings*, *97*(5), 951–990. doi: 10.1016/j.mayocp.2022.02.004.
Sebastiani, L., Simoni, A., Gemignani, A., Ghelarducci, B., & Santarcangelo, E. L. (2005). Relaxation as a cognitive task. *Archives Italiennes de Biologie*, *143*(1), 1–12.
Sebastiani L., Simoni A., Gemignani A., Ghelarducci, B., & Santarcangelo E. L. (2003). Autonomic and EEG correlates of emotional imagery in subjects with different hypnotic susceptibility. *Brain Research Bulletin*, *60*, 151–160.
Spiegel, D., & Albert, L. H. (1983). Naloxone fails to reverse hypnotic alleviation of chronic pain. *Psychopharmacology*, *81*, 140–143.
Spina, V., Chisari, C., & Santarcangelo, E. L. (2020). High motor cortex excitability in highly hypnotizable individuals: A favourable factor for neuroplasticity? *Neuroscience*, *430*, 125–130. 10.1016/j.neuroscience.2020.01.042
Storozheva, Z. I., Kirenskaya, A. V., Gordeev, M. N., Kovaleva, M. E., & Novototsky-Vlasov, V. Y. (2018). COMT genotype and sensory and sensorimotor gating in high and low hypnotizable subjects. *International Journal of Clinical and Experimental Hypnosis*, *66*(1), 83–105. doi: 10.1080/00207144.2018.13961.

Tellegen, A. (1981). Practicing the two disciplines for relaxation and enlightenment: Comment on "Role of the feedback signal in electromyograph biofeedback: the relevance of attention" by Qualls and Sheehan, *Journal of Experimental Psychology, General*, *110*, 217–231. https://pubmed.ncbi.nlm.nih.gov/6454759/

Tellegen, A., & Atkinson, G. (1974). Openness to absorbing and self-altering experiences ("absorption"), a trait related to hypnotic susceptibility *Journal of Abnormal Psychology*, *83*, 268–277. 10.1037/h0036681

Tzvi, E., Loens, S., & Donchin, O. (2022). Mini review: The role of the cerebellum in visuomotor adaptation. *Cerebellum*, *21*(2), 306–313. doi: 10.1007/s12311-021-01281-4

Vanhaudenhuyse, A., Ledoux, D., Gosseries, O., Demertzi, A., Laureys, S., & Faymonville, M. E. (2019). Can subjective ratings of absorption, dissociation and time perception during neutral hypnosis predict hypnotizability?: An exploratory study. *International Journal of Clinical and Experimental Hypnosis*, *67*(1), 28–38. doi: 10.1080/00207144.2019.1553765.

Varanini, M., Balocchi, R., Carli, G., Paoletti, G., & Santarcangelo, E. L. (2018). Hypnotizability and pain modulation: A body-mind perspective. *International Journal of Clinical and Experimental Hypnosis*, *66*(3), 265–281. doi: 10.1080/00207144.2018.1460561.

Varga, K., & Kekecs, Z. (2014). Oxytocin and cortisol in the hypnotic interaction. *International Journal of Clinical and Experimental Hypnosis*, *62*(1), 111–128. doi: 10.1080/00207144.2013.841494.

Varga, K., Németh, Z., & Szekely, A. (2011). Lack of correlation between hypnotic susceptibility and various components of attention. *Consciousness & Cognition*, *20*, 1872–1881. 10.1016/j.concog.2011.09.008

Vase, L., Robinson, M. E., Verne, N. G., Price, D. D. (2005). Increased placebo analgesia over time in irritable bowel syndrome (IBS) patients is associated with desire and expectation but not endogenous opioid mechanisms. *Pain*, *115*, 338–347. doi: 10.1016/j.pain.2005.03.014.

Xue, Y. T., Tan, Q. W., Li, P., Mou, S. F., Liu, S. J., Bao, Y.,. Jiao, H. C., & Su, W. G. (2015). Investigating the role of acute mental stress on endothelial dysfunction: a systematic review and meta-analysis. *Clinical Research in Cardiology*, *104*(4), 310–319. doi: 10.100s00392-014-0782-3.

Yao, J., Li, X., Zhang, W., Lin, X., Lyu, X., Lou, W., & Peng, W. (2021). Analgesia induced by anodal tDCS and high-frequency tRNS over the motor cortex: Immediate and sustained effects on pain perception. *Brain Stimulation*, *14*(5),1174–1183. doi: 10.1016/j.brs.2021.07.011.

Yargholi, E., & Nasrabadi, A. M. (2015). Chaos-chaos transition of left hemisphere EEGs during standard tasks of Waterloo-Stanford Group Scale of hypnotic susceptibility. *Journal of Medical Engineering & Technology*, *39*(5), 281–285. doi: 10.3109/03091902.2015.1048317.

Zachariae, R., Hansen, J. B., Andersen,M. A., Jinquan, T., Petersen, K. S., Simonsen, C., Zachariae, C., Thestrup-Pedersen, K. (1994). Changes in cellular immune function after immune specific guided imagery and relaxation in high and low hypnotizable healthy subjects. *Psychotherapy and Psychosomatics*, *61*, 74–92 10.1159/000288872,

Zachariae, R., Andersen, O. K., Bjerring, P., Jørgensen, M. M., & Arendt-Nielsen L. (1998). Effects of an opioid antagonist on pain intensity and withdrawal reflexes during induction of hypnotic analgesia in high- and low-hypnotizable volunteers. *European Journal of Pain*, 2(1), 25–34. doi: 10.1016/s1090-3801(98)90043-x.

Zarei, S. P., Briscese, L., Capitani, S., Rossi, B., Carboncini, M. C., Santarcangelo, E. L., & Nasrabadi, A. M. (2020). Hypnotizability-related effects of pain expectation on the later modulation of cortical connectivity. *International Journal of Clinical and Experimental Hypnosis*, 68(3), 306–326. doi: 10.1080/00207144.2020.1762196.

22
TYPES OF HIGH HYPNOTIZABLES

Deirdre Barrett

Department of Psychiatry, Harvard Medical School

This chapter summarizes traits that predict response to hypnotic induction and distinct clusters of traits which may represent different types of hypnotizability. The author defines hypnosis in accordance with the American Psychological Association Division 30 definition which she co-authored (Green et al., 2005), "A state of consciousness involving focused attention and reduced peripheral awareness characterized by an enhanced capacity for response to suggestion."

Through the late 20th century, studies on what predicted hypnotizability, as measured by formal tests such as Stanford Hypnotic Susceptibility Scales (Weitzenhoffer, & Hilgard, 1962) and the Harvard Group Scale of Hypnotic Susceptibility (Shor & Orne, 1962), began to converge on a trait—or group of closely linked traits—representing a preexisting disposition to informal trance: vividness of imagination, absorption in imagination, and ability to block out external stimuli. Josephine Hilgard (1970, 1979) found the childhood histories of her deep trance subjects were more likely than less hypnotizable subjects to involve imaginary playmates, parental encouragement of fantasy play, and a hearty appetite for fiction. As adults, the high susceptibles were more likely than others to be avid consumers of drama, film, and fiction, to daydream more, and to be more creative.

Hypnotic susceptibility also correlates with Tellegen and Atkinson's (1974) scale of absorption in imaginative activity, containing questions about vividness of imagery, intensity of emotional involvement in fantasy, tendency to tune out external stimuli when imaging, and experiences of synesthesia. Absorption has also been found by multiple regression analyses to account for factors such as positive attitudes toward hypnosis, which in turn have been linked to hypnotic susceptibility (Spanos & McPeake, 1977). More recent studies (Ott, 2016) support the strong correlation between absorption and hypnotic susceptibility, but only when assessed in the hypnotic context (Council et al., 1986).

Wilson and Barber (1981, 1983) studied 27 women who scored as the 4% most hypnotically responsive on several of the standard inventories plus their own criteria of being able to enter a trance with an instant re-hypnosis cue. They reported that all but one of them were distinguished by a constellation of fantasy-related characteristics: (1) They spent much of their waking time engaged in fantasy; most fantasized at least 90% of their waking time simultaneous with carrying on real-life activities. (2) They reported their imagery to be

DOI: 10.4324/9781003449126-30

every bit as vivid as their perceptions of reality; 65% said this was the case with their eyes open while 35% had to close their eyes for the visual component of their imagery to look completely real. (3) They experienced physiologic responses to their images such as needing a blanket to watch *Dr. Zhivago* on TV in a warm room, vomiting when they (mistakenly) thought they had eaten spoiled food, and being able to reach orgasm through fantasy with no physical stimulation. The majority of their female subjects had experienced physiological symptoms of false pregnancy at least once when they had reason to suspect they might be pregnant. (4) They had unusually early ages for their reported first memory, many dating back to infancy. Only one of Wilson and Barber's high hypnotizable subjects did not display this constellation of fantasy-related characteristics, and only a small minority of their low and medium susceptible subjects displayed any of them.

Several other studies examined the relationship between fantasy and hypnotizability—all finding a positive correlation but to varying degrees. Lynn and Rhue (1986) developed a "fantasy-proneness" scale based closely on the characteristics Wilson and Barber had described. They found that 80% of fantasy-prone subjects scored highly hypnotizable, while only about 35% of the non-fantasizers did so. Lynn and Rhue (1988) and Council and Huff (1990) found that high and medium fantasizers did not differ in hypnotic responsiveness, while low fantasizers were less hypnotically susceptible. Spanos (1989) found an even lower degree of correlation between fantasy proneness and hypnotic susceptibility.

Fantasizers Versus Other Types of High Hypnotizables

In two further studies that I describe in detail in this chapter (Barrett, 1992, 1996), I examined to what extent other highly hypnotizable people resembled Wilson and Barber's fantasizers and what traits might characterize deep trance subjects who were not extreme fantasizers. As being able to enter a trance instantly was the most idiosyncratic of Barber and Wilson's criteria, it was hypothesized that this might distinguish fantasizers from other deep trance subjects. In addition to exploring the replicability of Wilson and Barber's findings about fantasy activity among high hypnotizables, other points of interest were characteristics of hypnotic experience and how these interact with a person's waking fantasy style.

For the first of these studies (Barrett, 1992), 34 extremely hypnotizable subjects were selected from among approximately 1,200 undergraduate subject volunteers who had been hypnotized in the course of other research projects and demonstrations in classroom and dormitory settings over a several year period. They were selected using two standard scales: The Harvard Group Scale of Hypnotic Susceptibility, Form A (Shor and Orne, 1962); and The Stanford Scale of Hypnotic Susceptibility, Form C (Weitzenhoffer & Hilgard, 1962). All subjects scored either 11 or 12 on both scales. This constituted a very similar criterion for hypnotic susceptibility to Wilson and Barber's with the exception of not requiring instant or rapid hypnotic induction.

Subjects were hypnotized a total of three to four times, depending on what the protocol in the screening project had been. Their hypnotic experiences included both ones in which an amnesia suggestion and removal cue were given and ones in which they were not, age regression suggestions, a hypnotic hallucination of a candle that they were asked to blow out, a post-hypnotic hallucination of a person they knew arriving at the experimental room to talk with them, and an attempted instant re-hypnosis followed by several measures of trance depth.

Table 22.1 Waking Imagery and Hypnotic Characteristics of Fantasizers Compared with Dissociaters

Characteristic	*Fantasizers (12 Women, 7 Men)* Yes	No	*Dissociaters (10 Women, 5 Men)* Yes	No	*Chi Square df = 1 X =*
Waking image less than real	3	16	15	0	20.05**
Daydream amnesia	3	16	14	1	15.22**
Earliest memory > 3	0	19	11	4	14.44**
Absorption score low	0	19	7	8	6.19**
Need time to reach deep trance	0	19	15	0	30.06**
Spontaneous amnesia for trance details	0	1	9	6	11.61**
Suggested amnesia total	5	14	15	0	15.06**
Hypnosis very different from other experiences	2	17	15	0	22.99**
Field score high	11	8	15	0	6.08*

* p < .02, ** p < .001 Fantasizers.

For that first study, these high-hypnotizable subjects were interviewed from two and a half to four hours and were asked about the fantasy-related phenomena that Wilson, Barber, and J. Hilgard reported. They were also asked about the "dreamlike" qualities of surrealism, abrupt transitions within daydreams, startling out of them, and occasional amnesia for content that my earlier research had found (Barrett 1979, 1990). They were then asked about the "daymare" phenomena that Hartmann (1984) found among nightmare sufferers. They were also asked about how real and/or involuntary the hypnotic phenomena they experienced felt and about how much hypnosis was like other experiences (Table 22.1).

The first subgroup of deep trance subjects was selected by their ability to enter trance instantly, since Wilson and Barber had used this as a criteria for the group they characterized. These 19 people, 7 male and 12 female, also had a number of other characteristics that distinguished them from subjects who did not achieve their deep trances immediately. Most of these characteristics clustered around vividness of fantasy processes, so they are referred to for the rest of this chapter by Wilson and Barber's term *fantasizers*.

Vivid Imagery and Fantasies

Fantasizers scored extremely high on Tellegen and Atkinson's Absorption Scale: 32–37 of 37 items, with a mean of .34. During their interviews, they described five related characteristics of fantasy proneness that Wilson and Barber found most characteristic of their group: extensive history of childhood fantasy play, majority of adult time devoted to fantasizing, hallucinatory vividness of imagery, physiological effects from their imaging, and a variety of "psychic" experiences.

They all described rich fantasy life as children. They had a least one imaginary companion, but most had many. These included a real playmate who had moved out of state, a princess, an entire herd of wild horses, and space aliens among others. The fantasizers greatly enjoyed stories, movies, and drama; they tended to prolong their experience of these by incorporating them into their fantasy lives, providing another source of imaginary companions. For example, one subject described that, after seeing the movie *Camelot*, he had spent two years engaging daily in an elaborate scenario in which he was the son of Arthur and Guinevere and commanded the king's court. Periodically he would appoint new knights of his own invention to the Roundtable. His real-life brother was cast in the role of Mordred, but all the other characters were either from the film, or completely from his own imagination. The fantasizers described these imaginary companions as every bit as vivid as real persons. In addition to ongoing fantasies, these subjects described a wide variety of brief fantasy as children, such as watching a friend blow soap bubbles and suddenly developing a fantasy about there being a fairy that lived inside one of the bubbles. Seventeen of them found this changing of realities at will so compelling that before encountering its formal philosophical discussions they had formulated their own versions of the famous musings of Chuang-tzu: "One night, I dreamed I was a butterfly, fluttering here and there, content with my lot. Suddenly I awoke and was Chuang-tzu again. Who am I in reality: A butterfly dreaming that I am Chuang-tzu, or Chuang-tzu dreaming that I was a butterfly?" (trans. 1970).

Parents of 15 of the fantasizers were remembered as explicitly encouraging their fantasy. On a rainy day when one boy was bored, his mother would begin play suggestions with, "You could pretend to be ..." Another said her parents' formula response to her requests for expensive toys was, "You could take this ... (household object) and with a little imagination, it would look just like ... (that $200-whatever-Susie-just-got)." And she reported, "this worked for me—although Susie couldn't quite always see it." One mother very specifically trained hypnotic ability by reading trance exercises about age regression, being an animal, speeding up time, and so forth to her son from the book *Mind Games* (Masters & Houston, 1972).

Their adult fantasy continued to occupy the majority of their waking hours. They all fantasized throughout the performance of routine tasks and during any unoccupied time. Six of them said they did not "fantasize" or "daydream" when dealing with the most demanding tasks but still continued to have vivid images in response to any sensory words. The other 13 said they continued to have elaborate ongoing fantasy scenarios. Some experienced them superimposed and intertwined with the ongoing tasks: "I'm listening to my boss's directions carefully, but I'm seeing the *Saturday Night* live character 'Mockman' next to him mocking all his gestures." Others experienced the fantasies as simultaneous or separate, happening "on a side state," as one subject described it: "somehow I'm seeing the real world and experiencing my fantasy one at the same time."

Fantasizers also continued to have momentary vivid fantasies inspired by ongoing events. One young man had come to the interview directly from an archery class where he described that as he shot arrows at a target and watched others do so, he would briefly experience himself as the arrow being hurled by the force of the string through the air and felt himself piercing the fiberboard target. Another described that while passing up chocolate cake at lunch because of a diet, she momentarily "became" a microbe burrowing through the cake, tasting and smelling it as she devoured it, and feeling it squish around her body. She reported experiencing a sense of satiation with this fantasy indulgence.

All of these subjects described some of the dreamlike, surreal content, sudden transitions, and surprise that two earlier studies had reported for deep trance subjects' daydreams (Barrett, 1979, 1990, 1991). When asked whether they "startled" out of daydreams that they could not recall, four said they experienced this occasionally, although usually they had a "tip of the tongue" feeling about the fantasy and its memory would "come back" to them shortly.

Seven of them reported that they occasionally had frightening content that seemed not to be under their control as in the "daymares" reported by Hartmann's nightmare sufferers.

Like Wilson and Barber's subjects, they experienced physical effects from their imagery. Seven of the 12 female fantasizers had experienced false pregnancy symptoms. Even more of Wilson's subjects had experienced some such symptoms and full-blown cases (so to speak) presenting for treatment have been linked to high hypnotic susceptibility (Barrett, 1989). All of the fantasizers, male and female, described sometimes experiencing physical sensations to visual stimuli such as shivering when seeing a painting of the Alps; feeling hot, dry, and impulsively getting something to drink in response to looking at desert photos; and getting nauseated from motion sickness at a film set on a tossing submarine. Ten of them said they tried to avoid either fictional depictions or real newsreel footage of violence and injuries because they experienced pain akin to real injuries. For four of them, this might precipitate ill feelings for hours or days. One such subject who had long ago learned to avoid television news described several weeks previously that she had been watching a nationally televised swim meet in which a diver had unexpectedly been injured. As she described the scene, she clutched herself tightly, grimaced as if in pain, tears came to her eyes, and she described this as minimal compared to her reaction when watching the scene that had left her shaken and physically aching for hours.

Fourteen of the fantasizers could experience orgasm through fantasy in the absence of any physical stimulation, and all of them reported frequent, vivid, and varied sexual fantasies. Although most of them tended to have fairly active and varied sex lives, all of them had fantasies of many more variations than they actually engaged in. Seventeen of this group were exclusively heterosexual, and two males were predominantly homosexual with a bit of heterosexual experience. However, all of the women and two of the heterosexual men mentioned homosexual fantasies. Other fantasy partners included animals, children, statues, and a variety of suggestively shaped inanimate objects.

Wilson and Barber reported that their subjects often obtained greater enjoyment from their fantasized sex than their actual sexual relationships. When our group was queried, they said this was not a meaningful comparison as their two categories of sexual experience were fantasy only versus fantasy superimposed on real activity, of which the latter was often preferred. Real partners were heard to utter imaginary sexy comments, were dressed in hallucinatory erotic attire, had movie stars' faces (and occasionally other parts) superimposed onto theirs, were joined by additional imaginary partners, and were transformed into science-fiction creatures and circus animals. Only two subjects (one male, one female) said they tried not to fantasize during real sex, and both of them said they often failed.

Fantasizers all had some experiences that they considered "psychic": 14 had premonitions about events that were going to happen, 12 said that they could sometimes sense what significant others were thinking or feeling at a distance, 9 had dreams that came true, 13 had out-of-body experiences, and 8 had seen ghosts. Fifteen firmly believed these experiences were real paranormal phenomena, and the remaining four said they were undecided about their reality.

Early Memories and Parental Discipline

The earliest memories of the fantasizers were all identified as being before the age of three, and before the age of two for 11 subjects. For the purposes of this study, subjectively believed age and detail of first memories were compared. This study was not set up to definitely check whether the ages were accurate or whether indeed the memory was directly recalled rather than fantasized from stories told by parents. For randomly selected college students, the average of subjectively recalled first memory is about three and a half and 2–6 is the usual range (Barrett, 1980, 1983). The youngest memory that had a specific time estimate was of age eight months. This subject remembered two scenes: one in which he was being carried by his father down a hospital corridor and another in which he was lying on his back with one green-gowned man prodding his stomach while another pressed a plastic mask over his nose and mouth. He remembered excruciating pain in both scenes. He was quite convinced that these were memories of an appendectomy he had undergone at eight months, and that he had remembered details of this, which surprised his parents the first time they discussed it with him.

More typically, the incidents were too minor to be remembered by parents or to be tied to an exact date but sounded like those of a preverbal or early verbal child—for example, one incident that the subject estimated as before age two: "I remember being in my crib, which was pushed against a wall with a window above it. I was looking up at the window and it must have been raining outside because water drops were running down the outside of it. I was fascinated because I'd never noticed the window doing this before. This was a stage when I would point at things and ask 'whah?' and my mother would say the name for it. I pointed at the water drops and said 'shah?' and my mother said 'window.' I already knew this word so I frustratedly pointed again at the glass with the drops on the outside and repeated 'whah?' I guess she thought I meant the pane of glass—or maybe she even said 'rain' and I misunderstood—because what I heard her say was 'pain.' I thought I recognized the word for when I hurt myself and I realized that the drops were like the tears that ran down my face at those times. I watched amazed that the window could cry with pain like me. I think it was a long time before I corrected this impression and came to connect the drops with the 'rain' that fell when I was outside and that could also run down the window's 'pane.'"

Several of this group's earliest memories were of surreal events, most likely memories of fantasies or dreams such as this one: "I remember waking up in the middle of the night. In the air over me there were these big neon letters of the alphabet, maybe eight inches tall dancing around. They looked so wonderful. I recognized an 'A' and a 'D' because I knew the first few letters, but most of them were shapes I didn't know from later in the alphabet. They seemed to be floating into my room from the hall. I got out of bed and went into the hall where there were more neon letters in a line coming from my parents' room. I followed the line into my parents' bedroom. They were coming out of the drain on the floor; one by one they would pop up out of the drain and dance out of the room. I watched them there for a while and then I went back to my room and watched them in bed until I fell asleep again. Remember thinking I must tell my parents about this in the morning, but I don't know if I did. I must have been about to turn three because I could say the alphabet by three years old."

When asked about how their parents had disciplined them, 11 of the subjects said that their parent had disciplined them solely by some combination of two strategies: (1) rewards or withholding of rewards, and (2) reasoning with them, often emphasizing empathy: "One time I'd gotten in a fight at nursery school with another little girl because there was this doll there that was her favorite or regular toy to play with. I'd gotten it first that day; she tried to take it away from me and I pushed her down. The teacher called my mother and told her about it. Mother told me I should think about what she had felt like when she fell down, and it became like I really was her hitting the floor scraping one knee, and crying. I could also feel her desperation and thinking it really was her doll (even though it was the school's); she had named it and everything. After that, I wouldn't have done that again."

Eight of this group reported discipline that they experienced as harsh such as spankings, being locked in their rooms for extended periods, and verbal belittling. They typically used fantasy and imaginary companions to restore self-esteem after these incidents. Wilson and Barber (1978) reported that their subjects' fantasies in these situations did not revolve around retaliation except indirectly toward other objects. In the present sample, more than half of these fantasies were of retaliation against parents, albeit tempered by leniency on the part of the offended child. One child fantasized producing electric shocks to repel spankings. More typically, some other powerful being intervened against the parent sometimes because of punishing the child, sometimes for some other reason. Parents were kidnapped by aliens, chained in King Arthur's dungeon, arrested by the police, or sent back to grade school. In most cases, however, the next step was that the child intervened on the parents' behalf and the parents were released feeling repentant and/or indebted.

Fantasizers' Experience of Hypnosis

Despite being such deep trance subjects, these 19 people scored only just above average (mean = 18) on the Field Inventory (Field, 1965) and very low on the subgroup of Field Items that reported surprise at hypnotic phenomena. Nine of the 19 described hypnosis as not different than what they experienced in their waking fantasy activity, and the remaining ten found hypnosis mildly different by being somewhat more intense in some aspects but still similar to their other imagery experiences. These differences included hypnotic imagery being more consistently hallucinatory for six subjects, and two saying they felt much more subjective time had gone by in hypnosis than it would if they were fantasizing for a similar amount of real time. One drama major said, "Hypnosis is a lot like what I do with method acting only you can get more into it. When I'm doing an acting exercise, I can only get so far into the experience because some part of me has to keep watching that I don't become the character so much that I'd just walk out of the class if he was mad, but with the hypnosis you don't have to watch that sort of thing at all. During the age regression, I could leave my adult self behind completely."

These subjects were all quite aware that what they experienced during hypnosis were phenomena they produced themselves. None of them conceptualized it at all in terms of something the hypnotist was doing to them. "Hypnosis was a lot like what I do when I'm daydreaming or experiencing something from the past except it's even easier because your voice conjures up the images automatically," said one subject. The fantasizers generally seemed proud of their ability at hypnosis. All of them enjoyed the hypnotic experiences, although several remarked that the lengthy interviews about fantasy and memory were more personally significant to them. "Seeing the things you described in hypnosis is nice but pretty much like my daydreaming all the time, but talking about what my daydreams are like and how big a part of my life they are isn't something I've ever gotten to do before in this much detail."

Fantasizers experienced hypnotic amnesia only when it was specifically suggested—and not always absolutely then. Six of the eight fantasizers scoring 11 rather than 12 on the HGSHS-A had the amnesia suggestion as their only failed item. Some had partial recall although they had formally passed it. Others described that it seemed not as completely real an effect as the other hypnotic phenomena, citing working to keep items out of consciousness or being very aware they could counter the suggestion if they chose.

The fantasizers were also likely to know hypnotic hallucinations were not real without needing to be told this. When asked how they were sure they knew there had not been a real candle lit in the room for instance, 14 of them cited some cognitive strategy that they had long practiced for differentiating the hallucinations of their waking fantasies from reality. Nine of them also usually retained the knowledge that the hypnotist had given verbal suggestions to hallucinate what they then experienced, which made the deduction simple. In response to the HGSHS-A suggestion about hallucinating a fly during his first group induction, one subject had the following experience: "When you told us there was a fly buzzing around us, one appeared circling my head. Then I realized you had suggested it to everyone, and I saw and heard fifty of them circling around each student in unison. At the same time, the rock group Kansas' song *The Gnat Attack* began to play as if there was a stereo in the room. I thought all this was delightful and very funny. As soon as you said we could shoo the flies away, the music stopped too."

This group showed a moderate degree of muscular relaxation during hypnosis akin to what an average person might look like awake but at rest. There was not a dramatic loss of muscle tone, all of them remained seated in their chair without problem, and most shifted position occasionally during the trance. They only moved easily when asked to do so for candle-blowing and for tasks while age regressed. When asked to, they also talked readily in trance, some of them with a bit softer or more monotone voice than awake, but no one in the group was difficult to understand. All subjects in this subgroup woke from the trance immediately alert. Some began talking about their trance experience before the experimenter asked questions. The most immediate response upon awakening from hypnosis for the fantasizers was a big smile.

Dissociation Group

The other subgroup of 15 subjects was selected for scoring as very highly hypnotizable on standard measures of hypnosis (scores of 11 or 12 on the HGSHS-A and SSHS-C) but not meeting Wilson and Barber's additional criteria of being able to enter a trance instantly. They scored about average (range 16–33, mean = 26) on the Absorption Scale and did not display many of Wilson and Barber's fantasizers' characteristics.

In fact, the most distinctive quality of this subgroup's descriptions of fantasizing was the amnesia that had been noted for some subjects in a previous study (Barrett, 1989). The majority of them said their fantasizing was often characterized by inability to remember some or all of the content. Six of them said the only reason they knew they just daydream was that they were often startled to be spoken to, or otherwise have their attention summoned to the real world, with a sense that their mind had been occupied elsewhere. The reports of this group were quite dissimilar to most characterizations of "fantasy proneness" and "high absorption." They had so much more in common with the dissociative phenomena emphasized in Ernest Hilgard's (1977) neodissociation theory of hypnotic susceptibility that this subgroup is referred to as the *dissociaters* for the remainder of this discussion.

Fantasies, Early Memory, and Parental Discipline

The fantasies that the dissociaters did recall from both childhood and the present were more mundane than the other subgroup's. They tended to be pleasant, realistic scenarios about events they would like to happen in the near future. None of them said these fantasies were as real as in their sensory imagery as their perception of reality. Dissociaters were somewhat more like the fantasizers in how they reacted to external drama. They described that as both children and adults, they could become so absorbed in books, films, plays, and stories being told to them that they could lose track of time, surroundings, or their usual sense of identity. Their lack of equal vividness in self-directed fantasy seemed to stem partly from an external locus of control. It just did not seem to them that vivid images could be their own production, and so they tended to experience them mainly in response to others' lead as in hypnosis or in listening to stories. Sometimes this absorption in external stimuli was intertwined with amnestic phenomena; several subjects commented that they thought they got very caught up in horror movies, but then could not remember their content shortly afterwards.

One of the most dramatic incidents of amnesia was recounted in answer to a routine inquiry of one of the dissociaters as to whether she had ever been hypnotized before. She answered "maybe" and described the following experience: "One time, my boyfriend and I were watching a police show on TV. There was this scene where they were going to use hypnosis with a witness. The detective began to swing a watch and tell the witness that he was going to go into deep sleep. I don't remember anything after that until I started awake and said 'what happened' about twenty minutes later. My boyfriend says the show continued with questions during the hypnosis, several scenes of what other characters were doing, commercial break, and then came back to the scene where the detective was waking the witness up. But I don't remember any of that. I guess I was hypnotized by the watch."

Other amnestic experiences seemed to be triggered by more personal associations. One suggestion subjects were given in hypnosis was that they would see a book "... with something important for you in it. You may take it down from the bookshelf and open it." One woman reported the book she saw was *Sybil*. She had opened it in the trance but couldn't recall anything she had read then. She also said that in reality, she had bought the book two years before and was sure she had read it but could not remember anything about it. When asked if she could produce even a single sentence about the main topic of the book, she insisted she had no idea. The obvious diagnostic questions suggested by this will be discussed later in the section on dissociative disorders.

The way in which the dissociaters appeared most like the fantasizers was in the frequency of their dramatic psychophysiological reactions. Five of the ten women had experienced symptoms of false pregnancy. They reported getting cold watching arctic scenes and becoming nauseated after eating supposedly spoiled food that they later learned was fine. One developed a rash after being told by a prankster friend that a vine she had handled was poison ivy. Three of them also reported feeling pain when witnessing others' traumas. This might have been true of more of them, as six remarked that they often could not remember moments around witnessing injuries. After a swine flu vaccination (back in the scare of the 1970s), one subject had a hysterical conversion-like episode of ascending paralysis that mimicked Guillain-Barré syndrome, but which had remitted after a few minutes of reassurance from her physician about the safety of the vaccine.

None of this group said they achieved orgasms solely from fantasy. All of them reported sexual fantasies, but six subjects remarked that they sometimes couldn't remember them afterward. The interview did not specifically ask for examples of sexual fantasies. The fantasizer subgroup, as already described, volunteered voluminous content in the course of answering questions about frequency and vividness of these fantasies. The dissociaters rarely volunteered much detail, so less characterization was possible of their fantasy content. Most of the ones that were mentioned were mundane. The few who volunteered details consistently seemed to do so in the context of wanting reassurance about their normality. One subject was worried that she fantasized about anyone besides her boyfriend, and a male was bothered by thoughts of his girlfriend's attractive mother. A woman who in her early teens had been a victim of sexual abuse, now in her early twenties, found herself fantasizing about the abuse in an arousing manner during masturbation and intercourse. She seemed reassured to hear that was not uncommon among abuse and rape victims and that it did not invalidate her perception that the sexual contact had been predominantly frightening and unwanted at the time it occurred. Childhood sexual abuse may have been a common event as will be discussed later in the section on abuse.

Fewer subjects in this subgroup believed they had psychic experiences, and for nine of the 11 who did so, these experiences were confined solely to altered states of consciousness—dreams most commonly for several of them, automatic writing for two, and trance-like séance phenomena for two. One subject reported that the spirit of her father, who had died when she was nine, regularly appeared to her in dreams dressed in the uniform in which he was buried and gave her advice on current problems. During hypnosis, when she was told that she could open her eyes and "see someone that you know and like" seated across from her, she had opened her eyes and seen her father. She felt certain that her nocturnal visitations were real but was not certain whether the hypnotic hallucination was her father's spirit or not.

The earliest memories of the dissociaters were later than average (mean = 5 and for six subjects between the ages of 6 and 8). This was the opposite trend away from the general population mean than for the fantasizers. When asked about parental discipline, seven of the fantasizers recalled spankings and other corporal punishment, and five more of the others said they could not recall. Abuse and other clearly traumatic incidents will be discussed further in a subsequent section.

Dissociaters' Experience of Hypnosis

This subgroup scored very high on the Field questionnaire, mean = 33, usually answering "true" to all six items that express surprise and amazement at hypnotic phenomena. They were much likelier to conceptualize hypnotic phenomena due to some amazing talent of the hypnotist rather than as produced by themselves. They were resistant to hearing that it was something within their control, and in some sense this may really be less true for this group, for them, it is less consciously controlled. Six of them asked many questions seeking reassurance that their hypnotic susceptibility was normal. Two described hypnosis as partially unpleasant, not in terms of any specific content being negative but they did not like the concept that they were hallucinating. All described hypnosis as the more striking and interesting part of the experimental process; much of the interview about fantasy and imagery was not of great personal relevance. These subjects frequently experienced spontaneous amnesia for hypnotic events. Amnesia was consistent and total for them whenever it was suggested, and it sometimes persisted even once removal cues had been given. Half of them experienced some degree of spontaneous amnesia for trance events when it had not been suggested.

Dissociaters were often surprised at some of their hypnotic experiences, especially hypnotic hallucinations. They were much likelier than fantasizers to believe their hypnotic hallucinations were real until told otherwise. The few who realized they were not real distinguished themselves on the basis of their implausibility rather than by any other method for telling hallucinations from reality. They almost never remembered the verbal suggestions for the hallucinations, and when they did still ignored the association with their perceptions. One subject remained convinced that, coincidentally at the moment that I suggested the HGSHS-A fly hallucination to a roomful of subjects, a real fly happened to begin buzzing around him.

The dissociaters exhibited an extreme loss of muscle tone during trance, often slumping; two needed to be propped up so they did not fall out of their chairs. When asked to move or speak during the trance, their voices and movements were markedly subdued; four were partially inaudible. Six reported that their trance had to lighten for them to be able to move or speak at all.

When they were instructed to awaken, they would usually open their eyes, but most blinked and looked confused at first. Four asked disoriented questions such as "What happened?" or "Where was I?" They appeared to need almost to struggle to talk, and were slow to begin to answer questions. All these behaviors were transient, and all subjects were fully alert within a couple of minutes.

Follow-up: Comparison with Hidden Observer Distinction, Dream Phenomena, and Dissociative Disorders

In a later follow-up study (Barrett, 1996) with 24 subjects who were still geographically available (15 women, 9 men), they were hypnotized again, given suggestions of hypnotic deafness before the first four lines of a recorded nursery rhyme were played at a clear volume, and then tested for the Hilgard's hidden observer phenomena (Hilgard, 1979). These 24 were then interviewed with detailed queries about childhood trauma, dream content, and diagnostic questions for dissociative disorders. Chi square analyses were employed where expected cell size allowed. For smaller subsamples, significance was computed by Fisher's exact probability test.

All of both groups still tested as highly hypnotizable. Two of the dissociater group reported more-consciously controlled and better-recalled imagery than they had at the time of the first study. However, even these two did not show the fantasizer trait of instant-trance-entry and no one in either group had totally shifted group characteristics.

The hidden observer phenomenon was slightly more common in dissociaters (see Table 22.2). Seven of nine dissociaters manifested a hidden observer, while seven of 15 fantasizers did. What was much more clearly pronounced was the difference in content of hidden observers for dissociaters versus fantasizers. All dissociaters who manifested a hidden observer gave accurate descriptions of the stimulus. Four recited it flawlessly, two first named it or said "nursery rhyme," and when asked for the complete rhyme recited it with only minor mistakes. Three dissociaters gave hidden observer responses in a flat monotone similar to all other requested vocalizations they had ever made in trance. Two spoke in a more childlike voice than usually characterized these waking or trance vocalizations.

The final dissociater with a hidden observer responded quite dramatically to the suggestion: opening her eyes (not suggested), saying "Hi, I think I'm who you want to talk to" in a much more aggressive demeanor than the subject's usual waking or hypnotized style, reciting the rhyme in a sarcastic tone, glaring for about 15 seconds, and then closing her eyes again. This response will be discussed later in the section on dissociative diagnoses.

None of the seven dissociaters manifesting a hidden observer remembered the rhyme or their hidden observer responses upon awakening, nor did the three who failed to exhibit a hidden observer recall the rhyme upon awakening.

Table 22.2 Hidden Observers, Nightmares, and Trauma of Fantasizers Compared with Dissociaters

Characteristic	*Fantasizers (9 Women, 6 Men)*		*Dissociaters (6 Women, 3 Men)*		*Fischer Exact Probability Test*
	Yes	*No*	*Yes*	*No*	*p <*
Some hidden observer response	7	8	7	2	.10
Hidden observer with detailed accuracy	7	8	4	5	.85
Recurring nightmares	0	15	6	3	.005
Trauma known	2	13	5	4	.05
Trauma known or suspected	2	13	9	0	.005

The four fantasizers who gave fairly realistic accounts also describe an intentional strategy of "not listening." A typical response was, "It was the rhyme 'Twinkle, Twinkle, Little Star.' The voice was there but I kept telling myself I didn't hear it."

Three fantasizers said something additional in response to hidden observer suggestions that did not contain the majority of the poem. All of these contained some confabulated, visual, or dream-like content either related or unrelated to the poem. One contained a star in the night sky, one heard a "nursery rhyme" that they could not name or recite while experiencing apparently unrelated rich visual imagery, and the third heard "... something about diamonds; I know I could have heard more but I tried not to listen."

After awakening from hypnosis, all seven of the fantasizers had some memory of the rhyme and their hidden observer responses. They appeared integrated with the hidden observer identity although they could also still recall the point in time at which they had been unable to recall the stimulus. For them, the hidden observer seemed to have much the same effect as a simple amnesia removal cue.

Dreams

When asked to recount the most recent dream that they could recall clearly, 11 of the 15 fantasizers gave a dream from the previous night. All others were from the previous four days. They were typically lengthy, fantastic accounts.

There was one out-of-body account, one lucid dream, and a false awakening. All of these are very rare categories, albeit ones that I had found to correlate with hypnotizability in another study on a different sample (Zamore & Barrett, 1989). Three of the dreams were sexual (another rare category), most were pleasant, and none were nightmares. When asked if they had nightmares, four fantasizers reported that they had at least one a month. None of them reported any recurring nightmares.

In contrast, when dissociaters were asked to recount the most recent dream they could recall, many had trouble thinking of one. Although two recalled dreams from the previous night, several dated the last dream they could recall as years before. One gave a recurring nightmare that had happened only a few times as the only dream she believed she had ever recalled in her lifetime. Two more dissociaters gave a recurring nightmare as their most recent well-recalled dream, and three others reported they experienced recurring nightmares at least once a month. All of these subjects also reported nonrecurring nightmares, and one additional dissociater reported nonrecurring nightmares only. Three reported sexual content in their most recent dreams, but these were all within the context of nightmares or other unpleasant dreams. Their nightmares had even more obviously disturbing content than those of the fantasizers including things such as suffocating, the dreamer's body coming apart, and horribly injured babies and children.

Trauma Histories

None of the 15 fantasizers reported any severe beatings or sexual abuse by immediate family or caretakers. Two female subjects in this group did report abusive sexual behavior on the part of other adults, in one case a social acquaintance of the family, and in the other, a stranger. Fantasizers in this study actually reported less physical and sexual abuse than the approximately 20–25% rate reported in general college populations (Tdjan & Thoennes, 1998). Their higher-than-average recollection for early childhood events would make it unlikely they are underreporting, although this finding is inconsistent with Lynn and Rhue's finding that a history of abuse correlates with their fantasy-proneness questionnaire (Lynn & Rhue, 1988).

Four of the 15 dissociaters initially remembered abusive behavior. For three of them, this involved physical violence, and for two of them, it involved sexual abuse. In addition to these four with direct memories, two subjects said they didn't remember but had been told that they had been battered as children (in one case, an older sibling remembered witnessing this; in another case, a social worker had monitored the parents following a teacher's report of abuse). One additional subject in the group described a severe history of early childhood multiple fractures and burns for which his parents presented improbable explanations to others—and which he did not recall the origins of. Another subject experienced nausea and vomiting whenever anyone touched a certain portion of her thigh. Six of the remaining seven subjects reported some signs such as the recurring nightmares outlined in the previous section and the lack of recollections before the ages of 7 or 8 described earlier. These signs have been associated with an increased likelihood of childhood abuse (Belicki & Cuddy, 1996; Barrett & Fine, 1980). Two of the dissociaters reported regaining abuse memories in the four years between the initial and follow-up interviews, which further suggests the rate for this group may approach 100%.

In addition to this suggestion that between 6 and 14 of the dissociaters had been abused by parents, three of them reported other major traumas in childhood—in one case a very painful and extended medical condition, and for two the deaths of a parent when they were under 10.

Dissociative Diagnoses and Post-Traumatic Stress Disorder

No fantasizer came close to meeting DSM3-R (revised) Dissociative Disorder or Post Traumatic Stress Disorder, although 100% of the fantasizers fit what would constitute Dissociative Disorder Not Otherwise Specified: "trance states, i.e., altered states of consciousness with markedly diminished or selectively focused responsiveness to environmental stimuli" (APA, 1987, p. 277). However, DSM defines mental disorders to be diagnosed as "A psychological syndrome with present distress or disability ... or increased risk of suffering" (APA, 1987, p. xxii). The fantasizers do not appear to be distressed by their ability for selectively focused responsiveness.

Although the interview did not include all diagnostic questions for every other possible disorder less obviously related to the content of the study, fantasizers did not obviously meet any other diagnoses. Two fantasizers did demonstrate some bipolar tendencies, and one some schizotypal ones; however, in no case did they exhibit enough of the criteria and/or the severity of distress or impairment necessary for the formal diagnosis. Overall, the fantasizers appeared to be a mentally healthy group of people. Four dissociaters met Dissociative Disorder-Not Otherwise Specified criteria, one with features of multiple personality—the person whose hidden observer exhibited such autonomy and distinctness had other brief amnestic episodes of speaking as a very different persona. A fifth dissociater met formal criteria for Psychogenic Amnesia. Again, most of the remaining dissociaters could be seen as meeting the symptom criteria for this disorder by their daydream amnesia alone except that they did not appear to experience distress or impairment from their amnestic tendencies.

Even the five dissociaters with enough distress to qualify for dissociative diagnoses were toward the mild level of impairment from these disorders. Only one of them had sought long-term psychotherapy or therapy directed at trauma and dissociative symptoms. One of the other four with diagnoses and two others in this study have married abusive spouses, been unable to hold a job, made serious suicide attempts, or been hospitalized in psychiatric settings. However, all these events are common for other people with a serious trauma history and/or dissociative disorders.

Barber's "Positively Set" Hypnotizables

After I published the results of my two studies, T. X. Barber wrote of observing hypnotic subjects that fit my dissociater category and went on to describe what he viewed as a third group: "positively set" hypnotizables (Barber, 1999). He characterized these subjects as cooperative and trusting. He further described them as holding strongly positive attitudes and expectancies about hypnosis and being highly motivated to perform well on tests of hypnotic susceptibility. These subjects, Barber said, because of their cultural beliefs, and response biases, follow rather automatically with hypnotically suggested responses. For example, their cooperative predisposition leads them to supply cognitions compatible with stiffening their arm when that is suggested rather than to question or resist it. Barber says that positively set hypnotic subjects, unlike either fantasizers or dissociaters, typically do not perceive hypnosis as an altered state of consciousness but rather a situation in which they perform suggested behaviors. He suggested that his three-type model could unify the conflicting "state" versus "nonstate" debate about the nature of hypnosis as fantasizers and dissociaters were indeed experiencing a "state of hypnosis" while positively set subjects were "nonstate" responders.

Conclusions

In summary, there seem to be at least two—and perhaps three—distinct subgroups of people who are highly hypnotizable. Wilson and Barber's concept of the majority of highly hypnotizable people having vivid fantasy and imagery ability is sound. However, it appears there is another, somewhat similar group characterized by amnesia and dissociative phenomena, who do not achieve trance as rapidly but are nevertheless capable of eventually reaching as deep a trance as do fantasizers. These two subgoups seem to report altered state of consciousness—albeit different ones—in response to hypnotic inductions and suggestions. As someone who tends toward defining hypnosis from the "state" side, I view these two subsets as more relevant to the phenomena of hypnosis. However, this is largely a semantic distinction as Barber's positively set group also score very high on the standard scales. Therefore, it seems most accurate to think of those high on scales of hypnotizability as composed of three groups whose life histories have specialized them primarily toward one of these major phenomena: hallucinatory imagery, dissociative abilities, or cooperation and a positive response bias.

I do not have any conflicts of interest to disclose.

References

American Psychiatric Association (1987). *Diagnostic and statistical manual of mental disorders* (third edition-revised), Washington, DC: American Psychiatric Press. 10.1017/s0790966700015767

Barber, T. X. (1999). A comprehensive three-dimensional theory of hypnosis. In I. Kirsch, A. Capafons, E. Cardeña-Buelna, & S. Amigó (Eds.), *Clinical hypnosis and self-regulation: Cognitive-behavioral perspectives* (pp. 21–48). American Psychological Association. 10.1037/10282-001

Barber, T. X., & Wilson, S. C. (1978). The Barber Suggestibility Scale and the Creative Imagination Scale: Experimental and clinical applications. *American Journal of Clinical Hypnosis*, *21*, 84–108. 10.1080/00029157.1978.10403966

Barrett, D. L. (1979). The hypnotic dream: Its content in comparison to nocturnal dreams and waking fantasy. *Journal of Abnormal Psychology ,88*, 584–591. 10.1037/0021-843x.88.5.584

Barrett, D. L. (1980). The first memory as a predictor of personality traits. *Journal of Individual Psychology*, *36*, 136–149.

Barrett, D. L. (1983). Early recollections as predictors of self-disclosure and interpersonal style. *Journal of Individual Psychology*, *39*, 92–98.

Barrett, D. L. (1988). Trance-related pseudocyesis in a male. *International Journal of Clinical and Experimental Hypnosis*, *36*, 256–261. 10.1080/00207148808410516

Barrett (1989). Thick vs. thin boundaries: A concept related to hypnotic susceptibility. Paper presented at Eastern Psychological Association Meeting, Boston, MA, March.

Barrett, D. L. (1990). Daydreams of deep trance subjects: They strikingly resemble night time dreams. Paper presented at APA, Div. 30. August.

Barrett, D. L. (1991). Deep trance subjects: A schema of two distinct subgroups. In R. Kunzendorf (Ed.), *Imagery: Recent Developments* (pp. 101–112). New York: Plenum Press. 10.1007/978-1-4899-2623-4_12

Barrett, D. L. (1992). Fantasizers and dissociaters: An empirically based schema of two types of deep trance subjects. *Psychological Reports*, *71*, 1011–1014. 10.2466/pr0.71.7.1011-1014

Barrett, D. L. (1996). Fantasizers and dissociaters: Two types of high hypnotizables, two imagery styles. In R. Kusendorf, N. Spanos, & B. Wallace (Eds.), *Hypnosis and imagination*, New York: Baywood. 10.4324/9781315224374

Barrett, D. L. (1996a). Dreams in multiple personality. In D. Barrett (Ed.), *Trauma and dreams* (pp. 68-81). Cambridge, MA: Harvard University Press. 10.2307/j.ctv1ns7nqg.9

Barrett, D. L. (1998). *The pregnant man: Tales from a hypnotherapist's couch*. New York: Times Books/Random House.

Barrett, D. L., & Fine, H. J. (1980) A child was being beaten: The therapy of battered children as adults. *Psychotherapy: Theory, Practice, and Research*, *17*, 285–293. 10.1037/h0085925

Belicki, K., & Cuddy, M. (1996). Identifying sexual trauma histories from patterns of sleep and dreams. In D. Barrett (Ed.), *Trauma and dreams* (pp. 46–55). Cambridge, MA: Harvard University Press. 10.2307/j.ctv1ns7nqg.7

Council, J. R., Kirsch, I., & Hafner, L. P. (1986). Expectancy versus absorption in the prediction of hypnotic responding. *Journal of Personality and Social Psychology*, *50*(1), 182. 10.1037/0022-3514.50.1.182

Council, J. R., & Huff, K. D. (1990). Hypnosis, fantasy activity and reports of paranormal experiences in high, medium and low fantasizers. *British Journal of Experimental & Clinical Hypnosis*, 915–923. 10.1080/00207146508412946

Field, P. (1965). An inventory scale of hypnotic depth. *International Journal of Clinical and Experimental Hypnosis*, *13*, 238–249. 10.1080/00207146508412946

Green, J. P., Barabasz, A. F., Barrett, D., & Montgomery, G. H. (2005). Forging ahead: The 2003 APA Division 30 definition of hypnosis. *International Journal of Clinical and Experimental Hypnosis*, *53*(3), 259–264. 10.1080/00207140590961321

Hartmann, E. (1984). *The nightmare: The psychology and biology of terrifying dreams*. Basic Books.

Hilgard, E. R. (1977). *Divided consciousness: Multiple controls in human thought and action*. New York: John Wiley.

Hilgard, E. R. (1979). Divided consciousness in hypnosis: The implications of the hidden observer. In E. Fromm, & R. E. Shor (Eds.), *Hypnosis: Developments in research and new perspectives* (2nd ed.). Chicago: Aldine.

Hilgard, J. (1970). *Personality and hypnosis: A study of imaginative involvement*. Chicago: University of Chicago Press.

Hilgard, J. (1979). Imaginative and sensory-affective involvements: In everyday life and in hypnosis. In E. Fromm, & R. E. Shor (Eds.), *Hypnosis: Developments in research and new perspectives* (pp. 519–565). New York: Aldine.

Lynn, S. J., & Rhue, J. W. (1986). The fantasy prone person: Hypnosis, imagination and creativity. *Journal of Personality and Social Psychology*, *51*, 404–408. 10.1037/0022-3514.51.2.404

Lynn,.S. J., & Rhue, J. W. (1988). Fantasy proneness: Hypnosis, developmental antecedents, and psychopathology. *American Psychologist*,*43*, 35–44. 10.1037/0003-066x.43.1.35

Masters, R., & Houston, J. (1972). *Mind games: The guide to exploring inner space*. New York: Viking Press.

Ott, U. (2016). Absorption in hypnotic trance and meditation. In A. Raz, & M. Lifshitz (Eds.), *Hypnosis and meditation: Towards an integrative science of conscious planes* (pp. 269–278). Oxford University Press.

Shor, R. E., & Orne, E. C. (1962). *Harvard Group Scale of Hypnotic Susceptibility, Form A*. Palo Alto, CA: Consulting Psychologists Press. 10.1037/t02246-000

Spanos, N. P. (1989) Imaginal dispositions and situation-specific expectations in strategy-induced pain reductions. *Imagination, Cognition and Personality*, 9(2), 147. 10.2190/dgxk-hp82-ax61-p7tj

Spanos, N. P., & McPeake, J. D. (1977). Cognitive strategies, goal-directed fantasy, and response to suggestions in hypnotic subjects. *American Journal of Clinical Hypnosis*, *20*, 114–123. 10.1080/00029157.1975.10403751

Tdjan, P., & Thoennes, N. (1998). Prevalence, incidence, and consequences of violence against women survey. *National Institute of Justice & Centers for Disease Control & Prevention Research Brief*, Nov. https://doi.org/10.1037/e491852006-001

Tellegen, A., & Atkinson, G. (1974). Openness to absorbing and self-altering experiences ("absorption"), a trait related to hypnotic susceptibility. *Journal of Abnormal Psychology*, *83*, 268–277. 10.1037/h0036681

Weitzenhoffer, A. M., & Hilgard, E. R. (1962). *Stanford Hypnotic Susceptibility Scale, Form C* (Vol. 27). Palo Alto, CA: Consulting Psychologists Press.

Wilson, S. C., & Barber, T. X. (1981). Vivid fantasy and hallucinatory abilities in the life histories of excellent 1,981 hypnotic subjects (somnambules): A preliminary report. In E. Klinger (Ed.). *Imagery: Vol. 2: Concepts, results., and applications* (pp. 133–149). New York: Plenum Press. 10.1007/978-1-4684-3974-8_10

Wilson, S. C., & Barber, T. X. (1983). The fantasy-prone personality: Implications for understanding imagery, hypnosis, and parapsychological phenomena. In A. A. Sheik (Ed.), *Imagery—Current theory, research, and application* (pp. 327–339). New York: John Wiley & Sons, Inc.

Zamore, N., & Barrett, D. L. (1989). Hypnotic susceptibility and dream characteristics. *Psychiatric Journal of The University of Ottawa*, *14*, 572–574.

23

ALTERATION OF HYPNOTIC PHENOMENA AND HYPNOTIZABILITY WITH NON-INVASIVE BRAIN STIMULATION (NIBS)

State of the Art and Future Perspectives

Rinaldo L. Perri

University Niccolò Cusano, Rome, Italy

Non-Invasive Brain Stimulation

Non-invasive brain stimulation (NIBS) techniques have been adopted to modify brain functions and observe consequent effects at a perceptual, cognitive, or phenomenological level. In other words, they allow researchers to adopt a causal approach to assess the brain–behavior relationship in humans in a non-invasive way.

Since the 18th-century experiments of Luigi Galvani, scientists have observed that administration of electric currents can excite the nerves and produce muscular contractions. However, the first demonstration of NIBS dates back to more than 40 years ago when Merton and Morton (1980) showed that application of brief electric pulses to the motor cortex through the intact scalp produced behavioral effects mediated by cortical excitability with no need for surgery. The current intensity however was very high (in the order of 1–1.5 kV), uncomfortable, and poorly tolerated. A few years later, Barker and colleagues (1985) demonstrated that stimulation of the motor cortex was also possible using a brief external magnetic field through a circular wire coil, and that the muscle twitches did not produce pain or distress. Since then, painless and safe methods of NIBS have been developed for experimental and clinical applications: the main technologies are transcranial magnetic stimulation (TMS) and transcranial electrical stimulation, which rely on the administration of magnetic pulses and electric currents, respectively. Among the main limitation of NIBS is spatial resolution as they act over a large surface neural population with sometimes unpredictable consequences for the secondary effects on the neural network.

DOI: 10.4324/9781003449126-31

Transcranial Magnetic Stimulation

TMS consists of a wire coil placed over the scalp: it generates a magnetic field that penetrates the cranium, eliciting action potentials in the neuronal cells of the neocortex. Different approaches of TMS are possible such as single or repetitive magnetic pulses (rTMS). Depending on the stimulation frequency, rTMS has been associated with excitation or inhibition of the synaptic transmission as reflected by long-term potentiation (LTP) and long-term depression (LTD) (Bhattacharya et al., 2022). These after-effects last around 30–60 min and reflect mainly the rTMS influences on the glutamatergic synapses via NMDA receptors (Polanía et al., 2018). One of the best known applications of TMS is for the investigation of cortico-spinal excitability by triggering involuntary twitches of muscles in the region (usually the index finger) contralateral to the stimulated primary motor cortex. The behavioral response can be quantified by recording the latency and amplitude of the motor evoked potential through electromyography.

Transcranial Direct Current Stimulation

A typical transcranial direct current stimulation (tDCS) device consists of a saline-soaked pair of surface sponge electrodes (9–30 cm^2 surface) placed over the scalp and delivering current (1–2 mA) through a battery-driven constant current stimulator. tDCS can deliver positive (anode) or negative (cathode) current, respectively, associated with enhanced and reduced cortical excitability. In particular, it has been demonstrated that anodal tDCS increases the spontaneous neuronal firing by the depolarization of the resting membrane potential, while cathodal tDCS reduces cortical excitability likely due to hyperpolarization of the resting membrane potential (Bhattacharya et al., 2022). It is supposed that the generation of LTP and LTD is mediated mainly by the tDCS effects on NMDA receptors and the consequent influx of calcium ions (Ca^{2+}) into the cells. In fact, pharmacological studies demonstrated that the NMDA receptor agonist dextromethorphan reduced the tDCS effects on brain plasticity (Nitsche et al., 2003), while the NMDA agonist D-cycloserine increased the cortical excitability induced by anodal tDCS (Nitsche et al., 2004). tDCS effects on neural plasticity depend on different aspects such as intensity and duration of stimulation (usually 20 min) and are estimated to last approximately 30 minutes to 3 hours after a single session. Multiple sessions of tDCS stimulation are needed to get more stable modifications of neural plasticity, and its clinical efficacy was established especially for the mood and addiction disorders (for reviews see Razza et al., 2020; Yadollahpour & Yuan, 2018). A variant of tDCS is the transcranial alternating current stimulation (tACS), which is supposed to modulate the spontaneous cortical oscillatory activity through sinusoidal current applied at any frequency. As a confirmation, a primate study showed tACS-induced effects on the timing of neuron spiking activity (Krause et al., 2019).

Application of NIBS in Hypnosis Research: The "God Helmet"

The first documented attempt to alter hypnotic suggestibility through brain stimulation was that of De Sano and Persinger (1987) through burst-firing magnetic fields. As a director of Laurentian University's Consciousness Research Lab, Dr. Michael Persinger became famous for his studies with the so-called Koren helmet (built by Stan Koren), later known to the public as the "God helmet." The name was coined by a journalist to indicate the spiritual and religious experiences following the helmet stimulation of the brain. In fact, Persinger claimed that the sensed presence of a "Sentient Being" (e.g., vision of voids, meetings with God) can be reliably evoked by temporal patterns of weak magnetic fields applied across the temporoparietal region of the brain (Pierre & Persinger, 2006). The "God helmet" was then called *transcerebral magnetic stimulation:* it was adopted almost exclusively by Persinger's group and consisted of a modified motorcycle helmet placed over the head. Along both sides of the helmet, four small solenoids were embedded so that the magnetic field penetrated through the temporoparietal areas (for more details on equipment and stimulation parameters, see Richards et al., 1993). The device produced a field strength of approximately 1 micro Tesla (microT), that is a million times weaker than TMS. For this reason, some authors have argued that the experiential effects of these studies were due to suggestibility much more than to the stimulation (Granqvist et al., 2005). It is however interesting to know that the Persinger's group conducted different studies of hypnosis with the Koren helmet. In 1987, De Sano and Persinger measured the hypnotic susceptibility of 24 volunteers utilizing the hypnotic induction profile (HIP; Spiegel et al., 1976) before and after exposure to either sham, 1 Hz, or 4 Hz magnetic fields. During stimulation, subjects were instructed to view a green light that was pulsating at the same frequency as the magnetic field. Results indicated that all participants increased their susceptibility after the active stimulation, but with a sex difference: men enhanced their scores when exposed to the 4 Hz field while women to the 1 Hz. The study, however, presented some methodological issues, and a new investigation in this field came a few years later when Tiller and Persinger (1994) reported an effect for the weak (1 microT) magnetic field stimulation of the bilateral temporal lobes; only subjects who received the right hemisphere stimulation before the left reported an enhancement on the HIP scale. With a slightly different paradigm, the study was replicated a few years later (Healey et al., 1996): results indicated that 20 min of burst-firing magnetic fields over the right temporoparietal lobe increased hypnotizability by about 30% on the HIP. No differences emerged following left, bilateral, or sham stimulation.

Persinger died in 2018 and no one else has ever used the same device that has been supplanted by TMS. The only attempt to replicate Persinger's studies on mystical experiences was made by a Swedish group (Granqvist et al., 2005) which, however, failed to obtain similar results and seriously questioned the helmet's effects. Anyway, beyond the technical and methodological issues, these preliminary investigations have paved the way for the hypothesis of modulating brain activity to modify hypnotic behavior.

Application of NIBS in Hypnosis Research: TMS Studies

Nowadays, NIBS is widely used for the stimulation of high-order cognitive areas, such as the dorsolateral prefrontal cortex (DLPFC), for several goals such as cognitive training (Bakulin et al., 2020) and the treatment of psychological (Sagliano et al., 2019) and neurological diseases (Hara et al., 2021). Together with evidence of the DLPFC contribution to hypnosis (for a review see Landry et al., 2017), this background led the proponents of the cold control theory of hypnosis (Dienes et al., 2012; Dienes & Perner, 2007) to test the hypothesis of altering hypnotic suggestibility through TMS of frontal areas. In a few words, the cold control theory describes hypnosis as a metacognitive phenomenon leading to the subject being unaware of his/her intention in motor and cognitive actions.

The awareness of the intentions is defined as "high order thought" or HOTs, and hypnotic response would reflect intentional control without accurate HOTs: cold control. The reduction of conscious awareness of executive control has been associated with the deactivation of the left DLPFC, that is the hypothetical HOTs' site (Lau & Passingham, 2006). Accordingly, Dienes and Hutton (2013) disrupted left DLPFC activity through low frequency (1 Hz) rTMS when assessing the response of medium hypnotizable subjects to four suggestions: magnetic hands, arm levitation, rigid arm, and taste hallucination. The response to suggestions was measured both subjectively (self-rating) and objectively (behavioral evaluation) after TMS of the left DLPFC and the control site identified over the vertex of the scalp. Results indicated a slight increase in the hypnotic response when measured subjectively. Conversely, no results emerged on the objective assessment of hypnotic suggestibility. Based on these findings, authors concluded that disruption of frontal function enhanced the hypnotic response in accordance with predictions of cold control. However, it is not trivial to note that alteration of hypnotic response was modest (a mean difference of 0.3 points on a 0–5 scale) and related to only a few suggestions when assessed subjectively.

A replication of the study was made by an Australian group (Coltheart et al., 2018) which adopted exactly the same methods as the Dienes and Hutton (2013) investigation. Authors did not observe significant results either on subjective or objective measures of suggestibility, questioning the findings described above. In the same study, a second experiment with 39 medium hypnotizables was described, with the only difference being that the right (instead of the left) DLPFC was targeted by the rTMS. Again, analyses indicated no effects of stimulation on the subjective measures, while significant results emerged on the objective score of hypnotic suggestibility. In particular, hypnotizability increased by 14.95% with the effects being larger for the Taste and Levitation suggestions than for the other two. Authors concluded that disruption of the right but not the left DLPFC enhanced hypnotizability when this is measured objectively (Coltheart et al., 2018).

As with Dienes and Hutton's (2013) study, the findings of Coltheart's group were also innovative and relevant to the field, but it is the writer's opinion that their so-called "objective" measurement of suggestibility should be taken with caution. In particular, it consisted of the experimenter's rating of the magnitude of individual hypnotic response to each suggestion. If this approach shows evident limits for assessing ideomotor suggestions in the absence of physical measures, it is even more so for the perceptive ones. In fact, the "objective" measure of taste hallucination reflected the percentage of maximum possible facial expression, that is a rather vague and operator-dependent method of assessment.

These TMS studies were the first demonstrating the possibility of altering the hypnotic response through recent techniques of NIBS. Moreover, both investigations provided new and important evidence to the contribution of the DLPFC in hypnotic susceptibility. On the other hand, the two studies shared exactly the same methods, so a lot of questions remain about the contribution of different areas and frequency of stimulation on the observed phenomena, the specific role of the left and right DLPFC, and the effective magnitude of the TMS-induced effects on the behavioral and subjective hypnotic responses. Unfortunately, no other TMS studies have been published to date, so there is still a lot to know about the efficacy of different TMS parameters and montages on hypnotic phenomena. More research is needed in this field, but an issue to consider when using the TMS is the difficulty of stimulating during hypnosis (i.e., the online approach) as well as the short duration of the after-effects (estimated at a few minutes for a single 1 Hz rTMS session; Torii et al., 2012).

In fact, this latter aspect could also limit the offline approach (i.e., TMS before hypnosis) due to the timing of the hypnotic procedures.

Application of NIBS in Hypnosis Research: tDCS Studies

As is true for TMS, tDCS has been widely adopted for clinical (Perrotta & Perri, 2022) and experimental applications (Galli et al., 2019). The low spatial resolution of tDCS does not allow stimulation of precisely restricted portions of the cerebral cortex. However, the tDCS device is comfortable and easy to wear, allowing ecological applications with neuromodulatory after-effects lasting up to several hours (Nitsche & Paulus, 2001).

tDCS effects were compared to hypnotic analgesia suggestions in a study on pain perception and the descending pain modulating system (Beltran Serrano et al., 2019): authors reported a differential effect between the two approaches on the pain measures in 24 healthy females. They suggest that the impact of the interventions has differential neural mechanisms, since the hypnotic suggestion improved pain perception, whereas the transcranial direct-current stimulation increased inhibition of the descending pain modulating system. On the other hand, only two studies adopted the tDCS during hypnosis, and both with the aim to alter hypnotizability and the hypnotic experience. The first study by Perri and colleagues (2022) adopted a bilateral cathodal (i.e., inhibitory) stimulation of the DLPFC, with the target electrode over the left hemisphere (F3 site of the 10/20 international system) and the return electrode over the contralateral site. Participants were hypnosis naive subjects enrolled in a double-blind study with a pre-post design in which hypnotic assessment was administered both before and after the tDCS stimulation. The hypnotic experience was measured through the *Phenomenology of Consciousness Inventory: The Hypnotic Assessment Procedure* (PCI-HAP; Pekala et al., 2010) in order to assess subjective variations in consciousness, in addition to the canonical hypnotizability index, as operationalized by the Hypnoidal State Score (HSS). The HSS correlates about 0.60 (Forbes & Pekala, 1993) with scores on the Harvard Group Scale of Hypnotic Susceptibility (Shor & Orne, 1962), but it is based on a regression equation consisting of ten of the PCI (sub)dimensions. The HSS may be the only quantifiable, phenomenological, or "noetic" measure of hypnosis available to date (Pekala et al., 2017). The main findings of the study revealed that active tDCS enhanced the hypnotic depth by 11% ($p < 0.05$, $\eta^2p = 0.13$) and reduced the volitional control (subdimension of the PCI) by 30% ($p < 0.05$, $\eta^2p = 0.14$), while no differences emerged in the control group receiving sham stimulation. The volitional control corresponds to the sense of agency reflecting the awareness of one's intentions in cognitive and motor actions, and results were interpreted in terms of executive control-mediated reduction of conscious awareness that was associated with the deactivation of the left DLPFC (Dienes & Hutton, 2013). However, the bilateral montage of the tDCS did not allow the researchers to exclude with certainty the contribution of the right DLPFC. In fact, it is possible for the return electrode to have opposite physiological effects when put over the cranium (for a review see DaSilva et al., 2011); accordingly the possible contribution of the enhanced right DLPFC activity (in addition to the left decrease) cannot be excluded. For these reasons, Perri and Di Filippo (2023) planned a new experiment with the same paradigm as the previous one, but by adopting an extracephalic tDCS montage (F3/right deltoid) providing a unilateral stimulation of the left DLPFC. The main findings revealed that the inhibitory tDCS enhanced the hypnotizability by 15.4% with $\eta^2p = 0.26$ (i.e., greater percentage and effect size than the previous study) and altered a few dimensions of consciousness such as self-awareness and absorption, while no changes emerged on the feeling of agency and the pass rates for suggestions.

The two tDCS studies yielded similar results for the hypnotizability increase, but different for the sense of agency and self-awareness. The reasons for these differences could lie in the different neurophysiological effects of the two montages: in fact, as indicated by the electric field modeling, the bifrontal stimulation of Perri et al. (2022) spread the current to the dorsal-medial cortical areas while the extracephalic montage of Perri and Di Filippo (2023) targeted a more lateral region corresponding to the left middle frontal gyrus (MFG). As a confirmation, previous literature associated the medial frontal cortex with explicit assignments of agency (Spengler et al., 2009) and feeling of control of movements (Walsh et al., 2015), while activity of the DLPFC correlated with the self-rated level of hypnotic "depth" (Deeley et al., 2012), and it was also associated with metacognition (Dienes & Perner, 2007) and conscious judgments about the self (Miele et al., 2011).

Findings from tDCS studies were congruent and robust in terms of statistical power and corroborated the key role of the DLPFC in hypnosis.

The longer lasting after-effects of tDCS make this technique probably more suitable than the TMS for enhancing hypnotizability, also allowing for more ecological investigations. However, statistically significant changes in hypnotic experience do not mean they are also clinically significant: in fact, no effects of stimulation emerged on the responsivity to the hypnotic suggestions in these studies (note however that only three items were considered). This was likely due to the fact that suggestions-related brain areas have to be stimulated to produce behavioral effects (e.g., by stimulating the motor areas during an ideomotor suggestion). More research is still needed to translate experimental findings into clinical procedures to boost susceptibility.

Future Studies and Possible Implications for Hypnosis Research and Practice

With the aim of increasing responsiveness to suggestions, researchers have tested different methods of hypnotizability enhancement. Most of these investigations proposed psychological (see Lynn, 2004 for a review) and pharmacological approaches (Bryant et al., 2012; Whalley & Brooks, 2009) with questionable results or invasive methods. After decades of research, the NIBS interventions were also proposed and they currently show up as the most promising approach in this field. Experimental findings are still not enough to indicate NIBS as the ultimate strategy, but it is undoubtedly one of the best methods to modulate neural activity during hypnosis. In fact, NIBS allows the intriguing opportunity to adopt a causal approach to increase hypnotizability with the aim of modifying behaviors, perceptions, and cognitions in a non-invasive and operator-independent way.

Currently, all the published NIBS studies on hypnosis targeted the PFC because of its key role in the hypnotic experience (for a meta-analysis see Landry et al., 2017). However, the PFC is an associative area recruited for executive and supramodal processes, and it is not directly associated with any specific response to hypnotic suggestions. This could probably explain why the above reviewed NIBS studies altered the phenomenological experience of hypnosis but affected little (e.g., Dienes & Hutton, 2013) or no (e.g., Perri et al., 2022) responsiveness to suggestions. A further aspect to consider is that all stimulations were applied in inhibitory mode. Nevertheless, even though PFC deactivation was identified as a sign of the neutral hypnosis (Landry et al., 2017), greater engagement was observed when suggestions required increased executive control (Huber et al., 2013; Perri et al., 2020;

Zahedi et al., 2017, 2019). These findings suggest that cognitive flexibility (and not the PFC suppression) is a core aspect of hypnotic abilities. As a consequence, future studies should also consider the enhancement of the PFC activity to investigate if this leads to increased pass rates for hypnotic suggestions. Also, stimulation of other areas such as the agency brain network (e.g., Khalighinejad & Haggard, 2015), sensory, and motor cortices could clarify whether neural fluctuations in these regions can affect the feeling of control or the behavioral response to different classes of suggestions (ideomotor, perceptual, etc.). Moreover, protocols adopting online stimulation could be tested with the aim of maximizing the tDCS after-effects on hypnotic procedures, while tACS stimulation could be proposed to direct the cortical oscillatory activity toward neural patterns associated with higher susceptibility.

Whatever the specific goals and methods of future studies, it is the writer's opinion that accurate phenomenological measures are mandatory when investigating hypnotic phenomena: this is a fundamental principle of the most authoritative studies on consciousness (e.g., Oizumi et al., 2014), while most hypnosis research still suffers from a mainly behavioral approach (Perri, 2022).

In conclusion, the introduction of NIBS in hypnosis research represents a potential key step toward deepening knowledge on the neurophysiology of hypnosis, as well as on the brain–behavior relationship that underlies suggestibility. However, we are at the very beginning of this exciting course, so further research including larger samples and recruiting subjects with high or low hypnotizability is needed. As for the clinical implications, the possibility of boosting hypnotic responsiveness could be translated into better outcomes for hypnotic interventions like pain management and cognitive and emotional regulation. If so, all forms of hypnotherapy could theoretically benefit from neuromodulation with consequent benefits for patients. Also, it may be possible to broaden the audience of potential hypnotic clients by including subjects who would otherwise be considered refractory to hypnosis.

References

Bakulin, I., Zabirova, A., Lagoda, D., Poydasheva, A., Cherkasova, A., Pavlov, N., Kopnin, P., Sinitsyn, D., Kremneva, E., & Fedorov, M. (2020). Combining HF rTMS over the left DLPFC with concurrent cognitive activity for the offline modulation of working memory in healthy volunteers: A proof-of-concept study. *Brain Sciences*, *10*(2), 83. DOI: 10.3390/brainsci10020083

Barker, A. T., Jalinous, R., & Freeston, I. L. (1985). Non-invasive magnetic stimulation of human motor cortex. *The Lancet*, *325*(8437), 1106–1107. DOI: 10.1016/s0140-6736(85)92413-4

Beltran Serrano, G., Rodrigues, L. P., Schein, B., Souza, A., Torres, I. L., da Conceição Antunes, L., Fregni, F., & Caumo, W. (2019). Comparison of hypnotic suggestion and transcranial direct-current stimulation effects on pain perception and the descending pain modulating system: A crossover randomized clinical trial. *Frontiers in Neuroscience*, *13*, 662. DOI: 10.3389/fnins.2019.00662

Bhattacharya, A., Mrudula, K., Sreepada, S. S., Sathyaprabha, T. N., Pal, P. K., Chen, R., & Udupa, K. (2022). An overview of noninvasive brain stimulation: Basic principles and clinical applications. *Canadian Journal of Neurological Sciences*, *49*(4), 479–492. DOI: 10.1017/cjn.2021.158

Bryant, R. A., Hung, L., Guastella, A. J., & Mitchell, P. B. (2012). Oxytocin as a moderator of hypnotizability. *Psychoneuroendocrinology*, *37*(1), 162–166. DOI: 10.1016/j.psyneuen.2011.05.010

Coltheart, M., Cox, R., Sowman, P., Morgan, H., Barnier, A., Langdon, R., Connaughton, E., Teichmann, L., Williams, N., & Polito, V. (2018). Belief, delusion, hypnosis, and the right dorsolateral prefrontal cortex: A transcranial magnetic stimulation study. *Cortex*, *101*, 234–248. DOI: 10.1016/j.cortex.2018.01.001

DaSilva, A. F., Volz, M. S., Bikson, M., & Fregni, F. (2011). Electrode positioning and montage in transcranial direct current stimulation. *JoVE (Journal of Visualized Experiments)*, *51*, e2744. DOI: 10.3791/2744

De Sano, C. F., & Persinger, M. A. (1987). Geophysical variables and behavior: XXXIX. Alterations in imaginings and suggestibility during brief magnetic field exposures. *Perceptual and Motor Skills*, *64*(3), 968–970. 10.2466/pms.1987.64.3.968

Deeley, Q., Oakley, D. A., Toone, B., Giampietro, V., Brammer, M. J., Williams, S. C., & Halligan, P. W. (2012). Modulating the default mode network using hypnosis. *International Journal of Clinical and Experimental Hypnosis*, *60*(2), 206–228. DOI: 10.1080/00207144.2012.648070

Dienes, Z., Beran, M., Brandl, J. L., Perner, J., & Proust, J. (2012). Is hypnotic responding the strategic relinquishment of metacognition. In M. J. Beran (Ed.), *Foundations of Metacognition* (pp. 267–278). 10.1093/acprof:oso/9780199646739.003.0017

Dienes, Z., & Hutton, S. (2013). Understanding hypnosis metacognitively: RTMS applied to left DLPFC increases hypnotic suggestibility. *Cortex*, *49*(2), 386–392. DOI: 10.1016/j.cortex.2012.07.009

Dienes, Z., & Perner, J. (2007). Executive control without conscious awareness: The cold control theory of hypnosis. In Jamieson, G. A. (Ed.), *Hypnosis and conscious states: The cognitive neuroscience perspective* (pp. 293–314). Oxford University Press.

Forbes, E. J., & Pekala, R. J. (1993). Predicting hypnotic susceptibility via a phenomenological approach. *Psychological Reports*, *73*(3_suppl), 1251–1256. DOI: 10.2466/pr0.1993.73.3f.1251

Galli, G., Vadillo, M. A., Sirota, M., Feurra, M., & Medvedeva, A. (2019). A systematic review and meta-analysis of the effects of transcranial direct current stimulation (tDCS) on episodic memory. *Brain Stimulation*, *12*(2), 231–241. DOI: 10.1002/da.23004

Granqvist, P., Fredrikson, M., Unge, P., Hagenfeldt, A., Valind, S., Larhammar, D., & Larsson, M. (2005). Sensed presence and mystical experiences are predicted by suggestibility, not by the application of transcranial weak complex magnetic fields. *Neuroscience Letters*, *379*(1), 1–6. DOI: 10.1016/j.neulet.2004.10.057

Hara, T., Shanmugalingam, A., McIntyre, A., & Burhan, A. M. (2021). The effect of non-invasive brain stimulation (NIBS) on executive functioning, attention and memory in rehabilitation patients with traumatic brain injury: A systematic review. *Diagnostics*, *11*(4), 627. DOI: 10.3390/diagnostics11040627

Healey, F., Persinger, M. A., & Koren, S. A. (1996). Enhanced hypnotic suggestibility following application of burst-firing magnetic fields over the right temporoparietal lobes: A replication. *International Journal of Neuroscience*, *87*(3–4), 201–207. DOI: 10.3109/00207459609070838

Huber, A., Lui, F., & Porro, C. A. (2013). Hypnotic susceptibility modulates brain activity related to experimental placebo analgesia. *PAIN®*, *154*(9), 1509–1518. DOI: 10.1016/j.pain.2013.03.031

Khalighinejad, N., & Haggard, P. (2015). Modulating human sense of agency with non-invasive brain stimulation. *Cortex*, *69*, 93–103. DOI: 10.1016/j.cortex.2015.04.015

Krause, M. R., Vieira, P. G., Csorba, B. A., Pilly, P. K., & Pack, C. C. (2019). Transcranial alternating current stimulation entrains single-neuron activity in the primate brain. *Proceedings of the National Academy of Sciences*, *116*(12), 5747–5755. 10.1073/pnas.1815958116

Landry, M., Lifshitz, M., & Raz, A. (2017). Brain correlates of hypnosis: A systematic review and meta-analytic exploration. *Neuroscience & Biobehavioral Reviews*, *81*, 75–98. DOI: 10.1016/j.neubiorev.2017.02.020

Lau, H. C., & Passingham, R. E. (2006). Relative blindsight in normal observers and the neural correlate of visual consciousness. *Proceedings of the National Academy of Sciences*, *103*(49), 18763–18768. DOI: 10.1073/pnas.0607716103

Lynn, S. J. (2004). Enhancing suggestibility: The effects of compliance vs. imagery. *American Journal of Clinical Hypnosis*, *47*(2), 117–128.DOI: 10.1080/00029157.2004.10403630

Merton, P. A., & Morton, H. B. (1980). Stimulation of the cerebral cortex in the intact human subject. *Nature*, *285*(5762), 227–227. 10.1038/285227a0

Miele, D. B., Wager, T. D., Mitchell, J. P., & Metcalfe, J. (2011). Dissociating neural correlates of action monitoring and metacognition of agency. *Journal of Cognitive Neuroscience*, *23*(11), 3620–3636. DOI: 10.1162/jocn_a_00052

Nitsche, M. A., Fricke, K., Henschke, U., Schlitterlau, A., Liebetanz, D., Lang, N., Henning, S., Tergau, F., & Paulus, W. (2003). Pharmacological modulation of cortical excitability shifts induced by transcranial direct current stimulation in humans. *Journal of Physiology*, *553*(1), 293–301. DOI: 10.1113/jphysiol.2003.049916

Nitsche, M. A., Jaussi, W., Liebetanz, D., Lang, N., Tergau, F., & Paulus, W. (2004). Consolidation of human motor cortical neuroplasticity by D-cycloserine. *Neuropsychopharmacology*, *29*(8), 1573–1578. DOI: 10.1038/sj.npp.1300517

Nitsche, M. A., & Paulus, W. (2001). Sustained excitability elevations induced by transcranial DC motor cortex stimulation in humans. *Neurology*, *57*(10), 1899–1901. DOI: 10.1212/wnl.57.10.1899

Oizumi, M., Albantakis, L., & Tononi, G. (2014). From the phenomenology to the mechanisms of consciousness: Integrated information theory 3.0. *PLoS Computational Biology*, *10*(5), e1003588. 10.1371/journal.pcbi.1003588

Pekala, R. J., Baglio, F., Cabinio, M., Lipari, S., Baglio, G., Mendozzi, L., Cecconi, P., Pugnetti, L., & Sciaky, R. (2017). Hypnotism as a function of trance state effects, expectancy, and suggestibility: An Italian replication. *International Journal of Clinical and Experimental Hypnosis*, *65*(2), 210–240. DOI: 10.1080/00207144.2017.1276365

Pekala, R. J., Kumar, V. K., Maurer, R., Elliott-Carter, N., Moon, E., & Mullen, K. (2010). Suggestibility, expectancy, trance state effects, and hypnotic depth: I. Implications for understanding hypnotism. *American Journal of Clinical Hypnosis*, *52*(4), 275–290. 10.1080/00029157.2010.10401732

Perri, R. L. (2022). In medio stat virtus: The importance of studying mediums in hypnosis research. *American Journal of Clinical Hypnosis*, *64*(1), 4–11. 10.1080/00029157.2020.1859980

Perri, R. L., & Di Filippo, G. (2023). Alteration of hypnotic experience following transcranial electrical stimulation of the left prefrontal cortex. *International Journal of Clinical and Health Psychology*, *23*(2), 100346. 10.1016/j.ijchp.2022.100346

Perri, R. L., Facco, E., Quinzi, F., Bianco, V., Berchicci, M., Rossani, F., & Di Russo, F. (2020). Cerebral mechanisms of hypnotic hypoesthesia. An ERP investigation on the expectancy stage of perception. *Psychophysiology*, *57*(11), e13657. DOI: 10.1111/psyp.13657

Perri, R. L., Perrotta, D., Rossani, F., & Pekala, R. J. (2022). Boosting the hypnotic experience. Inhibition of the dorsolateral prefrontal cortex alters hypnotizability and sense of agency. A randomized, double-blind and sham-controlled tDCS study. *Behavioural Brain Research*, *425*, 113833. DOI: 10.1016/j.bbr.2022.113833

Perrotta, D., & Perri, R. L. (2022). Mini-review: When neurostimulation joins cognitive-behavioral therapy. On the need of combining evidence-based treatments for addiction disorders. *Neuroscience Letters*, 136588. 10.1016/j.neulet.2022.136588

Pierre, L. S.-, & Persinger, M. A. (2006). Experimental facilitation of the sensed presence is predicted by the specific patterns of the applied magnetic fields, not by suggestibility: Re-analyses of 19 experiments. *International Journal of Neuroscience*, *116*(19), 1079–1096. DOI: 10.1080/00207450600808800

Polanía, R., Nitsche, M. A., & Ruff, C. C. (2018). Studying and modifying brain function with non-invasive brain stimulation. *Nature Neuroscience*, *21*(2), 174–187. 10.1038/s41593-017-0054-4

Razza, L. B., Palumbo, P., Moffa, A. H., Carvalho, A. F., Solmi, M., Loo, C. K., & Brunoni, A. R. (2020). A systematic review and meta-analysis on the effects of transcranial direct current stimulation in depressive episodes. *Depression and Anxiety*, *37*(7), 594–608. DOI: 10.1002/da.23004

Richards, P. M., Persinger, M. A., & Koren, S. A. (1993). Modification of activation and evaluation properties of narratives by weak complex magnetic field patterns that simulate limbic burst firing. *International Journal of Neuroscience*, *71*(1–4), 71–85. DOI: 10.3109/00207459309000594

Sagliano, L., Atripaldi, D., De Vita, D., D'Olimpio, F., & Trojano, L. (2019). Non-invasive brain stimulation in generalized anxiety disorder: A systematic review. *Progress in Neuro-Psychopharmacology and Biological Psychiatry*, *93*, 31–38. DOI: 10.1016/j.pnpbp.2019.03.002

Shor, R. E., & Orne, E. C. (1962). Harvard Group Scale of Hypnotic Susceptibility, Form A.Consulting Psychologists Press.

Spengler, S., von Cramon, D. Y., & Brass, M. (2009). Was it me or was it you? How the sense of agency originates from ideomotor learning revealed by fMRI. *Neuroimage*, *46*(1), 290–298. DOI: 10.1016/j.neuroimage.2009.01.047

Spiegel, H., Aronson, M., Fleiss, J. L., & Haber, J. (1976). Psychometric analysis of the hypnotic induction profile. *The International Journal of Clinical and Experimental Hypnosis*, *24*(3–4), 300–315. DOI: 10.1080/00207147608416210

Tiller, S. G., & Persinger, M. A. (1994). Enhanced hypnotizability by cerebrally applied magnetic fields depends upon the order of hemispheric presentation: An anistropic effect. *International Journal of Neuroscience*, *79*(3–4), 157–163. DOI: 10.3109/00207459408986076

Torii, T., Sato, A., Iwahashi, M., & Iramina, K. (2012). Transition of after effect on P300 by short-term rTMS to prefrontal cortex. *IEEE Transactions on Magnetics*, *48*(11), 2873–2876. DOI: 10.1109/TMAG.2012.2204432

Walsh, E., Oakley, D. A., Halligan, P. W., Mehta, M. A., & Deeley, Q. (2015). The functional anatomy and connectivity of thought insertion and alien control of movement. *Cortex*, *64*, 380–393. 10.1016/j.cortex.2014.09.012

Whalley, M. G., & Brooks, G. B. (2009). Enhancement of suggestibility and imaginative ability with nitrous oxide. *Psychopharmacology*, *203*(4), 745–752. DOI: 10.1007/s00213-008-1424-0

Yadollahpour, A., & Yuan, T. (2018). Transcranial direct current stimulation for the treatment of addictions: A systematic review of clinical trials. *Current Psychiatry Reviews*, *14*(4), 221–229. DOI: 10.2174/1573400514666181008123358

Zahedi, A., Abdel Rahman, R., Stürmer, B., & Sommer, W. (2019). Common and specific loci of Stroop effects in vocal and manual tasks, revealed by event-related brain potentials and post-hypnotic suggestions. *Journal of Experimental Psychology: General*, *148*(9), 1575. 10.1037/xge0000574

Zahedi, A., Stuermer, B., Hatami, J., Rostami, R., & Sommer, W. (2017). Eliminating stroop effects with post-hypnotic instructions: Brain mechanisms inferred from EEG. *Neuropsychologia*, *96*, 70–77. DOI: 10.1016/j.neuropsychologia.2017.01.006

Mechanisms of Hypnotic Analgesia

24

HOW CAN WE BETTER UNDERSTAND HYPNOSIS AND ITS MODULATION OF PAIN WITH NEUROIMAGING?

Aminata Bicego[1], *Charlotte Grégoire*[1], *Floriane Rousseaux*[1], *Marie-Elisabeth Faymonville*[1,2], *and Audrey Vanhaudenhuyse*[1,3]

[1]Sensation and Perception Research Group, GIGA Consciousness, Liège University, Liège, Belgium; [2]Arsène Burny Cancerology Institute, Liège University Hospital, Liège, Belgium; [3]Interdisciplinary Algology Center, Liège University Hospital, Liège, Belgium

Introduction

This chapter will begin with an analysis of the most commonly accepted definition of hypnosis. To do so, we will divide it into three parts and present evidence supporting it from phenomenological and neuroimaging studies. We will then present evidence supporting the value of hypnosis in acute pain by summarizing the findings from experimental studies, including those studying hypnosedation. We then discuss the benefits of hypnosis for the management of two chronic conditions, chronic pain and oncology. Finally, we describe a contemporary use of hypnosis through virtual reality and finish with a general conclusion.

What Is Hypnosis? Phenomenological and Neuroimaging Accounts

The definition of hypnosis accepted by the majority is the one presented by the American Psychological Association Division 30: "a state of consciousness involving focused attention and reduced peripheral awareness characterized by an enhanced capacity for response to suggestion" (Elkins et al., 2015). This definition can be divided into three parts: (1) hypnosis as a specific state of consciousness, (2) integrative perspective of the neurophysiology of hypnosis and consciousness, and (3) suggestibility. We discuss each part below.

Part 1. Hypnosis, a Specific State of Consciousness

The first part of this definition emphasizes that hypnosis is a peculiar state of consciousness i.e., a *non-ordinary state of consciousness*. This perspective, still in development, was first

DOI: 10.4324/9781003449126-33

supported in the late 1980s (Ulrich et al., 1987) and 1990s (Crawford et al., 1993; Maquet et al., 1999) through rigorous studies relying on neuroimaging. During hypnosis, an increase by 16% of the global cerebral blood flow (CBF) was observed with specific increases in occipital and right temporal regions (Ulrich et al., 1987). However, one can argue that the results of this study should be interpreted with caution because of the unclear hypnotic condition description. Later, Crawford et al. (1993) showed that highly hypnotizable persons demonstrated a significant increase in overall CBF, as compared to low hypnotizable participants, suggesting that hypnosis requires a specific cognitive effort. In addition, compared to mental imagery, hypnosis was related to the activation of cortical areas involved in sight (i.e., occipital regions), emotion (i.e., anterior cingulate cortex; ACC), thought, and movement (i.e., frontal regions) that one experiences when living a real situation, suggesting that hypnosis allows reliving an experience as if it was real (Maquet et al., 1999). Other studies showed that participants felt significantly more relaxed, absorbed, dissociated, less distracted, and had less analytical, cluttered, and environment-oriented thoughts during hypnosis (Deeley et al., 2012; Demertzi et al., 2011). In addition, compared to mental imagery, the hypnotic subjective experience was shown to result in a greater top-down activation of sensory processing in the right hemisphere (Lanfranco et al., 2021). These studies are consistent with the conclusion that hypnosis is a specific state of consciousness that has its own neurophenomenology (Vanhaudenhuyse et al., 2020).

In accordance with these findings, an explanatory model of hypnosis was proposed based on qualitative analyses of 21 reports of participants' hypnotic experiences (Rainville & Price, 2003). Five dimensions seem to explain the process of hypnotic depth: feeling mentally (and physically) relaxed, increased absorption, decreased monitoring, disorientation (i.e., suspension of spatial-temporal cues), and automaticity (i.e., altered agency). All these dimensions are proposed to contribute to hypnotic depth through mutual reinforcement (Rainville & Price, 2003). Nevertheless, this model needs to be evaluated further with additional studies using larger samples in order to be validated.

Part 2. Neurophysiology of Hypnosis and Consciousness, an Integrative Perspective

The second part of the definition is also linked to consciousness through two of its components: (1) internal or self-awareness, which is involved in self-related processes; and (2) external awareness or awareness of the environment, which is related to cognitive processes of external sensory input (Vanhaudenhuyse et al., 2011). The internal awareness is mainly supported by the ACC, the mesiofrontal cortex, the precuneus, and the posterior cingulate cortex (PCC), the three last being regions of the default mode network[1] (DMN, Raichle, 2015; Vanhaudenhuyse et al., 2011). External awareness is subtended by a fronto-parietal lateral neural network involved in maintaining a focused attention, anticipating and responding adequately to stimuli coming from the environment (Landry et al., 2017; Vanhaudenhuyse et al., 2011). In ordinary consciousness, activity in these two components has a negative correlation, meaning that when one is self-oriented, one is less aware of the environment and vice versa. This is linked to a negatively correlated activation of the two related brain networks (Vanhaudenhuyse et al., 2011). In this study, and during hypnosis, participants reported having significantly more self-referential cognitions and less environmental-oriented thoughts compared to ordinary consciousness. This increase was linked to reduced functional connectivity of the external consciousness network, while results for the internal consciousness network were less straightforward. Some studies have shown reduced connectivity between the PCC and parahippocampal structures, and an increased connectivity between its middle prefrontal cortex and lateral parietal areas during hypnosis (Demertzi et al., 2011). Others have found a decrease in activation of both posterior and anterior parts of the DMN (Deeley et al., 2012; McGeown et al., 2009), but also a positive correlation between the connectivity within the dorsal ACC and hypnotic depth (McGeown et al., 2015). Conversely, a decreased connectivity has also been described in the left insula and areas of the right dorsolateral prefrontal, medial frontal, and superior temporal cortex (McGeown et al., 2015). These results suggest that hypnosis engenders modifications of functional connectivity in regions involved with spontaneous thought and environmental processing, supporting hypnosis's particular phenomenology.

An integrated framework of neural correlates of hypnosis proposed that the salience network (i.e., insula and ACC; responsible for the modified awareness of internal and external events) regulated both the central executive network (i.e., posterior parietal cortex and dorsolateral prefrontal cortex) and the DMN (i.e., medial prefrontal cortex and PCC) (Landry et al., 2017; Landry & Raz, 2015). The central executive network, which maintains attentional focus of relevant information and selects mental strategies that produce an adequate hypnotic response, acts upon the DMN. The latter is responsible for the decrease in self-referential processes. Both the executive and the DMN interact with the salience network which ultimately reinforces their mutual influence and produces a neurophenomenology specific to the hypnotic state (Landry et al., 2017).

Part 3. Suggestibility/hypnotizability

The third part of the definition concerns one of the four main characteristics of hypnosis, i.e., suggestibility, also referred to as hypnotizability. In the hypnotic context, suggestibility is the tendency to comply with suggestions and to exhibit reduced critical thinking (Spiegel, 1991). It is considered different from placebo response, conformity, or persuasibility (Elkins, 2021). We will rely on the term hypnotizability to address the ability of an individual to experience changes in physiology, sensations, emotions, thoughts, or behavior during hypnosis assessed by a standardized tool. In addition to hypnotizability, hypnosis has also been found to be associated with dissociation, absorption, and automaticity (Spiegel, 1991; Weitzenhoffer, 2002). Dissociation is the splitting of mental processes and bodily awareness and perceptions; absorption is the tendency to be fully involved in a perceptive or imaginary experience (Spiegel, 1991); and automaticity corresponds to an altered sense of agency which is lived as a non-voluntary response to a suggestion (Weitzenhoffer, 2002). Although the neural correlates of non-pathological hypnotically induced dissociation have not yet been identified, some hypotheses can be drawn from studies assessing pathological dissociation. Sierra and Berrios (1998) proposed that symptoms of depersonalization may be associated with a "disconnection" of a cortico-limbic brain system (i.e., amygdala, ACC) and prefrontal structures. In this model, depersonalization is more broadly conceptualized as a state of subjective detachment, involving emotional numbing, emptiness of thoughts, analgesia, and hypervigilance. Increased recruitment of the prefrontal cortex (PFC) may (both directly and indirectly via the ACC) inhibit the amygdala resulting in dampened autonomic output, hypoemotionality, and lack of emotional coloring that would in turn be reported as feelings of "unreality or detachment." Other studies showed that hippocampal volume was 19.2% smaller and amygdala volume was 31.6% smaller in the patients with dissociative identity disorder, compared to the healthy participants (Vermetten et al., 2006). Finally, the regional CBF ratio was decreased in the orbitofrontal region bilaterally and increased in median and superior frontal regions, and occipital regions bilaterally in patients with dissociative identity disorder as compared to healthy participants. The neurophysiology of dissociative psychopathology suggests a comprehensive model of interaction between anterior and posterior brain regions (Sar et al., 2007). Absorption appears to rely on regions involved in executive and attentional functions such as the thalamus, the ACC (Rainville et al., 2002), and the ventrolateral PFC (Deeley et al., 2012). Automaticity seems to correlate with activation of the right parietal operculum (Rainville et al., 2019) which is involved in awareness of involuntary actions (Deeley et al., 2013) and automatic responding (Deeley, 2003).

Hypnotizability is typically measured by standardized scales developed decades ago that are time-consuming, taking from 60 to 90 minutes to complete. More recently, the Sussex Waterloo Scale of Hypnotizability (Lush et al., 2018) and the Elkins Hypnotizability Scale (Kekecs et al., 2016) have been developed to decrease the administration time to 40 minutes or less. Individuals with a high score (8–11/12) are considered highly hypnotizable (HH), those with a low score (0–3/12) as low hypnotizable (LH). We recently reported that it is feasible to identify the degree of hypnotizability without a specific suggestion (i.e., in neutral hypnosis) and with a single self-reported dissociation score (Vanhaudenhuyse et al., 2019).

While it is assumed that hypnotizability is a stable trait (Piccione et al., 1989), some authors have shown that training in self-hypnosis (SH), relaxation, neurofeedback, transcranial magnetic stimulation, or transcranial direct current stimulation may improve hypnotizability scores (Batty et al., 2006; Dienes & Hutton, 2013; Perri & Di Filippo, 2023). Others highlighted that hypnotizability can vary between different assessments sessions (Fassler et al., 2008) and even throughout the same day (Green et al., 2015), rendering complicated rigorous research on the role that hypnotizability plays in hypnosis (Halsband & Wolf, 2021). Moreover, it is known that 70% of the population has moderate hypnotizability, leaving only 30% in the high or low proportion of the continuum (Landry et al., 2017). However, hypnosis has historically been studied by comparing HHs with LHs only.

Regarding brain structure, studies have shown differences in the brain of HHs compared to LHs. Greater hypnotizability was shown to be positively associated with larger gray matter volumes in the left middle occipital, the middle and superior temporal gyri, the left insula, the right inferior parietal lobule (McGeown et al., 2015), and the rostrum of the corpus callosum (Horton et al., 2004), while lower gray matter volumes were found in the left cerebellar lobules (Picerni et al., 2019). Depth of hypnosis has been shown to be associated with larger gray matter volumes in the medial and superior gyri bilaterally, and the ACC (McGeown et al., 2015). McGeown and colleagues argue that the ease of attaining hypnosis depth seemed to be the result of more developed ACC, dorsolateral PFC, ventromedial PFC, and insula, which are involved in attention, executive, and affective processing skills (McGeown et al., 2015). Recently, a study highlighted the links between hypnotizability and executive functions, suggesting that those links might influence the response to a suggestion during hypnosis (Faerman & Spiegel, 2021).

HHs individuals showed increased ACC activation during a congruent/incongruent attentional task after hypnotic induction (Egner et al., 2005). During hypnosis, HHs compared to LHs had greater functional connectivity between regions of the executive (i.e., dorsolateral PFC; DLPF) and salience (i.e., insula) networks and reduced functional connectivity between regions of the DMN (i.e., DLPF and PCC) (Hoeft et al., 2012; Jiang et al., 2017). Other investigators have found a positive association between hypnotizability and functional connectivity between the PCC and the precuneus, the lateral visual network and the left frontoparietal network, and the network underlying executive control and the right postcentral parietal cortex, while negative associations were observed between the right frontoparietal network and the right lateral thalamus (Huber et al., 2014). Outside of hypnosis, HHs have been shown to recruit more of the right inferior frontal gyrus and less of the ACC and intraparietal sulcus, whereas the LHs recruit more of their parietal cortex and ACC, during selective attention conditions (Cojan et al., 2015).

Concerning electroencephalographical (EEG) studies, no consensus yet exists with regard to the hypnotic state (Wolf et al., 2022). Indeed, some researchers have reported a global increase in alpha activity while others found no activation of alpha bands during the hypnotic state (Wolf et al., 2022). Despite contradictory findings concerning EEG studies, increased theta activity in HH has been consistently reported in a substantial series of studies (De Benedittis, 2015; De Pascalis, 2023; Jensen et al., 2015; Wolf et al., 2022).

Hypnosis and Pain Modulation: From Experimental Studies to Hypnosedation

Pain is a universal subjective phenomenon that incorporates perceptions, emotions, cognition, and behaviors, and defined as "an unpleasant sensory and emotional experience associate with, or resembling that associated with, actual or potential tissue damage" (Raja et al., 2020, p. 1977). When pain is processed, the primary and secondary somatosensory cortices address the sensory characteristics of the stimulus, and the medial PFC, the ACC, and insula treat the unpleasantness, providing affective and motivational responses to pain (Bushnell et al., 2013). Activation of the ACC modulates the perception of pain by receiving signals from limbic regions (amygdala, thalamus, and hippocampus) and selecting specific attentional functions in response to pain characteristics (Moriarty et al., 2011). In addition, the medial PFC is responsible for cognitive top-down control, particularly for emotionally driven behaviors such as control of the unpleasantness of pain or the fear behaviors associated with it (Thompson & Neugebauer, 2019). Hypnosis is an efficient technique to reduce pain intensity and unpleasantness, and increase pain tolerance and threshold (Thompson et al., 2019). In addition, hypnosis can reduce or increase (depending on the suggestion) early (N20) and late (P100, P150, P250) components in brain areas involved in sensory and cognitive/affective nociceptive processing suggesting that hypnosis acts upon early (sensitive) and late (cognitive) pain processing (De Pascalis et al., 2015; Perri et al., 2019). While applying painful stimulation during hypnosis, studies either showed no activation of brain regions related to pain processing (Vanhaudenhuyse et al., 2009) or deactivation of regions involved in the sensory processing of pain

(Casiglia et al., 2020). The ACC modulation plays a specific role in pain modulation, and particularly pain unpleasantness during hypnosis (Rainville et al., 1997), combined with cortical and subcortical networks (i.e., PFC, superior frontal gyrus, insula, pregenual cortices, pre-supplementary motor area, thalami, striatum, and brainstem) (Del Casale et al., 2015).

The interest of hypnosis in acute pain can also be studied through hypnosedation, a combination of local anesthesia, conscious sedation, and hypnosis (Faymonville et al., 1999). Hypnosedation has been used for a variety of conditions such as breast and prostate biopsy, and thyroid surgery (for a review, see Vanhaudenhuyse et al., 2020). Compared to general anesthesia, it has been shown to result in better peri- and post-operative comfort, decreased anxiety, emotional distress, pain, nausea, and reduced use of intraoperative anxiolytic and analgesic drugs. Physiological parameters, surgical time, and recovery were also enhanced when using hypnosedation (for a review, see Tefikow et al., 2013). In addition, the majority of the patients who have received hypnosedation treatment reported they would opt for this approach again and recommend it to others (Chapet et al., 2019). It is noteworthy that the clinical application of hypnosis for painful contexts is wide and not limited to surgical practice. Indeed, hypnosis has been successfully used during childbirth, dental procedures, and in burn units to cite a few (Gueguen et al., 2021; Merz et al., 2022; Provençal et al., 2018).

Hypnosis for Chronic Conditions

Although we recognize that hypnosis is used in many chronic contexts, this section will only focus on chronic pain and oncology. Those fields are the ones we are studying at the University and the University Hospital of Liege.

Chronic Pain

Chronic pain is a persistent and/or recurrent pain that lasts for more than three months (Merskey et al., 1994). Both the emotional and cognitive dimensions play an important role in the development and modulation of chronic pain. Studies underline the important contribution of cortico-limbic regions (i.e., contributing to the affective and cognitive aspects of pain) in the development and maintenance of chronic pain, suggesting the role of emotional and motivational processes, as well as sensory processing to a lesser extent, in the experience of chronic pain (Simons et al., 2014).

Individuals with chronic pain report higher levels of anxiety, depression, altered cognition, loss of perceived control, and sleep disturbance than individuals who do not have chronic pain (Bicego et al., 2022). Thus, for individual with chronic pain, hypnosis can be used to address all of these secondary symptoms and conditions in addition to helping them learn to modulate pain intensity. The literature on hypnosis for chronic pain is relatively rich, including studies focusing on hypnosis, SH, or the combination of SH with other complementary approaches (e.g., cognitive behavioral therapy (CBT), psychoeducation, or physiotherapy). In this section, we will present studies without claiming to be exhaustive. Studies focusing on comparing SH to another treatment (i.e., physiotherapy, meditation, biofeedback, usual care) or a control group have shown decrease in pain intensity (Aravena et al., 2020; Billot et al., 2020; Brugnoli et al., 2018; Dumain et al., 2022; Hosseinzadegan et al., 2017; McKernan et al., 2020; Wallen et al., 2021) and pain interference (Aravena et al., 2020; Billot et al., 2020; Dumain et al., 2022; McKernan et al., 2020) up to one-year follow-up in favor of SH (Dumain et al., 2022). Decreases in fatigue/sleeping problems (Aravena et al., 2020; Wallen et al., 2021), depression (Aravena et al., 2020), and anxiety up to two-year follow-up (Brugnoli et al., 2018) in favor of SH are also observed. It should be noted that all these studies used analgesia suggestions. However, a recent study comparing SH training to meditation and psychoeducation highlighted that SH and meditation allowed for similar reduction in pain intensity, pain interference, and depressive symptoms at three- and six-months follow-up (Williams et al., 2022). Other studies proposed combination of SH with CBT, self-care (SC),[2] or psychoeducation to patients with chronic pain (Bicego et al., 2021a,b; Castel et al., 2012; Rizzo et al., 2018; Vanhaudenhuyse et al., 2015, 2018). Some of them revealed decreases in pain intensity, pain interference, catastrophizing, psychological distress, sleep difficulties, anxiety, depression, mental quality of life, perceived control, perceived disability, and hope in medical cure (Bicego et al., 2021a,b; Castel et al., 2012; Rizzo et al., 2018; Vanhaudenhuyse et al., 2015, 2018). However, other studies did not corroborate these results as no significant difference emerged whether patients had received SH/SC or SH/SC and psychoeducation (Bicego et al., 2021a), music/SC, SC, or psychoeducation alone (Bicego et al., 2021b). Results indicated decreases in pain intensity, benefits in dysfunctional cognitions, increases in physical quality of life, and internal health locus of control up to one-year follow-up independent of the intervention (Bicego et al., 2021b)[3]. In these studies, analgesia suggestions (Bicego et al., 2021a,b; Castel et al., 2012; Vanhaudenhuyse et al., 2015, 2018), dissociation and previous pleasant event suggestions (Rizzo et al., 2018), safe place, sleep restauration, and comfort suggestions (Bicego et al., 2021a,b; Vanhaudenhuyse et al., 2015, 2018) were proposed. Using the same suggestions, decreases in pain perception, anxiety, and sleeping problems were observed in patients with phantom limb pain (Bicego et al., 2022). This emphasizes the importance of using suggestions that cover different issues that patients with chronic pain may encounter. We believe that it is by considering the full complexity of chronic pain that clinicians will provide the most appropriate help to patients.

Concerning the neurophysiology of hypnosis in chronic pain, the literature is rather limited. Overall, studies agree that hypnosis particularly targets the emotional network related to pain while acting to a lesser extent on the purely perceptual aspect of it (Bicego et al., 2022b). Indeed, in hypnosis suggestions of analgesia (direct) and general comfort (indirect) decrease pain perception by acting on the cognitive-sensory pain network (fronto-temporal regions, insula, somatosensory cortex, cerebellum) and on regions of the cortico-limbic circuit (caudate, accumbens, lenticular nuclei, and ACC) (Nusbaum et al., 2010). This highlights the fact that hypnotic suggestions are not linear and unidirectional but rather act in a dynamic and multidirectional manner on the person as a whole (De Benedittis, 2015, 2020).

Oncology

Cancer generates a number of physical and psychological repercussions such as fatigue (Ma et al., 2020) and emotional distress (i.e., anxiety and depression) which considerably undermine patients' quality of life (Wang et al., 2020). Hypnosis is increasingly used in oncology to deal with the adverse effects of cancer and its treatments. Common effective uses of hypnosis for patients with cancer include the management of pain and painful procedures, anxiety, emotional distress, sleep difficulties, and fatigue (Carlson et al., 2018; Sine et al., 2022). Nevertheless, most of the early studies on hypnosis for cancer care lacked rigorous designs, making it difficult to draw firm conclusions from this research (Montgomery et al., 2017). A non-randomized study investigating the efficacy of SH/SC compared to yoga and CBT up to nine-month follow-up indicated that SH/SC reduced psychological distress and improved quality of life, sleeping problems, and mental adjustment compared to yoga or CBT in women with breast cancer (Bragard et al., 2017; Grégoire et al., 2017). These encouraging results urged researchers to rely on evidence-based medicine guidelines to carry out clinical trials. A randomized controlled trial also showed positive results in favor of SH/SC on fatigue, sleep difficulties, emotional distress, self-esteem, and mindfulness in women with a variety of cancer diagnoses that were maintained at one-year follow-up (Grégoire et al., 2020, 2021, 2022). However, no significant effects of SH/SC on a population of patients with prostate cancer were observed (Grégoire et al., 2018). These results highlight the importance of adapting management according to the type of cancer, the type of procedures received by patients, and the treatment status of the patients (i.e., on- or off-treatment, beginning or end of the treatment).

Recently, we proposed to 23 patients with different cancer diagnoses (n =17 breast; n = 3 hematologic; n = 2 brain; n = 1 prostate), in- and off-treatment, to participate in a six-session group intervention (2 h each) of SH/SC (delay between session varied from two weeks to one month). Directly after the intervention, results showed an improvement of anxiety, depression, and sleep difficulties for all 23 patients. Even though the study had a small sample size and was not controlled, the results suggest the possibility that SH/SC may be effective regardless of diagnosis, treatment progress, and sex, highlighting the clinical relevance of proposing SH learning to patients when it is adapted. However, these observations should be reproduced with a larger sample to be confirmed. Finally, pilot studies have demonstrated the feasibility and benefits of proposing SH/SC for children with cancer and their parents (Gregoire et al., 2019). Parents reported the utility of sharing their experience, and an increased regulation of emotion and well-being. Children reported that SH/SC helped them to cope with negative emotions, to respect themselves more, to be more assertive, and to relax.

To our knowledge, only one case study has investigated the neural correlates of hypnosedation in a 57-year-old patient with breast cancer (Prinsloo et al., 2019). Results showed an increase in occipital regions that are involved in mental imagery and a decrease in parietal, somatosensory, and frontal regions (subtending convergence between vision and proprioception, sensory-motor movement, and attention respectively), as well as in the ACC (involved in pain modulation). During the follow-up session, the patient reported minimal pain and was happy to have avoided general anesthesia.

Overall, the extant research supports the conclusion that patients with cancer are interested in complementary interventions such as hypnosis and provides preliminary support for the benefits of such approaches on their quality of life.

Toward Contemporary Hypnosis? Virtual Reality Hypnosis

In recent years, virtual reality hypnosis (VRH) has gained ground in the hospital setting. VRH was initially defined as "a hypnotic induction and analgesic suggestion delivered through customized virtual reality hardware/software" (Patterson et al., 2010, p. 1). Nowadays, VRH devices contain various suggestions such as general comfort and relaxation for example. In virtual reality, hypnosis can be proposed before, during, or after the session and can be done live by the therapist or via a standardized audio format (Rousseaux et al., 2020a). While VRH has been proposed to facilitate hypnosis's induction (Patterson et al., 2010), the results of research to date have not confirmed this hypothesis (Rousseaux, et al., 2020a). We recently highlighted that studies on VRH lack homogeneity and thus prevent us from drawing any conclusions (Rousseaux et al., 2020a).

Research at the University and University Hospital of Liege has pioneered in the development of rigorous VRH research methods in experimental (i.e., painful stimulation, Figure 24.1) (Rousseaux et al., 2022a) and clinical settings (i.e., intensive care units, Figure 24.2) (Rousseaux et al., 2022b). Concerning experimental pain, we demonstrated that VRH, compared to ordinary consciousness, decreased pain perception and the brain response related to it in healthy volunteers (Rousseaux et al., 2022a). This suggests that VRH is a promising tool for the modulation of procedural/acute pain. Regarding the clinical study, the results did not demonstrate a superiority of VRH over hypnosis alone, music, or a control group on pain, anxiety, relaxation, and comfort in patients undergoing a cardiac surgery (Rousseaux, et al., 2022b). We discussed that the simple presence of a psychologist could probably partly explain these results and that an adequate therapeutic relation with the patient is a necessary condition for the good use of these techniques. These results have been replicated in other medical settings (Wiechman et al., 2022). There is a need to continue research in this area in order to

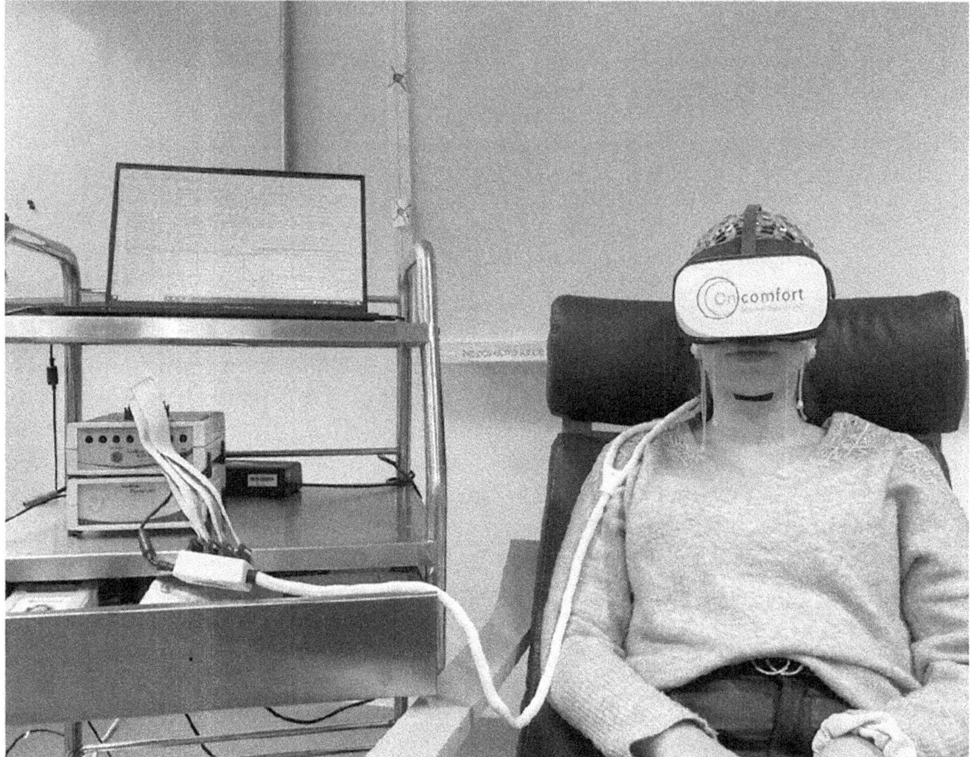

Figure 24.1 Healthy participant with an EEG cap and the virtual reality hypnosis device.

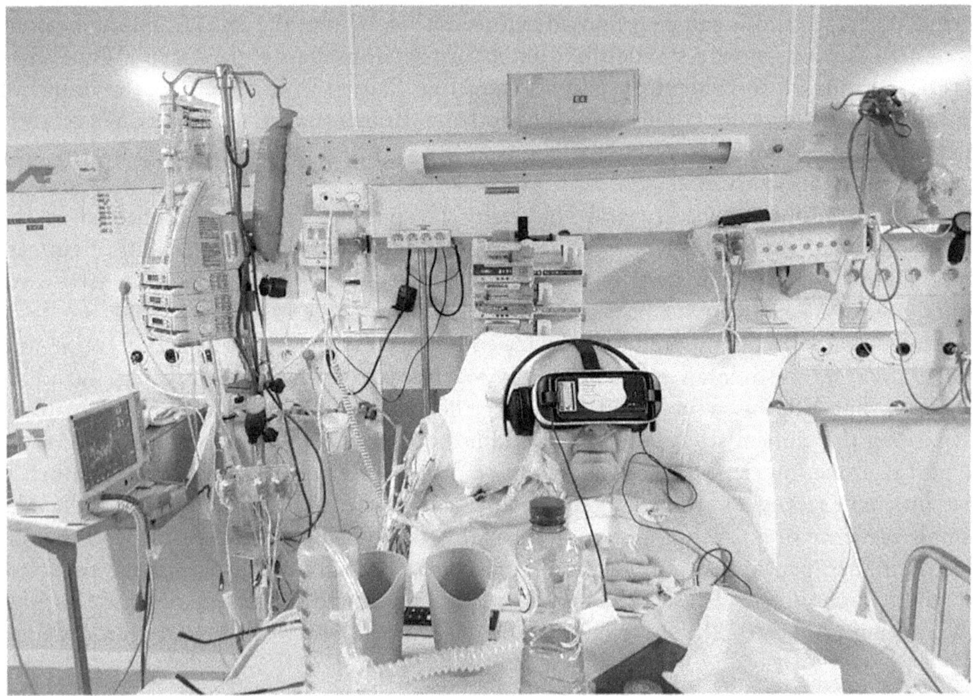

Figure 24.2 Patient in the intensive care unit with the virtual reality hypnosis device.

develop specific guidelines that would help understand for whom, why, when, and how to use VRH.

Conclusion

This chapter discussed hypnosis as a non-ordinary state of consciousness with a specific neurophenomenology. Hypnotizability is not a stable trait, but rather an inherent capacity that can evolve, which complicates the study of hypnotizability in hypnosis research. We summarized empirical findings supporting the conclusion that hypnosis is effective for the management of acute pain, surgery, chronic pain, and the many side effects of cancer and its treatments. We believe that the significant benefits of hypnosis result in large part from the fact that it allows individuals to discover and use their resources and thus to be actors in their recovery. Once mastered, people can apply hypnosis to many difficulties. Furthermore, hypnosis enables an understanding of neurophysiological and psychological mechanisms underlying pain, attentional processes, and consciousness. Finally, while we recognize that neuroscience is important because it allows us to better understand hypnosis, we also acknowledge the fact that understanding human behavior and its brain function is challenging and that only relying on neuroscience is simplistic. We believe that it is important to endorse a holistic vision of the human being, by combining disciplines (e.g., psychology, sociology, medicine, neurosciences, philosophy), methods (e.g., quantitative, qualitative, mixed), and cultures (e.g., occidental, oriental, African, Latin American), that only then will we effectively increase our understanding of hypnosis.

Acknowledgment

We are grateful to all the patients who participated in the studies. We also thank all the health professionals working at the CHU of Liège or elsewhere in Belgium who are helping, and Alain Collinet, who composed the musical records used in various studies we cited. Thanks to the University and University Hospital of Liege, "Plan National Cancer" of Belgium (Grant Number 138), Belgium Foundation Against Cancer (Grant Numbers: 2017064 and C/2020/1357), the Télévie (from the Belgian National Funds for Scientific Research, FRS-FNRS), the Benoit Foundation (Bruxelles), Wallonia as part of a program of the BioWin Health Cluster framework, the fund Geert Noël of the King Baudouin Foundation, and AstraZeneca Foundation.

Notes

1 The DMN is a neuronal network that is activated when one does not carry out any particular task (Raichle, 2015). It is involved in self-referential cognition (Landry et al., 2017).
2 Self-care is an approach developed by M-E F based on her clinical experience. It is inspired by CBT and acceptance and commitment therapy (Hayes et al., 2011). It consists of concrete tasks aiming at increasing the general well-being according to the values and goals of each individual.
3 These results are interesting though not surprising. They outline the role of unspecific effects or common factors in psychotherapy outcome, supporting the so-called Dodo bird verdict, a controversial topic in psychotherapy, referring to the claim that all empirically validated psychotherapies regardless of their specific components, are equally effective (Budd & Hughes, 2009).

References

Aravena, V., García, F. E., Téllez, A., & Arias, P. R. (2020). Hypnotic intervention in people with fibromyalgia: A randomized controlled trial. *The American Journal of Clinical Hypnosis*, *63*(1), 49–61. 10.1080/00029157.2020.1742088

Batty, M. J., Bonnington, S., Tang, B.-K., Hawken, M. B., & Gruzelier, J. H. (2006). Relaxation strategies and enhancement of hypnotic susceptibility: EEG neurofeedback, progressive muscle relaxation and self-hypnosis. *Brain Research Bulletin*, *71*(1–3), 83–90. 10.1016/j.brainresbull.2006.08.005

Bicego, A., Delmal, P., Ledoux, D., Faymonville, M.-E., Noordhout, B., Cerasoli, A., Cassol, H., Gosseries, O., & Vanhaudenhuyse, A. (2022b). Self-hypnosis for phantom limb pain: A multiple-case study. *OBM Integrative and Complementary Medicine*, *7*, 1-1. 10.21926/obm.icm.2203040

Bicego, A., Monseur, J., Collinet, A., Donneau, A.-F., Fontaine, R., Libbrecht, D., Malaise, N., Nyssen, A.-S., Raaf, M., Rousseaux, F., Salamun, I., Staquet, C., Teuwis, S., Tomasella, M., Faymonville, M.-E., & Vanhaudenhuyse, A. (2021b). Complementary treatment comparison for chronic pain management: A randomized longitudinal study. *PloS One*, *16*(8), e0256001. 10.1371/journal.pone.0256001

Bicego, A., Rémy, H., Diep, A. N., Donneau, A.-F., Faymonville, M.-E., Nyssen, A.-S., Malaise, N., Salamun, I., & Vanhaudenhuyse, A. (2021a). Psychological interventions influence patients' attitudes and beliefs about their chronic pain: A 6-month follow-up. *Chronic Pain & Management*. *5*, 135. 10.29011/2576-957X.100035

Bicego, A., Rousseaux, F., Faymonville, M.-E., Nyssen, A.-S., & Vanhaudenhuyse, A. (2022a). Neurophysiology of hypnosis in chronic pain: A review of recent literature. *The American Journal of Clinical Hypnosis*, *64*(1), 62–80. 10.1080/00029157.2020.1869517

Billot, M., Jaglin, P., Rainville, P., Rigoard, P., Langlois, P., Cardinaud, N., Tchalla, A., & Wood, C. (2020). Hypnosis program effectiveness in a 12-week home care intervention to manage chronic pain in elderly women: A pilot trial. *Clinical Therapeutics*, *42*(1), 221–229. 10.1016/j.clinthera.2019.11.007

Bragard, I., Etienne, A.-M., Faymonville, M.-E., Coucke, P., Lifrange, E., Schroeder, H., Wagener, A., Dupuis, G., & Jerusalem, G. (2017). A nonrandomized comparison study of self-hypnosis, yoga, and cognitive-behavioral therapy to reduce emotional distress in breast cancer patients. *International Journal of Clinical and Experimental Hypnosis*, *65*, 189–209. 10.1080/00207144.2017.1276363

Brugnoli, M. P., Pesce, G., Pasin, E., Basile, M. F., Tamburin, S., & Polati, E. (2018). The role of clinical hypnosis and self-hypnosis to relief pain and anxiety in severe chronic diseases in palliative care: A 2-year long-term follow-up of treatment in a nonrandomized clinical trial. *Annals of Palliative Medicine*, *7*(1), 17–31. 10.21037/apm.2017.10.03

Budd, R., & Hughes, I. (2009). The Dodo Bird Verdict—Controversial, inevitable and important: A commentary on 30 years of meta-analyses. *Clinical Psychology & Psychotherapy*, *16*, 510–522. 10.1002/cpp.648

Bushnell, M. C., Čeko, M., & Low, L. A. (2013). Cognitive and emotional control of pain and its disruption in chronic pain. *Nature Reviews. Neuroscience*, *14*(7), 502–511. 10.1038/nrn3516

Carlson, L. E., Toivonen, K., Flynn, M., Deleemans, J., Piedalue, K.-A., Tolsdorf, E., & Subnis, U. (2018). The role of hypnosis in cancer care. *Current Oncology Reports*, *20*(12), 93. 10.1007/s11912-018-0739-1

Casiglia, E., Finatti, F., Tikhonoff, V., Stabile, M. R., Mitolo, M., Albertini, F., Gasparotti, F., Facco, E., Lapenta, A. M., & Venneri, A. (2020). Mechanisms of hypnotic analgesia explained by functional magnetic resonance (fMRI). *International Journal of Clinical and Experimental Hypnosis*, *68*(1), 1–15. 10.1080/00207144.2020.1685331

Castel, A., Cascón, R., Padrol, A., Sala, J., & Rull, M. (2012). Multicomponent cognitive-behavioral group therapy with hypnosis for the treatment of fibromyalgia: Long-term outcome. *The Journal of Pain: Official Journal of the American Pain Society*, *13*(3), 255–265. 10.1016/j.jpain.2011.11.005

Chapet, O., Udrescu, C., Horn, S., Ruffion, A., Lorchel, F., Gaudioz, S., Clamens, C., Piriou, V., & Rigal, E. (2019). Prostate brachytherapy under hypnosedation: A prospective evaluation. *Brachytherapy*, *18*(1), 22–28. 10.1016/j.brachy.2018.10.004

Cojan, Y., Piguet, C., & Vuilleumier, P. (2015). What makes your brain suggestible? Hypnotizability is associated with differential brain activity during attention outside hypnosis. *NeuroImage*, *117*, 367–374. 10.1016/j.neuroimage.2015.05.076

Crawford, H. J., Gur, R. C., Skolnick, B., Gur, R. E., & Benson, D. M. (1993). Effects of hypnosis on regional cerebral blood flow during ischemic pain with and without suggested hypnotic analgesia. *International Journal of Psychophysiology*, *15*(3), 181–195. 10.1016/0167-8760(93)90002-7

De Benedittis, G. (2015). Neural mechanisms of hypnosis and meditation. *Journal of Physiology-Paris*, *109*(4–6), 152–164. 10.1016/j.jphysparis.2015.11.001

De Benedittis, G. (2020). Neural mechanisms of hypnotic analgesia. *OBM Integrative and Complementary Medicine*, *5*, 1–14. 10.21926/obm.icm.2002023

De Pascalis, V., Varriale, V., & Cacace, I. (2015). Pain modulation in waking and hypnosis in women: Event-related potentials and sources of cortical activity. *PloS One*, *10*(6), e0128474. 10.1371/journal.pone.0128474

De Pascalis, V. (2023). EEG oscillatory activity concomitant with hypnosis and hypnotizability. (in press, this volume)

Deeley, P. Q. (2003). Social, cognitive, and neural constraints on subjectivity and agency: Implications for dissociative identity disorder. *Philosophy, Psychiatry, and Psychology*, *10*(2), 161–167. 10.1353/ppp.2003.0095

Deeley, Q., Oakley, D. A., Toone, B., Giampietro, V., Brammer, M. J., Williams, S. C. R., & Halligan, P. W. (2013). Modulating the default mode network using hypnosis. *International Journal of Clinical and Experimental Hypnosis*, *60*(2), 206–228. 10.1080/00207144.2012.648070

Deeley, Q., Walsh, E., Oakley, D. A., Bell, V., Koppel, C., Mehta, M. A., & Halligan, P. W. (2013). Using hypnotic suggestion to model loss of control and awareness of movements: An exploratory fMRI study. *PLoS ONE*, *8*, e78324. 10.1371/journal.pone.0078324

Del Casale, A., Ferracuti, S., Rapinesi, C., Serata, D., Caltagirone, S. S., Savoja, V., Piacentino, D., Callovini, G., Manfredi, G., Sani, G., Kotzalidis, G. D., & Girardi, P. (2015). Pain perception and hypnosis: Findings from recent functional neuroimaging studies. *International Journal of Clinical and Experimental Hypnosis*, *63*(2), 144–170. 10.1080/00207144.2015.1002371

Demertzi, A., Soddu, A., Faymonville, M.-E., Bahri, M. A., Gosseries, O., Vanhaudenhuyse, A., Phillips, C., Maquet, P., Noirhomme, Q., Luxen, A., & Laureys, S. (2011). Hypnotic modulation of resting state fMRI default mode and extrinsic network connectivity. In *Progress in Brain Research* (Vol. 193, pp. 309–322). Elsevier. 10.1016/B978-0-444-53839-0.00020-X

Dienes, Z., & Hutton, S. (2013). Understanding hypnosis metacognitively: RTMS applied to left DLPFC increases hypnotic suggestibility. *Cortex: A Journal Devoted to the Study of the Nervous System and Behavior*, *49*, 386–392. 10.1016/j.cortex.2012.07.009

Dumain, M., Jaglin, P., Wood, C., Rainville, P., Pageaux, B., Perrochon, A., Lavallière, M., Vendeuvre, T., David, R., Langlois, P., Cardinaud, N., Tchalla, A., Rigoard, P., & Billot, M. (2022). Long-term efficacy of a home-care hypnosis program in elderly persons suffering from chronic pain: A 12-month follow-up. *Pain Management Nursing: Official Journal of the American Society of Pain Management Nurses*, *23*(3), 330–337. 10.1016/j.pmn.2021.06.005

Egner, T., Jamieson, G., & Gruzelier, J. (2005). Hypnosis decouples cognitive control from conflict monitoring processes of the frontal lobe. *NeuroImage*, *27*(4), 969–978. 10.1016/j.neuroimage.2005.05.002

Elkins, G. (2021). Hypnotizability: Emerging perspectives and research. *International Journal of Clinical and Experimental Hypnosis*, *69*(1), 1–6. 10.1080/00207144.2021.1836934

Elkins, G. R., Barabasz, A. F., Council, J. R., & Spiegel, D. (2015). Advancing research and practice: The revised APA Division 30 definition of hypnosis. *American Journal of Clinical Hypnosis*, *57*(4), 378–385. 10.1080/00029157.2015.1011465

Faerman, A., & Spiegel, D. (2021). Shared cognitive mechanisms of hypnotizability with executive functioning and information salience. *Scientific Reports*, *11*(1), 5704. 10.1038/s41598-021-84954-8

Fassler, O., Lynn, S. J., & Knox, J. (2008). Is hypnotic suggestibility a stable trait? *Consciousness and Cognition: An International Journal*, *17*, 240–253. 10.1016/j.concog.2007.05.004

Faymonville, M. E., Meurisse, M., & Fissette, J. (1999). Hypnosedation: A valuable alternative to traditional anaesthetic techniques. *Acta Chirurgica Belgica*, *99*(4), 141–146.

Green, J. P., Smith, R. J., & Kromer, M. (2015). Diurnal variations in hypnotic responsiveness: Is there an optimal time to be hypnotized? *International Journal of Clinical and Experimental Hypnosis*, *63*, 171–181. 10.1080/00207144.2015.1002675

Grégoire, C., Bragard, I., Jerusalem, G., Etienne, A.-M., Coucke, P., Dupuis, G., Lanctôt, D., & Faymonville, M.-E. (2017). Group interventions to reduce emotional distress and fatigue in breast cancer patients: A 9-month follow-up pragmatic trial. *British Journal of Cancer*, *117*(10), 1442–1449. 10.1038/bjc.2017.326

Grégoire, C., Chantrain, C., Faymonville, M.-E., Marini, J., & Bragard, I. (2019). A hypnosis-based group intervention to improve quality of life in children with cancer and their parents. *International Journal of Clinical and Experimental Hypnosis*, *67*, 117–135. 10.1080/00207144.2019.1580965

Grégoire, C., Faymonville, M.-E., Vanhaudenhuyse, A., Charland-Verville, V., Jerusalem, G., Willems, S., & Bragard, I. (2020). Effects of an intervention combining self-care and self-hypnosis on fatigue and associated symptoms in post-treatment cancer patients: A randomized-controlled trial. *Psycho-Oncology*, *29*(7), 1165–1173. 10.1002/pon.5395

Grégoire, C., Faymonville, M.-E., Vanhaudenhuyse, A., Jerusalem, G., Willems, S., & Bragard, I. (2021). Randomized controlled trial of a group intervention combining self-hypnosis and self-care: Secondary results on self-esteem, emotional distress and regulation, and mindfulness in post-treatment cancer patients. *Quality of Life Research: An International Journal of Quality of Life Aspects of Treatment, Care and Rehabilitation*, *30*(2), 425–436. 10.1007/s11136-020-02655-7

Grégoire, C., Faymonville, M.-E., Vanhaudenhuyse, A., Jerusalem, G., Willems, S., & Bragard, I. (2022). Randomized, controlled trial of an intervention combining self-care and self-hypnosis on fatigue, sleep, and emotional distress in posttreatment cancer patients: 1-Year follow-up. *International Journal of Clinical and Experimental Hypnosis*, *70*(2), 136–155. 10.1080/00207144.2022.2049973

Grégoire, C., Nicolas, H., Bragard, I., Delevallez, F., Merckaert, I., Razavi, D., Waltregny, D., Faymonville, M.-E., & Vanhaudenhuyse, A. (2018). Efficacy of a hypnosis-based intervention to improve well-being during cancer: A comparison between prostate and breast cancer patients. *BMC Cancer*, *18*(1), 677. 10.1186/s12885-018-4607-z

Gueguen, J., Huas, C., Orri, M., & Falissard, B. (2021). Hypnosis for labour and childbirth: A meta-integration of qualitative and quantitative studies. *Complementary Therapies in Clinical Practice*, *43*, 101380. 10.1016/j.ctcp.2021.101380

Halsband, U., & Wolf, T. G. (2021). Current neuroscientific research database findings of brain activity changes after hypnosis. *The American Journal of Clinical Hypnosis*, *63*(4), 372–388. 10.1080/00029157.2020.1863185

Hayes, S., Strosahl, K., & Wilson, K. (2011). *Acceptance and commitment therapy: The process and practice of mindful change*. Guilford Press.

Hoeft, F., Gabrieli, J. D. E., Whitfield-Gabrieli, S., Haas, B. W., Bammer, R., Menon, V., & Spiegel, D. (2012). Functional brain basis of hypnotizability. *Archives of General Psychiatry*, *69*(10), 1064–1072. 10.1001/archgenpsychiatry.2011.2190

Horton, J. E., Crawford, H. J., Harrington, G., & Downs, J. H. (2004). Increased anterior corpus callosum size associated positively with hypnotizability and the ability to control pain. *Brain: A Journal of Neurology*, *127*(Pt 8), 1741–1747. 10.1093/brain/awh196

Hosseinzadegan, F., Radfar, M., Shafiee-Kandjani, A. R., & Sheikh, N. (2017). Efficacy of self-hypnosis in pain management in female patients with multiple sclerosis. *International Journal of Clinical and Experimental Hypnosis*, *65*(1), 86–97. 10.1080/00207144.2017.1246878

Huber, A., Lui, F., Duzzi, D., Pagnoni, G., & Porro, C. A. (2014). Structural and functional cerebral correlates of hypnotic suggestibility. *PLOS One*, *9*(3), e93187. 10.1371/journal.pone.0093187

Jensen, M. P., Adachi, T., Tomé-Pires, C., Lee, J., Osman, Z. J., & Miró, J. (2015). Mechanisms of hypnosis: Toward the development of a biopsychosocial model. *International Journal of Clinical and Experimental Hypnosis*, *63*(1), 34–75. 10.1080/00207144.2014.961875

Jiang, H., White, M. P., Greicius, M. D., Waelde, L. C., & Spiegel, D. (2017). Brain activity and functional connectivity associated with hypnosis. *Cerebral Cortex (New York, N.Y.: 1991)*, *27*(8), 4083–4093. 10.1093/cercor/bhw220

Kekecs, Z., Bowers, J., Johnson, A., Kendrick, C., & Elkins, G. (2016). The Elkins Hypnotizability Scale: Assessment of reliability and validity. *International Journal of Clinical and Experimental Hypnosis*, *64*(3), 285–304. 10.1080/00207144.2016.1171089

Landry, M., Lifshitz, M., & Raz, A. (2017). Brain correlates of hypnosis: A systematic review and meta-analytic exploration. *Neuroscience & Biobehavioral Reviews*, *81*, 75–98. 10.1016/j.neubiorev.2017.02.020

Landry, M., & Raz, A. (2015). Hypnosis and imaging of the living human brain. *The American Journal of Clinical Hypnosis*, *57*(3), 285–313. 10.1080/00029157.2014.978496

Lanfranco, R. C., Rivera-Rei, Á., Huepe, D., Ibáñez, A., & Canales-Johnson, A. (2021). Beyond imagination: Hypnotic visual hallucination induces greater lateralised brain activity than visual mental imagery. *NeuroImage*, *239*, 118282. 10.1016/j.neuroimage.2021.118282

Lush, P., Moga, G., McLatchie, N., & Dienes, Z. (2018). The Sussex-Waterloo Scale of Hypnotizability (SWASH): Measuring capacity for altering conscious experience. *Neuroscience of Consciousness*, *2018*(1), niy006. 10.1093/nc/niy006

Ma, Y., He, B., Jiang, M., Yang, Y., Wang, C., Huang, C., & Han, L. (2020). Prevalence and risk factors of cancer-related fatigue: A systematic review and meta-analysis. *International Journal of Nursing Studies*, *111*, 103707. 10.1016/j.ijnurstu.2020.103707

Maquet, P., Faymonville, M. E., Degueldre, C., Delfiore, G., Franck, G., Luxen, A., & Lamy, M. (1999). Functional neuroanatomy of hypnotic state. *Biological Psychiatry*, *45*(3), 327–333. 10.1016/s0006-3223(97)00546-5

McGeown, W. J., Mazzoni, G., Vannucci, M., & Venneri, A. (2015). Structural and functional correlates of hypnotic depth and suggestibility. *Psychiatry Research*, *231*(2), 151–159. 10.1016/j.pscychresns.2014.11.015

McGeown, W. J., Mazzoni, G., Venneri, A., & Kirsch, I. (2009). Hypnotic induction decreases anterior default mode activity. *Consciousness and Cognition*, *18*(4), 848–855. 10.1016/j.concog.2009.09.001

McKernan, L. C., Finn, M. T. M., Patterson, D. R., Williams, R. M., & Jensen, M. P. (2020). Clinical hypnosis for chronic pain in outpatient integrative medicine: An implementation and training model. *Journal of Alternative and Complementary Medicine (New York, N.Y.)*, *26*(2), 107–112. 10.1089/acm.2019.0259

Merskey, H., Bogduk, N., & International Association for the Study of Pain (Éds.). (1994). *Classification of chronic pain: Descriptions of chronic pain syndromes and definitions of pain terms* (2nd ed). IASP Press.

Merz, A. E., Campus, G., Abrahamsen, R., & Wolf, T. G. (2022). Hypnosis on acute dental and maxillofacial pain relief: A systematic review and meta-analysis. *Journal of Dentistry*, *123*, 104184. 10.1016/j.jdent.2022.104184

Montgomery, G. H., Sucala, M., Baum, T., & Schnur, J. B. (2017). Hypnosis for symptom control in cancer patients at the end-of-life: A systematic review. *International Journal of Clinical and Experimental Hypnosis*, *65*(3), 296–307. 10.1080/00207144.2017.1314728

Moriarty, O., McGuire, B. E., & Finn, D. P. (2011). The effect of pain on cognitive function: A review of clinical and preclinical research. *Progress in Neurobiology*, *93*(3), 385–404. 10.1016/j.pneurobio.2011.01.002

Nusbaum, F., Redouté, J., Le Bars, D., Volckmann, P., Simon, F., Hannoun, S., Ribes, G., Gaucher, J., Laurent, B., & Sappey-Marinier, D. (2010). Chronic low-back pain modulation is enhanced by hypnotic analgesic suggestion by recruiting an emotional network: A PET imaging study. *International Journal of Clinical and Experimental Hypnosis*, *59*(1), 27–44. 10.1080/00207144.2011.522874

Patterson, D. R., Jensen, M. P., Wiechman, S. A., & Sharar, S. R. (2010). Virtual reality hypnosis for pain associated with recovery from physical trauma. *International Journal of Clinical and Experimental Hypnosis*, *58*(3), 288–300. 10.1080/00207141003760595

Perri, R. L., & Di Filippo, G. (2023). Alteration of hypnotic experience following transcranial electrical stimulation of the left prefrontal cortex. *International Journal of Clinical and Health Psychology: IJCHP*, *23*(2), 100346. 10.1016/j.ijchp.2022.100346

Perri, R. L., Rossani, F., & Di Russo, F. (2019). Neuroelectric evidences of top-down hypnotic modulation associated with somatosensory processing of sensory and limbic regions. *NeuroImage*, *202*, 116104. 10.1016/j.neuroimage.2019.116104

Piccione, C., Hilgard, E., & Zimbardo, P. (1989). On the degree of stability of measured hypnotizability over a 25-year period. *Journal of Personality and Social Psychology*, *56*, 289–295. 10.1037//0022-3514.56.2.289

Picerni, E., Santarcangelo, E. L., Laricchiuta, D., Cutuli, D., Petrosini, L., Spalletta, G., & Piras, F. (2019). Cerebellar structural variations in subjects with different hypnotizability. *Cerebellum (London, England)*, *18*(1), 109–118. 10.1007/s12311-018-0965-y

Prinsloo, S., Rebello, E., Cata, J. P., Black, D., DeSnyder, S. M., & Cohen, L. (2019). Electroencephalographic correlates of hypnosedation during breast cancer surgery. *The Breast Journal*, *25*(4), 786–787. 10.1111/tbj.13328

Provençal, S.-C., Bond, S., Rizkallah, E., & El-Baalbaki, G. (2018). Hypnosis for burn wound care pain and anxiety: A systematic review and meta-analysis. *Burns: Journal of the International Society for Burn Injuries*, *44*(8), 1870–1881. 10.1016/j.burns.2018.04.017

Raichle, M. E. (2015). The brain's default mode network. *Annual Review of Neuroscience*, *38*(1), 433–447. 10.1146/annurev-neuro-071013-014030

Rainville, P., Duncan, G. H., Price, D. D., Carrier, B., & Bushnell, M. C. (1997). Pain affect encoded in human anterior cingulate but not somatosensory cortex. *Science (New York, N.Y.)*, *277*(5328), 968–971. 10.1126/science.277.5328.968

Rainville, P., Hofbauer, R. K., Bushnell, M. C., Duncan, G. H., & Price, D. D. (2002). Hypnosis modulates activity in brain structures involved in the regulation of consciousness. *Journal of Cognitive Neuroscience*, *14*(6), 887–901. 10.1162/089892902760191117

Rainville, P., & Price, D. D. (2003). Hypnosis phenomenology and the neurobiology of consciousness. *International Journal of Clinical and Experimental Hypnosis*, *51*(2), 105–129. 10.1076/iceh.51.2.105.14613

Rainville, P., Streff, A., Chen, J.-I., Houzé, B., Desmarteaux, C., & Piché, M. (2019). Hypnotic automaticity in the brain at rest: An arterial spin labelling study. *International Journal of Clinical and Experimental Hypnosis*, *67*(4), 512–542. 10.1080/00207144.2019.1650578

Raja, S. N., Carr, D. B., Cohen, M., Finnerup, N. B., Flor, H., Gibson, S., Keefe, F. J., Mogil, J. S., Ringkamp, M., Sluka, K. A., Song, X.-J., Stevens, B., Sullivan, M. D., Tutelman, P. R., Ushida, T., & Vader, K. (2020). The revised International Association for the Study of Pain definition of pain: Concepts, challenges, and compromises. *Pain*, *161*(9), 1976–1982. 10.1097/j.pain.0000000000001939

Rizzo, R. R. N., Medeiros, F. C., Pires, L. G., Pimenta, R. M., McAuley, J. H., Jensen, M. P., & Costa, L. O. P. (2018). Hypnosis enhances the effects of pain education in patients with chronic nonspecific low back pain: A randomized controlled trial. *The Journal of Pain: Official Journal of the American Pain Society*, *19*(10), 1103.e1–1103.e9. 10.1016/j.jpain.2018.03.013

Rousseaux, F., Bicego, A. Y., Ledoux, D., Massion, P., Nyssen, A.-S., Faymonville, M.-E., Laureys, S., & Vanhaudenhuyse, A. (2020). Hypnosis associated with 3D immersive virtual reality technology in the management of pain: A review of the literature. *Journal of Pain Research*. https://orbi.uliege.be/handle/2268/242546

Rousseaux, F., Dardenne, N., Massion, P. B., Ledoux, D., Bicego, A., Donneau, A.-F., Faymonville, M.-E., Nyssen, A.-S., & Vanhaudenhuyse, A. (2022b). Virtual reality and hypnosis for anxiety and pain management in intensive care units: A prospective randomised trial among cardiac surgery patients. *European Journal of Anaesthesiology*, *39*(1), 58–66. 10.1097/EJA.0000000000001633

Rousseaux, F., Panda, R., Toussaint, C., Bicego, A., Niimi, M., Faymonville, M.-E., Nyssen, A.-S., Laureys, S., Gosseries, O., & Vanhaudenhuyse, A. (2022a). Virtual reality hypnosis in the management of pain: Self-reported and neurophysiological measures in healthy subjects. *European Journal of Pain (London, England)*. 10.1002/ejp.2045

Sar, V., Unal, S. N., & Ozturk, E. (2007). Frontal and occipital perfusion changes in dissociative identity disorder. *Psychiatry Research*, *156*(3), 217–223. 10.1016/j.pscychresns.2006.12.017

Sierra, M., & Berrios, G. E. (1998). Depersonalization: Neurobiological perspectives. *Biological Psychiatry*, *44*(9), 898–908. 10.1016/s0006-3223(98)00015-8

Simons, L. E., Elman, I., & Borsook, D. (2014). Psychological processing in chronic pain: A neural systems approach. *Neuroscience & Biobehavioral Reviews*, *39*, 61–78. 10.1016/j.neubiorev.2013.12.006

Sine, H., Achbani, A., & Filali, K. (2022). The effect of hypnosis on the intensity of pain and anxiety in cancer patients: A systematic review of controlled experimental trials. *Cancer Investigation*, *40*(3), 235–253. 10.1080/07357907.2021.1998520

Spiegel, D. (1991). Neurophysiological correlates of hypnosis and dissociation. *The Journal of Neuropsychiatry and Clinical Neurosciences*, *3*(4), 440–445. 10.1176/jnp.3.4.440

Tefikow, S., Barth, J., Maichrowitz, S., Beelmann, A., Strauss, B., & Rosendahl, J. (2013). Efficacy of hypnosis in adults undergoing surgery or medical procedures: A meta-analysis of randomized controlled trials. *Clinical Psychology Review*, *33*(5), 623–636. 10.1016/j.cpr.2013.03.005

Thompson, J. M., & Neugebauer, V. (2019). Cortico-limbic pain mechanisms. *Neuroscience Letters*, *702*, 15–23. 10.1016/j.neulet.2018.11.037

Thompson, T., Terhune, D. B., Oram, C., Sharangparni, J., Rouf, R., Solmi, M., Veronese, N., & Stubbs, B. (2019). The effectiveness of hypnosis for pain relief: A systematic review and meta-analysis of 85 controlled experimental trials. *Neuroscience and Biobehavioral Reviews*, *99*, 298–310. 10.1016/j.neubiorev.2019.02.013

Ulrich, P., Meyer, H. J., Diehl, B., & Meinig, G. (1987). Cerebral blood flow in autogenic training and hypnosis. *Neurosurgical Review*, *10*(4), 305–307. 10.1007/BF01781956

Vanhaudenhuyse, A., Boly, M., Balteau, E., Schnakers, C., Moonen, G., Luxen, A., Lamy, M., Degueldre, C., Brichant, J. F., Maquet, P., Laureys, S., & Faymonville, M. E. (2009). Pain and non-pain processing during hypnosis: A thulium-YAG event-related fMRI study. *NeuroImage*, *47*(3), 1047–1054. 10.1016/j.neuroimage.2009.05.031

Vanhaudenhuyse, A., Demertzi, A., Schabus, M., Noirhomme, Q., Bredart, S., Boly, M., Phillips, C., Soddu, A., Luxen, A., Moonen, G., & Laureys, S. (2011). Two distinct neuronal networks mediate the awareness of environment and of self. *Journal of Cognitive Neuroscience*, *23*(3), 570–578. 10.1162/jocn.2010.21488

Vanhaudenhuyse, A., Gillet, A., Malaise, N., Salamun, I., Barsics, C., Grosdent, S., Maquet, D., Nyssen, A.-S., & Faymonville, M.-E. (2015). Efficacy and cost-effectiveness: A study of different treatment approaches in a tertiary pain centre. *European Journal of Pain (London, England)*, *19*(10), 1437–1446. 10.1002/ejp.674

Vanhaudenhuyse, A., Gillet, A., Malaise, N., Salamun, I., Grosdent, S., Maquet, D., Nyssen, A.-S., & Faymonville, M.-E. (2018). Psychological interventions influence patients' attitudes and beliefs about their chronic pain. *Journal of Traditional and Complementary Medicine*, *8*(2), 296–302. 10.1016/j.jtcme.2016.09.001

Vanhaudenhuyse, A., ledoux, D., Gosseries, O., Demertzi, A., Laureys, S., & Faymonville, M.-E. (2019). Can subjective ratings of absorption, dissociation, and time perception during "neutral hypnosis" predict hypnotizability?: An exploratory study. *International Journal of Clinical and Experimental Hypnosis*, *67*(1), 28–38. 10.1080/00207144.2019.1553765

Vanhaudenhuyse, A., Nyssen, A.-S., Faymonville, M.-E., (2020). Recent insight on how the neuro-scientific approach helps clinicians. *OBM Integrative and Complementary Medicine*, *5*(2), 1–20. 10.21926/obm.icm.2002028

Vermetten, E., Schmahl, C., Lindner, S., Loewenstein, R. J., & Bremner, J. D. (2006). Hippocampal and amygdalar volumes in dissociative identity disorder. *The American Journal of Psychiatry*, *163*(4), 630–636. 10.1176/ajp.2006.163.4.630

Wallen, G. R., Middleton, K. R., Kazmi, N. B., Yang, L., & Brooks, A. T. (2021). A randomized clinical hypnosis pilot study: Improvements in self-reported pain impact in adults with sickle cell disease. *Evidence-Based Complementary and Alternative Medicine: ECAM*, *2021*, 5539004. 10.1155/2021/5539004

Wang, Y.-H., Li, J.-Q., Shi, J.-F., Que, J.-Y., Liu, J.-J., Lappin, J. M., Leung, J., Ravindran, A. V., Chen, W.-Q., Qiao, Y.-L., Shi, J., Lu, L., & Bao, Y.-P. (2020). Depression and anxiety in relation to cancer incidence and mortality: A systematic review and meta-analysis of cohort studies. *Molecular Psychiatry*, *25*(7), 1487–1499. 10.1038/s41380-019-0595-x

Weitzenhoffer, A. M. (2002). Scales, scales and more scales. *The American Journal of Clinical Hypnosis*, *44*(3-4), 209–219. 10.1080/00029157.2002.10403481

Wiechman, S. A., Jensen, M. P., Sharar, S. R., Barber, J. K., Soltani, M., & Patterson, D. R. (2022). The impact of virtual reality hypnosis on pain and anxiety caused by trauma: Lessons learned from a clinical trial. *International Journal of Clinical and Experimental Hypnosis*, *70*(2), 156–173. 10.1080/00207144.2022.2052296

Williams, R. M., Day, M. A., Ehde, D. M., Turner, A. P., Ciol, M. A., Gertz, K. J., Patterson, D., Hakimian, S., Suri, P., & Jensen, M. P. (2022). Effects of hypnosis vs mindfulness meditation vs education on chronic pain intensity and secondary outcomes in veterans: A randomized clinical trial. *Pain*, *163*, 1905–1981. 10.1097/j.pain.0000000000002586

Wolf, T. G., Faerber, K. A., Rummel, C., Halsband, U., & Campus, G. (2022). Functional changes in brain activity using hypnosis: A systematic review. *Brain Sciences*, *12*(1), 108. 10.3390/brainsci12 010108

25

EEG-ASSESSED BANDWIDTH POWER AND HYPNOTIC ANALGESIA

Mark P. Jensen

DEPARTMENT OF REHABILITATION MEDICINE UNIVERSITY OF WASHINGTON, SEATTLE, WA, USA

Mediation and Moderation

Emerging research findings based on carefully designed laboratory studies and clinical trials support the conclusion that hypnosis can reduce both acute and chronic pain (Milling et al., 2021; Thompson et al., 2019). Although the findings from efficacy studies are important for policy makers and those who manage health care plans in order to determine whether or not to pay for hypnosis treatment, this research does not provide evidence regarding the *mechanisms* that underlie hypnosis's effects on pain. In short, although we know that hypnosis can reduce pain, we do not yet know *how* it reduces pain and we have very limited knowledge regarding *for whom* hypnosis has its greatest benefits.

The "How does the treatment work?" question can be addressed by research that identifies the *mediators* of a treatment's beneficial effects (Baron & Kenny, 1986; Breitborde et al., 2010). A variable can be considered a mediator if there is evidence that the beneficial effects of a treatment are explained, at least in part, via its effects on that variable. For example, many psychological pain treatments known to be effective for reducing pain intensity are hypothesized to have their beneficial effects, at least in part, via their effects on pain-related beliefs. Changing pain beliefs is thought to impact pain intensity because such beliefs are hypothesized to influence how much attention a person pays to sensory information (Jensen, 2011). In this example, pain-related beliefs (including beliefs thought to be adaptive such as the belief that one can control pain, as well as beliefs thought to be maladaptive such as viewing pain as a catastrophe) are hypothesized as treatment mediators. This hypothesis can be directly tested in clinical trials that include measures of the potential mediator(s) at multiple outcome assessment points. Statistical analyses can then be conducted that test the extent to which the effects of treatment on the mediators and subsequent effects of the mediators on outcome explain the beneficial effects of the treatment (Preacher, 2015).

The "For whom does the treatment work?" question can be addressed with research that identifies the *predictors* and *moderators* of treatment outcome. A variable can be considered a predictor if it is assessed before treatment and analyses indicate that it is significantly associated with subsequent treatment outcome for a treatment or group of

DOI: 10.4324/9781003449126-34

treatments. On the other hand, a variable can be considered a treatment moderator if it predicts treatment outcome more for one treatment than another (Baron & Kenny, 1986; Breitborde et al., 2010). For example, trait hypnotizability is hypothesized to be a predictor of response to hypnosis treatments, and evidence supports this hypothesis for hypnosis treatments of pain induced in laboratory settings (Thompson et al., 2019) as well as for clinical pain (Milling et al., 2021), although the effects of trait hypnotizability on pain outcomes in clinical populations tend to be weak and inconsistent (Patterson & Jensen, 2003). If the results of analyses indicate that hypnotizability predicts response to a variety of treatments in addition to hypnosis treatments, it can be labeled as a general treatment outcome predictor. But if hypnotizability is shown to predict response to hypnosis treatments more than other pain treatments, it can be labeled as a treatment outcome moderator; its ability to predict treatment response is specific to hypnosis treatments only.

Alan Kazdin has noted a number of compelling arguments supporting the need for research addressing questions of treatment mechanisms (Kazdin, 2009). First, he points out that an increased understanding of treatment mechanisms can bring order to the field. If a variety of different treatments with proven efficacy are found to be effective because they influence a small subset of key mediators, treatments could be understood with respect to their relative effects on these variables. This can help to develop an overall understanding of how different treatments may be similar with respect to their impact on these key mechanisms (Jensen, 2011). Second, by identifying the most important change mechanisms, treatment efficacy could be maximized by focusing treatment more on the most important mechanism variables and less on variables that are unrelated to outcome. For example, if what people believe about their pain turns out to be more important than what they do to cope with their pain, then treatments that focus more on changing beliefs would be more effective than treatments that focus on teaching pain coping strategies. Third, knowledge regarding mechanisms can help translate research to practice by identifying specific treatment components that are essential when adapting pain treatments for specific clinical settings. Finally, an understanding of the mechanisms of treatment can help identify potential treatment moderators, permitting better matching of patients to treatment. If a specific pain coping response emerges as a key mediator, then individuals who are not currently using that pain coping response would be more likely than individuals who are using that coping response to benefit from a treatment that teaches and encourages that response (Day et al., 2015).

Electroencephalography-Assessed Bandwidth Power as a Possible Mediator, Predictor, and Moderator of General Hypnosis Treatment

What Does Electroencephalography Measure?

Electroencephalography (EEG) measures of power in different bandwidths are being increasingly studied as potential mediators, predictors, and moderators of hypnotic analgesia. EEG measures the electrical activity—the "firing"—of cortical neurons via electrodes placed directly on the scalp. Groups of these neurons fire together at different frequencies, from extremely slow (less than once per second, or < 1 Hz) to very fast (more than 100 s of times per second, or > 100 Hz). The combined firing of tens of thousands of neurons as a group (known as neuronal assemblies, Gerstein et al., 1989) in the same frequency has been hypothesized to be the physiological representation underlying the work of the brain such as movement or the experience of a feeling, an image, or idea (Hebb, 1949). According to this model, one neuronal assembly would fire as a group when we see or experience a very specific color; another assembly or group of assemblies would fire when we see or imagine a chair.

The raw EEG signal essentially assesses the number of neurons that are firing across all frequencies within the sensor range of the electrodes placed on the scalp. The overall magnitude or amplitude of this signal is referred to as *power* in the EEG literature. The raw EEG signal is usually grouped or classified into different frequency bandwidths, with the most common being labeled delta (e.g., 0–4 times/second [or 0–4 Hz]), theta (4–8 Hz), alpha (8–12 Hz), beta (12–30 Hz), and gamma (>30 Hz), although these bands are sometimes further classified into smaller bandwidths (e.g., low [4–6 Hz] versus high [6–8 Hz] theta).

One of the most interesting things about EEG measures of bandwidth power is that they are associated with different states or phenomenological experiences (Wahbeh et al., 2018). For example, a preponderance of delta power is seen in individuals with "diminished" consciousness, while a markedly high preponderance is observed during deep sleep (Emmons & Simon, 1956; Frohlich et al., 2021). A higher level of theta power can occur when people are either (or both) very sleepy or are engaged in a task requiring focused attention, depending on how awake the individual is or feels (Ishii et al., 2014; Zhang et al., 2019). More alpha activity occurs when people are physically or mentally relaxed (Ehrhardt et al., 2022; Tarrant et al., 2018) as well as when they have "creative ideation" (Fink & Benedek, 2014). More beta power is associated with perceived stress (Hall et al., 2007), and both beta and gamma power occur with information processing (Karakas & Basar, 1998; Spitzer & Haegens, 2017).

EEG-Assessed Bandwidth Power and General Hypnosis

Perhaps in part because early models of hypnosis viewed hypnosis as a specific "state" of consciousness distinct from normal waking states, and also because, as noted in the previous section of this chapter, measures of bandwidth power are known to be associated with different states of consciousness, there was an early interest in examining the role of bandwidth power as a potential mechanism underlying or explaining the effects of hypnosis (cf. Barker & Burgwin, 1949; Chertok & Kramarz, 1959; Dynes, 1947). This research has continued to the present day; a PubMed search conducted on October 22, 2022 using the words "EEG" and "hypnosis" as keywords yielded 832 articles. The findings from this research have been summarized by a number of researchers (De Benedittis, 2021; Jensen et al., 2015; Wolf et al., Campus, 2022) and a state-of-the-science review of this research is presented De Pascalis in Chapter 17 of this volume. Although all of these reviews have noted that there remains much to learn, a number of tentative conclusions can be drawn from this body of research:

1 Beta power is rarely found to be associated with hypnosis or response to hypnotic suggestions. Based on this evidence, it would appear that activity in the beta bandwidth is unlikely to be a significant mediator or predictor of response to hypnosis treatments.
2 Delta power has rarely been examined in hypnosis research. Additional research is needed to determine the effects of hypnosis on delta power, and if baseline levels of delta power predict response to hypnosis.

3 Although significant associations are not always found, when significant effects emerge, the bandwidth most commonly associated with hypnosis and response to hypnotic suggestions is theta, with higher levels of theta (i.e., more theta power) associated with a greater response to hypnosis treatments.
4 Although alpha and gamma power are not always found to be significantly associated with response to hypnosis, when significant effects do emerge, more alpha power tends to be associated with more response to hypnosis, while gamma power shows significant effects in both directions.

As a group, these findings have led us to develop what we refer to as the "slow wave" (i.e., mostly theta but also sometimes low alpha) hypothesis (Jensen et al., 2015, 2018). This hypothesis proposes that: (1) greater slower wave power assessed just before or during hypnotic suggestions—which can occur because someone has a trait tendency to have higher than average theta power or because a hypnotic induction or other technique was used to increase theta power—facilitates an enhanced response to hypnotic suggestions; and (2) neuronal assemblies that fire in slower wave power control neuronal assemblies throughout the brain that fire in faster bandwidths (e.g., gamma) to create the response to the hypnotic suggestions. This idea is based in part on the known role that theta and alpha activity plays in memory recall and recording (de Vries et al., 2020; Klimesch, 1999).

How, exactly, might theta and alpha bandwidth activity transmitted from frontal (control) centers activate or inhibit beta and gamma activity in other parts of the brain, including those that underlie motor activity (e.g., arm levitation), emotions, thoughts, and sensory experiences? This is thought to occur as a result of the fact that when they fire, they release neurotransmitters that inhibit the activity of the receptor neurons (Buzsáki, 2006). Thus, the release of inhibitory neurotransmitters at a specific frequency in the visual cortex would inhibit activity in *all* neuronal assemblies that would fire in faster frequencies *except* for any that were exactly in phase with the controlling (slower wave) frequency. For example, if inhibitory neurotransmitters are released exactly six times per section (i.e., 6.00 Hz, theta) in the area of the visual cortex that underlies the experience of color, then only neuronal assemblies that fire exactly at a frequency that is a multiple of 6.00 (e.g., 42.00 Hz, gamma) are able to fire when the controlling frequency is active; they are able to "fit" exactly into the envelop of 6.00 Hz (Buzsáki, 2006). If the group of neurons that fire when we experience the color blue are entrained to fire at exactly 42.00 Hz in the visual cortex, the controlling neurons need only fire at exactly 6.00 Hz. The experience of all other colors is inhibited; what is left is blue. If the neuronal assembly that underlies the experience of green fires at 42.70 Hz, then the controlling neurons need only fire at a rate of 6.10 Hz for green to be experienced, as seven 42.70 Hz firings fit exactly into a 6.10 Hz envelop. In this way, theta and alpha frequencies can inhibit the firing of many neuronal assemblies while allowing only very specific ones to become active, allowing the individual to have different thoughts, images, ideas, motor responses, and sensory experiences. This process of allowing for specific response while inhibiting all others can explain not only how we are able to recreate memories ("experience yourself in your favorite place") but also have negative hallucinations (i.e., by inhibiting the processing of visual input). In short, neurons that fire in the theta and alpha frequencies are hypothesized to be critical for controlling the activity of neurons that fire in the beta and gamma frequencies. Changes that occur in neuron assemblies that fire in faster frequencies (increases or decreases, depending on what is needed to respond to the hypnotic suggestion) then underlie the actual hypnotic response.

The slow wave hypothesis as an explanation for hypnotic responding has yet to be definitively confirmed. However, preliminary support for this hypothesis comes from a study that examined differences in hypnotizability as a function of time of day (Green et al., 2015). Using two large databases that contained hypnotizability scores assessed in samples of undergraduates, these investigators found higher hypnotic responsiveness scores when the hypnotizability measures were administered in the late morning and early evening. They also noted that other researchers have found similar patterns when measures were administered to the same individuals over time (Aldrich & Bernstein, 1987; Wallace, 1993). Although the finding appeared reliable, Green et al. did not have an explanation for the finding. However, the finding is consistent with the slow wave hypothesis (Jensen, 2016). Bandwidth power changes in a reliable way in 24-hour cycles. Specifically, most oscillation bandwidths are at their nadir in the early morning, increase during the day, and peak in the afternoon or evening (Cacot et al., 1995). The exception to this rule is theta power and the low end of alpha (e.g., 8 Hz), both of which peak at two times during the day: late morning and early evening.

Bandwidth Power and Hypnotic Analgesia

In this section, I will review the findings from the EEG research studies that have been conducted in light of the slow wave hypothesis. To identify the articles to review, I conducted a search of PubMed conducted on October 22, 2022 using the keywords ("hypnosis" and "EEG" and "pain" and ["delta" or "theta" or "alpha" or "beta" or "gamma"]). This search yielded 29 articles. I then read the titles and abstracts of these articles to identify any that examined bandwidth power as a potential predictor, moderator, or mediator of the effects of hypnotic analgesia. This screen yielded seven articles, the findings from which are described and discussed below. The articles are classified into three types: (1) those that examine baseline or trait power in different bandwidths as predictors of response to hypnotic analgesia; (2) those that examine the effects of techniques that increase slow wave bandwidth power as a strategy for enhancing subsequent response to hypnotic analgesia; and (3) those that examine the mediation effects of EEG bandwidth power on the effects of hypnotic analgesia. With respect to the first two types of studies, the slow wave hypothesis predicts that higher slow wave activity assessed before hypnosis and strategies that effectively increase slow wave activity would both be associated with greater response to hypnotic analgesia. With respect to mediation studies, the slow wave hypothesis predicts that the pain reduction effects of hypnotic analgesic would be mediated by the effects of hypnosis on increasing slower oscillation (theta and alpha) power and decreasing faster oscillation (beta and gamma) power, given the evidence that faster bandwidth activity is associated with more pain intensity (e.g., Chouchou et al., 2021; May et al., 2019; Simis et al., 2022).

Baseline Power as a Predictor of Subsequent Response to Hypnotic Analgesia

Two of the seven articles identified examined how baseline or trait bandwidth power predicts response to hypnotic analgesia. Both of these were pilot studies with low sample sizes. In the first study, Freeman and colleagues (Freeman et al., 2000) measured pain intensity in response to a cold pressor task (i.e., placing one's hand in ice water, which is usually experienced as painful soon after the hand placement) and both low theta (3.5–5.5 Hz) and high theta (5.5–7.5 Hz) bandwidth power from 19 electrodes in ten individuals scoring in the "high hypnotizable" range and ten individuals scoring in the "low hypnotizable" range on the Stanford Hypnotic Clinical Scale (Hilgard & Hilgard, 1975) in three conditions: waking relaxation, distraction, and hypnosis. They found that the highs reported more pain reduction in the hypnosis condition than the two control conditions and also reported more pain reduction than the lows. They also found that highs evidenced significantly (using an alpha of 0.10 given the low sample size) greater high theta power as assessed from two electrodes (a parietal and occipital electrode) during both the waking relaxation and hypnosis conditions.

In another study, our group examined the ability of bandwidth power assessed just before five different conditions: an audio recording of hypnotic analgesia, an audio recording of a meditation exercise, neurofeedback to increase alpha power (8–12 Hz) and decrease high beta power (18–30 Hz) over the temporal lobes, transcranial direct stimulation (tDCS) to activate activity in the motor cortex, and sham tDCS (Jensen et al., 2014). We found that more baseline theta power at 16 of 19 electrode sites (with 11 of these being statistically significant) was associated with more pain reduction in the hypnosis condition. Baseline theta power did not predict response to any of the other conditions, with the exception of less theta power at two posterior sites being significantly associated with response to neurofeedback. The only other significant predictor of response to hypnosis was that having *less* gamma activity as assessed from two electrodes over the left anterior sites predicted response to hypnosis (i.e., reflecting less information processing in the dorsolateral prefrontal cortex, consistent with the findings that reducing activity in this area using repetitive transcranial magnetic stimulation increases hypnotizability, Dienes & Hutton, 2013; Perri et al., Pekala, 2022). In short, and despite the low sample size, baseline theta power across the majority of electrodes evidenced an ability to predict response to hypnosis, and this ability was unique to hypnosis.

We cannot conclude that the findings from these two pilot studies provide strong confirmatory support for the slow wave hypothesis. However, the results are consistent with the hypothesis that theta power is associated with a positive response to hypnotic analgesia, specifically, and indicate that more research is to examine baseline and trait theta activity—perhaps high theta more than low theta (Freeman et al., 2000)—as a predictor of response to hypnotic analgesia is warranted.

Enhancing Response to Hypnotic Analgesia by Enhancing Theta

Three studies were identified that sought to examine the potential effects of enhancing slow wave activity as a strategy for enhancing response to hypnotic analgesia. All three of these studies combined neurofeedback with hypnosis. With neurofeedback, bandwidth power is assessed in real time, and when criteria are met that indicate a change in that bandwidth power—for purposes of the slow way hypothesis, the goal would be to increase slow wave power—the individual is provided with feedback about that change, usually in the form of a sound (e.g., music or the sound of water) or an image on a computer screen (e.g., changes in the height of a colored bar that reflect the power in the bandwidth of interest). Participants in neurofeedback studies are invited to relax, listen to (or watch) the feedback, and do whatever is needed to change that feedback. Because the changes in the feedback reflect changes in bandwidth power, the process teaches the participants to be able to increase or decrease, depending on the goal, actual bandwidth power.

In the first of the three studies identified, Melzack and Perry assigned 24 individuals with chronic pain to one of three conditions that included: (1) alpha bandwidth neurofeedback plus an audio recording of hypnosis (12 participants), (2) an audio recording of hypnosis sessions only (six participants), or (3) neurofeedback alone (six participants; Melzack & Perry, 1975). The participants in the combined condition received two sessions of hypnosis, two sessions of alpha neurofeedback with hypnosis, six sessions of alpha neurofeedback, and two practice sessions when they were invited to practice the techniques they had learned (i.e., 12 treatment sessions). The participants in the hypnosis condition received four sessions of listening to the hypnosis audio recording plus two practice sessions (i.e., six treatment sessions total), and the participants in the neurofeedback condition received eight sessions of neurofeedback plus two practice sessions (i.e., ten treatment sessions). Outcome was assessed with the McGill Pain Questionnaire, which assesses both pain intensity and quality (Melzack, 1975). Although the small sample size did not provide adequate power to test for statistically significant effects, and the differences in the number of sessions between the conditions may have biased the results in favor of the combined group relative to the other groups, the investigators found larger improvement (i.e., reductions) in both the sensory and affective dimensions of pain in the participants who participated in the combined treatment than in those who received hypnosis only. Those who received hypnosis only reported larger improvements than those who received neurofeedback only.

More recently, we conducted two pilot studies to evaluate the potential for theta power neurofeedback to enhance response to hypnotic analgesia. In the first of these, 20 individuals with multiple sclerosis and chronic pain were given one in-person hypnosis session followed by four pre-recorded hypnosis sessions, with each session providing different suggestions thought to help with pain management (Jensen et al., 2016). The participants were randomly assigned to receive 20 minutes of theta neurofeedback training or 20 minutes of relaxation training just before the four audio recording sessions. Pain intensity was assessed at pre-treatment, post-treatment, and at one-month follow-up. Eighteen participants completed all sessions. As the sample size was too small to allow for adequate power to test for statistically significant differences between the two conditions, we estimated and compared the effect sizes for change in pain from pre-treatment to both post-treatment and one-month follow-up. Consistent with the slow wave hypothesis, participants in the neurofeedback plus hypnosis condition reported larger effect size improvements in pain intensity from pre-treatment to post-treatment (Cohen's $d = 0.70$, medium to large effect) and from pre-treatment to follow-up ($d = 1.04$, large effect) than participants in the relaxation plus hypnosis condition (both *d*'s = 0.47, medium effect).

In a second study, we examined the potential hypnosis-enhancing effects of both neurofeedback and training in mindfulness (Jensen et al., 2018), with the rationale that mindfulness training might enhance hypnosis because it has been shown to increase both alpha and theta power (e.g., Cahn & Polich, 2006; Lomas et al., 2015). In this study, 32 individuals with multiple sclerosis and chronic pain, fatigue, or both, were randomly assigned to receive six sessions of theta neurofeedback, six sessions of mindfulness training, or no enhancing intervention. Fifteen of these participants reported bothersome pain when they were enrolled in the study. All participants then received five in-person hypnosis sessions that included suggestions for greater comfort and energy. Those assigned to the neurofeedback and mindfulness conditions received additional hypnosis and mindfulness training just before the last four hypnosis sessions. Outcomes were assessed at pre-treatment, pre-hypnosis treatment, post-treatment, and one-month follow-up. Of those participants with pain, those in the neurofeedback and hypnosis condition reported larger pain reductions, pre-treatment to follow-up (Cohen's *d* effect size = −1.01, large effect), than those in the mindfulness and hypnosis condition (*d* = −0.36, small effect) or hypnosis only condition (−0.43, small to medium effect).

Similar to the findings from the two studies examining bandwidth power as a moderator of treatment outcome, the three studies conducted to examine the treatment-enhancing effects of alpha and theta neurofeedback on response to hypnotic analgesia cannot be considered as providing definitive support for the slow wave hypotheses. However, the results are consistent with the hypothesis, suggesting that individuals who receive neurofeedback training to increase alpha or theta power prior to receiving hypnosis treatment will ultimately experience greater pain reductions once they start hypnosis treatment (see also Batty et al., 2006 for evidence supporting the idea that increasing theta activity can increase general hypnotizability, a finding also consistent with the slow wave hypothesis). It appears possible that neurofeedback training may enhance the longer-term benefits of hypnosis treatment.

Bandwidth Power as a Mediator of Hypnotic Analgesia

I was only able to identify two articles published that have examined the extent to which EEG-assessed bandwidth power may serve as a mediator of the beneficial effects of hypnosis on pain. In the first of these, De Pascalis and colleagues studied, among other things, the mediating effects of alpha power on both hypnotic analgesia and a placebo cream on pain intensity (De Pascalis et al., 2021). In 65 healthy women, these investigators assessed pain intensity, perceived involuntariness of experiencing hypnotic analgesia, low alpha (alpha1; 7–10 Hz), and high alpha (alpha2; 10–12 Hz) during four conditions: (1) while the participants were awake and during (a) aversive cold stimulation and (b) aversive cold stimulation after application of a placebo cream and (2) following hypnosis and during the aversive cold stimulation and aversive cold stimulation after application of a placebo cream. They found that higher levels of left-temporoparietal alpha2 power (but not alpha1 power) influenced pain reduction in the hypnosis condition, and that these effects were mediated by perceived involuntariness. The power of other bandwidths, including delta, theta, beta, or gamma power, was not assessed in this study.

Finally, in a large (*N* = 173) randomized clinical trial comparing the effects of four individual sessions of four pain treatments (hypnosis targeting pain reduction, hypnosis targeting changes in pain-related maladaptive thoughts, cognitive therapy targeting changes in pain-related maladaptive thoughts, and pain education), we examined the potential mediation effects of pre- to post-treatment changes in resting state bandwidth power on pre- to post-treatment reductions in pain intensity (Jensen et al., 2021). We found that none of the four treatments had a significant effect on resting state EEG activity for any of the five bandwidths examined (i.e., delta, theta, alpha, beta, and gamma). Consistent with this lack of effect on resting state EEG activity, changes in the resting state bandwidth power measures were not associated with pain reduction, nor were any of these changes found to mediate the beneficial effects of any of the treatments examined, including the two hypnosis treatments.

As with the first two types of studies evaluated here, given the fact that only two studies have been published regarding the mediation effects of slower or faster wave oscillations on hypnotic analgesia, definitive conclusions regarding the slow wave hypothesis based on the available mediation study findings cannot be made. However, the findings reported by De Pascalis and colleagues, cited above, regarding the effects of alpha2 as a mediator of the beneficial effects of hypnotic analgesia in response to aversive stimulation in healthy women are consistent with the slow wave (i.e., theta and/or alpha) hypothesis. Moreover, the lack of any mediation effects of either slower or faster oscillation power during a resting state (i.e., not during hypnosis) on the beneficial effects of hypnosis in a fully powered clinical trial suggests the possibility that any mediation, when it occurs, may be more likely to be observed during hypnosis and not outside of the hypnotic context.

Overall, the findings from the seven studies identified are generally consistent with the slow wave hypothesis for (1) identifying people might be more likely to respond to hypnotic analgesia (i.e., those with greater theta or alpha power before treatment), (2) identifying strategies that could enhance response to hypnotic analgesia treatments (i.e., interventions or approaches that increase theta or alpha power), and (3) understanding how hypnosis reduces pain (i.e., by increasing slower wave power *during hypnosis*). However, as noted previously, most of the few studies that have been published to date that provide data regarding the slow wave hypothesis are pilot studies conducted with very few subjects. More research, including more research with larger sample sizes, is needed to determine whether (and under what conditions) the slow wave hypothesis can be confirmed.

Research Implications

The primary research implication of the findings from the extant studies is clear: more research to test the slow wave hypothesis is warranted. That said, caution needs to be made with respect to interpreting the findings from this research. Given the complexities of EEG assessment and the many factors that can impact EEG-assessed brain activity, it is important to understand that there is a significant risk for type II errors in this research. That is, statistically significant effects, even when such effects are present in the population, will not always emerge.

As one example, higher levels of theta power can reflect either or both a lack of sleep and focused attention (Vogel et al., 1968). Higher levels of theta and low alpha can also be found in some individuals with chronic neuropathic pain, which has been attributed to a condition called thalamocortical dysrhythmia (Di Pietro et al., 2018). In short, even if the slow wave hypothesis is accurate, and higher level of slow wave activity can enhance response to hypnosis suggestions (perhaps labeled "hypnosis enhancing" slow oscillation power), there is most certainly another slow wave activity that is *not* related to response to hypnotic analgesia suggestions, or that could potentially even interfere with response to hypnotic analgesia (perhaps in this context labeled "hypnosis inhibiting" slow oscillation power). Thus, even if there are neuronal assemblies that fire in theta and alpha that play an important role in hypnotic responding, a statistically significant positive association between theta or alpha power assessed at baseline and response to hypnotic suggestions will not always be found, depending on the specific population being studied, the sample size, and the study procedures (see, for example, Hiltunen et al., 2021). As a result, it would be more important to examine *trends* in the findings from multiple studies, anticipating that although statistically significant effects will not always emerge, when they do, if the overall trend is that the majority of the significant findings are consistent with the slow wave hypotheses (as is the case for the studies reviewed in this chapter), the slow wave hypothesis can be considered to remain viable. On the other hand, if among the significant effects found, about half indicate positive associations and half indicate negative associations between measures of slow wave activity and response to hypnotic suggestions, this would indicate a clear lack of support for the slow wave hypothesis.

Clinical Implications

If research continues to emerge that is consistent with the slow wave hypothesis, then this research has important clinical implications. First and foremost, the findings would suggest that clinicians could potentially enhance a positive response to hypnosis treatment by facilitating more slow wave activity. Among the most obvious, of course, is to precede hypnotic suggestions with hypnotic inductions, as the latter have been shown to increase both theta and alpha power (see Chapter 17 in this volume, De Pascalis et al., 2021). For those clinicians who have training and experience in neurofeedback, they can consider combining neurofeedback with hypnosis as a strategy for enhancing the beneficial effects of the latter (Fukui et al., 2020; Jensen et al., 2016, 2018). It is also possible that music might be used to enhance theta power and therefore enhance response to hypnosis (e.g., Ramos & Corsi-Cabrera, 1989; Sandler et al., 2016).

A second implication is to be aware that the patient's theta and alpha power will likely ebb and flow, like all other biological phenomena. To the extent that the slow wave hypothesis is accurate, this means that there are going to be moments when patients will be more or less likely to respond to hypnotic suggestions as a function of their slow wave power at any one point in time. Two practical implications of this are to (1) seek to identify the signs that a patient or client is, in fact, ready to respond to hypnotic suggestions, and then provide those suggestions during a period of higher than average responsivity, and (2) plan to repeat the most important suggestions a number of times, under the assumption that the suggestion will be heard at least once during a time of relatively high responsivity. The potentially beneficial effects of hearing suggestions more than once may be one of the reasons that response to hypnosis treatment for clinical pain conditions—-which usually involves asking patients to listen to audio recordings of suggestions daily—may be less strongly associated with trait hypnotizability than in response to hypnotic suggestions for laboratory or induced pain. Individuals receiving hypnosis treatment for clinical pain conditions may hear suggestions dozens or even hundreds of times, whereas individuals participating in acute pain laboratory studies typically only hear a suggestion once.

Finally, given that EEG patterns are known to evidence specific time patterns over the course of a day, with theta power evidencing a "bump" in power relative to other bandwidths in the late morning and early evening (Cacot et al., 1995), clinicians working with patients who are struggling with responding to hypnosis treatment could consider scheduling those patients for a 10 am appointment, and recommend that the patient listen to their practice audio recordings around 10:30 am and/or 6:30 pm on a daily basis.

Summary and Conclusions

In this chapter, I described the slow wave hypothesis, which proposes that the beneficial effects of hypnotic analgesia rely on slower oscillations to control the neuronal assemblies that underlie the experience of pain. Specifically, more theta or alpha power is hypothesized to enhance the beneficial effects of hypnotic analgesia, which, when effective, would be expected to reduce beta and in particular gamma power of neuronal assemblies in the sensory cortex and perhaps other areas that make up the pain matrix. The hypothesis is based on what is known regarding the effects of hypnosis on, and the associations between, pain and bandwidth power. Preliminary evidence from a number of published studies is consistent with the slow wave hypothesis. However, more research is needed to provide enough evidence to draw firm conclusions regarding its accuracy. In the meantime, to the extent that the slow wave hypothesis is accurate, clinicians can use this information to enhance the efficacy of their hypnosis treatment by (1) providing treatments or strategies for enhancing slower wave power prior to hypnosis treatment; (2) closely observing patients for the moments when they may be more likely to respond to hypnotic suggestions; (3) ensuring that key or central hypnotic suggestions are repeated not only during the session but also between sessions, by encouraging patients to listen to an audio recording of the suggestions; and (4) scheduling patients who might need extra help for a 10 am appointment, and/or encourage patients to listen to audio recordings around 10:30 am and/or 6:30 pm. As more is learned about the mechanisms underlying effective hypnosis pain treatment, including mechanisms related to brain activity, more specific and effective clinical approaches will likely follow. Ultimately, this research and these ideas will result in more individuals benefiting from hypnosis treatment.

References

Aldrich, K. J., & Bernstein, D. A. (1987). The effect of time of day on hypnotizability: A brief communication. *International Journal of Clinical and Experimental Hypnosis*, *35*(3), 141–145. doi: 10.1080/00207148708416049

Barker, W., & Burgwin, S. (1949). Brain wave patterns during hypnosis, hypnotic sleep and normal sleep. *Archives of Neurology and Psychiatry*, *62*(4), 412–420. doi: 10.1001/archneurpsyc.1949.02310160032002

Baron, R. M., & Kenny, D. A. (1986). The moderator-mediator variable distinction in social psychological research: Conceptual, strategic, and statistical considerations. *Journal of Personal and Social Psychology*, *51*(6), 1173–1182. doi: 10.1037//0022-3514.51.6.1173

Batty, M. J., Bonnington, S., Tang, B. K., Hawken, M. B., & Gruzelier, J. H. (2006). Relaxation strategies and enhancement of hypnotic susceptibility: EEG neurofeedback, progressive muscle relaxation and self-hypnosis. *Brain Research Bulletin*, *71*(1-3), 83–90. doi: 10.1016/j.brainresbull.2006.08.005

Breitborde, N. J., Srihari, V. H., Pollard, J. M., Addington, D. N., & Woods, S. W. (2010). Mediators and moderators in early intervention research. *Early Intervention in Psychiatry*, *4*(2), 143–152. doi: 10.1111/j.1751-7893.2010.00177.x

Buzsáki, G. (2006). *Rhythms of the brain*. New York: Oxford University Press.

Cacot, P., Tesolin, B., & Sebban, C. (1995). Diurnal variations of EEG power in healthy adults. *Electroencephalography and Clinical Neurophysiology*, *94*(5), 305–312. doi: 10.1016/0013-4694(94)00298-y

Cahn, B. R., & Polich, J. (2006). Meditation states and traits: EEG, ERP, and neuroimaging studies. *Psychological Bulletin*, *132*(2), 180–211. doi: 10.1037/0033-2909.132.2.180

Chertok, L., & Kramarz, P. (1959). Hypnosis, sleep and electro-encephalography. *Journal of Nervous and Mental Diseases*, *128*(3), 227–238.

Chouchou, F., Perchet, C., & Garcia-Larrea, L. (2021). EEG changes reflecting pain: Is alpha suppression better than gamma enhancement? *Neurophysiologie Clinique*, *51*(3), 209–218. doi: 10.1016/j.neucli.2021.03.001

Day, M. A., Ehde, D. M., & Jensen, M. P. (2015). Psychosocial pain management moderation: The limit, activate, and enhance Model. *Journal of Pain*, *16*(10), 947–960. doi: 10.1016/j.jpain.2015.07.003

De Benedittis, G. (2021). Neural mechanisms of hypnosis and meditation-induced analgesia: A narrative review. *International Journal of Clinical and Experimental Hypnosis*, *69*(3), 363–382. doi: 10.1080/00207144.2021.1917294

De Pascalis, V., Scacchia, P., & Vecchio, A. (2021). Influences of hypnotic suggestibility, contextual factors, and EEG alpha on placebo analgesia. *American Journal of Clinical Hypnosis*, *63*(4), 302–328. doi: 10.1080/00029157.2020.1863182

de Vries, I. E. J., Slagter, H. A., & Olivers, C. N. L. (2020). Oscillatory control over representational states in working memory. *Trends in Cognitive Science*, *24*(2), 150–162. doi: 10.1016/j.tics.2019.11.006

Di Pietro, F., Macey, P. M., Rae, C. D., Alshelh, Z., Macefield, V. G., Vickers, E. R., & Henderson, L. A. (2018). The relationship between thalamic GABA content and resting cortical rhythm in neuropathic pain. *Human Brain Mapping*, *39*(5), 1945–1956. doi: 10.1002/hbm.23973

Dienes, Z., & Hutton, S. (2013). Understanding hypnosis metacognitively: rTMS applied to left DLPFC increases hypnotic suggestibility. *Cortex*, *49*(2), 386–392. doi: 10.1016/j.cortex.2012.07.009

Dynes, J. B. (1947). Objective method for distinguishing sleep from the hypnotic trance. *Archives of Neurology and Psychiatry*, *57*(1), 84–93. doi: 10.1001/archneurpsyc.1947.02300240100006

Ehrhardt, N. M., Fietz, J., Kopf-Beck, J., Kappelmann, N., & Brem, A. K. (2022). Separating EEG correlates of stress: Cognitive effort, time pressure, and social-evaluative threat. *European Journal of Neuroscience*, *55*(9–10), 2464–2473. doi: 10.1111/ejn.15211

Emmons, W. H., & Simon, C. W. (1956). EEG, consciousness, and sleep. *Science*, *124*(3231), 1066–1069. doi: 10.1126/science.124.3231.1066

Fink, A., & Benedek, M. (2014). EEG alpha power and creative ideation. Neuroscience *and Biobehavioral Reviews*, *44*, 111–123. doi: 10.1016/j.neubiorev.2012.12.002

Freeman, R., Barabasz, A., Barabasz, M., & Warner, D. (2000). Hypnosis and distraction differ in their effects on cold pressor pain. *American Journal of Clinical Hypnosis*, *43*(2), 137–148. doi: 10.1080/00029157.2000.10404266

Frohlich, J., Toker, D., & Monti, M. M. (2021). Consciousness among delta waves: A paradox? *Brain*, *144*(8), 2257–2277. doi: 10.1093/brain/awab095

Fukui, T., Williams, W., Tan, G., & Jensen, M. P. (2020). Combining hypnosis with biofeedback to enhance chronic pain management. *Australian Journal of Clinical Hypnotherapy and Hypnosis*, *41*, 3–15.

Gerstein, G. L., Bedenbaugh, P., & Aertsen, M. H. (1989). Neuronal assemblies. *IEEE Transactions on Biomedical Engineering*, *36*(1), 4–14. doi: 10.1109/10.16444

Green, J. P., Smith, R. J., & Kromer, M. (2015). Diurnal variations in hypnotic responsiveness: Is there an optimal time to be hypnotized? *International Journal of Clinical and Experimental Hypnosis*, *63*(2), 171–181. doi: 10.1080/00207144.2015.1002675

Hall, M., Thayer, J. F., Germain, A., Moul, D., Vasko, R., Puhl, M., Miewald, M., & Buysse, D. J. (2007). Psychological stress is associated with heightened physiological arousal during NREM sleep in primary insomnia. *Behavioral Sleep Medicine*, *5*(3), 178–193. doi:10.1080/15402000701263221

Hebb, D. O. (1949). *The organization of behavior: A neuropsychological theory*. New York: Wiley.

Hilgard, E. R., & Hilgard, J. R. (1975). *Hypnosis in the relief of pain*. Los Altos, CA: Kaufman.

Hiltunen, S., Karevaara, M., Virta, M., Makkonen, T., Kallio, S., & Paavilainen, P. (2021). No evidence for theta power as a marker of hypnotic state in highly hypnotizable subjects. *Heliyon*, *7*(4), e06871. doi: 10.1016/j.heliyon.2021.e06871

Ishii, R., Canuet, L., Ishihara, T., Aoki, Y., Ikeda, S., Hata, M., Katsimichas, T., Gunji, A., Takahashi, H., TNakahachi, T., Iwase, M., & Takeda, M. (2014). Frontal midline theta rhythm and gamma power changes during focused attention on mental calculation: An MEG beamformer analysis. *Frontiers in Human Neuroscience*, *8*, 406. doi: 10.3389/fnhum.2014.00406

Jensen, M. P. (2011). Psychosocial approaches to pain management: An organizational framework. *Pain*, *152*(4), 717–725. doi: 10.1016/j.pain.2010.09.002

Jensen, M. P. (2016). Brain oscillations and diurnal variations in hypnotic responsiveness: A commentary on "Diurnal variations in hypnotic responsiveness: Is there an optimal time to be hypnotized?" *International Journal of Clinical and Experimental Hypnosis*, *64*(1), 137–145. doi: 10.1080/00207144.2015.1099408

Jensen, M. P., Adachi, T., & Hakimian, S. (2015). Brain oscillations, hypnosis, and hypnotizability. *American Journal of Clinical Hypnosis*, *57*(3), 230–253. doi: 10.1080/00029157.2015.985573

Jensen, M. P., Battalio, S. L., Chan, J. F., Edwards, K. A., Day, M. A., Sherlin, L. H., & Ehde, D. M. (2018). Use of neurofeedback and mindfulness to enhance response to hypnosis treatment in individuals withmultiple sclerosis: Results from a pilot randomized clinical trial. *International Journal of Clinical and Experimental Hypnosis*, *66*(3), 231–264. doi: 10.1080/00207144.2018.1460546

Jensen, M. P., Gianas, A., George, H. R., Sherlin, L. H., Kraft, G. H., & Ehde, D. M. (2016). Use of neurofeedback to enhance response to hypnotic analgesia in individuals with multiple sclerosis. *International Journal of Clinical and Experimental Hypnosis*, *64*(1), 1–23. doi: 10.1080/00207144.2015.1099400

Jensen, M. P., Hakimian, S., Ehde, D. M., Day, M. A., Pettet, M. W., Yoshino, A., & Ciol, M. A. (2021). Pain-related beliefs, cognitive processes, and electroencephalography band power as predictors and mediators of the effects of psychological chronic pain interventions. *Pain*, *162*(7), 2036–2050. doi: 10.1097/j.pain.0000000000002201

Jensen, M. P., Sherlin, L. H., Fregni, F., Gianas, A., Howe, J. D., & Hakimian, S. (2014). Baseline brain activity predicts response to neuromodulatory pain treatment. *Pain Medicine*, *15*(12), 2055–2063. doi: 10.1111/pme.12546

Karakas, S., & Basar, E. (1998). Early gamma response is sensory in origin: A conclusion based on cross-comparison of results from multiple experimental paradigms. *International Journal of Psychophysiology*, *31*(1), 13–31. doi: 10.1016/s0167-8760(98)00030-0

Kazdin, A. E. (2009). Understanding how and why psychotherapy leads to change. *Psychotherapy Research*, *19*(4-5), 418–428. doi: 10.1080/10503300802448899

Klimesch, W. (1999). EEG alpha and theta oscillations reflect cognitive and memory performance: A review and analysis. *Brain Research Reviews*, *29*(2–3), 169–195. doi: 10.1016/s0165-0173(98)00056-3

Lomas, T., Ivtzan, I., & Fu, C. H. (2015). A systematic review of the neurophysiology of mindfulness on EEG oscillations. *Neuroscience & Biobehavioral Reviews*, *57*, 401–410. doi: 10.1016/j.neubiorev.2015.09.018

May, E. S., Nickel, M. M., Ta Dinh, S., Tiemann, L., Heitmann, H., Voth, I., Tölle, T. R., Gross, J., & Ploner, M. (2019). Prefrontal gamma oscillations reflect ongoing pain intensity in chronic back pain patients. *Human Brain Mapping*, *40*(1), 293–305. doi: 10.1002/hbm.24373

Melzack, R. (1975). The McGill Pain Questionnaire: Major properties and scoring methods. *Pain*, *1*(3), 277–299. doi: 10.1016/0304-3959(75)90044-5

Melzack, R., & Perry, C. (1975). Self-regulation of pain: The use of alpha-feedback and hypnotic training for the control of chronic pain. *Experimental Neurology*, *46*(3), 452–469. doi: 10.1016/0014-4886(75)90119-3

Milling, L. S., Valentine, K. E., LoStimolo, L. M., Nett, A. M., & McCarley, H. S. (2021). Hypnosis and the alleviation of clinical pain: A comprehensive meta-analysis. *International Journal of Clinical and Experimental Hypnosis*, *69*(3), 297–322. doi: 10.1080/00207144.2021.1920330

Patterson, D. R., & Jensen, M. P. (2003). Hypnosis and clinical pain. *Psychological Bulletin*, *129*(4), 495–521. doi: 10.1037/0033-2909.129.4.495

Perri, R. L., Perrotta, D., Rossani, F., & Pekala, R. J. (2022). Boosting the hypnotic experience. Inhibition of the dorsolateral prefrontal cortex alters hypnotizability and sense of agency. A randomized, double-blind and sham-controlled tDCS study. *Behavioural Brain Research*, *425*, 113833. doi: 10.1016/j.bbr.2022.113833

Preacher, K. J. (2015). Advances in mediation analysis: A survey and synthesis of new developments. *Annual Review of Psychology*, *66*, 825–852. doi: 10.1146/annurev-psych-010814-015258

Ramos, J., & Corsi-Cabrera, M. (1989). Does brain electrical activity react to music? *International Journal of Neuroscience*, *47*(3-4), 351–357. doi: 10.3109/00207458908987449

Sandler, H., Tamm, S., Fendel, U., Rose, M., Klapp, B. F., & Bosel, R. (2016). Positive emotional experience induced by vibroacoustic stimulation using a body monochord in patients with psychosomatic disorders is associated with an increase in EEG-theta and a decrease in EEG-alpha power. *Brain Topography*, *29*(4), 524–538. doi: 10.1007/s10548-016-0480-8

Simis, M., Imamura, M., Pacheco-Barrios, K., Marduy, A., de Melo, P. S., Mendes, A. J., Teixeira, P. E. P., Battistella, L., & Fregni, F. (2022). EEG theta and beta bands as brain oscillations for different knee osteoarthritis phenotypes according to disease severity. *Scientific Reports*, *12*(1), 1480. doi: 10.1038/s41598-022-04957-x

Spitzer, B., & Haegens, S. (2017). Beyond the status quo: A role for beta oscillations in endogenous content (re)activation. *eNeuro*, *4*(4). doi: 10.1523/ENEURO.0170-17.2017

Tarrant, J., Viczko, J., & Cope, H. (2018). Virtual reality for anxiety reduction demonstrated by quantitative EEG: A pilot study. *Frontiers in Psychology*, *9*, 1280. doi: 10.3389/fpsyg.2018.01280

Thompson, T., Terhune, D. B., Oram, C., Sharangparni, J., Rouf, R., Solmi, M., Veronese, N., & Stubbs, B. (2019). The effectiveness of hypnosis for pain relief: A systematic review and meta-analysis of 85 controlled experimental trials. *Neuroscience & Biobehavioral Reviews*, *99*, 298–310. doi: 10.1016/j.neubiorev.2019.02.013

Vogel, W., Broverman, D. M., & Klaiber, E. L. (1968). EEG and mental abilities. *Electroencephalography and Clinical Neurophysiology*, *24*(2), 166–175. doi: 10.1016/0013-4694(68)90122-3

Wahbeh, H., Sagher, A., Back, W., Pundhir, P., & Travis, F. (2018). A systematic review of transcendent states across meditation and contemplative traditions. *Explore: The Journal of Science and Healing*, *14*(1), 19–35. doi: 10.1016/j.explore.2017.07.007

Wallace, B. (1993). Day persons, night persons, and variability in hypnotic susceptibility. *Journal of Personal and Social Psychology*, *64*(5), 827–833. doi: 10.1037//0022-3514.64.5.827

Wolf, T. G., Faerber, K. A., Rummel, C., Halsband, U., & Campus, G. (2022). Functional changes in brain activity using hypnosis: A systematic review. *Brain Sciences*, *12*(1), 108. doi: 10.3390/brainsci12010108

Zhang, J., Lau, E. Y. Y., & Hsiao, J. H. (2019). Sleep deprivation compromises resting-state emotional regulatory processes: An EEG study. *Journal of Sleep Research*, *28*(3), e12671. doi: 10.1111/jsr.12671

Research in Hypnosis

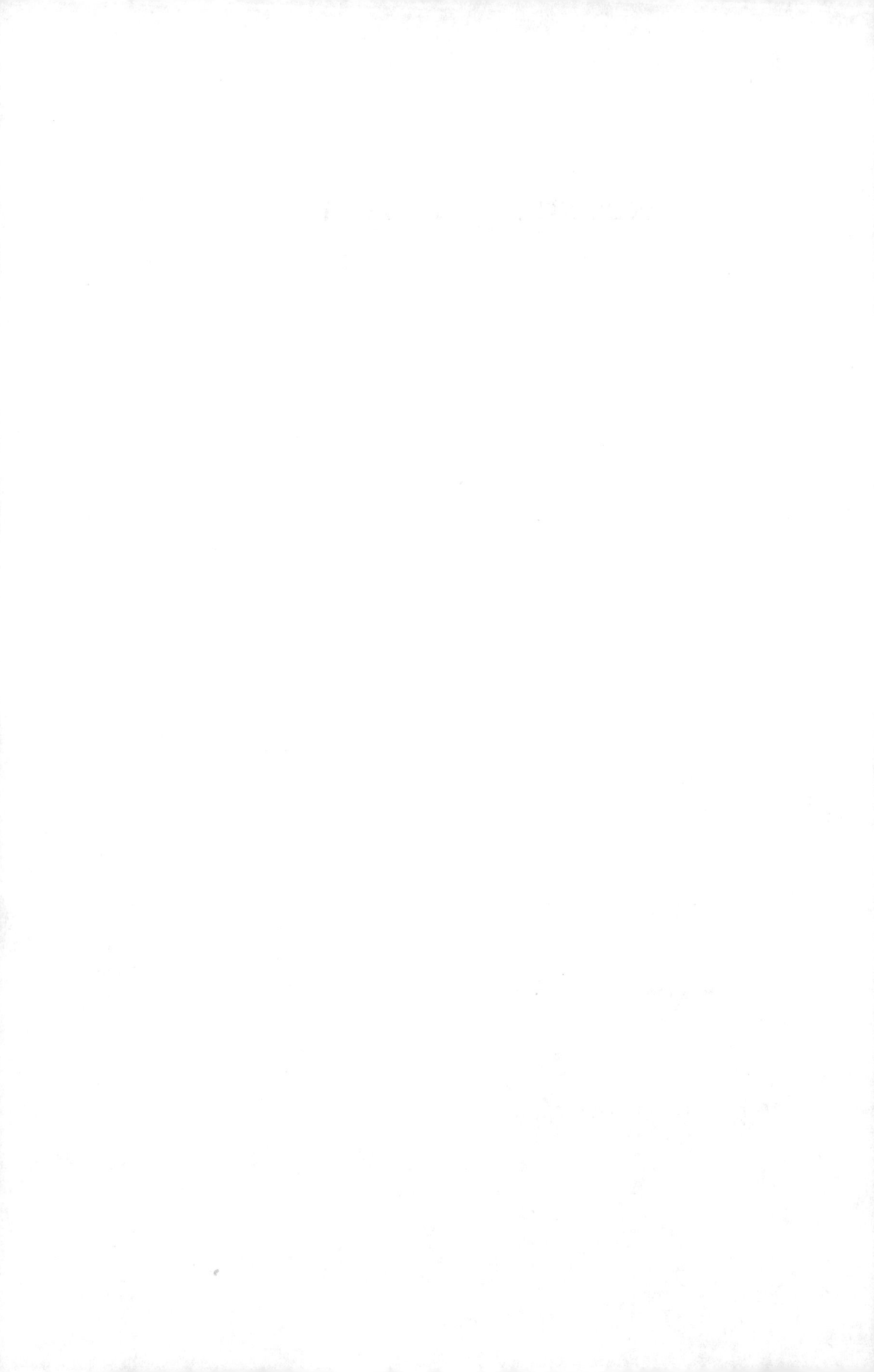

26

CONDUCTING RESEARCH IN CLINICAL HYPNOSIS

Donald Moss[1], *Olafur Palsson*[2], *and Zoltan Kekecs*[3]

[1]College of Integrative Medicine and Health Sciences, Saybrook University, CA, USA; [2]Department of Medicine, University of North Carolina at Chapel Hill, USA; [3]Institute of Psychology, ELTE Eötvös Loránd University, Budapest, Hungary

Research in Hypnosis History

Hypnosis has a rich basis in pure and applied research, with thousands of published studies. Early pioneers in hypnosis established scholarly journals to share knowledge about hypnosis practice. Gravitz (1987) determined that there have been at least 139 scholarly journals established from 1786 to the present, to publish research and clinical reports on mesmerism and hypnosis. He provided details on many early journals and books in hypnotism. Willmarth (2014) also provides much fascinating detail on early scholarly activity in hypnosis.

The first known scholarly journal on hypnosis, *Annales de la Sociète Harmonique des Amis-Rèunis de Strasbourg*, was published in Strasbourg, France in 1786 by Anton Mesmer's Society of Harmony (Society of Harmony, 1786–1789). Other more familiar examples emerged in the 19th century: John Elliotson, a British physician, began publishing the *Zoist* in England 1843, to publish articles about "animal magnetism" (Elliotson & Engeldue, 1843–1856). Baron du Potet, a French mesmerist, founded *The Journal of Magnetism* in France in 1845. Later the *Journal of Medical Hypnotism* was founded in Chicago in 1897 and a second journal, *Suggestive Therapeutics*, was founded in Chicago in 1898.

Early leaders also published books and monographs introducing hypnotic techniques and theoretical concepts about the mechanisms of hypnosis. An unknown editor published *Recueil des Pièces les Plus Intèressantes sur le Magnètisme Animal* in Paris in 1784. James Braid, an Edinburgh educated surgeon, published a treatise on hypnosis under the name *Neuroypnology*, in 1843, which moved away from Mesmer's concept of animal magnetism (Braid, 1843). James Esdaile, a Scottish physician, conducted 345 surgeries in India under anesthesia, and described his experiences in a monograph, *Mesmerism in India* (Esdaile, 1847).

Research in Modern Hypnosis

If we fast forward to the 20th century, research investigation strove to become more rigorously scientific, following evolving standards of science. Hypnosis research emerged in

DOI: 10.4324/9781003449126-36

abundance, including research by Ernest and Josephine Hilgard, Martin Orne, Nicholas Spanos, Theodore Xenophon Barber, Andre Weitzenhoffer, and David Spiegel (Hilgard, 1987). In the early to mid-twentieth century, the development of empirically derived and validated hypnotizability measures (Friedlander & Sarbin, 1938; Hilgard, 1970; Shor & Orne, 1962; Stern et al., 1978; Weitzenhoffer & Hilgard, 1959) made possible the study of individual differences in hypnotizability (also called hypnotic susceptibility, hypnotic ability, and hypnotic suggestibility) and its relationship to hypnotic effects and experiences. As one example, a study that followed a sample of research participants over a 25-year period suggested that hypnotizability scores remain stable over that extensive period of time (Weitzenhoffer & Hilgard, 1959; Piccione et al., 1989). Similarly, Morgan (1973) conducted a twin study of hypnotic susceptibility and calculated a heritability index of 0.64. These research studies suggested that hypnotic ability is a stable trait in humans, and that its heritability is comparable to that of chronic medical conditions such as type 2 diabetes, whose heritability has been reported as between 0.30 and 0.70 (Laakso & Fernandes Silva, 2022). Numerous laboratory studies in the 1950s–1970s illustrated the potential influence of hypnosis and hypnotizability on physiological parameters and pain modulation (Hilgard & Hilgard 1975), and identified various phenomenological characteristics associated with hypnosis.[1]

After the advances in laboratory hypnosis research in the 1950s–1970s, the field saw an influx of research on clinical applications of hypnosis and treatment modalities based on hypnotic techniques (Brown, 1992). Likewise, starting from the 1980s, there has been an ever-increasing stream of research identifying neural mechanisms underlying hypnotic phenomenon. This effort first started with peripheral neurophysiology and brain electrophysiology (EEG) studies (Gruzelier, 1998), and later expanded to neuroimaging using PET, fMRI, MEG, and other techniques (Landry et al., 2017; Rainville et al., 1997). Recently this has been supplemented by minimally invasive brain stimulation experiments such as transcranial magnetic stimulation to experimentally test predictions of psychophysiological models of hypnosis (Dienes & Hutton, 2013).

In August 2015, the International Society of Hypnosis (ISH) held a one-day gathering of researchers in hypnosis, prior to the ISH conference in Paris. An article by Jensen et al. (2017) summarizes the conclusions of that meeting. First, the authors recognized advances in three areas in hypnosis research in recent decades, including:

1 Clinical research supporting the efficacy of hypnosis for managing a number of clinical symptoms and conditions,
2 Research supporting the role of various divisions in the anterior cingulate and prefrontal cortices in hypnotic responding, and
3 An emerging finding that high hypnotic suggestibility is associated with atypical brain connectivity profiles.

The ISH conclave identified significant challenges to hypnosis research, including: (a) some loss of momentum in empirical research in the field, as a generation of research pioneers retires or dies, (b) some lingering prejudice that hypnosis is a taboo or unscientific topic for research, and (c) a lack of organized collaboration and communication among researchers globally, creating some fragmentation in focus and approach in research. The group proposed approaches for addressing the above-mentioned challenges in hypnosis research. They recommended that future research: (a) highlight the biological and neurobiological underpinnings of hypnotic suggestion and suggestibility, (b) examine the role and impact of specific hypnotic inductions, and (c) examine the similarity and differences between hypnotic interventions and related interventions such as mindfulness.

Finally, the ISH group formulated recommendations for improving the methodological rigor in future hypnosis research:

1 Include well-documented reliable assessment of hypnotic ability in research studies.
2 Include participants representing the full spectrum of hypnotic ability, not just groups of highs and lows.
3 Utilize research designs that carefully delineate the role and impact of specific inductions and suggestions.
4 Increase the practice of data sharing among research groups.
5 Shift research resources to studies examining the neurophysiological underpinnings of hypnotic phenomena.

Meta-Analyses of Hypnosis Research and Critiques of Research Design

In spite of acknowledged advances in research in the 20th and 21st centuries, outcomes research applying hypnosis to clinical disorders in medicine and mental health is often inconsistent and displays many methodological lapses. The emphasis in healthcare today is on the use of evidence-based interventions, and the methodological standards in outcomes research have advanced dramatically, with expectations of randomized controlled trials, pre-registration of research protocols, careful controls for risk of bias, and research designs of adequate power.

Recent meta-analyses in some respects show the efficacy of hypnotic interventions yet also highlight methodological inconsistencies and weaknesses in current outcome research in hypnosis. Two examples will be provided here.

Thompson et al. (2019) conducted a systematic review and meta-analysis of hypnosis for pain relief. The authors searched six major databases, using four clear eligibility criteria and two exclusion criteria. Researchers rated each study for methodological quality on a 15-item validity scale assessing methodological rigor, selection, and reporting bias. They identified only 85 studies with 3,632 participants that met inclusion and exclusion criteria. The authors concluded that hypnotic interventions produced a reduced pain intensity with a large effect size, lower affective pain ratings but with highly inconsistent effect sizes, higher pain tolerance but with moderately inconsistent effect sizes, and higher pain threshold but with highly inconsistent effect sizes. Varying numbers of studies were included in each of these calculations, because of differences in factors measured and reported in the 85 studies. Statistical analysis of asymmetry in reported findings on pain intensity, tolerance, and threshold suggested possible publication bias, but had only minimal impact on effect sizes.

The researchers were also able to analyze factors that mediated effect size and concluded that hypnotic effects were greater for participants with high or medium hypnotic susceptibility and in interventions with direct suggestions of pain relief. The authors reported significant evidence that hypnosis is efficacious for pain relief. On the other hand, they also concluded that "limited high quality data with numerous design biases prohibits reliable conclusions" (Thompson et al., 2019, p. 308).

Valentine et al. (2019) conducted a meta-analysis of hypnosis as a treatment for anxiety. The authors searched two major databases and identified 15 articles and dissertations that were eligible for the meta-analysis. Two of the studies included two differing hypnosis interventions compared to a control condition, so the researchers included 17 "trials" of hypnosis in the analysis of the 15 articles.

The authors assessed the risk of bias in the studies in five bias domains, using the Cochrane Risk of Bias Tool, and rated each type of bias as high, low, or unclear. They also calculated the effect sizes for all studies and again for those studies that included follow-up. Interestingly, there was little relationship between the calculated risk of bias indices and effect sizes. In other words, more rigorous studies that better controlled for the risk of bias did not show lower effects. Similarly, Milling et al. (2021, p. 312) reported higher effect sizes for methodologically more rigorous studies, which may indicate that more experienced researchers who design more rigorous studies can also produce more potent interventions, or are better at identifying good intervention opportunities and targets. Valentine et al. (2019) concluded that hypnosis is a highly effective treatment for anxiety. The mean weighted effect size for the 17 trials was 0.79, which falls in the large range for effect size. Studies that combined hypnosis with other interventions, such as cognitive behavioral therapy, showed larger effect sizes than hypnosis applied as a solo treatment.

In spite of positive conclusions about the efficacy of hypnosis for anxiety, Valentine et al. were critical of the lack of detail about the intervention in many studies, the lack of sufficient information to clearly assess risk of bias, and the inclusion of follow-up in only seven studies.

The Task Force for Efficacy Standards in Hypnosis Research

In 2018, then SCEH President Donald Moss reached out to representatives of ASCH, APA Division 30, the Milton H. Erickson Foundation, the National Pediatric Hypnosis Training Institute, and the International Society for Hypnosis, and proposed an international Task Force for Efficacy Standards in Hypnosis Research (the Task Force). All of the professional groups agreed on the need for such a Task Force. Zoltan Kekecs and Donald Moss agreed to co-convene the Task Force, and nine researchers from the US, Great Britain, Hungary, Italy, and Belgium committed to participate in the Task Force discussions. The participants in the first two years of deliberation were: Giuseppe De Benedittis (Italy), Gary Elkins (US), Marie Faymonville (Belgium), Zoltan Kekecs (Hungary), Donald Moss (US), Olafur Palsson (US), Phil Shenefelt (US), Eric Spiegel (US), Devin Terhune (United Kingdom), Katalin Varga (Hungary), David Wark (US), and Peter Whorwell (United Kingdom). In addition, six additional researchers agreed to serve as consultants to the Task Force: Walter Bongartz (Germany), Mark Jensen (US), Krjis Klajs (Poland), Elvira Lang (US), David Patterson (US), and Dirk Revenstorf (Germany). The Task Force began its work in February 2019 and continues to meet on a monthly basis.

One limitation of the Task Force's work and of this chapter should be emphasized. The Task Force did not examine the many specific challenges of research on pediatric hypnosis. The Task Force did not formulate recommendations specific to research on hypnosis applications for pediatric populations. There have been systematic reviews of specific pediatric applications of hypnosis (Birnie et al., 2014; Richardson et al., 2006; Uman et al., 2013), and hypnosis applications for children's problems are promising. In general, however, the published research remains limited and the researchers conducting systematic reviews have called for increased rigor in methodology. Development of guidelines for research on pediatric hypnosis is a priority for the future.

Recommendations for Best Practices in Research

The Task Force began by affirming existing standards and guidelines available to support rigorous research design. Researchers should follow the many already existing guidelines for empirical research: the Cochrane handbook for systematic reviews of interventions, the Risk of Bias 2 tool, the CONSORT statement, the STROBE checklist, the SPIRIT checklist, the TIDieR checklist, and papers and handbooks on clinical psychology research (Chan et al., 2013; Higgins et al., 2011; Knottnerus & Tugwell, 2008; Miles & Gilbert, 2005; Roberts & Ilardi, 2008; Schulz et al., 2010; Shadish & Cook, 2002, Sterne et al., 2019).

The Task Force next focused on formulating both essential and preferred guidelines specific to research on hypnosis (Kekecs et al., in preparation).

Essential Recommendations for Research Design

The following essential recommendations communicate standards for rigorous research in hypnosis. In designing research studies, researchers should:

1 Adopt detailed research protocols and treatment manuals, intervention scripts, and/or recorded interventions for the experimental and control group. This enables better meta-analytic comparison of studies and more effective replication of research studies.
2 Standardize and provide detailed plans on how participants will be educated about hypnosis. This should include specific detail on how the interventions will be described and labeled for the participants.
3 Select well-validated hypnotic ability scales, supported by research.

Essential Recommendations for Research Reporting

Deficiencies in reporting detail obstruct meta-analyses and undermine the possibility of effective replication of studies. Often it is lapses in reporting as much as lapses in the research design that lower meta-analytic efficacy ratings. Guidelines for reporting mirror the recommendations above for research design. In reporting research, authors should:

1 Include the detailed protocols, treatment manuals, intervention scripts, and/or recorded interventions in the published reports, or provide information or links for accessing them.
2 Include the procedures that were used for participant education.
3 Specify the hypnotic induction techniques in detail, including any manual, and make available recorded interventions.
4 Specify how the hypnotic intervention was labeled and explained for the participants. In addition, the reports should provide the researchers' rationale for categorizing the intervention as hypnosis.
5 Clearly stipulate how, when, and by whom hypnotic ability was assessed, along with psychometric properties of any instrument(s) used.

Preferred Recommendations for Research Design

The Task Force authors also included a series of recommended but not essential guidelines for hypnosis research. When possible, researchers should optimally:

1 Measure adherence to any home practice included in the intervention. Real-time online logging of home practice may improve accuracy in participants' reporting.
2 Assess hypnotic ability.
3 Utilize someone other than the interventionist to assess hypnotizability, to reduce experimenter bias.
4 Selecting hypnotizability measures that utilize both subjective and behavioral measures of responsiveness is best.
5 Include participants from the entire hypnotizability spectrum, not just lows and highs, to increase generalizability.
6 Assess the participants' expectancy about hypnotic effects, using well-validated measures.
7 Measure the level of rapport, therapeutic alliance, or therapeutic relationship between the client and the therapist (if any).
8 Include in research design measurement of specific variables that might identify the potential mechanisms of action of hypnosis.

Preferred Recommendations on Research Reporting

In addition, the Task Force authors suggested that when possible, researchers should:

1 Report participants' prior experience with hypnosis.
2 Report response expectancies for particular outcomes separately for different intervention groups, and when feasible, for different levels of hypnotizability.
3 Report the statistical association between response expectancies and the study outcomes.

Guidelines for Assessing Efficacy of Clinical Hypnosis Applications

The Task Force also formulated recommendations specific to rating the efficacy of various clinical applications of hypnosis (Kekecs et al., 2022). These recommendations were intended to guide researchers who want to assess the accumulated evidence about the efficacy of various hypnosis applications. The Task Force recommendations appeared in the *International Journal of Clinical and Experimental Hypnosis*, as "Guidelines for the Assessment of Efficacy of Clinical Hypnosis Applications" (Kekecs et al., 2022).

The Task Force authors began by recommending that efficacy reviewers implement existing systems already available for grading evidence on efficacy. For example, several grading systems have emerged in medical research such as the Grading of Recommendations Assessment, Development and Evaluation (GRADE), and the Oxford Centre for Evidence-Based Medicine (OCEBM): Levels of Evidence Table (Atkins et al., 2004; OCEBM Working Group, 2011). The Task Force authors specifically recommended the GRADE systems as applicable for efficacy research in clinical hypnosis (Kekecs et al., 2022).

These medical grading systems were not designed to deal with some of the nuances and complexities of behavioral and psycho-social interventions, so the Task Force authors went on to formulate additional recommendations for efficacy research in hypnosis. The guidelines were designed to be applied to bodies of research, not individual studies. Accordingly, a research team assessing the efficacy of hypnosis treatment for headache would examine the accumulated evidence, based on multiple studies, about this specific application of hypnosis.

1 First, the assessment of the efficacy of any hypnosis application should be based on a recent systematic review, implementing the highest quality standards, including multiple studies documenting the effectiveness of this application.
2 When possible, the review should utilize a meta-analytic quantitative synthesis of the evidence across studies.
3 The Task Force team endorses the application of the GRADE system, or a similar system of comparable rigor, to rate efficacy.
4 In assessing a body of research, the researchers should take into account sample size, effect sizes and confidence intervals, and clinical significance when assessing efficacy. An intervention can have statistically significant effects, without demonstrating clinical significance and clinical usefulness.
5 The Task Force authors recommend including assessment of hypnotizability in hypnosis outcome studies, because such assessment can support the hypnotic mechanism of the intervention. Nevertheless, the assessment of hypnotizability is not essential in rating efficacy.
6 Blinding of research participants and the interventionist as to the group assignment is optimal but not essential.
7 When possible, at least partial blinding is recommended. For example, it is best for the research staff who collect data or analyze the results to be blinded as to group assignments.
8 The rating of efficacy should only include studies in which the researchers label the intervention as hypnosis or hypnotic treatment. The intervention should be clearly described and should comprise an intervention that an expert reviewer would regard as hypnosis. It is not necessary that the intervention be described to the participants as hypnosis.
9 The highest levels of efficacy rating should be reserved for applications in which two or more independent research groups have conducted methodologically rigorous research, or in which one of the supporting studies is a well-designed multi-center trial.
10 When the application involves a chronic condition, ratings of efficacy should emphasize research designs with adequate follow-up measurements. For chronic conditions such as chronic pain, a follow-up of six months is appropriate to demonstrate lasting efficacy.

Survey on Current Practices in Clinical Hypnosis

In 2020–2021, the Task Force for Efficacy Standards in Hypnosis Research conducted an international survey under the leadership of Olafur Palsson, of hypnosis practitioners and researchers on current practices in hypnosis (Palsson et al., 2023). This project was undertaken due to the recognition by the Task Force of the general lack of information about real-world practices and outlook of both researchers and clinicians in the field of hypnosis. Therefore, the survey was designed to examine and document current practices, experiences, and perspectives of hypnosis clinicians and researchers (Palsson et al., 2023).

An international recruitment drive was conducted with the assistance of the major professional organizations in hypnosis, including the Society for Clinical and Experimental Hypnosis, the American Society of Clinical Hypnosis and its component societies, the ISH, the European Society of Hypnosis, the American Psychological Association's Division 30 (Society of Psychological Hypnosis), the Italian Society of Hypnosis, the Hungarian Association of Hypnosis, and the British Society of Clinical and Academic Hypnosis. A total of 775 hypnosis professionals in 32 countries completed the survey, including 691 clinicians and 133 researchers; these were overlapping groups as many of the researchers were also in clinical practice.

Readers are referred to the Palsson et al. (2023) article for a detailed description of the survey results. For this chapter, we will confine ourselves to reporting the respondents' answers regarding principles for conducting high-quality clinical hypnosis research, their views of hypnosis research priorities, and their perception regarding the effectiveness of common hypnosis applications.

The survey assessed the views of the 133 researchers in the sample regarding the importance of 14 different methodological factors for conducting high-quality clinical hypnosis research. Ratings were made on a five-point scale from "not at all important" to "extremely important." The results are summarized in Table 26.1. All the 14 methodological aspects presented in the survey were rated as very or extremely important by about half or more of the participating researchers. As many of these items were those recommended by the Task Force for Efficacy Standards in Hypnosis Research paper on

Table 26.1 Ratings by 133 Hypnosis Researchers of the Importance of Different Methodological Aspects for Conducting High-Quality Hypnosis Research

Survey question: *"In your best judgment, how important are each of the following for conducting high-quality clinical hypnosis research?"*

	% Giving Rating of Very or Extremely Important
Using highly reliable and valid measures	91.0
Using multiple outcome measure types (self-report, behavioral, observational, physiological, etc.)	85.7
Standardized and detailed training of study staff administering hypnosis intervention and testing	85.0
Documenting protocol violations systematically	75.9
Standardizing education/instructions of subjects about the intervention or study tasks	75.2
Systematically evaluating adherence of hypnotists and study staff to treatment protocol	74.4
Randomized allocation to intervention groups	73.7
Measuring expectancy of the subjects before and during intervention	69.2
Blinding of assessors/analysts to group assignment of subjects	66.1
Blinding of experimenters to hypnotizability level of subjects	63.9
Blinding study participants to the nature of the intervention they receive	59.4
Following a detailed manual in administering the interventions	58.6
Pre-registration of studies, on websites such as ClinicalTrials.org or OSF	56.4
Assessing hypnotizability of subjects	48.9

conducting high-quality hypnosis research, this validated the Task Force's guidelines as being generally in harmony with the current views of researchers in the field regarding best practices. Most highly endorsed as very or extremely important were the use of valid and reliable measures, applying multiple different types of measures, and using standardized training for research personnel conducting treatment and testing in hypnosis studies.

The survey also asked both hypnosis researchers and clinicians to rate the importance of 19 different priorities for the next ten years in clinical hypnosis research, based on the recent hypnosis literature and discussions at scientific hypnosis research meetings. The ratings were on a five-point scale from "not at all important" to "extremely important." The results are presented in Table 26.2 for both researchers and non-researcher clinicians (survey participants who had both professional roles were excluded from this analysis for better contrast). Most of the listed priority areas were rated as being very or extremely important by the majority of both the researchers and clinicians, suggesting that hypnosis professionals broadly believe that hypnosis research needs to divide its efforts among these many different clinical topics in the near future.

Table 26.2 Ratings by 133 Hypnosis Researchers and 593 Non-Researcher Hypnosis Clinicians of the Importance of Various Methodological Aspects for Conducting High-Quality Hypnosis Research

Survey question: *"In your best judgment, how important are each of these research priorities for clinical hypnosis in the next 10 years?"*

	% Giving a Rating of Very or Extremely Important:	
	Hypnosis Researchers (n = 133)	*Hypnosis Clinicians (n = 593)*
Stress management applications	88.0	87.0
Preparing individuals for, or producing beneficial effects during, medical procedures	86.5	81.1
Application for treating psychological trauma	76.7	88.4
Treatment of pain (acute and chronic)	75.9	81.5
Anxiety applications	75.2	83.5
Psychotherapy applications	74.4	80.9
Enhancing immune function with hypnosis	72.2	79.3
Cancer treatment applications	69.9	79.6
Treatment of psychosomatic disorders (such as irritable bowel syndrome)	69.9	78.3
Depression applications	66.9	78.8
Treatment of sleep problems	65.4	80.1
Well-being applications	63.9	70.5
Eliminating maladaptive habits	57.9	74.2
Benefits of combining hypnosis and medications for treatment of health problems	56.4	56.7
Supporting/enhancing physical activity with hypnosis	53.4	58.2
Weight loss/diet applications	51.1	62.2
Mindfulness applications of hypnosis	43.6	53.8
Developing more reliable methods to screen people for suitability for hypnosis treatment	36.8	23.4
Treatment of hot flashes	30.8	34.6

Table 26.3 Ratings by 133 Hypnosis Researchers of the Importance of Various Research Priorities for the Field of Experimental (Non-Clinical) Hypnosis

Survey question: *"In your best judgment, how important are each of these research priorities for experimental (non-clinical) hypnosis in the next 10 years?"*

	% Giving a Rating of Very or Extremely Important
Psychological mechanisms of hypnosis	79.7
Biological/physiological effects of hypnosis	78.2
Clarifying the brain functions underlying hypnosis	69.9
Effects of hypnotic suggestions on perception	65.4
Effects of specific suggestions on brain regions	61.7
Relationship between hypnosis/hypnotizability and other suggestion-based phenomena	51.9
Placebo effects and hypnosis/hypnotizability	51.1
Parallel investigation of hypnotist & hypnotized person – interactional	51.1
Sociocognitive effects on hypnotic responding (e.g., expectancy, social compliance, rapport)	49.7
Sleep and hypnosis	49.6
Techniques for modifying hypnotizability	45.9
Personality and cognitive correlates of hypnotizability	45.9
Hypnosis and access to, or modulation of, memories	41.3
Genetics of hypnotizability	29.3
Clarifying whether hypnosis is a state	24.8
Animal models of hypnosis	9.8

Similar ratings were obtained in the survey about the perceptions of the participating researchers regarding experimental (non-clinical) hypnosis priorities, using the same five-point importance rating scale, and a list of 15 current academic or laboratory research focus areas. While most of those topics were considered important priority areas by a substantial proportion of the researchers (see Table 26.3), the ones most commonly rated as very or extremely important were psychological mechanisms of hypnosis, biological or physiological effects of hypnosis, brain functions underlying hypnosis, and effects of hypnotic suggestions on perception and on brain regions; all of these were rated as highly or extremely important by more than 60% of the researchers. Only research on animal models of hypnosis received low endorsement (9.8%) as an important research priority among the ones rated.

One approach to assessing the clinical effectiveness of hypnosis for various disorders is to assess consensus experience among a group of hypnosis practitioners who regularly treat those disorders. This has not been used much in the field of hypnosis to date, as published efficacy findings are usually from more formal clinical research studies. However, ratings by practicing clinicians of the success of their interventions for specific problems can provide useful supplemental insights to formal research results, as the specifics of the interventions and patient populations in routine clinical practice in the community may be different from those in formal trials. The Task Force utilized the opportunity of its large international survey of clinicians to assess their perceptions of the effectiveness of 36 common applications of clinical hypnosis, based on their own personal experience with their clients. These were reported on a four-point rating scale with the response options of "not effective," "minimally effective," "moderately effective," or "highly effective." The

Table 26.4 Ratings by 691 Hypnosis Clinicians of the Effectiveness of Common Applications of Clinical Hypnosis, Based on Their Own Practice Experience

A. Hypnosis Applications Rated as Highly Effective by 70% or More of Respondents	
Stress reduction	Mindfulness
Enhancing well-being	Labor and childbirth
Preparing for surgery	Enhancing confidence/self-esteem
Anxiety	
B. Hypnosis Applications Rated as Highly Effective by 50 to 69% of Respondents	
Pain during medical procedures	Enhancing health-supporting behaviorsEnhancing health-supporting behaviors
Phobias	Irritable bowel syndromeIrritable bowel syndrome
Panic disorder	Tension headaches
Facilitating insight	Burn pain
Post-traumatic stress disorder	Insomnia
C. Hypnosis Applications Rated as Highly Effective by 30 to 49% of Respondents	
Dissociative disorders	Recovering important memories
Abdominal pain	Hypertension
Removing warts	Back pain
Cancer pain	Sexual dysfunction
Removing unwanted habits	Migraine headaches
Smoking cessation	Hot flashes
Chronic pain	Depression
D. Hypnosis Applications Rated as Highly Effective by Less Than 30% of Respondents	
Cardiac rehabilitation	Eating disorders
Fibromyalgia	Excessive weight (helping weight loss)
Obsessive-compulsive disorder	

clinicians did not rate applications with which they felt they had insufficient experience to judge the effectiveness. As seen in Table 26.4, seven of the listed applications were rated highly effective by the great majority (70% or more) of the clinicians, and another set of ten applications received high effectiveness ratings from at least 50% of the respondents. These results demonstrate the wide range of applications that are highly effective in the routine work of clinical practitioners. Fourteen additional applications were rated as highly effective by 30–49%, and five applications by less than 30% of the respondents.

It should be noted that the fact that some applications were rated highly effective by less clinicians does not necessarily mean that those interventions are less efficacious than other psychological interventions for the same disorders. The less highly rated items include a number of applications, for which well-designed studies report clinical efficacy (Flynn, 2018; Jensen et al., 2020; Johnson et al., 2019; Valentine et al., 2019; Zech et al., 2017). Furthermore, it is also important to note that the fact that some hypnosis applications were viewed as effective by less people than other applications does not mean that these applications would be worse than other interventions for the same condition. For example, excessive weight is notoriously resistant to treatment in the long term, regardless of the intervention (Norris et al., 2005).

Summary and Conclusions

From the earliest days of clinical hypnosis practice, leading researchers have sought to establish scholarly and research-based reporting on hypnosis techniques and hypnosis applications. The 20th century saw dramatic advances in research on hypnosis, with hypnosis laboratories reporting an abundance of studies on hypnotic phenomena and clinical applications of hypnosis. Nevertheless, with the recent emergence of highly rigorous standards of evidence in clinical research, an increasing number of systematic reviews have highlighted deficiencies and lapses in published research on hypnosis.

This chapter reported primarily on the recommendations and findings of the Task Force for Efficacy Standards in Hypnosis Research. The Task Force was an international initiative supported by many of the major professional organizations in hypnosis. The outcomes of the Task Force's work were reported in three areas: guidelines for best practices in research in hypnosis, guidelines for assessing efficacy in clinical hypnosis, and a survey-based report on the perspectives of hypnosis professionals on different clinical applications of hypnosis, standards for conducting high-quality clinical hypnosis research, and priorities for hypnosis research over the next decade. It is hoped that this report on the Task Force recommendations will encourage researchers to improve research design and reporting in hypnosis research, further establishing that clinical hypnosis deserves a respected place in evidence-based healthcare.

Note

1 It should be noted that, in spite of the impressive longitudinal studies by Weitzenhoffer, Hilgard, and Piccione, further research has suggested that hypnotizability may depend in part on demand characteristics (Orne, 1962), may be subject to some modification by behavioral training (Gorassini & Spanos, 1986), and in one study decreased significantly in a second measurement session (Fassler et al., 2008). A more recent study found that the choice of measures affects stability; the researchers found decreases in a second measurement session when using the Stanford Hypnotic Susceptibility Scale, Form C, but not using the Elkins Hypnotizability Scale (Kekecs et al., 2021). Measures of subjective experiences and expectancies appear to account for a significant portion in the variance in hypnotic responding. Some evidence also suggests that hypnotizability is associated with power in theta band EEG activity, as well as with gamma band activity (Jensen et al., 2015), with preliminary findings suggesting theta EEG biofeedback enhances responsiveness to hypno-analgesia (Jensen et al., 2016). Some other recent studies reported that inhibition of activity in the dorsolateral prefrontal cortex could alter hypnotizability (Coltheart et al., 2018; Dienes & Hutton, 2013; Faerman et al., 2021; Perri et al., 2022). In summary, hypnotizability may be relatively stable over time, yet is subject to fluctuation in response to behavioral, sociocognitive, and neurophysiological variables.

References

Atkins, D., Eccles, M., Flottorp, S., Guyatt, G. H., Henry, D., Hill, S., Liberati, A., O'Connell, D., Oxman, A. D., Phillips, B., Schünemann, H., Edejer, T. T.-T., Vist, G. E., Williams, J. W., & GRADE Working Group (2004). Systems for grading the quality of evidence and the strength of recommendations. I. Critical appraisal of existing approaches. The GRADE Working Group. *BMC Health Services Research*, *4*(1), 38.10.1186/1472-6963-4-38.

Birnie, K. A., Noel, M., Parker, J. A., Chambers, C. T., Uman, L. S., Kisely, S. R., & McGrath, P. J. (2014). Systematic review and meta-analysis of distraction and hypnosis for needle-related pain and distress in children and adolescents. *Journal of Pediatric Psychology*, *39*(8), 783–808. 10.1093/jpepsy/jsu029

Braid, J. (1843). *Neuroypnology: Or the rationale of nervous sleep, considered in relation with animal magnetism*. John Churchill.

Brown, D. P. (1992). Clinical hypnosis research since 1986. In E. Fromm, & M. R. Nash (Eds.), *Contemporary hypnosis research* (pp. 427–458). The Guilford Press.

Chan, A.-W., Tetzlaff, J. M., Altman, D. G., Dickersin, K., & Moher, D. (2013). SPIRIT 2013: New guidance for content of clinical trial protocols. *The Lancet*, *381*(9861), 91–92. 10.1016/S0140-6736(12)62160-6

Coltheart, M., Cox, R., Sowman, P., Morgan, H., Barnier, A., Langdon, R., Connaughton, E., Teichmann, L., Williams, N., & Polito, V. (2018). Belief, delusion, hypnosis, and the right dorsolateral prefrontal cortex: A transcranial magnetic stimulation study. *Cortex*, *101*, 234–248. 10.1016/j.cortex.2018.01.001

Dienes, Z., & Hutton, S. (2013). Understanding hypnosis metacognitively: rTMS applied to left DLPFC increases hypnotic suggestibility. *Cortex*, *49*(2), 386–392. 10.1016/j.cortex.2012.07.009

Elliotson, J., & Engledue, W. C. (Eds.). (1843–1856). *The Zoist: A journal of cerebral physiology & mesmerism, and their applications to human welfare.*

Esdaile, J. (1847). *Mesmerism in India, and its practical applications in surgery and medicine*. Silus Andrus and Sons.

Faerman, A., Bishop, J. H., Stimpson, K. H., Phillips, A., Gülser, M., Amin, H., Nejad, R., DeSouza, D. D., Geoly, A. D., Kallioniemi. E., Booil, J., Williams, N. R., & Spiegel, D. (2021). Modulation of a stable neurobehavioral trait using repetitive transcranial magnetic stimulation: A preregistered randomized controlled trial. *medRxiv*. 10.1101/2021.07.08.21260222

Fassler, O., Lynn, S. J., & Knox, J. (2008). Is hypnotic suggestibility a stable trait? *Consciousness and Cognition*, *17*(1), 240–253. 10.1016/j.concog.2007.05.004

Flynn N. (2018). Systematic review of the effectiveness of hypnosis for the management of headache. *The International Journal of Clinical and Experimental Hypnosis*, *66*(4), 343–352. 10.1080/00207144.2018.1494432

Friedlander, J. W., & Sarbin, T. R. (1938). The depth of hypnosis. *Journal of Abnormal and Social Psychology*, *33*(4), 453–475. 10.1037/h0056229

Gorassini, D. R., & Spanos, N. P. (1986). A social-cognitive skills approach to the successful modification of hypnotic susceptibility. *Journal of Personality and Social Psychology*, *50*(5), 1004–1012. 10.1037/0022-3514.50.5.1004

Gravitz, M. A. (1987). Two centuries of hypnosis specialty journals. *International Journal of Clinical and Experimental Hypnosis*, *35*(4), 265–276. 10.1080/00207148708416059

Gruzelier, J. (1998). A working model of the neurophysiology of hypnosis: A review of evidence. *Contemporary Hypnosis*, *15*(1), 3–21. 10.1002/ch.112

Higgins, J. P. T., Altman, D. G., Gotzsche, P. C., Juni, P., Moher, D., Oxman, A. D., Savovic, J., Schulz, K. F., Weeks, L., Sterne, J. A. C., Cochrane Bias Methods Group, & Cochrane Statistical Methods Group (2011). The Cochrane Collaboration's tool for assessing risk of bias in randomised trials. *BMJ*, *343*, d5928. 10.1136/bmj.d5928

Hilgard, E. R. (1970). *Personality and hypnosis: A study of imaginative involvement*. University of Chicago Press.

Hilgard, E. (1987). Research advances in hypnosis: Issues and methods, *International Journal of Clinical and Experimental Hypnosis*, *35*(4), 248–264. 10.1080/00207148708416058

Hilgard, E. R., & Hilgard, J. R. (1975). *Hypnosis in the relief of pain.* William Kaufmann.

Jensen, M. P., Adachi, T., & Hakimian, S. (2015). Brain oscillations, hypnosis, and hypnotizability. *American Journal of Clinical Hypnosis*, *57*(3), 230–253. 10.1080/00029157.2014.976786

Jensen, M. P., Gianas, A., George, H. R., Sherlin, L. H., Kraft, G. H., & Ehde, D. M. (2016). Use of neurofeedback to enhance response to hypnotic analgesia in individuals with multiple sclerosis. *International Journal of Clinical and Experimental Hypnosis*, *64*(1), 1–23. 10.1080/00207144.2015.1099400

Jensen, M. P., Jamieson, G. A., Lutz, A., Mazzoni, G., McGeown, W. J., Santarcangelo, E. L., Demertzi, A., De Pascalis, V., Bányai, É. I., Rominger, C., Vuilleumier, P., Faymonville, M. E., & Terhune, D. B. (2017). New directions in hypnosis research: Strategies for advancing the cognitive and clinical neuroscience of hypnosis. *Neuroscience of Consciousness*, *3*(1), nix004. 10.1093/nc/nix004

Jensen, M. P., Mendoza, M. E., Ehde, D. M., Patterson, D. R., Molton, I. R., Dillworth, T. M., Gertz, K. J., Chan, J., Hakimian, S., Battalio, S. L., & Ciol, M. A. (2020). Effects of hypnosis, cognitive therapy, hypnotic cognitive therapy, and pain education in adults with chronic pain: A randomized clinical trial. *Pain*, *161*(10), 2284–2298 10.1097/j.pain.0000000000001943

Johnson, A., Roberts, L., & Elkins, G. (2019). Complementary and alternative medicine for menopause. *Journal of Evidence-Based Integrative Medicine*, *24*, 2515690X19829380. 10.1177/2515690X19829380

Kekecs, Z., Roberts, L., Na, H., Yek, M. H., Slonena, E. E., Racelis, E., Voor, T. A., Johansson, R., Rizzo, P., Csikos, E., Vizkievicz, V., & Elkins, G. (2021). Test–retest reliability of the Stanford Hypnotic Susceptibility Scale, Form C and the Elkins Hypnotizability Scale. *International Journal of Clinical and Experimental Hypnosis*, *69*(1), 142–161. 10.1080/00207144.2021.1834858

Kekecs, Z., Moss, D., Elkins, G., De Benedettis, G., Pallson, O., Shenefelt, P., Terhune, D., Varga, K., & Whorwell, P. (2022). Guidelines for the assessment of efficacy of clinical hypnosis applications. *International Journal of Clinical and Experimental Hypnosis*, *70*(2), 104–122. 10.1080/00207144.2022.2049446

Kekecs, Z., Moss, D., Whorwell, P., Varga, K., Terhune, D. B., Shenefelt, P. D., Palsson, O. S., De Benedittis, G., & Elkins, G. (in preparation). Best practice recommendations for conducting controlled trials in clinical hypnosis research.

Knottnerus, A., & Tugwell, P. (2008). STROBE—A checklist to STrengthen the Reporting of OBservational studies in Epidemiology. *Journal of Clinical Epidemiology*, *61*(4), 323. 10.1016/j.jclinepi.2007.11.006

Laakso, M., & Fernandes Silva, L. (2022). Genetics of type 2 diabetes: Past, present, and future. Nutrients; *14*(15), 3201. 10.3390/nu14153201

Landry, M., Lifshitz, M., & Raz, A. (2017). Brain correlates of hypnosis: A systematic review and meta-analytic exploration. *Neuroscience & Biobehavioral Reviews*, *81*(Pt A), 75–98. 10.1016/j.neubiorev.2017.02.020

Miles, J., & Gilbert, P. (2005). *A handbook of research methods for clinical and health psychology*. Oxford University Press.

Milling, L. S., Valentine, K. E., LoStimolo, L. M., Nett, A. M., & McCarley, H. S. (2021). Hypnosis and the alleviation of clinical pain: A comprehensive meta-analysis. *International Journal of Clinical and Experimental Hypnosis*, *69*(3), 297–322. 10.1080/00207144.2021.1920330

Morgan, A. H. (1973). The heritability of hypnotic susceptibility in twins. *Journal of Abnormal Psychology*, *82*(1), 55–61. 10.1037/h0034854

Norris, S. L., Zhang, X., Avenell, A., Gregg, E., Brown, T. J., Schmid, C. H., & Lau, J. (2005). Long-term non-pharmacologic weight loss interventions for adults with type 2 diabetes. *The Cochrane Database of Systematic Reviews*, *2005*(2), CD004095. 10.1002/14651858.CD004095.pub2

OCEBM Working Group (2011). The Oxford 2011 Levels of Evidence Table. Oxford Centre for Evidence-Based Medicine. https://www.cebm.ox.ac.uk/resources/levels-of-evidence/ocebm-levels-of-evidence

Orne, M. T. (1962). On the social psychology of the psychological experiment: With particular reference to demand characteristics and their implications *American Psychologist*, *17*, 776–783. 10.1037/h0043424

Palsson, O. S., Kekecs, Z., De Benedittis, G., Moss, D., Elkins, G.y R., Terhune, D. B., Varga, K., Shenefelt, P. D., & Whorwell, P. J. (2023). Current Practices, Experiences, and Views in Clinical Hypnosis: Findings of an International Survey. *International Journal of Clinical and Experimental Hypnosis*, *71*, 92–114. 10.1080/00207144.2023.2183862

Perri, R. L., Perrotta, D., Rossani, F. & Pekala, R. J. (2022). Boosting the hypnotic experience. Inhibition of the dorsolateral prefrontal cortex alters hypnotizability and sense of agency. A randomized, double-blind and sham-controlled tDCS study. *Behavioral Brain Research*, *3*(425), 113833. 10.1016/j.bbr.2022.113833

Piccione, C., Hilgard, E. R., & Zimbardo, P. G. (1989). On the degree of stability of measured hypnotizability over a 25-year period. *Journal of Personality and Social Psychology*, *56*(2), 289–295. 10.1037/0022-3514.56.2.289

Rainville, P., Duncan, G. H., Price, D. D., Carrier, B., & Bushnell, M. C. (1997). Pain affect encoded in human anterior cingulate but not somatosensory cortex. *Science*, *277*(5328), 968–971. 10.1126/science.277.5328.968

Richardson, J., Smith, J. E., McCall, G., & Pilkington, K. (2006). *Hypnosis for procedure-related pain and distress in pediatric cancer patients: A systematic review of effectiveness and methodology related to hypnosis interventions. Database of Abstracts of Reviews of Effects (DARE):*

Quality-assessed reviews [Internet]. York, UK: Centre for Reviews and Dissemination (UK). https://www.ncbi.nlm.nih.gov/books/NBK72827/

Roberts, M. C., & Ilardi, S. S. (2008). *Handbook of research methods in clinical psychology*. John Wiley & Sons.

Schulz, K. F., Altman, D. G., Moher, D., & CONSORT Group (2010). CONSORT 2010 statement: Updated guidelines for reporting parallel group randomized trials. *Annals of Internal Medicine, 152*(11), 726–732. 10.7326/0003-4819-152-11-201006010-00232

Shadish, W. R., & Cook, T. D. (2002). *Experimental and quasi-experimental designs for generalized causal inference*. Houghton Mifflin and Company.

Shor, R. E., & Orne, E. C. (1962). *Harvard Group Scale of Hypnotic Susceptibility: Form A*. Consulting Psychologists Press.

Society of Harmony (1786–1789). *Annales de la Societe Harmonique des Amis-Reunis de Strasbourg*.

Stern, D. B., Spiegel, H., & Nee, J. C. (1978). The Hypnotic Induction Profile: Normative observations, reliability, and validity. *American Journal of Clinical Hypnosis, 21*(2–3), 109–133. 10.1080/00029157.1978.10403967

Sterne, J. A. C., Savović, J., Page, M. J., Elbers, R. G., Blencowe, N. S., Boutron, I., Cates, C. J., Cheng, H.-Y., Corbett, M. S., Eldridge, S. M., Emberson, J. R., Hernán, M. A., Hopewell, S., Hróbjartsson, A., Junqueira, D. R., Jüni, P., Kirkham, J. J., Lasserson, T., Li, T., McAleenan, A., Reeves, B. C., Shepperd, S., Shrier, I., Stewart, L. A., Tilling, K., White, I. R., Whiting, P. F., & Higgins, J. P. T. (2019). RoB 2: A revised tool for assessing risk of bias in randomised trials. *BMJ, 366*, l4898. 10.1136/bmj.l4898

Thompson, T., Terhune, D. B., Oram, C., Sharangparni, J., Rouf, R., Solmi, M., Veronese, N., & Stubbs, B. (2019). The effectiveness of hypnosis for pain relief: A systematic review and meta-analysis of 85 controlled experimental trials. *Neuroscience and Biobehavioral Reviews, 99*, 298–310. 10.1016/j.neubiorev.2019.02.013

Uman, L. S., Birnie, K. A., Noel, M., Parker, J. A., Chambers, C. T., McGrath, P. J., & Kisely, S. R. (2013). Psychological interventions for needle-related procedural pain and distress in children and adolescents. *The Cochrane Database of Systematic Reviews*, (10), CD005179. 10.1002/14651858.CD005179.pub3

Valentine, K. E., Milling, L. S., Clark, L. J., & Moriarty, C. L. (2019). The efficacy of hypnosis as a treatment for anxiety: A meta-analysis. *The International Journal of Clinical and Experimental Hypnosis, 67*(3), 336–363. 10.1080/00207144.2019.1613863

Weitzenhoffer, A. M., & Hilgard, E. R. (1959). *Stanford Hypnotic Susceptibility Scale, Form A*. Consulting Psychologists Press.

Willmarth, E. K. (2014). Hypnosis and the birth of clinical psychology. In T. H. Leihey, S. Greer, G. R. Lefrancois, T. W. Reiner, J. L. Spencer, I. E. Wickramasekera, & E. K. Willmarth (Eds.), *History of psychology* (pp. 75–100). Bridgepoint Education, Inc.

Zech, N., Hansen, E., Bernardy, K., & Häuser, W. (2017). Efficacy, acceptability and safety of guided imagery/hypnosis in fibromyalgia: A systematic review and meta-analysis of randomized controlled trials. *European Journal of Pain, 21*(2), 217–227. 10.1002/ejp.933

27

THE POTENTIAL ROLE OF HYPNOSIS AND NEUROFEEDBACK IN LINKING NEUROSCIENCE TO PSYCHOTHERAPY

Giuseppe De Benedittis

Associate Professor of Neurosurgery, University of Milano, Italy

Introduction

Hypnosis has long been an elusive concept for science, mainly due to the lack of objective neurobiological markers of the state of trance. Further, the definition of hypnosis is fundamental to scientific inquiry, but the endeavor to define hypnosis from differing theoretical perspectives has given rise to controversy as to the "real" essence of hypnosis. Disagreements are to be expected for two reasons (Elkins et al., 2015). First, the nature and mechanisms that underlie the effects of hypnosis are as yet not fully known. Second, definitions with theoretical bias will inevitably result in arguments about their accuracy. Throughout most of the last decades, the theoretical landscape of hypnosis has been dominated by the state versus nonstate controversy, or, in other words, whether hypnosis is a "process" or a "state", or both (Heap, 2017; Cox & Bryant, 2008).

Given the ontological uncertainty related to hypnosis, the operative definition of APA Division 30 (Elkins et al., 2015) has been adopted, despite its limitations. According to this definition, hypnosis is "a state of consciousness involving focused attention and reduced peripheral awareness characterized by an enhanced capacity for response to suggestion."

From a neurobiological perspective, the relentless advances of neuroscience in the last decades (largely due to the introduction and refinement of sophisticated electrophysiological and neuroimaging techniques) have opened up a "bridge of knowledge" between the classic neurophysiological studies and psychophysiological studies of cognitive, emotional, and sensory systems.

Of course, a bridge is designed to connect two realities bidirectionally. This holds true also for the " hypnotic brain" (De Benedittis, 2012). The term "hypnotic brain" refers to the discrete neurofunctional network in hypnosis and the use of hypnosis as a tool in brain research and clinical practice.

 DOI: 10.4324/9781003449126-37

While the remarkable progress of neuroscience has undoubtedly contributed to unravel the essence of the hypnotic reality, i.e., its neurocognitive structure, (Oakley & Halligan, 2009), on the other hand, hypnosis is increasingly recognized by the international scientific community as a physiological, valid, and flexible tool to explore the central and peripheral nervous system. This overlooked, striking effect, seems really a Copernican revolution in the field (De Benedittis, 2004).

Experimental Neuropsychopathology

A novel, wide array of electrophysiological and neuroimaging techniques contributed to significant advances of our knowledge of hypnotic phenomena, including functional neuroanatomy of neutral hypnosis and neural mechanisms underlying hypnotic processes and responses. These include (a) electrophysiological studies (e.g., bispectral analysis), (b) neuroimaging (e.g., SPECT, fMRI, PET); (c) advanced neuroimaging (e.g., real-time fMRI) and brain–computer interface (BCI), and (d) neurofeedback (NFB).

The most intriguing and advanced frontier of the hypnotic brain is possibly represented by the use of hypnosis as a neuropsychobiological investigation tool in psychotherapy (e.g., assessing psychobiological correlates of experimental unconscious conflicts with electrophysiological and/or neuroimaging techniques).

Experimental neuropsychopathology aims to elucidate the neurocognitive processes that contribute, in whole or in part, to the etiology, exacerbation, or maintenance of abnormal behavior (Zvolensky et al., 2001).

Hypnotic suggestions can serve as an experimental tool for the creation of hypnotic clinical analogues *(virtual patients)* (Oakley & Halligan, 2009) of neurological or psychiatric diseases, in order to gain insights into psychophysiopathological mechanisms and eventual being used appropriately in the therapeutic setting. The instrumental use of hypnotic suggestion provides a powerful methodological approach for cognitive/affective neuroscience to establish both the causal relevance of the specific brain areas activated during the hypnotically induced symptom presentation while comparing those activations in the same subject when performing the task normally (Oakley & Halligan, 2009).

Several studies have demonstrated the feasibility of generating hypnotic analogues for established functional disorders. Hypnotically suggested blindness is a striking phenomenon that provides evidence of congruence with its functional clinical equivalent in conversion disorder (Cox & Bryant, 2008). Neuroanatomical and behavioral observations have been used to identify post-hypnotic memory loss as a viable analogue for functional amnesia (Mendelsohn et al., 2008).

Derbyshire et al. (2004) have used hypnotically suggested pain in normal, pain-free individuals to create a clinical analogue of functional pain. What they found was that the hypnotic pain experience was associated with widespread activation in classic pain areas (thalamus, anterior cingulate cortex, insula, prefrontal cortex, and parietal cortex), similar to that seen with a comparable physically induced pain and proportionate to the level of subjective pain reported. Interestingly, this activation pattern was not seen when participants were asked to imagine the same pain experience in the waking state.

The psychophysiological and behavioral changes observed during the recall of memories in patients who have suffered psychological trauma often resemble the phenomena observed in a trance. Activation of identical brain structures has been observed in studies of strong emotional recall as well as in studies of neuroimaging in hypnosis: thalamus, hippocampus, amygdala, medial prefrontal cortex, anterior cingulate cortex (Bremner & Vermetten, 2004). Therefore, it is plausible that the neural circuits activated in recall of traumatic memories in patients with post-traumatic stress disorder (PTSD) may overlap to some extent with those observed in trance for the recovery of unconscious memories/conflicts.

Hypnotic Modulation of Conflicts in the Human Brain

Increasing evidence suggests that cognitive-emotional conflicts involve the activity of the anterior cingulate cortex (ACC) (Raz et al., 2005). The ACC monitors the occurrence of conflict between incompatible response tendencies and signals this information to a cognitive control system in dorsolateral prefrontal cortex (Raz et al., 2005). Cognitive control is thought to resolve conflict through the attentional biasing of perceptual processing, emphasizing task-relevant stimulus information.

Egner and Hirsch (2005) manipulated levels of conflict and control during a Stroop task using face stimuli, while recording hemodynamic responses from human visual cortex specialized for face processing. They showed that, in response to high conflict, cognitive control mechanisms enhance performance by transiently amplifying cortical responses to task-relevant information rather than by inhibiting responses to task-irrelevant information. These results implicate attentional target-feature amplification as the primary mechanism for conflict resolution through cognitive control and hypnotic state is likely to decouple cognitive control from conflict monitoring processes of the frontal lobe.

Hypothesizing that conflict reduction would be associated with decreased ACC activation, Raz et al. (2005) combined neuroimaging methods and studied highly and less-hypnotizable participants both with and without a suggestion to interpret visual words *(Stroop interference test)* as nonsense strings. The associated increase in activity in ACC in the absence of compensatory changes in left frontal cortical areas has been interpreted as evidence that hypnosis acts to decouple the normal relationship between conflict monitoring and cognitive control, thus confirming previous studies.

Neural Correlates of Psychotherapy (Neuro-Psychotherapy)

In the last decades, Kandel's innovative experiments (Kandel et al., 2021) have demonstrated that brain structures and synaptic connections are dynamic (Mundo, 2006). Synapses can be modified by a wide variety of environmental factors, including learning and memory processes. The hypothesis that psychotherapy process involves memory and learning processes has opened the possibility of a dialogue between neuroscience and related psychotherapy techniques (including hypnosis) (Mundo, 2006).

Preliminary evidence in electrophysiological and neuroimaging studies suggests that dynamic psychotherapy has significant, measurable impact on brain function and metabolism in specific brain areas. These changes can be long-lasting.

Conversely, neurodynamic changes may produce, enhance, and mirror subjective (cognitive/affective) and behavioral changes in the therapeutic setting. Mostly important, BCI allows a real-time therapeutic NFB. This can be the beginning of a new neuro-psychotherapy. NFB, one of the primary examples of self-regulation, designates a collection of techniques that train the brain and help to improve its function in physiological and pathological conditions. NFB is a type of biofeedback that presents real-time feedback from brain activity in order to reinforce or modulate brain function through operant conditioning. Main NFB techniques include EEG-NFB and rtfMRI-NFB.

EEG-NFB

Electroencephalography-neurofeedback (EEG-NFB) involves feedback of real-time EEG recordings of the patient. Typically, electrical activity from the brain is collected via sensors placed on the scalp using electroencephalography (EEG), with feedback presented using video displays or sound (Patel et al., 2021).

EEG measures neural activity on a millisecond timescale allowing us to access the rapidly changing dynamics of neuronal populations. This has made EEG a valuable research tool for understanding brain function for almost a century (Warbrick, 2022). The EEG signal is traditionally analyzed in terms of the power of rhythms in the spontaneous EEG or stimulus or task-specific event-related potentials (ERPs). The most relevant brain oscillations are found in the following frequency bands: delta (0.5–4 Hz), theta (4–8 Hz), alpha (8–13 Hz), beta (13–30 Hz), and gamma (above 30 Hz). ERPs are usually described in terms of the amplitude and latency of the peaks and troughs in the waveform and represent time-locked and/or phase-locked activation of neuronal populations in response to external stimuli, for example, sensory stimulation or cognitive tasks (Patel et al., 2021). Another oscillation which has been widely investigated was sensorimotor rhythm (SMR). SMR refers to oscillations in the 12–15 Hz range which appear in a spindle-like pattern over the sensorimotor cortex during idling of the motor cortex (Timmers, 2014). Since coming on the scene in the 1960s, EEG-NFB has become a treatment vehicle for a host of mental disorders (Omejc et al., 2019); however, its clinical effectiveness remains controversial (Thibault, 2015).

Several NFB protocols exist, with additional benefit from the use of quantitative electroencephalography (Arns et al., 2012). Main clinical applications of EEG-NFB include attention deficit hyperactivity disorder (ADHD), depressive and anxiety disorders, post-brain injury/stroke rehabilitation, epilepsy, and performance enhancement.

EEG-NFB in ADHD

Since the first reports of EEG-NFB treatment in ADHD in 1976, many studies have investigated the effects of NFB on different symptoms of ADHD such as inattention, impulsivity, and hyperactivity. Standard NFB protocols for ADHD including theta/beta, SMR, and slow cortical potentials are well investigated and have demonstrated specificity (Arns et al., 2014). Treatment outcomes have been controversial. Though an investigation into the effectiveness of NFB for ADHD has found NFB to have durable effects following treatment (Van Doren et al., 2019), two other studies (Lansberger et al., 2011; Rahmani, 2022) have contradicted this conclusion, showing that there is no significant benefit of NFB treatment compared with other treatments or control conditions. The results provide preliminary evidence that NFB treatment is not an effective clinical method for ADHD and suggest that more RTCs are needed to compare common treatment.

EEG-NFB in Psychiatric Disorders

NFB training has been found to be beneficial for patients for depression and self- regulation (Mehler et al., 2018). Individuals with PTSD also have been found to benefit from EEG-NFB.

A systematic review (Steingrimmson et al., 2020) aimed to assess whether EEG-NFB, compared with sham NFB, other treatment, or no treatment, is effective for PTSD. Four randomized controlled trials (RCTs) were included (123 participants). Results were consistently in favor of EEG-NFB with large effect sizes. The certainty of evidence was assessed as very low for the four assessed outcomes. Based on four RCTs, it is uncertain whether EEG-NFB reduces suicidal thoughts, PTSD symptoms, medication use, or improves function. Although all studies showed promising results, further investigations are needed to increase the certainty of evidence. Zafarmand (2022) recently provided preliminary evidence that EEG-NFB is an efficacious method for obsessive-compulsive disorder and suggests that more clinical trials are needed to compare common treatment such as medication, neurological, and behavioral interventions.

EEG-NFB in Epilepsy

About one third of patients with epilepsy do not benefit from medical treatment. For these patients, EEG biofeedback is a viable alternative (Tan, 2009). While dozens of scientific reports have been published on NFB for seizure disorder, most have been case series with too few subjects to establish efficacy. The most common protocol for seizure control was SMR, which was found to significantly reduce weekly seizures (Tan et al., 2009). In a meta-analysis on the role of EEG-NFB on epilepsy treatment, Tan et al. (2009) reported an overall mean decreased seizure incidence following treatment, and 64 out of 87 patients (74%) reported fewer weekly seizures in response to EEG biofeedback. Based on this meta-analysis, EEG operant conditioning was found to produce a significant reduction in seizure frequency. This finding is especially noteworthy given the patient group, individuals who had been unable to control their seizures with medical treatment.

EEG-NFB in Chronic Pain

A meta-analysis (Patel et al., 2020) investigated on the efficacy of EEG-NFB in chronic pain patients. Twenty-one studies were included. Reduction in pain following NFB was reported by one high-quality RCT, five of six low-quality RCT or NRCT, and 13 of 14 case series. Pain reduction reported by studies ranged from 6% to 82%, with ten studies reporting a clinically significant reduction in pain of >30%. The overall effect size was medium. These findings were confirmed by a more recent study by Hesam-Shariati (2022). The NFB protocols in both RCTs and non-randomized studies mainly involved the conventional EEG NFB approach, which targeted reinforcing either alpha or SMRs and suppressing theta and/or beta bands on one brain region at a time. A post-hoc analysis of RCTs utilizing the conventional approach resulted in a clinically meaningful effect estimate for pain intensity.

EEG-NFB in Neurorehabilitation

NFB has also been used to treat traumatic brain injury (May et al., 2013). It has also been found to be generally positive for stroke recovery, with improvements found in motor function and behavior comparable with conventional occupational therapy (Rayegani et al., 2014). In a systematic review, Renton (2017) showed that majority of studies identified improvements in participant cognitive deficits following the initiation of therapy, though limited study quality and strength of evidence restricted generalizability of conclusions regarding the use of this therapy to the greater stroke population.

EEG-NFB and Performance Enhancement

Finally, the applications of NFB to enhance performance extend to the arts in fields such as music, dance, and acting. Historically, alpha-theta training, a form of NFB, was created to assist creativity by inducing "hypnagogia", a "borderline waking state associated with creative insights", through facilitation of neural connectivity (Gruzelier, 2011).

rtfMRI-NFB

BOLD (blood oxygen level dependent) fMRI can be considered a correlate of neural activity rather than a measure of neural activity since it represents the complex process of neurovascular coupling and the interaction of circulatory and metabolic demands (Warbrick, 2022). These changes in blood flow occur seconds after neural activity changes, much more slowly than the millisecond timescale on which we measure EEG. Therefore, the temporal resolution of BOLD fMRI is limited by the slow hemodynamic response (Logothetis et al., 2001); however, fMRI provides a sub-millimetre spatial resolution that can be achieved, thus allowing the spatial localization of brain activity that we cannot achieve with EEG.

Neuroimaging can contribute to cognitive training in a number of ways (Cramer et al., 2011). fMRI can help to identify the neural correlates of various core mental processes that can be targeted by cognitive training and that are relevant for a number of psychiatric disorders (Dahlin et al., 2008; Persson & Reuter-Lorenz, 2008). fMRI has been limited by time-consuming data analysis and a low signal-to-noise ratio, impeding online analysis. Recent advances in acquisition techniques, computational power, and algorithms increased the sensitivity and speed of fMRI significantly, making real-time fMRI (rtfMRI) feasible and reliable (Cox et al., 1995). rtfMRI allows for BCI with a high spatial and temporal resolution and whole-brain coverage, while adding a high level of interactivity. Recent studies have shown that such BCI can be used to provide online feedback of the BOLD signal (Caria et al., 2007; deCharms, 2008; Weiskopf et al., 2007). Proof-of-concept for rtfMRI as a potential tool for harnessing plasticity in brain function, cognition, and behavior as well as for the treatment of brain disorders was demonstrated in 2005 by deCharms et al.

It has now become possible to image the functioning of the human brain in real time using rtfMRI, and thereby to access both sides of the mind–brain interface – subjective experience (that is, one's mind) and objective observations (that is, external, quantitative measurements of one's brain activity) – simultaneously. Developments in neuroimaging have undergone a rapid development since then, now being translated into many new potential practical applications, including the reading of brain states and learning self-control over local brain activity to modulate cognitive regions in response to intrinsic or extrinsic stimuli as well to evaluate the effects of various interventions (Caria et al., 2007; deCharms, 2008; Weiskopf et al., 2007). Behavioral effects such as modulation of pain, reaction time, cognitive or emotional processing have been shown in healthy and/or patient populations (Weiskopf, 2012).

RtfMRI NFB presents a new paradigm for studying the relationship between brain behavior, physiology, and pathology (Weiskopf, 2012). The rationale of this approach is quite obvious: if an individual can learn to directly control activation of localized regions within the brain, this might provide control over the neurophysiological mechanisms that mediate behavior and cognition and could potentially provide a different route for treating disease. Various regions of interest (ROI) have been studied with rtfMRI NFB. Studies investigated self-regulation in the primary motor (M1), somatosensory (S1) cortex, left Broca area together with the auditory association areas which are related to speech generation and the parahippocampal place area which is known to process visual information. Moreover, higher cognitive areas such as the affective/cognitive (ACad/ACcd) subdivision of the ACC, and the amygdala (Amygdala) involved in affective processing were chosen as target regions (Weiskopf et al., 2004). These brain areas have a wide range of functions, including movement, tactile sensation, visual perception, hearing, emotion, and pain.

A central goal of psychotherapy is that the patient and the therapist better understand and ultimately change the patient's cognitive processes and its neurophysiological correlates. Patients and clinicians might benefit from watching the brain as it functions during this process. Preliminary evidence suggests that local self-regulation can be used as a new paradigm in cognitive/affective neuroscience to study brain plasticity and the functional relevance of brain areas, even being potentially applicable for psychophysiological treatment (Cozolino, 2010; Weiskopf, 2012). In fact, potential therapeutic application for rtfMRI is in augmenting psychotherapy and in measuring the effects of psychotherapy on the brain. rtfMRI data can potentially be used as a quantitative endpoint to objectively measure the impact on the brain of individuals before, during, and after therapeutic interventions.

rtfMRI-NFB Self-Regulation of ROIs

Several studies have set out to determine the extent to which someone can learn to control activation in individual brain regions, initially focusing on the somatomotor cortex as this region seemed likely to be particularly easy to control (deCharms, 2008) by imagining moving the part of their body that corresponds to the area of the somatomotor cortex that is being monitored. After repeated training using the rtfMRI signal from a brain region to learn to guide the strategies they use to alter the activity of that brain region, most subjects succeed in learning increased control over activation in the targeted brain region.

rtfMRI-NFB Self-Regulation of Pain

By using rtfMRI, deCharms et al. (2005, 2008) found that subjects were able to learn to control activation in the rostral anterior cingulate cortex (rACC), a region putatively involved in pain perception and regulation. When subjects deliberately induced increases or decreases in rACC rtfMRI activation, there was a corresponding change in the perception of pain caused by an applied noxious thermal stimulus. These findings show that individuals can gain voluntary control over activation in rACC, concomitantly leading to control over pain perception, and that these effects were powerful enough to impact severe, chronic clinical pain. This effect was not observed after similar training conducted without rtfMRI information, or using rtfMRI information derived from a different brain region, or sham rtfMRI information derived previously from a different subject. rtfMRI feedback was used to train both healthy controls and chronic pain patients to modulate ACC activation for the purposes of altering pain experience (Chapin, 2012). Both groups improved in their ability to control ACC activation and modulate their pain with rtfMRI feedback training. Furthermore, the degree to which participants were able to modulate their pain correlated with the degree of control over ACC activation.

rtfMRI-NFB Self-Regulation in Affective and Anxiety Disorders

Experiments have shown that participants, while lying inside a scanner, can be trained to control their emotions while viewing real-time activation from areas that are involved in emotional processing. Caria et al. (2007) investigated whether healthy subjects could voluntarily gain control over right anterior insular activity. All participants were able to successfully regulate the activity in the right anterior insular cortex within three sessions of 4 min each. Training resulted in a significantly increased activation cluster in the anterior portion of the right insula across sessions. The increased activity in the right anterior insula during training demonstrates that the effects observed are anatomically specific and self-regulation of right anterior insula only is achievable. This was the first study investigating the volitional control of emotionally relevant brain regions by using rtfMRI training.

Traumatic memories are diagnostic symptoms of PTSD, and the dual representation theory posits separate memory systems subserving vivid re-experiencing (non-hippocampally dependent) versus declarative autobiographical memories (AM) of trauma (hippocampally dependent) (Kim & Diamond, 2002). But the psychopathological signs of trauma are not static over time, nor is the expression of traumatic memories. Multiple memory systems are activated simultaneously and in parallel on various occasions. Neural circuitry interaction is a crucial aspect in the development of a psychotherapeutic approach that may favor an integrative translation of the sensory fragments of the traumatic memory into a declarative memory system. The relationship between neuroimaging findings and psychological approaches may be relevant for greater efficacy in the treatment of psychologically traumatized patients (see review in Peres & Nasello, 2008). Traumatic experiences are associated with neurofunctional dysregulations in key regions of the emotion regulation (ER) circuits. In particular, amygdala responsivity to negative stimuli is exaggerated while engagement of prefrontal regulatory control regions is attenuated. Zweerings (2020) hypothesized that a single session of real-time fMRI-guided upregulation of prefrontal regions during an ER task enhances self-control during exposure to negative stimuli and facilitates transfer of the learned ER skills to daily life. Their findings suggest beneficial effects of the NF training indicated by reduced amygdala responses that were associated with improved symptom severity and affective state four weeks after the NF training as well as patient-centered perceived control during the training, helpfulness, and application of strategies in daily life.

deCharms (2008) performed a pilot study demonstrating the use of rtfMRI during cognitive behavioral therapy for an anxiety disorder as a potential means for measuring and augmenting the technique using rtfMRI during a psychiatric treatment session disorder, In this study, patients with obsessive–compulsive disorder received a specially adapted form of cognitive therapy while lying inside a scanner and watching the activation in brain regions that are associated with anxiety disorder. The patients were primarily asked to monitor and learn to control their own brain activation while they also interacted with their therapist through a two-way audio system.

rtfMRI-NFB left amygdala (LA) training is a promising intervention for major depressive disorder (MDD) (Tsuchiyagaito et al., 2021). The authors have previously proposed that rtfMRI-NFB LA training may reverse depression-associated regional impairments in neuroplasticity and restore information flow within emotion-regulating neural circuits. A recent systematic review (Young et al., 2018) shows that both healthy individuals and unmedicated patients with MDD can significantly increase their amygdala response to positive AM recall via rtfMRI-NFB training. Furthermore, they are able to maintain this response following training and in the absence of NFB information suggesting both short term and long-term transference of learning/ability to maintain this learned response in the absence of NFB information. In patients with MDD, significant improvements in clinical symptoms were observed, along with improvements in memory and attention for positive stimuli. Though changes in the processing of negative stimuli were also evident following NFB training, only changes to positive stimuli were associated with measures of clinical improvement and NFB success. This suggests the enhancement of the processing of positive emotional information, rather than suppression of the processing of negative, that underlies the clinical effects of our amygdala NFB paradigm.

rtfMRI-NFB has gained popularity as an experimental treatment for a variety of psychiatric illnesses. However, there has yet to be a quantitative review regarding its efficacy. Dudek and Dodell-Feder (2021) presented the first meta-analysis of rtfMRI-NFB for psychiatric disorders. Literature review identified 17 studies. The neural effects of rtfMRI-NFB were often evaluated in two contexts: (a) when participants were regulating while receiving NFB ("training sessions"), and (b) when participants were regulating in the absence of NFB ("transfer sessions") toward evaluating whether regulation can be sustained in a context without receiving a feedback signal, as in one's daily life. They found that rtfMRI-NFB produces a medium-sized effect on neural activity during training, a large-sized effect after training when no NFB is provided and small-sized effects for behavioral outcomes Together, these data suggest a positive impact of rtfMRI-NFB on brain and behavioral outcomes, although more research is needed to determine how rtfMRI-NFB works, for whom, and under what circumstances.

rtfMRI-NFB Self-Regulation in ADHD Patients

ADHD is characterized by poor cognitive control/attention and hypofunctioning of the dorsal anterior cingulate cortex (dACC). In a recent study, Zilverstand (2017) investigated for the first time whether rtfMRI training targeted at increasing activation levels within dACC in adults with ADHD leads to a reduction of clinical symptoms and improved cognitive functioning. Results showed that both groups achieved a significant increase in dACC activation levels over sessions. While there was no significant difference between the NFB and control group in clinical outcome, NFB participants showed stronger improvement on cognitive functioning. This study demonstrates the general feasibility of the suggested rt-fMRI NFB training approach as a potential novel treatment option for ADHD patients.

Unsolved Issues

Though promising on many aspects, a number of issues remain to be addressed to maximize the impact of neuroimaging on cognitive training (Cramer et al., 2011). Most imaging studies have been performed on small samples, with differing approaches, such as in relation to the underlying hypotheses of mechanisms of training-induced change, and further studies are needed regarding the validity and reliability of neuroimaging data. Critically important is the question of whether changes in circuit strength demonstrated using neuroimaging are paralleled by meaningful behavioral changes and determine whether they are replicable and are truly due to control over brain activation on the basis of rtfMRI rather than due to other unspecific moderators such as expectation or placebo effects. Another important challenge for the application of rtfMRI NFB for any clinical or other training purposes is the transfer (Brühl, 2015). Transfer means two things: (1) transferring the control acquired while receiving fMRI feedback into a situation without feedback (task in fMRI without feedback, task outside the MRI without feedback), and (2) transferring the learned skill onto other tasks or processes, at best into reality and into a function where the learned skill will be helpful in everyday life. Transfer is necessary for rtfMRI NFB training to be applied in reality, because the skill should also be applicable outside the scanner without the feedback to be useful. At the moment, many studies show good acquisition of control inside the scanner, but the evidence for ongoing behavioral changes in real life after the training is limited (Stoeckel et al., 2014). Most studies are still at the level of pilot studies, testing the feasibility of such methods in patients, and were not designed with the same rigorous design and measures as in clinical trials (e.g., no placebo treatment, no comparison with gold-standard therapy, only completers reported, no intention to treat analysis, no clinical outcome measures reported, no transfer/generalization reported). Therefore, the clinical application of rtfMRI NFB should still be considered to be at an experimental stage, requiring more research at the preclinical stage.

Limitations

NFB studies are still in their infancy. The complex relationships between subjective experience (cognitive, affective, relational), behavioral patterns, and objective neural correlates can be better approached with a neurophenomenological perspective (Varela, 1999), but very little research has been done so far, due to methodological and technical problems (e.g., limited availability of rtfMRI for clinical practice). Future clinical and experimental research should address this crucial issue, that might advance our understanding of these complex relationships (Cardeña et al., 2013; Lifshitz et al., 2013).

Therapy during brain imaging has obvious challenges: the patient and therapist have far less direct interaction than is typically desired and the setting is confining, foreign, and possibly frightening. As rtfMRI requires expensive equipment, cost is an important factor in considering whether rtfMRI-based treatments are feasible for any particular condition. The focus should be on severe conditions for which less-expensive forms of therapy are not available. In addition, manufacturers are developing new technologies to make MRI scanners smaller, cheaper, and increasingly suitable for the physician's office (deCharms, 2008).

Simultaneous EEG and rtfMRI NFB

rtfMRI with high spatial resolution does not provide adequate temporal sampling due to the slow BOLD response (in order of seconds) unlike EEG instead offers a high temporal resolution (in the order of milliseconds), but with a poor localization of signal sources (Mele et al., 2019). Given the strengths and deficits of both EEG and rtfMRI NFB, combining them has the potential to provide insight into brain function that cannot be measured by one modality on its own. Though both EEG and rtfMRI have been used separately in NFB, their combination in this context is relatively new. Simultaneous real-time fMRI and EEG NFB combines real-time NFB from both modalities to simultaneously regulate both hemodynamic and electrophysiological brain activities (Mele et al., 2019). Furthermore, the concurrent measurement of EEG-fMRI has demonstrated the potential of the technique to facilitate the development of clinical interventions, holding great promise for the future. The first application of rtfMRI-EEG-NFB for emotion self-regulation training in patients with MDD has been reported by Zotev et al. (2020). The experimental group participants reported significant mood improvements after the training. Results suggest that the rtfMRI-EEG-NFB may have potential for treatment of MDD.

The Potential Role of Hypnosis in Self-Regulatory Techniques

Hypnosis has been shown to foster brain neuroplasticity possibly by inducing epigenetic changes (Doidge, 2015). Further, it offers powerful techniques to isolate psychological processes in order to gain insights into their neural bases, thus optimizing clinical approaches (Barnier & McConkey, 2003; Woody & Szechtman, 2011). Given the established "greater cognitive flexibility" of hypnosis and self-hypnosis in self-regulatory processes and strategies (De Benedittis, 2015), it is plausible that the hypnotic approach can be similar to other processes of self-regulation using real-time technology (i.e., NFB). Whereas cognitive neuroscience has scantily fostered hypnosis as a manipulation, NFB techniques, namely EEG-NFB and rtfMRI-NFB, offer new opportunities to use hypnosis and posthypnotic suggestion as probes into brain mechanisms and, reciprocally, provide a means of studying hypnosis itself. In addition, these new innovative tools can be the neurophenomenological link between neuroscience and psychotherapy in the hypnotic setting.

This chapter advocates the potential role of hypnosis in self-regulatory strategies (hypno-NFB) and how the hypnotic state can serve as a way to tap neurocognitive questions and how cognitive assays can in turn shed new light on the neural bases of hypnosis. This cross talk should enhance research and clinical applications (Raz & Shapiro, 2002).

Conclusions and Future Directions

A new ambitious area of research is focusing to map the core processes of psychotherapy and the neurobiology underlying them. Practitioners should consider adding this perspective to their toolkits, because data show that only 15% of therapy success is related to the type of therapy you practice (specific effect); the therapeutic alliance, environmental factors, and even the placebo effect play a far greater role (Beitman, 2005).

The next target is clear: let's figure out the common denominators of effective therapy, what is actually going on in the neurocircuitry of patients and therapists during psychotherapy. Hypnosis may be the appropriate tool to bridging the gap between neuroscience and psychotherapy.

Eventually practitioners will be able to use information gleaned about affected brain circuitry and tailor treatments to modify those circuits through the most efficient means, whether via psychotherapy, medication, or other interventions.

Examples of the use of hypnotic suggestion to create analogues of functional, quasi-neurological (conversion) disorders such as limb paralysis, "hysterical" blindness, and functional pain, and of psychiatric symptoms such as auditory hallucinations and PTSD have been presented. A similar approach could be profitably extended in future research to other neuropsychological and psychiatric disorders.

The ultimate goal of cognitive training is to improve behavior by systematically harnessing neuroplasticity and driving adaptive changes in dysfunctional neural systems through carefully designed training (Cramer et al., 2011). Systems neuroscience-informed cognitive training appears to be a promising treatment approach for a number of brain disorders. A key future direction for this field will be to investigate whether hypnosis might maximize the extent to which cognitive training in one domain generalizes to others, and the extent to which such training has a meaningful impact on real-world functioning as well as the subjective experience of the individual (Green & Bavelier, 2008).

References

Arns, M., Drinkenburg, W., & Leon Kenemans, J. (2012). The effects of QEEG-informed neurofeedback in ADHD: An open-label pilot study. *Applied Psychophysiology and Biofeedback*, *37*(3), 171–180. 10.1007/s10484-012-9191-4

Arns, M., Heinrich, H., & Strehl, U. (2014). Evaluation of neurofeedback in ADHD: The long and winding road. *Biological Psychology*, *95*, 108–115. 10.1016/j.biopsycho.2013.11.013

Barnier, A. J., & McConkey, K. M. (2003). Hypnosis, human nature, and complexity: Integrating neuroscience approaches into hypnosis research. *International Journal of Clinical and Experimental Hypnosis*, *51*(3), 282–308. 10.1076/iceh.51.3.282.15524

Beitman, B. D. (2005). Defining the core processes of psychotherapy. *The American Journal of Psychiatry*, *162*(8), 1549–1550; author reply 1550. 10.1176/appi.ajp.162.8.1549-a

Bremner, J. D., & Vermetten, E. (2004). Neuroanatomical changes associated with pharmacotherapy in posttraumatic stress disorder. *Annals of the New York Academy of Sciences*, *1032*, 154–157. 10.1196/annals.1314.012

Brühl, A. B. (2015). Making sense of real-time functional magnetic resonance imaging (rtfMRI) and rtfMRI neurofeedback. *International Journal of Neuropsychopharmacology*, *18*(6), pyv020. 10.1093/ijnp/pyv020

Cardeña, E., Jönsson, P., Terhune, D. B., Marcusson-Clavertz, D. (2013). The neurophenomenology of neutral hypnosis. *Cortex*, *49*(2), 375–385. doi: 10.1016/j.cortex.2012.04.001. Epub 2012 Apr 11. PMID: 22579225.

Caria, A., Veit, R., Sitaram, R., Lotze, M., Weiskopf, N., Grodd, W., & Birbaumer, N. (2007). Regulation of anterior insular cortex activity using real-time fMRI. *NeuroImage*, *35*(3), 1238–1246. 10.1016/j.neuroimage.2007.01.018

Chapin, H., Bagarinao, E., & Mackey, S. (2012). Real-time fMRI applied to pain management. *Neuroscience Letters*, *520*(2), 174–181. 10.1016/j.neulet.2012.02.076

Cox, R. E. , & Bryant, R. A. (2008). Advances in hypnosis research: Methods, designs and contributions of intrinsic and instrumental hypnosis. In M. R. Nash, & A. J. Barnier (Eds), *The Oxford handbook of hypnosis: Theory, research, and practice* (pp. 311-336). Oxford University Press.

Cox, R. W., Jesmanowicz, A., & Hyde, J. S. (1995). Real-time functional magnetic resonance imaging. *Magnetic Resonance in Medicine*, *33*(2), 230–236. 10.1002/mrm.1910330213

Cozolino, L. J. (2010). *The neuroscience of psychotherapy: Healing the social brain* (2nd ed). W.W. Norton & Co.

Cramer, S. C., Sur, M., Dobkin, B. H., O'Brien, C., Sanger, T. D., Trojanowski, J. Q., Rumsey, J. M., Hicks, R., Cameron, J., Chen, D., Chen, W. G., Cohen, L. G., deCharms, C., Duffy, C. J., Eden, G. F., Fetz, E. E., Filart, R., Freund, M., Grant, S. J.,& Vinogradov, S. (2011). Harnessing neuroplasticity for clinical applications. *Brain: A Journal of Neurology, 134*(Pt 6), 1591–1609. 10.1093/brain/awr039

Dahlin, E., Neely, A. S., Larsson, A., Bäckman, L., & Nyberg, L. (2008). Transfer of learning after updating training mediated by the striatum. *Science, 320*, 1510–1512.

De Benedittis, G. (2004). Introduzione: Una rivoluzione copernicana? *Editoriale*. Ipnosi, *1*, 9–13.

De Benedittis, G. (2012). The hypnotic brain: Linking neuroscience to psychotherapy. *Contemporary Hypnosis and Integrative Therapy, 29*(1), 103–115.

De Benedittis, G. (2015). Neural mechanisms of hypnosis and meditation. *Journal of Physiology-Paris, 109*, 152–164. 10.1016/j.jphysparis.2015.11.001

deCharms, R. C. (2008). Applications of real-time fMRI. *Nature Reviews. Neuroscience, 9*(9), 720–729. 10.1038/nrn2414

deCharms, R. C., Maeda, F., Glover, G. H., Ludlow, D., Pauly, J. M., Soneji, D., Gabrieli, J. D. E., & Mackey, S. C. (2005). Control over brain activation and pain learned by using real-time functional MRI. *Proceedings of the National Academy of Sciences, 102*(51), 18626–18631. 10.1073/pnas.0505210102

Derbyshire, S. W. G., Whalley, M. G., Stenger, V. A., & Oakley, D. A. (2004). Cerebral activation during hypnotically induced and imagined pain. *NeuroImage, 23*(1), 392–401. 10.1016/j.neuroimage.2004.04.033

Doidge, N. (2015). Hypnosis, neuroplasticity, and the plastic paradox. *American Journal of Clinical Hypnosis. 57*(3), 349–354. doi: 10.1080/00029157.2015.985572. PMID: 25928683.

Dudek, E., & Dodell-Feder, D. (2021). The efficacy of real-time functional magnetic resonance imaging neurofeedback for psychiatric illness: A meta-analysis of brain and behavioral outcomes. *Neuroscience and Biobehavioral Reviews, 121*, 291–306. 10.1016/j.neubiorev.2020.12.020

Egner, T., & Hirsch, J. (2005). Where memory meets attention: Neural substrates of negative priming. *Journal of Cognitive Neuroscience, 17*(11), 1774–1784. 10.1162/089892905774589226

Elkins, G. R., Barabasz, A. F., Council, J. R., Spiegel D. (2015). Advancing research and practice: The revised APA Division 30 definition of hypnosis. *International Journal of Clinical and Experimental Hypnosis, 63*(1), 1–9. doi: 10.1080/00207144.2014.961870. PMID: 25365125.

Green, C. S., & Bavelier, D. (2008). Exercising your brain: A review of human brain plasticity and training-induced learning. *Psychology and Aging, 23*(4), 692–701. 10.1037/a0014345

Gruzelier, J. (2011). Neurofeedback and the performing arts. *Neuroscience Letters, 500*, e15. 10.1016/j.neulet.2011.05.106

Heap, M. (2017). Theories of hypnosis. In Elkins, G. T. (ed.), *Handbook of medical and psychological hypnosis* (pp. 9–18). Springer Publishing.

Hesam-Shariati, N., Chang, W.-J., Wewege, M. A., McAuley, J. H., Booth, A., Trost, Z., Lin, C.-T., Newton-John, T., & Gustin, S. M. (2022). The analgesic effect of electroencephalographic neurofeedback for people with chronic pain: A systematic review and meta-analysis. *European Journal of Neurology, 29*(3), 921–936. 10.1111/ene.15189

Kandel, E. R., Koester, J. G., Mack, S. H., Siegelbaum, S. A. (2021). *Principles of neural science*, 6th ed., McGraw-Hill.

Kim, J. J. & Diamond, D. M. (2002). The stressed hippocampus, synaptic plasticity and lost memories. *Nature Reviews Neuroscience, 3*(6), 453–462. doi: 10.1038/nrn849. PMID: 12042880.

Lansbergen, M. M., van Dongen-Boomsma, M., Buitelaar, J. K., & Slaats-Willemse, D. (2011). ADHD and EEG-neurofeedback: A double-blind randomized placebo-controlled feasibility study. *Journal of Neural Transmission, 118*(2), 275–284. 10.1007/s00702-010-0524-2

Lifshitz, M., Cusumano, E. P., & Raz, A. (2013). Hypnosis as neurophenomenology. *Frontiers in Human Neuroscience, 7*, 469. doi: 10.3389/fnhum.2013.00469. PMID: 23966930; PMCID: PMC3744032.

Logothetis, N. K., Pauls, J., Augath, M., Trinath, T., & Oeltermann, A. (2001). Neurophysiological investigation of the basis of the fMRI signal. *Nature, 412*(6843), 150–157. 10.1038/35084005

May, G., Benson, R., Balon, R., & Boutros, N. (2013). Neurofeedback and traumatic brain injury: A literature review. *Annals of Clinical Psychiatry: Official Journal of the American Academy of Clinical Psychiatrists, 25*(4), 289–296.

Mehler, D. M. A., Sokunbi, M. O., Habes, I., Barawi, K., Subramanian, L., Range, M., Evans, J., Hood, K., Lührs, M., Keedwell, P., Goebel, R., & Linden, D. E. J. (2018). Targeting the affective brain—A randomized controlled trial of real-time fMRI neurofeedback in patients with depression. *Neuropsychopharmacology*, *43*(13), 2578–2585. 10.1038/s41386-018-0126-5

Mele, G., Cavaliere, C., Alfano, V., Orsini, M., Salvatore, M., & Aiello, M. (2019). Simultaneous EEG-fMRI for functional neurological assessment. *Frontiers in Neurology*, *10*, 848. 10.3389/fneur.2019.00848

Mendelsohn, A., Chalamish, Y., Solomonovich, A., & Dudai, Y. (2008). Mesmerizing memories: Brain substrates of episodic memory suppression in posthypnotic amnesia. *Neuron*, *57*(1), 159–170. 10.1016/j.neuron.2007.11.022

Mundo, E. (2006). Neurobiology of dynamic psychotherapy: An integration possible? *The Journal of the American Academy of Psychoanalysis and Dynamic Psychiatry*, *34*(4), 679–691. 10.1521/jaap.2006.34.4.679

Oakley, D. A., & Halligan, P. W. (2009). Hypnotic suggestion and cognitive neuroscience. *Trends in Cognitive Sciences*, *13*(6), 264–270. 10.1016/j.tics.2009.03.004

Omejc, N., Rojc, B., Battaglini, P. P., & Marusic, U. (2019). Review of the therapeutic neurofeedback method using electroencephalography: EEG Neurofeedback. *Bosnian Journal of Basic Medical Sciences*, *19*, 213–220. 10.17305/bjbms.2018.3785

Patel, K., Henshaw, J., Sutherland, H., Taylor, J. R., Casson, A. J., Lopez-Diaz, K., Brown, C. A., Jones, A. K. P., Sivan, M., & Trujillo-Barreto, N. J. (2021). Using EEG alpha states to understand learning during alpha neurofeedback training for chronic pain. *Frontiers in Neuroscience*, *14*, 620666. 10.3389/fnins.2020.620666

Peres, J., & Nasello, A. G. (2008). Psychotherapy and neuroscience: Towards closer integration. *International Journal of Psychology: Journal International De Psychologie*, *43*(6), 943–957. 10.1080/00207590701248487

Persson, J., & Reuter-Lorenz, P. A. (2008). Gaining control: Training executive function and far transfer of the ability to resolve interference. *Psychological Science*, *19*(9), 881–888. 10.1111/j.1467-9280.2008.02172.x

Rahmani, E., Mahvelati, A., Alizadeh, A., Mokhayeri, Y., Rahmani, M., Zarabi, H., & Hassanvandi, S. (2022). Is neurofeedback effective in children with ADHD? A systematic review and meta-analysis. *Neurocase*, *28*(1), 84–95. 10.1080/13554794.2022.2027456

Rayegani, S. M., Raeissadat, S. A., Sedighipour, L., Rezazadeh, I. M., Bahrami, M. H., Eliaspour, D., & Khosrawi, S. (2014). Effect of neurofeedback and electromyographic-biofeedback therapy on improving hand function in stroke patients. *Topics in Stroke Rehabilitation*, *21*(2), 137–151. 10.1310/tsr2102-137

Raz, A., & Shapiro, T. (2002). Hypnosis and neuroscience. *Archives of General Psychiatry*, *59*, 85. 10.1001/archpsyc.59.1.85

Raz, A., Fan, J., & Posner, M. I. (2005). Hypnotic suggestion reduces conflict in the human brain. *Proceedings of the National Academy of Sciences of the United States of America*, *102*(28), 9978–9983. 10.1073/pnas.0503064102

Renton, T., Tibbles, A., & Topolovec-Vranic, J. (2017). Neurofeedback as a form of cognitive rehabilitation therapy following stroke: A systematic review. *PloS One*, *12*(5), e0177290. 10.1371/journal.pone.0177290

Steingrimsson, S., Bilonic, G., Ekelund, A.-C., Larson, T., Stadig, I., Svensson, M., Vukovic, I. S., Wartenberg, C., Wrede, O., & Bernhardsson, S. (2020). Electroencephalography-based neurofeedback as treatment for post-traumatic stress disorder: A systematic review and meta-analysis. *European Psychiatry: The Journal of the Association of European Psychiatrists*, *63*(1), e7. 10.1192/j.eurpsy.2019.7

Stoeckel, L. E., Garrison, K. A., Ghosh, S., Wighton, P., Hanlon, C. A., Gilman, J. M., Greer, S., Turk-Browne, N. B., deBettencourt, M. T., Scheinost, D., Craddock, C., Thompson, T., Calderon, V., Bauer, C. C., George, M., Breiter, H. C., Whitfield-Gabrieli, S., Gabrieli, J. D., LaConte, S. M., … Evins, A. E. (2014). Optimizing real time fMRI neurofeedback for therapeutic discovery and development. *NeuroImage. Clinical*, *5*, 245–255. 10.1016/j.nicl.2014.07.002

Tan, G., Thornby, J., Hammond, D. C., Strehl, U., Canady, B., Arnemann, K., & Kaiser, D. A. (2009). Meta-analysis of EEG biofeedback in treating epilepsy. *Clinical EEG and Neuroscience*, *40*(3), 173–179. 10.1177/155005940904000310

Thibault, R. T., Lifshitz, M., Birbaumer, N., & Raz, A. (2015). Neurofeedback, self-regulation, and brain imaging: Clinical science and Fad in the service of mental disorders. *Psychotherapy and Psychosomatics*, *84*(4), 193–207. 10.1159/000371714

Timmers, D. (2014). Treating attention deficits and impulse control. In D. S. Cantor , & J. R. Evans (Eds.), *Clinical neurotherapy* (pp. 139–169). Elsevier. 10.1016/B978-0-12-396988-0.00006-4

Tsuchiyagaito, A., Smith, J. L., El-Sabbagh, N., Zotev, V., Misaki, M., Al Zoubi, O., Kent Teague, T., Paulus, M. P., Bodurka, J., & Savitz, J. (2021). Real-time fMRI neurofeedback amygdala training may influence kynurenine pathway metabolism in major depressive disorder. *NeuroImage. Clinical*, *29*, 102559. 10.1016/j.nicl.2021.102559

Van Doren, J., Arns, M., Heinrich, H., Vollebregt, M. A., Strehl, U., & K Loo, S. (2019). Sustained effects of neurofeedback in ADHD: A systematic review and meta-analysis. *European Child & Adolescent Psychiatry*, *28*(3), 293–305. 10.1007/s00787-018-1121-4

Varela, F. J. (1999). The specious present: A neurophenomenology of time consciousness. In J. Petitot, F. J. Varela, B. Pachoud, & J.-M. Roy (Eds.), *Naturalizing phenomenology: Issues in contemporary phenomenology and cognitive science* (pp. 266–314). Stanford University Press.

Warbrick, T. (2022). Simultaneous EEG-fMRI: What have we learned and what does the future hold? *Sensors (Basel, Switzerland)*, *22*(6), 2262. 10.3390/s22062262

Weiskopf, N. (2012). Real-time fMRI and its application to neurofeedback. *NeuroImage*, *62*(2), 682–692. 10.1016/j.neuroimage.2011.10.009

Weiskopf, N., Scharnowski, F., Veit, R., Goebel, R., Birbaumer, N., & Mathiak, K. (2004). Self-regulation of local brain activity using real-time functional magnetic resonance imaging (fMRI). *Journal of Physiology, Paris*, *98*(4–6), 357–373. 10.1016/j.jphysparis.2005.09.019

Weiskopf, N., Sitaram, R., Josephs, O., Veit, R., Scharnowski, F., Goebel, R., Birbaumer, N., Deichmann, R., & Mathiak, K. (2007). Real-time functional magnetic resonance imaging: Methods and applications. *Magnetic Resonance Imaging*, *25*(6), 989–1003. 10.1016/j.mri.2007.02.007

Woody, E.& Szechtman, H. (2011). Using hypnosis to develop and test models of psychopathology, *The Journal of Mind-Body Regulation*, https://www.researchgate.net/publication/267386132

Young, K. D., Zotev, V., Phillips, R., Misaki, M., Drevets, W. C., & Bodurka, J. (2018). Amygdala real-time functional magnetic resonance imaging neurofeedback for major depressive disorder: A review. *Psychiatry and Clinical Neurosciences*, *72*(7), 466–481. 10.1111/pcn.12665

Zafarmand, M., Farahmand, Z., & Otared, N. (2022). A systematic literature review and meta-analysis on effectiveness of neurofeedback for obsessive-compulsive disorder. *Neurocase*, *28*(1), 29–36. 10.1080/13554794.2021.2019790

Zilverstand, A., Parvaz, M. A., & Goldstein, R. Z. (2017). Neuroimaging cognitive reappraisal in clinical populations to define neural targets for enhancing emotion regulation. A systematic review. *NeuroImage*, *151*, 105–116. 10.1016/j.neuroimage.2016.06.009

Zotev, V., & Bodurka, J. (2020). Effects of simultaneous real-time fMRI and EEG neurofeedback in major depressive disorder evaluated with brain electromagnetic tomography. *NeuroImage. Clinical*, *28*, 102459. 10.1016/j.nicl.2020.102459

Zvolensky, M. J., Lejuez, C. W., Stuart, G. L., & Curtin, J. J. (2001). Experimental psychopathology in psychological science. *Review of General Psychology*, *5*, 371–381.

Zweerings, J., Sarkheil, P., Keller, M., Dyck, M., Klasen, M., Becker, B., Gaebler, A. J., Ibrahim, C. N., Turetsky, B. I., Zvyagintsev, M., Flatten, G., & Mathiak, K. (2020). Rt-fMRI neurofeedback-guided cognitive reappraisal training modulates amygdala responsivity in posttraumatic stress disorder. *NeuroImage. Clinical*, *28*, 102483. 10.1016/j.nicl.2020.102483

SECTION III

Clinical Hypnosis in Practice

Behavioral and Affective Change

28
CLINICAL HYPNOSIS AND ANXIETY

David B. Reid[1] *and Ciara Christensen*[2]

[1]College of Integrative Medicine and Health Sciences, Saybrook University, USA; [2]Private Practice

Introduction

Limitless sources of worry and angst consume human beings on a daily basis. If it isn't our personal finances, challenges to our physical health and mental well-being, or our safety and security, some stressor lurking somewhere out there in our uncertain future seems to generate some sense of doom and gloom.

Fear is a universal human emotion alerting us to potential threats while motivating us to prepare for anticipated life challenges. Anxiety is a diffuse mood state that involves unpleasant emotional experiences marked by a significant degree of apprehension about future aversive or harmful events, whether they are real or imagined (Barlow & Cerny, 1988).

Anxiety disorders are the most common mental illness in the general population and frequently co-occur with other mental or medical disorders including alcohol or substance use that potentiate physical, cognitive, and emotional complications (American Psychiatric Association, DSM-5 Task Force, 2013). Females are 1.5–2 times more likely than males to meet criteria for an anxiety disorder (Thibaut, 2017) and research suggests that psychosocial contributors including reported childhood sexual abuse or chronic stressors, and genetic and neurobiological factors, may explain possible causes for the higher prevalence of anxiety in women (Bandelow & Michaelis, 2015). Several studies have also described high rates of anxiety disorders and symptoms of anxiety in the transgender population (Millet et al., 2017). Each of the five anxiety disorders identified below – specific phobia, social anxiety disorder, panic disorder, agoraphobia, and generalized anxiety disorder (GAD) – is diagnosed per criteria established by the Diagnostic and Statistical Manual of Mental Disorders, 5th Edition (American Psychiatric Association, DSM-5 Task Force, 2013) only when symptoms cannot be attributed to the physiological effects of a substance/medication or another medical condition or not better explained by another mental disorder.

A specific phobia is an intense and irrational fear of a specified object or situation that results in avoidance or extreme distress. Anxiety symptoms almost always immediately manifest after exposure to the phobic situation, to a degree that is persistent and out of

DOI: 10.4324/9781003449126-40

proportion to any actual risk. Frequently, phobic individuals avoid having contact with the objects or situations they fear (e.g., dogs, heights, or textures), without major restrictions in reported quality of life. Consequently, individuals diagnosed with specific phobias infrequently seek professional help (Bandelow & Michaelis, 2015). Social anxiety disorder (aka social phobia) involves fear and avoidance of social interactions and situations usually associated with concerns of being scrutinized by others and fear of being negatively evaluated by others, embarrassed, humiliated, rejected, or offending to others. Individuals struggling with social anxiety rarely consult with a medical provider. Panic disorder is diagnosed when an individual experiences recurrent, unexpected panic attacks and persistent fear of having future panic attacks. Panic attacks include abrupt surges of intense fear associated with intense physical discomfort that rapidly escalates within a matter of minutes. They may occur with or without identified precipitators that bring about panic. Individuals with agoraphobia typically experience heightened worry about an inability to escape a situation, especially if panic-like symptoms manifest or other embarrassing symptoms arise. Feared situations can include the use of public transportation, being in open spaces, being in enclosed places, waiting in line, being in a crowd, or being away from home alone, and in other situations. Generalized anxiety typically involves persistent and excessive worry that interferes with daily academic and vocational responsibilities. Individuals diagnosed with GAD are usually restless, on edge, tense, easily fatigued, and irritable.

In the United States, a 29% lifetime prevalence for anxiety disorders has been reported, with an estimated 40 million American adults suffering from an anxiety-related disorder within a given year (Kessler et al., 2005). Accordingly, anxiety disorders in the United States account for a staggering estimated annual economic burden of $42.3–$46.6 billion with nearly 75% of these costs attributable to morbidity, mortality, and reduced productivity (DuPont et al., 1996; Greenberg et al., 1999).

Hypnosis and Anxiety

Several narrative reviews suggest that hypnosis is effective for treating anxiety and anxiety-related disorders (Flory et al., 2007; Hammond, 2010). Case studies have frequently demonstrated the benefits of hypnosis for treating dental anxiety (Eitner et al., 2006; Goodman, 2019), needle phobia (Abramowitz & Lichtenberg, 2009), fear of flying (Hirsch, 2012), fear of swallowing or choking (Epstein & Deyoub, 1981; Reid, 2016), blood phobia (Noble, 2002), claustrophobia (Simon, 1999; Steggles, 1999), and panic disorder (Reid, 2017).

More importantly, and of relevance to this text, a number of controlled studies (including randomized controlled studies) have provided ample data for clinical hypnosis as an evidence-based intervention for treating anxiety associated with dental procedures (Dilmahomed & Jovani-Sancho, 2019; Eitner et al., 2011; Glaesmer et al., 2015; Huet et al., 2011), surgical and other medical interventions (Akgul et al., 2016; de Klerk et al., 2004; Lang et al., 2008; Saadat et al., 2006), test-taking and performance situations (Boutin & Tosi, 1983; Stanton, 1988). Wojcikiewicz & Orlick, 1987), and general anxiety (Allen, 1998; Stanton, 1978; Whitehouse et al., 1996).

In their meta-analysis quantifying the efficacy of hypnosis for treating anxiety, Valentine et al. (2019) demonstrated that hypnosis improved symptoms of anxiety to an extent that was greater than approximately 79% of control subjects. An overall mean weighted effect size of 0.79 (95% CI = 0.61–0.97) was reported when comparing hypnosis with contact (i.e., standard care and attention controls) to no-contact (i.e., no-treatment and waitlist controls) control conditions, as well as a mean weighted effect size of 1.12 (95% CI = 0.83–1.41) when hypnosis was compared with only no-contact control conditions. These findings compared with meta-analyses of other common therapeutic interventions determined that hypnosis was as effective as cognitive behavioral therapy (CBT), progressive muscle relaxation (PMR), and psychodynamic therapy for treating anxiety disorders.

Valentine et al. (2019) concluded that hypnosis was more effective in reducing anxiety symptoms when combined with other psychotherapeutic interventions including cognitive behavioral therapy (Schoenberger et al., 1997) and biofeedback (Allen, 1998). The meta-analysis reported a mean weighted effect size of 1.25 (95% CI = 0.82–1.68) when combining hypnosis with other treatments versus a mean weighted effect size of 0.70 (95% CI = 0.52–0.88) when hypnosis was the only intervention. These results support those reported by Milling et al. (2018) who determined that hypnosis was significantly more effective in treating obesity when combined with CBT than when utilized as a stand-alone intervention.

Mindfulness, an alternative intervention for treating anxiety, has steadily gained interest and attention in recent years within general mental health and hypnosis communities (Grover et al., 2018; Otani, 2016, 2020; Shenefelt, 2018). Some have encouraged the inclusion of mindfulness within hypnosis treatment protocols for treating anxiety and other conditions including depression (Olendzki & Elkins, 2017; Yapko, 2011). Hofmann et al. (2010) reported an effect size of 0.41 (CI = 0.23–0.59) when mindfulness was compared with contact and no-contact control groups for treating individuals with a variety of medical and psychological conditions. Blanck et al. (2018) reported an effect size of 0.39 (CI = 0.22–0.56) when mindfulness was compared with no-contact control conditions in reducing anxiety experienced by student volunteers. In contrast, Valentine et al. (2019) obtained an effect size of 0.79 (CI = 0.61–0.97) when hypnosis was compared with contact and no-contact control conditions. The implication being that hypnosis may be more effective than mindfulness in treating anxiety.

Self-hypnosis (e.g., use of audio-recorded assisted and self-directed guidance) has been repeatedly espoused as a beneficial ancillary intervention to hetero-hypnosis for enhancing treatment outcomes (American Society of Clinical Hypnosis, 2019; Elkins, 2017) despite equivocal findings reported in clinical literature. Valentine et al. (2019) reported that the outcome of hypnosis interventions that incorporated self-hypnosis training was no different from those that did not. A recent meta-analysis may help to explain the inconsistency of findings and opinions regarding the benefits of self-hypnosis. Eason and Parris (2019) recently reported a systematic review and meta-analysis of the efficacy of 22 trials of self-hypnosis for a range of concerns including anxiety. They concluded that self-hypnosis was more likely to be effective when taught as an independent self-directed skill and when it involved at least three practice sessions.

Treating anxiety should generally begin by educating a patient about their anxious symptoms and how they involve an adaptive response to what usually amounts to a *perceived* threat. When one's well-being is threatened (real or imagined), the body responds in predictable physiological ways (e.g., rapid heartbeat, tightness in the chest, perspiration) once adrenaline and cortisol enter the blood stream. Persistent anxiety eventually disrupts daily functioning, an anxiety disorder becomes evident, and professional intervention is warranted.

Explaining how bothersome anxiety symptoms are natural responses to certain life circumstances may mitigate secondary fears about losing control of emotions, managing behaviors, and even regulating cognitions. Helping patients appreciate *how* anxiety symptoms are the byproduct of natural unconscious processes can foster an understanding that their body is actually not losing control, but behaving predictably, as it should. Informing someone that their fight-or-flight system is intact and functioning fine but unfortunately "acting out" at inappropriate and inconvenient times can encourage an appreciation that control to some extent is possible, and that learning more adaptive ways of managing stress and anxiety can be personally empowering.

Clinical Hypnosis: A Set of Skills

We maintain that it is insufficient (if not inappropriate) when using hypnosis to help someone minimize anxiety symptoms to simply "put them in trance" and offer suggestions for relaxation and posthypnotic suggestions to "just relax." Doing so offers simple solutions to complex problems that are unlikely to yield therapeutic results.

Hypnosis has been identified and considered by some as an adjunctive tool among other therapeutic tools (e.g., cognitive-behavioral therapy, psychodynamic therapy) within a metaphorical therapeutic toolbox (Daitch, 2018; Saadat & Kain, 2007; Yapko, 2014; Zarren & Eimer, 2002). Hypnosis is a malleable skill set that does not require formal inductions, scripted guidance, or a linear step-wise process otherwise known as the Legacy Model (see Alter & Sugarman, 2017; Sugarman et al., 2018; Sugarman et al., 2020). We conceptualize hypnosis, as applied in our outpatient practices, as a set of versatile tools within a therapeutic toolbox including numerous hypnotic interventions at our disposal for helping patients manage anxiety. Our intention in this chapter is to help clinicians consider which tools to use (and perhaps when to use them) that can guide relevant hypnotic suggestions aligning with the patient's values, and can be readily integrated into their daily living.

Several hypnotic interventions are available to the clinician assisting patients seeking help with managing anxiety, including, but not limited to, fractionation (shifting depth of trance experiences), permissiveness (offering multiple options for trance experiences), ego strengthening (reinforcing confidence, esteem, personal value), linking (pairing experiences during trance), interspersal (embedding suggestive messages into the trancework), silence (an under-appreciated hypnosis intervention for empowering a sense of self-control and regulation of physiology), ratification (verifying and validating that therapeutic trance occurred and is/will be helpful), metaphors (indirect hypnotic strategy conveying personally useful information and help bypass resistance to change[s]), posthypnotic suggestions (strategy to counter problematic behaviors and emotions, irrational thinking, etc., helping to create a framework for envisioning the future and different ways of responding), and anchors (offering suggestive possibilities for bolstering confidence, affect regulation, and distress tolerance).

Clinical hypnosis interventions can be inserted into a more "formal," stepwise, or "Legacy" approach, or strategically employed during a naturalistic and at times conversational intervention. In our view, the latter approach promotes a greater sense of personal control, mastery of skills, and confidence in a patient's ability to better manage symptoms of anxiety. As Milton Erickson frequently claimed, hypnosis is not a "cure," but instead a method for cultivating a climate for therapeutic change (Rossi, 1993). Like Erickson, we contend that hypnosis helps "drive," facilitate, and promote therapeutic change through the utilization of a trance experience that is already present within a patient. Utilizing hypnosis adjunctively offers the patient an opportunity to have a realization of empowerment and being able to transition in an adaptive state (Zeig, 2018). Experientially, via hypnosis, the patient learns different ways to manage anxiety and the associated symptoms adversely impacting their physiology.

Introducing Hypnosis: A Trance Forming Opportunity

It has been our experience that introducing hypnosis and describing what it is (and isn't) permits an opportunity for a beneficial trance experience. After explaining how trance (i.e., an altered and altering state of consciousness) is a natural human experience (e.g., day-dreaming, losing track of time) and it essentially involves a set of skills and interventions that utilize trance to help people empower themselves, patients frequently express a sense of intrigue and curiosity.

This seeding of curiosity could be followed by an intended verbalized recognition of some observed spontaneous behavior that evolves into a more conversational approach to hypnosis, absent any kind of formal "induction." For instance, responding to a patient's deep inhalation by saying: "Wow, that was a deep breath!" or noting a shifting of their position sitting in a chair: "I noticed how you shifted in your chair and uncrossed your legs right before you answered that question." This intervention, referred to as "kneading," one of the four "Basic Skills" of hypnosis espoused by Alter and Sugarman (2017), initiates some disruption and perhaps disorientation for the patient. Doing so also introduces a sense of novelty (and maybe confusion), which has been considered an initial stage for promoting healing (Rossi, 2002), as well as the generator of "trance openings" (Sugarman et al., 2020). This kneading process, warranting no further dynamic analysis typical of a psychotherapy session (e.g., "Why did you do that?"), also serves as an initial, implied (perhaps unconscious) message that the helped individual is the keeper of the solutions to that which may restrict or burden them (i.e., anxiety).

Respectful kneading, according to Alter and Sugarman (2017) followed by "wondering" queries, builds on associations conveying an increased sense of personal control and self-mastery. For instance, saying, "I wonder how that deep breath helped you ... not only now, but I don't know, how that deep breath may also help you later ...." Or perhaps posing questions about their anxiety experiences: "Do you ever wonder how you managed these kinds of things before? What was that like? .... I wonder ... how did you do that?" This line of curious wondering, regardless of whether a person's eyes are closed, staring off into the distance, fixed on some arbitrary spot, or darting about, ultimately reinforces and presumes a sense of personal mastery over one's experiences.

These wonderings may be familiar to some as "age regression" and perhaps "ego strengthening" interventions and involve an exploration, recognition, and appreciation of experiences in one's life that have been productive, beneficial, successful, and contrary to behaviors, thoughts, and perceptions that perpetuate current anxiety. Wondering can also include future-focused interventions (i.e., "age progression" and "posthypnotic suggestions") like, "Perhaps you can wonder how this experience that you are creating at this time will remain with you, and help you later ... whether it is later today, tomorrow, or some other time. Just how that will happen? And how you will know? And even wonder what will happen after that happens." Ultimately, the implied message is: "You really know how to take care of yourself, don't you?"

Numerous individually tailored hypnosis interventions can help patients minimize anxiety symptoms including metaphors, anchors, imbedded opportunities for silence, instruction using self-hypnosis, and an empowering permissive conclusion of the hypnosis intervention.

Metaphors

Metaphors, given their relatively non-threatening, indirect, and powerful history of associative learning messages, can also be appealing to the unconscious mind and provide "an altered framework in which novel experiences can be entertained" (Lankton & Lankton, 1983, p. 90).

When helping patients manage and mitigate anxiety, using hypnosis, I (DBR) frequently share a personal story that relates their symptoms to a smoke alarm. The story goes something like this: One Thanksgiving morning while preheating my oven in preparation for the big feast, I noticed smoke seeping from the oven door. I pulled the door open as black smoke filled the kitchen, prompting other family members to throw open nearby windows. The fire alarm screeched and did its job. But there was no fire. The alarm, however, had no way of knowing if the smoke billowing from the oven was benign, or life threatening. A critical threshold was met and an alarm sounded.

I (CC) appreciate the value of sharing this story with patients because I think it also illustrates an important dilemma which emerges in therapy, that is, assimilating facts and recognizing adaptive concepts are not the same (Zeig, 2018) and both are important to attend to. Patients often know their responses to stress (e.g., sudden rapid heart rate, shortness of breath, feeling lightheaded) and anxiety are quite similar to smoke detectors. They may know what to do to reduce responding to these "false alarms," although frequently the challenge is realizing and putting into practice what they know (Zeig, 2018). Using hypnosis for facilitating a healthier and more adaptive trance experience can help manage and perhaps mitigate unwanted symptoms. It offers patients a bridge between knowing which self-care interventions to practice that promote healthier responses and realizing (over time) the more they practice, the greater their ability to self-regulate responses to triggering stimuli provoking anxiety.

Anchors

Anchors though typically "prescribed" by the clinician during hypnosis provide opportunities for managing anxiety. Repeated and frequent pairing of calm, comforting, soothing relaxation with a conditioned stimulus like a smooth rock or gemstone, or comfortable positioning of fingers, can generate a sense of calm and comfort when future stressful experiences arise.

I (DBR) prefer to introduce the concept of anchors during therapeutic conversation. After reviewing basic tenets of classical conditioning, I encourage the consideration of a possible anchor that could accompany personal experiences of comfort and calm. Encouraging the selection of a personal anchor reinforces a sense of personal engagement and promotes self-care. Once an anchor has been selected, instruction for "feeling" or "holding" the anchor is offered with suggestions for increased comfort. Posthypnotic suggestions encouraging anchors and expected successful experiences with practice should also be encouraged.

Silence

Scottish historian, Thomas Carlyle opined, "Under all speech that is good for anything, there lies a silence that is better" (Carlyle, 1869, p. 218). During hypnosis interventions, there are times when what we *do not* say is more impactful than what we *do* say. Offering prescribed (or spontaneous) silent time promotes opportunities for processing, reflecting, ratifying, and reinforcing a sense of self-control and personal mastery.

Silence whether following a question posed by the clinician promoting a sense of kneading, wondering, or invited in the midst of a session, or after eyes reopen and scan the room offers wonderful opportunities that foster respect for patient autonomy and their ability to promote change from within. At times, I (DBR) introduce ego-strengthening and reinforcement of self-care after a brief period of silence by saying, "How nice that you took this time to take care of yourself ... just like that. And how you can wonder and be curious (also in the silence) right now ... and how taking this time can take care of you later (age progression)."

As the session concludes, and the patient shifts into a more conscious state of alertness, it can be tempting to break a moment of silence and probe the client for information regarding the efficacy of the session. Doing so can be disruptive, and some would contend, disrespectful. We suggest you linger a bit in that silent moment, providing interpersonal space, a continued sense of calm, and an opportunity for the patient to take care of themselves as they conclude their personal experience.

Prescribed silence also permits time for the clinician to momentarily reflect, gain some composure (if needed), and strategize hypnotic interventions, especially when considering what to say next.

Self-Hypnosis

"Self-hypnosis" (i.e., "auto-hypnosis") implies that hypnosis is conducted exclusively with one's self. That is, without another. It has been posited, however, that as individuals we are often being influenced by others in manners that preserve our autonomy and that *all* hypnosis is both auto and hetero hypnosis (see Sugarman et al., 2020). For this chapter, we refer to self-hypnosis as hypnosis that one implements for oneself and does not involve interventions from another.

It is the rule, not the exception, that we teach and encourage the use of self-hypnosis for treating anxiety. In combination with personally selected anchors (see above), paired with calming and comforting physiological interventions (e.g., breath-work), patients can gain a greater sense of control over their emotional, physical, and spiritual well-being. Interspersed moments of silence during hetero-hypnosis sessions also serve as opportunities to reinforce self-hypnosis benefits. These opportunities should be capitalized upon through the inclusion of ego-strengthening suggestions that in turn can also serve as posthypnotic suggestions for continued and expanded benefit of using self-hypnosis to reduce symptoms of anxiety.

Permissive Conclusions

Counting down the final seconds of a year while ringing in the next with fireworks and noise-makers can be a celebratory event. Many sport events conclude as the clock winds down to zero. Some respected clinical hypnosis societies introduce attendees to the concept of counting (up and down). Proposed hypnotic inductions begin with an imagined descent down a set of stairs, directed by a counting clinician who simultaneously suggests a "deeper state of relaxation" accompanying the contrived decent. And since we count down in the beginning, according to these societies, so must we count up (though sometimes it is once again a count down) to conclude the session.

I (DBR) have previously proposed that we minimize counting and promote respect for our patient's autonomy by employing a more permissive and naturalistic opportunity for concluding a hypnosis experience (Reid, 2022). After all, if our clinical objective is to promote self-care and enhance the management of one's physiology and regulation of the autonomic nervous system (i.e., fight-or-flight response) for minimizing anxiety, why would we not hand over the control of a hypnotic experience to our patients rather than keeping control of the session ourselves? Provided that the clinician has managed time adequately and ensures that there is ample time for a respectful, naturalistic re-alert, there is little need for a guided ascent (or descent) on an imagined stairway.

A more permissive re-alert could go something like: "In a moment I will invite you to be more alert and aware of your surroundings. For now, take a moment and realize that you created this experience ... your unconscious mind has become more available to help and assist ... and when you are confident that you have internalized this experience in a way that it remains with you and is available for you, allow yourself to become more alert ... eventually as alert as you were before you walked into my office."

There's no final count down. No stairs. No finger snapping or need to raise one's voice beyond that of conversational speech. In the silence of the moment, it promotes a "simmering" of the plasticity of a naturalistic experience that continues beyond the bounds of the hypnosis session. And in the silence, with perhaps an approving and supportive nod from the clinician, inferred messages are delivered: "Wow, you just did that. How did you do that?" and "Isn't it nice to know that you can do that?"

Conclusion

Most clinicians familiar with clinical hypnosis have likely appreciated its benefits for treating individuals with anxiety and anxiety-related disorders. As noted in this chapter and throughout this book, the gold standard for the "approval/acceptance" of medical and mental health treatment interventions requires support of established empirically validated evidence-based research. There is ample empirical data derived from randomized controlled studies and published in peer-reviewed journals, to classify clinical hypnosis as an evidence-based treatment intervention for anxiety and anxiety-related disorders (Christensen et al., 2022). The literature supporting hypnosis for treating anxiety associated with numerous medical, dental, mental health concerns, athletic and scholastic performance demonstrates considerable efficacy that persists over time.

Reading traditional "standardized scripts" or using pre-recorded inductions and interventions though warranted in research studies have no business in the interpersonal and synchronized hypnotic interaction between a clinician and a person in their care. Script reading is the antithesis of individualized and personalized care. Tailoring treatment interventions with hypnosis for treating anxiety enhances treatment outcomes and therapeutic benefits beyond that demonstrated in controlled studies.

Whether employed in isolation or as an adjunctive therapeutic intervention, clinical hypnosis has been shown to effectively alleviate anxiety by facilitating adaptive coping skills, enhancing realistic thinking, improving stress management, strengthening control of one's physiology, and improving effective problem-solving skills. Clinical hypnosis can be conceptualized as a set of skills or tools (i.e., metaphors, anchors, silence, post-hypnotic suggestions, ego strengthening, permissive re-alerting) available within a therapeutic toolbox that when used properly and creatively can empower individuals to help themselves to reduce symptoms of anxiety which interfere with activities for daily living.

References

Abramowitz, E. G., & Lichtenberg, P. (2009). Hypnotherapeutic olfactory conditioning (HOC): Case studies of needle phobia, panic disorder, and combat-induced PTSD. *International Journal of Clinical and Experimental Hypnosis*, *57*(2), 184–197. 10.1080/00207140802665450

Akgul, A., Guner, B., Çirak, M., Çelik, D., Hergünsel, O., & Bedirhan, S. (2016). The beneficial effect of hypnosis in elective cardiac surgery: A preliminary study. *Thoracic and Cardiovascular Surgeon*, *64*(7), 581–588. 10.1055/s-0036-1580623

Allen, B. T. (1998). *A design of a combined cognitive-behavioral, biofeedback, and hypnosis training protocol (CBHT) for the reduction of generalized anxiety disorder* [Unpublished Doctoral Dissertation]. Adler School of Professional Psychology.

Alter, D. S., & Sugarman, L. I. (2017). Reorienting hypnosis education. *American Journal of Clinical Hypnosis*, *59*(3), 235–259. 10.1080/00029157.2016.1231657

American Psychiatric Association, DSM-5 Task Force (2013). *Diagnostic and statistical manual of mental disorders: DSM-5™* (5th ed.). American Psychiatric Publishing, Inc. 10.1176/appi.books.9780890425596

American Society of Clinical Hypnosis (2019). *Standards of training. Level 1: Fundamentals of clinical hypnosis workshop*. American Society of Clinical Hypnosis Education and Research Foundation.

Bandelow, B., & Michaelis, S. (2015). Epidemiology of anxiety disorders in the 21st century. *Dialogues in Clinical Neuroscience*, *17*(3), 327–335. 10.31887/DCNS.2015.17.3/bbandelow

Barlow, D. H., & Cerny, J. A. (1988). *Psychological treatment of panic*. Guilford Press.

Blanck, P., Perleth, S., Heidenreich, T., Kröger, P., Ditzen, B., Bents, H., & Mander, J. (2018). Effects of mindfulness exercises as stand-alone intervention on symptoms of anxiety and depression: Systematic review and meta-analysis. *Behaviour Research and Therapy*, *102*, 25–35. 10.1016/j.brat.2017.12.002

Boutin, G. E., & Tosi, D. J. (1983). Modification of irrational ideas and test anxiety through rational stage directed hypnotherapy [RSDH]. *Journal of Clinical Psychology*, *39*(3), 382–391. 10.1002/1097-4679(198305)39:3

Carlyle, T. (1869). *Critical and miscellaneous essays* (Vol. 5). Chapman and Hall.

Christensen, C., Finley, A., & Connor, K. (2022). Integrating hypnosis into clinical practice and applications. In G. R. Elkins (Ed.), *Introduction to clinical hypnosis: The basics and beyond* (pp. 349–392). Independently Published.

Daitch, C. (2018). Cognitive behavioral therapy, mindfulness, and hypnosis as treatment methods for generalized anxiety disorder. *American Journal of Clinical Hypnosis*, *61*(1), 57–69. 10.1080/00029157.2018.1458594

de Klerk, J. E., du Plessis, W. F., Steyn, H. S., & Botha, M. (2004). Hypnotherapeutic ego strengthening with male South African coronary artery bypass patients. *American Journal of Clinical Hypnosis*, *47*(2), 79–92. 10.1080/00029157.2004.10403627

Dilmahomed, H., & Jovani-Sancho, M. (2019). Hypnoanalgesia in dentistry: A literature review. *American Journal of Clinical Hypnosis*, *61*(3), 258–275. 10.1080/00029157.2017.1409613

DuPont, R. L., Rice, D. P., Miller, L. S., Shiraki, S. S., Rowland, C. R., & Harwood, H. J. (1996). Economic costs of anxiety disorders. *Anxiety*, *2*(4), 167–172. 10.1002/(sici)1522-7154(1996)2:4

Eason, A. D., & Parris, B. A. (2019). Clinical applications of self-hypnosis: A systematic review and meta-analysis of randomized controlled trials. *Psychology of Consciousness: Theory, Research, and Practice*, *6*(3), 262–278. 10.1037/cns0000173

Eitner, S., Schultze-Mosgau, S., Heckmann, J., Wichmann, M., & Holst, S. (2006). Changes in neurophysiologic parameters in a patient with dental anxiety by hypnosis during surgical treatment. *Journal of Oral Rehabilitation*, *33*(7), 496–500. 10.1111/j.1365-2842.2005.01578.x

Eitner, S., Sokol, B., Wichmann, M., Bauer, J., & Engels, D. (2011). Clinical use of a novel audio pillow with recorded hypnotherapy instructions and music for anxiolysis during dental implant surgery: A prospective study. *International Journal of Clinical and Experimental Hypnosis*, *59*(2), 180–197. 10.1080/00207144.2011.546196

Elkins, G. (2017). Hypnotic relaxation therapy. In G. R. Elkins (Ed.), *Handbook of medical and psychological hypnosis: Foundations, applications, and professional issues* (1st ed., pp. 83–97). Springer Publishing Company.

Epstein, S. J., & Deyoub, P. L. (1981). Hypnotherapy for fear of choking: Treatment implications of a case report. *International Journal of Clinical and Experimental Hypnosis*, *29*(2), 117–127. 10.1080/00207148108409152

Flory, N., Martinez Salazar, G. M., & Lang, E. V. (2007). Hypnosis for acute distress management during medical procedures. *International Journal of Clinical and Experimental Hypnosis*, *55*(3), 303–317. 10.1080/00207140701338670

Glaesmer, H., Geupel, H., & Haak, R. (2015). A controlled trial on the effect of hypnosis on dental anxiety in tooth removal patients. *Patient Education and Counseling*, *98*(9), 1112–1115. 10.1016/j.pec.2015.05.007

Goodman, A. A. (2019). Cases: Clinical hypnosis in dentistry. *American Journal of Clinical Hypnosis*, *61*(3), 290–294. 10.1080/00029157.2018.1544435

Greenberg, P. B., Sisitsky, T., Kessler, R. C., Finkelstein, S. N., Berndt, E. R., Davidson, J. R. T., Ballenger, J. C., & Fyer, A. J. (1999). The economic burden of anxiety disorders in the 1990s. *Journal of Clinical Psychiatry*, *60*(7), 427–435. 10.4088/jcp.v60n0702

Grover, M. P., Jensen, M. P., Patterson, D. R., Gertz, K. J., & Day, M. A. (2018). The association between mindfulness and hypnotizability: Clinical and theoretical implications. *American Journal of Clinical Hypnosis*, *61*(1), 4–17. 10.1080/00029157.2017.1419458

Hammond, D. C. (2010). Hypnosis in the treatment of anxiety- and stress-related disorders. *Expert Review of Neurotherapeutics*, *10*(2), 263–273. 10.1586/ern.09.140

Hirsch, J. A. (2012). Virtual reality exposure therapy and hypnosis for flying phobia in a treatment-resistant patient: A case report. *American Journal of Clinical Hypnosis*, *55*(2), 168–173. 10.1080/00029157.2011.639587

Hofmann, S. G., Sawyer, A. T., Witt, A. A., & Oh, D. (2010). The effect of mindfulness-based therapy on anxiety and depression: A meta-analytic review. *Journal of Consulting and Clinical Psychology*, *78*(2), 169–183. 10.1037/a0018555

Huet, A., Lucas-Polomeni, M.-M., Robert, J.-C., Sixou, J.-L., & Wodey, E. (2011). Hypnosis and dental anesthesia in children: A prospective controlled study. *International Journal of Clinical and Experimental Hypnosis*, *59*(4), 424–440. 10.1080/00207144.2011.594740

Kessler, R. C., Chiu, W. T., Demler, O., & Walters, E. E. (2005). Prevalence, severity, and comorbidity of 12-month DSM-IV disorders in the National Comorbidity Survey replication. *Archives of General Psychiatry*, *62*(6), 617–627. 10.1001/archpsyc.62.6.617

Lang, E. V., Berbaum, K. S., Pauker, S. G., Faintuch, S., Salazar, G. M., Lutgendorf, S., Laser, E., Logan, H., & Spiegel, D. (2008). Beneficial effects of hypnosis and adverse effects of empathic attention during percutaneous tumor treatment: When being nice does not suffice. *Journal of Vascular and Interventional Radiology*, *19*(6), 897–905. 10.1016/j.jvir.2008.01.027

Lankton, S. R., & Lankton, C. H. (1983). *The answer within: A clinical framework of Ericksonian hypnotherapy*. Crown House Publishing.

Millet, N., Longworth, J., & Arcelus, J. (2017). Prevalence of anxiety symptoms and disorders in the transgender population: A systematic review of the literature. *International Journal of Transgenderism*, *18*(1), 27–38. 10.1080/15532739.2016.1258353

Milling, L. S., Gover, M. C., & Moriarty, C. L. (2018). The effectiveness of hypnosis as an intervention for obesity: A meta-analytic review. *Psychology of Consciousness: Theory, Research, and Practice*, *5*(1), 29–45. 10.1037/cns0000139

Noble, S. (2002). The management of blood phobia and a hypersensitive gag reflex by hypnotherapy: A case report. *Dental Update*, *29*(2), 70–74. 10.12968/denu.2002.29.2.70

Olendzki, N., & Elkins, G. (2017). Mindfulness and hypnosis. In G. R. Elkins (Ed.), *Handbook of Medical and psychological hypnosis: Foundations, applications, and professional issues* (1st ed., pp. 579–588). Springer Publishing Company.

Otani, A. (2016). Hypnosis and mindfulness: The twain finally meet. *American Journal of Clinical Hypnosis*, *58*(4), 383–398. 10.1080/00029157.2015.1085364

Otani, A. (2020). The mindfulness-based phase-oriented trauma therapy (MB-POTT): Hypnosis-informed mindfulness approach to trauma. *American Journal of Clinical Hypnosis*, *63*(2), 95–111. 10.1080/00029157.2020.1765726

Reid, D. B. (2016). A case study of hypnosis for phagophobia: It's no choking matter. *American Journal of Clinical Hypnosis*, *58*(4), 357–367. 10.1080/00029157.2015.1048544

Reid, D. B. (2017). Treating panic disorder hypnotically. *American Journal of Clinical Hypnosis*, *60*(2), 137–148. 10.1080/00029157.2017.1288608

Reid, D. B. (2022). *Realerting: You can count on it without counting* [Presidential Address to Division 30 (Society of Psychological Hypnosis)]. American Psychological Association Annual Convention, August 2022, Minneapolis, MN, USA.

Rossi, E. L. (1993). *The psychobiology of mind-body healing: New concepts of therapeutic hypnosis* (2nd ed.). W. W. Norton.

Rossi, E. L. (2002). *The psychobiology of gene expression: Neuroscience and neurogenesis in hypnosis and the healing arts.* W. W. Norton & Company.

Saadat, H., Drummond-Lewis, J., Maranets, I., Kaplan, D., Saadat, A., Wang, S.-M., & Kain, Z. N. (2006). Hypnosis reduces preoperative anxiety in adult patients. *Anesthesia & Analgesia*, *102*(5), 1394–1396. 10.1213/01.ane.0000204355.36015.54

Saadat, H., & Kain, Z. N. (2007). Hypnosis as a therapeutic tool in pediatrics. *Pediatrics*, *120*(1), 179–181. 10.1542/peds.2007-1082

Schoenberger, N. E., Kirsch, I., Gearan, P., Montgomery, G., & Pastyrnak, S. L. (1997). Hypnotic enhancement of a cognitive behavioral treatment for public speaking anxiety. *Behavior Therapy*, *28*(1), 127–140. 10.1016/s0005-7894(97)80038-x

Shenefelt, P. D. (2018). Mindfulness-based cognitive hypnotherapy and skin disorders. *American Journal of Clinical Hypnosis*, *61*(1), 34–44. 10.1080/00029157.2017.1419457

Simon, E. P. (1999). Hypnosis using a communication device to increase magnetic resonance imaging tolerance with a claustrophobic patient. *Military Medicine*, *164*(1), 71–72. 10.1093/milmed/164.1.71

Stanton, H. E. (1978). A simple hypnotic technique to reduce anxiety. *Australian Journal of Clinical and Experimental Hypnosis*, *6*(1), 35–38.

Stanton, H. E. (1988). Improving examination performance through the clenched fist technique. *Contemporary Educational Psychology*, *12*(4), 309–315. 10.1016/0361-476X(88)90029-X

Steggles, S. (1999). The use of cognitive-behavioral treatment including hypnosis for claustrophobia in cancer patients. *American Journal of Clinical Hypnosis*, *41*(4), 319–326. 10.1080/00029157.1999.10404231

Sugarman, L. I., Schafer, P. M., Alter, D. S., & Reid, D. B. (2018). Learning clinical hypnosis wide awake: Can we teach hypnosis hypnotically? *American Journal of Clinical Hypnosis*, *61*(2), 140–158. 10.1080/00029157.2018.1437710

Sugarman, L. I., Linden, J. H., & Brooks, L. W. (2020). *Changing minds with clinical hypnosis: Narratives and discourse for a new health care paradigm* (1st ed.). Routledge.

Thibaut, F. (2017). Anxiety disorders: A review of current literature. *Dialogues in Clinical Neuroscience*, *19*(2), 87–88. 10.31887/dcns.2017.19.2/fthibaut

Valentine, K. E., Milling, L. S., Clark, L. J., & Moriarty, C. L. (2019). The efficacy of hypnosis as a treatment for anxiety: A meta-analysis. *International Journal of Clinical and Experimental Hypnosis*, *67*(3), 336–363. 10.1080/00207144.2019.1613863

Whitehouse, W. G., Dinges, D. F., Orne, E. C., Keller, S. E., Bates, B. L., Bauer, N. K., Morahan, P., Haupt, B. A., Carlin, M. M., Bloom, P. B., Zaugg, L., & Orne, M. T. (1996). Psychosocial and immune effects of Self-Hypnosis training for stress management throughout the first semester of medical school. *Psychosomatic Medicine*, *58*(3), 249–263. 10.1097/00006842-199605000-00009

Wojcikiewicz, A., & Orlick, T. (1987). The effects of posthypnotic suggestion and relaxation with suggestion on competitive fencing anxiety and performance. *International Journal of Sport Psychology*, *18*(4), 303–313.

Yapko, M. D. (2011). *Mindfulness and hypnosis: The power of suggestion to transform experience* (1st ed.). W. W. Norton Company.

Yapko, M. D. (2014). *Essentials of hypnosis* (2nd ed.). Routledge.

Zarren, J. I., & Eimer, B. N. (2002). *Brief cognitive hypnosis: Facilitating the change of dysfunctional behavior*. Springer Publishing Company.

Zeig, J. K. (2018). *The anatomy of experiential impact through Ericksonian psychotherapy: Seeing, doing, being*. Milton H. Erickson Foundation Press.

29

APPLYING HYPNOSIS STRATEGICALLY IN TREATING DEPRESSION

Michael D. Yapko
PRIVATE PRACTICE, FALLBROOK, CA, USA

About the Author: Background and Perspectives

I'm a clinical psychologist residing in Southern California. I've been in the mental health field for almost five decades. At the age of 19, when I was an undergraduate student, I witnessed my first demonstration of clinical hypnosis featuring the treatment of a woman suffering chronic and severe pain. I was deeply impressed by the rapid and dramatically successful session and committed myself then to study and develop some expertise with hypnosis as a treatment tool. Around the same time, as my studies in clinical psychology progressed, I became aware that major depression was a widespread and debilitating condition. Despite it being a highly prevalent disorder then, even more so now, it seemed to me that treatment was poorly conceived and practiced. Depressed clients made it clear that unless progress could be made quickly, it was too easy for them to continue to feel hopeless and helpless, often leading them to prematurely drop out of treatment. I made depression my clinical focus and it became my professional ambition to help develop more efficient and efficacious strategies of intervention.

I had the good fortune to have ample time studying depression with many such pioneering figures as Aaron Beck and Albert Ellis, among others. I was also especially fortunate to have had the opportunity to study hypnosis in depth with such luminaries as William Kroger and Jay Haley as well as many other key figures in the field. My strategic orientation to both hypnosis and therapy was greatly influenced by Jay Haley and, through him, Milton Erickson. I learned early on that while each one of the many experts I studied with had a personally preferred approach to the practice of hypnosis and psychotherapy, these experts routinely contradicted each other. It became clear to me early on that there wasn't a single "right" way to do either hypnosis or psychotherapy, changing my initial priority from doing it "right" to instead striving to do it *effectively*. I recognized that I would need to develop and follow my own path as a clinician, as we each must, acknowledging the influence of others but, hopefully, seeing further by standing on the shoulders of these giants.

Now the author of 16 books and editor of three others, I am especially gratified for the widespread interest in my work. To date I have been invited to teach in more than

DOI: 10.4324/9781003449126-41

30 countries and to serve as keynote speaker in major conferences. My "flagship" book, the widely used hypnosis textbook *Trancework: An Introduction to the Practice of Clinical Hypnosis* (Yapko, 2019), is now in its fifth edition, the first hypnosis textbook to go to five editions. It's a comprehensive text that gives interested readers a broad overview of the field by introducing its pioneers, summarizing its varied theoretical foundations, and especially emphasizing scientifically informed, practical clinical applications. In the book, I not only share other expert definitions of hypnosis but also provide my own:

> Hypnosis is a focused experience of attentional absorption that invites people to respond experientially on multiple levels in order to amplify and utilize their personal resources in a goal-directed fashion. When employed in the clinical context, hypnosis involves paying greater attention to the essential skills of using words and gestures in particular ways to achieve specific therapeutic outcomes, acknowledging and utilizing the many complex personal, interpersonal, and contextual factors that combine in varying degrees to influence client responsiveness.
>
> *(Yapko, 2019, p. 8)*

My definition is, of course, inevitably incomplete, but places greater emphasis on the interpersonal aspects and goal-oriented nature of hypnosis than do other definitions. This more interpersonally based perspective contrasts with more traditional viewpoints of the hypnotic experience commonly referred to as "trance." The term trance reflects a subjective experience within the patient. If the quality of the patient's "trance state" is the only focus of consideration, thinking only or primarily of the patient's capacities for generating a suitable "trance" as the determining factor of their clinical response, then the role of the clinician in guiding the experience in an obviously interpersonal interaction is de-emphasized. However, one's style for eliciting hypnosis and offering therapeutic suggestions is a core component of successful hypnosis sessions.

While there are tendencies of brain measures of hypnotic responses described in the neuroscientific literature, a "trance state" has yet to be either reliably defined or measured. A primary reason for the difficulty in identifying a "trance state" is because what brain scans reveal is entirely dependent on the direction and content of a patient's focus. Simply put, scans of people will look quite different when remembering a traumatic event than when focusing on some pleasant fantasy imagery despite presumably being in hypnosis under both conditions (Holroyd, 2003; Yapko, 2011, 2020).

Rather than employ the term "trance," I favor using the phrase "attentional processes." My emphasis in hypnosis, as well as in psychotherapy, is on catalyzing the process of therapeutic change through focused attention and deliberate strategies of hypnotic intervention. These are based entirely on individual patient profiles and range from direct to indirect and from content-oriented to process-oriented (Yapko, 2019, 2021). This orientation will be further elaborated later in this chapter on applying hypnosis strategically in the treatment of depression.

Empirical Support for Hypnosis in the Treatment of Depression

I was acutely aware when I began my work that depression was widely considered a disorder for which hypnosis was contraindicated. Many hypnosis experts said so in no uncertain terms in their writings and trainings despite having no credible supportive evidence for their opinions. In 1992, I wrote what I believe was the very first book ever written specifically on the subject of using hypnosis to treat depression (Yapko, 1992), a fact which helps explain why the volume of research literature on this subject is less than desired. In that book, I reviewed the outdated perspectives about both hypnosis and depression that gave rise to the myth that hypnosis would likely generate iatrogenic consequences for patients. Then I attempted to correct those myths by providing more current understandings of both hypnosis and depression that were long overdue. This book and subsequent books (Yapko, 2001, 2006) on the same subject made the point convincingly that hypnosis was, indeed, a valuable means of providing treatment for those suffering depression.

The merits of applying hypnosis in treating depression have been empirically validated by clinicians and researchers many times since then. Alladin and Alibhai (2007) integrated hypnosis with cognitive behavioral therapy (CBT) and demonstrated a clear benefit to depression treatment results in doing so. A meta-analysis regarding the use of hypnosis in the treatment of depressive symptoms concluded that hypnosis appeared to significantly improve symptoms of depression (Shih et al., 2009). Another meta-analysis by Milling and his colleagues (2019) involving ten studies incorporating 13 trials of hypnosis showed effect sizes comparable to those of other established treatments such as CBT and interpersonal therapy (IPT). From these and other meta-analytic studies that show hypnosis enhances the use of CBT (Kirsch et al., 1995; Ramondo et al., 2021), the evidence is formidable that there are good reasons to integrate hypnosis into treatments for depression.

As the evidence grew for the merits of integrating hypnosis in treatment, I was pleased to see that the previously discouraged topic of treating depression with hypnosis gradually became a common and even popular one at conferences. I was honored when then-editor Arreed Barabasz, EdD, PhD, asked me to guest-edit the first-ever special issue on "Hypnosis and Treating Depression" for the April–June 2010 issue of the *International Journal of Clinical and Experimental Hypnosis*, further amplifying professional awareness for the therapeutic possibilities for treating this pervasive and debilitating disorder (Yapko, 2010a, 2010b).

Overview: The Scope of the Problem

Major depressive disorder, more commonly referred to simply as "depression," is the most common mood disorder in the world. To highlight both the seriousness and prevalence of depression, the World Health Organization (2017) recently declared depression as the leading cause of disability around the world adversely affecting more than 300 million people. It is estimated that the rate of prevalence is 3.8% of the global population, 5.0% among adults, and 5.7% among adults older than age 60.

Depression is much more than a mood disorder, however. Its destructive tentacles reach into virtually every aspect of one's life including physical health, productivity, and the quality of one's relationships. The devastating impact on individual lives cannot be overstated and include suffering with many debilitating symptoms, the inability to work or be productive, the undeveloped human potentials, and even the loss of life when people take their own lives.

The impact of depression goes well beyond the lives of individual sufferers, however. It includes the destruction of marriages and families from the stresses of trying to cope, the economic costs to businesses that deal with depressed employee absenteeism and higher rates of costly accidents caused by distracted workers, the social costs of depressed people coping poorly when they engage in a variety of antisocial behaviors (such as driving while under the influence of alcohol and drugs), and the substantial costs to the health care system when treating depression as well as the many medical conditions associated with depression such as cardiovascular disease and diabetes.

Despite the fact that there are treatments for depression that are known to be effective, the World Health Organization claims that more than 75% of people living in low- and middle-income countries do not receive any treatment (Evans-Lacko et al., 2018; Moitra et al., 2022). Even in higher income countries such as the United States, the percentage of people who seek treatment is relatively low. The primary reasons for undertreatment are a lack of available resources, a shortage of trained clinicians skilled in treating depression, the stigma of seeking help for perceived personal weaknesses, and the negative expectations associated with the belief that help is unlikely to succeed (World Health Organization, 2017, 2022; Yapko, 2019, 2022). We as health care professionals clearly need to do more outreach to people struggling with depression.

The Medical Model Dominates Treatment ... But *Should* It?

As new antidepressant medications came to market, the conceptualization of depression as a "medical illness" dramatically increased in popularity such that antidepressant medications became the most common form of treatment (Marasine et al., 2021). Beyond antidepressants, many new biological approaches to treatment are currently being investigated, including the use of psychedelics (such as ketamine, psilocybin, and others), probiotic and macrobiotic diets, magnetic e-resonance therapy, Stanford neuromodulation therapy, EEG-assisted transcranial magnetic stimulation, and cryotherapy.

As promising as new medications and new biological treatments for depression might seem to be, they are generally based on the belief that depression is best thought of as a medical illness. However, the medical model has been roundly criticized for not being the most suitable framework for conceptualizing depression and its treatment. One recent study of about 50,000 people failed to find *any* genes that influenced "mental illness" (Curtis, 2021). The view of depression as caused by a "biochemical imbalance" has received little supportive evidence and, to the contrary, has received considerable contradictory evidence (Harrington, 2019; Maes & Stoyanov, 2022). An explosive and extraordinarily widely disseminated study by Joanna Moncrieff and her colleagues (2022) dealt what many consider a "death blow" to the notion of depression's cause being a "biochemical imbalance" featuring a "shortage of serotonin."

The framing of depression as a medical illness or brain disease may have had the intention of reducing the stigma associated with seeking treatment. However, that perspective appears to have had a negative effect on those who actually do seek treatment. Two recent studies have provided convincing evidence that telling people they have a "brain disease" that needs biological intervention is not only misleading but also demotivates people from learning the cognitive and social skills known to not only reduce but even *prevent* depression. The consequence is demonstrably poorer treatment outcomes (Lebowitz et al., 2021; Schroder et al., 2020). It is unsurprising that a recent study concluded that overall, people who use antidepressant medications to manage their depression did *not* have a better quality of life in the long run than people who did not use these medications (Almohammed et al., 2022).

In an earlier article concerning the overprescribing of antidepressants (Yapko, 2013), I described eight considerations beyond treatment efficacy alone that should lead those who reflexively prescribe antidepressant medications reasons to re-consider that practice. These include adverse side-effects, difficulty withdrawing from their use, diminished sense of personal agency, and ecological concerns.

The COVID-19 Global Pandemic and Depression

Despite the predominance of biological views and treatments of depression, evidence has grown steadily that depression is more a social than medical problem (Harrington, 2019; Moncrieff et al., 2022; Yapko, 2009) The strongest risk factors for depression are largely acquired socially, highlighting the influence of both psychological and social factors in the onset and course of depression. Simply put, viewing the problem as exclusively in your biochemistry rather than your circumstances has become an increasingly untenable perspective.

The COVID-19 pandemic has turned the world into a living laboratory relative to depression, giving us a clear view of how a significant change in circumstances affects people's mood. World Health Organization (2022) indicated that the worldwide rate of depression increased by 25% in just the first year of the pandemic. Recent research indicates that the rates of depression and its most common co-morbid condition anxiety have at least *doubled* since the onset of the pandemic in early 2020 (COVID-19 Mental Disorders Collaborators, 2021).

The COVID-19 pandemic has highlighted key points relevant to the aims of this chapter's emphasis on psychotherapy in general and the use of clinical hypnosis in particular. It has shown us: (1) How predisposing risk factors can become activated when circumstances change; (2) How strongly connected anxiety and depression really are; (3) How easily people can make bad decisions that make matters worse; (4) How powerful the drive for social connection is and how costly any disruptions to connection can be (e.g., the pain of loneliness); and (5) How global thinking and the inability to make key distinctions such as perceived restrictions to personal freedom versus one's sense of social responsibility in the wearing of masks or the ability to distinguish levels of risk in one's behavior.

Why Hypnosis for Treating Depression?

It is apparent there are many different pathways to depression. Fortunately, there are many different pathways out as well. Hypnosis is valuable in its ability to address any or all of the multiple dimensions of a problem (e.g., physiological, cognitive, affective, behavioral, contextual, temporal). Thus, clinicians can easily incorporate hypnosis into their preferred style of intervention. The primary purpose of hypnosis is to *absorb* the person in a frame of mind that is consistent with the therapeutic objectives, empowering them to address and resolve whatever issues they may be dealing with in deliberate and skillful ways.

Hypnosis as a treatment tool offers many clear advantages in treatment. Hypnosis:

- Helps people focus, a great advantage since depression often disrupts focus
- Models flexibility within the therapy relationship by inter-relating on multiple levels
- Encourages a shift in direction of focus to new possibilities, thereby building hope
- Facilitates the acquisition of new skills, thereby building greater self-efficacy

- Encourages people to re-define themselves as resourceful rather than "a failure"
- Eases the transfer of information across contexts, helping generalize gains across contexts
- Intensifies useful subjective associations, amplifying the concepts and phrases that help
- Provides experiential learning on multiple levels rather than only one
- Defines people as active managers of themselves rather than victims of a disease

Does hypnosis cure people? No. What holds the potential to be therapeutic is what happens *during* hypnotic experiences, namely the new and beneficial associations the client forms through the shift in focus and absorption in new possibilities. The general goal of hypnosis is to target patient rigidities, i.e., those patterns that simply do not change even though circumstances have. Such rigidities may be addressed in hypnosis through education and re-education, de-framing and reframing, pattern interruptions, and any of the scores of other growth-oriented approaches. There are many different forms of rigidity a clinician could identify and target for intervention, including:

- Cognitive rigidity (entrenched patterns of unhelpful thinking)
- Behavioral rigidity (persistent ways of behaving that lead to negative outcomes)
- Emotional rigidity (fixed emotional responses that lead to emotional distress)
- Perceptual rigidity (enduring self-injurious ways of perceiving situations or people)
- Identity rigidity (an ongoing way of defining oneself as if incapable of changing)
- Relational rigidity (a consistent and self-defeating way of relating to others)

Setting the Stage for Applying Hypnosis Strategically in Psychotherapy

Adopting a view of depression that places greater emphasis on "skills over pills" is a means of empowering those people who are among the most disempowered people we treat, typically feeling both helpless and hopeless. For those approaches to therapy with the highest treatment success rates, most notably CBT, IPT, and behavioral activation therapy, the emphasis is on teaching specific skills. These commonly include critical thinking and problem-solving skills, teaching social skills necessary for building positive relationships, and ways to be proactive in developing positive behaviors in such key areas as goal setting, time management, and coping with stress. In my own clinical practice, therefore, treatment is individualized; there is no fixed number of sessions or schedule for delivering them. Each client is different with different goals and different approaches to achieving those goals, and each has a different rate of learning and mastering those skills.

How one thinks about depression and how one thinks about hypnosis directly shape one's type and style of intervention. It is important to acknowledge that many approaches to treatment can generate positive results. However, it is important to distinguish between approaches that merely help people *feel* better versus those that help people to *be* better. Thus, any hypnosis session is only going to be as good as the defined targets of treatments allow.

Common Targets of Depression Treatment

There are many subjective patterns of self-organization that may serve as pre-existing risk factors for depression. These patterns may also become entrenched (i.e., rigid) features of the disorder. The more common ones include:

- Negative expectancy (giving rise to feelings of hopelessness and apathy)
- Global cognitive style (thinking in over-general terms)
- Rigidity (the reflexive use of ineffective strategies for attaining desired goals)
- Low tolerance for ambiguity (wanting certainty when none is forthcoming)
- Low frustration tolerance (quickly giving up when facing a challenge)
- Internal orientation (using one's subjective and often erroneous beliefs to form perceptions or make decisions)
- Past temporal orientation (hashing and re-hashing the unchangeable negative past)
- External locus of control (reactive rather than proactive on one's own behalf)
- Negative coping styles (rumination and avoidance)

Addressing these and other such patterns well described in the depression literature represents a core component of effective treatments. Which patterns most influence the onset and course of a specific person's depression is essential to hypnosis session design and delivery. Any strategies of hypnosis, though, will likely strive to affirm the positive value of those patterns in *some* contexts while encouraging the client to utilizing more adaptive ones in contexts where that pattern is ineffective at least, destructive at most.

In the following section, I will present two such strategies as examples of ways hypnosis might be structured and ways suggestions might be delivered when countering patterns of negative expectancy and rigidity. (Many more such strategies and sample transcripts can be found in Yapko, 2001, 2006, 2010a, 2016, 2019, 2021b, 2022, and Yapko & Criswell, in press.)

Two Key Strategies of Applied Hypnosis: Structures and Representative Verbiage

Hypnotically Building Positive Expectancy

Given the power of negative expectations to derail *any* form of treatment and given the power of positive expectations to inspire new possibilities, a focus on the issue of expectancy is a vitally important component of effective treatment. Even when hypnosis is not employed formally, a therapeutic conversation that inspires hope and positive expectations in a patient feeling hopeless is most important. Given the high response rate of depression to placebo-based interventions, where treatments that probably shouldn't have any therapeutic impact do, using hypnosis to orient depressed individuals to positive possibilities is simply common sense. The many ways a positive orientation to the future can serve the aims of therapy are described in detail in an earlier article (Yapko, 2022).

An elaborate hypnosis session structure for this strategy was presented in detail in *Treating Depression with Hypnosis* (Yapko, 2001). A second version of this approach is provided in *Process-Oriented Hypnosis* (Yapko, 2021). An abbreviated third version is presented here along with sample statements to highlight the primary aims of each stage of the process. The generic strategy structure is provided in Table 29.1.

As one considers the use of hypnosis in treatment, a good starting point is to consider what the therapeutic message the therapist hopes to convey. In essence, the message of the building expectancy session is this: "Your future holds many positive possibilities." The sequence of steps for getting this message across to someone is flexible, of course, but there are certain key messages one would likely want to get across during the course of the hypnosis session. These are the "themes" that are the heart of the session. Next, I provide

Table 29.1 A Generic Strategy for Hypnotically Building Positive Expectancy

- Induction
- Response set regarding possibilities
- Theme #1: The past doesn't necessarily predict the future
- Theme #2: Take sensible action now with tomorrow in mind
- Theme #3: Try and try again, but vary approaches
- Check-in with the client
- Post-hypnotic suggestion: Integrating optimism
- Closure and disengagement

some representative suggestions for each step of the sequence. It bears repeating that even when a formal hypnosis session is not employed, these messages for inspiring hope can be part of any therapeutic conversation.

Induction

("You can *look forward* to a comfortable and meaningful experience as you let your eyes close and begin to focus internally")

Response Set

("There are so many possibilities of where to focus your attention ... on the comfort of your body as it relaxes ... on the quality of your thoughts as you form new understandings ... on the pleasure of discovering abilities you didn't even know you had ...")

Theme #1

("So often people make the mistake of thinking that the way things were is the way things are going to be ... yet history isn't a very reliable indicator of what is to come ... who could have known a hundred years ago that humans would land on the moon? ... it was science fiction then but it's real now ... and who could have known just a few years ago how much we'd come to rely on the internet to get our news and build relationships?... It's a safe prediction that your life is going to change ... in ways that can happily surprise you ...")

Theme #2

("The actions you take today will have a huge influence on what you experience tomorrow ... there is a wonderful African proverb that is worth giving serious thought to ... It says 'tomorrow belongs to those who prepare today' ... and when you think about what you want for yourself ... the way you'd like to feel ... the way you'd like to live ... you might well feel energized to take a step in that direction ...")

Theme #3

("There are things you have wanted for yourself ... things you have tried in the past that didn't go the way you'd hoped ... and you're now coming to realize it isn't because you're a failure ... or you're undeserving ... it's because the way you approached it not only didn't work but *couldn't* have worked ... the problem isn't you, it was your strategy ... and now you're in the comfortable position of being willing to experiment with new approaches ... learning and using new and better ways of going after the things you want for yourself ... and enjoying the consequences ...")

Check-In

("And in just a moment I'd like you to describe out loud what you're aware of right now ... and you can describe it easily ... even deepening your experience as you speak ...")

Post-Hypnotic Suggestion

("The future hasn't happened yet ... and the choices you make now ... and the actions that you take now ... can allow you to look forward with a realistic and motivating optimism ...")

Closure and Disengagement

("Take your time in bringing this experience to a comfortable close ... and then slowly begin to re-orient ... re-alerting yourself now and opening your eyes")

Hypnotically Facilitating Flexibility

Rigidity has been identified as the foundation of maladaptive responses, whether they are persistent cognitive distortions, retreats into passivity, conflict avoidance, or any of the diverse content-based issues a patient might present for therapy. The main message of the facilitating flexibility session is this: "There are many different approaches to managing some situation well or achieving a goal. Your way of doing things can be effective in some contexts but not others, and that's when it will be helpful to you to have other ways of responding."

The generic strategy structure is provided in Table 29.2.

As before, the sequence of steps for getting the main message across to someone is flexible, but there are certain key messages (i.e., themes) one would likely want to get across during the course of the formal hypnosis session or therapeutic conversation. Next, I provide some representative suggestions for each step of the sequence.

Table 29.2 A Generic Strategy for Hypnotically Facilitating Flexibility

- Induction
- Build response set re: alternatives
- Theme #1: Multiple ways to do or view something
- Theme #2: Exploring and discovering new possibilities
- Theme #3: Trying something different just to see what happens
- Check-in with the client
- Post-hypnotic suggestion: Evolving flexibility
- Closure and disengagement

Induction

("There are so *many different ways of getting absorbed* in the comfort of hypnosis ... and how you deepen your comfort this time ... and how you build greater focus this time ... might be similar to other times ... or quite different from other times ...")

Response Set

("There is no one right way to sit ... you can choose what's comfortable for you ... and there is no single right way to begin exploring different options for achieving what you want for yourself ...")

Theme #1

("If you want to travel to another part of the country ... how many different ways are there to get there?... Fly? Drive? Take a train? Ride a bicycle? Walk?... And if you want to be a good parent ... how many different ways are there to do that?... Be loving and affectionate? Be clear and firm in the positions you take?... Be patient and supportive?... Be tolerant and accepting?... And for almost anything you might want ... there are many different pathways, not just one ...")

Theme #2

("You can appreciate the courage of the pioneering explorers of long ago ... those who saw the distant horizon and wanted to know what was out there ... and when curiosity grows stronger than fear or doubt ... people set out to explore ... not knowing what they might discover ... not unlike what you're doing now as you explore your inner horizons ... not knowing what you'll discover inside that will be so valuable to you ...")

Theme #3

("And as your curiosity builds ... and your willingness to do something different builds along with it ... you can enjoy discovering that when you approach that challenging situation differently ... in a way that's far more likely to succeed ... your willingness to experiment can give rise to new possibilities that are wonderfully satisfying ...")

Check-In

("And in just a moment I'd like you to describe out loud what you're aware of right now ... and you can describe it easily ... even deepening your experience as you speak ...")

Post-Hypnotic Suggestion

("There's so much you've learned in your lifetime ... and as you continue to grow as a person ... it gets easier to reach inside and make good use of the parts of you that can best respond in a given situation ...")

Closure and Disengagement

("Take your time in bringing this experience to a comfortable close ... and then slowly begin to re-orient ... re-alerting yourself now and opening your eyes")

Conclusion

Perhaps the first principle one learns in studying hypnosis is that *what you focus on you amplify*. Thus, a clinician must be deliberate about choosing focal points for hypnotic interventions. In this chapter, many different factors contributing to and exacerbating depression have been identified. The point was made emphatically that what a clinician focuses on should be determined according to the specific patterns and rigidities that give rise an individual's quality of depression. There is no "one-size-fits-all" approach nor is there a "best" treatment for depression. There are, however, common characteristics of effective interventions, namely active and experiential treatments that help build specific skills for managing one's mood ... and one's *life*. Hypnosis is an active and experiential approach, and the evidence is growing steadily that skillfully applied hypnosis can do a great many things to help enrich and empower some of the most disempowered and despairing people we hope to help.

References

Alladin, A., & Alibhai, A. (2007). Cognitive hypnotherapy for depression: An empirical investigation. *International Journal of Clinical and Experimental Hypnosis*, *55*(2), 147–166. 10.1080/00207140601177897

Almohammed, O. A., Alsalem, A. A., Almangour, A. A., Alotaibi, L. H., Al Yami, M. S., & Lai, L. (2022). Antidepressants and health-related quality of life (HRQoL) for patients with depression: Analysis of the medical expenditure panel survey from the United States. *PLOS One*, *17*(4), e0265928. 10.1371/journal.pone.0265928

COVID-19 Mental Disorders Collaborators (2021). Global prevalence and burden of depressive and anxiety disorders in 204 countries and territories in 2020 due to the COVID-19 pandemic. *The Lancet*, *398*(10312), 1700–1712. 10.1016/s0140-6736(21)02143-7

Curtis, D. (2021). Analysis of 50,000 exome-sequenced UK Biobank subjects fails to identify genes influencing probability of developing a mood disorder resulting in psychiatric referral. *Journal of Affective Disorders*, *281*, 216–219. 10.1016/j.jad.2020.12.025

Evans-Lacko, S., Aguilar-Gaxiola, S., Al-Hamzawi, A., Alonso, J. A., Benjet, C., Bruffaerts, R., ... Thornicroft, G. (2018). Socio-economic variations in the mental health treatment gap for people with anxiety, mood, and substance use disorders: Results from the WHO World Mental Health (WMH) surveys. *Psychological Medicine*, *48*(9), 1560–1571. 10.1017/s0033291717003336

Harrington, A. (2019). *Mind fixers: Psychiatry's troubled search for the biology of mental illness*. W. W. Norton & Company.

Holroyd, J. (2003). The science of meditation and the state of hypnosis. *American Journal of Clinical Hypnosis*, *46*(2), 109–128. 10.1080/00029157.2003.10403582

Kirsch, I., Montgomery, G., & Sapirstein, G. (1995). Hypnosis as an adjunct to cognitive-behavioral psychotherapy: A meta-analysis. *Journal of Consulting and Clinical Psychology*, *63*(2), 214–220. 10.1037/0022-006x.63.2.214

Lebowitz, M. S., Dolev-Amit, T., & Zilcha-Mano, S. (2021). Relationships of biomedical beliefs about depression to treatment-related expectancies in a treatment-seeking sample. *Psychotherapy (Chicago, Ill.)*, *58*(3), 366–371. 10.1037/pst0000320

Maes, M., & Stoyanov, D. (2022). False dogmas in mood disorders research: Towards a nomothetic network approach. *World Journal of Psychiatry*, *12*(5), 651–667. 10.5498/wjp.v12.i5.651

Marasine, N. R., Sankhi, S., Lamichhane, R., Marasini, N. R., & Dangi, N. B. (2021). Use of antidepressants among patients diagnosed with depression: A scoping review. *BioMed Research International*, *2021*, 1–8. 10.1155/2021/6699028

Milling, L. S., Valentine, K. E., McCarley, H. S., & LoStimolo, L. M. (2019). A meta-analysis of hypnotic interventions for depression symptoms: High hopes for hypnosis? *American Journal of Clinical Hypnosis*, *61*(3), 227–243. 10.1080/00029157.2018.1489777

Moncrieff, J., Cooper, R. E., Stockmann, T., Amendola, S., Hengartner, M. P., & Horowitz, M. A. (2022). The serotonin theory of depression: A systematic umbrella review of the evidence. *Molecular Psychiatry*. 10.1038/s41380-022-01661-0

Moitra, M., Santomauro, D., Collins, P. Y., Vos, T., Whiteford, H., Saxena, S., & Ferrari, A. J. (2022). The global gap in treatment coverage for major depressive disorder in 84 countries from 2000–2019: A systematic review and Bayesian meta-regression analysis. *PLOS Medicine*, *19*(2), e1003901. 10.1371/journal.pmed.1003901

Ramondo, N., Gignac, G. E., Pestell, C. F., & Byrne, S. M. (2021). Clinical hypnosis as an adjunct to cognitive behavior therapy: An updated meta-analysis. *International Journal of Clinical and Experimental Hypnosis*, *69*(2), 169–202. 10.1080/00207144.2021.1877549

Schroder, H. S., Duda, J. M., Christensen, K., Beard, C., & Björgvinsson, T. (2020). Stressors and chemical imbalances: Beliefs about the causes of depression in an acute psychiatric treatment sample. *Journal of Affective Disorders*, *276*, 537–545. 10.1016/j.jad.2020.07.061

Shih, M., Yang, Y.-H., & Koo, M. (2009). A meta-analysis of hypnosis in the treatment of depressive symptoms: A brief communication. *International Journal of Clinical and Experimental Hypnosis*, *57*(4), 431–442. 10.1080/00207140903099039

World Health Organization (2017). *Depression and other common mental disorders: Global health estimates*. World Health Organization. https://apps.who.int/iris/handle/10665/254610

World Health Organization (2022, March 2). *COVID-19 pandemic triggers 25% increase in prevalence of anxiety and depression worldwide*. World Health Organization. Retrieved March 20, 2023, from https://www.who.int/news/item/02-03-2022-covid-19-pandemic-triggers-25-increase-in-prevalence-of-anxiety-and-depression-worldwide

Yapko, M. D. (1992). *Hypnosis and the treatment of depressions: Strategies for change*. Brunner-Mazel.

Yapko, M. D. (2001). *Treating depression with hypnosis: Integrating cognitive-behavioral and strategic approaches* (1st ed.). Routledge.

Yapko, M. D. (Ed.). (2006). *Hypnosis and treating depression: Applications in clinical practice* (1st ed.). Routledge.

Yapko, M. D. (2009). *Depression is contagious: How the most common mood disorder is spreading around the world and how to stop it* (1st ed.). The Free Press.

Yapko, M. D. (2010a). Hypnosis in the treatment of depression: An overdue approach for encouraging skillful mood management. *International Journal of Clinical and Experimental Hypnosis*, *58*(2), 137–146. 10.1080/00207140903523137

Yapko, M. D. (2010b). Hypnotically catalyzing experiential learning across treatments for depression: Actions can speak louder than moods. *International Journal of Clinical and Experimental Hypnosis*, *58*(2), 186–201. 10.1080/00207140903523228

Yapko, M. D. (2011). *Mindfulness and hypnosis: The power of suggestion to transform experience* (1st ed.). W. W. Norton Company.

Yapko, M. D. (2013). Treating depression with antidepressants: Drug-placebo efficacy debates limit broader considerations. *American Journal of Clinical Hypnosis*, *55*(3), 272–290. 10.1080/00029157.2012.707156

Yapko, M. D. (2016). *The discriminating therapist: Asking "how" questions, making distinctions, and finding direction in therapy* (1st ed.). Yapko Publications.

Yapko, M. D. (2019). *Trancework: An introduction to the practice of clinical hypnosis* (5th ed.). Routledge.

Yapko, M. D. (2020). Contemplating… the obvious: What you focus on, you amplify. *International Journal of Clinical and Experimental Hypnosis*, *68*(2), 144–150. 10.1080/00207144.2020.1719841

Yapko, M. D. (2021). *Process-oriented hypnosis: Focusing on the forest, not the trees*. W. W. Norton & Company.

Yapko, M. D. (2022). Encouraging hindsight in advance: Age progression in therapy - and life. *American Journal of Clinical Hypnosis*, *65*(1), 4–17. 10.1080/00029157.2022.2038067

Yapko, M. D., & Criswell, S. R. (In Press). Hypnosis and depression. In L. S. Milling (Ed.), *Evidence-Based Practice in Clinical Hypnosis*. American Psychological Association.

30

THE HYPNOTIC LENS ON TRAUMA AND TREATMENT

Julie H. Linden
PRIVATE PRACTICE OQUOSSOC, ME, USA

Background Perspectives

Hypnosis, defined in a variety of ways in this volume, was missing from my clinical psychology training. Instead, it was a treatment modality introduced to me when I became a consultant to the first burn center in my city of origin in the early 1970s. The director who offered me this new role reasoned that no amount of medication would be enough for severely burned individuals and they would need other ways to manage their pain, in particular, hypnosis.

This was an astonishing notion, a contrast to my psychoanalytical background, and one to which I was open. I was introduced to Dabney Ewin (1925–2020), a pioneer in the use of hypnosis for burn treatment and a wise mentor for my new study. This approach paved the way for my next 50 years of exploring the relationship between all forms of traumatic experiences and what was termed *hypnosis*. I worked with people managing chronic illnesses (Linden, 1995, 1996), people who had survived war (Linden, 2002), and people who had experienced physical, verbal, and sexual abuse. They ranged from 1 ½ to 80 years of age. These cumulative clinical encounters have influenced and shaped my understanding of psychology, clinical hypnosis, and trauma. I was integrative in my theoretical orientations, and person-centered in my approach, looking for skills that fit the patient's need, not vice versa. Today I would describe myself as following a biopsychosocial person-centered model (Jensen et al., 2015; Sugarman et al., 2020) applying hypnotic principles and communication skills to psychotherapy grounded in current neuroscience, a description increasingly shared by many in the field of clinical hypnosis.

Brief History of Trauma Awareness in Health Care

To understand the close relationship between trauma and hypnosis, a brief history of the entrance of trauma into our mental health nomenclature and the public's awareness is required. It is a bumpy road on which the sequelae of war trauma (Kapor-Stanulovic, 1999), awareness of child abuse, and the women's movement coalesced with neuroscience research.

DOI: 10.4324/9781003449126-42

Humanity is affected by traumatic events. Wars may have the most devastating effects, as they destroy trust, relationships, and social order. Shell shock, traumatic neurosis, traumatic hysteria, and battle fatigue were a few of the older terms for the debilitating symptoms observed in those who had experienced the ravages of war (Barker, 1996; Kapor-Stanulovic, 1999; Watkins, 2000). Physicians from the French Nancy school, Liébeault and Bernheim experimented with hypnosis, as did Charcot from the Salpêtriere school looking for ways to treat the tenacious, trauma-related symptoms that impaired functioning (see Facco, in this handbook). Pierre Janet, French neurologist and psychologist, and student of Charcot's, developed the dissociation theory of hypnosis, searching to understand ailments in soldiers and the mentally ill in which no physical evidence of disability was present (see van der Hart & Horst, 1989). Posting unconscious causes, his work highlighted dissociative processes and the possible mechanisms of conversion disorders in the care of soldiers during World War I. His stages of treatment and underlying principles are foundational to our understanding and treatment of PTSD.

Interest in hypnosis briefly waned as Freud further developed treatment approaches involving the unconscious, only to resurge with World War II when it was widely employed to manage the pain of the wounded (Kluft, 1985, 1988; Watkins, 2000).

Prior to the introduction of modern, safe general anesthesia in 1956, physicians and surgeons on the battlefield used hypnosis for analgesia and pain management, reviving interest in its utility. Modern hypnosis societies and research began with the end of that war, and again, the challenges of recalcitrant symptoms (Watkins, 2000).

In 1952, the first Diagnostic and Statistical Manual (DSM-1) was published. It included the diagnosis Gross Stress Reaction resulting from combat or civilian catastrophes (American Psychiatric Association, 1952). Mostly, soldiers suffered in silence with little public understanding (Barker, 1996).

Then, in the United States, pediatric radiologist C. Henry Kempe (1962) introduced the term "battered child syndrome" in his scholarly article and galvanized awareness of abuse of children (Kempe et al, 1962). This served to lessen the silence and denial that had proliferated in the medical community prior to its courageous publication. Or perhaps the dissociated emotions of pain and horror in the medical community finally surfaced. While an in-depth exploration of this topic surpasses the scope of this chapter, the abuse of children also fostered both more understanding of how hypnosis could be helpful with the young and developmental awareness in trauma nomenclature (Linden, 2014).

The public's increased grasp of the sequelae of trauma was further amplified by soldiers returning from Vietnam exhibiting symptoms reminiscent of those studied after both World Wars.

In the 1970s, psychiatrist Bessel van der Kolk (1987) was instrumental in researching treatment for Vietnam veterans who were so disabled by their war experiences. A pattern of turning to clinical hypnosis as a research paradigm and treatment option emerged with the trauma of war, highlighting both the fixed attention to ideas and images and dissociation characteristic of trauma and hypnosis responses (Cardeña, 2000; Putnam, 1997).

And finally, the women's movement galvanized females to seek their places in the scholarly debates on violence and trauma. This raised awareness of domestic violence, the long-term effects of childhood sexual abuse, and of the unique coping strategies of females. For example, Taylor et. al. (2000) developed the theory of Tend and Befriend contrasting it with male responses to stress. She addressed the hormonal response of women under stress, incorporating the increasing awareness of neurophysiological components of trauma.

Women release the pituitary hormone oxytocin, which downregulates the sympathetic nervous system activation characteristic of the fight-flight response. Oxytocin is released when women engage in nurturing and affiliative behavior. Estrogen amplifies the calming effect of the hormone. In men, who also produce oxytocin, androgens lessen its effect. Éva Bányai's research on active alert hypnosis (Bányai, 2018) began years of research in her laboratory that yielded information on the interactive effects of hypnosis between and within the genders of therapist and client. Varga and Kekecs (2014) have researched the effect of oxytocin during hypnosis interactions that align with these gender differences in stress responses.

The "false memory wars" of the 1990s (mostly in the United States; Schacter, 1995) were an interesting coalescence of raised awareness of abuse, women's increasing agency, and efforts to use hypnosis to access the unconscious to resolve or lessen symptoms. An explosion of research on the practice and effects of hypnosis touted as creating false memories paradoxically led to our increasing understanding of memory (Loftus, 1997), dissociative phenomena (Freyd, 1997), and suggestion. However, hypnosis is often portrayed as the villain in memory theory, rather than the more complex issues of the interplay of its application, dissociative responses, and nascent neurophysiological models of memory.

Labels and Diagnostic Terms

With this confluence of events, psychology amplified its research into trauma.

Post-traumatic stress disorder was introduced to the DSM in 1980 in its third edition (American Psychiatric Association, 1980).

After several decades of intense research on trauma through the 1980s and 1990s (Friedman, 2014; van der Kolk et al., 1996), PTSD became the preferred term to describe the recognized symptoms of hyper and hypo arousal, intrusive thoughts, flashbacks, and avoidance. This change was reflected in the DSM revisions from 1987 to 2000. Initially, diagnosis required a recognizable stressor, one outside the range of normal human experience. Later the individual's *perception* of the event became the primary feature (Daly, 2004). PTSD is now recognized globally in the diagnostic nomenclature having been added to the International Classification of Diseases in 1992 (WHO, 1992).

The diagnostic symptoms of PTSD reflected the nervous system's reactions of avoidance and arousal. However, focusing on the post responses did not provide a comprehensive understanding of the response to traumatic experiences. *Acute stress disorder* (ASD), introduced in 1994, was defined as symptoms of anxiety and dissociation that occurred within one month of a traumatic event. When ASD does not resolve by six months, it becomes longer term (PTSD) and sometimes chronic. *Trauma by proxy* (Brooks & Siegel, 1996), a further delineation of types and causes of trauma, is the term used to describes our reaction to a trauma experienced by someone else. This diagnostic addition expanded awareness of trauma as a relational experience. Children are particularly vulnerable to this as they may identify with the victim due to less mature self-boundaries and confuse reality and fantasy (Linden, 2014, 2019).

Vicarious traumatization, sometimes called secondary traumatic stress (Figley, 1995), refers to the toxic effects of violent behavior on observers and this includes the caregivers and clinicians treating those who are traumatized (McCann & Pearlman, 1990b).

Attachment theory tells us we generate empathy toward others. We cannot observe abuse and violence and not be affected if we have healthy attachments. We may bear witness (Bloom & Reichert, 1998) but when we do not act, then our sense of efficacy is undermined, we feel helpless, powerless, guilty, and ashamed. This idea becomes important when we apply clinical hypnosis skills, because we can imagine acting, and the preparation to act releases undischarged energy (Levine & Kline, 2007).

Simple Versus Complicated Trauma

Trauma can be further defined as simple or complicated (Brown & Fromm, 1986), single or repetitive (De Zulueta, 1993), one car accident, or repeated molestation. A single event of brief duration occurring later in life without man-made violence can resolve more quickly, than ongoing traumatization such as that experienced in war.

Herman (1992b) introduced the notion of complex PTSD which addressed the relational, repetitive, and developmental qualities of trauma. Van der Kolk (2005) prefers the term Developmental Trauma Disorder (DTD) for children noting the impact of trauma on development. The term *Continuous Traumatic Stress* was introduced in the 1980s by Straker (Straker, 2013; Eagle & Kaminer, 2013) to describe those seeking treatment who were living under ongoing conditions of risk to their safety. Another label variation is *Anticipatory Trauma*, descriptive of what one does with terrorism, gun violence, sexual abuse, and other interpersonal violence (Ziss, 2020) with chronic consequences. The array of terms to describe trauma will likely continue to grow, as research and clinical experience contribute more understanding to its biopsychosocial genesis and treatment.

The increased research on hypnosis and trauma developed in tandem (Perry, 2001, 2009) and have been intertwined in time, definitions, and treatment. *Dissociative Identity Disorder,* (DID) was also introduced as the preferred diagnosis for multiple personality disorder in the American Psychiatric Association nomenclature, DSM-IV (1994). This change in name reflected the growing recognition of role of dissociative response to trauma (Kluft, 1985, 1996; van der Hart et al, 2005).

Definitions of Trauma

As the research on trauma was underway, definitions ranged widely (Gil, 1998; Herman, 1992b; Perry, 2001; Pynoos, 1994; Van der Kolk, 1987). Sensitive to our earliest fears as infants and reminding us that trauma is a relational process, Lindemann (1944) defined it as "the sudden cessation of human interaction". As with child abuse, the medical community was hesitant to see the relationship between behaviors and symptoms and traumatic events (Anbar & Linden, 2010).

Current practice recognizes trauma as a universal phenomenon that involves events and the person's capacity to manage them (McCann & Pearlman 1990a). The nervous system's response, once oversimplified as a fight or flight reaction, is increasingly defined with the polyvagal language of Porges (2011). Neurological forces, largely unconscious, provide protection through interoception (internal sensing by organs) and social mediating (mirror neurons, orienting responses). The range of events is wide: from nature's floods, to chronic illness, to man's war. The impact of trauma is mediated by age and social response and its effects are specific. What is traumatic for one person may not be for another. Viewed through the neurobiological lens, trauma is anything that alerts the organism to experience its survival as threatened.

This perspective of trauma provides a more fluid developmental model that integrates the innate wiring of the autonomic nervous system with individual experience and meaning given to any threatening experience, and changing throughout one's life. Our previous life experiences, particular sensitivities of our nervous systems, quality of attachment, developmental stage, temperament, personality, and cognitive style, influence both our experience and interpretation of what we call traumatic (Bonanno, 2004; Self-Brown et al., 2004). Trauma may simply be when it is too much for the embodied mind to manage that flow of information and energy across the brain (Doidge, 2007, 2015; Siegel, 2010, Siegel et al., 2019).

This understanding of trauma is the reason that van der Kolk (2014) describes it as a somatic experience. His research has shown that many systems of the body, neurological, endocrinological, muscular, and immunological, are activated under stress. We experience trauma in the body. The conscious mind works to forget, to suppress, to avoid remembering trauma but as van der Kolk's reasons the body does not forget. Instead, the brain's alarm system recalibrates, stress hormones increase, and our filtering of information is altered. Peter Levine (2010) developed a treatment approach called Somatic Experience to train therapists in ways to identify and release trauma stored in the body. His work and that of Ogden's sensorimotor psychotherapy (Ogden & Fisher, 2015) stemmed from an understanding of the unconscious and dissociation. Dissociation is embedded in hypnosis practice.

Dissociation and Hypnosis

Dissociation is observed in and reported by those experiencing clinical hypnosis. Pierre Janet (1907) studied the concept of dissociation in psychopathology and elaborated on its relationship to hypnosis and ego states (van der Kolk & van der Hart, 1989). Definitions of dissociation vary by those who have contributed to its place in psychological treatment and ego state therapy (Cardeña, 1994; Dell, 2019; Leutner & Piedfort-Marin, 2021; Watkins & Watkins, 1997). Ernest Hilgard (Hilgard & Hilgard, 1975) in his hypnosis research lab at Stanford University chose "hidden observer" to explain the phenomena of his studies in which a person had achieved hypnotic comfort, and yet, reported pain with ideomotor signaling. He used the term "neodissociation", separating his concept from that of Janet (van der Hart & Horst, 1989). Phillips and Frederick (1995) offer a practical model describing dissociation on a continuum from the mundane automaticity of daily activities like driving, to daydreams, lucid dreams, fugue states, and DID. It allows people to distance, compartmentalize, and remove themselves from the trauma in order to gain control (Anbar & Linden, 2010) and to function.

Other changes in consciousness include a narrowing in focus of attention, numbing, out of body, "spacey" descriptions, with an alteration in sense of time and sensory perceptions (Cardeña, 2000) all of which are observed in someone in the plastic trance process. One can distance, have discontinuity, and compartmentalize in order to maintain, gain, or regain control (Anbar & Linden, 2010). As noted, this lets the body handle some of the responses. In the short term dissociating can be helpful.

One problem with chronic dissociating is that it may inhibit our ability to put the experience into words or to make meaning of an event, and then dissociation is more harmful than helpful. A disadvantage of dissociation (van der Hart et al., 1993) is that the coping method may become hardened and inflexible. Van der Hart et al. (2006) introduced the theory of structural dissociation of the personality (TSDP) offering new terminology for the trauma-fractured development of self. Ego state therapy developed by Watkins and Watkins (1997) considered hypnosis a form of dissociation. Hypnosis research into dissociation, clinical observations using hypnosis procedures, and traumatized clients are a triumvirate of overlaid concepts.

These findings of the phenomenological experiences of clinical hypnosis exemplify the similarities and overlap of responses to trauma and hypnosis. It is these parallels that make clinical hypnosis an effective treatment for trauma. The structured and therapeutic use of hypnotic dissociation can activate and then alter these same pathways to resolve debilitating symptoms (Linden & Sugarman, 2021). This disruption of embodied learning and cognitive conditioning with the use of dissociative language loosens engrams of learning often associated with traumatic responses.

Applying Hypnosis

Historically, clinicians have applied hypnosis to treat trauma (Brown & Fromm, 1986; Hilgard & LeBaron, 1984; Watkins, 2000) and research has shown this to be an effective therapeutic skill set (O'Toole et al., 2016). Elkins (2017, 2022) notes its far-ranging application in medical and psychological disorders, most of which relate to traumatic experiences. Chronic illnesses, painful disorders, anxiety, and depression, to name a few, are traumatic experiences (with a range of intensity) that respond to hypnosis communication skills.

Once recognized as a valuable tool by the British Medical Association in 1955, and the American Medical Association's (AMA) Council on Mental Health in 1958 (Kroger, 1977), in 1987 the AMA rescinded its 1881–1958 policies and has no official position on hypnosis. Lacking medical support, hypnosis has come in and out of fashion as a treatment method, been reconfigured (systematic desensitization, eye movement desensitization, and reprocessing), and elements of it borrowed from and incorporated into other treatment approaches (mindfulness) (Wolpe, 1996; Yapko, 2011).

The lack of consensus on how to define it and how to apply its principles has not interfered with its adoption by clinicians, as observed in the size of membership in clinical hypnosis organizations globally. Hypnosis can both relax the aroused nervous system and work within a "window of tolerance" (Siegel, 1999) and can get to the original affective state required for successful treatment (James, 1989). The response to something traumatic can take our rational thinking "offline". Through relational neuroscience, calm, soothing, melodic, rhythmic techniques can restore cognitive functioning and autonomic regulation (Banks & Hirschman, 2015). We are calm in the face of another's calm (Linden, 2014). The establishment of safety, trust, predictability, and resonance supplied in the relational hypnotic context eases the way to the suppressed emotions that are inhibiting healing. In addition, one can achieve corrective orienting, completing a defensive orientation interrupted by a trauma, which often occur in accidents (Heller & Heller, 2001).

Since the explosion of knowledge of the brain and nervous system, augmented by instruments of research such as fMRIs, there is a growing understanding of where emotions, cognitions, memory, sensory perceptions reside and interact – and how working hypnotically, verbally and nonverbally, permits those to change and bring relief of traumatic symptoms. The field of hypnosis has an evidence-based practice and research base more robust than most treatment modalities (Barabasz & Barabasz, 2013). It continues to be both an experimental probe and a clinical skill in a range of disciplines (Sugarman, et al., 2020) and is well suited to trauma treatment.

Developmental Variation and Vulnerability

Aligned with van der Kolk's previously noted term DTD (van der Kolk, 2005), one cannot discuss trauma without tending to developmental variation (Terr, 1990). Trauma is experienced diversely with age just as hypnosis is utilized differently across the lifespan (Kohen & Olness 2011; Linden, 2003, 2004, 2014). Children are undoubtedly more significantly shaped by traumatic experiences as their denominator of life experiences is smaller. Their critical developmental periods are altered, internal coping strategies are nascent, they have undeveloped abstract reasoning, and their caregivers are often simultaneously traumatized. And identifying signs of trauma in children can be more challenging. Perception is more basic and primitive than cognition, so for the preverbal youngster, the traumatic perception may remain indigestible (Eth & Pynoos, 1984). As we assess behavior and signs of trauma, there are some critical items to consider.

Preschoolers (3–6 years) have a hard time distinguishing between reality and fantasy. They also have difficulty with sense of time, distance, and geography which in addition to porous boundaries makes them vulnerable to trauma by proxy. They lack a vocabulary to express feelings and may say they are having fun but instead look sad or intense. Like adults, they too regress in the face of trauma becoming clingy or losing skills they had acquired. Their play may be repetitive or aggressive, and they have trouble with narrating a story in sequence. Young children do not understand the concept of death or its permanence, and they tend to use magical thinking to explain events. Keeping these elements in mind will enable age-appropriate hypnotic techniques such as movement, drawing pictures, and simple language.

Primary school-aged children (6–12 years) do understand death but usually will not talk about it; they hide their feelings to protect others and like the preschooler prefer nonverbal modes of expression. There is a need for control, as they grow more independent and thus they may blame themselves for something traumatic, e.g., a traffic accident. They have a need for rules but will test the rules. Reckless behavior at this age often relates to being unsure of the future. There is a move from magical thinking to explaining the supernatural (from monsters to ghosts). Other signs of trauma at this age are changes in school performance, either difficulty concentrating or becoming more focused as well as interruptions in relating to friends.

With adolescents, the process of individuating leads young people to prefer their peers to adults and they may identify coping mechanisms through their friends. They often isolate, are depressed, and become suicidal, and are likely to engage in revenge fantasies. They are like adults in their use of hypnosis techniques but without fully developed frontal lobes and executive control. Psychiatrist Judith Herman called attention to adolescent vulnerability due to less power than adults, exposure to war, combat, and rape. The latter two are primarily experiences of adolescence and early adult life. "Rape and combat might thus be considered complementary social rites of initiation into the coercive violence at the foundation of adult society. They are the paradigmatic forms of trauma for women and men respectively" (Herman, 1992a, p. 61).

Owing to research on traumatic symptoms in children (Garbarino et al.,1991; Perry, 2001; Pynoos, 1994), theoretical rethinking (Levine, 2010; Levine & Kline, 2007; Siegel et al., 2019) has influenced a deeper understanding of the complex interaction of (1) early healthy attachment; (2) the neurophysiology of the alarm, fear, and survival systems; and (3) the somatosensory contributions to our response to and healing from traumatic events (Linden, 2014, 2019). Complex developmental trauma (Ford & Courtois, 2009) and DTD (van der Kolk et al., 2019) were terms introduced to address trauma across the lifespan. Key considerations for the development of PTSD include the age of the person at the time of trauma, personality factors, previous exposure to trauma, genetic predispositions (van der Kolk, 1987), family dynamics, and a host of other factors that make us who we are.

It is important to keep in mind that the focus of hypnotic treatment is both recovery and resilience and as developmental psychologist Masten notes "Resilience is made up of ordinary processes, rather than extraordinary ones" (Masten, 2001, p.227). Safe, containing relationships where suggestions are used to disrupt old patterns and create new possibilities for the future are the ordinary processes of healing, therapeutic communication. However, while hypnosis is successfully used for many forms of trauma, some trauma is much harder to treat such as torture. All therapies have their limitations. A strength of hypnotic communication is how easily it can be integrated with other therapies. Unfortunately, this includes more nefarious uses of hypnotic skills for undue influence and abusive mind control. Hassan and Shah (2019) describe how the very same skills applied to heal from trauma can produce identity-damaging effects.

Becoming Trauma-Informed

After decades of research, refining the understanding of the effects of trauma on humans (Klissourov, 2018), and the public's easy use of PTSD to describe a dizzying range of emotional responses to a wide range of events, many researchers and clinicians began advocating for all clinicians to become trauma-informed (Poole & Greaves, 2012). The idea to consider trauma when diagnosing and treating individuals receiving medical and mental health services at first glance seems obvious. However, like the movement to assess pain in the 2000s (JCAHO, 2001), it was not obvious, but once instituted it greatly increased both the care of and the attention to those suffering from hidden trauma.

Training in hypnosis procedures and communication for all medical and psychological clinicians is central to trauma-informed care. The concepts of dissociation, trauma, and hypnosis are a triumvirate waiting to be fully integrated into patient-centered care.

References

American Psychiatric Association (APA) (1952). *Diagnostic and statistical manual mental disorders.* (1st ed.) APA Press. Retrieved July 23, 2022 http://www.turkpsikiyatri.org/arsiv/dsm-1952.pdf

American Psychiatric Association (APA). (1980). *Diagnostic and statistical manual of mental health disorders* (3rd ed.). APA Press.

American Psychiatric Association. (1994). *Diagnostic and statistical manual of mental disorders* (4th ed.). American Psychiatric Publishing, Inc.

Anbar, R., & Linden, J. (2010). Understanding dissociation and insight in the treatment of shortness of breath with hypnosis: A case study. *American Journal of Clinical Hypnosis*, *52*(4), 263–274.

Banks, A., & Hirschman, L. A. (2015) *Wired to connect: The surprising link between brain science and strong, healthy, relationships.* Jeremy Trcher/Penguin.

Bányai, É. I. (2018). Active-alert hypnosis: History, research, and applications. *American Journal of Clinical Hypnosis*, *61*(2), 88–107. 10.1080/00029157.2018.1496318

Barabasz, A., & Barabasz, M. (2013). Hypnosis for PTSD: Evidence based placebo-controlled studies. *Journal of Trauma & Treatment*, *S4*, 1–5. 10.4172/2167-1222.s4-006

Barker, P. (1996). *The regeneration trilogy*. Viking Press.

Bloom, S. & Reichert, M. (1998). *Bearing witness: Violence and collective responsibility*. Haworth Press.

Bonanno, G. A. (2004). Loss, trauma, and human resilience: Have we underestimated the human capacity to thrive after extremely aversive events? *American Psychologist*, *59*(1), 20–28. 10.1037/0003-066x.59.1.20

Brooks, B., & Siegel, P. (1996). *The scared child*. Wiley & Sons, Inc.

Brown, D. P., & Fromm, E. (1986). *Hypnotherapy and hypnoanalysis*. Lawrence Erlbaum.

Cardeña, E. (1994). The domain of dissociation. In S. J. Lynn, & J. W. Rhue (Eds.), *Dissociation: Clinical and theoretical perspectives* (pp. 15–31). The Guilford Press.

Cardeña, E. (2000). Hypnosis in the treatment of trauma: A promising, but not fully supported, efficacious intervention. *International Journal of Clinical and Experimental Hypnosis*, *48*(2), 225–238. 10.1080/00207140008410049

Daly, O. (2004). Stresspoints. *Spring*, *18*(2), 4.

Dell, P. (2019). Reconsidering the autohypnotic model of the dissociative disorders. *Journal of Trauma & Dissociation*, *20*(1), 48–78, 10.1080/15299732.2018.1451806

De Zulueta, F. (1993). *From pain to violence*. Jason Aronson, Inc.

Doidge, N. (2007). *The brain that changes itself: Stories of personal triumph from the frontiers of brain science*. Penguin Group.

Doidge, N. (2015). Hypnosis, neuroplasticity, and the plastic paradox. *American Journal of Clinical Hypnosis*, *57*(3), 349–354. 10.1080/00029157.2015.985572

Eagle, G., & Kaminer, D. (2013). Continuous traumatic stress: Expanding the lexicon of traumatic stress. *Peace and Conflict: Journal of Peace Psychology*, *19*(2), 85–99. 10.1037/a0032485

Elkins, G. R. (2017). *Handbook of medical and psychological hypnosis: Foundations, applications, and professional issues*. Springer.

Elkins, G. R. (2022). Clinical hypnosis in health care and treatment. *International Journal of Clinical and Experimental Hypnosis*, *70*(1), 1–3. 10.1080/00207144.2022.2011112

Eth, S., & Pynoos, R. S. (1984). *Post-traumatic stress disorder in children*. American Psychiatric Publications, Inc.

Figley, C. R. (1995). Compassion fatigue as secondary traumatic stress disorder: An overview. In C. R. Figley (Ed.), *Compassion fatigue: Coping with secondary traumatic stress disorder in those who treat the traumatized* (pp. 1–20). Brunner/Mazel.

Ford, J. D., & Courtois, C. A. (2009). Defining and understanding complex trauma and complex traumatic stress disorders. In C. A. Courtois, & J. D. Ford (Eds.), *Treating complex traumatic stress disorders: An evidence-based guide* (pp. 13–30). The Guilford Press.

Freyd, J. J. (1997). *Betrayal trauma: The logic of forgetting childhood abuse*. Harvard University Press.

Friedman, M. J. (2014). *PTSD history and overview*. U.S. Department of Veterans Affairs; PTSD: National Center For PTSD. Retrieved February 12, 2023, from https://www.ptsd.va.gov/professional/treat/essentials/history_ptsd.asp

Garbarino, J., Kostelny, K., & Dubrow, N. (1991). *No place to be a child: Growing up in a war zone*. Jossey-Bass Publishers.

Gil, E. (1998). *Play therapy for severe psychological trauma* (videotape and manual). Guilford Press.

Hassan, S., & Shah, M. (2019). The anatomy of undue influence used by terrorist cults and traffickers to induce helplessness and trauma, so creating false identities. *Ethics, Medicine and Public Health*, *8*, 97–107. 10.1016/j.jemep.2019.03.002

Heller, D. P., & Heller, L. S. (2001). *Crash course: A self-healing guide to auto accident trauma and recovery*. North Atlantic Books.

Herman, J. L. (1992a). *Trauma and recovery: The aftermath of violence – from domestic abuse to political terror* (1st ed.). Basic Books.

Herman, J. L. (1992b). Complex PTSD: A syndrome in survivors of prolonged and repeated trauma. *Journal of Traumatic Stress*, *5*(3), 377–391. 10.1002/jts.2490050305

Hilgard, E. R., & Hilgard, J. R. (1975). *Hypnosis in the relief of pain* (1st ed.). William Kaufmann, Inc.

Hilgard, J. R., & LeBaron, S. (1984). *Hypnotherapy of pain in children with cancer*. William Kaufmann, Inc.

Janet, P. (1907). *The major symptoms of hysteria.* Macmillan Publishing. 10.1037/10008-000

James, B. (1989). *Treating traumatized children: New insights and creative interventions.* Lexington Books (D. C. Heath & Co.).

Joint Commission on the Accreditation of Healthcare Organizations (JCAHO) (2001). *Pain standards for 2001.* Retrieved February 16, 2023, from https://www.jointcommission.org/-/media/tjc/documents/resources/pain-management/2001_pain_standardspdf.pdf

Jensen, M. P., Adachi, T., Tomé-Pires, C., Lee, J., Osman, Z. J., & Miró, J. (2015). Mechanisms of hypnosis: Toward the development of a biopsychosocial model. *International Journal of Clinical and Experimental Hypnosis, 63*(1), 34–75. 10.1080/00207144.2014.961875

Kapor-Stanulovic, N. (1999). Encounter with suffering: Socioeconomic transition, wars, and children – A reminder. *American Psychologist, 54*(11), 1020–1027.

Kempe, C. H., Silverman, F. N., Steele, B. F., Droegemueller, W., & Silver, H. K. (1962). The battered-child syndrome. *Journal of the American Medical Association, 181*(1), 17–24. 10.1001/jama.1962.03050270019004

Klissourov, G. (2018). *Meta-analysis of the effectiveness magnitude of hypnosis on posttraumatic stress disorder treatment.* Doctoral Dissertation. Walden University, Retrieved July 23, 2022, from Walden Dissertations and Doctoral Studies https://scholarworks.waldenu.edu/cgi/viewcontent.cgi?article=7333&context=dissertations

Kroger, W. S. (1977). *Clinical and experimental hypnosis: In medicine, dentistry, and psychology.* (2nd ed.). Lippincott Co., Retrieved September 22, 2022, from https://doctorlib.info/psychiatry/hypnosis/index.html

Kohen, D. P., & Olness, K. (2011). *Hypnosis and hypnotherapy with children* (4th ed.). Taylor & Francis.

Kluft, R. P. (Ed.). (1985). *Childhood antecedents of multiple personality disorders: Clinical insights* (1st ed.). American Psychiatric Association Publishing.

Kluft, R. P. (1988). The dissociative disorders. In: J. A. Talbott, R. E. Hales, & S. C. Yudofsky (Eds.), *The American psychiatric publishing textbook of psychiatry* (pp.557–584). American Psychiatric Press.

Kluft, R. P. (1996). Dissociative identity disorder: Perspectives on recent findings and current controversies. In B. Peter, B. Trenkle, F. C. Kinzel, C. Duffner, & A. Iost-Peter (Eds.), *Munich lectures on hypnosis and psychotherapy* (hypnosis international monographs (HIM), No. 2) (pp. 45–67). M.E.G. Stifftung.

Leutner, S. & Piedfort-Marin, O. (2021) The concept of ego state: From historical background to future perspectives. *European Journal of Trauma & Dissociation, 5*(4), 100184. 10.1016/j.ejtd.2020.100184.

Levine, P. A. (2010). *In an unspoken voice: How the body releases trauma and restores goodness.* North Atlantic Books.

Levine, P. A., & Kline, M. (2007). *Trauma through a child's eyes: Awakening the ordinary miracle of healing.* North Atlantic Books.

Lindemann, E. (1944). Symptomology and management of acute grief. *American Journal of Psychiatry, 101*, 141–148.

Linden, J. H. (1995). When mind-body integrity is traumatized by problems with physical health: The women's response. In G. Burrows, & R. Stanley (Eds.), *Contemporary international hypnosis* (pp. 169–175). Wiley.

Linden, J. H. (1996). Trauma prevention: Hypnoidal techniques with the chronically ill child. In B. Peter, B. Trenkle, F. C. Kinzel, C. Duffner, & A. Iost-Peter (Eds.), *Munich lectures on hypnosis and psychotherapy* (hypnosis international monographs (HIM), No. 2 (pp. 15–26). M.E.G. Stifftung.

Linden, J. H. (2002). The application of hypnosis to children and adolescents traumatized by war. In B. Peter, W. Bongartz, D. Revenstorf, & W. Butollo (Eds.), *Munich 2000 – The 15th International Congress of Hypnosis (Proceedings of the "15th International Congress of Hypnosis" at the University of Munich, Germany). Hypnosis international monographs (HIM), No. 6* (pp. 21–29). M.E.G. Stifftung.

Linden, J. H. (2003). Playful metaphors. *American Journal of Clinical Hypnosis, 45*(3), 245–250. 10.1080/00029157.2003.10403530

Linden, J. H. (2004). Making hypnotic interventions more powerful with a developmental perspective. *Psychological Hypnosis, 13*(3), 7–9.

Linden, J. H. (2014). Hypnosis in childhood trauma. In L. I. Sugarman, & W. C. Wester (Eds.), *Therapeutic hypnosis with children and adolescents* (2nd ed., pp. 143–166). Crown House Publishing.
Linden, J. H. (2019). Relationship factors in the theater of the imagination: Hypnosis with children and adolescents. *American Journal of Clinical Hypnosis*, *62*(1–2), 60–73. 10.1080/00029157.2019.1568961
Linden, J. H., & Sugarman, L. I. (2021). The hypnosis skill set: Four principles for evoking the plasticity of the embodied mind. In M. P. Jensen (ed.), *Handbook of hypnotic techniques, Vol. 2: Favorite methods of master clinicians. Voices of experience series* (pp. 9–34). Denny Creek Press.
Loftus, E. F. (1997). Creating false memories. *Scientific American*, *277*(3), 70–75. 10.1038/scientificamerican0997-70
Masten, A. S. (2001). Ordinary magic: Resilience processes in development. *American Psychologist*, *56*(3), 227–238. 10.1037/0003-066x.56.3.227
McCann, I. L., & Pearlman, L. A. (1990a). *Psychological trauma and the adult survivor: Theory, therapy, and transformation*. Brunner/Mazel.
McCann, I. L., & Pearlman, L. A. (1990b). Vicarious traumatization: A framework for understanding the psychological effects of working with victims. *Journal of Traumatic Stress*, *3*(1), 131–149. 10.1007/bf00975140
Ogden, P., & Fisher, J. (2015). *Sensorimotor psychotherapy: Interventions for trauma and attachment*. W. W. Norton & Co.
O'Toole, S. K., Solomon, S. L., & Bergdahl, S. A. (2016). A meta-analysis of hypnotherapeutic techniques in the treatment of PTSD symptoms. *Journal of Traumatic Stress*, *29*(1), 97–100. 10.1002/jts.22077
Perry, B. D. (2001) The neurodevelopmental impact of violence in childhood. In D. Schetky, & E. P. Benedek, (Eds.), *Textbook of child and adolescent forensic psychiatry* (pp. 221–238). American Psychiatric Press, Inc. https://www.researchgate.net/publication/253039874_The_Neurodevelopmental_Impact_of_Violence_in_Childhood/references#fullTextFileContent
Perry, B. D. (2009). Examining child maltreatment through a neurodevelopmental lens: Clinical applications of the neurosequential model of therapeutics. *Journal of Loss & Trauma*, *14*(4), 240–255. 10.1080/15325020903004350
Phillips, M., & Frederick, C. (1995). *Healing the divided self: Clinical and Ericksonian hypnotherapy for dissociative conditions (Norton professional book)* (1st ed.). W. W. Norton & Co.
Poole, N., & Greaves, L. (2012). *Becoming trauma informed*. Centre for Addiction and Mental Health.
Porges, S. W. (2011). *The polyvagal theory: Neurophysiological foundations of emotions, attachment, communication, and self-regulation* (1st ed.). W. W. Norton & Co.
Putnam, F. W. (1997). *Dissociation in children and adolescents: A developmental perspective* (1st ed.). The Guilford Press.
Pynoos, R. S. (Ed.). (1994). *Posttraumatic stress disorder: A clinical review*. Sidran Press.
Schacter, D. L. (1995). Memory wars. *Scientific American*, *272*(4), 135–139.
Schore, A. N. (1994). *Affect regulation and the origin of the self: The neurobiology of emotional development* (1st ed.). Lawrence Erlbaum Associates.
Self-Brown, S., LeBlanc, M., & Kelley, M. L. (2004). Effects of violence exposure and daily stressors on psychological outcomes in urban adolescents. *Journal of Traumatic Stress*, *17*(6), 519–527. 10.1007/s10960-004-5801-0
Siegel, D. J. (1999). *The developing mind: How relationships and the brain interact to shape who we are* (1st ed.). The Guilford Press.
Siegel, D. J. (2010). *Mindsight: The new science of personal transformation*. Bantam.
Siegel, D., Ogden, P., Lanius, R., Schore, A. & van der Kolk, B. (2019). *The neurobiology of attachment* (National Institute for the Clinical Application of Behavioral Medicine (NICABM), [Video]. The Treating Trauma Master Series. Retrieved February 15, 2023, from https://www.nicabm.com/program/treating-trauma-master
Straker, G. (2013). Continuous traumatic stress: Personal reflections 25 years on. *Peace and Conflict: Journal of Peace Psychology*, *19*(2), 209–217. 10.1037/a0032532
Sugarman, L. I., Linden, J. H., & Brooks, L. (2020) *Changing minds with clinical hypnosis: Narratives and discourse for a new health care paradigm*. Routledge.

Taylor, S. E., Klein, L. C., Lewis, B. P., Gruenewald, T. L., Gurung, R. a. R., & Updegraff, J. A. (2000). Biobehavioral responses to stress in females: Tend-and-befriend, not fight-or-flight. *Psychological Review*, *107*(3), 411–429. 10.1037/0033-295x.107.3.411

Terr, L. (1990). *Too scared to cry: Psychic trauma in childhood* (1st ed.). Harper & Row Publishers.

van der Hart, O., & Horst, R. (1989). The dissociation theory of Pierre Janet. *Journal of Traumatic Stress*, *2*(4), 397–412. 10.1002/jts.2490020405

van der Hart, O., Steele, K., Boon, S., & Brown, P. D. (1993). The treatment of traumatic memories: Synthesis, realization, and integration. *Dissociation: Progress in the Dissociative Disorders*, *6*(2–3), 162–180.

van der Hart, O., Nijenhuis, E. R. S., & Steele, K. (2005). Dissociation: An insufficiently recognized major feature of complex posttraumatic stress disorder. *Journal of Traumatic Stress*, *18*(5), 413–423. 10.1002/jts.20049

van der Hart, O., Nijenhuis, E., & Steele, K. (2006). *The haunted self: Structural dissociation and the treatment of chronic traumatization (Norton series on interpersonal neurobiology)*. W. W. Norton & Co.

van der Kolk, B. A. (1987). *Psychological trauma* (1st ed.). American Psychiatric Publications, Inc.

van der Kolk, B. A., & van der Hart, O. (1989). Pierre Janet and the breakdown of adaptation in psychological trauma. *American Journal of Psychiatry*, *146*(12), 1530–1540. 10.1176/ajp.146.12.1530

van der Kolk, B. A., McFarlane, A. C., & Weisaeth, L. (Eds.). (1996). *Traumatic Stress: The effects of overwhelming experience on mind, body, and society*. The Guilford Press.

van der Kolk, B. (2005). Developmental trauma disorder: Toward a rational diagnosis for children with complex trauma histories. *Psychiatric Annals*, *35*(5), 401–408. 10.3928/00485713-20050501-06

van der Kolk, B. A. (2014). *The body keeps the score: Brain, mind, and body in the healing of trauma*. Viking.

van der Kolk, B., Ogden, P., Lanius, R., Siegel, D., & Porges, S. (2019). *The neurobiology of trauma – What's going on in the brain when someone experiences trauma?* National Institute for the Clinical Application of Behavioral Medicine (NICABM). [Video]. The Treating Trauma Master Series. Retrieved February 15, 2023, from https://www.nicabm.com/program/treating-trauma-master

Varga, K., & Kekecs, Z. (2014). Oxytocin and cortisol in the hypnotic interaction. *International Journal of Clinical and Experimental Hypnosis*, *62*(1), 111–128. 10.1080/00207144.2013.841494

Watkins, J. G. (2000). The psychodynamic treatment of combat neuroses (PTSD) with hypnosis during World War II. *International Journal of Clinical and Experimental Hypnosis*, *48*(3), 324–335. 10.1080/00207140008415250

Watkins, J. G., & Watkins, J. G. (1997). *Ego states: Theory and therapy* (1st ed.). W. W. Norton & Co.

World Health Organization (1992). *The ICD-10 classification of mental and behavioural disorders: Clinical descriptions and diagnostic guidelines*. World Health Organization. https://apps.who.int/iris/handle/10665/37958

Wolpe, J. (1996). Hypnosis and the evolution of behavior therapy. In B. Peter, B. Trenkle, F. C. Kinzel, C. Duffner, & A. Iost-Peter (Eds.), *Munich lectures on hypnosis and psychotherapy* (hypnosis international monographs (HIM), No. 2) (pp. 137–139). M.E.G. Stifftung.

Yapko, M. D. (2011). *Mindfulness and hypnosis: The power of suggestion to transform experience*. W. W. Norton & Co.

Ziss, M. (2020) Pre-trauma growth under terror threat: Suggestive communication method in anticipatory trauma. *International Journal of Clinical and Experimental Hypnosis*, *68*(4), 475–482, DOI: 10.1080/00207144.2020.1799712

31

EATING DISORDERS

Using Hypnotic Techniques and Rapport to Treat Anorexia and Bulimia Nervosa

Camillo Loriedo[1] *and Carlotta Di Giusto*[2]

[1]Sapienza University of Rome and Italian School for Hypnosis, Rome, Italy; [2]Italian School for Hypnosis, Rome, Italy

Distinctive Issues in the Treatment of ED

Eating disorders (ED) are complex disorders characterized by dysfunctional eating behavior, excessive preoccupation with weight, and an altered perception of body image. According to DSM-5 (American Psychiatric Association, DSM-5 Task Force, 2013), the major ED are:

Anorexia nervosa is characterized by underweight, fear of gaining weight, and excessive evaluation of weight and body shape. In DSM-5, the amenorrhea criterion was removed, as this disorder also affects prepubertal girls, menopausal women, and men.

Bulimia nervosa is characterized by binge eating episodes, with a frequency of at least three times a week for three consecutive months, and subsequent compensatory behaviors such as exercising, vomiting, and laxative use.

Binge eating disorder is characterized by binge eating episodes, as in bulimia, but without compensatory conducts. For this reason, it is frequently associated with serious obesity.

Anorexia nervosa (AN) is linked with a mortality rate 5–10 times higher than that of healthy same age and sex people. These disorders are increasingly common in pre-adolescence and childhood. Early onset, interfering with a healthy developmental process both biologically and psychologically, is associated with much more serious consequences to the body and mind. Notably, early onset can lead to a higher risk of permanent damage secondary to malnutrition, especially to tissues that have not yet reached full maturation such as bones and central nervous system (Wentz et al., 2009).

A recent multicenter survey (Monteleone et al., 2021) conducted on ED during the COVID lockdown showed an 18 percent increase in insomnia, 20 percent increase in anxiety and depression, 30 percent increase in panic, and 16 percent increase in post-traumatic symptoms. Notably, at the end of the lockdown, the symptoms did not show any decrease, though there was an additional 10 percent increase in the level of anxiety,

DOI: 10.4324/9781003449126-43

possibly related to the overall sense of malaise, uncertainty about the future, and insecurity generated by the pandemic.

Devoe et al. (2022) examined 56 research studies on COVID and ED, finding 36% increase in ED symptoms and 48% increase in ED hospitalizations.

Hypnosis as a Treatment

This chapter's objective is to solve the consequences of a singular paradoxical situation: although it has been a long time since (Pettinati et al., 1985) high levels of hypnotizability were found for AN and bulimia nervosa, a careful review of ED literature, including anorexia and bulimia nervosa, confirms a "remarkable scarcity in the use of hypnosis" as a form of treatment (Torem, 2017, p. 523).

Furthermore, the senior author of this paper who spent about 30 years serving as Director of the Center for Diagnosis and Treatment of Eating Disorders of the Psychiatric Clinic of Sapienza University of Rome had the opportunity to realize how ED are the clearest example of how the mind and body can be involved together in a complex form of disorder. After some initial hesitation, since hypnosis can be considered one of the most, if not the most, appropriate treatment for disorders that involve both body and mind components to apply it to ED was a natural consequence.

Another observation of great interest was to discover that alexithymia, one of the central issues present in the greatest part of ED, can be significantly reduced through some targeted hypnotic interventions, as also confirmed by studies of Gay, Hanin, and Luminet (2008), and of Suzuki (2005).

The loss or reduction of "body awareness" (Sciortino & Kayser, 2022) and "body ownership" (Fiorio et al., 2020), and loss of "sense of agency", i.e., the sense we have of controlling or initiating our actions (Polito et al., 2013), that represent other relevant areas of impairment in EDs scarcely accessible to other forms of treatment, have been demonstrated to be sensitive to hypnotic intervention.

Even if they represent an important part of the discomfort caused by ED, these aspects are very often not considered in most known forms of treatment. Being able to work also on them, and not only on the impressive alimentary part of the disorders, is certainly an important contribution that hypnosis offers to avoid, chronicity and the greater risk in this arena.

ED frequently compromises physical health due to altered eating behaviors (e.g., food restriction, excessive eating, purging, and/or compensatory behaviors) leading to altered nutritional condition. Unless treated through a timely and clinically apt protocol, ED may become a chronic state, seriously jeopardizing systemic organic health (cardiovascular, gastrointestinal, endocrine, hematologic, skeletal, central nervous system, dermatologic, etc.) and, in severe cases, leading to death.

Theoretical Framework

We adopted a "naturalistic" approach to hypnosis (Erickson 1964), an approach in which the notion of *rapport* emerges as a selective and exclusive relationship taking place in a context where a modified focused state of consciousness allows the development of increased mutual responsiveness between the subject and the hypnotist. According to naturalistic hypnosis, *trance* may be defined as a spontaneous or induced natural highly focused state of consciousness. More than from hypnotic suggestions, therapeutic outcomes are spawned by the therapist's aptitude to recognize and utilize *minimal cues*, little behavior details, and spontaneous phenomena that can generate in a subject "the loss of orientation toward external reality and the establishment of a new orientation toward an abstract conceptual reality" (Erickson, 1964, p. 152). Teaching self-hypnosis to the subject is also a highly relevant technique in the context of ED treatment.

A Multifactorial Approach

In 80% of cases, ED occur in association with other psychological disorders. Almost all psychic disorders may accompany the course of ED, but the most frequent comorbidities are: (a) *Personality Disorders* and in particular *Borderline Personality Disorder*; (b) *Obsessive-Compulsive Disorders*, with a peculiar emphasis on ritual behavioral rigidity and high levels of perfectionism; (c) *Depressive Disorders*, with reduced self-esteem, social isolation, and guilt; (d) *Dissociative Disorders* with *Depersonalization, Derealization*, and *Dissociative Identity Disorder*; and (e) *Impulse-control disorders* that may lead to substance addictions, sexual promiscuity, and self-injury.

Since ED etiology is determined by a *plurality of factors* intermingling with a subject's genetic vulnerability, this chapter elucidates, following Garfinkel and Garner (1982), how their treatment requires a *multifactorial approach*. Garfinkel and Garner propose a classification of *risk*, *triggering*, and *maintaining factors* of ED.

Genetic Factors

Among risk factors, the role of genetic factors in the development of ED has been highlighted in several studies. A promising study focuses on the influence and polymorphism of the gene encoding serotonin transporter (5-HTTLPR), which appears to be a marker for AN (Calati et al., 2011). Research on twins points to a genetic predisposition to AN (Stice et al., 2011) though results appear mixed.

An association between the 5-HTTLPR polymorphism and the intimacy subjects felt in hypnotic sessions was proved (Katonai et al., 2017).

Traumatic Experiences

Risk factors include familiarity with ED, depression, substance abuse, and unresolved past trauma. Many authors consider histories of childhood sexual abuse, childhood physical abuse, and childhood emotional abuse as nonspecific risk factors for the development of ED (Racine & Wildes, 2015; Sanci et al., 2008). Furthermore, many studies have tested the hypothesis that traumatic experiences occurring in childhood, adolescence, and adulthood may be related to the severity of ED symptoms (Vanderlinden et al., 2018).

The role of *Neglect* that has been defined as "the colossus of traumas of patients with eating disorders" (Piacentino et al., 2016, p. 165.), both in the form of *childhood emotional neglect and childhood physical neglect (CPN)* in ED susceptibility has been scrutinized, too (Jaite et al., 2012; Kong & Bernstein, 2009). CPN is a type of trauma that is often "hidden" and can include seemingly small yet painful and cumulative events such as bereavement and loss, attachment injuries, and/or bullying experiences (Pignatelli, et al., 2017).

Sociocultural Factors

Other risk factors include early difficulties in achieving membership to social groups with greater sociocultural pressure toward a positive lean physicality (such as models, gymnasts, dancers). Others include the internalization of the ideal of a lean body, dissatisfaction with one's body image, low self-esteem, perfectionism (Loriedo & Mirigliani, 2016), and negative emotional states.

Included in the multifactorial etiological model of ED are sociocultural factors, typical of Western societies with high industrialization and standard of living. Western sociocultural factors may also explain the new ED symptomatic dimensions that include intense gaining weight fear and body image issues, the emergence of a tubular beauty ideal, and the increased susceptibility of women to mocking within their peer groups.

Brain-Based Neuroscience

Among *risk factors*, predisposing elements include the distortion of one's body image, related to neurobiological, psychological, and cultural aspects. At the brain level, the areas involved in body perception distortion are the dorsal occipital cortex, right temporal-parietal-occipital junction, fusiform gyrus, inferior parietal lobe, and dorsolateral prefrontal cortex, while the right parahippocampal gyrus appears to be involved in incongruous self-evaluations about one's appearance.

The anorexics' brain shows alterations in the white matter bundles, linking the brain's areas of cognitive control and body image perception. In a study of 14 female adolescents who had been diagnosed with ED less than six months earlier, researchers observed alterations in the bundles, which were already present in the very early stages of anorexia (Gaudio, 2017). This might explain why the patients think obsessively about the food they eat and their own bodies, of which they have a distorted image.

Indeed, ED population is unable to perceive their true size and the severity of their state of malnutrition. On a psychological and social level, some researchers have pointed out that continuous exposure to unattainable beauty models proposed by the mass media promotes body image distortion.

Myers and Biocca (1992) found that a group of female students overestimated their body size by 16 percent after watching 30 minutes of commercials.

Triggering Factors

These involve events occurring in the year preceding the onset of the ED such as house or city relocations, illness or death of a loved one, failure in school or sports, breakup of romantic relationships, teasing, and negative comments about weight and body shape.

Maintaining Factors

Among these factors, we find unconscious collusion of family members, blaming the disease, high family conflict, and secondary benefits derived from the disease state, e.g., a history of conflictual family issues, patient blaming by relatives, and secondary benefits, such as preventing parents from divorcing, showcase an anorexic condition.

Applications of Hypnosis

Literature on hypnosis as an independent treatment for ED remains scant, notwithstanding the distinguished history of hypnosis as a potential therapy for body-related disorders. Notably, since the beginning of the last century, Pierre Janet (1919) called attention to the use of hypnosis to treat patients' dissociative states and "fixed ideas" concerning eating and body image. Milton Erickson (Erickson & Rossi, 1979) mentions treating anorexic patients by using indirect suggestions and paradoxical interventions. In treating patients with AN, Yapko (1986) used direct and indirect suggestions that strengthened self-esteem, improved body image, and addressed delayed maturity issues.

Since the 1990s, several authors (Torem, 1986; Vanderlinden et al., 1993) showed increased interest toward the study of dissociative symptoms affecting ED and correlations between these symptoms and levels of hypnotizability. Notably, in 1985, Pettinati, Horne, and Staats examined hypnotizability among females with bulimia, purging, and not purging anorexia by comparing them with age-matched control groups. The group with bulimia was found to be highly hypnotizable, to a statistically significant extent compared with anorexic patients and age-matched control groups. In particular, the study found that those with purging-type anorexia had significantly higher hypnotizability than those without purging. Barabasz (1991) and Covino et al., (1994) confirmed high hypnotizability of women with bulimia and enthused research and clinical interest in the use of hypnosis in the treatment of bulimia.

Pettinati et al. (1989) found that women with bulimia scored significantly higher on Factor III of the *Stanford Hypnotic Susceptibility Scale: Form C*, a factor representing the ability to dissociate (Weitzenhoffer & Hilgard, 1962), compared to both the purging and non-purging anorexics groups.

After reviewing the literature on hypnosis as a supported clinical intervention, Lynn et al. (2000) concluded that "as a whole, the clinical research, to date, generally substantiates the claim that hypnotic procedures can ameliorate some psychological and medical conditions, as judged against the Chambless and Hollon (1998) methodological guidelines" (p. 239).

Crucially, hypnosis, from a review of the literature, is frequently used as a supplement and amplifier of therapeutic processes (Griffiths et al., 1994). Griffiths (1995) has employed hypnosis with positive suggestions in an eight-week cognitive-behavioral therapy (CBT)-based protocol to improve self-control, reinforce changes, acquire new and healthier eating habits, increase control in binge and purge triggering situations, improve self-esteem, and encourage participation in social situations. The results of this study show a significant reduction in binge eating and vomiting, both in the short term and in a follow-up, two years later. A study by Barabasz (2007) compared a CBT protocol for treating bulimia with a CBT protocol integrated with hypnosis and self-hypnosis techniques: the results show a greater reduction in binge eating and coping behaviors in the CBT and hypnosis group. Nash and Baker (1993) showed how hypnosis strengthens the ego and reduces the characteristic body image distortion that plagues ED patients. Results show significant remission of symptoms in 76% of subjects. Vanderlinden and Vandereyken (1990) have dealt extensively with the application of hypnosis in conjunction with CBT to facilitate the therapeutic process, both for the treatment of bulimia nervosa and AN. Hypnosis proved to be an effective tool to strengthen therapeutic alliance and enhance the reintegration of dissociative states underlying bulimic disorders (Vanderlinden et al., 1993).

Despite the promising studies outlined above, hypnosis is not yet fully recommended and scientifically validated due to methodological hurdles. As a case in point, Ericksonian hypnosis is based on *tailoring* and *utilization* principles, an approach that considers personal idiosyncrasies and resources, a *person-centered* rather than a pathology-centered approach.

Hypnotic Approaches to ED: Distinctive Features and Complementarity

ED patients have experienced neglect, abuse, and emotional betrayal, and this explains why treating ED proves to be highly effective only if a solid therapeutic alliance and a corrective emotional experience are established. It is necessary to generate a safe place within the therapeutic setting: traumatic memories are cautiously activated, and the patient's own pacing is valued. Indirect and especially bodily communication may lower tension and emotional suffering, as well as feedback about minimal body cues may also prove useful to cope with ED patients' alexithymia.

New Perspectives in the Treatment of EDs

Ericksonian hypnotherapy may be employed successfully in the treatment of eating symptoms and the dissociative states underlying them.

Given the strong association between trauma and the development of ED (Seubert & Virdi, 2018), hypnotic techniques may be used successfully in the treatment of trauma (Loriedo & Di Giusto, 2021) and regressive hypnosis may be proposed especially in those patients in whom the underlying dynamic of the ED is related to past trauma. Often *trauma abreaction* leads to an improvement in eating symptoms (Torem & Curdue, 1988). Before using regressive hypnosis, however, it is imperative to propose stabilizing hypnotic techniques, such as *safe place* induction, and then to cautiously summon the patient's traumatic memories (Loriedo & Di Giusto, 2021). The most commonly used techniques are the *affect bridge* (Watkins, 1971) and *screen techniques* (Maldonado & Spiegel, 1994; Michelson et al., 1996).

Affect bridge consists of asking patients to recollect the earliest memory of a specific emotion and re-experience the concomitant event. The purpose is to employ an emotional impression as a sort of *bridge* across time to regress patients to an "initial sensitizing event" until the acknowledgment that those sentiments belong to the past and are no longer required to be faced in the present.

Screen techniques require the patient, in trance, to project a visual representation of a disturbing memory onto a virtual screen, placed at some distance from him. Viewing the traumatic events from a state of safety allows the patient to access negative memories and react to them with new emotional, cognitive, procedural, and relational responses; the goal is to reduce state-dependent memory activation and integrate traumatic memories in a safe state (Dietrich, 2000). In the split-screen technique (Spiegel & Spiegel, 1987), for example, designed to render traumatic memories more tolerable, the patient projects traumatic memories onto the left side of a screen, while images of reassurance and protection are projected onto the right side of the screen. The patients may then be invited to summon images of a safe place, or visualize a reaction to the traumatic event, for example, screaming or defending themselves.

In the hypnotic treatment of EDs, the use of self-hypnosis as a therapeutic modality is highly recommended, given its reassuring component, a key element in the early stages of ED therapy (see the chapter on self-hypnosis). Self-hypnosis is especially suitable for patients who display the need to reestablish control with food and other critical situations, and those requiring confidence in their own resources and self-efficacy. The learning phase is usually carried out in a therapeutic setting and may consist of one or more sessions to teach patients to achieve trance. A conditioning phase where the patient achieves trance through a conditioned command agreed upon in advance (e.g., closing the fist) may be added. A training phase allows the patient to experience outside the therapeutic setting the acquired learnings following a mutually agreed schedule (e.g., daily, for 15 days).

Ego-strengthening techniques, first proposed by Hartland (1971) and later elaborated by other authors (Frederick & McNeal, 2013), promote feelings of strength, efficacy, and a sense of well-being in the patient. Nature metaphors may be employed, such as the tree as a symbol of strength or a secret garden with flowers and plants. The patient is thus invited to cultivate them as a metaphor for nurturing and caring for oneself.

Projection-to-the-future techniques (Erickson, 1980; Yapko, 1984) seem to be particularly apt to treat adolescent patients, as adolescence is a time of great physical and psychological transformation and focuses on one's "future identity". Through hypnosis, the patient is encouraged to experience a future when eating issues have been successfully dealt with and personal goals have been achieved. This imagery promotes confidence, self-esteem, and trust in a conceivable and feasible healing process (Torem, 1992).

Body-related techniques are another crucial hypnotic tool. Given that patients with ED often exhibit alexithymia, hypnotic techniques, unlike purely verbal approaches, may bypass this limitation through somatic work, capturing minimal cues, e.g., changes in breathing, perception of more relaxed or tense body parts, and using them to improve self-perception and promote new, healthier ways of self-control.

Clinical Illustration

The following is an inductive technique adopted by us, with small variations, in a good number of other cases. Its relevance with respect to what is explicated in this chapter is due to the demonstration of the great hypnotic susceptibility of bulimic patients and the great ease of clinical application. Its use is facilitated by two particular forms of minimal cues that will be described together with the case.

A young woman of 28 years, bulimic, asks for help because she can't control her diet and is constantly at risk of a major overweight that she contains only by resorting to wearying physical activity. She maintains her main complaint is the presence of a series of "horrendous pimples" on her face caused in her opinion by her irrepressible binges that oblige her consuming every night five jars of Nutella, a chocolate hazelnut sugary spread.

Despite a clear tendency to obesity, she claims that losing weight isn't of any interest to her since all she wants is to get rid of those "horrendous pimples" on her face.

Gustative-Olfactive Induction. Her inability to resist when facing the jars of Nutella is particularly evident. The first important minimal cue that strikes the therapist's observation is that the simple word "Nutella" is enough to produce in a few seconds an intense swallowing reflex. Talking about Nutella is sufficient to make her mouth water and describing the jar content increases further her imaginative representation making her desire dramatic.

In similar cases, the utilization of spontaneous gustatory responses (frequent in subjects with EDs, even in restrictive forms of anorexia) allows the incorporation of them in a particular *gustatory-olfactory induction technique.*

In this specific induction, the therapist suggests the subject close her eyes and begins to describe the presence on the table of a nice jar of Nutella, still closed, that will soon be at her complete disposal, but *only if she can imagine it in all its details.*

A progressive-conditioned mode of induction. When the subject succeeds in giving a perfect description of the jar, the hypnotist invites her to look at it again, to get closer, and to take it. Only after grasping it, the subject can feel the contact perfectly well and, if she succeeds in doing so, she can begin to unscrew the lid. The hypnotist continues here with the very effective method we propose here as *progressive-conditioned mode of induction:* the subject is exposed to a long series of passages, but each passage activates an intense expectation for the next one, and the next is only allowed if the previous passage has been completed in a satisfactory manner.

The subject is told to unscrew the cap slowly and calmly, because only in this way can she smell its seductive Nutella scent. And when fully satisfied, she will be able to notice the presence of a small spoon, but she will not be able to use it, until she has chosen how deep she wants to immerse it into the cream.

After this passage, she will bring the cream to her mouth slowly and savor it carefully because only in this way will she be able to fully discover the difference with the old Nutella flavor she knew.

"You feel that the cream taste is particularly pleasant, and you will soon understand why. But your understanding will be really clear only when the jar will be completely emptied and well cleaned by your spoon.

At that moment you will realize why that special taste can be so deep: because for the first time emptying of the jar *is not accompanied by any sense of guilt, nor by the fear that it can cause those horrendous pimples on your face".*

Here the second minimum signal is used, the word "horrendous pimples", which the patient had already accentuated with particular emphasis during the first interview, clearly suggesting how important it was to meet her fundamental motivation. Now the same words returned with equal emphasis by the therapist, but this time the patient, who suddenly seems to perceive the important advantage contained in the jar offered by the therapist, accompanies it is with an amused smile.

Only after she fully understands the reason for that *special flavor*, she is told: "Now after feeling that new special flavor, you will be able to feel a *special sweet heaviness.* And when you feel both these special sensations, you can discover a new jar of the same type on the table. And, *if you feel the need*, you can start the procedure again. Even every night at home, following these special sensations, you can repeat this same experience ... if you need ... several times, but never more than five.

Jars of this type, which will serve for your daily use, will appear on the shelf of your kitchen every evening, and you will be able to use them day after day, without problems and, when the *horrendous pimples* begin to disappear, *you will realize you are able to get rid of what you don't need*, and it will be a great satisfaction for you to discover you can obtain it *without any particular sacrifice ...*".

In the next session, the young woman returns reporting she had quietly tasted all five jars of Nutella that she had found on the shelf on the first night. Starting from the second night she had begun to reduce their number because, according to her, these new jars *were particularly satisfying and gave her a sense of sweet heaviness,* and these sensations diminished her need for too many.

To her surprise, after a month she discovered that his new Nutella supply had no longer produced the horrendous pimples, and her weight had surprisingly shrunk. She wanted to clarify once again that reducing her weight was not her goal; nevertheless, she was not at all sorry about this secondary effect, since she had achieved it *without any particular sacrifice.*

Future Orientation

Past research on ED therapy consigned hypnosis as an ancillary or enhancing approach, complementary to other therapies, especially CBT. For the authors, it is mandatory to investigate further hypnosis effectiveness as a therapy in its own right by developing protocols reconciling the centrality of the therapeutic relationship with a *naturalistic* approach focusing on the patient's unique subjectivity and resources. Studies concerning the clinical efficacy of Ericksonian hypnotherapy are not easily replicable due to the lack of standardized approaches that can be followed and fulfill the criteria for "evidence-based" treatments (Barabasz, 2007).

References

American Psychiatric Association, DSM-5 Task Force. (2013). *Diagnostic and statistical manual of mental disorders: DSM-5^{TM}* (5th ed.). American Psychiatric Publishing, Inc. 10.1176/appi.books.9780890425596

Barabasz, M. (1991). Hypnotizability in bulimia: Brief report. *International Journal of Eating Disorders*, *10*(1), 117–120. 10.1002/1098-108X(199101)10:1<117::AID-EAT2260100113>3.0.CO;2-T

Barabasz, M. (2007). Efficacy of hypnotherapy in the treatment of eating disorders. *International Journal of Clinical and Experimental Hypnosis*, *55*(3), 318–335. 10.1080/00207140701338688

Calati, R., De Ronchi, D., Bellini, M., & Serretti, A. (2011). The 5-HTTLPR polymorphism and eating disorders: A meta-analysis. *International Journal of Eating Disorders*, *44*(3), 191–199. 10.1002/eat.20811

Chambless, D. L., & Hollon, S. D. (1998). Defining empirically supported therapies. *Journal of Consulting and Clinical Psychology*, *66*(1), 7–18. 10.1037/0022-006x.66.1.7

Covino, N. A., Jimerson, D. C., Wolfe, B., Franko, D. L., & Frankel, F. (1994). Hypnotizability, dissociation, and bulimia nervosa. *Journal of Abnormal Psychology*, *103*(3), 455–459. 10.1037/0021-843x.103.3.455

Devoe, D. J., Han, A., Anderson, A., Katzman, D. K., Patten, S. B., Soumbasis, A., Flanagan, J., Paslakis, G., Vyver, E., Marcoux, G., & Dimitropoulos, G. (2022). The impact of the COVID-19 pandemic on eating disorders: A systematic review. *International Journal of Eating Disorders*, *56*(1), 5–25. 10.1002/eat.23704

Dietrich, A. (2000). A review of visual/kinesthetic disassociation in the treatment of posttraumatic disorders: Theory, efficacy and practice recommendations. *Traumatology*, *6*(2), 85–107. 10.1177/153476560000600203

Erickson, M. H. (1964). Initial experiments investigating the nature of hypnosis. *American Journal of Clinical Hypnosis*, *7*(2), 152–162. 10.1080/00029157.1964.10402410

Erickson, M. H. (1980). The case of Barbie: An Ericksonian approach to the treatment of anorexia nervosa. In J. K. Zeig (Ed.), *Teaching seminar with Milton H. Erickson* (pp. 133–143). Brunner/Mazel.

Erickson, M. H., & Rossi, E. L. (1979). *Hypnotherapy: An exploratory casebook* (1st ed.). Irvington Publishers.

Fiorio, M., Modenese, M., & Cesari, P. (2020). The rubber hand illusion in hypnosis provides new insights into the sense of body ownership. *Scientific Reports*, *10*(1). Article number 5706. 10.1038/s41598-020-62745-x

Frederick, C., & McNeal, S. (2013). *Inner strengths: Contemporary psychotherapy and hypnosis for ego-strengthening*. Routledge.

Garfinkel, P. E., & Garner, D. M. (1982). *Anorexia nervosa: A multidimensional perspective* (1st ed.). Bruner Meisel U.

Gaudio, S., Quattrocchi, C. C., Piervincenzi, C., Zobel, B. B., Montecchi, F. R., Dakanalis, A., Riva, G., & Carducci, F. (2017). White matter abnormalities in treatment-naive adolescents at the earliest stages of anorexia nervosa: A diffusion tensor imaging study. *Psychiatry Research: Neuroimaging*, *266*, 138–145. 10.1016/j.pscychresns.2017.06.011

Gay, M.-C., Hanin, D., & Luminet, O. (2008). Effectiveness of an hypnotic imagery intervention on reducing alexithymia. *Contemporary Hypnosis*, *25*(1), 1–13. 10.1002/ch.344

Griffiths, R. A. (1995) Hypnobehavioral treatment for bulimia nervosa: A treatment manual. *Australian Journal of Clinical and Experimental Hypnosis*, *21*, 25–40.
Griffiths, R. A., Hadzi-Pavlovic, D., & Channon-Little, L. (1994). A controlled evaluation of hypnobehavioural treatment for bulimia nervosa: Immediate pre-post treatment effects. *European Eating Disorders Review*, *2*(4), 202–220. 10.1002/erv.2400020405
Hartland, J. (1971). Further observations on the use of "ego-strengthening" techniques. *American Journal of Clinical Hypnosis*, *14*(1), 1–8. 10.1080/00029157.1971.10402136
Jaite, C., Schneider, N., Hilbert, A., Pfeiffer, E., Lehmkuhl, U., & Salbach-Andrae, H. (2012). Etiological role of childhood emotional trauma and neglect in adolescent anorexia nervosa: A cross-sectional questionnaire analysis. *Psychopathology*, *45*(1), 61–66. 10.1159/000328580
Janet, P. (1919). *Les médications psychologiques, Vol. 3. Les acquisitions psychologiques: [Psychological medications, Vol. 3. Psychological acquisitions]*. Felix Alcan.
Katonai, E. R., Szekely, A., Vereczkei, A., Sasvari-Szekely, M., Bányai, É. I., & Varga, K. (2017). Dopaminergic and serotonergic genotypes and the subjective experiences of hypnosis. *International Journal of Clinical and Experimental Hypnosis*, *65*(4), 379–397. 10.1080/00207144.2017.1348848
Kong, S., & Bernstein, K. (2009). Childhood trauma as a predictor of eating psychopathology and its mediating variables in patients with eating disorders. *Journal of Clinical Nursing*, *18*(13), 1897–1907. 10.1111/j.1365-2702.2008.02740.x
Loriedo, C., & Mirigliani, A. (2016). Disturbi della nutrizione e del comportamento alimentare [Nutrition and eating behavior disorders]. In M. Bondi (a cura di [Ed.]), *Compendio di psichiatria e salute mentale [Compendium of psychiatry and mental health]* (pp. 515–528). Alpes Italia.
Loriedo, C., Di Giusto, C., & Frau, C. (2021). Disturbi correlati a traumi e a fattori di stress [Trauma-related disorders and stressors]. In G. De Benedittis, C. Loriedo, C. Mammini, & N. Rago (Eds.), *Trattato di ipnosi: Dai fondamenti teorici alla pratica clinica [Treatise on hypnosis: From theoretical foundations to clinical practice]* (pp. 560–579). Franco Angeli.
Lynn, S., Kirsch, I. Barabasz, A., Cardena, E., & Patterson, D. (2000). Hypnosis as an empirically supported clinical intervention: The state of the evidence and a look to the future, *International Journal of Clinical and Experimental Hypnosis*, *48*(2), 239–259 DOI: 10.1080/0020714000841 0050
Maldonado, J. R., & Spiegel, D. (1994). The treatment of post-traumatic stress disorder. In S. J. Lynn & J. W. Rhue (Eds.), *Dissociation: Clinical and theoretical perspectives* (1st ed., pp. 215–241). The Guilford Press.
Michelson, L. K., Ray, W. J., & Peterson, J. A. (Eds.). (1996). Hypnotherapeutic techniques to facilitate psychotherapy with PTSD and dissociative clients. In *Handbook of dissociation* (pp. 449–474). Springer. 10.1007/978-1-4899-0310-5_22
Monteleone, A. M., Marciello, F., Cascino, G., Abbate-Daga, G., Anselmetti, S., Baiano, M., Rucci, P., Barone, E., Bertelli, S., Carpiniello, B., Castellini, G., Corrivetti, G., De Giorgi, S., Favaro, A., Gramaglia, C., Marzola, E., Meneguzzo, P., Monaco, F., Oriani, M. G., … Monteleone, P. (2021). The impact of COVID-19 lockdown and of the following "re-opening" period on specific and general psychopathology in people with eating disorders: The emergent role of internalizing symptoms. *Journal of Affective Disorders*, *285*, 77–83. 10.1016/j.jad.2021.02.037
Myers, P. C., & Biocca, F. (1992). The elastic body image: The effect of television advertising and programming on body image distortions in young women. *Journal of Communication*, *42*(3), 108–133. 10.1111/j.1460-2466.1992.tb00802.x
Nash, M. R., & Baker, E. L. (1993). Hypnosis in the treatment of anorexia nervosa. In J. W. Rhue, S. J. Lynn, & I. Kirsch (Eds.), *Handbook of clinical hypnosis* (pp. 383–394). American Psychological Association. 10.1037/10274-018
Pettinati, H. M., Kogan, L. G., Margolis, C., Shrier, L., & Wade, J. H. (1989). Hypnosis, hypnotizability, and the bulimic patients. In L. M. Hornyak & E. K. Baker (Eds.), *Experiential therapies for eating disorders* (1st ed., pp. 34–59). The Guilford Press.
Pettinati, H. M., Horne, R., & Staats, J. M. (1985). Hypnotizability in patients with anorexia nervosa and bulimia. *Archives of General Psychiatry*, *42*(10), 1014–1016. 10.1001/archpsyc.1985.01790330094011
Piacentino, D., Loriedo, C., Biondi, M., Girardi, P., Vanderlinden, J., & Pignatelli, A. M. (2016). Emotional neglect as the colossus among traumas in patients with eating disorders: A case-control study. *European Psychiatry*, *33*(S1), S165. 10.1016/j.eurpsy.2016.01.331

Pignatelli, A. M., Wampers, M., Loriedo, C., Biondi, M., & Vanderlinden, J. (2017). Childhood neglect in eating disorders: A systematic review and meta-analysis. *Journal of Trauma & Dissociation*, *18*(1), 100–115. 10.1080/15299732.2016.1198951

Polito, V., Barnier, A. J., & Woody, E. Z. (2013). Developing the Sense of Agency Rating Scale (SOARS): An empirical measure of agency disruption in hypnosis. *Consciousness and Cognition*, *22*(3), 684–696. 10.1016/j.concog.2013.04.003

Racine, S. E., & Wildes, J. E. (2015). Emotion dysregulation and anorexia nervosa: An exploration of the role of childhood abuse. *International Journal of Eating Disorders*, *48*(1), 55–58. 10.1002/eat.22364

Sanci, L., Coffey, C., Olsson, C. A., Reid, S., Carlin, J. B., & Patton, G. (2008). Childhood sexual abuse and eating disorders in females. *Archives of Pediatrics & Adolescent Medicine*, *162*(3), 261–267. 10.1001/archpediatrics.2007.58

Sciortino, P., & Kayser, C. (2022). The rubber hand illusion is accompanied by a distributed reduction of alpha and beta power in the EEG. *PloS One*, *17*(7), e0271659. 10.1371/journal.pone.0271659

Seubert, A. J., & Virdi, P. (2018). *Trauma-Informed approaches to eating disorders*. Springer Publishing Company.

Spiegel, H., & Spiegel, D. (1987). *Trance and treatment: Clinical uses of hypnosis*. American Psychiatric Publications.

Stice, E., Marti, C. N., & Durant, S. (2011). Risk factors for onset of eating disorders: Evidence of multiple risk pathways from an 8-year prospective study. *Behaviour Research and Therapy*, *49*(10), 622–627. 10.1016/j.brat.2011.06.009

Suzuki, T. (2005). Hypnotic imagery: Therapy for a hives patient with alexithymic characteristics. *Contemporary Hypnosis*, *22*(2), 94–98. 10.1002/ch.28

Torem, M. S. (1986). Dissociative states presenting as an eating disorder. *American Journal of Clinical Hypnosis*, *29*(2), 137–142. 10.1080/00029157.1986.10402697

Torem, M. S. (1992). "Back from the future": A powerful age-progression technique. *American Journal of Clinical Hypnosis*, *35*(2), 81–88. 10.1080/00029157.1992.10402990

Torem, M. S. (2017). Eating disorders. In G. R. Elkins (Ed.), *Handbook of medical and psychological hypnosis: Foundations, applications, and professional issues* (pp. 523–534). Springer Publishing Company.

Torem, M. S., & Curdue, K. J. (1988). PTSD presenting as an eating disorder. *Stress Medicine*, *4*(3), 139–142. 10.1002/smi.2460040305

Vanderlinden, J., & Palmisano, G. L. (2018). Trauma and eating disorders: The state of the art. In A. J. Seubert & P. Virdi (Eds.), *Trauma-informed approaches to eating disorders* (pp. 15–32). Springer Publishing Company.

Vanderlinden, J., & Vandereycken, W. (1990). The use of hypnosis in the treatment of bulimia nervosa. *International Journal of Clinical and Experimental Hypnosis*, *38*(2), 101–111. 10.1080/00207149008414505

Vanderlinden, J., Vandereycken, W., Van Dyck, R., & Vertommen, H. (1993). Dissociative experiences and trauma in eating disorders. *International Journal of Eating Disorders*, *13*(2), 187–193. 10.1002/1098-108X(199303)13:2<187::AID-EAT2260130206>3.0.CO;2-9

Watkins, J. (1971). The affect bridge: A hypnoanalytic technique. *International Journal of Clinical and Experimental Hypnosis*, *19*(1), 21–27. 10.1080/00207147108407148

Weitzenhoffer, A. M., & Hilgard, E. R. (1962). *Stanford Hypnotic Susceptibility Scale: Form C*. Consulting Psychologists Press.

Wentz, E., Gillberg, I. C., Anckarsäter, H., Gillberg, C., & Råstam, M. (2009). Adolescent-onset anorexia nervosa: 18-year outcome. *British Journal of Psychiatry*, *194*(2), 168–174. 10.1192/bjp.bp.107.048686

Yapko, M. D. (1984). *Trancework: An introduction to the practice of clinical hypnosis*. Irvington Press.

Yapko, M. D. (1986). Hypnotic and strategic interventions in the treatment of anorexia nervosa. *American Journal of Clinical Hypnosis*, *28*(4), 224–232. 10.1080/00029157.1986.10402658

32

THE PROMISE OF HYPNOSIS WITHIN CBT FOR SMOKING CESSATION

Joseph P. Green[1] *and Steven Jay Lynn*[2]

[1]The Ohio State University, Lima, Ohio, USA; [2]Binghamton University, Binghamton, New York, USA

Smoking damages nearly every organ and physiological system within the human body, leading to preventable disease, disability, and premature death. For example, the vast majority (e.g., 80–90%) of lung cancer and chronic obstructive pulmonary disease-related deaths are attributed to smoking (US Department of Health and Human Services (USDHHS, 2014); Hartmann-Boyce et al., 2021). In addition, smoking increases the risk of stroke and coronary heart disease by a factor of four; enhances the risk of diabetes, arthritis, and cataracts; complicates treatment and survival from tuberculosis, emphysema, and bronchitis; impairs wound healing; heightens the risk of tooth and gum disease; and is linked with sleep disruptions (USDHHS, 2010, 2014). Smokers face elevated risk of severe complications and death following Covid-19 infection and behavioral patterns associated with smoking, such as gathering with other smokers and sharing tobacco products, may contribute to the increased risk of Covid-19 infection (Ahmed et al., 2020). Smoking shortens life on average of upwards of ten years (Jha et al., 2013). Worldwide, smoking results in more than 7 million deaths, with an additional 1.2 million deaths attributable to diseases stemming from exposure to second-hand smoke (World Health Organization (WHO), 2022).

Smoking may compromise sexual functioning and lead to fertility problems in men and women (Choi et al., 2015). Male smokers have lower sperm counts and higher rates of morphological defects (Bundhun et al., 2019). Long-term smoking is associated with erectile dysfunction (ED), with smokers 1.5–2 times more likely to suffer from ED (Harte & Meston, 2008). Even young, healthy, nonsmoking men can be adversely affected by nicotine. After conducting a randomized, double-blind investigation of the effect of nicotine on physiological and subjective reports of sexual arousal, Harte and Meston (2008) concluded, "Isolated nicotine can significantly attenuate physiological sexual arousal in healthy nonsmoking men" (p. 110).

Connections between smoking and sexual functioning are less clear among women (see Costa & Peres, 2015), although smoking has a negative impact on female sexual functioning in terms of increased frequency of sexual arousal and orgasmic disorders, and decreased sexual satisfaction among women smokers (Ju et al., 2021). Moreover, a dose-effect relation exists between smoking and the rate of sexual dysfunction (Choi et al., 2015). Even second-hand

DOI: 10.4324/9781003449126-44

smoke can contribute to female sexual dysfunction (Ju et al., 2021). Both active and passive (i.e., second hand) smoking has been linked to primary female infertility, is harmful to a growing fetus, and increases the risk of miscarriage and birth defects (USDHHS, 2010, 2014).

Nicotine increases blood pressure and heart rate and may, by itself, impair vascular functioning, even among adolescents (Guo et al., 2022). The acute effects of nicotine on the cardiovascular system vary, with faster delivery associated with stronger effects. For example, the nicotine nasal spray produces a quicker delivery than the patch. Rapid delivery is associated with greater pleasure associated with smoking and a quicker reduction in craving intensity, thereby increasing the potential for abuse and dependence (see Jensen, 2020).

Why do people smoke? Initial experimentation with smoking may reflect psychosocial motives to appear cool, tough, independent, defiant, or to fit in with peers. The appeal of a rebellious persona may override the aversive taste commonly experienced when people first smoke (Jarvis, 2004). For many, pharmacological factors are the principal reason to continue smoking. Nicotine is a psychomotor stimulant and is highly addictive. People report improved attention and concentration after smoking, but benefits are temporary, requiring regular dosing of more nicotine to stave off withdrawal. Indeed, the reinforcing effects of smoking likely stem from alleviating or postponing withdrawal symptoms (Jarvis, 2004).

For some, smoking may alleviate or modify pain signals. Bakhshaie et al. (2016) reported higher rates of smoking dependence among individuals suffering from chronic and severe pain, implying that people may smoke to attenuate pain. Schmelzer et al. (2016) found an association between smoking, stress, and back pain such that smokers were 1.5 times more likely than never-smokers to report persistent back pain, even after accounting for body mass, age, race, education, and employment status. Bakhshaie et al. (2016) recommend that clinicians conduct thorough pain histories and offer treatment options to address underlying pain symptomatology for those trying to quit smoking.

Although smoking rates in the United States have declined since the Surgeon General's 1964 proclamation that smoking causes cancer, nearly 31 million U.S. adults continue to smoke and over 47 million report using tobacco products (Cornelius et al., 2022). Analyzing data from the 2020 U.S. National Health Interview Survey, Cornelius and colleagues (2022) reported that cigarette smoking (12.5%) was the most common method of tobacco consumption followed by e-cigarettes (3.7%), cigars (3.5%), smokeless tobacco (2.3%), and pipes (1.1%). Men (14.1%) reported higher rates of smoking than women (11.0%). Globally, around 22% of the world's population use tobacco (WHO, 2022). Smoking disproportionately impacts residents of low-income countries. Of the worldwide estimate of 1.3 billion people who smoke, more than 80% live in low- or middle-income countries (WHO, 2022).

The good news is that interest in smoking cessation is high. U.S. surveys suggest that approximately seven out of ten smokers wish they could stop, and a majority of smokers report attempting to quit within the past year (Hartmann-Boyce et al., 2021; USDHHS, 2014). Yet, achieving smoking cessation and maintaining gains is difficult, with less than 10% of unassisted initial quit attempts being successful (Brose et al., 2011). Fortunately, stopping smoking may reverse the negative health impacts of smoking (Hartmann-Boyce et al., 2021). For example, stopping smoking for five years returns the risk of cardiovascular disease to that of those who never smoked, and ten years of smoking abstinence halves the risk of lung cancer compared to those who continue smoking (USDHHS, 2010).

Stopping smoking prior to age 40 may reduce the risk of dying from a smoking-related disease by 90% (Jha et al., 2013). The USDHHS (2010) estimates that one-third of all cancer-related deaths could be eliminated via smoking cessation.

There's more good news. A number of treatment protocols including medication, nicotine replacement therapies (NRT), and counseling-based programs have demonstrated efficacy for smoking cessation (see Green & Lynn, 2019; 2023). For example, Tonnesen (2009) noted 12-month success rates of the nicotine patch, combined NRT approaches, and medication to range from 26.5% to 36.5%. In a large-scale investigation, Baker (2016) contrasted NRT with medication for smoking cessation and found no advantage for one approach over the other with 27% and 20% of participants successfully stopping at 6 and 12 months, respectively. These rates are similar to those reported decades earlier for stand-alone behavioral interventions. Baker (2016) and others (e.g., Hartmann-Boyce et al., 2021) recommend adding counseling or behavioral-based interventions to pharmacotherapy approaches to improve success rates. Indeed, the combination of behavioral counseling with NRT or medication may double response rates and are consistent with current U.S. Clinical Practice Guidelines (Fiore et al., 2008).

Hypnosis holds promise as a popular and cost-effective treatment for smoking (see Green & Lynn, 2017, 2019, 2023; Lynn et al., 2010, 2019). We view hypnosis as a tool, a technique, or strategy rather than a complete therapy and prominently feature it within a broader cognitive-behavioral treatment for smoking. Public opinion on the use of hypnosis for achieving smoking cessation is good (e.g., Sood et al., 2006). Reviews and meta-analyses support hypnosis for smoking with success rates typically within the 25–35% range (e.g., Green & Lynn, 2000; Green et al., 2006a, 2008; Tahiri et al., 2012; Viswesvaran & Schmidt, 1992). However, the empirical foundation for the claim that "hypnosis works for smoking" is limited by overreliance on case studies and narrative reviews, use of non-standardized treatment protocols, reliance on self-report of smoking abstinence, inconsistent classification of dropouts as treatment failures, and lack of randomized clinical trials (Barnes et al., 2019; Green & Lynn, 2000, 2019, 2023). Because hypnosis is commonly embedded within cognitive and behavioral treatments for smoking, it is often difficult to determine the independent efficacy of any one ingredient. In their Cochrane Review, Barnes and colleagues (2019) cited limited evidence supporting hypnosis for smoking cessation; however, they concluded that the totality of the evidence failed to convincingly show that "hypnotherapy is more effective for smoking cessation than other forms of behavioural support or unassisted quitting" (p. 2).

In a rigorous investigation, Carmody et al. (2008) conducted a randomized trial contrasting an early version of our protocol against a standard counseling approach. In addition to psychological intervention, all participants received NRT. Smoking abstinence rates, confirmed by biochemical tests, were higher (but not statistically different) among hypnosis vs. counseling participants at 6 (26% vs. 18%) and 12 months (18% vs. 14%) post treatment. Two additional studies not included in the Cochrane review (Barnes et al., 2019) are worthy of mention. Hasan and colleagues (2014) considered treatment preferences for smoking cessation among cardiac and pulmonary hospital patients. Those interested in NRT or hypnosis were randomly assigned to one of three approaches involving a 90-minute hypnosis session, NRT, or a combination of the two. Those uninterested in hypnosis or NRT were assigned to a self-help condition. All active treatment participants received supportive counseling after discharge. Six-month abstinence rates were highest among those who received hypnosis (36.6%) in addition to supportive counseling, followed by self-help (27%) and NRT (18%). Adding NRT to hypnosis failed to meaningfully affect the success of hypnosis and supportive counseling alone. Whereas the comparisons failed to reach statistical significance, results suggested that hypnosis can potentiate gains from counseling approaches for smoking cessation. Finally, Elkins et al. (2006) randomly assigned 20 smokers to receive hypnosis, supportive counseling, or be wait-listed (control). Biochemical confirmed reports of smoking abstinence at six months were 40% for hypnosis compared with 0% for control participants. The authors concluded that "the overall results of the present study support the efficacy of an intensive approach to hypnotherapy for adult smokers" (p. 309). In short, whereas we currently lack large-scale and methodologically rigorous studies to establish hypnosis as an empirically supported treatment for smoking, hypnosis is favorably perceived by the public and holds promise as an adjunctive treatment for smoking cessation. We next describe our view of the role of hypnosis within a larger framework of psychological and medical interventions for smoking cessation and outline components of our multimodal treatment for smoking.

Pitching Hypnosis and Debunking Myths

It is important to establish positive yet realistic expectancies. As part of the educational component of our program (detailed later), we frame the general utility of hypnosis by citing research showing that hypnosis may potentiate gains achieved by medical and psychological therapies (e.g., Kirsch et al., 1995; Valentine et al., 2019). We acknowledge that the empirical evidence for hypnosis for the treatment of smoking is inconclusive and needs further study. Hypnosis – especially if used alone – is not a magic bullet or a guarantee of success. We emphasize that our approach incorporates hypnosis into a larger framework of a multidimensional cognitive-behavioral approach. We convey excitement about hypnosis to help participants focus attention, maintain concentration, keep their goal of not smoking foremost in their mind, implement effective change strategies, and redefine themselves as a nonsmoker.

We stress committing to the goal of not smoking, actively working the program, and maintaining motivation to persevere in the face of difficulties. We discuss health risks and benefits of stopping smoking to capitalize on clients' motivation to avoid or minimize health problems and to achieve a better overall quality of life. We inform clients that smoking cessation is difficult but doable, as many people stop smoking every day. We reinforce clients' decision to stop smoking and express optimism about their chances of success.

We debunk myths and discuss common misconceptions about hypnosis. Informed by sociocognitive and response set theory (e.g., Lynn et al., 2017; Lynn et al., 2023), we define hypnosis as "an interpersonal situation in which a person designated as a hypnotist conveys communications that are intended to enhance experiential involvement and responsiveness to imaginative suggestions in a context that is construed to be *hypnotic*" (Lynn et al., 2022, p. 1; see also Lynn et al., 2015, 2017). We steer clear from presenting hypnosis as a "trance" or as necessarily involving an "altered state of consciousness" for several reasons. First, critics of the term argue that it is vague, lacks specificity, and is rarely operationalized (e.g., Lynn et al., 2020). Additionally, conceptualizing hypnosis as "falling into trance" is consonant with other fears and misplaced concerns about losing control, being unable to resist suggestions, or getting stuck and unable to exit hypnosis (see Green et al., 2006b; Green et al., 2012; Lynn et al., 2010). Further, conceptualizing hypnosis as trance promotes a passive response set whereby participants anticipate that something will *happen to them,* even if they are not engaged, opposed to, or uninterested in experiencing a suggestion (see Lynn et al., 2020). Accordingly, we view defining hypnosis as *trance* as both unnecessary and potentially detrimental to establishing an active response set of open and willing engagement with suggested material (Kirsch & Lynn, 1995; Lynn et al., 2020). Indeed, Lynn and colleagues (2002) found that participants who believed that hypnotic responsiveness relied on achieving a trance or altered state of consciousness scored lower on standardized assessments of hypnotizability relative to those who believed that responsiveness stemmed from a willingness to cooperate with suggestions.

The Winning Edge Program

In what follows, we present the core components of our approach. Our protocol can be delivered in group or individual format distributed over two or three weekly sessions of around 1.5–2.5 hours (e.g., Green, 1999, 2010; Green & Lynn, 2019, 2023). While providing structured guidance for beginning clinicians or those new to hypnosis, we intentionally provide latitude for clinicians to tailor language to the needs of their clients, incorporate additional strategies as they see fit, and offer client-specific reassurances along the way. We stress that our approach is a 'work in progress' as we strive to continually update, modify, and improve our protocol by including evidence-based and promising techniques into our suite of treatment options that include motivational interviewing (e.g., Miller & Rose, 2009); work on decisional balance (Krigel et al., 2017); use of implementation instructions (e.g., Gollwitzer, 1999); and insights gained from self-determination theory (Ryan & Deci, 2000).

Our protocol rests on cognitive-behavioral therapy (CBT) techniques for habit control and incorporates mindfulness, acceptance, and hypnosis-based strategies to achieve smoking cessation and live according to best values. A treatment manual detailing the various components of our program is presented in our volume, *Cognitive-behavioral therapy, mindfulness, and hypnosis for smoking cessation: a scientifically informed intervention* (Green & Lynn, 2019). Materials include a clinician's guide for program delivery; our hypnosis scripts and video-based educational program; handouts and worksheets. We also present case illustrations, along with tips for individualizing treatment and handling common questions (e.g., use of NRT, medication, e-cigarettes; comorbidity concerns).

General Overview

We begin by welcoming participants and congratulating them on their decision to stop smoking. After brief introductions, participants discuss their smoking history, prior successful periods of abstinence, and top concerns about trying to stop smoking. We recommend that facilitators adopt a warm, encouraging, and non-judgmental tone while empathically recognizing the difficulty of the challenge. We start with a description of our multidimensional approach, noting that hypnosis is one of many techniques to move clients toward a smoke-free life. After answering questions, we obtain consent.

We have dubbed our collection of techniques as, "The Winning Edge". We present each strategy and discuss implementation. We regularly revisit the value of employing this arsenal of tactics as we respond to questions and during follow-up conversations. Within the group, we present a one-hour, narrated video presentation of our approach featuring animated slides and video clips. We provide a copy of the video for participants to watch a second time at home, ideally with a supportive family member or friend. Next, we briefly describe the main strategies and tactics comprising our approach.

Introducing CBT

We facilitate a short discussion of CBT, the foundation of our approach. We note that CBT is an empirically supported treatment for many conditions and problematic behaviors, is the gold standard of psychological therapies, and can be effective for treating smoking. Our program offers clear guidance to "unlearn" the habit of smoking.

The Educational Component

We empower participants with knowledge about how behaviors are learned, reinforced, and automatized. To illustrate the strength of the habit, we instruct participants to calculate the number of times they have raised a cigarette to their mouth. We detail a number of poisons and toxic chemicals found within burning tobacco (e.g., benzene, arsenic, formaldehyde). We play a video-taped presentation by a health professional discussing risks association with smoking and the benefits of stopping smoking. We highlight the financial cost of cigarette consumption. We discuss NRT and encourage its use for those willing to incorporate it into their plan.

The Motivation Piece and the Importance of Social Support

We devote considerable time addressing ambivalence and instruct participants to conduct a cost-benefit analysis of continuing versus stopping (see Green & Lynn, 2017). We inquire if participants would be willing to stop for one million dollars. Invariably, everyone agrees and confidently states that they could stop in exchange for such a reward. To harness and mold motivation, we then ask, "What is your life worth? What is your health worth?" We share the fact that progress is rarely linear and that participants should anticipate temporary setbacks along their journey to freedom from smoking. We encourage participants to remain committed to their goal, and we praise any progress no matter how small.

Social support is another important ingredient. We encourage participants to inform others of their goal to not smoke and to actively seek support from friends and family. We also provide the opportunity for group members to pair-up as part of a "buddy system". We instruct participants to place goal reminders throughout their homes and to regularly review their reasons to stop smoking. We present a visualization exercise in which participants imagine the benefits of stopping and costs of continuing smoking. We invite participants to anchor their motivation and desire to become a nonsmoker by making a circle with their thumb and forefinger and to enact this gesture regularly as a reminder of their goal and to crystallize motivation.

The Cognitive Piece

We address dysfunctional and counter-productive beliefs associated with smoking both within the group and on handouts. Examples include negative self-predictions (e.g., "I just can't stop"), emotional reasoning (e.g., "I *feel* like I won't succeed, therefore I won't be able to"), over-generalization (e.g., "My parents smoked, so I guess I have no choice"), catastrophic thinking (e.g., "Withdrawal will be unbearable"), and labeling (e.g., "I can't quit because I'm an addict"). We frankly discuss nicotine withdrawal symptoms and offer ways to cope. We acknowledge the possibility of weight gain following cessation, offer weight control strategies, and stress that the health benefits of stopping smoking far outweigh risks associated with gaining a few pounds (Clair et al., 2013). We review misconceptions that smoking cessation invariably leads to weight gain or withdrawal symptoms that are necessarily strong and unavoidable. Finally, we discuss the importance of staying confident and continuing to work on the program.

The All-Important Behavioral Ingredients

Smoking is a learned behavior that has been reinforced many times. The *Identifying Triggers* handout helps participants increase awareness of times, situations, acquaintances, and emotions associated with the desire to smoke and plan alternative behaviors to smoking. We discuss stimulus control whereby participants make small but meaningful changes to their physical environment to increase awareness of high-risk situations. For example, participants might place goal reminder cards throughout their home; move their "smoking chair" to a different location; place a picture of a child or grandchild next to their ashtray; or place an unusual object in a conspicuous place on their porch where they previously smoked as a reminder of their goal. We discuss the importance of monitoring snacking patterns, drinking plenty of water, getting enough sleep, and maintaining regular exercise.

Managing the Urge

We stress that the habit of smoking is undermined with each and every action taken in light of the urge and decision to smoke. Small victories accumulate into larger gains. Participants discuss their prior smoking cessation attempts, and we collectively draw on strategies and behavioral substitutions that previously worked. We ask participants to imagine themselves in a tug of war with a *smoking monster* with a vast abyss in-between. While the temptation is to pull harder and harder, the solution is to drop the rope. By *dropping the rope*, participants disengage from the struggle and maintain some distance from the temptation to smoke. The urge may persist, but they no longer have to struggle or expend energy to battle it. Our instructions to "surf the urge" include recognizing the urge, positive self-talk, goal awareness (e.g., reviewing reasons not to smoke), and behavioral substitution. We provide a list of alternative behaviors to smoking and encourage participants to fortify this inventory with their own ideas. We stress that most cravings pass, or at least greatly diminish, within a few minutes, so distraction techniques or substitution strategies can be quite helpful.

Incorporating Mindfulness and Acceptance-Based Strategies

We encourage participants to be aware, acknowledge, and accept the fact that they will likely experience cravings and that these feelings may intensify over the first few days following cessation. Indeed, even after long-term abstinence, urges to smoke may emerge from time to time. Participants learn to decouple the desire to smoke from smoking behavior. We use a variety of strategies including mindfulness, acceptance, relaxation, and hypnosis, and build upon knowledge gained to give participants *the winning edge* to divert attention away from smoking cues; maintain their focus on their goal; and refrain from engaging in smoking behavior (i.e., "surf the urge"). Within our hypnosis scripts, we weave in suggestions for increasing tolerance and acceptance of self and others, accepting feelings and cravings without judging them as good or bad, and appreciating the critical distinction between feelings (of wanting to smoke) and actions (choosing to do something other than smoking).

Incentivizing Success and Preventing Relapse

We invite participants to celebrate their success by establishing near and longer term goals (e.g., 1, 3, and 6 month rewards) and regularly reviewing them. Rewards might range from buying something new to taking a vacation to simply having dinner and spending time with a loved one to celebrate the achievement.

While complete abstinence is the ostensible goal, we recognize that smoking reduction is beneficial for many participants. Many need more time beyond the weeks of our group meetings to achieve full abstinence. We encourage participants to continue to *work on the program* and to *redouble their resolve* as needed. We discuss the role of stress and negative emotions in triggering relapse. We plan for difficult moments, anticipate obstacles, and detail plans for avoiding the resumption of smoking. General stress management strategies and sustained social support are fundamental to maintaining gains.

The Boost from Self-Hypnosis

Hypnosis is the chief ingredient of our program. We present hypnosis as a skill to be learned and stress the importance of active participation to experience the suggestions. We debunk common myths and misconceptions about hypnosis (e.g., people lose control, get stuck, cannot resist suggestions, or that hypnosis is powerful mind control characterized by spectacular shifts in consciousness; see Green, 2003; Green et al., 2006b; Lynn et al., 2020). Consistent with our sociocognitive perspective, we characterize all hypnosis as *self-hypnosis*, as the participant does the work and success depends on their cooperation. We stress that being an imagination superstar or having prior experience is not required to use hypnosis to advantage. Additionally, we stress that initial hypnotic responsiveness does not predict the ultimate benefit of hypnosis and that responsiveness often improves with practice.

Prior to administering hypnosis, we present a video of a model discussing her experience with hypnosis. Within our hypnosis scripts, we review the numerous and varied elements comprising our overall approach. We include suggestions to realize smoking abstinence, visualize oneself as a nonsmoker overcoming obstacles and challenges, maintain motivation and focus, and successfully manage urges to smoke. We wrap our suggestions for smoking cessation around the overarching goal of living in accord with one's highest values, promoting overall health, and increasing happiness, tolerance, and feelings of well-being.

We provide two hypnosis scripts. The first includes general suggestions for relaxation, focusing attention, crystallizing goals, and living a purpose-driven life. While revisiting these themes, the second script recapitulates all the elements comprising our winning edge strategy as applied to smoking cessation. In short, we reinforce and rehearse behavioral change strategies that we taught and discussed in the first session. In the latest iteration of our scripts, we crafted suggestions to include implementation instructions by using "if-then" statements to enhance responsiveness and realize goals (Gallo et al., 2012; see Green & Lynn, 2019). For example: *If you fully commit to all of the strategies and tactics within our program, and if you allow yourself to get fully absorbed in your hypnosis and go just as deep as you'd like to go, then you will maximize the chances of achieving your goal, becoming a nonsmoker, and living your life in accordance with your highest values. Wouldn't that be great?*

Success Ceremony and Continued Support

A highlight of our second session is a "success ceremony" during which participants announce their principal reason(s) for stopping smoking, tear or crumble up a paper picturing cigarettes, and confidently proclaim that they are "done with smoking forever!" We instruct participants to listen daily to the hypnosis recordings, complete the worksheets, and regularly review program materials. Participants continue to monitor progress by recording their smoking frequency. We provide additional support via telephone and follow-up sessions at two and four weeks posttreatment.

Conclusions

In this chapter, we outlined the components of our multifaceted smoking cessation program. We presented hypnosis as a promising intervention complementing cognitive-behavioral, mindfulness, and acceptance-based strategies to achieving smoking abstinence. While we are encouraged and optimistic about the utility of adding hypnosis to CBT, much work remains to establish hypnosis as an empirically supported treatment for smoking. Regardless of outcomes associated with randomized control trials, individual applications appear useful with patients intrinsically interested in using hypnosis to overcome smoking.

References

Ahmed, N., Maqsood, A., Abduljabbar, T., & Vohra, F. (2020). Tobacco smoking a potential risk factor in transmission of COVID-19 infection. *Pakistani Journal of Medical Sciences*, *36*, S1–S4. 10.12669/pjms.36.COVID19-S4.2739

Baker, T. B., Piper, M. E., Stein, J. H., Smith, S. S., Bolt, D. M., Fraser, D. L., & Fiore, M. C. (2016). Effects of nicotine patch vs varenicline vs combination nicotine replacement therapy on smoking cessation at 26 weeks. *JAMA*, *315*(4), 371. 10.1001/jama.2015.19284

Bakhshaie, J., Ditre, J. W., Langdon, K. J., Asmundson, G. J., Paulus, D. J., & Zvolensky, M. J. (2016). Pain intensity and smoking behavior among treatment seeking smokers. *Psychiatry Research*, *237*, 67–71. 10.1016/j.psychres.2016.01.073

Barnes, J., McRobbie, H., Dong, C. Y., Walker, N., & Hartmann-Boyce, J. (2019). *Hypnotherapy for smoking cessation*. Cochrane Systematic Reviews, Issue 6. Art. No.: CD001008. 10.1002/14651858.cd001008.pub3

Brose, L. S., West, R., McDermott, M. S., Fidler, J. A., Croghan, E., & McEwen, A. (2011). What makes for an effective stop-smoking service? *Thorax*, *66*(10), 924–926. 10.1136/thoraxjnl-2011-200251

Bundhun, P. K., Janoo, G., Bhurtu, A., Teeluck, A. R., Soogund, M. Z. S., Pursun, M., & Huang, F. (2019). Tobacco smoking and semen quality in infertile males: A systematic review and meta-analysis. *BMC Public Health*, *19*(1). Article number: 36. 10.1186/s12889-018-6319-3

Carmody, T., Duncan, C., Simon, J., Solkowitz, S., Huggins, J., Lee, S., & Delucchi, K. (2008). Hypnosis for smoking cessation: A randomized trial. *Nicotine & Tobacco Research*, *10*(5), 811–818. 10.1080/14622200802023833

Clair, C., Rigotti, N. A., Porneala, B., Fox, C. S., D'Agostino, R. B., Pencina, M. J., & Meigs, J. B. (2013). Association of smoking cessation and weight change with cardiovascular disease among adults with and without diabetes. *JAMA*, *309*(10), 1014. 10.1001/jama.2013.1644

Choi, J., Shin, D. W., Lee, S., Jeon, M. J., Kim, S. M., Cho, B., & Lee, S. M. (2015). Dose-response relationship between cigarette smoking and female sexual dysfunction. *Obstetrics & Gynecology Science*, *58*(4), 302–308. 10.5468/ogs.2015.58.4.302

Cornelius, M. E., Loretan, C. G., Wang, T. W., Jamal, A., & Homa, D. M. (2022). Tobacco product use among adults – United States, 2020. *MMWR. Morbidity and Mortality Weekly Report*, *71*(11), 397–405. 10.15585/mmwr.mm7111a1

Costa, R. M., & Peres, L. (2015). Smoking is unrelated to female sexual function. *Substance Use & Misuse*, *50*(2), 189–194. 10.3109/10826084.2014.962054

Elkins, G., Marcus, J., Bates, J., Hasan Rajab, M., & Cook, T. (2006). Intensive hypnotherapy for smoking cessation: A prospective study. *International Journal of Clinical and Experimental Hypnosis*, *54*(3), 303–315. 10.1080/00207140600689512

Fiore, M. C., Jaén, C. R., Baker, T. B., Bailey, W. C., Benowitz, N. L., Curry, S. J., et al. (2008). *Treating tobacco use and dependence: 2008 update.* Clinical practice guideline. Agency for Health Care Policy and Research (US). 10.1037/e481882008-001

Gallo, I. S., Pfau, F., & Gollwitzer, P. M. (2012). Furnishing hypnotic instructions with implementation intentions enhances hypnotic responsiveness. *Consciousness and Cognition*, *21*(2), 1023–1030. 10.1016/j.concog.2012.03.007

Gollwitzer, P. M. (1999). Implementation instructions: strong effects of simple plans. *American Psychologist*, *54*(7), 493–503. 10.1037/0003-066X.54.7.493

Green, J. P. (1999). Hypnosis and the treatment of smoking cessation and weight loss. In I. Kirsch, A. Capafons, E. Cardeña-Buelna, & S. Amigo, (Eds.), *Clinical hypnosis and self-regulation: Cognitive-behavioral perspectives* (pp. 249–276). American Psychological Association.

Green, J. P. (2003). Beliefs about hypnosis: Popular beliefs, misconceptions, and the importance of experience. *International Journal of Clinical and Experimental Hypnosis*, *51*(4), 369–381. 10. 1076/iceh.51.4.369.16408

Green, J. P. (2010). Hypnosis and smoking cessation: Research and application. In S. J. Lynn, J. W. Rhue, & I. Kirsch (Eds.), *Handbook of clinical hypnosis, II* (pp. 593–614). American Psychological Association.

Green, J. P., Houts, C. R., & Capafons, A. (2012). Attitudes about hypnosis: Factor analyzing the VSABTH-C with an American sample. *American Journal of Clinical Hypnosis*, *54*(3), 167–178. 10.1080/00029157.2011.616823

Green, J. P., & Lynn, S. J. (2000). Hypnosis and suggestion-based approaches to smoking cessation: An examination of the evidence. *International Journal of Clinical and Experimental Hypnosis*, *48*(2), 195–224. 10.1080/00207140008410048

Green, J. P., & Lynn, S. J. (2017). A multifaceted hypnosis smoking cessation program: Enhancing motivation and goal attainment. *International Journal of Clinical and Experimental Hypnosis*, *65*(3), 308–335. 10.1080/00207144.2017.1314740

Green, J. P., & Lynn, S. J. (2019). *Cognitive-behavioral therapy, mindfulness, and hypnosis for smoking cessation: A scientifically informed intervention.* Wiley Blackwell. 10.1002/9781119139676

Green, J. P., & Lynn, S. J. (2023). Hypnosis for the treatment of smoking. In L. Milling (Ed.), *Evidence-based practice in clinical hypnosis* (pp. xx-xx). American Psychological Association.

Green, J. P., Lynn, S. J., & Montgomery, G. H. (2006a). A meta-analysis of gender, smoking cessation, and hypnosis: A brief communication. *International Journal of Clinical and Experimental Hypnosis*, *54*(2), 224–233. 10.1080/00207140500528497

Green, J. P., Lynn, S. J., & Montgomery, G. H. (2008). Gender-related differences in hypnosis-based treatments for smoking: A follow-up meta-analysis. *American Journal of Clinical Hypnosis*, *50*(3), 259–271. 10.1080/00029157.2008.10401628

Green, J. P., Page, R. A., Rasekhy, R., Johnson, L. K., & Bernhardt, S. E. (2006b). Cultural views and attitudes about hypnosis: A survey of college students across four countries. *International Journal of Clinical and Experimental Hypnosis*, *54*(3), 263–280. 10.1080/00207140600689439

Guo, Q. N., Wang, J., Liu, H. Y., Wu, D., & Liao, S. X. (2022). Nicotine ingestion reduces heart rate variability in young healthy adults. *BioMed Research International*, *2022*, 1–7. 10.1155/2022/ 4286621

Harte, C. B., & Meston, C. M. (2008). Acute effects of nicotine on physiological and subjective sexual arousal in nonsmoking men: A randomized, double-blind, placebo-controlled trial. *Journal of Sexual Medicine*, *5*(1), 110–121. 10.1111/j.1743-6109.2007.00637.x

Hartmann-Boyce, J., Livingstone-Bank, J., Ordóñez-Mena, J. M., Fanshawe, T. R., Lindson, N., Freeman, S. C., Sutton A. J., Theodoulou, A., & Aveyard, P. (2021). *Behavioural interventions for smoking cessation: an overview and network meta-analysis*. Cochrane Database of Systematic Reviews, Issue 1. Art. No.: CD013229. 10.1002/14651858.cd013229.pub2

Hasan, F. M., Zagarins, S. E., Pischke, K. M., Saiyed, S., Bettencourt, A. M., Beal, L., Macys, D., Aurora, S., & McCleary, N. (2014). Hypnotherapy is more effective than nicotine replacement therapy for smoking cessation: Results of a randomized controlled trial. *Complementary Therapies in Medicine*, *22*(1), 1–8. 10.1016/j.ctim.2013.12.012

Jarvis, M. J. (2004). ABC of smoking cessation: Why people smoke. *BMJ, British Medical Journal*, *328*(7434), 277–279. 10.1136/bmj.328.7434.277

Jensen, K. P., Valentine, G., Gueorguieva, R., & Sofuoglu, M. (2020). Differential effects of nicotine delivery rate on subjective drug effects, urges to smoke, heart rate and blood pressure in tobacco smokers. *Psychopharmacology*, *237*, 1359–1369. 10.1007/s00213-020-05463-6

Jha, P., Ramasundarahettige, C., Landsman, V., Rostron, B., Thun, M., Anderson, R. N., McAfee, T., & Peto, R. (2013). 21st-Century hazards of smoking and benefits of cessation in the United States. *New England Journal of Medicine*, *368*(4), 341–350. 10.1056/nejmsa1211128

Ju, R., Ruan, X., Xu, X., Yang, Y., Cheng, J., Zhang, L., Wang, B., Qin, S., Dou, Z., & Mueck, A. O. (2021). Importance of active and passive smoking as one of the risk factors for female sexual dysfunction in Chinese women. *Gynecological Endocrinology*, *37*(6), 541–545. 10.1080/09513590.2021.1913115

Kirsch, I., & Lynn, S. J. (1995). Altered state of hypnosis: Changes in the theoretical landscape. *American Psychologist*, *50*(10), 846. 10.1037/0003-066X.50.10.846

Kirsch, I., Montgomery, G., & Sapirstein, G. (1995). Hypnosis as an adjunct to cognitive behavioral psychotherapy: A meta-analysis. *Journal of Consulting and Clinical Psychology*, *63*(2), 214–220. 10.1037/0022-006x.63.2.214

Krigel, S. W., Grobe, J. E., Goggin, K., Harris, K. J., Moreno, J. L., & Catley, D. (2017). Motivational interviewing and the decisional balance procedure for cessation induction in smokers not intending to quit. *Addictive Behaviors*, *64*, 171–178. 10.1016/j.addbeh.2016.08.036

Lynn, S. J., Cardeña, E., Green, J. P., & Laurence, J. R. (2022). The case for clinical hypnosis: Theory and research-based do's and don'ts for clinical practice. *Psychology of Consciousness: Theory, Research, and Practice*, *9*(2), 187–200. 10.1037/cns0000257

Lynn, S. J., Green, J. P., Kirsch, I., Capafons, A., Lilienfeld, S. O., Laurence, J. R., & Montgomery, G. H. (2015). Grounding hypnosis in science: The "new" APA Division 30 definition of hypnosis as a step backward. *American Journal of Clinical Hypnosis*, *57*(4), 390–401. 10.1080/00029157.2015.1011472

Lynn, S. J., Green, J. P., Polizzi, C. P., Ellenberg, S., Guatam, A., & Aksen, D. (2019). Hypnosis, hypnotic phenomena, and hypnotic responsiveness: Clinical and research foundations – A 40 year perspective. *International Journal of Clinical and Experimental Hypnosis*, *67*(4), 475–511. 10.1080/00207144.2019.1649541

Lynn, S. J., Green, J. P., Zahedi, A., & Apelian, C. (2023). The response set theory of hypnosis reconsidered: Toward an integrative model. *American Journal of Clinical Hypnosis*, *65*(3), 186–210. 10.1080/00029157.2022.2117680

Lynn, S. J., Kirsch, I., Terhune, D. B., & Green, J. P. (2020). Myths and misconceptions about hypnosis and suggestion: Separating fact and fiction. *Applied Cognitive Psychology*, *34*(6), 1253–1264. 10.1002/acp.3730

Lynn, S. J., Maxwell, R., & Green, J. P. (2017). The hypnotic induction in the broad scheme of hypnosis: A sociocognitive perspective. *American Journal of Clinical Hypnosis*, *59*(4), 363–384. 10.1080/00029157.2016.1233093

Lynn, S. J., Rhue, J. W., & Kirsch, I. (2010). *Handbook of clinical hypnosis* (2nd ed.). American Psychological Association.

Lynn, S. J., Vanderhoff, H., Shindler, K., & Stafford, J. (2002). Defining hypnosis as a trance vs. cooperation: Hypnotic inductions, suggestibility, and performance standards. *American Journal of Clinical Hypnosis*, *44*(3-4), 231–240. 10.1080/00029157.2002.10403483

Miller, W. R., & Rose, G. S. (2009). Toward a theory of motivational interviewing. *American Psychologist*, *64*(6), 527–537. 10.1037/a0016830

Ryan, R. M., & Deci, E. L. (2000). Self-determination theory and the facilitation of intrinsic motivation, social development, and well-being. *American Psychologist*, *55*(1), 68–78. 10.1037/0003-066x.55.1.68

Schmelzer, A. C., Salt, E., Wiggins, A., Crofford, L. J., Bush, H., & Mannino, D. M. (2016). Role of stress and smoking as modifiable risk factors for nonpersistent and persistent back pain in women. *The Clinical Journal of Pain*, *32*(3), 232–237. 10.1097/ajp.0000000000000245

Sood, A., Ebbert, J., Sood, R., & Stevens, S. (2006). Complementary treatments for tobacco cessation: A survey. *Nicotine & Tobacco Research*, *8*(6), 767–771. 10.1080/14622200601004109

Tahiri, M., Mottillo, S., Joseph, L., Pilote, L., & Eisenberg, M. J. (2012). Alternative smoking cessation aids: A meta-analysis of randomized controlled trials. *The American Journal of Medicine*, *125*(6), 576–584. 10.1016/j.amjmed.2011.09.028

Tønnesen, P. (2009). Smoking cessation: How compelling is the evidence? A review. *Health Policy*, *91*(S1), S15–S25. 10.1016/s0168-8510(09)70004-1

U.S. Department of Health and Human Services (USDHHS) (2010). *How tobacco smoke causes disease: The biology and behavioral basis for smoking attributable disease: A report of the Surgeon General*. U.S. Department of Health and Human Services, Centers for Disease Control and Prevention, National Center for Chronic Disease Prevention and Health Promotion, Office on Smoking and Health.

U.S. Department of Health and Human Services (USDHHS) (2014). The health consequences of smoking – 50 Years of progress: A report of the Surgeon General, Executive Summary. U.S. Department of Health and Human Services, Centers for Disease Control and Prevention, National Center for Chronic Disease Prevention and Health Promotion, Office on Smoking and Health. 10.1037/e510072014-001

Valentine, K. E., Milling, L. S., Clark, L. J., & Moriarty, C. L. (2019). The efficacy of hypnosis as a treatment for anxiety: A meta-analysis. *International Journal of Clinical and Experimental Hypnosis*, *67*(3), 336–363. 10.1080/00207144.2019.1613863

Viswesvaran, C., & Schmidt, F. L. (1992). A meta-analytic comparison of the effectiveness of smoking cessation methods. *Journal of Applied Psychology*, *77*(4), 554–561. 10.1037/0021-9010.77.4.554

World Health Organization (WHO). (2022, May 25). *Tobacco*. World Health Organization. Retrieved March 3, 2023, from https://www.who.int/news-room/fact-sheets/detail/tobacco

33
SYSTEMIC HYPNOSIS
How to Develop and Use Systemic Trances with Couples and Families

Camillo Loriedo, Nicolino Rago, and Ilaria Genovesi

SII Società Italiana Ipnosi – SIIPE Scuola Italiana di Ipnosi e Psicoterapia Ericksoniana

Outline

The family is the main context in which the psychic and emotional development of an individual takes place. Later, in the course of life, the person becomes part of different systems of relationship: from the couple to the family, to friendships, to the world of work. In this chapter, hypnosis will be treated from a systemic perspective, i.e., as a form of circular and evolutionary interaction within systems. After briefly covering the history of systemic hypnosis through its main protagonists, the general principles, the hypnotic process with the family system, the typical phenomena that develop in the hypnotic interaction, and some direct, and indirect techniques of systemic hypnotic intervention will be illustrated. Finally, in the paragraph dedicated to the clinical examples of the application of systemic hypnosis, *Integrative Inductions* (Loriedo, 2017) and their use in family forms of dissociation will be described, and a clinical case treated with the Hypnotic Induction of Dancing Hands technique (Loriedo et al., 2018) will be presented.

Theoretical Framework and History

Milton Erickson was one of the pillars on which both hypnosis and family therapy were built (Haley, 1973).

The reciprocal interest between family therapy and hypnosis arose between 1952 and 1956, the years in which Gregory Bateson and the Palo Alto colleagues, Jay Haley, John Weakland, and Don Jackson were engaged in a study on schizophrenia (Bateson et al, 1956). Scientists found that hospitalized schizophrenics worsened whenever they returned to the family, a phenomenon that the individual psychoanalytic model was not able to explain. To study these family interactions, paradoxes, and double bind-based communication, a new frame of reference was needed.

Gregory Bateson asked his colleagues to visit Milton Erickson once a week, who, while mainly involved with individual hypnosis, was already meeting with families

 DOI: 10.4324/9781003449126-45

(Haley, 1985). Weakland and Haley took from Erickson's therapy work a number of important contributions for the newborn family therapy: the strategic approach, use of directives, paradoxical interventions (encouraging resistance), several techniques, the illusion of alternatives, and the use of ordeals (Rago & Rivelli, 2021). Erickson frequently used hypnosis with families and couples and was the first to combine hypnosis and family therapy in a way that today we can define as systemic. In most reported cases, he preferred an indirect hypnotic approach (47 times out of 65 total clinical situations reported, of which 32 were couples and 33 were families). From the cases presented in his works, we only found two interventions out of 65, equal to about 3%, in which formal direct hypnosis was simultaneously applied to more than one member of a system. Direct hypnotic-systemic interventions were carried out on two couples, while there is no evidence of a direct induction performed by Erickson with a whole family (Rago & Rivelli, 2021).

The use of hypnosis in systemic family therapy was proposed later by other authors, and above all by Michele Ritterman (1983) who also favored indirect inductions, without a clear, formal induction of trance.

Ritterman (1983) conceptualized the information flow among family members as exchanges of hypnotic suggestions. For example, if a family member is too suggestible to some indirect family stimuli, or is unable to escape from these stimuli, the therapist may access the trance state to immunize that member against these "invisible" family directives. Utilizing hypnosis in family therapy, Ritterman (1983) develops a therapeutic counter-induction, traveling the same roads of the family suggestions to deliver new messages and activate new internal processes. Consistent with her perspective, the author tends not to make a formal induction with the whole family, and when working with couples she prefers to make a direct induction on one member while working indirectly with the other. In other words, for Ritterman (1983), the use of hypnosis with the entire family system is unusual.

In addition to Erickson (1967) and Ritterman (1983), other important studies about the use of hypnosis applied to family systems are the ones of Lankton and Lankton (1983), Lankton et al. (1995), Kershaw (1992), and Schmidt (2004).

Orientation: Direct Versus Indirect and Systemic Versus Individual

In comparing how these authors use hypnosis with families, we can conclude that not all of them openly declare to the family they will use hypnosis.

The approach we have proposed since the 1980s (Loriedo & Zeig, 1986; Loriedo et al., 1987) is centered on a formal or direct hypnotic induction and includes all the family system members. Hypnosis is used explicitly with the goal of creating a hypnotic context shared by the whole family system, which we consider a core element of this type of intervention. The presupposition of this approach can be ascribed to the work of Gregory Bateson (1979) who has described families and other human systems as a mind, able to develop its evolutionary processes. Another important part of the approach consists of clearly notifying the family members that the hypnotic trance will be applied to the entire family. This is done not only because informed consent is now considered a prerequisite for a correct therapeutic relationship but also because we strongly believe that when family members accept to be part of the hypnotic session, their individual and shared expectation of change will intensify the therapeutic effect.

General Principles and Goals of Systemic Hypnosis

Working with an entire family is different from working with single individuals. The following are the general principles concerning the use of hypnosis from a systemic point of view (Loriedo & Torti, 2010):

1. *The individual hypnotic experience is amplified in a shared hypnotic context.* When a family member enters hypnosis, the other participants in the session are facilitated to do the same.
2. *Each family member has a different quality of hypnotic experience, but the individual experiences of each family member contain meanings that are shared with the rest of the family.* A systemic approach is based on a "both/and" perspective and tends to be inclusive rather than dichotomous. Consequently, the individual and the larger system are both considered the center of therapeutic interventions.
3. *The family system includes all family members.* If we follow a systemic approach, then every single family member should be, directly or indirectly, part of the therapeutic experience and have a direct and meaningful interaction with the therapist.
4. *The therapist speaks indirectly to the whole system even when directly addressing only one family member.* That means that when suggestions are directed at one person, they may have indirect effects on others.
5. *Hypnosis can elicit different hypnotic phenomena in family members.* Each member of the family can generate a different hypnotic phenomenon and thus report to the others a qualitatively different experience, but systemic hypnosis is able to activate at the same time some common pattern among the different family members.

According to these principles, the hypnotic systemic interventions develop along the following therapeutic steps (Loriedo et al., 2011):

1. *Transform the hypnotic induction into a shared experience.* Sharing a deep hypnotic experience produces by itself therapeutic effects and offers the members of the family or couple a unique form of closeness.
2. *Develop some joint activity.* Carrying out in hypnosis some special activity together is an experience that allows the interruption or even substitution of the usual rigid patterns.
3. *Intersperse the need and the expectation for change.* The conjoint hypnotic experience opens the door to the need for novelty and to the pleasure of being free from conflict and symptomatic behavior.
4. *Deal with ambivalence and conflicts.* In terms of systems theory, ambivalence and conflicts arise in subjects who cannot succeed to think in terms of complexity. Complex systems imply the presence of multiple levels, and when ambiguity, contradictions, or interpersonal conflicts emerge on one level, they can be resolved by referring to a higher (meta) level. In dysfunctional systems, the shared experience of trance produces a deep sense of collaboration and synchronicity among the system's members. This facilitates access to the meta-level and more complexity. It also makes opposites compatible, thus reducing ambiguity and conflicts in an individual, couple or family.
5. *Find a metaphor that can be used to describe the interpersonal stalemate and used as a meta concept that can offer a way out to the symptom.*

6 *Prepare interactive sequences that introduce change and ask of the family members some form of ideomotor signaling to confirm it.* We have found that in family systems, minimal details given as a signal of positive emotional state prove to be more effective than the habitual verbal communication.
7 *Protect family members or partners, preventing unexpected risks.* It is important for the therapist to recognize change but also to demonstrate a deep interest in preventing possible risks.
8 *Support the development of the authentic person that family relationships tend to hide.*

In problematic families or couples, we often see one or more members assuming full-time function or role, while the real person seems to be missing. The therapist should be able to activate and support the emerging self, respecting as well the function played in service of the system.

Trance Phenomena Produced by a Systemic Family Induction

In families, situations occur spontaneously that facilitate or determine the state of trance. An example of family skills to develop induced spontaneous trances are lullabies, anecdotes, stories, fables, truisms, common places, and some redundant educational techniques.

We have never been too convinced by the classic separation of induction from trance, as if induction should just be considered as a preparation or introduction to the hypnotic experience, a sort of anesthesia to be obtained before surgery in order to make hypnosis possible. In our experience, induction *is* therapy. We consider it a fundamental part of hypnotic treatment with a key role in the therapeutic process. Moreover, induction is the most important means of creating rapport. The way in which the therapist guides the patient within the hypnotic reality, and the way in which the patient responds to the hypnotist's guidance, gives the hypnotic relationship its peculiar form. When hypnosis is applied to family systems, the process of induction seems to be even more useful and relevant. The simple fact of inducing a trance in the entire system will produce several meaningful phenomena.

Below we summarize the new behavioral and relational patterns that develop out of a systemic trance induction (Loriedo & Torti, 2010; Loriedo et al., 2011):

Reduction of Spontaneous Interactive Exchanges

The number of exchanges decreases, and the interaction becomes less intense than it usually is, encouraging greater focus on oneself.

Slower Interactive Rhythm

The speed of exchanges is also reduced and, as a secondary effect, automatic interactions that are part of dysfunctional family communication tend to decrease or even disappear.

Conjoint Activity and Increased Sense of Belonging

When family members are invited by the hypnotist to develop shared activities, they often report having experienced a new sense of connection that probably is rooted in both behavioral synchronism and emotional attunement. Families who shared a hypnotic experience demonstrated a greater sense of connection and a greater ability to work together as a team than in previous non-hypnotic sessions. This mutual collaboration, which family members develop when performing tasks, proves to be a great support for systemic interventions.

Physical Synchronism

The effect of movements, postural and breathing rhythm synchronization, due to the shared participation of the family system in an unusual experience, will later facilitate the execution of other additional conjoint tasks.

Emotional Synchronism

The sense of physical harmony is reinforced by the synchronization of emotions and feelings. Synchronic behaviors provide visual evidence of increased harmony, a phenomenon that facilitates further synchronization on an affective level. Interviews with the family after a shared hypnotic session reveal that the participants had experienced very similar emotions and sensations.

Interruption of Usual Interactive Patterns

The familiar trance has the power to disrupt by itself old interactive patterns and make new ones appear.

Increased Attention to Individual Patterns

Despite other family members presence, hypnosis allows individuals a greater tendency to seek meanings and explanations inside themselves much more than from the external environment. In this way, interpersonal boundaries are enforced, while individual autonomy tends to develop.

Reduced Attention to Family Relationships

The amount of attention devoted to the relationship level can be considered an indirect measure of the dysfunctionality of a family or couple (Watzlawick et al., 1967). According to the authors, the healthier a relationship is, the more the relational aspects recede in the background. Once again, systemic trance tends to produce a more functional family setting.

Increased Attention to the Content

This different value given to content and relationship by "healthy" and "sick" families was noted by Ruesch and Bateson (1951). Therefore, the fact that shared hypnotic trance favors a greater ability to pay attention to the content of communication is an additional advantage of hypnotic family induction. Trance state induces in individual family members an increased degree of attention to the content and an improved listening skill.

Reduced Responsiveness to Other Family Members

Being absorbed in hypnosis can decelerate mutual reactivity among family members. If hypnotic communication includes pauses, it can allow time for reflection to prepare a more weighted and appropriate response.

Increased Responsiveness to the Therapist

Once the trance state is induced, the subject becomes more sensitive to the therapist's suggestions. Erickson (1957) describes this process in individuals: "Another significant change occurs while the patient is hypnotized. He becomes much more responsive to ideas, is able to accept suggestions, and to act upon them more easily than in his ordinary state of awareness. The patient's increased responsiveness under hypnosis helps the doctor to secure the kind of cooperation that is essential to successful medical treatment" (p. 49).

The context of increased responsiveness toward the therapist also favors the subject compliance. Erickson and Rossi (1976) attribute this significant change in the subject's reactivity to a particular form of attention that they call "attentive responsiveness". This type of responsiveness can be observed in the form of a very high level of absorption of the subject when the hypnotist speaks. Systemic family trance produces attentive responsiveness in every single family member, and this shared induced quality improves both relationships within the family and their relationship with the therapist.

Forms of Systemic Induction with the Family

As with individuals, with families we also can have both direct and indirect forms of induction. Despite the therapeutic advantages it brings, the direct, in which the therapeutic context is explicitly and formally defined as hypnotic, is more rarely used with families. The indirect, informal induction of trance is achieved through a casual conversation, or narration, without making any specific reference to the term "hypnosis". As we have seen, Ritterman (1983) is the main representative of this systemic indirect approach. Since it is impossible to avoid an informal conversation with the therapist, this approach is facilitated by a low level of resistance.

We will now deal in more detail with both approaches starting with the indirect family induction.

Indirect Family Induction

Typically, it is done in the following ways.

The Family Trance Is Induced in an Indirect Way

Many renowned family therapists, even beyond their intention, are considered "indirect hypnotists"; families are fascinated by their intervention and deeply absorbed by listening to them. To name just a few: Virginia Satir, Carl Whitaker, Giancarlo Cecchin, Luigi Boscolo, Salvador Minuchin (1974). Indirect induction to the whole family is especially indicated with families who habitually use an indirect communication style, or for families who tend to reject the idea of hypnosis, because of their exaggerated rationality.

Utilization of the Natural Family Trance

Some families have a great inclination toward hypnosis, and in these cases, if the therapist observes spontaneous trance manifestations, he/she can reinforce and use them to achieve therapeutic goals.

Inducing Indirectly Part of the Family While Inducing Directly Other Family Members

When the resistance is not uniform in the family system, it is possible to combine in different proportions both indirect and direct. Indirect hypnosis will be more useful with the most resistant members, without losing the advantage of a direct induction with those who allow its use.

Indirect Induction Techniques with the Family

As stated, for family therapists the indirect form appears to be easy and natural. A simple speech, a story, or a metaphor, containing embedded suggestions are sufficient to elicit a hypnotic effect that will not be recognized as such.

Here are some specific indirect induction techniques that can be used with families and couples.

The Use of Space and Posture

"The space occupied by family members or assigned by the therapist is a factor that shapes the family system relationships. This way in which the family establishes its relationships is of the greatest importance; in fact, it is possible to make a diagnosis of a family by seeing how the family members are arranged in the available space" (Loriedo et al., 1987, p. 27). A therapist can then use the space and posture to change indirectly the family members' relationships.

Family Rituals

Rituals have the property of hypnotizing the family members: the family is engaged in a complex interactive mode in which everyone plays a part that is already set, and is automatically and repetitively carried out, as in some forms of hypnosis, particularly in somnambulistic hypnosis. Mara Selvini Palazzoli et al. (1978) similarly used ritual modalities to convert dysfunctional rituals into a therapeutic sense that limits the family potentials.

Interspersing Suggestions

Interspersal technique has been one of Erickson's most important discoveries (Erickson, 1966; Erickson et al., 1976) and has been proposed by him as a therapeutic modality of considerable effectiveness. The therapist embeds a suggestive therapeutic message in casual conversation.

Metaphors

Each family uses natural metaphors on its own. An example is the case of a couple who complained, among other conflicts, a rather evident sexual disagreement, to which, however, no explicit reference was made. Instead, their way of skiing was described. When they were in the mountains, the wife liked to make the descents very slowly, while the husband preferred to go directly to the valley, so when he arrived, she still was beginning the descent. A therapeutic intervention aimed at changing the metaphorical content allows to work with the couple without the need to openly mention the sexual problem, respecting their choice of not mentioning it, but obtaining equally valid results.

Confusion Technique

Confusion already exists in some family situations, and therefore constitutes another opportunity to transform the family trance into a therapeutic change. As in the case of a rather confused couple who came to therapy with the problem of not being able to decide whether they should separate or stay together. This type of attitude can often provoke in the therapist a position tending to suggest which the most suitable solution would be. But a similar indication, whether direct or indirect, would place on the shoulders of the therapist a responsibility that must correctly be returned to the couple. The use of confusion to resolve confusion may, in such cases, prove to be the most appropriate tool.

Direct Family System Induction

For many years, family therapists have considered direct hypnosis inappropriate to the family context. Our position (Loriedo et al., 2018) is that direct inductions imply several advantages: explicit informed consent, clearer definition of the context as hypnotic, more intense evocative effect, stronger expectation for change, and access to a variety of hypnotic phenomena.

Direct hypnosis can be applied in the following three configurations (Loriedo, 2008; Loriedo & Torti, 2010): (1) hypnosis with the index patient in the presence of the family, (2) direct hypnosis with another family member in the presence of the patient, and (3) direct hypnosis with the whole family.

Hypnosis with the Index Patient in the Presence of the Family

It is considered the best approach to use when there is a strong emphasis on the index patient, as often is the case with patients with psychosomatic, somatic, anorexic, substance, or alcohol abuse symptoms. It is the recommended approach when the family comes to therapy only for the index patient and does not want to take part in it directly.

In the current literature, this approach seems to be unique. Despite not using direct hypnosis with families, Ritterman (1983) theoretically admits it, only fearing the disclosure of more private aspects when hypnotizing the symptom bearer, but this problem will occur anyhow in all forms of family therapy.

Lankton et al. (1995), in the formal trance guidelines, categorically prohibit hypnosis for the index patient, following the principle to avoid further designating the "sick" subject.

Of course, we consider the protection of the personal aspects of the symptom bearer, as well as of other family members, a fundamental rule in every form of therapy, and we never consider acceptable the use of hypnosis to force a hypnotized subject to reveal personal material in front of the family. Systemic practice demonstrates that accepting the family together with the index patients does not activate family resistance, dropout, and other forms of opposing the treatment that could produce chronicity.

According to a basic systemic principle, accepting the existing system's rules is the best way to enter the system and produce change. Since all the other doors are not accessible in many dysfunctional families, the most natural access to these families is the index patient induction.

The more intense is the family designation, the more this procedure makes it simple for the family to accept the therapeutic intervention: putting the index patient at the center of the intervention does not question the rest of the family and their relationships. At the same time, the therapist can observe the indirect effects that hypnosis has on the family, and find the best favorable condition to send direct messages to the patient that also have an indirect effect on the family.

An example is the case of a girl who required hypnosis because all the previous therapies failed. Direct hypnotic suggestions to the girl, together with embedded indirect suggestions for the parents attending the session, were given.

"You are comfortably sitting in your armchair ... now you place all your attention on the right hand ... it gets lighter and lighter, and slowly begins to levitate.

While your hand slowly moves up, your parents can carefully observe it moving ... and as it moves up, they begin to understand many things they never understood before" (Loriedo et al., 1987, p. 31).

While apparently the speech is addressed to the girl, some suggestions are simultaneously addressed to parents, and they are delivered in a form that cannot be countered and therefore can produce an effect that then tends to be maintained over time. In this way, direct hypnosis with the index patient and indirect hypnosis with other family members can be used during the entire inductive process.

During and after the hypnotic induction, both the individual (directly) and the family (indirectly) attention becomes focused on the girl's hand levitation, and later, on other hypnotic phenomena. In this way, the therapist can develop both in the individual and in the family the attentive responsiveness that is the main basis for an effective therapeutic intervention that will involve the entire system.

Focusing attention on the little variations of the index patient, the family develops the implied value of an important ability to notice details of her behavior that they habitually neglect. At the same time, parents learn to give consideration not only to her symptomatic behavior but also to the new acts performed by the girl by virtue of her hypnotic experience.

As a confirmation of this new awareness reached by the family members that are present during the index patient induction is the fact that, in our experience after 2–3 sessions, over 50% of them ask to be included in the direct induction.

It is useful (and correct) to inform the whole family that taking part in the hypnotic session of the child will not only be useful for the hypnotized but could also produce a beneficial change for the attending participants.

Direct Hypnosis with Another Family Member in the Presence of the Patient

This configuration can be chosen when there are good reasons not to start with the index patient, while another family member turns out to be an easier way in. A typical situation that requires this choice as a solution is a presented symptom that involves a strong tendency to maintain control. In these cases, a serious obstacle to accepting hypnosis, even if hypnosis is requested by the same patient, is often implied. In these cases, direct induction with another family member will be helpful to prepare the index patient's formal induction. Often using hypnosis with another family member, not designated by the family as a patient, can serve to facilitate hypnosis in the index patient. For example, with a woman who was profoundly afraid of fainting and would never agree to undergo hypnosis, it was possible to obtain the induction when her husband agreed to undergo the trance first. When the woman realized that when her husband was hypnotized, he neither lost control nor fainted, she decided to experience hypnosis without difficulty.

Erickson's direct systemic interventions with family members pertain almost exclusively to this typology. In different clinical situations, always related to the hypnotic treatment of pain, he hypnotizes a daughter to induce a trance to the mother (Erickson, 1983, 1984).

Direct Hypnosis with the Whole Family

Finally, the case that seems more difficult to realize, but probably only for an emotional reason, is to use hypnosis with the whole family in a formal and explicit way, thus openly declaring: "we will do hypnosis in which all family members will experience a trance state". In reality, the opposition that might be expected in the face of such a proposal is often only an expectation of the therapist.

An example of the use of this modality is the case of an agoraphobic family. In this family, in addition to the agoraphobic index patient, other family members had something to do with this same symptom. The girl could never go out alone, she always had to go out with her mother, but in this way, her mother didn't go out except with her. Both suffered from the same type of problem although the mother's one was made less evident by the official designation of the daughter.

As for the father, it was discovered that he always went to work following very specific paths, and one path in particular was the only one that did not create intense anguish. After a few minutes of conversation, already in the first session, it was very clear that the whole family suffered from the same problem. The therapist proposed to the family a collective hypnotic experience. Families who have a good ability to recognize and discuss their problems usually gladly accept this type of hypnosis, as did this family.

When in trance everyone should have been required to solve his/her problem and to be able to go out alone without anguish. Unfortunately, at that time, such a possibility didn't correspond to the family members' available resources. Then the hypnotist decided to introduce the trance this way: "I would like each one of you to focus on the idea that one of the people next to you can leave the house and go quietly out without any problem, with perfect ease (Loriedo et al. 1987, p. 34)".

Accepting that another family member could go out of the house facing the situation that previously aroused a phobic response, each member of the family implicitly granted but also received permission to do something that the family culture considered forbidden. Then, thinking about the other ones who could face without fear the open spaces, each family member wondered, "Why couldn't I do the same?". When they alerted from the trance, not only the family members' relationships but also each one's point of view was changed.

In other cases, when the decision appears more difficult, specific techniques can be adopted to obtain a general consensus, as we will see in the next paragraph.

Specific Direct Techniques for Families

There are specific techniques that can be used to facilitate the whole family to enter hypnosis together and initiate change of their dysfunctional patterns (detailed explanations in Loriedo & Torti, 2010). (1) Require the family to focus on the index subject. (2) Repeat family history using their same language. (3) Recognize and summarize every member's point of view. This involves repeating perspectives and reframing each as a contribution to a better understanding of one another. (4) Each family member explains the problem with a story and these are used as part of an induction. (5) Generate fantasies through silence that can be used to guide a therapeutic intervention. (6) The imaginary journey. (7) To listen to the other members of the family in silence.

Other Therapeutic Factors Relevant to Systemic Hypnosis

During the family experience, general hypnotic phenomena can emerge, and can be used to improve both the relationships among the family members and the relationship with the therapist. The systemic hypnotic phenomena that we have described will always be part of the family systemic trance, and since their presence tends to improve the functional relationship, they will offer a powerful contribution to a successful therapeutic process.

A family that experiences joint trance induced in a direct form benefits from a clearly well-defined therapeutic context where the presence of trance is not hidden or unspoken, and every single family member openly participates. According to Peake et al. (1986), hypnosis brings with it an effect of change acceleration. We have observed that when hypnosis occurs in a clearly defined systemic context, this effect is further amplified.

Application of Systemic Hypnosis with Families and Couples

A model of systemic hypnosis, *Integrative Inductions Model* (Loriedo, 2017), discusses how to apply systemic hypnosis to different types of family systems.

According to the *Integrative Inductions Model* the therapist dedicates the first few sessions to observe and activate the family interactive patterns with the aim to discover the primary themes the family is presenting to therapy. The therapist observes the family connections/disconnections that represent the critical systemic dysfunctional interaction in order to choose the most appropriate systemic therapeutic induction tailored to each different family structure.

The identified themes will be used by the therapist as the basis for tailored metaphors that later will be converted into therapeutic family inductions or narratives. The key role played by these inductions is in their integrative function as they are designed to correct the dysfunctional family hyper-connections or disconnections.

We have divided families' interactional structure into five different non-harmonious or dysfunctional modes.

Segregating Families

In these families, one or more family members have not developed sufficient autonomy and appear to be segregated inside the family. To cover intense chronic conflicts, the index patient, frequently diagnosed as psychotic or depressed, is not allowed to access the outside world. The integrative intervention should (1) reduce family internal tension, (2) increase family flexibility, and (3) develop individual autonomy.

Individual Detachment

One (or more) family members are not considered as part of the family and tend to be excluded from the rest of the system. They find themselves detached and separated from the others by an intense emotional distancing. In this case, the family dysfunctional pattern consists mainly in an *emotional or physical neglect*, that tends to isolate the index patient like a foreign body, typically diagnosed as somatoform disorders, eating disorders (bulimia), or borderline personality disorder. The integrative objectives are to: (1) help the family to focus on the index patient; (2) allow the detached individual to be recognized and accepted by the family; (3) put the family in the condition of recognizing the value of and meaningful role of the excluded member.

Family Dissociation

There is a general disconnection or the presence of very weak connections in these families; the sense of isolation prevails, and the relationships are cold and distant. Salvador Minuchin (1974) described these families as "disengaged", and with rigid internal boundaries. Obsessive-compulsive disorder, phobias, and schizoid personality, disorder are the more common diagnosis. Integrative metaphors are to: (1) activate a sense of warmth and pleasure, (2) re-establish reciprocal involvement and connections, and (3) weaken the fear of reciprocal involvement.

Hyper-Connected Families

Hyper-connected families are dissociated from the rest of the world but strongly connected through their internal components. There is little or no interest in what is external to the system and family members behave as though they do not have permission to develop meaningful external relationships. External attempts to enter the family system are usually gently refused or strongly rejected. Such families are described by Minuchin (1974) as enmeshed, and their typical diagnostic categories include psychosomatic disorders, phobias, and eating disorders (anorexia nervosa). The integrative interventions are: (1) to reduce the reciprocal involvement, (2) re-connect with the outside world, and (3) guarantee to each individual permission for differentiation and autonomy.

Chaotic Families

Chaotic family systems (Olson, 2000) connect in a confused and disharmonic way. Dysfunctional triangles, transgenerational violation, surrogated roles, and altered hierarchical relationships are common to these systems. This family organization has been defined as *skewed* by Lidz et al. (1960) because of its dysfunctional structure. Common diagnostic categories are anti-social personality disorders and drug addiction. Intervention objectives are to: (1) reorganize the system structure, (2) reestablish functional roles and boundaries, and (3) increase a sense of togetherness and individual autonomy.

For a broader discussion and specific integrative interventions, see Loriedo (2017).

Clinical Illustration

The Dancing Hands Systemic Induction (Loriedo et al., 2018) is a technique developed by Loriedo that has proven to be particularly useful for dysfunctional families with structural problems facing the transition phases of the family life cycle.

The technique is a systemic extension of the Hand Levitation Technique (Erickson, 1961), modified for the family context. It is used with an entire family system which makes it particularly suitable for building an atmosphere of collaboration and synchronism that resemble a kind of dance, hence the name of Systemic Induction of Dancing Hands.

The therapist welcomes the family and asks for the name, age, work, and passion of each family member. There is a widowed, employed, 50-year-old father, with a hobby of cycling. He introduces his 29-year-old son and two daughters, 25- and 14-years old.

Then the therapist explores the family's expectations and goals. The father expresses his feelings of loneliness, and the children report a blocked anger, following an unprocessed mourning for the mother's loss. There is a climate of conflict and a lack of synchronicity.

All are available to enter hypnosis together except Luca, who with arms crossed, admits his perplexity, and says he doesn't know if wants to or not. In response to his posture, the therapist offers Luca the possibility not to enter at all, or to enter and exit the trance whenever he wants, and Luca finally accepts this special option reserved to him.

Focusing on the hands and understanding how they can represent the problem has the property of activating the family hands dance.

"Please focus on your hands wherever they are, in whatever position they are. And while you focus on your hands you try to understand how they can represent the problem you are living, a problem related to the loss of an important beloved person, a problem that has changed the family structure" (Loriedo et al., 2018, p. 319).

The therapist summarizes each member's point of view and the family develops a surprising synchronicity that had been absent.

The therapist continues to encourage the hand motions to represent the state of mind and makes comments on the movements, e.g., "The clenched fists of the father, seem to contain inside the anger hatched over time" (Loriedo et al., 2018, p. 320). Then the family members are asked to express with words how each one feels. The therapist suggests, "as hands have represented the present family impasse, they now can move again and suggest a possible evolution toward change" (Loriedo et al., 2018, p. 320).

Now the therapist enters the final stage of the intervention:

> Now, I ask each of you to imagine what is the gesture you would like to receive from the others. Imagine that the other family members can really make that gesture towards you, with hands or body posture. Just think for a moment and then tell me ..."
>
> *(Loriedo et al., 2018, p. 321)*

Each expresses their wishes and many mention receiving a hug from the others. So, the therapist asks if there is a possible willingness to respond to those desires. The father expresses the wish that Luca, who is so tough, can also be part of the family embrace. At that precise moment, Luca uncrosses his arms. The therapist concludes:

> Before concluding, we can now do one last important thing. I cannot ask you *now* to have a physical embrace, I prefer to leave each one of you in your comfortable

position, but you can give your body and mind the opportunity to experience and feel this warm and deep hug that extends to all the family members. I ask you to imagine a general embrace in which all present family members can participate, and if you desire it, even an absent member ... A hug that gives strength, courage, and possibilities for the future. I give you time to imagine it and to feel it. And although Luca initially seemed to want to stay out of it, let me say that he was the first to represent, participating in the family dance with his folded arms, the embrace that then inspired all of you. Since you all responded to that signal, now the embrace suggested by Luca seems to be too tight. Maybe this is the reason why he finally opened his arms. What we need now is a *wider hug that includes all of you together* and that allows you to feel each other's warmth and closeness. ...

(Loriedo et al., 2018, p. 330)

Finally, the therapist proceeds to re-orient the family by inserting a post-hypnotic suggestion: ".... in your memory will remain a *larger hug* that has changed a painful immobility into a small but profoundly significant movement" (Loriedo et al., 2018, p. 331).

Clinical experience reveals systemic hypnosis in family therapy to be a valuable, underutilized tool. There is scant research on its efficacy, cost effectiveness, or symptom reduction, true of most family therapeutic interventions, but our experience suggests this is a direction to pursue.

References

Bateson, G., Jackson, D. D., Haley, J., & Weakland, J. (1956). Toward a theory of schizophrenia. *Systems Research and Behavioral Science.*, *1*, 251–264. 10.1002/bs.3830010402

Bateson, G. (1979). *Mind and nature: A necessary unity*. Dutton Books.

Erickson, M. H. (1957). Hypnosis in general practice. In E. L. Rossi (Ed.), (1980) *The collected papers of Milton H. Erickson on hypnosis* (Vols. 4; Innovative hypnotherapy, (pp. 49–51). Irvington Publishers.

Erickson, M. H. (1961). Historical note on the hand levitation and other ideomotor techniques. *American Journal of Clinical Hypnosis*, *3*(3), 196–199. 10.1080/00029157.1961.10701715

Erickson, M. H. (1966). The interspersal hypnotic technique for symptom correction and pain control. *American Journal of Clinical Hypnosis*, *8*(3), 198–209. 10.1080/00029157.1966.10402492

Erickson, M. H., & Haley J. (1967). *Advanced techniques of hypnosis and therapy*. Grune & Stratton.

Erickson, M. H. (1983). *Healing in hypnosis: The seminars, workshops, and lectures of Milton H. Erickson* (E. L. Rossi, M. O. Ryan, & F. A. Sharp, Eds.; Vol. 1). Irvington Publishers.

Erickson, M. H. (1984). *Life reframing in hypnosis: The seminars, workshops, and lectures of Milton H. Erickson* (E. L. Rossi & M. O. Ryan, Eds.; Vol. 2). Irvington Publishers.

Erickson, M. H., & Rossi, E. L. (1976). Two level communication and the microdynamics of trance and suggestion. *American Journal of Clinical Hypnosis*, *18*(3), 153–171. 10.1080/00029157.1976.10403794

Erickson, M. H., Rossi, E. L., & Rossi, S. I. (1976). *Hypnotic realities: The induction of clinical hypnosis and indirect forms of suggestion*. Irvington Publishers.

Haley, J. (1973). *Uncommon therapy: The psychiatric techniques of Milton H. Erickson, M.D.* W. W. Norton.

Haley, J. (1985). *Conversations with Milton H. Erickson, Vol. II. Changing couples*. Triangle Press.

Kershaw, C. J. (1992). *The couple's hypnotic dance: Creating Ericksonian strategies in marital therapy* (1st ed.). Brunner/Mazel.

Lankton, S. R., & Lankton, C. H. (1983). *The answer within: A clinical framework of Ericksonian hypnotherapy* (1st ed.). Brunner/Mazel.

Lankton, S. R., Lankton, C. H., & Matthews, W. J. (1995). Ericksonian family therapy. In A. S. Gurman & D. P. Kniskern (Eds.), *Handbook of Family Therapy* (Vol. 2 (pp. 239–283). Brunner/Mazel.

Lidz, T., Cornelison, A. R., Fleck, S., & Terry, D. (1960). Schism and skew in the families of schizophrenics. In N. W. Bell & E. F. Vogel (Eds.), *A modern introduction to the family.* (pp. 650–662). The Free Press.

Loriedo, C. (2008). Systemic trances: Using hypnosis in family therapy. *Family Therapy Magazine*, 7(4), 27–30.

Loriedo, C. (2017). Hypnotic inductions for families. Integrating systemic disconnections in the family mind. In M. P. Jensen (Ed.), *The art and practice of hypnotic induction: Favorite methods of master clinicians.* Denny Creek Press.

Loriedo, C., Angiolari, C., & Martini, L. (Eds.). (1987). *Atti del Congresso internazionale di ipnosi e terapia della famiglia; 8. convegno della Società italiana di ipnosi clinica; Il modello terapeutico di Milton H. Erickson; Roma, 16-20 ottobre 1985: [Proceedings of the International Congress of Hypnosis and Family Therapy; 8th Conference of the Italian Society of Clinical Hypnosis; Milton H. Erickson's therapeutic model; Rome, October 16–20, 1985].* L'antologia, Napoli.

Loriedo, C., Di Leone, F. G., & Zullo, D. (2011). Integrating Ericksonian hypnosis and systemic couple therapy in the treatment of conversion disorders. *Contemporary Hypnosis and Integrative Therapy*, *28*(3), 204–223.

Loriedo, C., Rago, N., & Genovesi, I. (2018). Un abrazo más amplio: la inducción sistémica de las manos danzantes: [A wider embrace: The systemic induction of dancing hands]. In A. Téllez (Ed.), *Estrategias de Hipnosis Clínica y Terapia Breve [Clinical hypnosis and brief therapy strategies (Spanish edition)]* (pp. 315–334). Universitad Autonoma de Nuovo Leòn.

Loriedo, C., & Torti, C. (2010). Systemic hypnosis with depressed individuals and their families. *International Journal of Clinical and Experimental Hypnosis*, *58*(2), 222–246. 10.1080/00207140903523277

Loriedo, C., & Zeig, J. K. (1986). Intervista su "Ipnosi e terapia familiare" [Interview on "Hypnosis and family therapy"]. *Psychoobjective*, *1*(6), 2–4.

Minuchin, S. (1974). *Families and family therapy.* Harvard University Press.

Olson, D. (2000). Circumplex model of marital and family systems. *Journal of Family Therapy*, 22, 144–167. 10.1111/1467-6427.00144

Peake, T. H., Billups, A. J., & Trott, K. L. (1986). Inducing psychotherapy: Hypnotic analogue for brief psychotherapy. *Journal of Contemporary Psychotherapy*, *16*(2), 151–160. 10.1007/bf00947168

Rago, N., & Rivelli, M. C. (2021). Ipnosi sistemica con le famiglie e con le coppie [Systemic hypnosis with families and couples]. In G. De Benedittis, C. Loriedo, C. Mammini, & N. Rago (Eds.), *Trattato di ipnosi: Dai fondamenti teorici alla pratica clinica [Treatise on hypnosis: From theoretical foundations to clinical practice]* (pp. 773–788). Franco Angeli.

Ritterman, M. (1983). *Using hypnosis in family therapy.* Jossey-Bass Publishers.

Ruesch, J., & Bateson, G. (1951). *Communication: The social matrix of psychiatry* (1st ed.). W. W. Norton & Co.

Schmidt, G. (2004). Concetti di ipnoterapia sistemica per l'interazione con i clienti depressi e con i loro sistemi-relazionali: Dalla depressione ai mondi correlati.[Systemic hypnotherapy concepts for interacting with depressed clients and their relational systems: From depression to related worlds.] *Rivista Europea Di Terapia Breve Strategica E Sistemica*, *1*, 127–154. Retrieved March 13, 2023 http://www.brieftherapymalta.com/web_3.0/publications/ita/schmidt.pdf

Selvini Palazzoli, M., Boscolo L., Cecchin, G. F., & Prata G. (1978). *Paradox and counterparadox. A new model in the therapy of the family in schizophrenic transaction.* Jason Aronson, Lanham.

Watzlawick, P., Beavin, J. H., & Jackson, D. D. (1967). *Pragmatics of human communication.* Norton.

34

A SYSTEMIC VIEW

Hypnosis to Solve Problems of Overweight and Obesity

Cecilia Fabre Robles

Centro Ericksoniano de México Cancun, México

Introduction

In 2010, the World Health Organization defined obesity and overweight as an abnormal or excessive accumulation of fat that can be harmful to health (Tamayo & Restrepo, 2014).

Every handbook of hypnosis contains a chapter on eating disorders (see, e.g., Levitt, 1993, Sapp, 2017). Nevertheless, the reviews of the topic usually conclude that the reports are anectodal and without detailed results. Nor do they report follow-ups (Mott & Roberts, 1979), or that the effects can be attributed to nonhypnotic factors (Wadden & Anderton, 1982).

The meta-analyses of effectiveness of hypnotic treatment studies of obesity are sometimes promising (Kirsch et al., 1995), and other times debatable (Allison & Faith, 1996). In general, however, it seems that hypnosis is an effective tool in weight loss, especially in combination with cognitive-behavioral therapy (CBT; Milling et al., 2018) or with mindfulness (Pellegrini et al., 2021). Interestingly, some studies demonstrate that hypnotic arms of clinical studies keep the desired weight longer or continue to lose weight after the treatment period (Bolocofsky et al., 1985).

In this chapter, I propose a model for working in a group setting with overweight and obese issues in adults, using Ericksonian hypnosis, that is a natural alert hypnosis using indirect communication (Erickson, 2007). I present some theoretical ideas about a model and its origins that I have developed from my clinical experience in hypnosis, with people who have come to my private practice because they wanted to lose fat and maintain a healthy weight (Fabre, 2021).

I will also outline the advantages of working with Ericksonian psychotherapy and hypnosis over other models of psychotherapy. Ericksonian psychotherapy proposes that we all have the resources we need for solving whatever difficulty life presents us. The goal of this psychotherapy is to help clients recognize those resources in order to be able to continue their development. It offers a pleasant and healthy healing process, through natural, amplified states of consciousness (or altered states of consciousness), often resolving the origin of painful situations in an unconscious, safe, and secure way. In addition, I share how to use some ideas from the CBT and reinforce them with hypnosis.

DOI: 10.4324/9781003449126-46

The result of using this approach, in my professional experience, is that people lose weight in a healthy way, at a comfortable pace, feeling at ease, and they learn to stay at that healthy weight naturally, avoiding weight gain at the end or after the process.

Why Is the Issue of Overweight and Obesity Important?

The increase, year after year, in the number of people with obesity is worrisome in many countries; it represents a threat to people's health. Although socially the concern about obesity is mostly related to aesthetics, i.e., how one looks, medically, overweight and obesity substantially increase the risk of suffering from various health disorders. Obesity has become a global problem, much more serious in countries from North, Central, and South America (Samocha-Bonet et al., 2012).

It is important to understand this phenomenon from its psychological components, that is, the emotional origin and factors that lead a person to gain excessive weight, stay overweight, and to disconnect from their body, and lose emotional and physical health. The emotional health of those who suffer from obesity or overweight is partially the result of a socio-cultural demand to be thinner. This causes unhappiness with the body, deteriorates self-image and self-esteem, and compels people to stay on strict diets, which makes them feel different and punished. People generally expect and manage to lose weight quickly but then regain it quickly. This can put their physical health at risk. The consequences of cycles of fat loss and regaining weight can also lead to the development of psychopathologies (de la Rubia, 2002).

I consider the relationship with food to be a dependency or a habit, since people with obesity and overweight, in most cases, develop addictive behaviors of dependence on food or certain foods. I treat the food habits with hypnosis, as it would be done with any other habit.

According to the American Psychological Association's Div. 30 (Society of Psychological Hypnosis), hypnosis is a procedure during which a health professional or researcher suggests while treating someone that he or she experience changes in sensations, perceptions, thoughts, or behavior (Division 30 Executive Committee, 2014).

Hypnosis is very useful in these cases, since the problems of dependencies are created by many different factors, each of which can be addressed with hypnosis. Hypnosis can help to manage emotions, create new habits, and replace the symbolic level of the habit (Robles & Touyarot, 2018).

There are different types of approaches for working with food habits. In my experience, Ericksonian hypnosis is most useful because of its tenets that the problem is the solution and each person has the resources to be well. It is only a matter of finding how to use the resources. I began to develop my approach by inviting and gathering in a group of men and women who had weight issues. I asked them what their main difficulties were in achieving the goal of losing weight and staying at their ideal weight. From there, I tried to understand what the origins of their difficulties were, what universal emotional issues were foundational, and I discovered some themes that led me to structure my work. The topics worked on in the group are anxiety, compulsion, beliefs regarding your body, managing your sensations, painful life experiences, overweight as protection, distinguishing between hunger and anxiety, adjusting internal mechanisms for emotional control, self-confidence, self-esteem, self-love, the desire to move your body and exercise it, learning to take responsibility for your well-being into your own hands, working with fears and insecurity, fear of being well, and dissolving or minimizing the risks of relapse.

I successfully used this approach with different groups for about eight years. Then I wrote a manual for psychotherapists, which I titled *Lightening Your Soul, Lightening Your Body* (Fabre, 2021).

Stress is an important factor in the etiology of obesity. Both anxiety and stress are caused by the difficulty in managing emotions. Hypnosis facilitates the management of emotions, in addition to supporting the reconnection with our body (Bennett et al., 2013). For this reason, as well as my experience, I decided to formally use hypnosis in each session. Hypnosis has proven to be highly effective for stress and dependency management because it facilitates learning to feel and become aware of what is happening internally (Sinha & Jastreboff, 2013).

Ericksonian hypnosis proposes to put oneself in the other's shoes, to ask oneself, how I have felt in similar situations. This relational interaction helped me to understand what could be underneath the themes I propose. I designed the trance exercises, with universal themes that we all live, building on the ideas of Dr Teresa Robles (2016).

A triggering factor for overweight and its maintenance is referred to as emotional hunger (Mayo Clinic, 2012/2022). The person eats because he is disconnected from his emotions; he simply needs to calm something he is feeling but does not or cannot identify. Food becomes a way to stop feeling some emotions without identifying what is being experienced, e.g., anger, sadness, fear, boredom, or perhaps loneliness.

Emotional hunger can appear in the face of surprising or unexpected events in life, as well as everyday problems that trigger intense emotions that the person is not able to handle. The response is the need to put something in their mouth, to eat even though the body does not really need to do so.

Depression is associated with overweight. Although in some cases it may have existed previously, it can intensify when the person gains weight. This happens frequently in adolescents, because at this stage, being overweight causes ridicule from peers and affects their self-esteem.

What Happens When There Is Overweight or Obesity?

At the Behavioral Level

Obesity involves at least two significant behaviors: overeating high-calorie foods and sedentary lifestyles.

Several factors are involved in the origin of both behaviors, among them the external demands to comply and look good. For example, sitting still after finishing a job instead of going out to exercise or eating without hunger to please others.

Overeating is partly caused by this situation, since when a person prefers to spend hours working and instead of getting up and going to eat, they seek to eat anything quickly, without taking the time to nourish themselves in a healthy way.

The person stops doing what would help them to stay healthy, because caring others is more valuable than what one does for oneself. Ironically, he/she often feels that he/she is not sufficiently recognized or valued by others.

Ideas such as "cooking is difficult", "time is for work", or "time is money" reinforce this behavior. Our western culture participates in reinforcing this, for example, by creating facilities to eat quickly (e.g., fast foods), leaving food within reach all the time, and preparing food with additives, colorings, excessive calories, and sugars. These facilitate gaining weight and metabolic disorders but save time and effort and thus allow us to continue working and meeting the demands of the outside world.

The time for feeding ourselves is very valuable to connect with our physical needs and to be able to detect if we are hungry or thirsty, to give us the quality and quantity of food we need. When we were babies, things were different. We ate when we were hungry, we cried to ask for food, and as soon as we felt our body was satisfied, we took the breast out of our mouth or made a gesture spitting out the bottle or the food.

In my model, I seek to reconnect attendees with the wisdom of their bodies to generate healthy behaviors that allow them to look at themselves, to give themselves the time, love, and dedication they invest in others.

Disconnection from our body and excessive attention to external demands can lead to decreased rest and sleep because it seems more important to work than to sleep. Lack of sleep can disrupt appetite hormones, promote higher food intake, reduce energy expenditure, and change the body composition to favor fat storage (Knutson et al., 2007; Morselli et al., 2010; Shlisky et al., 2012). Thus, lack of sleep is another trigger for weight gain.

Becoming aware of the body's needs and reconnecting with it healthfully are important and are achieved through Ericksonian hypnosis exercises.

Sedentary lifestyles are an additional problem. Nowadays, more activities are done by sitting in front of a screen, whether for study, work, or recreation. Sedentary lifestyles accompanied by the intake of high-calorie foods of low nutritional value increase overweight.

Éva Bányai (2018) has recommended the use of Active Alert Hypnosis in psychotherapy. She states that the patients who can benefit most from this technique are those who suffer from depression or require ego reinforcement.

Active Alert Hypnosis increases motivation toward physical movement and reconnects people with the pleasure of moving the body. It is very important that the participants of the program become aware of the importance of exercise in their physical, mental, and emotional health, and that they experience it as viable, easy, and enjoyable. This increases their motivation to move.

The disconnection of people from their body and emotions leads them to eat automatically, sometimes without even realizing if they are hungry or not. They do not distinguish physical hunger from emotional hunger, i.e., unconscious emotion that they would like to stop feeling and that they cannot handle.

Frequently, when I ask group participants what they ate during the week, they only remember the meals where they sat down to eat at the table, but do not remember the ones they ate in front of the television, the computer, or driving in the car. This way of eating seems to operate without conscious awareness. It is an automatic and unconscious behavior, and therefore, often uncontrollable.

Cohen and Farley (2008) state that mastering an automatic behavior requires many resources because individuals are unaware of both the stimulus input that evokes the response and of the behavior itself. For this reason, the success of their control is very limited.

Developing conscious awareness is one solution to automatic eating. My model includes some practical exercises to be performed before eating any morsel. For example, whatever you are going to eat has to be done seated at the table; no eating in a resting place or at the work table; no eating while doing another activity, such as using the cell phone or watching television.

I ask them to become aware of the size of their hunger and what their body needs at that moment, also to reflect on how that food got into their hands or onto their plate, all that had to happen for them to be able to eat it. I ask them with this awareness, to be grateful for the whole process, to thank nature and everyone involved, including themselves, and I tell them to repeat it every time they are going to eat.

At the Emotional Level

The most common emotional effects of obesity are low self-esteem, lack of social skills, distorted view of the body, depression, suicidal thoughts, and self-punishment (Puhl et al., 2013). Cultural values praise the perfect body, both in women and men, and negatively affect self-esteem and perception of well-being (Carraça et al., 2011; Cash & Pruzinsky, 2002).

Social stigma plays an important role in the development of emotional effects; in my groups only 10% of the participants are male and 90% are female, who are clearly concerned about their self-image and generally have low self-esteem.

Why Ericksonian Hypnosis?

The idea that a problem holds (and hides) the solution to a problem is a basic tenet of Ericksonian hypnosis (Erickson, 2007). It uses nature, creativity, and universal metaphors to help people change.

We all have inner resources to solve situations that life presents us. These learnings are from our life experiences, stored in our unconscious mind. We can access this wisdom at the time we need them. For example, as a baby, we were connected with the needs of our body; if we were hungry, we ate; when we felt satiated, we stopped eating; if we were sleepy, we slept; when the rest was enough, we woke up with energy and the need to play, to move and exercise our body. And we did all this naturally, without question, feeling our needs. This is a resource to be used as a hypnotic suggestion.

Both Erickson's inductions (Short, et al., 2016) and the I Ching readings contain themes that are universal to all human beings (Robles, 1991/2021), e.g., healing the wounds, unconditional love, finding and following our "real" paths in life. My group work is based on universal themes related to the origins of overweight and obesity.

When a universal theme is presented in a group, whether in hypnotic conversation or in a formal trance, each participant listens to it and reflects on it, cuts it to size, experiences it from his or her own point of view, and finds the solution within.

Teresa Robles (1991/2021) wondered how is it that we start to feel badly? She proposed three cultural and social learnings that cause us symptoms, illnesses, and suffering. One is *rigidity*. We learn that there is only one way to solve things. Two, we learn that there are *only two options*, either something is right or wrong, there is no intermediate possibility that allows us to experience life without judgment. And three, we value that things are difficult or painful, we complain constantly, and we believe that everything is difficult or impossible. She calls this the culture of *suffering*. Ericksonian hypnosis suggests that our internal resources and capacities appear automatically when we enter trance. Bateson (1979) conceived the whole of nature as a (wise) mind and the interaction among living creatures as a connected pattern. Quantum Physics (Krause, 2021) proposes that in each part of universe there is the complete information of the universe just as in each cell, there is the complete information of the person. Robles (2021) calls the information of the universe within us, Universal Wisdom. It is everywhere and is all powerful. It is something different from rational intelligence and we share it with nature and with the whole universe; we are it and it acts in an automatic and healthy way. These are suggestions that can be used to initiate change in our clients.

Drawing from nature's wisdom, my model encourages people to go at their own pace and style and to live the process of losing weight without pressure, with acceptance and motivation. Losing weight ceases to be a punishment and becomes a pleasure (contrary to culture of *suffering*). Attendees do not feel obligated to follow a diet and do not feel limited; they decide how much they eat and what they eat (contrary to *rigidity* and *only two options*), from a different angle of observation, from the love of themselves and their body.

In my groups, people have tried many ways to lose weight. They believe that they will only achieve this by dieting and making a very big effort, and limiting themselves from foods they like. These beliefs can be challenged with cognitive and behavioral techniques (Robles & Touyarot, 2018). My model incorporates assignments and homework, registration of emotions and factors related, and analysis of all of them and then, reinforced in hypnosis.

Neuroscientific research is beginning to explain how hypnosis evokes brain plasticity and allows us to change behavioral patterns, attitudes, emotions, and even physiology in an efficient and lasting way. In this way, hypnosis helps us to function differently and acquire new habits.

My model provides tools and tasks, like those of Erickson (Short et al., 2016), that foster emotional growth, and independence from therapy while maintaining behavioral changes.

Research Model

My model arises from qualitative research that I did during more than eight years of work with people suffering from overweight and some obesity. I used the Action Research Model of applied research, which is aimed at directly producing a benefit to people (Baskerville & Myers, 2004).

O'Hanlon in (1993/2020) commented that while other therapies often establish rigid protocols for research or therapeutic practice, Erickson promoted the continuous revision of interventions, and the observation of improvement or positive change in the client. The therapist acts as the researcher who accompanies the client to achieve his goals, walking at his pace, like the rider of the horse who holds the reins and takes him to pasture, knowing that the horse is the one who knows the way and the destination where to go (O'Hanlon, 1993/2020).

Contrary to the neutral position of scientific researchers working with standardized protocols, Action Research is a clinical model that places the therapist as a researcher, in a helping or guiding role with respect to the practitioners, always searching together for the solution (Baskerville & Myers, 2004). In this research, the model responds to and is transformed by members' contributions. It is also a self-reflective scientific study that helps professionals to improve their practice (Muñoz et al., 2002).

Benefits of a Group Model

People are both unique and similar. We share similar life experiences as we grow up, but with our own unique responses and learnings. Similar experiences are the universal themes that resonate in a group.

I have learned that group hypnosis helps people to grow, especially because the images and sensations that each one shares help others to connect with other perspectives of the same situation. The symbols that appear represent the particular way of perceiving of each participant and when describing them in group, they share a metaphor of the same subject; when listening to it, the others receive new information, a different view of the same situation that allows them to form a more complete view, through different perspectives. If someone has difficulty imagining, the images of others help them to develop this possibility, exercising and activating their creativity, which is so important in hypnosis work.

Sharing their progress gives feedback to others, motivates them to continue advancing, they feel that it is possible to achieve a goal that many times, for them, was thought to be impossible, many of these people had been dieting for a long time, without very good results.

Finally, group work has allowed me to work with a greater number of participants simultaneously, and more and more people are benefiting from this work. My model is about losing weight "the other way around" from the usual way of losing weight. Lightening oneself emotionally first, before losing body weight, allows people to lose weight with peace of mind. Clinical hypnosis achieves this.

I am always improving my model. The pandemic encouraged the use of these techniques virtually. Feedback from participants led to the inclusion of a retreat. In this people had contact with planting, growing, and cooking food that proved therapeutic.

Finally, the 'Lightening Your Soul and Your Body' program, with its group sessions and retreat, has great benefits, not only in terms of weight loss but also in terms of changing people's relationship with life, with themselves, and with others.

Lightening the Soul and the Body Model

This model consists of ten weekly sessions and five more optional sessions of reinforcement and follow-up. It is important to be involved in the ten weekly sessions for at least six months, since losing weight quickly is not the solution.

The Process

Each topic is presented as a self-hypnotic suggestion.

1 Keep a diary. This usually involves collecting data on the eating problem and possible contributing factors (e.g., overeating, under-eating, where and when eating, inadequate nutrition, lifestyle problems) (Coman & Evans, 1995). In this I emphasize "the how" of their solution. For example, learning to connect with their body and asking themselves: "what am I hungry for that is not food?" what is my need right now? Then acknowledging this seeking to give it to themselves.
2 Instead of preparing them for the likelihood of relapse as is done with other techniques, I use hypnotic suggestions in trance. I begin by saying that we are not going on a diet and

suggesting that we are going to lighten the soul and that the body lightens as a consequence, as the soul lightens the body loses weight.

3 Unlike other weight loss programs, no weight loss goals are set. Everyone goes at their own healthy pace. Some participants begin to lose weight while in the group, others begin to notice that they are losing weight as they leave the group and over the months that follow.
4 Applying cognitive behavioral techniques involves identifying stimulus control difficulties and learning new control strategies, for example, controlling the act of eating by chewing the food a certain number of times. I emphasize connecting with their body between bites to feel their needs, to ask themselves if they are satisfied or if what they have eaten is enough. They learn to ask themselves what else their body needs. They can learn to nourish the soul with the moment, the place, the conviviality, the presence of those at the table, and any components that shift old patterns.

Program and Group Sessions

Session 1

We begin by asking the participants what they hope to achieve with this group, setting expectations. The therapist listens and integrates their expectations in a healthy way, while explaining what Ericksonian hypnosis is, how these techniques work, the power of imagination, and Universal Wisdom.

They work on renewing and reinforcing their expectations, their desire to lose weight and anxiety, and conclude the session with a picture of a future in which they feel how they want to feel.

They are asked not to go on restrictive diets and to eat what their body needs to be slim. They are asked to keep a notebook during this process, to write their soul's messages, reflections, feelings, perceptions, and learnings that make them feel good.

Session 2

After session 1, each session begins by asking how they felt and what they observed this week. The therapist makes positive suggestions based on what is shared.

For this second session, it is likely that anxiety and compulsion to eat have increased and therefore guilt, because as they feel freer with the permission to eat, they replicate what happened when they were doing restrictive dieting. Sometimes they eat as much as they can, as if it were a special permission or as if it were the last time to eat something before starting the diet. We work in a trance to help them to trust in their body and to transform anxiety into an amulet of healthy care that allows them to change.

They are taught to detect and distinguish between physical and emotional hunger. They learn to ask the body, before eating anything, what it needs. If it is emotional hunger, they are encouraged to write down what they are feeling to nourish their soul, before eating. If they continue to crave something, they can give it to themselves in a reduced portion.

Session 3

The control/discontrol mechanism is worked on in trance. People who eat with anxiety or who eat compulsively often get out of control with food and with themselves, while controlling themselves externally (Fabre, 2021).

A second exercise is done to let go of family conditioning and an exercise to commit to themselves to be well. Then they are given the task of pampering themselves three times a day with something different than food. These tasks should continue to be practiced throughout the ten sessions.

Session 4

Each person comments briefly on how the week has gone. We connote their positive efforts and reinforce the commitment they have made to themselves and their body.

I use the metaphor that diets are like oppressive and authoritarian parents; they teach us to distrust ourselves and place restrictions on us. Years of dieting lead us to distrust our body's messages. Sometimes we stop listening to it when it is hungry, we forget the importance of attending to its needs, and that our body knows and tells us perfectly what it needs. They are reminded in hypnotic conversation, that as babies we ate only when we were hungry, and then little by little we received messages that confused our ability to trust our physical sensations. For example, messages to eat on schedule and not always in sync with our body's needs, or if we ate a lot, we would get fat. Eating when hungry means trusting our body and its wisdom, and it is very important to regain that trust. In trance, we work on this topic.

Session 5

We work with a metaphor that represents body fat. I explain that it is like a "cast" that is heavy. We put it on because we got hurt, but it is likely that the wound has already healed, and if not, it needs air and light. We must gradually remove the plaster because when removed suddenly, it can make us feel vulnerable. I make the suggestion that the underlying wounds are healing, while they learn to take responsibility for their welfare in their hands.

Session 6

In this session, we talk about family, social, and cultural beliefs around food, which sometimes make us eat when we are not hungry. We work in trance with beliefs, often inherited, that manifest themselves in thoughts such as, "if I don't eat it now, it will run out later and I won't have enough", "it's today or never", etc. In this session, they are given the task to serve themselves a third less than what they visualize as the size of their hunger and observe if it is enough. Also, they are to throw away the food that is left on their plate, once. Throwing away food implies breaking with beliefs that make us overeat such as "there are starving children in the world, so eat what is on your plate".

Session 7

During this session, I work with Active Alert Hypnosis, to connect the movement of the body, and the enjoyment of physical activity to the desire to lose weight. The themes that I work on during this session are motivation and desire, in movement, we do a rehearsal for the future, to achieve the present goals, to lose weight and stay slim.

This activity is done by asking participants to stand up and begin to replicate the movement of walking; the therapist connects them with the energy of desire, their motivations, and goals, while suggesting that moving the body is easy and pleasurable.

From this session on, they are asked to keep moving their bodies and enjoy the activity. They are asked to bring a dish of their choice for the next session.

Session 8

We work at the table in front of the food they brought; in hypnotic conversation, the therapist reviews everything we have learned in previous sessions while suggesting to listen and take care of the body.

Session 9

This session seeks to regain self-confidence, and that they dare to ask for what they need, and that they can receive any answer, with peace of mind.

Session 10

During this session, participants are taught various self-hypnosis exercises to manage their emotions in different circumstances. Like for example simply, feel their breathing.

The group is offered five additional optional sessions to reinforce what need, to be scheduled with the participants.

Results

My clinical experience has shown that working in a group enhances the effect of the sessions. Hypnosis works effectively to meet the therapeutic objectives of the group: to lighten the Soul and then the Body, as well as to enhance the effectiveness of some cognitive and behavioral techniques.

I surveyed the patients who had participated to learn how it benefited them and if the results were maintained. About 90% responded. Of the responders, 30% were between 20 and 40 years old, 50% were between 41 and 60 years old, and 20% over 61 years old (see Table 34.1 for details).

Table 34.1 Feedback from the Participants About the Benefits of the Program

Feedback from the Participants	*Yes*
The program helped to lose weight	85%
Achieved a conscious and healthy diet	90%
Reduced their anxiety about eating certain foods	85%
Diminished their anxiety	85%
Said that the program helped them to avoid binge eating	80%
Decreased their food portions	77%
Reported that they started to enjoy different foods	85%
Report having acquired tools to manage their emotions	100%
Report that the way they relate to food has changed	96%
Have changed behavioral patterns that kept them overweight	80%
The way to love and take care of their body has changed	88%
Consider that it will be easy from this group to maintain an adequate eating regime	88%
Have started to enjoy moving their body and exercising	80%

This research was based on the responses of 56 people, who attended one of the ten groups I gave online during the pandemic. The exit evaluation was done two months after the conclusion of each group. The weight they lost ranged from a few grams to 7 kilos. All reported no weight gain since they completed the group program.

Conclusion

These results allow me to conclude that working with this model is effective for many people. In contrast to many diet programs, my model raises awareness of self-care for the body and soul and helps recovery of self-confidence and self-esteem. And the return to enjoying life.

For the future, research with a control group using only cognitive behavioral therapy is needed. Also, I would like to begin to apply my model with anorexia and bulimia, using action research, as I have already found that with modified suggestions persons with these disorders also benefit.

References

Allison, D. B., & Faith, M. S. (1996). Hypnosis as an adjunct to cognitive-behavioral psychotherapy for obesity: A meta-analytic reappraisal. *Journal of Consulting and Clinical Psychology, 64*(3), 513–516. 10.1037/0022-006x.64.3.513

Baskerville, R., & Myers, M. D. (2004). Special issue on action research in information systems: Making IS research relevant to practice foreword. *MIS Quarterly, 28*(3), 329–335.

Bányai, É. I. (2018). Active-alert hypnosis: History, research, and applications. *American Journal of Clinical Hypnosis, 61*(2), 88–107. 10.1080/00029157.2018.1496318

Bateson, G. (1979). *Mind and nature: A necessary unity*. Bantam Books.

Bennett, J., Greene, G., & Schwartz-Barcott, D. (2013). Perceptions of emotional eating behavior. A qualitative study of college students. *Appetite, 60*(1), 187–192. 10.1016/j.appet.2012.09.023

Bolocofsky, D. N., Spinler, D., & Coulthard-Morris, L. (1985). Effectiveness of hypnosis as an adjunct to behavioral weight management. *Journal of Clinical Psychology, 41*(1), 35–41. 10.1002/1097-4679(198501)41:1

Carraça, E. V., Markland, D., Silva, M. N., Coutinho, S. R., Vieira, P. N., Minderico, C. S., Sardinha, L. B., & Teixeira, P. J. (2011). Dysfunctional body investment versus body dissatisfaction: Relations with well-being and controlled motivations for obesity treatment. *Motivation and Emotion, 35*(4), 423–434. 10.1007/s11031-011-9230-0

Cash, T. F., & Pruzinsky, T. (Eds.). (2002). *Body image: A handbook of theory, research, and clinical practice* (1st ed.). The Guilford Press.

Cohen, D., & Farley, T. A. (2008). Eating as an automatic behavior. *Preventing Chronic Disease, 5*(1), A23.

Coman, G. J., & Evans, B. G. (1995). Clinical update on eating disorders and obesity: Implications for treatment with hypnosis. *Australian Journal of Clinical & Experimental Hypnosis, 23*(1), 1–13.

de la Rubia, J. M. (2002). Los trastornos de la conducta alimentaria, un complejo fenómeno biopsicosocial [Eating disorders, a complex biopsychosocial phenomenon]. *Revista De La Facultad De Salud Pública Y Nutrición, 3*(3). Retrieved March 24, 2023, from https://respyn.uanl.mx/index.php/respyn/article/view/89/76

Division 30 Executive Committee. (2014). Definition and description of hypnosis. *American Psychological Association – Division 30: Society of Psychological Hypnosis*. Retrieved February 25, 2023, from https://www.apadivisions.org/division-30/about#:~:text=30%20Executive%20Committee%20prepared%20the,procedure%20designed%20to%20induce%20hypnosis

Erickson, M. H. (2007). *Seminarios de introducción a la hipnosis: California, 1958* (Spanish edition). Alom Editores.

Fabre, C. (2021). *Aligerando tu alma y tu cuerpo: Manual de grupo para bajar de peso [Lightening your soul and your body: Group manual for weight loss]*. Alom Editores.

Kirsch, I., Montgomery, G., & Sapirstein, G. (1995). Hypnosis as an adjunct to cognitive-behavioral psychotherapy: A meta-analysis. *Journal of Consulting and Clinical Psychology*, *63*(2), 214–220. 10.1037/0022-006x.63.2.214

Knutson, K. L., Spiegel, K., Penev, P. D., & Van Cauter, E. (2007). The metabolic consequences of sleep deprivation. *Sleep Medicine Reviews*, *11*(3), 163–178. 10.1016/j.smrv.2007.01.002

Krause, G. (2021). *Tejiendo sueños y realidades: Aportaciones del paradigma holográfico a la psicoterapia ericksoniana. [Weaving dreams and realities: Contributions of the holographic paradigm to Ericksonian psychotherapy.]* Alom Editores.

Levitt, E. E. (1993). Hypnosis in the treatment of obesity. In J. W. Rhue, S. J. Lynn, & I. Kirsch (Eds.), *Handbook of clinical hypnosis* (1st ed., pp. 533–553). American Psychological Association. 10.1037/10274-024

Mayo Clinic. (2022, December 2). *Weight loss: Gain control of emotional eating*. Retrieved March 24, 2023, from https://www.mayoclinic.org/healthy-lifestyle/weight-loss/in-depth/weight-loss/art-20047342?pg=2 (Original article published 2012. Retrieved February 8, 2013, from http://www.mayoclinic.com/health/weight-loss/MH00025/NSECTIONGROUP=2)

Milling, L. S., Gover, M. C., & Moriarty, C. L. (2018). The effectiveness of hypnosis as an intervention for obesity: A meta-analytic review. *Psychology of Consciousness: Theory, Research, and Practice*, *5*(1), 29–45. 10.1037/cns0000139

Morselli, L., Leproult, R., Balbo, M., & Spiegel, K. (2010). Role of sleep duration in the regulation of glucose metabolism and appetite. *Best Practice & Research. Clinical Endocrinology & Metabolism*, *24*(5), 687–702. 10.1016/j.beem.2010.07.005

Mott, T., & Roberts, J. (1979). Obesity and hypnosis: A review of the literature. *American Journal of Clinical Hypnosis*, *22*(1), 3–7. 10.1080/00029157.1979.10403994

Muñoz, J. F., Quintero, J., & Munévar, R. A. (2002). Experiencias en investigación-acción-reflexión con educadores en proceso de formación en Colombia [Experiences from reflective action-research in a teacher education program in Colombia]. *Revista Electrónica De Investigación Educativa*, *4*(1). Retrieved March 24, 2023, from http://redie.ens.uabc.mx/vol4no1/contents-munevar.html

O'Hanlon, W. (2020). *Raíces profundas: Principios básicos de la terapia y de la hipnosis de Milton Erickson [Taproots: Underlying principles of Milton Erickson's therapy and hypnosis]* (J. Piatigorsky, Trans.; Spanish edition). Ediciones Paidós. (Original work published 1993)

Pellegrini, M., Carletto, S., Scumaci, E., Ponzo, V., Ostacoli, L., & Bo, S. (2021). The use of Self-Help strategies in obesity treatment: A narrative review focused on hypnosis and mindfulness. *Current Obesity Reports*, *10*, 351–364. 10.1007/s13679-021-00443-z

Puhl, R. M., Luedicke, J., & Heuer, C. A. (2013). The stigmatizing effect of visual media portrayals of obese persons on public attitudes: Does race or gender matter? *Journal of Health Communication*, *18*(7), 805–826. 10.1080/10810730.2012.757393

Robles, T. (2016). *Manual de grupo para aprender a manejar el estrés: y evitar el síndrome de fatiga crónica [Group manual to learn how to manage stress and avoid chronic fatigue syndrome]*. Alom Editores.

Robles, T. (2021). *Concierto para cuatro cerebros en psicoterapia: quince años después [A concert for four hemispheres in psychotherapy: Fifteen years later]* (2nd ed.). Alom Editores. (Original work published 1990)

Robles, T., & Touyarot, A. (2018). *Manual de grupo para terminar con las dependencias [Group manual for ending dependencies]*. Alom Editores.

Samocha-Bonet, D., Chisholm, D. J., Tonks, K., Campbell, L. V., & Greenfield, J. R. (2012). Insulin-sensitive obesity in humans – A 'favorable fat' phenotype? *Trends in Endocrinology & Metabolism*, *23*(3), 116–124. 10.1016/j.tem.2011.12.005

Sapp, M. (2017). Obesity and weight loss. In G. R. Elkins (Ed.), *Handbook of medical and psychological hypnosis: Foundations, applications, and professional issues* (1st ed., pp. 589–597). Springer Publishing Company.

Shlisky, J. D., Hartman, T. J., Kris-Etherton, P. M., Rogers, C. J., Sharkey, N. A., & Nickols-Richardson, S. M. (2012). Partial sleep deprivation and energy balance in adults: an emerging issue for consideration by dietetics practitioners. *Journal of the Academy of Nutrition and Dietetics*, *112*(11), 1785–1797. 10.1016/j.jand.2012.07.032

Short, D., Erickson, B. A., & Erickson Klein, R. (2016). *Hope & resiliency: Understanding the psychotherapeutic strategies of Milton H. Erickson*. Crown House Publishing.

Sinha, R., & Jastreboff, A. M. (2013). Stress as a common risk factor for obesity and addiction. *Biological Psychiatry*, *73*(9), 827–835. 10.1016/j.biopsych.2013.01.032

Tamayo, D., & Restrepo, M. (2014). Aspectos psicológicos de la obesidad en adultos [Psychological aspects of obesity in adults]. *Revista De Psicología Universidad De Antioquia*, 6(1), 91–112. Periódicos Eletrônicos De Psicologia (PePSIC). Retrieved March 24, 2023, from http://pepsic.bvsalud.org/scielo.php?script=sci_arttext&pid=S2145-48922014000100007&lng=pt&nrm=iso&tlng=es]

Wadden, T. A., & Anderton, C. H. (1982). The clinical use of hypnosis. *Psychological Bulletin*, *91*(2), 215–243. 10.1037/0033-2909.91.2.215

Children and Adolescents

35

HYPNOSIS IN THE TREATMENT OF FUNCTIONAL SOMATIC SYMPTOMS IN CHILDREN AND ADOLESCENTS

Helene Helgeland[1], *Blanche Savage*[2], *and Kasia Kozlowska*[3]

[1]Department of Child and Adolescent Mental Health in Hospitals, Oslo University Hospital, Oslo, Norway; [2]Department of Psychological Medicine, The Children's Hospital at Westmead, Sydney, Australia; [3]Department of Psychological Medicine, The Children's Hospital at Westmead, Westmead Research Institute, University of Sydney Medical School, Sydney, Australia

Introduction

What Are Functional Somatic Symptoms?

The term *functional somatic symptoms* (FSS) refers to a broad array of physical symptoms reflecting disturbances of neurophysiological regulation (Agorastos & Chrousos, 2021; Chrousos, 2009; Kozlowska et al., 2020). Symptoms range from physical discomfort (e.g., pain, dizziness, or nausea) to disruptions of bodily functions (e.g., irregular bowel or bladder function), disturbances of motor or sensory processes or capacities (e.g., paralysis, loss of vision, or seizure events), and loss of the sense of health and well-being (e.g., exhaustion, general malaise, or fatigue) (see Figure 35.1). In children (including adolescents), FSS emerge in the context of physical and psychological stressors that disrupt or dysregulate the stress system. Comorbid anxiety and depressive symptoms are common. Levels of functional and social disability sit along a spectrum, from mild to severe, compromising the child's capacity to engage in normal developmental tasks such as playing with friends, attending school, and attaining independence with activities of daily living. Because considerable progress in understanding the etiology of FSS has been made in the last decade, the long-term outcomes for pediatric FSS are currently being established. Prompt diagnosis, engagement, and treatment – using a holistic (biopsychosocial) approach – are associated with the best outcomes (Thapar et al., 2020; Vassilopoulos et al., 2022).

Assessment and Treatment of Functional Somatic Symptoms

The biopsychosocial model of illness is fundamental to understanding and effectively treating FSS in children (Førde et al., 2022; Garralda & Rask, 2015; Helgeland et al.,

DOI: 10.4324/9781003449126-48
This chapter has been made available under a CC-BY-NC-ND 4.0 license.

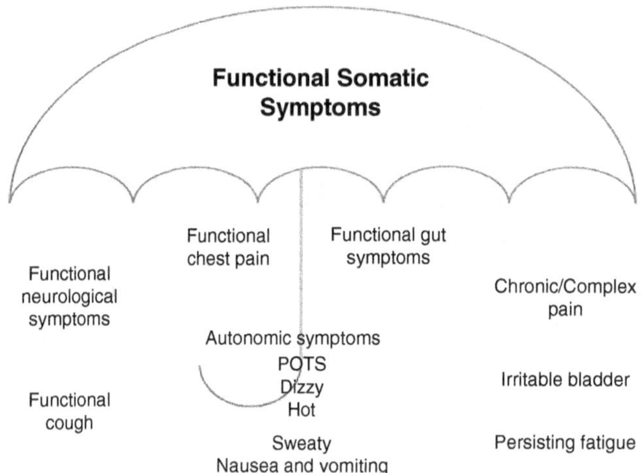

Figure 35.1 The umbrella term: functional somatic symptoms. The wide-ranging functional diagnoses that fall under the umbrella term. (© Kasia Kozlowska 2019).

2022; Savage et al., 2022). The biopsychosocial perspective challenges the clinician to identify the many different factors – the body, individual, family, school, and social and ecological system levels – that contribute to the child's presentation. It also challenges the clinician to co-construct a case formulation that synthesizes and integrates each child's medical history, developmental history, family history, life situation, and other relevant information provided by the child, caregivers, and teachers. The formulation should also include hypotheses about predisposing, triggering, maintaining, and protective factors. In children with FSS, the biopsychosocial approach pays particular attention to adverse childhood experiences, the manner in which these experiences are biologically embedded, and the cumulative effect of these experiences on the body systems and on health and well-being (Helgeland et al., 2022; Kozlowska et al., 2020).

A case formulation, collaboratively constructed with the patient and family, is a synergistic synthesis that merges the clinician's expertise and professional knowledge, the child's experiences, and the values and preferences of the child and family (Helgeland et al., 2022; Kozlowska et al., 2020). The therapeutic relationship that develops through this collaborative process contributes to mutual trust and to the acceptance of the formulation itself, both of which are important for engaging the family and securing their commitment to the course of treatment. For the patient and family, a clear understanding of the child's symptoms and situation can reduce worries, stimulate the development of good coping skills, and promote expectations for positive outcomes.

The clinician uses the formulation to guide treatment and as an ongoing framework for communicating with both the child and the family. What this means in practice is a stepped-care approach, where the treatment intervention is personalized to meet the clinical needs of each child and family (see Figure 35.2).

What Is Hypnosis?

Many of biopsychosocial treatment interventions for FSS can be considered as incorporating forms of hypnosis, "a unique form of top-down regulation [i.e., information

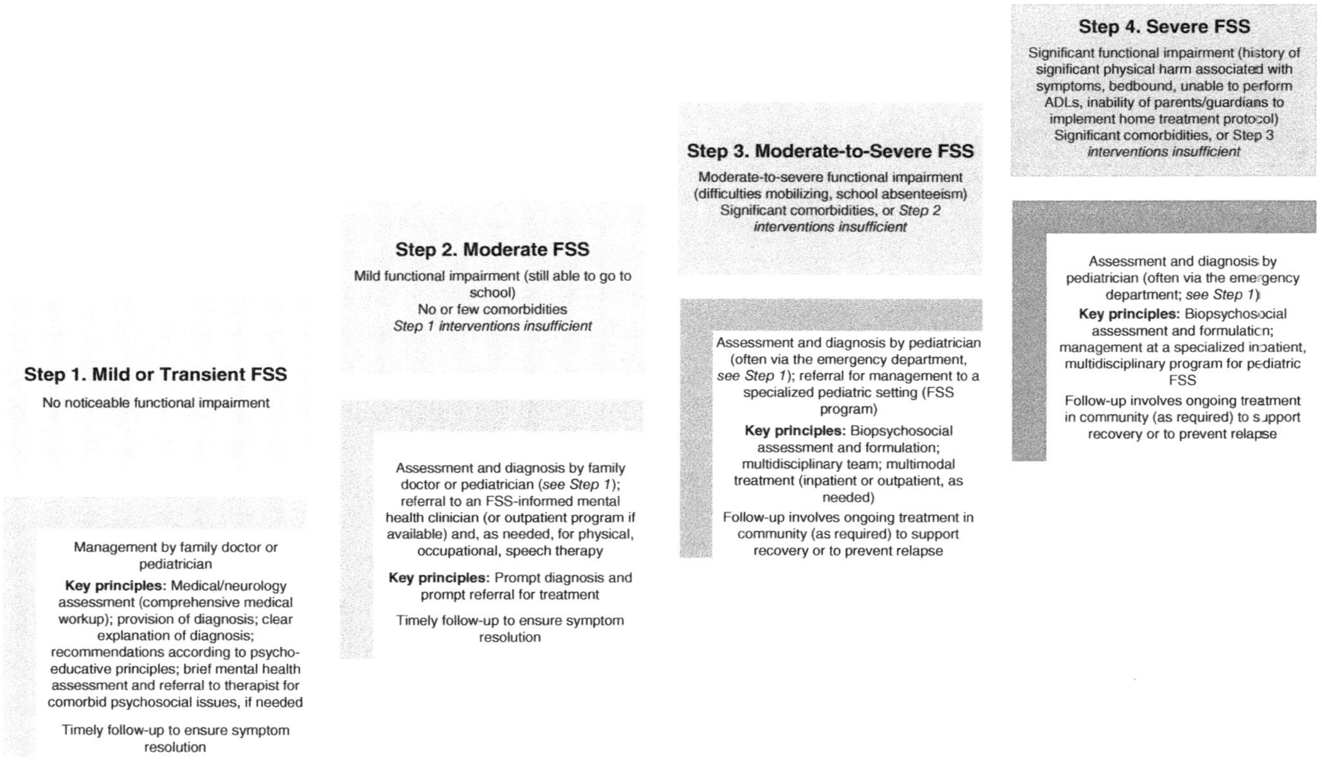

Step 1. Mild or Transient FSS
No noticeable functional impairment

Management by family doctor or pediatrician
Key principles: Medical/neurology assessment (comprehensive medical workup); provision of diagnosis; clear explanation of diagnosis; recommendations according to psycho-educative principles; brief mental health assessment and referral to therapist for comorbid psychosocial issues, if needed
Timely follow-up to ensure symptom resolution

Step 2. Moderate FSS
Mild functional impairment (still able to go to school)
No or few comorbidities
Step 1 interventions insufficient

Assessment and diagnosis by family doctor or pediatrician (*see Step 1*); referral to an FSS-informed mental health clinician (or outpatient program if available) and, as needed, for physical, occupational, speech therapy
Key principles: Prompt diagnosis and prompt referral for treatment
Timely follow-up to ensure symptom resolution

Step 3. Moderate-to-Severe FSS
Moderate-to-severe functional impairment (difficulties mobilizing, school absenteeism)
Significant comorbidities, or *Step 2 interventions insufficient*

Assessment and diagnosis by pediatrician (often via the emergency department, *see Step 1*); referral for management to a specialized pediatric setting (FSS program)
Key principles: Biopsychosocial assessment and formulation; multidisciplinary team; multimodal treatment (inpatient or outpatient, as needed)
Follow-up involves ongoing treatment in community (as required) to support recovery or to prevent relapse

Step 4. Severe FSS
Significant functional impairment (history of significant physical harm associated with symptoms, bedbound, unable to perform ADLs, inability of parents/guardians to implement home treatment protocol)
Significant comorbidities, or Step 3 *interventions insufficient*

Assessment and diagnosis by pediatrician (often via the emergency department; *see Step 1*)
Key principles: Biopsychosocial assessment and formulation; management at a specialized inpatient, multidisciplinary program for pediatric FSS
Follow-up involves ongoing treatment in community (as required) to support recovery or to prevent relapse

Figure 35.2 Stepped-care model for the management of pediatric functional somatic symptoms. Research on pediatric FSS treatment provides strong support for current clinical practice. It also offers a foundation for a stepped approach to treatment. Stepped care coupled with a biopsychosocial formulation serves as a framework for an individualized treatment process in pediatric FSS. Within the context of available health care resources, stepped care is initially tailored to the needs of the individual child (and family) based on the pattern and severity of FSS presentation. The level and type of intervention are then adjusted to take into account the child's response, over time, to particular treatments or treatment combinations. The hypnosis intervention – embedded in natural conversion or formal – can be integrated into all steps of the model. This model and legend is adapted from Vassilopoulos and colleagues (2022), © Kasia Kozlowska, Areti Vassilopoulos, & Aaron D. Fobian 2021. Adapted and used with permission.

processing] in which verbal suggestions are capable of eliciting pronounced changes" in neurophysiology, perception, and behavior (Terhune et al., 2017, p. 59). Top-down regulation strategies are those that involve use of the mind – involving the use of imagery and metaphor, as well as self-directed shifting of attention, thoughts, or feelings – to bring about change to brain and body states. From a neuroscience perspective, hypnosis is coming to be seen as involving neuroplasticity processes that harness "the ability of the nervous system to change its activity in response to intrinsic or extrinsic stimuli by reorganizing its structure, functions, or connections" (Mateos-Aparicio & Rodríguez-Moreno, 2019, p. 1).

According to Michael Yapko

> hypnosis is a focused experience of attentional absorption that invites people to respond experientially on multiple levels in order to amplify and utilize their personal resources in a goal directed fashion. When employed in the clinical context, hypnosis involves paying greater attention to the essential skills of using words and gestures in particular ways to achieve specific therapeutic outcomes, acknowledging and utilizing the many complex personal, interpersonal, and contextual factors that combine in varying degrees to influence client responsiveness.
>
> *(Yapko, 2019, p. 8)*

This focused experience of attention absorption is also referred to as trance.

Suggestions – verbal or nonverbal – invite the child to experience himself/herself or the world in a new way and can lead to changes in the child's physiology, sensations, perception, emotions, thoughts, and behaviors. Suggestions used within the frames of hypnosis are referred to as *hypnotic suggestions*, whereas *hypnotizability* – or *hypnotic suggestibility* – refers to an individual's proneness or ability to respond positively to hypnotic suggestions (Terhune et al., 2017).

There are no research studies looking at hypnotic suggestibility in children with FSS. Adult studies suggest that patients with functional neurological symptoms (a subtype of FSS) show increased hypnotic suggestibility (Terhune et al., 2017; Wieder et al., 2021), which is likely both a vulnerability factor and a strength. On one hand, patients (including children) with FSS may be vulnerable to negative suggestions from themselves (e.g., catastrophizing). On the other hand, patients may be receptive to health-promoting suggestions.

Sugarman and colleagues use the shorthand "changing minds" or "mind changing" to refer to these nonlinear processes that take place on multiple system levels (Sugarman et al., 2020). From a neuroscience perspective, the neuroplasticity processes hypothesized to underpin the therapeutic benefits of hypnosis are nonlinear, and they operate across multiple system levels (Mateos-Aparisio & Rodrigues-Moreno, 2019).

We – the authors – became interested in hypnosis early in our professional careers. During our family therapy training, we became increasingly aware of the power of words. We came to understand that the way that we communicated with children and their families had a powerful impact on the healing process. We were particularly intrigued by the work of Milton Erickson, an American psychiatrist who applied clinical hypnosis – stories, metaphors, and health-promoting suggestions – in his work with individuals and families. Inspired by senior colleagues who were skilled practitioners in clinical hypnosis, and also by the slowly mounting research evidence supporting the efficacy of clinical hypnosis in treating children with FSS, we undertook to start our own training in hypnosis.

Over time, we came to realize that *the hypnosis skillset* is an integral element of all healing traditions.

In our own clinical work with children with FSS, we use and adapt therapeutic elements of hypnosis from both traditional and more contemporary approaches. These elements may be

- integrated into the natural conversation with the child and family in the clinical encounter,
- integrated into the ritual of the treatment intervention,
- used to support medical or physical interventions or procedures,
- used to change focus of attention,
- used in connection with self-hypnosis, with or without the use of audio recordings of a hypnosis session,
- formally applied in a structured and more traditional way.

Every Clinical Encounter Counts

When children with FSS and their parents enter a clinician's office seeking an explanation for the child's worrisome symptoms, their focus of attention is on the symptoms. A clinician working from a contemporary hypnosis framework appreciates that the child and family are already in a state of narrowed attention and openness to suggestion.

Hence, what the clinician – doctor, therapist, nurse, physiotherapist, or pharmacist – communicates to the child and the parents in the initial clinical encounter may have a decisive impact on their understanding of the symptoms. The clinician's communication may shape expectations pertaining to the course of treatment, perceptions of risk (the symptoms being dangerous or not), possibilities of control and coping, and probable outcomes. The clinician's communication will also shape the child's illness behavior.

Below we provide examples of verbal suggestions. Negative suggestions communicate a lack of understanding or recognition of the child's experiences and set up negative expectations for the future. By contrast, positive suggestions communicate understanding and empathy and set up positive expectations for the future.

Negative verbal suggestions:

> "Don't be afraid. It's nothing dangerous. Don't cry!"
> "We can find no explanation for your pain. It must be all in your head."
> "You just have to learn to live with your nausea."

Positive verbal suggestions:

> "This will be fine. You can be calm and confident. We will manage this together!"
> "Many children experience symptoms like you have. The good news is that with proper treatment everyone gets better."
> "We'll work together to find the best treatment for you."

Children with FSS and their parents are also sensitive and vulnerable to the clinician's nonverbal communications, both positive and negative. Negative nonverbal communications signal the clinician's lack of interest, lack of knowledge, or own inner feelings of insecurity. Common examples of negative nonverbal communications include

- focusing attention on other things (e.g., focusing solely on the computer, answering the telephone),
- interrupting,
- coming late to the scheduled appointment,
- signaling little time (e.g., looking at the watch repetitively),
- speaking quickly and in a rushed manner.

By contrast, positive nonverbal communications signal interest, competence, familiarity with the subject matter, and knowledge of potential treatment options.

From our perspective, every clinical encounter provides an excellent opportunity to foster health-promoting experiences in the child and parents. Such experiences promote feelings of hope, coping possibilities, and positive outcome expectancies, all of which are important elements of treatment.

The Comprehensive Medical Assessment

How the doctor (or other health professional) carries out the medical assessment sends powerful signals to the child and the parents about how to perceive the child's symptoms. In a targeted medical history, the doctor collects information about the functional nature of the child's symptoms and about the presence of any indicators – red flags – that signal the possibility of an underlying disease process. As part of the holistic biopsychosocial assessment, the doctor also inquires about family, school, and other psychosocial stressors that could potentially be contributing to the child's presentation. Importantly, questions emerging from a biopsychosocial assessment function as powerful "suggestions" that facilitate and promote, in the patient and family, a holistic understanding of the child's symptoms. This is important for treatment success (Førde et al., 2022; Helgeland et al., 2022; Savage et al., 2022). Throughout the history-collecting process and the examination, the doctor has an excellent opportunity to build rapport, signal interest, respect, and knowledge. The doctor can also use the examination as a therapeutic ritual confirming strength and well-functioning of the child`s heart, lungs, tummy, muscles, and as a means of signaling expectations for a positive outcome, using such language as: So, now I can see that your heart and lungs and other parts of your body are healthy and doing fine – which will be helpful when it comes to treating your current symptoms, the ones that are disturbing you.

To complete a thorough assessment, the doctor may order any indicated supplementary tests to exclude concurrent medical problems that may potentially contribute to the child's presentation and symptom pattern. In the absence of "red flags," however, the doctor can – at this point of the first consultation, and before the results of any supplementary tests are known – convey that an organic disease is unlikely to explain the child`s symptoms.

An important part of the doctor's role is to give the illness a name, to provide the child (and family) with a *positive* diagnosis of FSS. For FSS that are neurological in nature, the positive diagnosis is based on positive rule-in neurological signs (Kozlowska & Mohammad, 2022; Stone, 2016). For example, functional tremor is characterized by changing frequency over time and settling or decrease of the tremor with contralateral body movements (called entrainment), with distraction, and when the child's attention is directed to another body part (see Kozlowska & Mohammad, 2022, for other functional neurological symptoms). For other FSS, diagnoses are based on criteria developed by expert consensus (Hyams et al., 2016; Kozlowska et al., 2020; Thapar et al., 2020).

The doctor will also need to provide the child and family with a credible explanation of the child's diagnosis, the treatment required, and the expectations of a good treatment outcome. The explanation – which functions as a therapeutic suggestion – makes the child's symptoms understandable and controllable, and sets up the expectation that, with treatment, the symptoms will be of limited duration. From the perspective of the child and the family, this optimistic frame nurtures hope, healing, and coping opportunities.

The following vignette provides an example of health-promoting language, in a case with no "red flags," used during the history-taking process and medical examination:

> "Your gut symptoms fall under the umbrella of functional disorders. This means that the structure of your organs is normal but that function has been disrupted. The formal medical names for your gut symptoms are *functional abdominal pain*, *functional nausea*, and *aerophagia* – aerophagia means bringing up air by belching. After listening carefully to your history and informed by my examination of your tummy, I'm confident that your body has the ability to get better, and it might even surprise you when I tell you that it has already started this work. It will be interesting to see how you will notice this in your body. I'm also confident that no serious disease is causing your symptoms. To make doubly sure, I will order some supplementary tests. But my expectation is that all the tests will come back normal, which is very good. At our next appointment, we will discuss your treatment options. My experience is that with good and prompt treatment, outcomes are excellent. Most children return to health and well-being. I look forward to seeing you next week."

When the Clinical Encounter Does Not Go Well: The Use of Negative Illness-Promoting Suggestions

Unfortunately, the clinical encounter does not always go well. Many patients with FSS tell stories about being misunderstood, distrusted, dismissed, and rejected in their clinical encounters with health care professionals in both medical and mental health settings (Kozlowska et al., 2021). Unfortunately, too many doctors use negative suggestions when communicating with the child and the parents. These experiences are "mind changing" in a negative way.

The absence of a credible explanation of the child's symptoms is particularly unfortunate. Instead of being of help, the doctor's comments may invalidate the child, the parents, and their experiences:

> "The tests are all normal. There is nothing wrong with you."
> "I don't see why you are not at school."
> "There is no medical explanation for your symptoms. Most likely, it's psychological."
> Or, in a report: "Mary presents with medically unexplained symptoms ...."

The lack of an explanation may also represent an uncontrollable threat. For some children (and families), the expectations become catastrophic – the opposite of having hope – and, thus, illness promoting. This will be reflected in the child's feelings (worry, anxiety, and sadness), thoughts (catastrophizing and negative thinking), and behavior (withdrawal, social isolation, and passivity), and in the upregulation of the stress system (Kozlowska et al., 2020). The outcome reflects an escalation of FSS and comorbid emotional symptoms (e.g., anxiety and depression).

The parents will also be affected. Many families become increasingly worried that the symptoms represent a threat to their child's health and well-being. Many parents become more and more focused on the child's symptoms and respond to the child with ever-increasing caregiving behaviors. Through their attention and solicitous responses, they unwittingly amplify the child's symptoms and contribute to a vicious cycle that aggravates and maintains the child's functional symptoms.

In the absence of a credible explanation, many children and families also become entangled in a process of never-ending medical assessments in search for an answer.

Some families come to be deeply offended, and they may bring negative expectations pertaining to past medical encounters to subsequent medical appointments with other medical professionals.

Starting Treatment

The treatment for FSS involves a multimodal biopsychosocial intervention (Førde et al., 2022; Garralda & Rask, 2015; Helgeland et al., 2022; Kozlowska et al., 2020). The components of this intervention are based on the biopsychosocial assessment and resulting formulation which help the clinician or clinical team and the family to identify the factors that contribute to and maintain the child's symptoms. These factors may arise not only at the system levels of the individual, family, peers, and school but also at the socioeconomic, political, and environmental levels.

In simple cases, the intervention may involve a small number of clinicians and system levels: provision of a diagnosis and explanation (doctor), and implementation of parental or family guidance (doctor or mental health clinician). In more complex cases, the intervention may involve a broader range of clinicians and system levels (see Figures 35.2 and 35.3).

Hypnosis Integrated into the Natural Conversation with the Child and Family in the Clinical Encounter

Hypnosis – as part of the natural conversation with the child and family in the clinical encounter – can be integrated into every component of the treatment intervention. In this section, we describe how we do this in our own practice.

Building Inner Agency and Mastery

Building a sense of agency and mastery is fundamental to all treatment interventions for children with FSS and their families. When the child discovers inner opportunities to self-regulate and to experience a sense of agency, the child is at the helm. Feelings of agency, control, and mastery engage the child as an active participant in the treatment process.

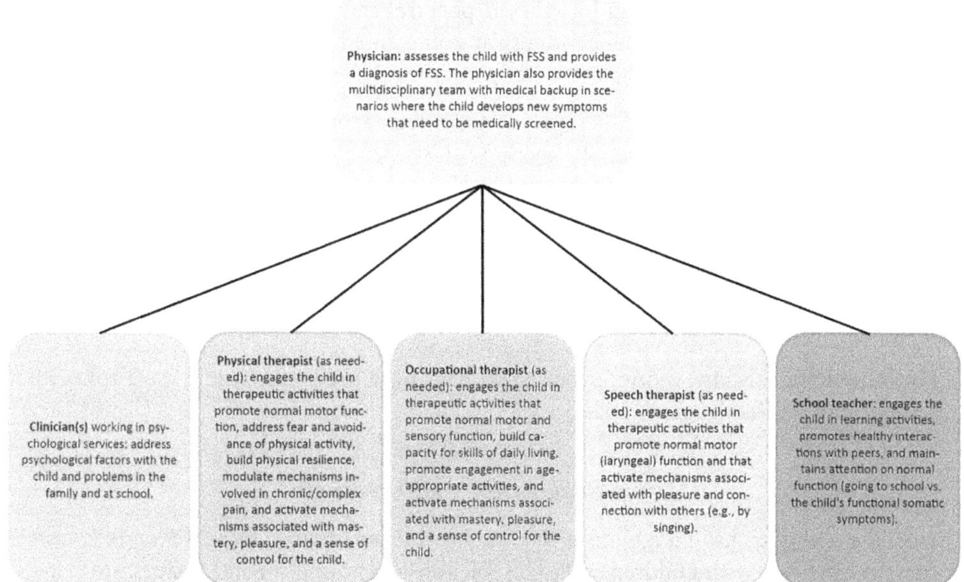

Figure 35.3 Multidisciplinary team. A physician, clinicians from psychological services, and staff from the child's school are included on every team. A physical therapist, occupational therapist, speech therapist, and other allied health professionals (e.g., art, music, and recreational therapists) join the team as required. © Kasia Kozlowska 2021.

This opens new "mind changing" experiences that nurture hope, mastery, and positive outcomes.

In the following vignette, in an individual therapy session, the therapist uses surprise and novelty in her conversation with a 16-year-old girl with chronic pain to introduce the adolescent to new ideas pertaining to her ability to self-regulate pain. The underlying idea is that a change in the child's information processing is stimulated by surprise and novelty. Surprise and novelty function as a disruption that shifts the child's focus of attention to suddenly pay attention to something that may be important ("What's in it for me?"). This intervention may lead to changes in the child's previous beliefs and expectancies. In family therapy, the described intervention would be viewed as a paradoxical intervention whose goal is to bring about change.

> Susan was suffering from an always-present headache that caused her significant functional and social disability. In the first therapy session, she told the therapist about her devastating symptoms. Her face was sad, her posture slumped, and she talked with a low voice. When asked to place her pain on a scale from 0 to 10, her usual pain rating was 6 – as now in the therapy session – and her top pain rating was a 10.
>
> "Oh, that is interesting. If I understand you right, you are rather good at turning your pain up. Can you turn it up right now?" the therapist said curiously.
>
> "No, I can't!" Susan replied and looked at him with surprise.
>
> Later in the same session, when the therapist had explored Susan's passion – dancing – the therapist noticed that Susan's body showed obvious signs of her feeling more and

more *well* and content. She had a relaxed posture, calm breathing, smiled, and was engaged in the conversation. The therapist commented on it, and Susan nodded in confirmation. When asked, she rated her pain to be a 3.

"How did you do that?" the therapist commented eagerly.
"I did nothing!" Susan answered – again with surprise.
"Yes, you did! Cool! How did you do that?"
"I actually don't know," Susan replied while thinking.
"Well, parts of you know. It will be interesting to find out more about this ability you have to control the headache that's bothering you," the therapist continued curiously. Susan replied with a smile.

For other hypnosis interventions that could have been used with Susan, see Yapko, 2019 and Sugarman and colleagues, 2020.

Using Imagination and Creativity

The child's ability to use imagination to create *health-promoting mental images* is central in clinical hypnosis with children with FSS. Health-promoting mental images are conceptualized as a powerful therapeutic tool, as a top-down self-regulation strategy (Kozlowska et al., 2020). This tool can be particularly helpful for children who habitually harbor *illness-promoting mental images* that function to activate the stress system and maintain the child's functional symptoms (Kozlowska et al., 2021). For example, images of negative past experiences may repeatedly come into the child's mind, or the child may anticipate and imagine future experiences in a negative way. The therapist supports the child to use imagination and creativity to rework or transform past unhealthy experiences, prepare the child to cope effectively with upcoming challenging situations, or experience present life challenges – including FSS – differently. This intervention helps the child to change focus of attention (see later section) and can break an ongoing vicious cycle in which cognitive processes – the images that the child brings (spontaneously) to mind – maintain the child's symptoms.

The following vignette highlights the use of imagination by a ten-year-old girl with functional abdominal pain during her individual therapy session:

Ann presented with a one-year history of increasing, recurrent abdominal pain and school absenteeism. Unrecognized learning difficulties were an important predisposing factor and also played a role in precipitating and perpetuating Ann's symptoms. Despite a thorough and fine-tuned readjustment of her educational program at school, Ann continued to experience abdominal pain, which was unpredictable and outside her control.

The therapist's evaluation was that Ann had developed heightened pain perception accompanied by fear and anticipatory anxiety regarding the pain, and that she had adopted protective responses in situations that she believed would trigger her pain.

The therapist invited Ann to explore how she could be the boss of her body. When the therapist drew a funny illustration of the brain-gut-axis and the two-way dialog between the brain and the gut, Ann exclaimed eagerly, "Like a tin-o-phone!" [a toy phone consisting of two cans attached to each other with a rope].

In the following therapy session, Ann used her imagination to create and occupy her favorite place using all her senses. Then, she practiced her self-regulatory skill by imagining herself sitting in a director's chair in her brain calling down to her gut, "It's time to calm down, gut, and please use your inside voice. You know, I'm the boss of this body." At the end of the session, Ann exclaimed, "So this is how my body feels when I am in control of my body!"

Using Metaphors

The use of metaphors in clinical hypnosis is common and is closely related to imagination and creativity (see previous section). "The essence of metaphor is understanding and experiencing one kind of thing in terms of another" or using elements from something known and pre-existing to describe something conceptual or abstract (Lakoff & Johnson, 2003, p. 5). Metaphors help children understand, structure, and communicate experiences that are difficult to communicate literally. The way that a child thinks of a concept can change the child's understanding of it and the way that the child approaches it. Paying attention to the child's use of metaphors in therapy gives the therapist valuable information about how the child sees the world and moves through it, and how the child relates to other people.

An appropriate metaphor can provide new understanding and guide the child's thinking and judgment. Most of the time, the most pertinent and powerful metaphor comes from the child – not the therapist. The therapist's job is to grasp the metaphor when it appears in the dialog with the child and to use it in therapy so it becomes a shared and meaningful symbol of understanding. The child is thus empowered to use the metaphor as a top-down regulation strategy, one that the child can access at any time to settle him- or herself and to facilitate a *transformative* experience.

The following vignette highlights the use of metaphor by a 11-year-old boy with dizziness, debilitating fatigue, and a myriad of other functional symptoms during his individual therapy sessions:

John lived with his parents and his older sister. One year earlier, at 10 years of age, he had developed enduring dizziness and lack of energy in the aftermath of a severe cold. Over the following month, he gradually developed widespread pain, pronounced fatigue, and lack of his usual enthusiasm. He had not been at school the last six months, and he had no energy for friends and his soccer practice. Even the slightest activity could knock him out completely. Since his energy and dizziness were unpredictable, he and his parents carefully assessed his "status" before engaging in any activity. Despite such efforts, John was on a downward spiral. He had seen a number of doctors and been through extensive medical assessments, but no one had given him an explanation or been able to help him. In one therapy session, John appeared lethargic and depressed. His conversation with the therapist proceeded as follows:

J: No one can help me – not even my parents.

T: Oh, that must be very difficult ... [pause] ... It seems that we have to find a way you can help yourself. I wonder how we can do that together.

J: That's impossible ... [He paused for a long time, and his eyes wandered around the room. He suddenly became aware of a withered flower in a vase with no water in the windowsill.] You see, I am like that flower now.

T: Thank you for telling me this important information. Now I know more about how your body is feeling, and now *we know* more about what you need. Like the flower, you need water ...*your* kind of water.
J: [His eyes widened, and he burst out in surprise:] Is it true?
T: [confirming pause]
J: I've believed that I never will get well again, ever ... in my entire life, but ... [He sighed in relief – a clear sign of calming self-regulation.]
T: Exactly. That's a good sigh. You know what you need.
J: [another deep sigh ... and a smile]

John had brought up the perfect metaphor – his metaphor. He was the withered flower in the empty vase. Like the vase, a container of water, his body was a container of energy. This metaphor clearly communicated his bodily sensation. In the next meeting, the therapist and John made accurate drawings of the vase. While drawing, the therapist curiously asked about his favorite activity: playing with his friends.

J: That was before ...
T: Yes, I understand, but still I am very curious about knowing more about the person you have been for most of your life ...

During the moments that the therapist curiously explored in great detail John's memory of playing with his friends, John's facial expression and posture became more eager and open, and his voice more energetic.

T: I wander how you will feel it in your body when it is refilled with refreshing water?
J: [paused, then sighed and smiled]

The flower vase became a central metaphor throughout the treatment process. John and the therapist introduced the vase to his parents and explained the "pathogenic mechanisms." In order to refill the vase with life-giving water, they *all* had to assist John in discovering and stopping the leakage holes in the vase, and *he* had to refill it – with the assistance of his parents, teacher, and therapist.

Embedding Positive Suggestions into the Conversation

Positive suggestions are embedded into all conversations with the child and family, both explicitly through direct language and implicitly through indirect language and behavior (e.g., the therapist's facial expression, tone of voice, and body language).

The following statements provide some other examples of explicit – or direct – suggestions through language:

> "When you follow this treatment, you will get better and better, and slowly and steadily you will build up your strength. You will start off going to school two days a week – as we agreed – and then, when your strength is coming back, you will go to school more and more often. You will start off doing a small amount of exercise, which will strengthen your body, and then you will be able to do more and more of your favorite things."

"When you practice your self-hypnosis skills before bedtime, your sleep will improve."

"Just take a nice deep breath, hold for a moment, then exhale slowly, and let your body calm down."

The following are examples of implicit – or indirect – suggestions embedded in the therapist's conversation and behavior:

"It will be interesting to know how you will feel in your body when your symptoms fade away [or when you are back in school playing with your friends]."

"I met a girl who made a bothersome headache go away, just by using her breathing technique [or practicing her self-hypnosis skills] once a day and whenever she needed it."

When a child is having a functional seizure, therapists need to sit calmly, ground themselves, and wait for the child to recover. They are sending the message that they are not panicked and that they trust the child's agency to recover from the seizure.

Use of the Treatment Ritual

In our clinical practice in Oslo and Sydney, we (the authors) participate in multidisciplinary teams of professionals who treat children and adolescents with complex FSS. In this section, we describe how we use the ritual of the multimodal treatment program to steer the child in the direction of health and well-being.

The Feeling of Being Part of an Effective Treatment Program

The ritual of the treatment intervention and the use of the psychosocial context – coupled with health-promoting hypnotic suggestions whether embedded in natural conversation or formal hypnosis – are important elements of the treatment intervention for children with FSS. We deliberately use the psychosocial context of the treatment program to communicate that effective care is available. We create a beneficial treatment ritual – ranging from simple rituals of prescribing medication (when indicated) to complex rituals of multimodal treatment. The name, structure, and psychosocial context of the treatment program convey an implicit, but powerful message to the child and the family: "You are now part of a special program that will help you get better."

Communicating Expertise and Providing Accurate Information

Communicating expertise and providing accurate information serve as positive suggestions that the child will actually get better. Parents of children with FSS – and the children themselves – respond with relief when clinicians communicate their knowledge and expertise. The family's anxiety reduces even further when they are given information about the beneficial outcomes of treatment. Communicating what the child and family need to do in order for the child to return to health and well-being increases the sense of hope, direction, and purpose. The power of the suggestion is amplified if the clinician's communication is clear, direct, and authoritative. The family come to recognize that the clinician understands FSS, knows what to do, and will work with the child and family in a collaborative way to bring the child back to health.

Therapeutic Rituals That Promote Predictability, a Sense of Control, and Mastery

One of the therapeutic rituals that we use is the child's *timetable* – scheduled for the day, week, or month, depending on the therapeutic context – to promote behavioral change and to provide a scaffold that the child can use to build physical and emotional strength. Co-constructing and applying a timetable adjusted to the individual child provides structure and predictability to the future, and contributes to the child's feeling of control and mastery. The timetable also implicitly communicates positive expectations to the child – about what we expect them to be able to achieve in a day, week, or month.

Other therapeutic rituals that we use in the inpatient setting are *daily morning ward rounds* to see the child and *regular meetings* – scheduled in the timetable – that include the complete interdisciplinary treatment team and the family. These encounters are imbued with suggestions that strengthen the ego, hope, and expectations for positive outcomes. They also provide a powerful message to the child that the treatment team and the family regularly recognize how important it is to create the space and time to think about the child and the child's health and well-being.

We also use the therapeutic ritual of *a personalized treatment plan* – depicted in visual form – with most of our patients. For example, when working with children with functional seizures, the therapeutic ritual of reading warning signs of neurophysiological activation and of then implementing a regulation strategy is depicted on the five steps of the Five-Step Plan or on a simpler, three-color Traffic Life Safety Plan (Savage et al., 2022). Each of these plans (rituals) involves daily practice (= practicing the ritual). The child knows – from our conversations with embedded implicit and explicit positive suggestions – that we expect that the child will, over time, be able to achieve mastery of the treatment plan and, in time, over the FSS. Individual therapy sessions involve practicing the therapeutic tools that are part of the treatment plan, thereby facilitating skill building and mastery. Over time, the child develops the capacity to implement the plan independently – that is, without help from a parent or other adult.

Using Hypnosis to Support Medical or Physical Interventions

The benefits of hypnosis on reducing pain and distress in children undergoing medical procedures are well known in the clinic (Birnie et al., 2018; Kuttner, 2012). In our practice, we use hypnosis to support children with FSS undergoing medical procedures. In this section, we focus on hypnosis as an adjunct to physiotherapy.

In some children with functional motor symptoms, we combine formal hypnosis with physiotherapy. This intervention can be very useful when physiotherapy cannot be implemented because of pain, a fixed dystonia, dizziness, or projectile vomiting secondary to overwhelming anxiety. In all these cases, suggestions embedded in the natural conversations with the child have failed to calm the child's dysregulated neurophysiological systems sufficiently, enabling the physiotherapist to begin treatment. In these difficult cases, the predictable, scaffolding frame of formal hypnosis – the use of a formal induction procedure – enhances the child's capacity to focus attention away from the symptoms and respond to hypnotic suggestions. The formal hypnosis ritual allows the child's neurophysiological systems to settle sufficiently for the physiotherapist to engage in the therapeutic work that needs to be done.

The two vignettes below are helpful examples.

> Jai, [a] 14-year-old boy[,] ... presented with painful fixed dystonia in the neck, motor weakness and lack of coordination in the legs, and a pain-related curve of the body to the left. He consequently both sat and slept in a C-shape. He could not walk, sit up straight in the wheelchair, or toilet or shower himself. After the clinical team determined that Jai was highly hypnotizable – he could enter the trance state easily – hypnosis was integrated into his occupational therapy and physiotherapy sessions. While Jai was in a trance state, his psychotherapist made suggestions to Jai about his body state – that his body was deeply relaxed, that he could disconnect from the pain, that he could image that his body was bendable like a reed, or that his body could sway like a tree. These suggestions enabled the physiotherapist and occupational therapists to straighten and reposition Jai in the wheelchair. At the end of each session, when Jai was guided out of the trance state, he would suddenly find himself in the non-C-shaped position, and he would panic. He reported that he perceived his body – temporarily straight in the wheelchair – as being bent and wrong. By contrast, his internal perception of the C-shaped position was that his body was straight. Jai was initially unable to use any interventions to manage his panic – including suggestions during the trance state that he stay calm – but the length and intensity of the panic gradually settled as he habituated himself to the process of emerging from a trance. (Reproduced from Kozlowska et al. 2020, p. 232)

> Clara was a 13-year-old girl who had extreme dizziness that prevented her from sitting or standing. Part of her treatment was to be strapped to a "tilt table" (a special bed that the child is strapped to, which moves from horizontal to vertical to allow the body to have the benefits of standing). Clara was unable to tolerate being on the tilt table and would become so dizzy that she would vomit. The team was becoming concerned about potential secondary complications due to Clara's being bed-bound for so many months.

> Clara's mother had told Clara about her own experiences with formal hypnosis, and Clara had requested that the therapist use an induction that was similar to the one described by her mother. Clara enjoyed the *trial* induction and reported that the hypnosis helped settle the pain she felt in her body and that it helped her feel less tense and tight (more calm).

> Subsequently, the team was able to use hypnosis in conjunction with Clara's physiotherapy sessions. Clara would lie on the tilt table, and her therapist would implement the following ritual: a formal induction with eye fixation and progressive muscle relaxation (Clara's choice), suggestions that Clara step away from her body while allowing her mind to go where it chose (in this case, she imagined herself doing her favorite activity – body surfing on waves in the sea), followed by calming and ego-strengthening suggestions of mastery and control. Clara

responded well. Her breathing slowed down, her body posture became relaxed, and her face expressed peace and harmony. In this situation – while still under formal hypnosis – the physiotherapist was able to raise the tilt table so that Clara was in a standing position. Clara was able to tolerate this for ten minutes – increased in subsequent sessions – without vomiting or dizziness.

Changing Focus of Attention

Attention to functional symptoms amplifies them (Kozlowska et al., 2020). Thus, shifting focus of attention is an essential component of the treatment intervention across system levels, guiding the child, clinicians, parents, and teachers in managing focus of attention.

In their individual therapies, children learn (and practice) hypnosis – the skill of shifting their attention away from distressing bodily symptoms and from illness-promoting cognitive processes and images. They learn to shift their attention to images, thoughts, therapeutic tasks, or activities that help their body's stress system (and symptoms) settle and that give them a sense of agency and control. When learning to manage functional seizures, the child learns how to shift focus of attention from the warning signs that herald a functional seizure to the therapeutic tools that settle the body and that help the child avert the seizure (Savage et al., 2022).

In family work, families practice conversing and interacting in ways that shift attention away from the symptoms and toward health-promoting interactions. In the classroom, teachers focus the child's attention on the task at hand. And in formal treatment, the programs are structured so that the child's attention is shifted away from the functional symptoms, onto activities of daily living, and also onto the therapeutic tools that will help the symptoms settle.

Self-Hypnosis With or Without the Use of Audio Recordings

The treatment of FSS involves the ongoing practice of self-regulation skills – regular exercise, bottom-up regulation skills, and top-down regulation skills (including hypnosis) – as part of the activities of daily living. In this context, in the child's individual therapy sessions, we often teach the children self-hypnosis so that they can subsequently practice their self-regulatory skills at home. Self-hypnosis can be used to target the child's FSS, sleep, or anxiety or to strengthen the ego. Some children easily grasp this opportunity of using their imagination and creativity to take control of their bodies. Other children prefer to practice self-hypnosis at home with assistance from their parents or using audio recordings of a hypnotic session.

A growing literature documents the beneficial effect of using hypnosis recordings for self-hypnosis practice at home to address FSS in children (Gillan, 2021). Many children are pleased to take home recordings with their therapist's voice. It is a way of taking an element of the treatment program – and the child's newfound skills, resources, mastery, and self-efficacy – back to the home setting. Recordings of the therapist's voice also provide familiarity and predictability, which, like bedtime stories, are soothing and signal connection and safety. The length and the content of the recording are adjusted to the individual child. Most children prefer short recordings of only a few minutes duration. In our clinical practice, we often co-construct a short hypnosis session to be recorded together with the child.

The vignette below presents an example.

> In the case of John – the boy with the flower vase metaphor – the therapist made a recording of a formal hypnosis session that they had designed together. Encouraged to practice at home, John used the recording as often as possible. On some days, however, he "did not feel like listening to the recording"; instead, he took a brief look at a nice drawing of a blue metallic bottle that he perceived as containing magic medicine [for further details, see vignette in section below]. "Just a glance is enough and my body remembers it's magic," John stated.

Use of Formal Hypnosis

In our work with children with FSS, we also use formal hypnosis where elements of hypnosis are applied in a structured and more traditional way during individual therapy sessions to address the child's symptoms.

The Hypnosis Session as a Therapeutic Ritual

Some children enjoy and benefit from the experience of formal hypnosis as a *therapeutic ritual* applied in a structured and traditional way. The vignette below presents an example.

> Jasmine was a 16-year-old girl who had functional dystonia in one leg: her leg would twist and cause her excruciating pain. Sometimes the pain would be so severe that she would faint. Jasmine had previously been chosen from the audience of a stage hypnotist to be hypnotized on stage. Jasmine found this an impressive experience and would talk repeatedly about how highly hypnotizable she was. It was clear to the therapist that Jasmine had very specific beliefs about what it was like to be hypnotized. Her strong belief in the power of the ritual of hypnosis led her to prefer hypnosis involving induction via eye fixation and counting backward as a means of treating her symptoms. Over time, with the support and guidance of the therapist during the hypnosis sessions, Jasmine became more engaged in how to use her imagination and self-regulatory skills to avert her pain and fainting episodes. Interestingly, Jasmine did not want to practice self-hypnosis; instead, she preferred to listen to a recording by her therapist verbally guiding her through her preferred hypnosis session.

When a therapist chooses to use formal hypnosis, the therapist and the child co-create the therapeutic ritual of a "hypnosis session." Through a process of reciprocal exploring and creative dialog, the therapist is particularly responsive to the child's wishes and suggestions. For example, the child and therapist can explore whether the child prefers an induction via slow breathing, eye fixation, progressive muscle relaxation, or something else. Some children prefer the therapist's assistance evoking and elaborating an inner image of the child's "good place to be," whereas others prefer to "go to" their inner "good place to be" right away.

Together, the child and the therapist may explore how the child imagines him- or herself taking control of the symptoms and the body. Examples include changing the size or the color of the child's pain or feelings of anxiety, so that they become something tiny or take on the child's favorite color; blowing the pain or fear into balloons and letting them disappear in the air; creating their own inner pain switch in a "convenient" place in the child's body; or putting on a very special magic glove that can be used to change the child's perceived sensations (Coogle et al., 2021).

For some children, *preparing* the "hypnosis session" is perhaps as important as actually *engaging* in it because the process of preparing the session includes health-promoting suggestions and expectations. In addition, in some particularly vulnerable children, the frame of more formal hypnosis may represent a scaffolding and predictable framework for the therapy itself – making it safe for the child to engage in therapy (see previous section).

> During the conversations with John, the 11-year-old boy with the flower vase metaphor, it became evident that he wanted to "refill" the vase with healing water – in accordance with his metaphor. John explained to the therapist that the water was "like a healing medicine!" – a new metaphor, signaling that John was now hopeful about the ultimate success of the treatment process. Through careful preparation, John and the therapist agreed on the ingredients of their ritual and on the details concerning John's medicine.
>
> John's imaginative "good place to be" was at the soccer field together with his best friends, on a sunny day (but not too hot), playing his best game ever, with both his parents and his favorite uncle watching and cheering. At half time, John picks up his brand new metallic blue drinking bottle without knowing that it contains the magic medicine – the healing water. When drinking, each sip sizzles pleasantly down his throat and into his tummy, giving a nice, warm sensation. The warm sensation then spreads throughout his body, making the body feel more and more energized, alert, and strong.
>
> After practicing the first session together, the therapist commented curiously, "It will be interesting to see when your body will notice the effect of this magic medicine of yours." "It already does," John replied. "Oh, that's a good thing! It will be interesting to see how many 'doses' of this magic medicine of yours your body will need!" the therapist continued. "I guess about five or six doses," John stated. "You sure know the best!" the therapist confirmed.

The Use of Scripts as Part of the Therapeutic Ritual

Some children with FSS like us to use a familiar hypnosis script because the repetition provides the child with a sense of predictability and safety. Some children like the script to be chosen by the therapist. Others enjoy composing the script with the therapist – a process that can increase the child's mastery and motivation, as well as strengthen the expectation for a positive outcome. Preparing a script together can also represent a hypnotic experience in itself. The *sensible use* of scripts can be a valuable support for clinicians who are in the process of learning hypnosis skills (Lindheim & Helgeland, 2017). As therapists become more practiced and confident, they are usually able to put scripts aside and to practice in a more natural and creative way. The decision to use a script – or not – needs to be decided on an individual basis, depending on what resonates with the individual child and the therapist.

Hypnosis Delivered in the Group Setting

Hypnosis delivered in a group setting is an important development that may make hypnosis available to a larger number of children with FSS (Gillan, 2021). The discussion of group hypnosis, however, is beyond the scope of this chapter.

Conclusion

Biopsychosocial interventions informed by hypnosis are an integral component in the treatment of FSS in children. They promote hope, predictability, sense of control, and mastery, thereby contributing to the healing process. Over the last decade, considerable progress has been made in understanding the neurobiology of FSS and in developing models that outline the hypothesized mechanisms that underpin the efficacy of hypnosis (Price, 2020; Terhune et al., 2017). Future research is needed on the underlying neurobiology and the most effective way of incorporating hypnosis-informed practice into the biopsychosocial intervention and the stepped care model for FSS.

References

Agorastos, A., & Chrousos, G. P. (2021). The neuroendocrinology of stress: The stress-related continuum of chronic disease development. *Molecular Psychiatry*. 10.1038/s41380-021-01224-9

Birnie, K. A., Noel, M., Chambers, C. T., Uman, L. S., & Parker, J. A. (2018). Psychological interventions for needle-related procedural pain and distress in children and adolescents. *Cochrane Database Systematic Review, CD005179-CD005179*. 10.1002/14651858.CD005179.pub4

Chrousos, G. P. (2009). Stress and disorders of the stress system. *Nature Reviews: Endocrinology*, *5*(7), 374–381. 10.1038/nrendo.2009.106

Coogle, J., Coogle, B., & Quezada, J. (2021). Hypnosis in the treatment of pediatric functional neurological disorder: The magic glove technique. *Pediatric Neurology*, *125*, 20–25. 10.1016/j.pediatrneurol.2021.08.011

Førde, S., Breen Herner, L., Helland, I. B., & Diseth, T. H. (2022). The biopsychosocial model in paediatric clinical practice; A multidisciplinary approach to somatic symptom disorders. *Acta Paediatrica*.

Garralda, E. M., & Rask, C. U. (2015). Somatoform and related disorders. In *Rutter's child and adolescent psychiatry: Sixth edition* (pp. 1035–1054). Wiley-Blackwell. 10.1002/9781118381953.ch72

Gillan, C. (2021). Review article: the effectiveness of group and self-help hypnotherapy for irritable bowel syndrome and the implications for improving patients' choice and access to treatment. *Alimentary Pharmacology and Therapeutics*, *54*(11–12), 1389–1404. 10.1111/apt.16623

Helgeland, H., Gjone, I. H., & Diseth, T. H. (2022). The biopsychosocial board: A conversation tool for broad diagnostic assessment and identification of effective treatment of children with functional somatic disorders. *Human Systems: Therapy, Culture and Attachments*. 10.1177/26344041221099644

Hyams, J. S., Di Lorenzo, C., Saps, M., Shulman, R. J., Staiano, A., & van Tilburg, M. (2016). Childhood functional gastrointestinal disorders: Child/adolescent gastroenterology (New York, N.Y. 1943), *150*(6), 1456–1468.e1452. 10.1053/j.gastro.2016.02.015

Kozlowska, K., & Mohammad, S. (2022). Functional neurological disorder in children and adolescents: Assessment and treatment. In L. Sivaswamy & D. Kamat (Eds.), *Symptom based approach to pediatric neurology* (683–724). Springer Nature.

Kozlowska, K., Sawchuk, T., Waugh, J. L., Helgeland, H., Baker, J., Scher, S., & Fobian, A. D. (2021). Changing the culture of care for children and adolescents with functional neurological disorder. *Epilepsy & Behavior Reports*, *16*, 100486. 10.1016/j.ebr.2021.100486

Kozlowska, K., Scher, S., & Helgeland, H. (2020). *Functional somatic symptoms in children and adolescents: The stress-system approach to assessment and treatment*. London: Palgrave Macmillan.

Kuttner, L. (2012). Pediatric hypnosis: pre-, peri-, and post-anesthesia: Pediatric hypnosis. *Pediatric Anesthesia*, *22*(6), 573–577. 10.1111/j.1460-9592.2012.03860.x

Lakoff, G., & Johnson, M. (2003). *Metaphors we live by*. University of Chicago Press.

Lindheim, M. Ø., & Helgeland, H. (2017). Hypnosis training and education: Experiences with a Norwegian one-year education course in clinical hypnosis for children and adolescents. *American Journal of Clinical Hypnosis*, *59*(3), 282–291. 10.1080/00029157.2016.1230728

Mateos-Aparicio, P., & Rodríguez-Moreno, A. (2019). The impact of studying brain plasticity. *Frontiers in Cellular Neuroscience*, *13*, 66-66. 10.3389/fncel.2019.00066

Price, J. (2020). Hypnosis & functional neurological symptom disorder (FND). *Neurodigest*, *5*, 12–14.

Savage, B., Chudeleigh, C., Hawkes, C., Scher, S., & Kozlowska, K. (2022). *Treatment of functional seizures in children and adolescents: A mind-body manual for health professionals (version 1)*. Australian Academic Press.

Stone, J. (2016). Functional neurological disorders: The neurological assessment as treatment. *Practical Neurology*, *16*(1), 7–17. 10.1136/practneurol-2015-001241

Sugarman, L. I., Brooks, L. W., & Linden, J. H. (2020). *Changing minds with clinical hypnosis: Narratives and discourse for a new health care paradigm*. Routledge.

Terhune, D. B., Cleeremans, A., Raz, A., & Lynn, S. J. (2017). Hypnosis and top-down regulation of consciousness. *Neuroscience and Biobehavioral Reviews*, *81*, 59–74. 10.1016/j.neubiorev.2017.02.002

Thapar, N., Benninga, M. A., Crowell, M. D., di Lorenzo, C., Mack, I., Nurko, S., Saps, M., Shulman, R. J., Szajewska, H., van Tilburg, M. A. L., & Enck, P. (2020). Paediatric functional abdominal pain disorders. *Nature Reviews. Disease Primers*, *6*(1), 89-89. 10.1038/s41572-020-00222-5

Vassilopoulos, A., Mohammad, S., Dure, L., Kozlowska, K., & Fobian, A. D. (2022). Treatment approaches for functional neurologic disorders in children. *Current Treatment Options in Neurology*, *24*, 77–97. 10.1007/s11940-022-00708-5

Wieder, L., Brown, R. J., Thompson, T., & Terhune, D. B. (2021). Suggestibility in fuctional neurological disorder: A meta-analysis. *Journal of Neurology Neurosurgery and Psychiatry*, *92*, 150–157. 10.1136/jnnp-2020-323706

Yapko, M. D. (2019). *Trancework. An introduction to the practice of clinical hypnosis*. (5th ed.). Routledge.

36

HYPNOSIS

Finding Relief for Children and Teens in Pain

Leora Kuttner[1] *and Adrienn Vargay*[2,3]

[1]Faculty of Medicine, Pediatric Department, BC Children's Hospital & University of British Columbia, Vancouver, Canada; [2]Institute of Psychology, ELTE Eötvös Loránd University, Budapest, Hungary; [3]Pediatric Pain Centre, HRC Bethesda, Budapest, Hungary

Introduction

It is said that "Pain is the only condition in which the patient is the diagnostician".

Historically, however, when children complained of pain, their pain was ignored (Schechter et al., 2003). The prevailing myth was they would get used to it, and it won't do them any harm. Consequently, children's pain was under-diagnosed, under-treated and newborn's pain completely dismissed pharmacologically, physically, and psychologically, until very recently. These harmful practices and myths persisted through the 1980s.

In the last 35 years, an international community of pain researchers and clinicians from many pediatric disciplines, nursing, psychology, neonatology, pharmacy, physiotherapy, anesthesiology, developmental and general pediatrics have been addressing this unconscionable neglect. As a result, we are now witnessing major changes in pediatric training and pain practices, pediatric guidelines and standard requirements. Painful procedures performed on infants now require analgesics and anesthetics, recognizing that despite the underdevelopment of their nervous system, infants experience more undifferentiated and intense pain, and inadequate analgesia has significant deleterious consequences on their long-term development (Anand et al., 1987; Grunau, 2002). Research shows that despite the myth "they tolerate discomfort well" (Swafford & Allan, 1968), children remember their painful procedures (Noel et al., 2015), become sensitized to pain, develop phobic responses and loose trust in their providers. The Joint Commission on Accreditation of Hospitals now requires that all established pain management standards be routinely implemented and maintained for pediatric hospitals' accreditation.

Psychological child-centered treatment methods were also developed to effectively treat pain and anxiety problems (Katz et al., 1980; Olmsted et al., 1982). Pediatric hypnosis emerged as a robust, effective and broad-spectrum treatment adapted to children's developmental and emotional/cognitive stages and has found an important place in pediatric clinics and hospitals worldwide for a range of pediatric pain problems (Fisher et al., 2018; Friedrichsdorf & Goubert, 2020; Rogovik & Goldman, 2007; Tsao & Zeltzer, 2005). We've determined that hypnosis can be beneficial for, pre- and post-surgery (Kuttner, 2012; Lobe, 2007), emergencies (Peebles-Kleiger, 2000), blood collection (Birnie et al., 2014;

DOI: 10.4324/9781003449126-49

Maxym, 2008), painful and invasive procedures (Butler et al., 2005; Liossi et al., 2009), abdominal pain management (Rutten et al., 2014; Vlieger et al., 2012), headache relief (Esparham et al., 2018; Kohen, 2011; Jong et al., 2019), complex pain management (Bastek et al., 2022) and pediatric palliative care and end of life (Friedrichsdorf & Kohen, 2018, Kuttner & Friedrichsdorf, 2007; Zernikow et al., 2009). In this chapter, we will examine how hypnosis has been used to provide pain and distress relief for children. We'll look at how, as an integrated mind-body intervention, the hypnosis experience naturally lends itself to the complex nature of managing pain, and how hypnotic child-centered interventions can have long-lasting benefits for chronic and complex pain. In these and in other respects, hypnosis is a "best-fit" intervention for children and teens for a wide range of pain experiences.

Who Are We?

- LK: Hypnosis has been and remains fundamental to my work in pediatric pain management. I value its creativity, flexibility, and power to effect rapid change and sustain hope and healing. Early in my career as a pediatric clinical psychologist (1979), knowing the unique potential of hypnosis, I felt compelled to find more effective and therapeutic pain treatments. I undertook research and program development at British Columbia's Children's Hospital Pediatric Oncology division in Vancouver and developed interventions for invasive procedures for outpatient and inpatient pain programs, training medical, nursing staff, children and their parents. For the next forty years I've enjoyed utilizing the multiplicity of hypnosis approaches to help children and teens in acute, recurrent, and chronic complex pain. I conveyed this clinical evidence through 50+ journal articles, two books, many book chapters and five documentary films, including "No Fears, No Tears–13 Years Later". Forty years later, I'm deeply heartened to see the increased awareness of children's pain, and significant increase in hypnosis training and implementation in pediatric centers worldwide.
- AV.: I got my first inspiration and knowledge of hypnosis techniques and research in prof. Dr. Éva Bányai's laboratory doing lab and clinical hypnosis research during my first years at Eötvös Loránt University, Budapest, Hungary. At the same time, I was volunteering with children with burns and accident rehabilitation, using suggestion and story therapy elements to treat their pain. It was here that I first became familiar with the complexities of pain management, realizing the potential of therapies working with different altered states of consciousness. I became committed both to hypnosis and the therapy of children with somatic problems. Later, I trained as a psychologist in palliative care and pediatric oncology. I worked in the orthopedic clinic with young people with cancer who had undergone amputation. I wrote my PhD in hypnotherapy of breast cancer patients under the supervision of Éva Bányai. I now work with children with chronic pain at the first pediatric pain clinic in Hungary.

Our Philosophical and Practice Approach

Our practice approach is strongly influenced by humanistic-existentialist philosophies and theories, Ericksonian hypnosis approaches, interpersonal and family systems theory, and the interpersonal aspect of hypnosis in the work.

We use hypnosis both as a formal trance experience and within a naturalistic conversation in a trusted safe relationship, knowing it's significant therapeutic potential to transform sensory, emotional and cognitive experience. Both forms of hypnosis, formal and informal, have benefits. However, combined the hypnotically oriented conversation serves as the lead up, preparing the child through informal suggestions to become oriented toward the need for therapeutic change – so when the formal, ritualized hypnotic process starts, it is a natural consequence. We've seen how with skilled application and dedication, hypnosis gains deeper potency and greater efficacy. To achieve this our interpersonal hypnotic process needs to be crafted and individually tailored to each child, his/her pain problem, the beliefs and convictions that sustain this pain, and physical habits developed to protect and guard it. Research has shown, and we've experienced, that hypnosis interventions can change pain experience as much as many analgesic medications, and far more than placebos (Spiegel & Albert, 1983).

A non-scripted hypnosis experience grounded in the therapeutic relationship and developed to navigate the patient's entrenched fears, dashed hopes, depression or accompanying anger is more relevant and effective than hypnosis that is "manualized" or scripted. We also know there is an ineffable therapeutic "something" that occurs when all the critical elements are being sensitively and adequately addressed that allows pain to down-modulate, and coping and mastery to emerge.

Definition of Pain

Pain is a function of the conscious brain. "You have to pay attention to pain for it to hurt" (Spiegel, 2007, p. 1281). Pain is more than a nociceptive or negative sensory signal; it's a culturally informed, psychophysiological, emotional, learned experience. Pain is thus an integrated, neurobiological, emotional and social phenomenon. As a mind-body noxious, distressing experience, pain involves the physical site of the pain, the emotional reaction to this pain, the social and cultural context for the pain, all integrated within the limbic and brain cortices, which then interprets the neuronal signals as *"pain!"* (Melzack, 1973).

The antiquated, simplistic approach that categorizes a child's pain as either physical or psychological; organic or functional; in the body or the mind, has no place in today's pediatric practice. Pain is both embodied in the mind and "painfully minded" in the body (Dienstfrey, 1991). As a biopsychosocial integrated phenomenon, pain is ultimately subjective. The observer assessing pain can only discern that the observed patient is in pain from behavior and physiological measures, e.g., increased heart rate and disrupted respiratory rate (Melzack, 1973). The amount of pain cannot be reliably or validly measured, standardized or determined. Therefore, McCaffery's (1968) definition first stated in 1968 that a patient's pain is *"whatever the experiencing person says it is, existing whenever and wherever the person says it does"* provides our therapeutic starting point (Rosdahl & Kowalsky, 2007).

Under-Treatment of Children's Pain and Consequent Institutional Changes

With research challenging the harmful beliefs that children with less developed nervous systems don't experience pain in the same way that adults do, medical and hospital practice began changing through the 1980s, 1990s and 2000s. Pediatric researchers and clinicians from many disciplines turned their attention to understanding and mitigating the damaging impact of pain on children – and pediatric hypnosis emerged in the forefront of interventions (Kuttner, 1986; Kuttner et al., 1988; Olmsted et al., 1982). Pioneering research with Leukemia patients, where both assessment and treatment require a long line of painful needles – IVs for chemotherapy, daily bloodwork, lumbar punctures and bone marrow aspirations – resulted in significant positive outcomes using behavioral and hypnosis interventions. Olmstead, Zeltzer and LeBaron's findings (1982) that 6–12-year-olds benefit from hypnosis during procedures; and Kuttner's subsequent year-long research into both 6–12 year olds and 3–6 year olds (who have the highest prevalence of leukemias), drew attention to the versatility of hypnotic techniques to manage children's procedural pain. These included hypnotic methods such as the child's favorite stories adapted to mitigate pain, providing anxiety and distress relief during lumbar punctures (Kuttner, Bowman & Teasdale, 1988); transferring hypno-analgesia from a finger to the child's iliac crest during a painful bone marrow aspiration (documented in "No Fears, No Tears – 13 years Later", Kuttner, 1998), using hypno-analgesia, *The Magic Glove* for IVs insertion for chemotherapy and cubital access for blood work (documented in "*No Fears, No Tears*", Kuttner, 1986), *The Magic Glove* (Kuttner, 2014), and *The Pain Switch* to access a child's scalp-port for intrathecal chemotherapy.

These hypnosis mind-body methods are now part of hospital-wide practice in many Canadian and US hospitals. Nurses, anesthesiologists, pediatricians and pain teams have been trained to use hypnosis as part of their clinical practice (BC Children's ChildKind Initiative; Alberta Children's Hospital, Carlson et al., 2018; UCSF Benioff Children's Hospital, San Francisco; Sick Kids Hospital, Toronto). Furthermore, over 1,000 pediatric clinicians have received pediatric hypnosis training through The National Pediatric Hypnosis Training Institute (NPHTI) annual training workshops in Minneapolis, USA.

Hypnosis Is a Good Fit for Treating Pain, Particularly Persistent Pain

Hypnosis is a natural, elegant fit with the unique problems of treating persistent pain. Hypnosis has the striking advantage of being able to address the pain experience simultaneously at sensory, cognitive and affective-emotion levels, and while the patient is in a relaxed and receptive physical state (Jensen, 2009; Wood & Bioy, 2008). This facilitates developing a very different relationship with the pain. Few other therapies address as much at one time.

Hypnosis is communication – verbal and nonverbal, conscious and subconscious. Careful and deliberate selection of language to create a climate of new possibilities from the moment of first contact with a patient is fundamental to achieving pain relief. This communication occurs not only in what is being said but also in what is implied between the words, by how the words are delivered and the elemental qualities of prosody, poetry and pauses. Furthermore, these multilayered messages are conveyed within a therapeutic relationship in which trust has been cultivated, enhancing potential patient responsiveness.

Therapeutically, hypnotic experience invites multiple aspects of experience to occur and change, simultaneously or sequentially. We invite the child to think differently about the pain experience, focus attention moment by moment on useful, desired or beneficial shifts in emotion and sensory experience, thereby cultivating an attentional focus to new patterns of pain processing and thereby developing new neurobiological networks. By tailoring the hypnotic experience to the unique pain presentation, the child learns to dissociate from suffering, open novel pathways that by-pass rational control, and create new sensory-emotional associations with the previously distressing pain. Over time and with self-hypnosis practice, new neuronal sensory networks patterns and habits develop for optimal functioning and pain reduction (Jensen, 2009; Kuttner, 2010).

Educating Patients on How Pain Is Processed

Explaining how pain is processed in the body and brain is key to setting up successful hypnosis treatment. This provides crucial information in a novel cognitive frame so that catastrophic thinking patterns, fears and misguided ideas can be addressed and changed. From clinical experience, we've found that a diagram [Figure 36.1] or sketching, while explaining the physiological pain pathway from the pain-site up into the brain, and from the brain back down to the pain-site, helps the child to envision the desired change (Kuttner, 2010; Lauder & Massey, 2010) Conversational hypnosis for a younger child or someone not scientifically oriented using suggestions and invitations could go like this:

"Do you know that the brain is the Boss of the Pain? Let me show you with this picture how this works. When you feel pain, this message travels very quickly through your nerves opening these gates [Figure 36.1] to the brain. Your brain is the boss and makes sense of this message: '*Ah the pain is in my leg from kicking too hard, or the wrong way. I know this pain' (says your brain). 'I've had it before. So, if I sit down and rub it, it helps'*. Brain then immediately starts closing the gates: '*J. is rubbing her leg so those gates need to close, making the pain smaller and smaller'*. So, your Brain helps pain go away when you use one of your helpers, that we figured out makes you feel better. Isn't that great to know!"

Discussion with an older scientifically oriented child or teen could go something like this: "*Let's look at how pain works in your brain and your body, and what needs to happen for you to experience relief. Did you know the pain signal moves very rapidly from that pain into your spine (here), up to the limbic system where the thalamus, your control center in the middle of your brain, sends signals throughout the brain, to make sense of it.* ***Your brain at this point interprets the signals as 'pain'". So, your Brain is truly the Boss of the Pain,*** *figuring out if the signal is important or not, and deciding what to do. Your brain's memory decides "Have I had this before? Where did it occur? What did I do before to help it settle?" So, you draw on previous experiences: "When I lie down, do my belly breathing and my hypnosis, that makes the discomfort go down"*.

"*The amazing thing is, once your brain makes sense of the pain signal, and uses your skills, that information instantly goes down your spine closing the pain gates, so you don't feel the pain as intensely. This is your* ***downward inhibitory system*** *easing pain. The more you learn to access working with your pain system, the quicker, easier and more relief you' ll get when turning down pain signals! Isn't that cool!" "We all have this inbuilt pain-relieving system, as well as a pain-alerting system. Both are needed. The alerting/alarm system keeps you safe, and the relieving, gating system brings you comfort and a return to activity.* ***Your pain-alerting system has been over-functioning and your pain-relieving system has not been activated.*** *Using hypnosis helps the relieving system to become active and strong, closing the gates allowing you to move more comfortable and confidently and pick up your life again"*.

Understanding pain mechanisms is a crucial first step to engaging the suffering child, creating a willingness to entertain change (motivation) and a map of how this previously inconceivable change can occur, since it's a physiological, scientifically proven option. Even

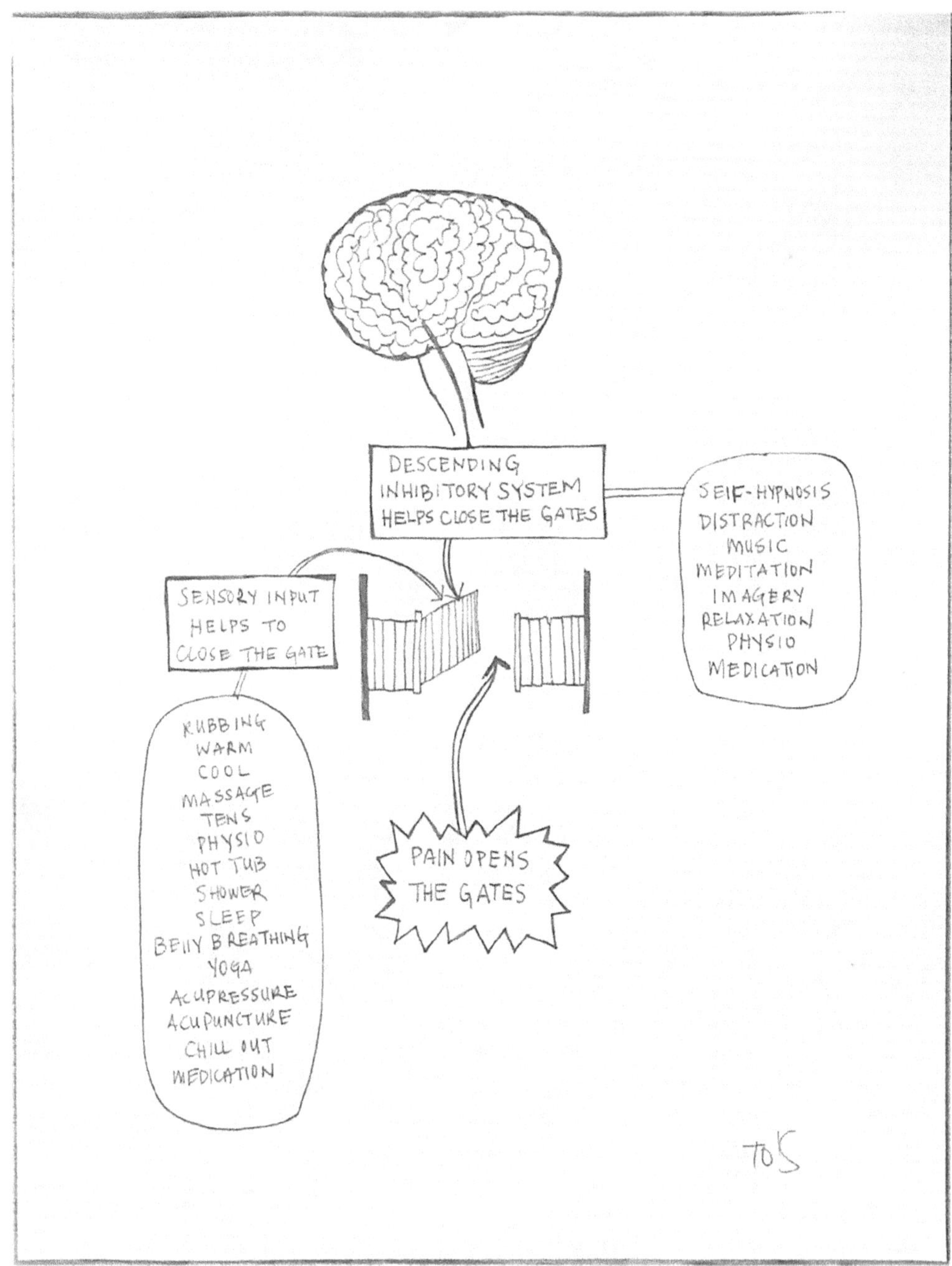

Figure 36.1 The brain's descending inhibitory influence on diminishing pain.

very young children prior to a procedure, when shown a picture of a castle with the gate open or closed can be drawn into discussing their feelings or factors that open the gate and how being absorbed into a story can close those gates, helping them cope better with the painful procedure.

Complex Chronic Pediatric Pain

Chronic and recurrent pain affects 20–25% of the child population and is commonly diagnosed when pain persists for at least three months, or when pain persists after the necessary healing period has elapsed (Treede et al., 2015). Pain clinics include the extent to which the child is not functioning and restricting activities such as school attendance, involvements with friends, sports and favorite hobbies.

The neurological process underlying the persistence of pain that occurs without injury is known as "*central sensitization*", and is now better understood as the process by which nerves become hypersensitive to minimally noxious stimulus (Woolf, 2011). Inadequately treated, severe acute pain can cause not only sensory receptors but also the central nervous system to change in structure and function. This leads to increased sensitivity so that even a small stimulus is sufficient to trigger a painful sensation. Recent research has increased our knowledge of the interacting roles of the descending inhibitory control, the neurochemistry and neurophysiology of nociceptive transmission, pain genetics and the immune and autonomic nervous systems. These factors, including trauma, depression, insomnia, create a vulnerability to pain that various triggers then amplify. Addressing and changing those factors and triggers using hypnotic metaphors within a trance and/or naturalistic hypnotic communication offer a new framework to provoke change, instill hope and provide a roadmap to recovery.

Hypnotic Metaphors Explain and Help Re-Pattern the Puzzle of Pain

Hypnotic metaphors make complex problems more accessible and understandable. They by-pass the linear rational mind, providing a creative inroad to challenging aspects of care, and reduce resistance to change, altering preconceived notions about pain (Coakley & Schechter, 2013). Most of all, metaphors provide explanatory analogies that illuminate many puzzling components.

For example:

> "That pain you're having is like a ...
>
> ... Car alarm that has become over-reactive and oversensitive despite no sign of danger. Frequently the original trigger for persisting pain has ceased or cannot be determined, but the pain system itself continues to react, transmitting pain signals".
>
> *"Have you ever noticed how some car alarms are so sensitive that when a truck or even a person walks by a parked car this sets off the car alarm? Now, the purpose of the alarm is to alert others that the car is in danger – but when there is no sign of danger it's a false alarm! Some children and teens have more sensitive nervous systems that produce false alarms that get triggered by unexpected movements or situations. Could that be the case with you?"*
>
> "That pain you're having is like a ...
>
> ... Software failure in the computer".
>
> *"Have you noticed that when your computer is not working properly, it usually has nothing to do with the inside, the hardware of the computer. Your body is your hardware, your muscles, ligaments, and bones. But it's the operating software that*

has a glitch, so we need to retrain your software system, and reboot it with hypnosis giving it new programs that work better for you".

"Maybe your pain gates are too open and we need to connect with your ...

... Pain gating system" (Melzack & Wall, 1965)

We have many gating opportunities in the spine, brain, and limbic system where pain gates can be closed so the pain signal is weakened, eased, or closed down. When the gates are open wide the signal flows through the spine up to the brain and that's where they're understood as "pain". We can close these gates physically, like rubbing the pain site, using a cold pack, taking medication, or using a TENS machine. Also focusing attention, like being in your favorite movie, traveling to a favorite place and using your imagination brain will close pain gates. We're going to practice closing these gates so that you get really good at reducing the pain, bringing comfort into your body".

This metaphor can be developed into the powerful *Pain Switch* technique discussed in the next section.

Hypnosis Techniques That Are a "Good-Fit" for Managing Pain

Favorite Place

This popular hypnotic technique relies on the process of dissociating away from the present distressing reality to a familiar/favorite place. Being absorbed into an alternate, preferred place, it becomes possible to shift sensory and emotional pain toward comfort, creating relief. This is achieved by targeting sensory experiences (visual, auditory, olfactory, sensory, and gustatory senses) so that the imaginal involvement modifies the pain sensation, creating some distance from it. In the film "*No Fears, No Tears*" 9-year-old Seana reports, "*When I go away on trips like this ... I forget about tummy pains or leg pains or feet pain, I just forget all about it!*" Children find traveling away to a favorite place, a natural effortless process. When absorbed in their favorite place, distress, pain and fatigue becomes less relevant or pressing. Providing post-hypnotic suggestions will ensure that this comfort and pain relief continues when the hypnotic trance concludes:

"You'll be surprised to notice as you return to the room, that the comfort in your favorite place comes back with you ... it's curious and feels so good ... you'll continue to feel the ease and well-being as your eyes open ... good ... so you can move-on comfortably with your day. It'll be so interesting to stay with this new experience, a sign of your new abilities to re-pattern your brain and body to create and maintain comfort".

Pain Switch (Kuttner, 2018)

This technique is body-centered. By teaming up focused, narrowed attention with deep diaphragmatic controlled breaths, the Pain Switch alters pain sensation, as the child learns to progressively "turn-down" the pain signal. In this way, patients learn to purposefully connect with their pain and create new empowering associations by regaining some control over distressing sensory experience.

Starting with an explanation of how pain is processed (Koechlin et al., 2020), the child is invited to travel into the control center in the middle of the brain (thalamus in the limbic system) where switches control different areas of the body. Once there, the child is invited to:

1 Locate the switch that controls this pain and report what number (0 ->10) the switch is on.
2 Note the "wire/nerve connections" from this switch to the pain area in the body, and from that area back up to the pain switch, while simultaneously,
3 Exhale deep belly breaths as the switch gets turned down, so body tension is released and pain signals progressively diminish.
4 Provide reports on these changing sensations, color and pain switch numbers. Importantly, the child is closely tracked by the clinician through this intense experience until arriving at a satisfactory place, *"as low as you are able, or wish to go at this time"* (Note, the goal is to achieve diminution in pain and not necessarily get to zero – which is often unrealistic with chronic pain). Variations such as using a lock to keep the switch in place can be utilized. Anecdotally, patients report that the hypnotic pain switch experience creates a different and more empowered relationship with their pain, decreasing feelings of helplessness and despair, and increasing their self-control in modulating pain and distress.

Hypnosis for Acute and Procedural Pain

The Magic Glove (Kuttner, 2014)

"Hypnotic analgesia is real, no less palpable an analgesic than medication, although the pathways are different and do not seem to involve endogenous opiates" (Spiegel, 2007, p. 1280).

Adapting "The Glove" technique to pediatrics, we've found using a warm, gentle stroking of the child or teen's hand beneficial, as the magic glove is put on, "so *that you know what's happening, and you're not bothered because you're protected by the magic glove*". The tactile hypnotic process soothes anticipatory anxiety and reduces skin sensitivity. Analgesia is tested with a pencil's sharp point, first on the non-glove hand (10/10 sensation) and then contrasted with the same pressure on the gloved hand to get a reading (10/10). If there isn't sufficient difference, the hypo-analgesia can be increased by re-applying the glove together with hypnotic suggestions, providing more time for sensory alteration, *"so that it's snug and protected, making you feel safe so that you're not bothered by anything"* (see Kuttner, 2014, ten-minute Youtube tutorial). The magic glove has a wide range of acute pain applications: IVs, IM injections, bloodwork and can be adapted to indwelling lines, Porta-caths, Hickman lines and drainage tubes.

The Meg Foundation Resources

"ImaginAction" and *"Boss of your Brain"* are animation-based, child and parent-focused using hypnotic communication to address acute and procedural pain, available online at https://www.megfoundationforpain.org

Recurrent and Chronic Pain Require Complex Approaches

As the development of chronic pain is the result of complex bio-psycho-socio processes, its therapy usually requires an equally complex approach to fully understand and successfully address the complex, multidimensional causes of the problem. Understandably, unilateral medical or invasive therapies are usually unsuccessful in the treatment of chronic pain and psychological therapies are an essential component with physical treatments for positive outcomes.

Substantial recent research evidence and case studies indicate that hypnosis is significantly effective for chronic pain-related conditions such as functional abdominal pain (FAPs) and irritable bowel syndrome (IBS) (Vlieger et al., 2012; Rutter et al., 2014; 2014), migraine and headaches (Anbar & Zoughbi, 2008; Jong et al., 2019; Kohen, 2010; Kohen, 2011; Kohen & Zajac, 2007), functional neurological disorders (Coogle et al., 2021) and multiple chronic and complex symptoms (Bastek et al., 2022).

Hypnosis, hand in hand with learning how sensitization develops, how chronic pain works on biological, psychological and social levels, and understanding the brain's ability to regulate bodily functions are the cornerstone of therapy. Usually, all hypnosis interventions start with the explanation of the nature of chronic pain (Bastek et al., 2022). Being complex, chronic pain is usually accompanied by diverse symptoms including sleep dysregulation, restricted normal physical activity, difficulties at school, reduced social relationships and mood problems.

Hypnosis can be delivered by targeting different layers of chronic pain. Treatment can focus on what's currently bothering the patient most, rather than focusing directly on pain (Delivet et al., 2018; Vlieger et al., 2007). Delivet et al.'s (2018) study taught children self-hypnosis for home practice. Clinician and child decide what most affects the child's quality of life and develop home hypnosis exercises to mitigate this. Most common problems were sleep quality, pain intensity and returning to normal physical activity. Focusing on interrelated symptoms seems to indirectly affect the intensity of the pain (Delivet et al., 2018). Bastek et al. (2022) found hypnosis intervention effective irrespective of type and number of symptoms.

Ego strengthening, increasing self-confidence and well-being with metaphors such as the "*rainbow planet*" where children choose colors from the rainbow for different needs like health, tranquility, courage or confidence, and the "*beach without worries*" where children engage with their beach and waves to release stress and strengthen their ego (Rutten et al, 2014). These general experiences target underlying psychosocial issues and related emotions. Gulewitsch and Schlarb (2017) found no significant difference between using symptom-driven or general hypnosis.

Gut-directed hypnosis, a popular intervention, directly addresses the primary symptom. Children with FAPs or IBS were taught to gain control over their gut function. Vlieger et al. (2007) utilized the metaphor of *"running your car at a smooth, normal speed through the tunnel enhancing your bowel's normal smooth function"*. Beneficial pain reduction effects of hypnosis endured for five years beyond the termination of therapy (Vlieger et al., 2012). In a follow-up study, researchers provided patients with self-hypnosis audio-recordings for home practice and found significant long-term benefits (Rutten et al., 2013, 2014). Recently these researchers reported that 80% of their patients had adequate abdominal relief at six-year follow-up (Rexwinkel et al., 2022). These long-term beneficial outcomes for chronic pain are highly encouraging.

Hypnosis for End of Life and Palliative Care

Hypnosis has been effectively integrated into advanced multimodal end-of-life therapies to support seriously ill children and teens dealing with loss and anticipatory loss. Often the therapeutic focus is to sustain and enhance their hope so that they can live fully, until death. Hypnosis also helps to address distressing symptoms at end of life such as dyspnea, nausea, vomiting, pain and anxiety (Friedrichsdorf & Kohen, 2018). Pain management, in all of its forms, together with using a variety of hypnotic phenomena provides relief from suffering, which is desperately desired by children whose disease and its treatments consume many, if not most waking hours of each day. Teaching a child self-hypnosis as part of a multimodal approach in end-of-life treatment provides a supportive technique to deal with life and death concerns, and can bolster the child's inner strength. Meaningful experiences can be rekindled within hypnotic imaginative engagement so that pain is lessened and anxiety diminished. Clinicians caring for seriously ill teens and children can benefit by adding hypnosis as a versatile intervention within their skill set.

Final Thoughts

Pediatric hypnosis is solution-focused, relationship-based and a fundamentally optimistic treatment for a wide range of acute, recurrent, complex chronic or end-of-life pediatric pain conditions (Kuttner, 2020). As treatment for pain relief, it requires developmental sensitivity and adaptability in approach, language and metaphors to create optimal hypnosis experiences.

Using hypnosis to treat pediatric pain is beyond the "quick-fix pill" solution and can therefore meet with some resistance by stressed parents and weary or despairing children. Building a collaborative framework in which the physiology of pain processing is explained helps engage more productively with this resistance. Beyond that, using pediatric hypnosis as an intervention requires a willingness to trust oneself as clinician, to take the time to creatively explore and develop solutions within a respectful relationship with a child. Pediatric hypnosis can be used to stir hope, motivate and provide essential education on the mind–body interaction. It demands we respect individual temperament and developmental needs and adapt techniques for a best fit with each child – all the time cultivating creative resilience and holding the conviction that there is a way through this pain to gain relief.

References

Anand, K. J. S., Sippell, W. G., & Aynsley-Green, A. (1987). Randomised trial of fentanyl anaesthesia in preterm babies undergoing surgery: Effects on the stress response. *The Lancet*, *329*(8524), 62–66. 10.1016/s0140-6736(87)91907-6

Anbar, R. D., & Zoughbi, G. G. (2008). Relationship of headache-associated stressors and hypnosis therapy outcome in children: A retrospective chart review. *American Journal of Clinical Hypnosis*, *50*(4), 335–341. 10.1080/00029157.2008.10404300

Bastek, V. B., Groeneveld, E. M., & Van Vliet, M. J. (2022). Medical hypnotherapy; even in a tertiary care setting a promising treatment. *International Journal of Contemporary Pediatrics*, *9*(5), 418. 10.18203/2349-3291.ijcp20221065

Birnie, K. A., Noel, M., Parker, J. D., Chambers, C. T., Uman, L. S., Kisely, S., & McGrath, P. J. (2014). Systematic review and meta-analysis of distraction and hypnosis for needle-related pain and distress in children and adolescents. *Journal of Pediatric Psychology*, *39*(8), 783–808. 10.1093/jpepsy/jsu029

Butler, L. M., Symons, B. K., Henderson, S. L., Shortliffe, L. D., & Spiegel, D. (2005). Hypnosis reduces distress and duration of an invasive medical procedure for children. *Pediatrics*, *115*(1), e77–e85. 10.1542/peds.2004-0818

Carlson, T., Kuttner, L., MacLeod, K., & Fletcher, B. (2018, August). Changing hospital culture: Training program in medical hypnosis for paediatric staff. Symposium presented at the *XXI World Congress of Medical and Clinical Hypnosis*, Montreal, Canada.

Coakley, R., & Schechter, N. (2013). Chronic pain is like … The clinical use of analogy and metaphor in the treatment of chronic pain in children. *Pediatric Pain Letter*, *15*(1), 1–8.

Coogle, J., Coogle, B., & Quezada, J. (2021). Hypnosis in the treatment of pediatric functional neurological disorder: The Magic Glove Technique. *Pediatric Neurology*, *125*, 20–25. 10.1016/j.pediatrneurol.2021.08.011

Delivet, H., Dugue, S., Ferrari, A., Postone, S., & Dahmani, S. (2018). Efficacy of self-hypnosis on quality of life for children with chronic pain syndrome. *International Journal of Clinical and Experimental Hypnosis*, *66*(1), 43–55. 10.1080/00207144.2018.1396109

Dienstfrey, H. (1991). *Where the mind meets the body: Type A, the relaxation response, psychoneuroimmunology, biofeedback, neuropeptides, hypnosis, imagery, and the search for the mind's effect on physical health* (1st ed.). HarperCollins Publishers.

Esparham, A., Herbert, A., Pierzchalski, E., Tran, C. G., Dilts, J. J., Boorigie, M., Wingert, T., Connelly, M. L., & Bickel, J. (2018). Pediatric headache clinic model: Implementation of integrative therapies in practice. *Children*, *5*(6), 74. 10.3390/children5060074

Fisher, E., Law, E. F., Dudeney, J., Palermo, T. M., Stewart, G. B., Eccleston, C., & Pain, P. C. (2018). Psychological therapies for the management of chronic and recurrent pain in children and adolescents. *The Cochrane Library – Cochrane Database of Systematic Reviews*. 10.1002/14651858.cd003968.pub5

Friedrichsdorf, S. J., & Goubert, L. (2020). Pediatric pain treatment and prevention for hospitalized children. *Pain Reports*, *5*(1), e804. 10.1097/pr9.0000000000000804

Friedrichsdorf, S. J., & Kohen, D. P. (2018). Integration of hypnosis into pediatric palliative care. *Annals of Palliative Medicine*, *7*(1), 136–150. 10.21037/apm.2017.05.02

Grunau, R. E. (2002). Early pain in preterm infants: A model of long-term effects. *Clinics in Perinatology*, *29*(3), 373–394. 10.1016/s0095-5108(02)00012-x

Gulewitsch, M. D., & Schlarb, A. (2017). Comparison of gut-directed hypnotherapy and unspecific hypnotherapy as self-help format in children and adolescents with functional abdominal pain or irritable bowel syndrome: A randomized pilot study. *European Journal of Gastroenterology & Hepatology*, *29*(12), 1351–1360. 10.1097/meg.0000000000000984

Jensen, M. P. (2009). Hypnosis for chronic pain management: A new hope. *Pain*, *146*(3), 235–237. 10.1016/j.pain.2009.06.027

Jong, M. C., Boers, I., Van Wietmarschen, H., Tromp, E., Busari, J. O., Wennekes, R., Snoeck, I. N., Bekhof, J., & Vlieger, A. M. (2019). Hypnotherapy or transcendental meditation versus progressive muscle relaxation exercises in the treatment of children with primary headaches: A multicentre, pragmatic, randomised clinical study. *European Journal of Pediatrics*, *178*(2), 147–154. 10.1007/s00431-018-3270-3

Katz, E. R., Kellerman, J., & Siegel, S. E. (1980). Behavioral distress in children with cancer undergoing medical procedures: Developmental considerations. *Journal of Consulting and Clinical Psychology*, *48*(3), 356–365. 10.1037/0022-006x.48.3.356

Kohen, D. P. (2010). Long-term follow-up of self-hypnosis training for recurrent headaches: What the children say. *International Journal of Clinical and Experimental Hypnosis*, *58*(4), 417–432. 10.1080/00207144.2010.499342

Kohen, D. P. (2011). Chronic daily headache: Helping adolescents help themselves with self-hypnosis. *American Journal of Clinical Hypnosis*, *54*(1), 32–46. 10.1080/00029157.2011.566767

Kohen, D. P., & Zajac, R. (2007). Self-hypnosis training for headaches in children and adolescents. *The Journal of Pediatrics*, *150*(6), 635–639. 10.1016/j.jpeds.2007.02.014

Koechlin, H., Locher, C., & Prchal, A. (2020). Talking to children and families about chronic pain: The importance of pain education – An introduction for pediatricians and other health care providers. *Children*, *7*(10), 179. 10.3390/children7100179

Kuttner, L. (1986). *No fears, no tears – Children with cancer coping with pain* [Video; DVD, 28 mins, Documentary]. Crown House Publishing. https://www.crownhouse.co.uk/no-fears-no-tears-dvd
Kuttner, L., Bowman, M., & Teasdale, M. (1988). Psychological treatment of distress, pain and anxiety for young children with cancer. *Journal of Developmental and Behavioral Pediatrics* 9(6), 374–381. DOI: 10.1097/00004703-198812000-00010
Kuttner, L. (1998). *No fears, no tears – 13 years later* [Video; DVD, 46 mins, Documentary]. Crown House Publishing. https://www.crownhouse.co.uk/no-fears-no-tears-13-years-later-dvd
Kuttner, L. (2010). *A child in pain: What health professionals can do to help* (1st ed.). Crown House Publishing.
Kuttner, L. (2012). Pediatric hypnosis: pre-, peri-, and post-anesthesia. *Pediatric Anesthesia, 22*(6), 573–577. 10.1111/j.1460-9592.2012.03860.x
Kuttner, L., (2014, January 20). *The magic glove: Hypnotic pain management for children* [Video]. YouTube. Retrieved March 9, 2023, from https://youtu.be/cyApK8Z_SQQ
Kuttner, L. (2018). The pain switch for teens with complex pain. Chapter 13. In M. P. Jensen (Ed.), *Hypnotic techniques for chronic pain management: Favorite methods of master clinicians (2) (Voices of experience)* (1st ed., np). Denny Creek Press.
Kuttner, L. (2020). Pediatric hypnosis: Treatment that adds and rarely subtracts. *International Journal of Clinical and Experimental Hypnosis, 68*(1), 16–28. 10.1080/00207144.2020.1685329
Kuttner, L., & Friedrichsdorf, S. J. (2007). Hypnosis and palliative care. In L. I. Sugarman & W. C. Wester (Eds.), *Therapeutic hypnosis with children and adolescents* (1st ed., pp. 491–509). Crown House Publishing.
Lauder, G. R., & Massey, R. (2010). *Complex regional pain syndrome (CRPS) explained: For teenagers, by teenagers.* Xlibris.
Liossi, C., White, P. D., & Hatira, P. (2009). A randomized clinical trial of a brief hypnosis intervention to control venepuncture-related pain of paediatric cancer patients. *Pain, 142*(3), 255–263. 10.1016/j.pain.2009.01.017
Lobe, T. E. (2007). Perioperative hypnosis. In L. I. Sugarman & W. C. Wester (Eds.), *Therapeutic hypnosis with children and adolescents* (1st ed., pp. 333–355). Crown House Publishing.
Maxym, M. (2008). *Hypnosis for relief of pain and anxiety in children receiving intravenous lines in the pediatric emergency department* [Open Access Thesis]. Yale Medicine Thesis Digital Library. 355. Retrieved March 9, 2023, from https://elischolar.library.yale.edu/ymtdl/355
McCaffery, M. (1968). *Nursing practice theories related to cognition, bodily pain, and man-environment interactions.* UCLA Students' Store.
Melzack, R. (1973). *The puzzle of pain.* Penguin Books.
Melzack, R., & Wall, P. D. (1965). Pain mechanisms: A new theory: A gate control system modulates sensory input from the skin before it evokes pain perception and response. *Science, 150*(3699), 971–979. 10.1126/science.150.3699.971
Noel, M., Palermo, T. M., Chambers, C. T., Taddio, A., & Hermann, C. (2015). Remembering the pain of childhood: Applying a developmental perspective to the study of pain memories. *Pain, 156*(1), 31–34. 10.1016/j.pain.0000000000000001
Olmsted, R. W., Zeltzer, L. K., & LeBaron, S. (1982). Hypnosis and nonhypnotic techniques for reduction of pain and anxiety during painful procedures in children and adolescents with cancer. *The Journal of Pediatrics, 101*(6), 1032–1035. 10.1016/s0022-3476(82)80040-1
Peebles-Kleiger, M. J. (2000). The use of hypnosis in emergency medicine. *Emergency Medicine Clinics of North America, 18*(2), 327–338. 10.1016/s0733-8627(05)70128-0
Rexwinkel, R., Bovendeert, J. F., Rutten, J. M. T. M., Frankenhuis, C., Benninga, M. A., & Vlieger, A. M. (2022). Long-term follow-up of individual therapist delivered and standardized hypnotherapy recordings in pediatric irritable bowel syndrome or functional abdominal pain. *Journal of Pediatric Gastroenterology and Nutrition, 75*(1), 24–29. 10.1097/mpg.0000000000003478
Rogovik, A. L., & Goldman, R. D. (2007). Hypnosis for treatment of pain in children. *Canadian Family Physician, 53*(5), 823–825. Retrieved March 10, 2023, from https://www.cfp.ca/content/53/5/823
Rosdahl, C. B., & Kowalski, M. T. (2007). *Textbook of basic nursing.* Lippincott Williams & Wilkins.
Rutten, J. M. T. M., Reitsma, J. B., Vlieger, A. M., & Benninga, M. A. (2013). Gut-directed hypnotherapy for functional abdominal pain or irritable bowel syndrome in children: A systematic review. *Archives of Disease in Childhood, 98*(4), 252–257. 10.1136/archdischild-2012-302906

Rutten, J. M., Vlieger, A. M., Frankenhuis, C., George, E. K., Groeneweg, M., Norbruis, O. F., Tjon a Ten, W., Van Wering, H., Dijkgraaf, M. G. W., Merkus, M. P. & Benninga, M. A. (2014). Gut-directed hypnotherapy in children with irritable bowel syndrome or functional abdominal pain (syndrome): A randomized controlled trial on self exercises at home using CD versus individual therapy by qualified therapists. *BMC Pediatrics*, *14*(1), 1–8 10.1186/1471-2431-14-140

Schechter, N. L., Berde, C. B., & Yaster, M. (Eds.). (2003). *Pain in infants, children, and adolescents.* Lippincott Williams & Wilkins.

Spiegel, D. (2007). The mind prepared: Hypnosis in surgery. *Journal of the National Cancer Institute*, *99*(17), 1280–1281. 10.1093/jnci/djm131

Spiegel, D., & Albert, L. H. (1983). Naloxone fails to reverse hypnotic alleviation of chronic pain. *Psychopharmacology*. 10.1007/bf00429008

Swafford, L. I., & Allan, D. S. (1968). Pain relief in the pediatric patient. *Medical Clinics of North America*, *52*(1), 131–136. 10.1016/s0025-7125(16)32952-2

Treede, R., Rief, W., Barke, A., Aziz, Q., Bennett, M. J., Benoliel, R., Cohen, M., Evers, S., Finnerup, N. B., First, M. B., Giamberardino, M. A., Kaasa, S., Kosek, E., Lavand'homme, P., Nicholas, M. K., Perrot, S., Scholz, J., Schug, S. A., Smith, B. H., ... Wang, S. J. (2015). A classification of chronic pain for ICD-11. *Pain*, *156*(6), 1003–1007. 10.1097/j.pain.0000000000000160

Tsao, J. C. I., & Zeltzer, L. K. (2005). Complementary and alternative medicine approaches for pediatric pain: A review of the state-of-the-science. *Evidence-Based Complementary and Alternative Medicine*, *2*(2), 149–159. 10.1093/ecam/neh092

Vlieger, A. M., Menko-Frankenhuis, C., Wolfkamp, S. C., Tromp, E., & Benninga, M. A. (2007). Hypnotherapy for children with functional abdominal pain or irritable bowel syndrome: A randomized controlled trial. *Gastroenterology*, *133*(5), 1430–1436. 10.1053/j.gastro.2007.08.072

Vlieger, A. M., Rutten, J. M., Govers, A. M., Frankenhuis, C., & Benninga, M. A. (2012). Long-term follow-up of gut-directed hypnotherapy vs. Standard care in children with functional abdominal pain or irritable bowel syndrome. *The American Journal of Gastroenterology*, *107*(4), 627–631. 10.1038/ajg.2011.487

Wood, C., & Bioy, A. (2008). Hypnosis and pain in children. *Journal of Pain and Symptom Management*, *35*(4), 437–446. 10.1016/j.jpainsymman.2007.05.009

Woolf, C. J. (2011). Central sensitization: Implications for the diagnosis and treatment of pain. *Pain*, *152*(3), S2–S15. 10.1016/j.pain.2010.09.030

Zernikow, B., Michel, E., Craig, F., & Anderson, B. D. (2009). Pediatric palliative care. *Pediatric Drugs*, *11*(2), 129–151. 10.2165/00148581-200911020-00004

37

CLINICAL USE OF HYPNOSIS IN PEDIATRIC DENTISTRY

Randi Abrahamsen

(Retired from), Section for Orofacial Pain and Jaw Function, Department of Dentistry and Oral Health, Aarhus University, Aarhus C, Denmark

Background

As a dentist I have used hypnosis in dentistry for more than 35 years providing private dental practice and also Community Dental Service care for children, adolescents, elderly, and people with physical and mental disabilities. I previously taught and lectured in the Section of Orofacial Pain and Jaw Function, Department of Dentistry and Oral Health, Aarhus University, where I was involved in orofacial pain research and hypnosis. My PhD thesis was entitled *Effect of Hypnosis on Persistent Orofacial Pain – in a Neurobiological Perspective* and I published articles in international journals. I am a teacher, trainer, supervisor, and past president of the Danish Society of Clinical Hypnosis. I give lectures and workshops and train health care staff in communication and hypnosis. I am the author of *Hypnosis and Communication in Dentistry* (Abrahamsen, 2020). I am a board member of the European Society of Hypnosis.

Theoretical Framework: Approaches and Principles in Pediatric Dentistry

This chapter will focus on hypnotic techniques that can help children develop their resources to overcome dental fear (DF), anxiety, phobia for dental treatment, and other significant problems. DF refers to an unpleasant emotional reaction to a specific threatening stimulus occurring in situations associated with dental treatment. In childhood, it is considered a normal adaptive response. Dental anxiety (DA) is a nonspecific, excessive, and unreasonable negative emotional reaction to the anticipation of a future threatening experience such as the dental treatment. Dental phobia (DP) denotes a severe type of DA and is characterized by marked and persistent anxiety in relation to either clearly discernible situations or objects (e.g., drilling, injections) or to the dental situation in general (Klingberg & Broberg, 2007). Children who suffer from these conditions are a common time-consuming problem in dentistry. Prevalence rates vary from 13.3% to 29.3% among countries and decrease with maturing (Cianetti et al., 2017). Children with psychological difficulties may have problems coping with dental treatment (Balian et al., 2021).

DOI: 10.4324/9781003449126-50

In several countries, nitrous oxide/oxygen inhalation sedation (N2O) is widely and effectively used to help the children cope with dental treatment (Veerkamp et al., 1993; Hennequin et al., 2012). However, when a child has major difficulties in coping with urgent dental treatment and shows behavioral management problems, other solutions may have to be used. One expensive option is to perform the dental treatment with general anesthesia (GA). A less costly option during conscious sedation (CS) is the use of, for example, Midazolam (Ashley et al., 2018). In some countries, the child might even be fixated protectively during the CS to lie still for the dental treatment (Davis et al., 2016). The use of Midazolam in higher doses may cause side effects, especially paradoxical reactions (Somri et al., 2012). GA will solve the dental problem, but the anxiety will remain or it might even be aggravated. In fact, it has been pointed out that dental treatment with GA does not enable the anxious child to return for normative dental care (Savanheimo et al., 2012).

Commonly Used Principles in Pediatric Dentistry

Principles that give the child a sense of control over the dental procedure and create predictability with every step in the treatment are commonly used to prevent DA. For children presenting with low levels of DF or DA, approaches would include tell-show-do (explain the procedure, show the instrument, rehearse the procedure), voice control, distraction, modeling, memory reconstruction, positive reinforcement, relaxation training, magic tricks, and positive images. Children with moderate levels of DF or DA may require more intensive interventions, such as providing them with information on coping strategies, while children who exhibit DP may benefit from the complementary use of pharmacological and psychological approaches, especially cognitive behavioral therapy (CBT) (Newton et al., 2012).

Intraoral injection phobia has been treated successfully in a setting with dentists, who have had a special training in CBT (Berge et al., 2017). A special chair-site psychological approach including behavioral interventions and CBT has been effective for children (including children with disabilities) suffering from DF at a two-year follow-up (Kankaala et al., 2019).

These studies suggest that the use of hypnosis in combination with these techniques could be even more beneficial for the child. The communication skills of the dentist seem to be the main factor in developing the ability of the anxious child to cope with dental treatment (Schouten et al., 2003; Ten Berge et al., 2002). A dentist trained in hypnosis develops great communication skills, is trained to establish rapport with the child, able to observe minimal cues of changes in the body language of the child. A benefit of hypnosis can be the ability to perform the dental treatment in an anxious child without medicines and eventually the anxiety would fade. It is very essential that we dentists consider expanding our role. We should not only treat the decayed teeth, but also be coaches, who help the child develop resources and overcome the anxiety of dental treatment.

Effect of Hypnosis on Children's Dental Fear and Anxiety

Unfortunately, the evidence of the clinical use of hypnosis in pediatric dentistry is limited to very few studies. Authors of case reports and narrative reviews recommend the use of hypnosis in pediatric dentistry (Peretz, 1996; Peretz et al., 2013). Elements from the use of hypnosis in children undergoing painful procedures in medical settings and from the use of hypnosis in dental settings for adults could be adapted to pediatric dentistry. Controlled studies have demonstrated the effectiveness of hypnosis on the acceptance of local anesthetic (LA) injection in children. Compared to control, use of hypnosis demonstrated fewer undesirable behaviors (i.e., movement, physical resistance, and leg movement) together with a lower pulse rate (Gokli et al., 1994) and reduced preoperative anxiety and pain (Huet et al., 2011).

Dental treatment under CS with a low dose Midazolam in combination with hypnosis has been shown to effectively reduce the anxiety level and to improve children's negative behavior in a larger retrospective longitudinal practice-based observational study (Rienhoff et al., 2022).

Approaches and Clinical Implications

When a child cannot cope with dental treatment, we can look for what resources they have in other areas of life. It is hard to access resources when anxious. With simple techniques dentists can help the child to get in contact with their resourceful part. I think this is what we all have been doing intuitively as dentists, when we meet our young nervous patients, asking them about friends, holidays, and sports to calm them down before dental treatment. But with hypnosis, we can take it a step further.

It has always been important to me that children would be able to have treatment with another dentist. The children should not be depending on me, but develop their own resources and sense of control with the dental treatment. Before performing the actual dental treatment, I play with the children according to their age and maturity. During the play, I use the *tell-show-do* principle to guide and familiarize the child with sounds and sensations throughout every step of the dental treatment.

I work with two elements:

1 *Desensitization* (not in hypnosis). Teach the children about the dental treatment. Step by step we enact each phase of the dental treatment: the injection, the drilling, and the filling. The child and I perform the dental treatment on a cast model. The children hold the instruments and I help them and support their hand, when they hold the syringe, use the drill on the tooth model, etc. In this way, the children become familiar with the process and instruments of the treatment. In every step, I read every little minimal cue of anxiety in the body language of the children (breathing, wrinkling of eyebrows, shrinking of shoulders, etc.) with the purpose of addressing the anxiety at that stage and preventing it from overwhelming the child. When the actual treatment is performed, the predictability of each step will help the child to cope with dental treatment.
2 *Develop resources in hypnosis.* With the use of ego-state methods (Watkins & Watkins,1978; Philips & Frederick, 1995), the resources of the children to cope with dental treatment are developed. In children, who have had a painful bad experience with the drill, a reframing of the sound of the drilling machine is used. (An example is given later.)

Invite Yourself to the Children's Universe

In this first playful interview with the child, I would notice and remember every word, that make the child's eye sparkle and use the words later in trance to develop resources.

I become familiar with the children's interest: friends, favorite sport, film, computer games, action heroes, songs, bedtime story, pets. These words are used to create a safe place with a favorite activity. With younger children, I often sit with them and ask them to make a drawing of things they like. It is a familiar situation for children and I can ask questions and praise the drawing. Later I might ask them to draw, what makes them feel afraid.

Case a 12-Year-Old Boy with Dental Anxiety

P was afraid of the drill and pain and refused to have dental treatment. He had some bad experiences with painful dental treatment, where local analgesia did not work. At our first meeting, he was very shy, just looking at his feet as he entered the room and sat in the chair. He said hello in a low voice and shook hands avoiding eye contact. But when I asked him, what he liked to do, he suddenly looked up finding my eyes and started to talk hesitantly at first, then vividly about football and a match he had played yesterday. I said: *I can hear football means a lot to you, tell me some more about it ... how do you fell when you play football?* He replied sitting up strong and forcefully in the chair: *Oh ... I like football so much. I feel strong, free, and fast. I feel the support of my friends when we are playing, I can tackle through everything.*

TRANCE

I used his words to create a nice hypnotic trance safe place is playing football ... *Where everything is just like you want it to be, where you can feel strong, free, and fast. You feel, that you can be so strong ... that you can tackle through everything with the support of your friends, you know you have the support ... you know you are so strong and can tackle everything.*

ANCHORING THE RESOURCEFUL FEELING IN THE BODY

P is now in contact with his powerful resources. We anchored this resource physically in his body. *Tell me about your powerful strong feeling tackling through everything. Where do you feel your strong feeling in your body?* He answered: *My strong feeling is all the way down in my spine.*

I asked P to remember his strong feeling in the body while suggesting different sensory modalities. *I would like you to find a way to remember your strong feeling, you can remember it as a color, a melody, a symbol or like the strong feeling down through your spine. Just find your own best way to remember it and let me know.* P replies soon: *I will remember my strong red ribbon down through my spine.*

FUTURE PACING

I asked P to imagine just like magic some situations, where it could be useful to have his red strong ribbon in his spine. I asked him to tackle through these situations just the way he wanted it to be with the feeling of his red strong ribbon through the spine. He imagined and changed a few unpleasant situations from school. P was trained in all the dental equipment and the sound of the drill was reframed in hypnosis (see later). P imagined that the sound of the drill was a moped he was riding going on a fun adventure. After this reframing he was able to cope with dental treatment.

Ego-States as Metaphors

The methods I use in the treatment of a dental phobic child have its roots in Ericksonian hypnosis and positive psychology. Learning the child's interests I build on them to develop the positive resources within the child. Together we work toward the common goal, i.e., to be able to cope with dental treatment. Sometimes it is enough that the children get in contact with their resources or strength, but other times I have to work with the inner part, that holds the anxiety in ego-states. Often an anxious child is unable to tell what he or she is afraid of and only says: "*I am so afraid*" and cannot remember any painful or traumatic experience. The traumatic experience might have been walled off from the memory.

Ego-state therapy was described in the 1970s by John and Helen Watkins (Watkins & Watkins, 1978). The aim of ego-state therapy is to make the boundaries between the different behavioral and experiential ego-states more permeable, serving the person by a greater unity by improving communication between the ego-states. Looking at a child suffering from DP, we can see that the child has a traumatic part, which has frozen in some experience related to anxiety for dental treatment. The traumatic part has boundaries and has no access to other parts of the child with, for example, courage and success in coping with difficult things in other aspects of life. With healing communication, the different parts can be integrated. The traumatic part can be healed and the anxiety dissolves. Philips and Frederick (1995) describe in their book *Healing the Divided Self* (Philips & Frederick, 1995) the SARI model, a four-step treatment. **SARI** stands for 1: **S**afety and stabilization. 2: **A**ccessing trauma material. 3: **R**esolving traumatic experiences. 4: **I**ntegration and new identity.

A dentist is not a psychologist and should therefore not do psychotherapy. On the other hand, we often have to solve acute pain problems. We should be able to save the tooth if it is treated soon, but this may lead to traumatizing the anxious child further. In my country, we have unfortunately long waiting lists to get psychological help for children. For more than 15 years, I have used this method and found it to be safe way to work with children. The method builds on the SARI model used in a metaphoric way.

Stage 1: Safety with Ego-Strengthening

In trance the child finds a safe, wonderful place: the good feeling in the body it gives the child being in the safe place is anchored with the modality suitable for the child. Positive age regression to a good experience with for example the feeling of being brave and overcome a challenging task is retrieved and anchored in a similar way. A symbol or a metaphor for a resourceful ego-state is created. At the safe place the child finds a *Helper, who is there somewhere ... in your special place only to help you.* The child might find a pet, a fairytale creature, an animal, a cartoon figure, a hero from computer game, a movie or sports star. In the following the Helper is a lion. The child gets in contact with the *lion*, plays with the lion, or even goes on an adventure with the *lion*. The *Lion* is always there for the child and will help and give the child all that is needed. The *lion* is anchored and the child is asked to think about the lion whenever it is needed and every evening at bedtime. At following sessions new *Helpers* might occur.

Stage 2: Accessing Trauma Material

The traumatic part in the child is symbolized by a special being who needs help (*a wounded part*). It could be a flower, a pet, a fairytale creature, an animal, a cartoon figure, a character from a computer game, movie, or sports. In the following an afraid, lonely, injured cat is the *Wounded Being.*

Stage 3: Resolving Traumatic Experiences

When the child finds the cat together with the *lion,* the child and the lion help the cat with everything it needs. Suggestions like the following are given: *It is like magic in a fairytale ... you have all the capacities, all the skills to do, whatever is needed to help the cat ...* The child and the lion might hold, comfort, and heal the cat and provide whatever is needed until the cat is healed and happy. The cat also receives the experience of courage or braveness the child senses in its body (previously found at the safe place or with the positive age regression).

The feelings carried by the traumatic ego-state as a result of a traumatic event symbolized by *Wounded Being* can be reconstructed and renegotiated. The traumatic part integrates with the resourceful ego-states *Helpers.* There could be several *Wounded Beings* that need to be taken care of and new Helpers occurring to help. When everything is fine in the child's hypnotic world, the treatment can move to stage 4.

Stage 4: Integration of New Identity

At this step, the child should also be familiar with all phases of the dental treatment, as explained in the desensitization above. The child should have no fear, when exposed to the different steps of the desensitization. The child is now helped to further develop skills to cope with treatment. A future progression (*pacing*) in trance is suggested, where a relaxed friend is having dental treatment. The child watches together with the *lion* or they may even participate in the treatment. *We have played through all the phases of repairing a tooth, you are the expert, now you use all your knowledge to help your friend have a nice experience repairing the tooth. A kind nice dentist is listening and helping with every wish to make things so easy.* In the following step, the child together with his friend watches the lion relaxed having dental treatment. At the last step, the child is relaxed while having the dental treatment with the support of the friend and the *lion.* Should any difficulties in coping occur during these progressions, I would go back and work with it in both desensitization and the ego-state in hypnosis.

Healing Metaphor Stories

Telling metaphor stories will engage the child, facilitate the child's identification with the problem, and have the child join the search for solution (Burns, 2004). Approaching end of the hypnotic session, I tell healing stories, which gives the child time to integrate the new skills learned during stages 2, 3, and 4 of ego-state work. *Just listen to a nice story, while you play with all the friends you made and helped today.* Healing stories by George W. Burns (2004) *101 Healing Stories for Kids and Teens* are recommendable.

The Pain Reflex Conditioned by the Sound of the Drill

Hypnosis is an effective way to create changes in the nervous system from sympathetic activation (activated during anxiety and pain) to parasympathetic (during relaxation). According to the theory of state-dependent learning, once a child has had a painful experience during the drilling of a tooth, the sympathetic system will be activated. The pain experience will be associated to the sound of the drill. As with Pavlov's dogs, a conditioned reflex is developed. When the child hears the sound of the drill at a later appointment, the memories of the unpleasant pain experience are triggered automatically and a feeling of pain starts to evolve. Often an expression like *I hate the sound of the drill. I feel the pain in my tooth immediately* would be a sign of a conditioned pain reflex that needs to be deconditioned with hypnosis.

Every dentist can desensitize the child to the sound of the drill, but when it is done in hypnosis it is easier and quicker. In hypnosis, a new conditioned reflex of staying relaxed and calm where the parasympathetic system is active can be created. The sound of the drill can be anchored to nice, wonderful, happy memories and feelings of being brave and strong.

Reframing of the Drill in Hypnosis

After developing a safe place and building resources, the child (P from the case above) is gradually introduced to the sound of the highspeed drill without the dental burr, preferably together with suction, while counting from 1 to 10 paired with the child's exhalation. I start with the drill at a distance, for example over P's abdomen, and gradually move closer to P's mouth. Stepwise in the following order still counting from 1 to 10 at each step: the drill at the chest, under his lower jaw, outside his mouth with the mouth closed, outside his mouth with the mouth open, in his mouth, next to his tooth, to finally let the drill head (still without burr in the hand piece) touch a tooth chosen by him. It is intended that the vibrations of the drill head be felt on the tooth. Each step must be acceptable for P before proceeding to the next step; otherwise, this step is repeated until full acceptance and comfortable reactions are seen in P. Positive, self-reinforcing, calm breathing suggestions are spoken on an ongoing basis. The desensitization might need to be repeated later. In this way, the reflexive response to the drill is deconditioned. The sound of the drill is no longer associated with pain and anxiety, but instead with relaxation and calm. In fact, it can be a posthypnotic cue to relaxation. The transition to the actual drilling of a cavity actually becomes almost imperceptible to the child.

Hypnosis and Management of Children's Digit Sucking

Case: A Seven-Year-Old Girl Sucking Her Thumb Excessively

R had a 10 mm overbite and insufficient lip closure. She sucked her thumb for many hours during the day, especially in school, when she was anxious and at bedtime. Her thumb was very sore. All the usual advice to stop the habit had been unsuccessful. Sometimes it would help to hold her father's hand, when she was falling asleep. He worked nightshifts so it wasn't always possible.

R was treated successfully in three sessions with hypnosis. Her dreamland was an Adventureland with castles and princesses. A good feeling in the stomach was anchored as pink balloon. The *Helper*, who could help her stop the habit, appeared as a big, good natured, calm black dog. She describes that the dog takes care of her and makes her feel safe. When she rests her hand in the dog's fur, there is no need to suck on the thumb. The feeling of the dad's hand at bedtime and the feeling of the dog's fur under her hand are anchored and used as cues to feel safe in stressful situations, where she usually would suck her thumb. During the sessions together with the dog, she finds, helps, and heals some *Wounded Beings:* a crying baby all alone, a cat with no one to play with, a squirrel afraid of the darkness, a baby bird fallen out of the nest, a flower in the need of water, and a lost princess. At the last session they all play happily together. The first session (with the exception of the *Wounded Being*) is recorded for the girl to help her practice her new skill. After six weeks, she manages to cope with difficulties without sucking her thump and her thump is fine again. At follow-up six months later, she can close her lips and the overjet is reduced.

Gagging Management in Children with the Use of Hypnosis

I have always considered the gagging reflex as an expression of an ego-state. Like in the other cases, working in hypnosis with externalization of the ego-state as metaphor is a safe and easy method to help children overcome the gagging.

Case: A Eight-Year-Old Girl with Severe Gagging

T always had difficulties with gagging. When her parents try to brush her teeth, it is often a big fight, T would usually end up gagging and crying. The dentist has only been able to look at the front teeth with a mirror and X-ray is impossible. Now T has pain and decayed teeth. The dentist is considering treatment in GA. T had an adeno- and tonsillectomy at age four and has had many problems with ear infections. T cannot remember anything that might have triggered the gagging. She had once a very bad experience with an angry dental nurse, who tried to force T to have an X-ray taken. T was treated successfully in two hypnosis sessions. After the first session, she was able to have her teeth brushed and after the second session, she was able to have dental treatment without any problems. Interestingly, T spontaneously healed two ego-states corresponding to traumatic experiences (X-ray and adenectomy) in her real life.

In hypnosis, T dreamed of a nice trip to Disneyland, where she was on a marvelous ride in the roller coaster. T anchored a feeling of happiness and courage in her stomach. I invited T to find a *Helper*, who would help T to examine, what it is, that controls the gagging. Minnie Mouse appeared as the helper and they went on the roller coaster in T's body to find out. In the throat they find some ugly, big, black vomiting trolls. Minnie Mouse grows very big and kicks the trolls out. T states that she now can breathe freely with plenty of air. I ask T to imagine her mother brushing her teeth while T is relaxing and feels she can breathe freely and have plenty of air. At the second session, she can have X-rays taken with a little gagging. In hypnosis, T again dreams of Disneyland, where Minnie gives T a magic drink. Two more trolls are found and kicked out. Suddenly T bursts into tears and tells about a tiny troll girl, who is crying and cannot breathe, because she has instruments in her throat and is bleeding. Minnie and R help the little troll girl till she is happy again. They find another tiny girl who is crying, because somebody is angry with her because of an X-ray. Again, they help and heal the tiny girl till she is happy. T puts a Minnie Mouse on guard at T's throat to ensure free passage and plenty of air.

Future Orientation

I cannot help but cite our Danish famous philosopher Søren Kierkegaard (1813–1855), who said the secret to the entire art of helping: "*If One Is Truly to Succeed in Leading a Person to a Specific Place, One Must First and Foremost Take Care to Find Him Where He is and Begin There. Anyone, who cannot do this, is himself under a delusion, if he thinks, he is able to help someone else. In order truly to help someone else, I must understand more than he, but certainly first and foremost understand, what he understands*" (Kierkegaard, [1855] 1962, pp. 96–97). I find this very important in the use of hypnosis and especially in the meeting with children. I love to work with children, they are openminded, without prejudices and have brilliant imaginations, and have often already the solution of how to make a change. Meeting them in their universe, understanding their resources, and their fears will help lead them to cope with the treatment. Children might not understand what they are afraid of, but during the desensitization I begin to understand the fears of the child and the child begins to feel familiar with the instruments and feels control of the situation. Training of the stop signal empowers the child develop confidence to the dentist. Often, I experience that the child only uses the stop signal once or twice, because they know that they can have a break anytime, they want to.

In my early years using hypnosis, I feared that I might provoke difficulties aggravating a problem. However, working with the ego-states as symbols or metaphors is a helpful way to work with the child's traumatic experiences. The child develops resources to overcome fear, heal the traumas, and become independent of the hypnosis dentist.

My vision is to include hypnosis at various levels of dentistry education and establish special hypnosis clinics for children suffering from DF, where staff have been educated with special skills in hypnosis. This would prevent the use of CS and GA and the aggravation of the DF into adulthood saving economic resources while improving care. Let us work for the widely use of hypnosis in pediatric dentistry to stop the suffering of children.

References

Abrahamsen, R. (2020). *Hypnose og kommunikation i tandplejen. [Hypnosis and communication in dentistry]*. Klim.

Ashley, P. F., Chaudhary, M., & Lourenço-Matharu, L. (2018). Sedation of children undergoing dental treatment. *Cochrane Database of Systematic Reviews, 2018*(12). 10.1002/14651858.cd003877.pub5

Balian, A., Cirio, S., Salerno, C., Wolf, T. G., Campus, G., & Cagetti, M. G. (2021). Is visual pedagogy effective in improving ocoperation towards oral hygiene and dental care in children with Autism spectrum disorder? A systematic review and meta-analysis. *International Journal of Environmental Research and Public Health, 18*(2), 789. 10.3390/ijerph18020789

Berge, K. G., Agdal, M. L., Vika, M., & Skeie, M. S. (2017). Treatment of intra-oral injection phobia: A randomized delayed intervention controlled trial among Norwegian 10- to 16-year-olds. *Acta Odontologica Scandinavica, 75*(4), 294–301. 10.1080/00016357.2017.1297849

Burns, G. W. (2004). *101 Healing stories for kids and teens: Using metaphors in therapy*. John Wiley & Sons.

Cianetti, S., Lombardo, G., Lupatelli, E., Pagano, S., Abraha, I., Montedori, A., Caruso, S., Gatto, R., De Giorgio, S., & Salvato, R. (2017). Dental fear/anxiety among children and adolescents. A systematic review. *European Journal of Paediatric Dentistry: Official Journal of European Academy of Paediatric Dentistry, 18*(2), 121–130. 10.23804/ejpd.2017.18.02.07

Davis, D. M., Fadavi, S., Kaste, L. M., Vergotine, R. J., & Rada, R. E. (2016). Acceptance and use of protective stabilization devices by pediatric dentistry diplomates in the United States. *Journal of Dentistry for Children*, *83*(2), 60–66.

Gokli, M. A., Wood, A. J., Mourino, A. P., Farrington, F. H., & Best, A. M. (1994). Hypnosis as an adjunct to the administration of local anesthetic in pediatric patients. *ASDC Journal of Dentistry for Children*, *61*(4), 272–275.

Hennequin, M., Collado, V., Faulks, D., Koscielny, S., Onody, P., & Nicolas, E. (2012). A clinical trial of efficacy and safety of inhalation sedation with a 50% nitrous oxide/oxygen premix (Kalinox™) in general practice. *Clinical Oral Investigations*, *16*(2), 633–642. 10.1007/s00784-011-0550-y

Huet, A., Lucas-Polomeni, M. M., Robert, J. C., Sixou, J. L., & Wodey, E. (2011). Hypnosis and dental anesthesia in children: A prospective controlled study. *International Journal of Clinical and Experimental Hypnosis*, *59*(4), 424–440. 10.1080/00207144.2011.594740

Kankaala, T., Määttä, T., Tolvanen, M., Lahti, S., & Anttonen, V. (2019). Outcome of chair-side dental fear treatment: Long-term follow-up in public health setting. *International Journal of Dentistry*, *2019*, 1–6. 10.1155/2019/5825067

Kierkegaard, S. A. (1962). *Synspunktet for min Forfatter-Virksomhed [The point of view for my work as an author]*. Gyldendal. (Original work published 1855)

Klinberg, G., & Broberg, A. G. (2007). Dental fear/anxiety and dental behaviour management problems in children and adolescents: A review of prevalence and concomitant psychological factors. *International Journal of Paediatric Dentistry*, *17*(6), 391–406. 10.1111/j.1365-263x.2007.00872.x

Newton, T., Asimakopoulou, K., Daly, B., Scambler, S., & Scott, S. (2012). The management of dental anxiety: Time for a sense of proportion? *British Dental Journal*, *213*(6), 271–274. 10.1038/sj.bdj.2012.830

Peretz, B. (1996). Relaxation and hypnosis in pediatric dental patients. *Journal of Clinical Pediatric Dentistry*, *20*(3), 205–207.

Peretz, B., Bercovich, R., & Blumer, S. (2013). Using elements of hypnosis prior to or during pediatric dental treatment. *Pediatric Dentistry*, *35*(1), 33–36.

Phillips, M., & Frederick, C. (1995). *Healing the divided self: Clinical and Ericksonian hypnotherapy for dissociative conditions (Norton professional book)* (1st ed.). W. W. Norton & Company.

Rienhoff, S., Splieth, C. H., Veerkamp, J. S. J., Rienhoff, J., Krikken, J. B., Campus, G., & Wolf, T. G. (2022). Hypnosis and sedation for anxious children undergoing dental treatment: A retrospective practice-based longitudinal study. *Children*, *9*(5), 611. 10.3390/children9050611

Savanheimo, N., Sundberg, S. A., Virtanen, J. I., & Vehkalahti, M. M. (2012). Dental care and treatments provided under general anaesthesia in the Helsinki Public Dental Service. *BMC Oral Health*, *12*(1). 10.1186/1472-6831-12-45

Schouten, B. C., Eijkman, M. a. J., & Hoogstraten, J. (2003). Dentists' and patients' communicative behaviour and their satisfaction with the dental encounter. *Community Dental Health*, *20*(1), 11–15.

Somri, M., Parisinos, C. A., Kharouba, J., Cherni, N., Smidt, A., Abu Ras, Z., Darawashi, G., & Gaitini, L. A. (2012). Optimising the dose of oral midazolam sedation for dental procedures in children: A prospective, randomised, and controlled study. *International Journal of Paediatric Dentistry*, *22*(4), 271–279. 10.1111/j.1365-263x.2011.01192.x

Ten Berge, M., Veerkamp, J., & Hoogstraten, J. (2002). The etiology of childhood dental fear: The role of dental and conditioning experiences. *Journal of Anxiety Disorders*, *16*(3), 321–329. 10.1016/s0887-6185(02)00103-2

Veerkamp, J., Gruythuysen, R., Van Amerongen, W., & Hoogstraten, J. (1993). Dental treatment of fearful children using nitrous oxide. Part 3: Anxiety during sequential visits. *ASDC Journal of Dentistry for Children*, *60*(3), 175–182.

Watkins, J. G., & Watkins, H. H. (1978). The theory and practice of ego-state therapy. In H. Grayson (Ed.), *Short-term approaches to psychotherapy* (1st ed., pp. 176–220). Human Sciences Press.

Medicine

38
HYPNODONTICS

Gabor Filo
DENTISTRY870, HAMILTON, ON, CANADA

Hypnodontics is defined in *The Dictionary of Hypnosis* as, "a new variety of dentistry which uses hypnosis" (Winn, 1965, p. 50). Aaron Moss (1953) coined the term in 1948 during a resurgence of interest in hypnosis specifically in dentistry. His intention was to coin a term with fewer negative connotations.

Dentists have historically been at the forefront of attempting to manage pain, for as the Bard so eloquently states, "there was never yet philosopher that could endure the toothache patiently" (Shakespeare, 1598). In the absence of dependable anesthesia, dental hypnosis has been one of these methods – the first *recorded* tooth extraction with hypnoanesthesia is considered to have been performed by Jean Victor Oudet on November 14, 1836 (Mehrstedt & Wikström, 1997).

Drs Ribaud and Kiaro of Portiers performed major orofacial surgery using hypnosis in 1847 when they removed a jaw tumor (Moss, 1953, p. 21). Dr W. A. Turner, of Leeds, in 1890 removed 40 teeth under hypnoanesthesia induced by J. M. Bramwell (author of *Hypnotism: Its History, Practice and Theory* (1906)), while a year later in Huddersfield, Dr Charles Rippon removed 20 teeth via a hypnosis note from Dr Draper (Frost, 1959, p. 2). Not to be left behind, the American Dr. Bonwill performed extractions with hypnoanesthesia in 1894 (Shaw, 1958).

Elliotson's *Zoist* journal, during its lifetime from 1843 to 1856, reported many dental and general surgical interventions employing hypnoanesthesia from around the globe (Gravitz, 1988). This dissemination by case study has predominated over time, but more research aimed at the dental context has come to the fore recently.

Dentists in North America allied themselves into two organizations roughly separating the continent geographically. These were the *American Hypnodontic Society* (New York and the North East) formally changing its name from The American Society for the Advancement of Hypnodontics in 1952 and the American Society of Psychosomatic Dentistry (the Midwest) founded in 1949 (Moss, 1953). Both organizations are now defunct and the few hypnodontists that remain are members of other clinical and lay hypnosis organizations.

An interesting historical tidbit about the degree to which dentists were a driving force for hypnosis was the composition of the original officers of the American Society of Clinical Hypnosis (ASCH). Of the seven officers listed in 1958, five were dentists as published in the first issue of their Journal ("Biographical Notes on Officers of the American Society of Clinical Hypnosis and the Academy of Applied Psychology in

DOI: 10.4324/9781003449126-52

Dentistry," 1958). Also noteworthy, one of the officers was a Canadian dentist underscoring ASCH's North American flavor.

In Europe, the German Dental Hypnosis Society (*Deutsche Gesellschaft für Zahnärztliche Hypnose e. V.* (DGZH)) was founded by Albrecht Schmierer in 1994 and is a thriving vibrant organization boasting a large dental membership. To my knowledge, there are at present no other exclusively dental hypnosis societies.

In 1959, the American Board of Hypnosis In Dentistry was formed as a component of the American Board of Clinical Hypnosis, Inc. to certify competence in dental hypnosis. The Board confers Diplomate status and has had notable international members over its lifespan such as Per-Olaf Wikström of Sweden and Albrecht Schmierer.

The domain of hypnodontics was best encapsulated by the legendary hypnodontist Kay F. Thompson (a student of Milton Erickson's and an integral member of the American Dental Association) as, "What we are doing is taking our words to tap into the physiological substrate so the individual can control, not only his mind, but his body, his responses, and his behaviors" (Kane & Olness, 2004, epigraph page). Giddon and Anderson (2006) eloquently summarized the dental therapeutic scope as, "the importance of the mouth may be conceptualized into three sequential levels, varying in biological and social significance: survival, socialization, and self-actualization" (Giddon & Anderson, 2006, p. 3). Stolzenberg (1950) quotes Weiss lamenting that "of all the branches of medicine, dentistry has perhaps been the one most separated from the psyche" (Stolzenberg, 1950, p. 105). We "*amalgam smiths*" may only be treating a tooth, but we address the whole person to whom it is attached.

Hypnodontics may be considered to entail the management of the following areas:

- Mind:
  - Dental fear, anxiety, phobia management
  - Pain
- Body:
  - Pain amelioration, analgesia, anesthesia
  - Bleeding management/ control
  - Salivation control and management
  - Gagging control and management
- Responses:
  - Stress management
  - Recurrent aphthous ulcer management
- Behaviors:
  - Smoking cessation
  - Habit control e.g., digit sucking, tongue thrusting
  - Bruxism

The items listed are merely a general overview and are not exhaustive. They are attributed to a category for convenience, but they are interrelated and could be listed under several categories.

Mind

Landa (1953) described the rise of the psychosomatic concept of disease, "as an antidote for the 'machine age' in medicine and dentistry." He found it, "astounding and at times frightening to realize that the high esteem in which modern society holds the machine is in inverse ratio to the value it puts on the human being" (Landa, 1953, p. 2). What would he think today? His contemporary Ryan (1946) noted, "We have been so emphatic on the physical values of dental treatment that we have ignored the psychic aspects of the dental experience" (Ryan, 1946, p. 63). Facco, three-quarters of a century later, reinforces that "dentistry has become more and more technological, leading professionals to focus on teeth only, rather than patients; accordingly, dental anxiety has been mainly faced seeking for the ideal sedative, an illusory target" (Facco & Zanette, 2017, p. 10).

Seventy years ago, dentistry had rudimentary drills, one class of local anesthetic (Novocaine™ i.e., procaine) when used, mostly silver mercury amalgam filling material and dentures seemed to be an inevitability. Contemporary dental care is synonymous with a modern dental operatory that may contain computerized body contoured chairs, intraoral cameras, surgical microscopes, hard and soft tissue lasers, digital radiography, amongst other technologies.

Television in the operatories and piped in music and virtual reality headsets are the prevalent trend to provide distraction (anxiolysis). *High tech is equated with high touch* in the consumer's mind.

My observation after 40 years of practice is that patient expectations, beliefs, and mindsets before, during, and after treatment are of paramount importance. Interactions in the dental setting are multidirectional, so the entire dental office staff's psychological situation also impacts the patient experience. Sadly, most dental schools gloss over this important area (Clarke, 1996; Rucker, 2019). The psychology of the dental experience is thus minimized or neglected.

Dental Fear, Anxiety, and Phobia

Historically most dental patients had trepidations about visiting the dentist. Usually, the visit was the culmination of days of excruciating dental pain; thus dental interventions reinforced the popular view of the dentist as an agent of the Inquisition.

Dental fear, anxiety, and phobias are still prevalent ranging from 40% of the trepidatious and white knucklers to 10% of the hard-core avoiders (Halsband & Wolf, 2015). These percentages vary depending on the study. The hierarchy of fear generated by studies usually puts needles and drills at the top.

Oosterink et al. (2008) generated a hierarchy from 67 dental anxiety provoking stimuli listing the top five as (1) dental surgery, (2) having some gum burned away, (3) a root canal treatment, (4) insufficient anesthetics, and (5) extraction of a tooth.

Before we pursue dental fear and anxiety, as hypnosis relates to it, we need a definition of hypnosis that is germane to the dental context. Reginald Humphreys and Kathleen Eagan proposed an Autonomic Model of Hypnosis in 1999. They state, "Trance in general, and hypnosis in particular, are understood as occasions of marked alteration of the individual's usual autonomic nervous system (ANS) balance, towards either sympathetic (SNS) or parasympathetic (PSNS) dominance" (Humphreys & Eagan, 1999). The alterations are along a continuum from mild to severe with the extremes of either pole being pathological. Dentists encounter this continuum on a daily basis with ample physiological indicators making the recognition of an altered state easy.

Frost considered, "The majority of dental patients who require the assistance of hypnosis do so because of fear of one or more aspects of treatment" (Frost, 1959, p. 71). Ryan (1946), another of the early dental psychosomatic therapists, enumerates: "First, a conscious fear is easier to approach than one that is buried below the threshold of consciousness. Second, a real threat to the organism can be handled better by the responsive bodily apparatus than an imaginal threat. Third, a fear of a more or less tangible thing, as a direct physical condition such as the dental experience, can be met more easily than can an anxiety state that is vague, indefinite, and ill-defined" (Ryan, 1946, p. 64).

All of the expressions of a patient's fear will be through the activation of the sympathetic nervous system fight or flight response. Gerschman and Burrows (1997) propose for a conscious patient, the dental fear-inducing stimuli are a peculiar characteristic of dental treatment: (1) forced immobility under threat of discomfort for long periods of time; (2) presence of a perceived danger of unsignaled, uncontrollable noxious simulation; and (3) interference with the most important modulation of communication.

All of the early pioneers of psychosomatic dentistry suggested the role of hypnosis was to engender relaxation (Moss, 1953). Translating this to clinical practice, you cannot have both the SNS or the PSNS simultaneously maximally activated. Hypnotically induced relaxation has the PSNS regain dominance over the SNS to damp down the fight or flight response, or preferentially preempting it through an antagonistic inhibition.

Dental fear, anxiety, and phobia are complex in their etiology, their evaluation, and their classification. Currently, five pathways are described in a 2014 literature review (Carter et al., 2014), that are thought to specifically relate to dental fear and anxiety generation:

> (1) Cognitive conditioning by personal stressful experiences in the dental context; (2) vicarious, garnered from granny's dental horror tales regaled to the grandchildren; (3) verbal threat, similar to the vicarious pathway in that an authority figure uses the dentist as a threat or "boogeyman" with children; (4) informative pathway in which children learn to fear the dental environment from dental phobic elders, negative connotations advertised by media (e.g., television, movies), and friends with personal negative experiences; and the (5) parental pathway, that is, parental modeling of fear to children under 12 years of age.

Each of these etiologies offers the potential for hypnotic interventions.

Screening for dental anxiety and phobia (odontophobia) has involved clinical interviews and the use of questionnaires. The use of these questionnaires is not widespread outside of those practices that specialize in anxiety patients and research centers (see Armfield & Heaton, 2013; Carter et al., 2014; Milgrom et al., 1995 for examples of these instruments).

The screening process has led to discussion about how to formally categorize a diagnosis for odontophobia. The ICD-11 (World Health Organization [WHO], 2022) considers it as a simple phobia. The DSM 5 (American Psychiatric Association [APA], DSM-5 Task Force, 2013) suggests it as a blood – injection – injury phobia type. Regardless of the formal diagnosis, screening is important to determine whether the patient should be referred to a mental health professional, before any dental interventions, conventional or hypnotically aided, are attempted.

Dental anxiety disorders, i.e., the dentally anxious and phobic patients, are also highly hypnotizable (Gerschman, 1989) which underscores the need for screening as there may be a causal relationship between hypnotizability and phobia (Gerschman & Burrows, 1997). This also requires the careful choice of words while caring for these patients so as not to inadvertently suggest something that will be taken out of context and lead to a negative outcome (the law of pessimistic interpretation, Ewin, 2009).

Hypnosis with the dentally anxious, fearful, and phobic is perhaps best utilized preventively as a stress inoculation (Gerschman, 1997).

We should keep in mind that hypnosis is not in itself a therapy; rather it facilitates treatments or may be an adjunct to treatments. Thompson considers it facilitative for behavior therapies such as systematic desensitization, gradual exposure (extinction), modeling, positive reinforcement, negative reinforcement, biofeedback, cognitive restructuring, distraction, and psychodynamic techniques. She considers hypnosis an adjunct to local anesthetic administration, relative analgesia (N_2O), intravenous sedation, and general anesthesia (Thompson, 1997).

Pain

Historically pain has been the reason dentists have been unloved, feared, and disliked. A physician is revered for making us better no matter how much it hurts, while dental interventions have been equated with torture. Dental pain, fear, and anxiety go hand in hand, especially when the anticipated pain induces fear and ultimately avoidance. Genetics may underscore this as well most notably in red haired folks who have a variant of the MC1R gene. They react less to local anesthetics and are more fearful of dental pain (Weiner, 2011).

Hypnosis and self-hypnosis have been utilized as an adjunctive treatment for both dental pain and anxiety yielding equivocal clinical results in various studies for anxiety management (Wolf et al., 2016a, 2016b). Hypnosis may not compare to the "gold standard" consistency of local anesthetic, but nevertheless it has effects equivalent to sedation. Interestingly, clinical anxiety may enhance the patient's hypnotic abilities in the relief of pain (Abrahamsen & Naish, 2021). Self-hypnosis can be quite impressive as Rausch (1980) demonstrated when having a cholecystectomy performed using only self-hypnosis.

Hypnosis on the whole has been shown to have beneficial effects including decreasing heart rates, rhythm, and blood pressure, modifying anxiety and pain perception. For the systemically debilitated that cannot tolerate sedation medications, hypnosis is a useful adjunct (Cozzolino et al., 2020; Silva et al., 2022).

Body

Hypnotic pain management techniques utilize individually or in combination direct suggestions of anesthesia (glove anesthesia), direct diminution of sensations (pain control dial imagery), sensory substitutions (pressure, heat, cold, etc.), displacement from one locale to another, dissociation, posthypnotic suggestions to extend relief as needed, and self-hypnosis as a convenient resource (Barber, 1996).

Dentists encounter patient's acute pain from infection, trauma, cracked teeth, dentinal sensitivity, iatrogenic injury, and post-treatment inflammation. Chronic orofacial pain involves temporomandibular disorders (see Chapter 37), neuropathic pain (e.g., trigeminal neuralgia, glossopharyngeal neuralgia, pre-herpetic and post-herpetic neuralgia), vascular headaches, and manifestations of systemic diseases. All of these have a physiological and a psychological component of suffering. They may also be tinged with anxiety and depression. Thus, any intervention should have a holistic approach, not merely symptomatic relief, for which hypnosis is ideal.

Casiglia and coworkers found, "that studying the unconscious cardiovascular effects of pain would help us to clarify whether, during hypnotic analgesia, pain was really blocked at a certain level of the nervous system, rather than simply dissociated from consciousness" (Casiglia et al., 2012b). Trigeminal and non-trigeminal pain was examined. They found that hypnotic analgesia blocked non-trigeminal nociceptive stimuli at the dorsal horn of the spinal column.

Trigeminal pain differs from non-trigeminal pain in that there is vasodilation and bradycardia, not the usual vasodilation and tachycardia. Casiglia's group found that when hypnosis facilitated analgesia was employed with both trigeminal and non-trigeminal pain, the painful stimuli were blocked at a certain level of the nervous system and were not limited to dissociation. They considered this as offering full protection to the brain and the heart (Casiglia et al., 2012a). Based on these findings, it would be prudent to adjunctively use hypnotic analgesia or anesthesia for invasive dental procedures.

Bleeding Management/Control

Dentistry being a surgical profession, bleeding has always been a concern whether intra-operatively, post-surgically, or during restorative procedures. Bleeding during dental treatments may be iatrogenic or pathological in nature.

Bleeding disorders, whether acquired or hereditary, are largely grouped as platelet disorders, coagulation disorders, and blood vessel defects (Moake, 2021).

Hemophilia is perhaps the best known disorder with the most frequent use of hypnosis as an intervention. Dubin describes using hypnosis with a diagnosed schizophrenic hemophiliac patient who required an extraction (Dubin & Shapiro, 1974).

Salivation Control and Management

Saliva is a physiological blessing and a clinical curse for the dentist. Navazesh referred to saliva as the "fountain of health information that reflects an individual's state of health and disease" (Navazesh, 2006, p. 37). Salivary functions include caries repair and prevention, digestion, and immune responses.

Salivary dysfunction may be caused iatrogenically, by medical conditions and infections. Dysfunction leads to xerostomia with a concomitant increase in caries that may cause the ultimate loss of the dentition. Should that occur, the prosthetic replacement with dentures will be impacted as retention requires a thin film of saliva. Eating dry foods will be difficult for a hypo-salivating patient. Xerostomia may also engender swollen salivary glands, burning sensations, and soreness; ulceration of the soft tissues may increase and there is an increased susceptibility to infection (Simons et al., 2007). Periodontal disease, exacerbated by the xerostomia induced decrease in the oral immune function, is impacted by emotions and stress (Stolzenberg, 1950) leading to a vicious cycle.

Hypersalivation is the bane of the restorative dentist. Today's filling materials are not very compatible with saliva. The dental rubber dam is used to isolate teeth during restorative procedures. Blessing as this may be, it is a negative stimulus to the claustrophobic odontophobe and is generally disliked by patients and dentists alike.

Salivation is impacted by the ANS. Parasympathetic dominance is characterized as watery thin saliva, while sympathetic dominance as dry thick ropy saliva (Landa, 1953). Restoratively speaking, PSNS dominance is preferred, which may be elicited and enhanced by hypnosis.

Before employing hypnosis to manage salivation, the etiology should be determined and treated conventionally where possible. Hypnosis is viable for the odontophobe's anxiety-induced xerostomia by addressing the ANS.

Gagging Control and Management

Dental interventions and preventive dental home care require uncomplicated entry into the oral cavity. Gagging is a major obstacle to both. It may range from mild to severe retching with vomiting in the extreme.

Evolutionarily gagging (pharyngeal reflex) is a protective reflex, a survival mechanism to stop us from inhaling or swallowing dangerous and noxious substances (Simons et al., 2007). Gagging involves the sensory limb of Cranial Nerve (CN) IX (glossopharyngeal nerve) and to a lesser extent the motor limb by CN X (vagus nerve). Touching the soft palate can lead to a similar reflex response involving the sensory limb of CN V (trigeminal nerve).

Gagging may also reflect the patient's fear and anxiety about dental care as well as a distrust of dentists. This is most evident when the gag is set off in the anterior regions of the oral cavity suggesting this is purely a behavioral response and not a reflexive one (Randall et al., 2014).

Hypnotic interventions range from waking hypnosis to deep trance. Various methods of management have been addressed by Moss (1953), Shaw (1958), and Simons et al. (2007).

Responses

Stress Management

The oral cavity is a barometer of systemic health. Deleterious changes will be apparent and impact the structures of the oral cavity (Mostofsky et al., 2006; Stolzenberg, 1950). "The stress of life" as Hans Selye (1956) named it laid the groundwork for our current appreciation of stress and its general and specific impact.

Stress induces an increase in the heart rate, blood pressure, and respiration which may cause fear, anxiety, and anger. Associated motor changes include tremor, increased muscle tension especially notable in facial expressions. There may be concomitant cognitive functional changes displayed as distortive unproductive thinking, indecisiveness, impaired perception, with impaired judgment and problem-solving skills (Eli, 1992).

Stress may manifest in the mouth as acute necrotizing ulcerative gingivitis, chronic periodontitis, recurrent herpes labialis, recurrent aphthous ulcers, and possibly caries. Local anesthesia induces stress which for some leads to anxiety. Paradoxically this may cause analgesia or hyperalgesia. Local anesthetic failure may cause a drastic hypotension, tachycardia, hyperventilation, and hysterical blindness (Eli, 1992).

The origins of stress during dental care may be in learned responses, environmental factors, or impaired communication with the dentist. Since dentistry is an intimate interaction, there is a reciprocal impact by the dentist's own stress levels. Landa (1953), to mitigate iatrogenic influences, developed his concept of *psychological asepsis and antisepsis* which is comparable to conventional infection prevention and control in dental practice. It also underscores an axiom I learned early on that the clinician enters trance before the patient.

Dentists should evaluate and or be aware of patients' intrapsychic and psychosocial situations referred for psychological-psychiatric support, stress management, or addiction counseling (Mostofsky et al., 2006). Moss, however, considered that "psychodental therapy is strictly within the province of dentistry. The elimination of fear and anxiety associated with drilling and surgery has been a constant problem for dentists" (Kroger, 1977, p. 324). It is worth stating here that there is a continuum of mental health concerns from stress to severe psychopathologies and the prudent dental practitioner refers to a mental health professional when appropriate.

Managing stress hypnotically is based on converting an SNS-driven trance state to a PSNS-driven one and then ensuring that the patient can engage their PSNS state on demand. This may be accomplished with any hypnotic induction and any depth of trance. On-demand control may be elicited with post hypnotic suggestions and appropriate re-induction cues. Teaching self-hypnosis as a life skill is invaluable for this.

Recurrent Aphthous Ulcer Management

Recurrent aphthous ulcers are extremely painful in relation to the size of the ulceration. They impede talking, eating, and drinking. Those that are afflicted may have serial ulcers one after the other. Aphthae are related to stress and induce stress in a vicious cycle. Stress in this circumstance implies precipitating factors of psychological stressors, trauma, chemical irritants, metabolic issues, and some foods (Simons et al., 2007) amongst them being chocolate, coffee, peanuts, eggs, cereals, almonds, strawberries, cheese, and tomatoes (Hennessy, 2022).

Conventional treatments include topical corticosteroids, non-steroidal anti-inflammatories, antibiotic mouth rinses, caustic chemical cauterization, low-level laser therapy, and laser ablation. The ultimate goals are pain relief to permit the functions of daily living and diminish the duration of the aphthae, possibly reducing the frequency, the severity, and maintaining periods of remission.

Hypnotic interventions focus on pain management via self-analgesia and anesthesia validating that patients have physiologic control. Stress management strategies in general should be taught and encouraged. Future pacing of a healthy resilient body image to minimize outbreaks should also be included in the strategy (Lehrer et al., 2007).

Behaviors

Smoking Cessation

Smoking has had a long cultural and historical impact on humanity. It has a decided negative impact on the oral cavity. Oral cancers (especially when mixed with alcohol use) and periodontal disease are the two most prevalent concerns (Mostofsky et al., 2006). Smoking also impacts the taste buds, causes halitosis, and has a decidedly negative impact on the aesthetics of the smile which carries a societal penalty in a youth and beauty-oriented society.

Management strategies are all predicated on the patient's volitional desire to stop smoking. See Chapter 32 for a discussion of hypnosis and smoking cessation.

Habit Control

Dentists are occasionally confronted by patient habits that have a detrimental impact on the oral cavity. These include digit sucking (usually the thumb), smoking, tongue thrust, chewing or sucking on objects (pens, pencils, ice cubes, etc.), lip sucking, and bruxism. Hypnosis has been utilized in the correction and elimination of habits (Harris, 1986; Secter, 1961; Simons et al., 2007).

Bruxism

Bruxism at its simplest is a parafunctional activity in which the teeth either clench or grind. Two distinct forms are currently defined – sleep bruxism and awake bruxism.

Sleep bruxism is masticatory activity during sleep that is characterized as rhythmic or non-rhythmic and is not a movement disorder or a sleep disorder in otherwise healthy individuals.

Awake bruxism is characterized by repetitive or sustained tooth contact and/or by bracing or thrusting of the mandible in otherwise healthy individuals. This is generally associated with psychosocial factors such as stress and anxiety.

Conventional treatment usually begins with a bruxism appliance or interocclusal appliance. Psycho-behavioral techniques for bruxism include relaxation, meditation, hypnosis, breathing exercises, massages, and behaviorally avoiding risk factors and triggers, where stress is the exacerbating factor. Pharmacological treatments address the symptoms of bruxism (Trottier, 2022).

Hypnosis interventions considered bruxism to have a habit-based etiology, an orthodontic one or a psychological one. Stolzenberg (1950) suggested it was a form of self-directed aggression. He quotes Boyens self-suggestion at bedtime, "I will awaken if I bite or clench my teeth" and Charles Miller, "Lips together, teeth apart" (Stolzenberg, 1950, p. 43).

Ironically, Landa (1953) held it to be a bad habit formation and considered it more prevalent among dentists than anyone else!

Inductions

Hypnotic induction may be classified in many ways. There is the authoritarian, direct (classic) and permissive (Ericksonian), indirect forms, as well as the passive (classical "sleep" appearing), passive-alert (David Wark's Active Hypnosis, Wark & Reid, 2018) and active-alert (Éva Bányai's stationary bicycle, Bányai, 2018) varieties. Each may be adapted for use in the dental setting.

When the patient presents with an acute emergency, a more authoritarian direct form will be successful where for all other dental interventions the permissive forms are more appropriate today (Rausch, 1990). Dabney Ewin (2009) explains this succinctly that in an emergency, rapport is unnecessary only credentials are necessary as the patient is already in a hypnoidal state.

Hypnodontists on the whole employ waking hypnotic suggestions (Wells, 1966; Rucker, 2019) more than formal inductions. When formal inductions are used, especially at chairside, the tendency is for rapid inductions (Schmierer et al., 2022) (see Chapter 11 on rapid inductions). Hypnotizability tests are easily converted into full inductions and can be quite rapid. Many of the more protracted inductions can also be modified for rapid use. The dental context also offers full sensorial stimuli for the induction: kinesthetic stimuli by way of the automatically reclining dental chair, auditory stimuli from the various sounds in a dental operatory, and visual stimuli by way of the overhead light that can all be incorporated into elicitation and intensification of the hypnotic experience.

More leisurely formal inductions are similar to medical and mental health utilized protracted inductions. Many hypnodontists utilize a private office or special room for hypnosis, especially if the patient is phobic, to avoid the operatory triggers.

Hypnodontics: Practice Integration

The model of practice that is most frequently encountered is mental health derived, one which may in part be one of the reasons that after initial training few dentists employ hypnosis. A germane piece of the puzzle as to why a very useful clinical modality is absent is practice management, that is, a pragmatic guide to implementation is lacking from most training (Rucker, 2019). The usual guidance is predicated on a specific mental health model.

Potential Models of Hypnodontics

When I took my first formal workshop, the premise of hypnodontics was a conventional session (mental health model). Today, this has evolved into consciously using therapeutic language (Bartlett, 1971; Holden, 2012; Thompson, 1963; Thompson, 1966) or what W. R. Wells (1966) termed waking hypnosis and Elman (1984) defined as achieving hypnotic effects without formal trance.

Effective therapeutic communication requires the entire team to be trained from the front office to the chairside assistant. Lang and Laser have written an auxiliary oriented book (Lang & Laser, 2009) as a guide, or Lang's Comfort Talk® (Lang, n.d.) is recommended for training. Regardless, patient communications must be consciously managed.

The auxiliary utilization model involves the staff members being sufficiently trained to assist patients during their dental care experiences after session(s) with the doctor (Schmierer, 2008). An interesting modification of this model is that of Schmierer's where he had a clinical psychologist in his practice.

If audio recordings have been made during their training sessions, patients may listen to them while in the dental chair (Eitner et al., 2011). Generic recordings may also be offered to the patient for use if they do not wish to avail themselves of bespoke care (Schmierer, 2008; Gow, 2017). Online applications are being utilized in assisting patients. Lang's Comfort Talk app now offers an accessible and very portable alternative in the age of the smart phone.

Today the use of online internet consultation has gained traction since the global pandemic shutdown. It offers many advantages, but ultimately, in a hands-on profession the patient must still be seen in vivo. Online intake appointments and hypnosis sessions, as a workup to the in vivo sessions, are convenient and cost-effective.

In Summary

Dental hypnosis today still has a place in a very technologically evolved profession. It eases the patients' experiences while giving them a life skill, eases the operations of clinics when well incorporated, and enhances the dental care providers clinical work and mental well-being.

References

Abrahamsen, R., & Naish, P. (2021). Studies in patients with temporomandibular disorders pain: Can scales of hypnotic susceptibility predict the outcome on pain relief? *American Journal of Clinical Hypnosis*, *64*(1), 12–19. 10.1080/00029157.2020.1863183

American Psychiatric Association [APA], DSM-5 Task Force. (2013). *Diagnostic and statistical manual of mental disorders: DSM-5™* (5th ed.). American Psychiatric Publishing, Inc., 10.1176/appi.books.9780890425596

Armfield, J., & Heaton, L. (2013). Management of fear and anxiety in the dental clinic: A review. *Australian Dental Journal*, *58*(4), 390–407. 10.1111/adj.12118

Bányai, É. I. (2018). Active-alert hypnosis: History, research, and applications. *American Journal of Clinical Hypnosis*, *61*(2), 88–107. 10.1080/00029157.2018.1496318

Barber, J. (1996). *Hypnosis and suggestion in the treatment of pain: A clinical guide* (1st ed.). W. W. Norton & Co.

Bartlett, E. E. (1971). The use of hypnotic techniques without hypnosis per se for temporary stress. *American Journal of Clinical Hypnosis*, *13*(4), 273–278. 10.1080/00029157.1971.10402124

Biographical Notes on Officers of the American Society of Clinical Hypnosis and the Academy of Applied Psychology in Dentistry. (1958). *American Journal of Clinical Hypnosis*, *1*(1), 31–34. 10.1080/00029157.1958.10401770

Carter, A. E., Carter, G., Boschen, M., AlShwaimi, E., & George, R. (2014). Pathways of fear and anxiety in dentistry: A review. *World Journal of Clinical Cases*, *2*(11), 642–653. 10.12998/wjcc.v2.i11.642

Casiglia, E., Tikhonoff, V., Giordano, N., Andreatta, E., Regaldo, G., Tosello, M. T., Rossi, A. M., Bordin, D., Giacomello, M., & Facco, E. (2012a). Measured outcomes with hypnosis as an experimental tool in a cardiovascular physiology laboratory. *International Journal of Clinical and Experimental Hypnosis*, *60*(2), 241–261. 10.1080/00207144.2012.648078

Casiglia, E., Tikhonoff, V., Giordano, N., Regaldo, G., Facco, E., Marchetti, P., Schiff, S., Tosello, M. T., Giacomello, M., Rossi, A. M., De Lazzari, F., Palatini, P., & Amodio, P. (2012b). Relaxation versus fractionation as hypnotic deepening: Do they differ in physiological changes? *International Journal of Clinical and Experimental Hypnosis*, *60*(3), 338–355. 10.1080/00207144.2012.675297

Clarke, J. H. (1996). Teaching clinical hypnosis in U.S. and Canadian dental schools. *American Journal of Clinical Hypnosis*, *39*(2), 89–92. 10.1080/00029157.1996.10403370

Cozzolino, M., Celia, G., Rossi, K. L., & Rossi, E. L. (2020). Hypnosis as sole anesthesia for dental removal in a patient with multiple chemical sensitivity. *International Journal of Clinical and Experimental Hypnosis*, *68*(3), 371–383. 10.1080/00207144.2020.1762494

Dubin, L. L., & Shapiro, S. S. (1974). Use of hypnosis to facilitate dental extraction and hemostasis in a classic hemophiliac with a high antibody titer to factor VIII. *American Journal of Clinical Hypnosis*, *17*(2), 79–83. 10.1080/00029157.1974.10403718

Eitner, S., Sokol, B., Wichmann, M., Bauer, J., & Engels, D. (2011). Clinical use of a novel audio pillow with recorded hypnotherapy instructions and music for anxiolysis during dental implant surgery: A prospective study. *International Journal of Clinical and Experimental Hypnosis*, *59*(2), 180–197. 10.1080/00207144.2011.546196

Eli, I. (1992). *Oral psychophysiology: Stress, pain, and behavior in dental care* (1st ed.). CRC Press.

Elman, D. (1984). *Hypnotherapy* (1st ed.). Westwood Publishing Co.

Ewin, D. M. (2009). *101 things I wish I'd known when I started using hypnosis* (1st ed.). Crown House Publishing.

Facco, E., & Zanette, G. (2017). The odyssey of dental anxiety: From prehistory to the present. A narrative review. *Frontiers in Psychology*, *11*(8), 1155. 10.3389/fpsyg.2017.01155

Frost, T. W. (1959). *Hypnosis in general dental practice*. The Year Book Publishers.

Gerschman, J. A. (1989). Hypnotizability and dental phobic disorders. *Anesthesia Progress*, *36*(4–5), 131–137. https://www.ncbi.nlm.nih.gov/pmc/articles/PMC2190685/

Gerschman, J. A., & Burrows, G. D. (1997). Dental anxiety disorders and hypnotizability. In M. Mehrstedt & P.-O. Wikström (Eds.), *Hypnosis in dentistry* (Hypnosis international monographs (HIM), Vol. 3, pp. 25–32). M.E.G. Stifftung. https://www.meg-stiftung.de/index.php/de/publikationen/3-hypnosis-international-monographs/18-hypnosis-in-dentistry

Giddon, D. B., & Anderson, N. K. (2006). The oral and craniofacial area and interpersonal attraction. In D. I. Mostofsky, A. G. Forgione, & D. B. Giddon (Eds.), *Behavioral dentistry* (1st ed., pp. 3–18). Wiley-Blackwell.

Gow, M. A. (23 Aug 2017). Personal communication.

Gravitz, M. A. (1988). Early uses of hypnosis as surgical anesthesia. *American Journal of Clinical Hypnosis, 30*(3), 201–208. 10.1080/00029157.1988.10402733

Halsband, U., & Wolf, T. G. (2015). Functional changes in brain activity after hypnosis in patients with dental phobia. *Journal of Physiology-Paris, 109*(4–6), 131–142. 10.1016/j.jphysparis.2016.10.001

Harris, G. M. (1986). Hypnotherapy for chronic tongue sucking: A case study. *American Journal of Clinical Hypnosis, 28*(4), 233–237. 10.1080/00029157.1986.10402659

Hennessy, B. J. (2022). Recurrent aphthous stomatitis. In *Merck Manual for the Professional.* Retrieved February 25, 2023, from https://www.merckmanuals.com/en-ca/professional/dental-disorders/symptoms-of-dental-and-oral-disorders/recurrent-aphthous-stomatitis

Holden, A. (2012). The art of suggestion: The use of hypnosis in dentistry. *British Dental Journal, 212*(11), 549–551. 10.1038/sj.bdj.2012.467

Humphreys, R., & Eagan, K. (1999). *The autonomic model of hypnosis and its application in treatment* [Paper presented]. Annual Meeting of the American Society of Clinical Hypnosis, 1999, Reno, NV, United States.

Kane, S., & Olnes, K. (2004). *The art of therapeutic communication: The collected works of Kay Thompson.* Crown House Publishing.

Kroger, W. S. (1977). *Clinical and experimental hypnosis in medicine, dentistry, and psychology* (2nd ed.). J. B. Lippincott.

Landa, J. S. (1953). *The dynamics of psychosomatic dentistry.* Dental Items of Interest Pub. Co.

Lang, E. (n.d.). *Comfort talk* [Video]. Comfort Talk. Retrieved February 25, 2023, from https://comforttalk.com/

Lang, E., & Laser, E. (2009). *Patient sedation without medication: Rapid rapport and quick hypnotic techniques: A resource guide for doctors, nurses, and technologists* (1st ed.). Trafford Publishing.

Lehrer, P. M., Woolfolk, R. L., Sime, W. E., & Barlow, D. H. (2007). *Principles and practice of stress management* (3rd ed.). The Guilford Press.

Mehrstedt, M., & Wikström, P.-O. (Eds.). (1997). *Hypnosis in dentistry, Volume 3, 1997, 112 Pages of the magazine HIM – Hypnosis international monographs.* Die MEG-Stiftung. Retrieved February 25, 2023, from https://www.meg-stiftung.de/index.php/de/publikationen/3-hypnosis-international-monographs/18-hypnosis-in-dentistry

Milgrom, P., Weinstein, P., & Getz, T. (Eds.). (1995). *Treating fearful dental patients: A patient management handbook* (2nd ed.). University of Washington, Continuing Dental Education.

Moake, J. L. (2021). Overview of hemostasis. In *MSD manual professional edition.* Retrieved February 25, 2023, from https://www.msdmanuals.com/professional/hematology-and-oncology/hemostasis/overview-of-hemostasis?query=Overview+of+Hemostasis

Moss, A. A. (1953). *Hypnodontics: Hypnosis in dentistry* (1st ed.). Dental Items of Interest Pub. Co.

Mostofsky, D. I., Forgione, A. G., & Giddon, D. B. (Eds.). (2006). *Behavioral dentistry.* Wiley-Blackwell.

Navazesh, M. (2006). Saliva in health and disease. In D. I. Mostofsky, A. G. Forgione, & D. B. Giddon (Eds.), *Behavioral dentistry* (1st ed., pp. 37–48). Wiley-Blackwell.

Oosterink, F. M. D., De Jongh, A., & Aartman, I. H. A. (2008). What are people afraid of during dental treatment? Anxiety-provoking capacity of 67 stimuli characteristic of the dental setting. *European Journal of Oral Sciences, 116*(1), 44–51. 10.1111/j.1600-0722.2007.00500.x

Randall, C. L., Shulman, G. P., Crout, R. J., & McNeil, D. W. (2014). Gagging and its associations with dental care-related fear, fear of pain and beliefs about treatment. *Journal of the American Dental Association, 145*(5), 452–458. 10.14219/jada.2013.50

Rausch, V. (1980). Cholecystectomy with self-hypnosis. *American Journal of Clinical Hypnosis, 22*(3), 124–129. 10.1080/00029157.1980.10403216

Rausch, V. (1990). Dental hypnosis. In D. C. Hammond (Ed.), *Handbook of hypnotic suggestions and metaphors* (1st ed., pp. 192–193). W. W. Norton & Co.

Rucker, L. M. (2019). Introducing clinical hypnosis to dentists: Special challenges and strategies. *American Journal of Clinical Hypnosis, 61*(3), 276–289. 10.1080/00029157.2017.1404961

Ryan, E. J. (1946). *Psychobiologic foundations in dentistry* (1st ed.). Charles C. Thomas Publisher.
Schmierer, A. (2008). Dental hypnosis. In D. Wark. (ed), Introduction to hypnosis for medical doctors, nurses, medical students, and selected health care workers, volume 2, health care applications of clinical hypnosis. *American Society of Clinical Hypnosis*. Retrieved from http://asch.net/Public/PublicLibrary/tabid/209/Default.aspx
Schmierer, A., De Col, L., Stöcker, T., & Wolf, T. G. (2022). A hypnotic turbo-induction technique for wisdom tooth extraction: Care report. *American Journal of Clinical Hypnosis*, 1–13. 10.1080/00029157.2022.2123774
Secter, I. I. (1961). Tongue thrust and nail biting simultaneously treated during hypnosis: A case report. *American Journal of Clinical Hypnosis*, *4*(1), 51–53. 10.1080/00029157.1961.10401867
Selye, H. (1956). *The stress of life*. McGraw Hill.
Shakespeare, W. (1598). *Much ado about nothing: Act 5, Scene 1, lines 35-36*. PlayShakespeare.com: The Ultimate Free Shakespeare Resource. Retrieved February 25, 2023, from https://www.playshakespeare.com/much-ado-about-nothing/scenes/act-v-scene-1
Shaw, S. I. (1958). *Clinical applications of hypnosis in dentistry* (1st ed.). W. B. Saunders Co.
Silva, J. J., Da Silva, J., Souza, L. F., Sá-Caputo, D., Cortez, C. M., Paineiras-Domingos, L. L., & Bernardo-Filho, M. (2022). Effectiveness of hypnosis on pain and anxiety in dentistry: Narrative review. *American Journal of Clinical Hypnosis*, *65*(2), 87–98. 10.1080/00029157.2021.2005528
Simons, D., Potter, C., & Temple, G. (2007). *Hypnosis and communication in dental practice* (1st ed.). Quintessence Publishing.
Stolzenberg, J. (1950). *Psychosomatics and suggestion therapy in dentistry*. Philosophical Library.
Thompson, K. F. (1963). A rationale for suggestion in dentistry. *American Journal of Clinical Hypnosis*, *5*, 181–186. 10.1080/00029157.1963.10402289
Thompson, K. F. (1966). Communicate to motivate. *American Journal of Clinical Hypnosis*, *9*(1), 26–30. 10.1080/00029157.1966.10402518
Thompson, S. (1997). Hypnosis in the modification of dental anxiety. In M. Mehrstedt & P.-O. Wikström (Eds.), *Hypnosis in dentistry* (Hypnosis international monographs (HIM), Vol. 3, pp. 33–47). M.E.G. Stifftung. https://www.meg-stiftung.de/index.php/de/publikationen/3-hypnosis-international-monographs/18-hypnosis-in-dentistry
Trottier, M. A. (2022). Analysis bruxism. *Ontario Dentist*, *99*(5), 24–29.
Wark, D. M., & Reid, D. B. (2018). Looking at alert, conversational hypnosis. *American Journal of Clinical Hypnosis*, *61*(2), 85–87. 10.1080/00029157.2018.1506636
Weiner, A. A. (2011). *The fearful dental patient: A guide to understanding and managing* (1st ed.). Wiley-Blackwell.
Wells, W. R. (1966). Experiments in waking hypnosis. In L. Kuhn & S. Russo (Eds.), *Modern hypnosis* (pp. 45–55). Wilshire Books.
Winn, R. B. (1965). *Dictionary of hypnosis* (1st ed.). Philosophical Library.
Wolf, T. G., Wolf, D., Below, D., D'Hoedt, B., Willershausen, B., & Daubländer, M. (2016a). Effectiveness of self-hypnosis on the relief of experimental dental pain: A randomized trial. *International Journal of Clinical and Experimental Hypnosis*, *64*(2), 187–199. 10.1080/00207144.2016.1131587
Wolf, T. G., Wolf, D., Callaway, A., Below, D., D'Hoedt, B., Willershausen, B., & Daubländer, M. (2016b). Hypnosis and local anesthesia for dental pain relief – Alternative or adjunct therapy? – A randomized, clinical-experimental crossover study. *International Journal of Clinical and Experimental Hypnosis*, *64*(4), 391–403. 10.1080/00207144.2016.1209033
World Health Organization [WHO]. (2022, February 11). *ICD-11 2022 release*. World Health Organization. Retrieved February 25, 2023, from https://www.who.int/news/item/11-02-2022-icd-11-2022-release

39

HYPNOSIS IN PEDIATRIC AND ADULT PULMONOLOGY

Ran D. Anbar

Center Point Medicine, La Jolla, CA, USA

Author's Background

Although I trained as a pediatric pulmonologist at Massachusetts General Hospital in the 1980s, I only encountered hypnosis in 1997. At that time, I met an 18-year-old patient with severe milk allergy, who developed significant respiratory distress by imagining eating a cheeseburger, which he could not do in real life. When I told him to stop imagining the scenario his breathing became normal.

I wondered if a patient could think his way into illness, could he think his way out? Soon thereafter, I understood this event to have been triggered by a hypnotic interaction.

After doing a lot of reading and taking several workshops in hypnosis, I learned that hypnosis can help anyone with chronic symptoms. Stress can cause physical symptoms, or patients with physical symptoms can develop psychological problems such as anxiety because of the difficulties with their health. In all cases, learning how to self-regulate with hypnosis can help patients improve their symptoms.

Theoretical Framework and Principles of My Approach from Which I Practice

The first step in meeting with a patient is to establish rapport, including through asking open-ended questions and exploring their motivation for change. For example, in situations when patients are only being seen at the urging of a family member, but are uninterested in change, I explain that hypnosis will not be beneficial.

Further, I invite the patients to direct their therapy, by choosing what issue they would like to tackle first. I follow their lead even if the issue appears to be a minor one. I believe that when engaged in psychological therapy, patients will lead the clinician to where they need to go. By learning skills to overcome one issue, patients often generalize the skill to other areas in their lives, including the ones of greatest importance to them.

This patient-led approach continues throughout their course of therapy. For example, when I teach them to interact with their subconscious (as described later), I ask their subconscious for advice regarding the next steps in therapy.

When I introduce the concept of hypnosis to my patients, I tell them that hypnosis involves a shift in their thinking patterns. For my pediatric patients, I define hypnosis as, "Using your imagination to help yourself."

 DOI: 10.4324/9781003449126-53

I emphasize that all hypnosis is self-hypnosis, and therefore in the same session when we complete the first guided hypnosis experience, I instruct patients, "Please use hypnosis again on your own just like we did together. Then, let me know whether it felt the same or better than when we did it together." By implying that they will be successful, patients are guided to perceive success with their efforts, and thus few report experiencing difficulties on their own.

Whether the patients respond that the hypnosis experience felt the same or better I reply, "Then, you don't need me to do hypnosis!" Thus, I immediately complete the transfer of the hypnosis experience and its associated empowerment to the patients.

Hypnosis Instruction

There are three basic parts to hypnosis instruction that I provide most of my patients who are older than eight years.

Part 1: Positive Talk. As a prelude to the use of hypnosis, I discuss the importance of positive self-talk. As a demonstration, I ask the patient to flex their biceps while I pull against their arm in two scenarios: after the patient has told themselves that they are strong, and after telling themselves they are weak. Their verbal declaration translates into increased or decreased muscle strength, respectively.

Next, I ask the patients to predict what will occur if they tell themselves that they are "not weak." Most are surprised to find out that their arm becomes weak in this circumstance as well (Anbar, 2021). I explain that the messages we tell ourselves affect our strength based on our subconscious response.

I explain that one of the reasons for the power of positive talk is that it helps the mind consider new possibilities. For example, a ten-year-old who had a falling out with some of his friends might react by saying to himself, "I'm always going to be alone. Nobody likes me." When his mind hears these thoughts, it reacts with agreement, and this causes the boy to feel even worse. On the other hand, the boy can be taught to say something that is absolutely true about the unfortunate situation: "I want to make more friends and for them to like me." When he thinks in this way, the boy's mind is prompted to ask itself, how is this going to be possible? Coaching patients to make a positive statement including an action often can be helpful: "I want to make more friends by going to the playground and playing with new kids."

When I work with children, I ask their permission to involve their parents in an exercise: I ask the parents to notice whether their children are using negative language, and if so, to tell them to rephrase their statements. If parents are invited to help in this manner, I also encourage the children to similarly alert the parents about any of their negative statements. In this way, the entire family works on applying positivity in their lives.

Part 2: Hypnotic Calming. I explain to patients that maintaining a calm state can help them better tackle life challenges, including dealing with stressful situations, interacting in a constructive way with others, and coping with illness or pain. Thus, I offer to teach them how to use hypnosis to achieve a state of relaxation.

I encourage the patients to choose a safe, calm place in which they can imagine relaxing. "You can activate multiple sites in your brain that will help achieve calmness by imagining what you might perceive in your place with each of your senses. What can you imagine seeing? Hearing? Smelling? Feeling? Tasting?"

Once patients become calm in the hypnotic state, I coach them to progressively relax their muscles from head to toe. I instruct patients to pick a hand gesture (e.g., making a peace sign) that can trigger a similar state of relaxation when they are not doing hypnosis (which is a post-hypnotic suggestion.) I encourage them to rehearse this "relaxation sign" while in hypnosis and to tell themselves, "From now on, whenever I make this sign, I can become this relaxed even when I am not doing hypnosis."

I then tell the patients, "You can imagine staying in hypnosis for the next few moments. When you are ready to come back, please raise your hand."

When they indicate they are ready, I instruct patients, "Remind yourself to practice hypnosis at least once a day for two weeks. Hypnosis is a mind/body skill. The more you practice it, the better you become."

Finally, my re-alerting instructions are brief. "When you are ready to come back, and you'll know exactly when that time will be, please return." I do not believe a formal re-alerting process is generally necessary in patients treated for pulmonary issues, when they have been instructed that "all hypnosis is self-hypnosis" and that they are in control of their imagination. Nonetheless, formal re-alerting is recommended for patients who have serious psychiatric illnesses.

Once patients are alert, I ask two questions in order to help frame their hypnosis experience:

1 "On a scale of 0–10, in which 0 means completely relaxed, and 10 means very stressed (I clench my fists when saying so), how would you rate your relaxation before hypnosis? How about now?" As long as they report being more relaxed, which is usually the case, I say, "Wow. How often have you been this relaxed?" After their response I say, "You can become this relaxed whenever you want to. You can either go back to your safe, calming place in your mind, or you can make your relaxation sign."
2 "Do you want to feel something neat?" The patients usually respond affirmatively. I respond, "Make your relaxation sign," while I show them that I am making their sign. I make sure to look at them after that instruction, as it seems that patients relax more when they believe I expect them to do so. Most patients report that their sign makes them relaxed, which I applaud.

Part 3: Subconscious. In my experience, a majority of patients with pulmonary issues improve significantly following instruction regarding positive talk and hypnotic calming. However, some patients benefit from exploration of the possible psychological reasons that have triggered or perpetuated their symptoms. Such psychological work should be undertaken by a healthcare provider with expertise in provision of mental health care.

An efficient way of identifying psychological issues using hypnosis involves interactions with the subconscious. I use the term "subconscious" because this is commonly understood by patients as the part of their mind outside of their conscious awareness. Examples of subconscious behaviors that can be cited include "The part of your mind that shows you dreams," or "The part of the mind that drives a car while you're thinking about something else."

Interactions with the subconscious can be accomplished through ideomotor signaling, muscle testing, automatic talking, automatic writing, automatic word processing, imagining the subconscious is writing on a whiteboard, or speaking to an inner advisor. A detailed discussion of these methods can be found in the 2021 chapter by Anbar & Cherry (2021), "Communicating with the Subconscious: Ideomotor and Visualization Techniques."

The subconscious can be extensively interviewed regarding the patients' symptoms, which sometimes becomes pivotal in helping to resolve their symptoms as discussed further in the Clinical Illustrations section later in this chapter.

Orientation

The approach presented in this chapter regarding treatment of pulmonary disorders with hypnosis involves dealing with:

1 Psychophysiology, given that all physical symptoms that improve with use of hypnosis have a psychological overlay.
2 A Relational Model, given the importance of establishing a strong, therapeutic relationship between clinician and patient in achieving the best clinical outcome.
3 Analytical Psychology, given the emphasis on helping patients identify and address the subconscious experiences, thoughts, and feelings that may have contributed to the onset or perpetuation of their physical symptoms.
4 Integrative Psychotherapy, as the therapy offered in the treatment of pulmonary disorders, can include elements of techniques from many psychotherapeutic orientations including cognitive behavioral therapy, psychodynamic therapy, client-centered therapy, and existential therapy.

Literature Review

There have been few published randomized clinical trials regarding the use of hypnosis for patients with pulmonary issues. Most of these have involved patients with asthma.

Asthma

Asthma can cause spasm of the small airways and also leads to airway inflammation that can obstruct breathing. Triggers of asthma flare-ups include upper airway infections, emotions, and exposure to inhaled allergens, pollution, or cigarette smoke.

In a study of 62 asthma patients who were randomized to receive three different hypnosis protocols or control intervention at three different sites, patients who were taught to use hypnosis reported less wheezing and use of short-acting medication. No significant changes were documented in pulmonary function (Maher-Loughnan et al., 1962).

In a multicenter year-long trial, 252 children and adults with moderate and severe asthma were randomized to monthly hypnosis sessions and daily self-hypnosis, or to a control group in which patients used daily relaxation and breathing exercises. Hypnosis was associated with an increased forced expiratory volume in one second (FEV1) of 4.3% ($p<0.05$). There were no significant differences between the groups in their incidence of wheezing or medication use (British Tuberculosis Association, 1968).

In another randomized, controlled study of 39 adults with mild to moderate asthma, patients who were highly hypnotizable demonstrated a significant reduction in reactivity to methacholine challenge testing (which is increased in patients with asthma, $p<0.01$), decreased short-acting asthma relief medication use ($p<0.05$), and decreased subjective scores for nocturnal symptoms ($p<0.05$), wheeze ($p<0.01$), and activity limitation ($p<0.01$).

In contrast, patients who were low hypnotizable or the control group demonstrated no significant changes in these parameters (Ewer & Stewart, 1986).

In a two-year randomized, controlled study of 28 children with asthma, those who were taught hypnosis had a significantly larger reduction in wheezing as compared to the control group ($p<0.05$), and fewer school absences related to wheezing ($p<0.001$) (Kohen, 1996).

In several anecdotal reports, hypnosis has been shown to help with the subjective aspects of asthma including symptom frequency and severity, coping with asthma-specific fears, managing acute exacerbations, frequency of medication use, and healthcare utilization (Anbar, 2016a; Brown, 2007).

As asthma is a disease that is triggered by physiological pathology, therapy with hypnosis can augment but generally not replace medical therapy. However, I have documented that in many patients who develop anxiety in association with their asthma, hypnosis can lead to a major decrease in their respiratory symptoms that have arisen because of anxiety, e.g., shortness of breath (Anbar, 2003).

***

Hypnosis has also been shown to augment therapy for patients with organic pulmonary disease other than asthma.

Chest Pain

Non-cardiac chest pain can be caused by gastroesophageal reflux, problems in the esophagus, musculoskeletal injuries, lung disease, stress, anxiety, or depression.

In a randomized study of 28 patients with non-cardiac chest pain, 80% of the 15 who received hypnotherapy improved as compared to 23% of controls, at 17 weeks follow-up. The improvement was maintained for two years in 14 of the 15 hypnotherapy patients, as compared to three of the 13 control patients (Jones et al., 2006).

Chronic Obstructive Pulmonary Disease

Chronic obstructive pulmonary disease (COPD) is a chronic lung disease caused by inflammation of the airways because of exposure to inhaled irritants. Most commonly it is caused by smoking cigarettes. Forms of COPD include chronic bronchitis and emphysema.

Use of a single, 15-minute hypnosis session improved anxiety and lowered the respiratory rate in 19 patients with COPD (Anló et al., 2020).

Cystic Fibrosis

Cystic fibrosis (CF) is a life-shortening genetic disease that causes progressive lung damage, pancreatic dysfunction, and affects other organ systems as well. Because of rapid medication development, between 1996 and 2021 the median age of survival for patient born with CF increased from the low 20s to 50 years (Anbar, 2016b).

A non-blinded controlled trial of 12 patients with CF demonstrated that self-hypnosis improved anxiety and peak expiratory flow rates (Belsky & Khanna, 1994.)

In a case series, 86% of 49 patients with CF at my CF Center reported that hypnosis was of benefit to them (Anbar, 2000a). The most frequent uses of hypnosis among these patients were to relax, improve their tolerance to medical procedures and treatments, and ease headaches. Some of the patients reported that hypnosis helped improve their adherence to their prescribed medications.

In a case series of three patients with CF, hypnosis was used for control of pain, anxiety, taste, and nausea, and modification of general disease perception (Friedrichsdorf & Kohen, 2018).

Interstitial Lung Disease

Interstitial lung disease (ILD) describes a large group of disorders that cause progressive scarring of lung tissue, which leads to increased breathing problems and often early death.

I published a case report regarding a 16-year-old with ILD that led to end-stage lung disease for which he was placed on a waiting list for lung transplantation. I taught him to use hypnosis that helped him successfully control his shortness of breath, pain associated with developing a pneumothorax (lung collapse), pain associated with medical procedures such as insertion of a chest tube, insomnia, and mood (Anbar, 2000b).

***

Functional respiratory disorders can be defined as occurring in patients who present with persistent physical symptoms lacking an identifiable organic basis, or symptoms in excess of what would be expected from their physiologic cause (Anbar & Hall, 2012, see Helgeland et al., this volume).

Several case series of patients using hypnosis for functional respiratory disorders including chronic dyspnea, habit cough, and vocal cord dysfunction have been reported.

Dyspnea (Shortness of Breath)

Dyspnea can be caused by lung disease, heart disease, poor physical conditioning, and anxiety. Dyspnea, and occasionally associated sighing, without an identifiable physical cause can be of functional origin.

We reported that following one or two sessions of hypnosis instruction, chronic dyspnea, including sighing dyspnea, which occurred with or without exercise, resolved in 81% and improved in the remaining 19% of 16 children who had normal pulmonary function testing at rest (Anbar, 2001a).

Habit Cough

Habit cough typically presents in childhood as a loud, disruptive cough, which nearly always resolves when patients are asleep. Hypnosis was reported to achieve resolution of habit cough in 90% of 51 children after 1–3 sessions of hypnosis (Anbar & Hall, 2004).

Vocal Cord Dysfunction

Vocal cord dysfunction (VCD), in which the vocal cords abnormally adduct during inhalation, tends to occur because of stress (Anbar & Fernandes, 2016). VCD often causes a noise during inhalation (stridor) and affected individuals typically report difficulty with inhalation. Most commonly, VCD occurs during exercise in high achieving, teenage athletes, because of self-imposed stress during competitions. Such VCD usually resolves immediately when the athlete learns to employ hypnotic relaxation. VCD can also be triggered by other stressors such as academic or social stress, in which case its resolution may require identification and addressing of the triggering stressor.

In two case series, we showed that VCD resolved in 54% and improved in an additional 38% of 37/51 children who returned for follow-up after receiving 1–3 sessions of instruction in self-hypnosis, provided by me or the social worker working at our Pediatric Pulmonary Center (Anbar, 2002; Anbar & Hummell, 2005).

Smoking Cessation

Case series and meta-analyses suggest that quit rate associated with hypnosis for smoking cessation is in the range of 25–35% (Green & Lynn, 2016).

A 2019 Cochrane review of 14 studies showed that smoking cessation approaches with hypnosis have included discussions of the patients' motivation to quit, imagery to help strengthen the patients' motivation, suggestions to prompt quitting and maintenance of abstinence from smoking including aversion techniques, and instruction in self-hypnosis techniques. The review concluded that there is insufficient evidence to determine whether hypnotherapy is more effective for smoking cessation as compared to other behavioral management approaches or unassisted quitting (Barnes et al., 2019).

* * *

Hypnosis has been reported to be useful in helping patients become more receptive to undergoing medical procedures or undergoing pulmonary therapy. There are no published studies comparing the efficacy of hypnosis in this setting with other forms of improving comfort or tolerability.

Bronchoscopy

Bronchoscopy involves giving patients either local or general anesthesia, and inserting a scope into their main airways (trachea and bronchi) in order to check for abnormalities.

In a prospective, randomized trial of 60 patients undergoing flexible bronchoscopy, clinical hypnosis helped reduce the anxiety, cough, shortness of breath, and amount of local anesthetic required as compared to a control group. Fourteen patients in the control group stated they would refuse another bronchoscopy with local anesthesia, as compared to seven patients in the hypnosis group (Portel et al., 2022).

Chest Physiotherapy

Chest physiotherapy involves percussing the chest to help clear lung mucous in certain diseases.

After being taught how to use self-hypnosis to help augment the effectiveness of their chest physiotherapy, 4/7 patients at our CF Center reported that they continued to use this technique at home on a regular basis (Anbar, 2014).

Noninvasive Positive Pressure Ventilation

Noninvasive positive pressure ventilation (NPPV) involves applying a tight-fitting mask over the nose, or the nose and mouth in order for air to be blown into patients' lungs, which helps patients with certain diseases breathe better.

Clinical hypnosis was shown to help nine children (ages 2–15 years) better accept and tolerate application of NPPV in a six-month trial (Delord et al. 2013). Despite their resistance to NPPV therapy before learning hypnosis, all the patients accepted the NPPV interface after the first hypnosis session, and a median of three sessions were required for them to tolerate the NPPV for more than six hours/night.

Laryngoscopy

Laryngoscopy involves inserting a thin scope into a patient's nose and into the back of the throat to examine the upper airway. This procedure typically is done with local anesthesia.

In two case reports involving children, hypnosis was used to improve tolerance of indirect laryngoscopy (Anbar & Hehir, 2000; Tubere, 1983).

Mechanical Ventilation

Patients with some lung diseases require being placed on a full-time ventilator (breathing machine) to stay alive. The mechanical ventilation can be temporary or permanent, depending on the patients' conditions.

In one case report, hypnotherapy was used to help reduce anxiety of a patient who was being weaned off mechanical ventilation (Treggiari-Venzi, et al., 2000). In another case, I reported that hypnotherapy was associated with an improvement in the oxygen saturation of a patient with pneumonia who was receiving chronic mechanical ventilation in treatment of a neuromuscular disorder (Anbar, 2013).

Radiotherapy

Radiotherapy involves exposing patients to radiation to treat their cancer.

In a case series of six patients with lung cancer, hypnosis was used to stabilize the patients' respiratory motion so that their radiotherapy could be administered more accurately (Li et al., 2013).

Phenomenology: New Directions

Most of the beneficial aspects of therapeutic hypnosis documented in the field of pulmonology are attributable to its efficacy with helping reduce anxiety through use of imagery and suggestions for relaxation, and occasional use of metaphors to help resolve specific pulmonary symptoms such as cough. An exception is the use of hypnotherapy for smoking cessation that consists of therapeutic suggestions directed at overcoming addiction and habit.

Through my work in pulmonology, I have found that accessing the patients' subconscious was key to helping resolve pulmonary issues that were triggered or perpetuated by psychological components other than anxiety related to their illness. For example, a patient with habit cough only improved once his conflict with his parents was identified and addressed (Anbar, 2007). Another patient only improved when his subconscious identified that he felt the cough was an essential part of his soul, and rather than learning how to let go of the cough, the solution involved having it remain but become silent (Anbar, 2021).

Further, little work has been published about helping patients achieve a spiritual perspective (defined as a feeling or sense that there is something greater than oneself) as part of their therapy for pulmonary conditions.

Spirituality can encompass faith in a guiding entity or simply be evoked by being in nature, entering an ornate lobby, or listening to inspiring music. Becoming aware of the great power of the subconscious mind usually leads to enhanced spiritual understanding.

Enhancement of the patients' spiritual state can be very beneficial for them and their family members in dealing with severe or terminal illness such as CF, COPD, or lung cancer. For example, a spiritual understanding can be used as a way of helping them cope with their fears about death or suffering. Some people explore in hypnosis what might occur after they die, while others gain relief by achieving an understanding that they have the inner strength to cope with their suffering and that it will only be short-lived.

Directions for Future Research

Most of the reported experiences with hypnosis in the field of pulmonology have been reported as individual case studies or case series. Thus, controlled studies would be beneficial to help determine:

1 Does routine use of hypnosis for anxiety relief and enhanced comfort in patients with chronic lung disease including asthma, CF, COPD, and ILD yield cost savings, in terms of decreased need for medications, utilization of health resources for exacerbations, or missed school or workdays?
2 As anxiety appears to play a significant role in development of respiratory symptoms, future research in this field might assess the level of anxiety as a separate risk factor and outcome variable.
3 The efficacy and cost-effectiveness of treatment with hypnosis for VCD could be compared to speech therapy, which is the most prescribed therapy for this condition (Anbar & Fernandes, 2016).
4 Different hypnosis protocols can be studied in terms of their efficacy in the treatment of pulmonary disorders. Variables can include how many sessions are conducted under supervision by a clinician, the types of suggestions and hypnotic phenomena used, and whether patients are expected to practice hypnosis at home, with or without a recording of hypnotherapy.
5 For patients who require psychological therapy beyond anxiety relief, the efficacy of use of interactions with the subconscious can be compared with other psychological therapy such as cognitive behavioral therapy.

Therapeutic Relevance

Healthcare providers frequently fail to recognize the overlap between organic and functional respiratory symptoms:

- Patients with asthma, CF, or COPD can develop increasing shortness of breath because of anxiety. Further, anxiety can trigger asthma-related tightening of the airways or cause VCD.

Table 39.1 Symptoms Suggestive That Psychological Issues May Be Related to Patients' Symptoms

Respiratory Symptoms
Chest pain in the absence of cardiac or gastrointestinal disease
Difficulty with inspiration
Disruptive cough
Dyspnea despite normal lung function
Hyperventilation (which patients may term breathing too fast)
Inspiratory noise (e.g., stridor, gasping, rasping, or squeak)
Localization of breathing problem to the neck or upper chest
Sighing
Other Symptoms
Anxious appearance
Dizziness
Feeling something is stuck in the throat
Palpitations
Paresthesias
Shakiness
Tics
Weakness
Symptom Characteristics
Absence during sleep or when patient is distracted
Associated with a particular location or activity
Emotional response to symptoms
Emotional trigger of symptoms
Exposure to traumatic life event
Incomplete response to medications

Adapted from Anbar, R.D., & Geisler, S.C. (2005).

- Patients with whooping cough (pertussis) can develop cough because of airway damage caused by this bacterial infection. Such cough is sometimes called the "100-day cough" since it can persist for over three months. However, I have found that two months after onset, the cough tends to resolve with use of hypnosis, which may indicate a habit component to the cough at that time.

Therefore, best medical practice should incorporate addressing possible psychological causes of pulmonary symptoms using hypnosis early in the course of therapy for pulmonary conditions, especially if patients fail to respond completely to therapy with medical treatment.

Clues that psychological issues are likely an important factor in individual patients can be reviewed in Table 39.1.

Clinical Illustrations

Habit Cough

A 12-year-old boy presented with a cough that started after he contracted an upper respiratory tract infection (Anbar, 2007). The cough was loud and honking and persisted for several weeks. Notably, the cough resolved when the patient slept. His physical examination and pulmonary function testing were normal. The patient was treated with prednisone, hydrocodone, metoclopramide, omeprazole, and over-the-counter cough suppressants without relief. As a result of the cough, the patient missed 50 days of sixth grade and received home tutoring. He said he liked his friends and teachers, and said he wanted to return to school.

I felt that the patient had habit cough, based on its characteristic presentation and its resolution during sleep, in the absence of any physiologic findings (Anbar & Hall, 2004). He was instructed in self-hypnosis techniques including imagery of playing a video game, and petting a ferret, based on the patient's profound interest in playing video games and wish that he could have a ferret for a pet. Use of hypnosis was associated with immediate resolution of the cough.

The cough recurred half a year later at the beginning of the next school year, in association with sore throat. However, the cough did not resolve with use of hypnosis at that time. Following discussion, it became apparent that the patient was upset with his parents for controlling when he could play his video games. I encouraged the patient and his parents to negotiate a contract in which he was allowed to do his homework when he wanted to, as long as he maintained his grades. Thus, the patient felt he had more control over his "free time." Once the contract was signed, use of hypnosis was again associated with immediate resolution of his cough.

This case illustrates that habit cough can resolve immediately after hypnosis, unless there is an underlying psychosocial stressor that is contributing to perpetuation of the cough. In the latter case, addressing the psychosocial stressor may be required to resolve the symptom.

Vocal Cord Dysfunction

A 13-year-old was in good health until she developed a sore throat associated with shortness of breath, inspiratory stridor, coughing, and chest tightness (Anbar, 2004). Notably, her stridor persisted while she slept. Also, she reported intermittent dizziness, headaches, and numbness and tingling of her extremities. Despite therapy with systemic steroids and nebulized bronchodilators, her symptoms persisted for ten days. A laryngoscopic examination of her upper airway demonstrated that her vocal cords were abnormally adducted during inspiration, which was diagnostic of VCD.

The patient's symptoms persisted for an additional two weeks despite employment of hypnotic imagery for general relaxation, as well as specific imagery to relax her vocal cords. At that point, she described a dream from the previous night during which she saw that her stepfather's eyes were bloodshot. She said she did not know what this dream meant, and that in "real life" his eyes often were bloodshot, for an unknown reason.

I taught the patient how to use automatic word processing (Anbar, 2001b) to allow her subconscious to explain what stressors might be underlying the perpetuation of her symptoms. Through typing, the subconscious explained that the patient had seen her stepfather smoking pot and that the subconscious did not want the patient to tell her mother about this, as this could disrupt their marriage. The subconscious explained that her breathing difficulties developed to help ensure the patient would not disclose this information. Equipped with his broader foundational understanding, I asked whether the patient could trust herself to maintain confidentiality without the symptomatic deterrent. She affirmed that she could, and her vocal cord dysfunction immediately ceased.

Clues that this patient's VCD was atypical included that the breathing issues occurred at rest, did not resolve during sleep, were associated with other symptoms suggestive of psychological issues (e.g., dizziness and numbness and tingling of her extremities), and did not improve easily with use of hypnotic relaxation. Given that the VCD in this case turned out to be related to psychological issues that patient was unable to express verbally, the patient could also have been diagnosed as having developed a conversion disorder.

This case illustrates the importance of interactions with the subconscious to identify psychological issues that might be underlying a functional disorder. In the absence of such identification, it is likely that the patient's symptoms would have persisted.

Future Orientation

We have a big opportunity to make a significant impact on the treatment of patients with pulmonary disease by raising awareness in the medical community and in the public eye regarding the importance of hypnotherapy in this setting. Ideally, on-going lectures regarding the efficacy of hypnotherapy should be given in undergraduate years, in medical schools, in nursing schools, in graduate programs involving mental health, and to the general public.

There is a shortage of mental health providers in the world, and they have difficulty keeping up with the needs of patients with psychiatric disturbance. In the ideal world, many patients with medical conditions will be offered psychological therapy in additional to medical therapy, which would add to the burden of mental health professionals. To ease this burden, I believe that primary care providers should be routinely trained in application of basic hypnosis techniques with their patients. Since the onset of COVID, we have learned that effective hypnosis training can be accomplished online. This can make training more accessible to primary care providers, and care more available to patients.

References

Anbar, R. D. (2000a). Self-hypnosis for patients with cystic fibrosis. *Pediatric Pulmonology*, *30*(6), 461–465. 10.1002/1099-0496(200012)30:6

Anbar, R. D. (2000b). Of mind, body, and modern technology. *Clinical Pediatrics*. 10.1177/000992280003900711

Anbar, R. D. (2001a). Self-hypnosis for management of chronic dyspnea in pediatric patients. *Pediatrics*, *107*(2), e21. 10.1542/peds.107.2.e21

Anbar, R. D. (2001b). Automatic word processing: A new forum for hypnotic expression. *American Journal of Clinical Hypnosis*, *44*(1), 27–36. 10.1080/00029157.2001.10403453

Anbar, R. D. (2002). Hypnosis in pediatrics: Applications at a pediatric pulmonary center. *BMC Pediatrics*, *2*(11). 10.1186/1471-2431-2-11

Anbar, R. D. (2003). Self-hypnosis for anxiety associated with severe asthma: A case report. *BMC Pediatrics*, *3*(7). 10.1186/1471-2431-3-7

Anbar, R. D. (2004). Stressors associated with dyspnea in childhood: Patients' insights and a case report. *American Journal of Clinical Hypnosis*, *47*(2), 93–101. 10.1080/00029157.2004.10403628

Anbar, R. D. (2007). User friendly hypnosis as an adjunct for treatment of habit cough: A case report. *American Journal of Clinical Hypnosis*, *50*(2), 171–175. 10.1080/00029157.2007.10401613

Anbar, R. D. (2013). Hypnosis for children with chronic disease. In L. I. Sugarman & W. C. Wester (Eds.), *Therapeutic hypnosis with children and adolescents* (2nd ed., pp. 403–431). Crown House Publishing.

Anbar, R. D. (2014). Self-hypnosis as a complementary airway clearance technique in patient with cystic fibrosis (abstract). *American Journal of Respiratory and Critical Care Medicine*,189, A4682.

Anbar, R. D. (2016a). Asthma. In G. R. Elkins (Ed.), *Handbook of medical and psychological hypnosis: Foundation, application, and professional issues* (pp. 161–167). Springer Publishing Company.

Anbar, R. D. (2016b). Cystic fibrosis. In G. R. Elkins (Ed.), *Handbook of medical and psychological hypnosis: Foundation, application, and professional issues* (pp. 199–203). Springer Publishing Company.

Anbar, R. D. (2021). *Changing children's lives with hypnosis: A journey to the center* (pp 129–139). Lanham, MD: Rowman & Littlefield.

Anbar, R. D., & Cherry, R. N. (2021). Communicating with the subconscious: Ideomotor and visualization techniques. In M. P. Jensen (Ed.), *Handbook of hypnotic techniques, Vol. 2* (pp. 196–231). Kirkland, WA: Denny Creek Press.

Anbar, R. D., & Fernandes, B. A. (2016). Vocal cord dysfunction. In G. R. Elkins (Ed.), *Handbook of medical and psychological hypnosis: Foundation, application, and professional issues* (pp. 429–433). New York, NY: Springer Publishing Company.

Anbar, R. D., & Geisler, S. C. (2005). Identification of children who may benefit from self-hypnosis at a pediatric pulmonary center. *BMC Pediatrics*, *5*(6). 10.1186/1471-2431-5-6

Anbar, R. D., & Hall, H. (2004). Childhood habit cough treated with self-hypnosis. *The Journal of Pediatrics*, *144*(2), 213–217. 10.1016/j.jpeds.2003.10.041

Anbar, R. D., & Hall, H. R. (2012). What is a functional respiratory disorder? In R. D. Anbar (Ed.), *Functional respiratory disorders: When respiratory symptoms do not respond to pulmonary treatment* (pp. 3–17). New York, NY: Humana Press.

Anbar, R. D., & Hehir, D. A. (2000). Hypnosis as a diagnostic modality for vocal cord dysfunction. *Pediatrics*. 10.1542/peds.106.6.e81

Anbar, R. D., & Hummell, K. E. (2005). Teamwork approach to clinical hypnosis at a pediatric pulmonary center. *American Journal of Clinical Hypnosis*, *48*(1), 45–49. 10.1080/00029157.2005.10401489

Anló, H., Herer, B., Delignières, A., Bocahu, Y., Segundo, I., Alingrin, V. M., Gilbert, M., & Larue, F. (2020). Hypnosis for the management of anxiety and dyspnea in COPD: A randomized, sham-controlled crossover trial. *International Journal of Chronic Obstructive Pulmonary Disease*, *15*,2609–2620. 10.2147/copd.s267019

Barnes, J., Dong, C., McRobbie, H., Walker, N., Mehta, M., & Stead, L. F. (2019). Hypnotherapy for smoking cessation. *The Cochrane Library*. 10.1002/14651858.cd001008.pub2

Belsky, J., & Khanna, P. (1994). The effects of self-hypnosis for children with cystic fibrosis: A pilot study. *American Journal of Clinical Hypnosis*, *36*(4), 282–292. 10.1080/00029157.1994.10403088

British Tuberculosis Association. (1968). Hypnosis for asthma – A controlled trial: A report to the Research Committee of the British Tuberculosis Association. *British Medical Journal*, *4*(5623), 71–76. 10.1136/bmj.4.5623.71

Brown, D. (2007). Evidence-based hypnotherapy for asthma: A critical review. *International Journal of Clinical and Experimental Hypnosis*, *55*(2), 220–249. 10.1080/00207140601177947

Delord, V., Khirani, S., Ramirez, A., Joseph, E. L., Gambier, C., Belson, M., Gajan, F., & Fauroux, B. (2013). Medical hypnosis as a tool to acclimatize children to noninvasive positive pressure ventilation. *Chest*, *144*(1), 87–91. 10.1378/chest.12-2259

Ewer, T. C., & Stewart, D. E. (1986). Improvement in bronchial hyper-responsiveness in patients with moderate asthma after treatment with a hypnotic technique: A randomised controlled trial. *British Medical Journal (Clinical Research Edition)*, *293*(6555), 1129–1132. 10.1136/bmj.293.6555.1129

Friedrichsdorf, S. J., & Kohen, D. P. (2018). Integration of hypnosis into pediatric palliative care. *Annals of Palliative Medicine*, *7*(1), 136–150. 10.21037/apm.2017.05.02

Green J. P., & Lynn, S. J. (2016). Smoking cessation. In G. R. Elkins (Ed.), *Handbook of medical and psychological hypnosis: Foundation, application, and professional issues* (pp. 621–627). New York, NY: Springer Publishing Company.

Jones, H., Cooper, P. A., Miller, V., Brooks, N. J., & Whorwell, P. J. (2006). Treatment of non-cardiac chest pain: A controlled trial of hypnotherapy. *Gut*, *55*(10), 1403–1408. 10.1136/gut.2005.086694

Kohen, D. P. (1996). Relaxation/mental imagery: Self-hypnosis for childhood asthma: Behavioral outcomes in a prospective, controlled study. *Australian Journal of Clinical and Experimental Hypnosis*, *24*(1), 12–28.

Li, R., Deng, J., & Xie, Y. (2013). Control of respiratory motion by hypnosis intervention during radiotherapy of lung cancer I. *BioMed Research International.* 10.1155/2013/574934

Maher-Loughnan, G. P., Macdonald, N., Mason, A. A., & Fry, L. (1962). Controlled trial of hypnosis in the symptomatic treatment of asthma. *British Medical Journal*, *2*(5301), 371–376. 10.1136/bmj.2.5301.371

Portel, L., Perel, A., Masson, L., Roy, C., & Mebs, S. (2022). Tolerance's improvement of flexible bronchoscopy by Ericksonian hypnosis: The BREATH study. *Respiratory Medicine and Research*, *81*, 100798. 10.1016/j.resmer.2020.100798

Treggiari-Venzi, M. M., Suter, P. M., De Tonnac, N., & Romand, J. (2000). Successful use of hypnosis as an adjunctive therapy for weaning from mechanical ventilation. *Anesthesiology*, *92*(3), 890–892. 10.1097/00000542-200003000-00042

Tubere, G. (1983). Suggestione ipnotica in anestesia. Un caso clinico: [Hypnotic suggestion in anesthesia. A clinical case]. *Minerva Medica*, *74*(37), 2157–2158.

40

HYPNOSIS IN NEUROLOGICAL DISORDERS AND NEUROREHABILITATION

Giuseppe De Benedittis
University of Milano, Italy

Introduction

Neurological diseases are the expression of an organic and/or dysfunctional disorders affecting the central nervous system (CNS), the peripheral nervous system, or the autonomic nervous system. In addition to the primarily organic injury or dysfunction, various psychological factors can significantly modulate neurological diseases, their therapeutic prognosis, and neurorehabilitation program.

Neurological patients frequently ask their physicians about complementary and alternative medicine as options for treatment, because of the excellent safety profile, the relatively low cost, and their ability to allow patients to take a more active role in their treatment.

The Role of Hypnosis in Neurological Disorders

Hypnosis has a significant, albeit underestimated, role in neurological disorders and neurorehabilitation. There have been numerous studies using hypnotic techniques in neurologic disorders (for a review, see De Benedittis, 2021). Despite the remarkable potential of the medium, hypnosis in neurology and neurorehabilitation is unfortunately underused in clinical practice, probably due to the erroneous belief that central and/or peripheral nervous pathologies are less responsive to cognitive modulations such as hypnosis. Consequently, the clinical indications are currently limited, though in progressive expansion. Most of the studies are not high quality, often due to lack of adequate controls and small case numbers.

The main clinical applications of hypnosis in neurology concern the following areas (De Benedittis, 2021): (a) pain (e.g., headaches, neuropathic pain); (b) movement disorders (e.g., spasmodic torticollis, psychogenic tremors, Parkinson's disease, Gilles de la Tourette syndrome); (c) multiple sclerosis (MS); (d) psychogenic non-epileptic seizures; (e) Raynaud syndrome; and (f) neurorehabilitation.

In addition to the aforementioned clinical indications, hypnosis is useful in (De Benedittis, 2021) (a) differential diagnostics between organic and functional pathologies (e.g., epilepsy versus psychogenic epileptiform syndromes); (b) optimization of functional

 DOI: 10.4324/9781003449126-54

skills even in clinical conditions in which complete and/or partial recovery is not possible; (c) control of pain and disability associated with neurological pathology; (d) implementation of motivations in neurorehabilitation; and (e) improvement of the quality of life.

Movement Disorders

Movement Disorders represent a heterogeneous category of neurological disorders, of the hypokinetic (e.g., Parkinson's disease) or hyperkinetic (e.g., spasmodic torticollis) type, often located at a border between neurology and psychiatry. They are the neurological disorders most commonly treated with hypnosis.

Flamand-Roze et al. (2016) reported a systematic review on the state of the art and on the prospects for the use of hypnosis in the treatment of different types of movement disorders. The treatments always associated hypnotherapy sessions with the practice of self-hypnosis and the sessions included relaxation procedures, visualizations, and exercises aimed at improving movement control through appropriate suggestions and metaphors. Due to the heterogeneity of clinical syndromes, the small patient sample, and methodological flaws, overall, there was insufficient evidence to determine whether hypnosis is effective in these patients, although some promising results warrant further investigations.

Dystonia

Dystonia is a neurological movement disorder, in which sustained muscle contractions can cause twisting and repetitive movements or abnormal postures (Donaldson et al., 2012; Evatt et al., 2011). The most frequent form of focal dystonia is referred to as spasmodic torticollis or *idiopathic cervical dystonia* (ICD) (Donaldson et al., 2012; Evatt et al., 2011).

Epidemiology

The incidence rate of spasmodic torticollis is approximately 1.2 per 100,000 person-years (Claypool et al., 1995), and a prevalence rate of 57 per million (The Epidemiological Study of Dystonia in Europe – ESDE – Collaborative Group, 2000).

Signs and Symptoms

Spasmodic torticollis is a chronic, painful movement disorder that results in involuntary rotation of the neck left, right, up, and/or down (Donaldson et al., 2012; Evatt et al., 2011). Both the agonist and antagonist muscles contract simultaneously during the dystonic movement. Over time, the involuntary spasm of the neck muscles increases in frequency and strength until it reaches a plateau. Symptoms can also worsen while standing or during times of increased stress. Other symptoms include muscle hypertrophy, neck pain, dysarthria, and tremors (Donaldson et al., 2012; Evatt et al., 2011). Studies have shown that over 75% of patients report neck pain, and 33% to 40% head tremors (Jankovic et al., 2007). The muscles most frequently involved are the sternocleidomastoid (SCM) and the trapezius, but excessive activity is not limited to these muscles and can extend to adjacent muscles.

ICD is affected by a variety of factors. As in other dyskinesias, emotional stress is the most common aggravating factor. Symptoms usually improve with sleep or supine, while worsening in sitting, standing, and walking positions (Balint & Bhatia, 2014; Donaldson et al., 2012).

Pathophysiology

The pathophysiology of spasmodic torticollis is still poorly understood. In many cases, it may involve some genetic predisposition toward the disorder combined with environmental conditions (Waddy et al., 1991). Furthermore, psychological factors may significantly modulate the disorder (De Benedittis, 2016). Although no specific identifiable causes or structural abnormalities are found, dysfunctional pathology of the CNS is suspected most likely in those brain areas associated with motor function such as the basal ganglia (Vacherot et al., 2007).

Diagnosis

The diagnosis of spasmodic torticollis is mainly based on physical objectivity, due to the lack of specific clinical criteria.

Principles of Treatment

Dystonia and particularly ICD are neuromuscular disorders extremely resistant to most therapies (physical, medical, and surgical), and the therapy is almost always symptomatic. This includes supportive and counseling therapy, physical therapies, drug therapies (e.g., levodopa, dopamine agonists), intrathecal infusion of baclofen, neurosurgical procedures (e.g., thalamotomy, pallidotomy, and deep brain stimulation) (see review in De Benedittis, 2016). Botulinum toxin (A and B) has become the standard of care in symptomatic management of this condition since the early 2000s (De Benedittis, 2016). Injected into the muscle, botulinum toxin acts by inhibiting the release of neurotransmitters at the neuromuscular junction and inducing a transient inhibition of the muscle. Due to the temporary nature of the effects of botulinum toxins, repeated and regular administration is required to maintain clinical improvement. Significant side effects are not uncommon, and the outcome is often uncertain (De Benedittis, 2016).

The Role of Hypnosis in ICD

Spasmodic torticollis is also one of the most challenging pathologies to treat with hypnosis (Crasilneck & Hall, 1985). Anecdotal reports of successful ICD treatment with hypnosis have been published (see review in De Benedittis, 2016). The author reported four cases of ICD successfully treated with hypnosis, two of which were in combination with EMG-Biofeedback (De Benedittis, 1996).

A history of major stressful events associated with a cognitive-emotional assessment of their negative impact on patterns of life seemed to herald the onset of stiff neck in all cases, probably acting as an antecedent or precursor of the disease (De Benedittis, 1996). Neurological examination and diagnostic studies such as MRI and EMG were normal in all cases. Psychometric evaluation revealed abnormal personality patterns in all cases. Most of them also mentioned difficulties in controlling their emotions, impulsiveness, irritability, and aggressive tendencies. Using the paradigm of "organ language" (Ewin & Eimer, 2006), the torticollis seems to be the symbolic expression of the subject's "distancing" from a relevant problem, with the head often turning to the left, understood in terms of symbolic avoidance of anxious-aggressive impulses. Obsessive-compulsive patterns were frequently observed in our patient group, providing further support for the theory of a link between basal ganglia disorders related to involuntary movements and psychiatric disorders, particularly obsessive-compulsive disorders (Bihari et al., 1992). All four patients reported significant improvement with hypnosis alone or with combined EMG-Biofeedback and hypnosis treatment. Significant changes in daily life activities have been observed, including return to work, improvement of social and civic life, and return of the ability to drive a car. A significant improvement in mood and emotional control was also noted, with concomitant reduction in anxiety levels. All subjects were followed for one year up to ten years. All cases maintained improvement over time, without significant relapses.

Hypnotic Techniques

The techniques for the treatment of cervical dystonias (*i.e.*, spasmodic torticollis) require prolonged, complex, and personalized treatments, aimed at controlling pain (often present and aggravated by limited movements of the neck and head), changing the postural structure and neuromuscular rehabilitation process, with anatomo-functional rebalancing of the muscles involved. "Postural hypnosis" (i.e., hypnosis in a standing position) is used, in order to counteract and minimize muscle spasms activated by cervical postural reflexes, responsible for lateroversion (De Benedittis, 1996, 2004, 2016). A hierarchical and progressive hypno-desensitization is introduced, depicting most aspects of stressful situations frequently associated with worsening of the symptoms, while the patient is relaxed and in hypnosis. Suggestions are formulated to displace somatized and unfocused anxiety from the cervical muscle districts to the right hand closed in a fist. Sensory-imagery conditioning is also used, with the subject being instructed to imagine pleasant events to be associated with a normal alignment of his or her head and neck. Hypnosis facilitates differential muscle retraining (i.e., decreasing the tone of the spasmodic SCM muscle and increasing the tone of the antagonist, contralateral muscle) and helps patients regain their former behavioral patterns through several sessions ("forgotten assets"). These patterns, strongly imprinted in every life situation, had been completely erased by the neuromuscular disorder. They are restored and positively extended.

Twice weekly hypnotic sessions are usually needed. Patients are encouraged to practice self-hypnosis twice a day for 20 minutes as a supporting device. Duration of the treatment is of crucial importance. The hypnotherapeutic process is usually gradual and slow, taking several months to induce and stabilize significant changes as well as to reverse the anatomo-functional imbalance of the neck muscles. Duration of treatment ranges from 6 to 12 months.

Case Example

The patient was a 44-year-old man, who had a seven-year history of torticollis to the left. His father died when he was 35 years old. He tried to get through this terrible loss by rushing headlong into his job, but during a period of severe work-related stress, the patient developed panic attacks. A few months later, spasmodic torticollis to the left began. The onset was associated with pain in the neck and head, concomitant with oscillatory movements. The involuntary movements became more intense with emotional stimuli, exertion, fatigue, and when in an upright position. The patient had to stop driving a car and often had difficulty in sleeping at night. A variety of medical and psychiatric treatment regimens proved totally ineffective. After 12 months of combined hypnotic and EMG-Biofeedback treatment, the patient achieved control of head and neck position, pain disappeared, sleep was undisturbed, and he could now drive a car again. He maintained good results during the ten-year follow-up after initial treatment.

Transcript

Postural Hypnosis for ICD (Spasmodic Torticollis)

While you're comfortably standing against the wall, I would like you to pay attention to the strong tension in all the muscles of your body, particularly those of your neck. And now you might want to release all that unsufferable tension. Relax, letting all the tension go ... focusing on these muscles as they just relax completely, noticing what it feels like as the muscles become more and more relaxed ... focusing all your attention on the pleasant feelings associated with relaxation owing into the muscles of your face and of your neck ... spreading into your shoulders and upper arms ... enjoy the feelings in the muscles as they loosen up, smooth out, unwind, and relax more and more deeply ... pay attention only to the sensations of relaxation as the relaxation process takes place.

Now close your hand and make a tight fist and let all the tension in your neck or those painful feelings flow into that hand ... and as the tension and those strong feelings flow into the hand, the fist will become tighter and tighter ... And now you can open your fist, slowly and safely, and let as much of the tension [or feelings] *as you want to get rid of flow away into the air ... and as the tension streams away from you, you will go deeper and deeper into trance.*

As you drift along, you feel yourself relaxed, deeper and deeper relaxed – way down – so that more and more you know that your body is getting under your complete control. You have the ability to control your neck muscles, stop your tension, and relax ... or just keeping it in a straight position ... that's okay. ... When you feel this happening, just relax ... and each time you practice, you get better and better, more and more relaxed and able to control your muscles and posture.

Parkinson's Disease

Epidemiology

Parkinson's is the second most common neurodegenerative disease after Alzheimer's, affecting 10 million people worldwide (Lisak et al., 2016).

Signs and Symptoms

Among the signs and symptoms of the disease, the most typical of a motor nature are tremor at rest, slowing of movement (bradykinesia), difficulty starting a movement (akinesia), muscle stiffness, postural instability, often associated with muscle pain (De Virgilio et al., 2016).

Pathophysiology

In Parkinson's, there is a progressive degeneration of the pigmented neurons of the compact part of the substantia nigra, of the locus coeruleus, and of other dopaminergic neuronal groups of the brainstem. The loss of neurons in the substantia nigra involves the depletion of dopamine in the dorsal region of the putamen, an integral part of the basal ganglia, causing the classic symptoms and motor signs. Parkinsonism can also be caused by taking drugs that block dopaminergic receptors in the striatum such as antipsychotics and antiemetics; vascular parkinsonism can be induced by multiple infarcts localized in the basal ganglia, while other forms of parkinsonism can be due to multiple systemic atrophy and progressive supranuclear palsy (Wilkinson & Lennox, 2005).

Principles of Treatment

The primary pharmacological treatment consists in the enhancement of dopaminergic activity within the nigrostriatal pathways, both by taking levodopa, which is transformed into dopamine in the surviving neurons of the substantia nigra, and by taking dopamine agonists, which mimic the effect of dopamine in the striatum. Unfortunately, these drug therapies have limited efficacy over time and significant side effects. Major non-drug therapies include surgery such as deep brain stimulation (DBS), consisting of the brain implantation (e.g., subthalamic nucleus) of an electrostimulation device, and physical therapies such as rehabilitation strategies (Witt et al., 2017).

The Role of Hypnosis in Parkinson Disease

Although large-scale studies have not yet been conducted, numerous case reports published over the years demonstrate the usefulness of hypnotherapy in the treatment of a wide range of symptoms associated with Parkinson's disease, not just of a motor nature (Elkins, 2016; Mozzoni, 2018).

Ajimsha et al. (2014) conducted a single-blind randomized controlled study on patients in the early development phase of Parkinson's disease, finding the greater efficacy of the combination of hypnosis and physical training, compared to physical training alone.

Schlesinger et al. (2009) conducted a study on patients in early and intermediate stages of Parkinson's disease, finding that a single hypnosis session was able to significantly reduce or even eliminate tremor not only during session but also in the following seven hours.

Hypnotic Techniques

After a standard hypnotic induction of relaxation, the patient is asked to focus on a spot on the ceiling and imagine himself at the top of a staircase leading to a comfortable room. Hypnotic cues aim to increase relaxation and reduce the intensity and frequency of resting tremors. Examples of suggestions provided (Mozzoni, 2018, p. 49):

> *"While in a deep, calm and relaxed state of trance, with each breath you take, you will be able to respond to any hypnotic suggestion. There is a relationship between mind*

and body ... and as you go into an even deeper trance state ... the dopamine levels will start to rise ... and the tremor becomes less and less ... the dopamine levels. ... increasing ... and decreasing tremors ..."

Post-hypnotic suggestions are also offered to reduce tremor, decrease pain, improve sleep, and libido. Hypnotic treatment is supported by self-hypnosis.

Psychogenic Movement Disorders or Functional Movement Disorders

Psychogenic movement disorder (PMD) or functional movement disorder is a movement disorder caused by a psychopathological state, rather than an organic disorder of the nervous system.

PMD presents a diagnostic and therapeutic challenge. The terminology for classifying this disorder is confusing and makes diagnosis difficult, which can be formulated on the basis of a probability or *ad excludendum* criterion, since psychogenic documentation is often difficult or impossible to pursue (Peckham & Hallett, 2009).

The treatments used are varied (psychotherapies, CBT, acupuncture, etc.) and of dubious efficacy. Hypnosis seems to play a significant role. In a randomized controlled clinical trial, 44 PMD patients were randomly assigned to a control group (waiting list) or an active treatment group (hypnosis) (Moene et al., 2003). The hypnotic group improved compared to the control group (90% versus 26.1% of the control group). The improvement was maintained at a six-month follow-up.

Gilles de la Tourette Syndrome

Gilles de la Tourette syndrome is a neurological disorder characterized by the presence of inconstant, sometimes fleeting, and other times chronic motor and phonatory tics, the severity of which can range from extremely mild to disabling (Olson, 2004).

"Tics" are sudden, repetitive, non-rhythmic ("motor tics") or expressive ("phonic tics") movements that involve certain muscle groups. Motor tics are based on movement, while speech tics are based on involuntary sounds produced by moving air through the nose, mouth, or throat.

Coprolalia (the involuntary expression of socially censurable or taboo words or phrases) is the best-known symptom of Tourette's syndrome, but it is neither sufficient nor necessary to make the diagnosis, as only about 10% of patients are affected, while the most common motor sign and initial tic are, respectively, closing the eyes and clearing the throat (Singer, 2005). The causes and origins of the syndrome are still uncertain. The etiology is multifactorial, genetic, and environmental factors are involved (Robertson, 2000).

However, tics are believed to result from dysfunction of the thalamus, basal ganglia, and frontal cortex, which results in abnormal dopamine activity (Singer & Walkup, 1991). Some manifestations of the syndrome may be related to obsessive compulsive disorder (Singer & Walkup, 1991).

Commonly prescribed drug treatments include (Kurlan, 2014) haloperidol, clonidine, clomipramine, and serotonergic SSRI drugs, which can be used effectively in reducing the motor effects of the syndrome (tics, uncontrolled movements, vocalizations, and screams) and obsessive ones. DBS neurosurgery interventions are also proposed for the most severe cases, with results that are still controversial (Kurlan, 2014).

As regards hypnosis, the literature presents limited case reports or studies of a few cases (Kohen & Kaiser, 2014), albeit with encouraging results regarding a reduction in tics and drugs taken.

Multiple Sclerosis

MS is a chronic demyelinating autoimmune disease that affects the white matter of the CNS causing a broad spectrum of signs and symptoms (Compston & Coles, 2002). Patients can experience a wide range of symptoms/signs, including reduced mobility, sensory disturbances, chronic pain, fatigue, bladder and bowel dysfunction, depression, and cognitive impairment. The disease has a prevalence that varies between 2 and 150 cases per 100,000 individuals (Rosati, 2001).

In the disease, the patient's immune defenses attack and damage the myelin sheath. When this happens, the axons are no longer able to effectively transmit signals (Compston & Coles, 2002). Although the mechanism by which the disease manifests itself has been well understood, the exact etiology is still unknown. The different theories propose both genetic and infectious causes; furthermore, correlations with environmental risk factors have been highlighted (Compston & Coles, 2002). The disease can manifest itself with a very wide range of neurological symptoms and can progress to physical and cognitive disability. MS can take various forms, including relapsing and progressive (Lublin et al., 1996). There is currently no known cure. The lack of effective standard treatments has led many patients to turn to alternative therapies including hypnosis (Senders et al., 2012; Wahbeh et al., 2008).

Although clinical evidence suggests a certain usefulness of hypnosis especially in controlling the main symptom, namely chronic pain, the literature on it is still modest.

Jensen et al. (2009) recruited 22 patients with MS and chronic pain in a semi-experimental study that compared the effects of self-hypnosis (HYP) with progressive muscle relaxation (PMR) on pain intensity and interference of pain. Participants in the HYP condition reported clinical improvement in pain and pain interference compared to participants in the PMR condition, and these results were maintained at a three-month follow-up.

Finally, 15 patients with MS (Jensen et al., 2011) received 16 treatment sessions for chronic pain which included four sessions each of four different treatment modules: (a) an educational control intervention; (b) self-hypnosis training (HYP); (c) cognitive restructuring (CR); and (d) a combined cognitive-hypnotic restructuring intervention (CR-HYP). CR-HYP treatment had beneficial effects outweighing the effects of CR and HYP alone.

Epilepsy and Non-Epileptic Psychogenic Crisis

Non-epileptic psychogenic crises represent approximately 20–40% of patients admitted to epilepsy centers (Asadi-Pooya & Sperling, 2015). Diagnosis is often challenging.

Hypnosis can be useful not only in the treatment of non-epileptic (epileptic) psychogenic seizures but also in the differential diagnosis between idiopathic epilepsy and epileptic psychogenic seizures (De Benedittis, 2021; Dickinson & Looper, 2012; Martinez-Taboas, 2002).

While it is well known that emotional and stressful stimuli can trigger both genuine and psychogenic epileptic attacks, hypnosis allows the two conditions to be differentiated, based on the following considerations (De Benedittis, 2021):

1 Unlike genuine epileptic seizures, psychogenic seizures can be reproduced in a trance state and interrupted with appropriate post-hypnotic commands.
2 In the case of a psychogenic crisis, the patient can remember the critical event, a condition that is never feasible in genuine generalized crises, characterized by complete interruption of the state of consciousness.
3 Patients with psychogenic crises are generally highly hypnotizable (Kuyk et al., 1995).

While the diagnostic and therapeutic role of hypnosis in non-epileptic psychogenic crises appears relatively well established, the use of hypnosis in epilepsy is generally contraindicated. The literature on the subject is virtually non-existent or limited to a few and controversial case reports or studies (De Benedittis, 2021).

Raynaud Syndrome

Raynaud syndrome, also known as Raynaud's phenomenon, is a medical condition in which the spasm of small arteries causes episodes of reduced blood flow to end arterioles. Typically, the fingers, and less commonly, the toes, are involved. The episodes result in the affected part turning white and then blue, often associated with numbness or pain.

Episodes are typically triggered by cold or emotional stress. Primary Raynaud's, also known as idiopathic, means that it is spontaneous, of unknown cause, and unrelated to another disease. Secondary Raynaud's can occur due to a connective-tissue disorder such as scleroderma or lupus, smoking, thyroid problems, and certain medications such as birth control pills. Diagnosis is typically based on the symptoms. About 4% of people have the condition (Wigley & Flagahan, 2016).

The primary treatment is avoiding the cold. Medications for treatment of cases that do not improve include calcium channel blockers and iloprost (Wigley & Flagahan, 2016).

Little evidence supports alternative medicine such as hypnosis. However, in reviewing the literature, Johnson (2016) reported that hypnosis and biofeedback offer promise for the treatment for Raynaud's symptomology (Johnson, 2016).

One patient with Raynaud phenomenon was trained to increase the temperature in his hands bilaterally, using combined hypnotic and operant techniques. An increase in temperature of as much as 4.3 C was observed in both hands, along with marked symptomatic improvement that was still in effect 7 1/2 months after the last treatment session (Jacobson et al., 1973). Hypnosis may also enhance the effects obtained by biofeedback of skin temperature (Shenefelt, 2003).

Neurorehabilitation

The restoration of the physical and psychological functional capacities of individuals who have suffered functional losses due to injuries or traumatic diseases is the essence of rehabilitation. The rehabilitation process is a bio-psychosocial endeavor and a model of holistic health through its interdisciplinary nature. Rehabilitation is also about learning to adapt to disability and gain accommodation for deficits.

Neurorehabilitation represents a fascinating but almost unexplored field of application of hypnosis (De Benedittis, 2021). The specific literature is very limited but encouraging. One of the main contributions of hypnosis to rehabilitation is its potential to facilitate change and accelerate learning (Appel, 2003, 2016). Hypnosis is able to enhance the patient's functional recovery, improving compliance with long and often exhausting physiatric treatments and significantly reducing the timing (De Benedittis, 2021).

Hypnotic techniques are aimed at implementing the motivations of patients with neurological lesions, often tired by physical disability and the frustrating sense of functional impotence, to counteract the associated psychopathological correlates (anxiety, depression), but also and above all to optimize functional recovery. Finally, hypnosis can improve the therapeutic response to physiatric rehabilitation maneuvers, reducing pain and spasticity, where present.

Hypnosis is increasingly used in the rehabilitation of patients with neurological problems. Indeed, neurological patients with a loss of motor skills achieve successful rehabilitation using motor images during hypnosis. The underlying mechanisms of "how" and "where" hypnosis works in the brain, however, are largely unknown. To identify brain areas involved in motor imagery under hypnosis, an fMRI study was conducted in which healthy subjects were required to both imagine and perform repetitive finger movements during a hypnotic trance (Müller et al., 2012). Increases in fMRI signal exclusively related to hypnosis were observed in the left superior frontal cortex, left anterior cingulate gyrus, and left thalamus. These areas represent the central nodes of the salience network that connects the primary and higher motor areas. Therefore, these data confirm the idea that hypnosis improves motor imaginations.

In a pilot clinical study of six post-stroke patients with motor deficits, Diamond et al. (2006) observed qualitative improvements in motor function related to increased range of motion, increased grip strength, and reduced spasticity of the paretic upper limb.

Another important rehabilitation area concerns memory. Impaired working memory is common in patients with brain injuries. Unfortunately, rehabilitation efforts for this impairment have so far produced little or no effect. A randomized, controlled study (Lindeløv et al., 2017) demonstrated that working memory performance can be effectively restored by prompting hypnotized patients to regain the pre-injury level of working memory functioning.

Contraindications, Precautions, and Safety Profile

In expert hands, hypnosis is a method with proven efficacy in selected cases, highly safe, and substantially free of side effects. There are no absolute contraindications to the use of hypnosis in neurology; instead, there are a number of relative contraindications. There is insufficient evidence to support the use of hypnosis in epilepsy and Parkinson's disease. Hypnosis is not recommended in cases of paroxysmal pain (e.g., trigeminal neuralgia, cluster headache) as patients with very acute pain are poorly responsive to the hypnotic means; in cases of patients who have inadequate motivations, dereistic expectations, and/or conspicuous "secondary gains" (for example, patients who derive a relational advantage from their illness, those who have applied for financial benefits). Another significant contraindication is represented by all those neurodegenerative diseases characterized by significant cognitive deficits as well as idiopathic or symptomatic epilepsy (De Benedittis, 2021).

In neurorehabilitation, the use of hypnosis is contraindicated in complete motor deficits (i.e., plegia) and sensory aphasia.

Conclusions

Despite its underuse in clinical practice, hypnosis has a significant role in neurological disorders and neurorehabilitation. A wide range of clinical syndromes (e.g., pain, movement disorders, Parkinson's disease, MS) may benefit from hypnotic interventions. In addition, hypnosis is able to enhance the patient's functional recovery in neurorehabilitation, improving compliance and significantly reducing the timing of recovery, thus optimizing the therapeutic outcome. However, more refined clinical studies and greater sample of patients are needed to establish the efficacy of hypnosis in neurology and neurorehabilitation.

References

Ajimsha, M., Majeed, N. A., Chinnavan, E., & Thulasyammal, R. P. (2014). Effectiveness of autogenic training in improving motor performances in Parkinson's disease. *Complementary Therapies in Medicine*, *22*(3), 419–425. 10.1016/j.ctim.2014.03.013

Appel, P. R. (2003). Clinical hypnosis in rehabilitation. *Seminars in Integrative Medicine*, *1*(2), 90–105. 10.1016/s1543-1150(03)00010-3

Appel, P. R. (2016). Rehabilitation: Amelioration of suffering and adjustment. In G. R. Elkins (Ed.), *Handbook of medical and psychological hypnosis: Foundations, applications, and professional issues* (1st ed., pp. 399–408). Springer Publishing Company.

Asadi-Pooya, A. A., & Sperling, M. R. (2015). Epidemiology of psychogenic nonepileptic seizures. *Epilepsy & Behavior*, *46*, 60–65. 10.1016/j.yebeh.2015.03.015

Balint, B., & Bhatia, K. P. (2014). Dystonia: An update on phenomenology, classification, pathogenesis and treatment. *Current Opinion in Neurology*, *27*(4), 468–476. 10.1097/wco.0000000000000114

Bihari, K., Hill, J. L., & Murphy, D. L. (1992). Obsessive-compulsive characteristics in patients with idiopathic spasmodic torticollis. *Psychiatry Research*, *42*(3), 267–272. 10.1016/0165-1781(92)90118-m

Claypool, D. W., Duane, D. D., Ilstrup, D. M., & Melton, L. J. (1995). Epidemiology and outcome of cervical dystonia (spasmodic torticollis) in Rochester, Minnesota. *Movement Disorders*, *10*(5), 608–614. 10.1002/mds.870100513

Compston, A., & Coles, A. (2002). Multiple sclerosis. *The Lancet*, *359*(9313), 1221–1231. 10.1016/s0140-6736(02)08220-x

Crasilneck, H. B., & Hall, J. A. (1985). *Clinical hypnosis: Principles and applications* (2nd ed.). Pearson.

De Benedittis, G. (1996). Hypnosis and spasmodic torticollis – Report of four cases: A brief communication. *International Journal of Clinical and Experimental Hypnosis*, *44*(4), 292–306. 10.1080/00207149608416094

De Benedittis, G. (2004). Postural hypnosis and EMG-biofeedback in idiopathic cervical dystonia. *Hypnos*, *31*(3), 136–145.

De Benedittis, G. (2016). Spasmodic torticollis. In G. R. Elkins (Ed.), *Handbook of medical and psychological hypnosis: Foundations, applications, and professional issues* (1st ed., pp. 419–427). Springer Publishing Company.

De Benedittis, G. (2021). Neurologia e neuroriabilitazione (Neurology and neurorehabilitation). In G. De Benedittis, C. Loriedo, C. Mammini, & N. Rago (Eds.), *Trattato di ipnosi: Dai fondamenti teorici alla pratica clinica (Italian Edition)* (pp. 381–399). Franco Angeli.

De Virgilio, A., Greco, A., Fabbrini, G., Inghilleri, M., Rizzo, M. I., Gallo, A., Conte, M., Rosato, C., Ciniglio Appiani, M., & De Vincentiis, M. (2016). Parkinson's disease: Autoimmunity and neuroinflammation. *Autoimmunity Reviews*, *15*(10), 1005–1011. 10.1016/j.autrev.2016.07.022

Diamond, S. G., Davis, O. C., Schaechter, J. D., & Howe, R. D. (2006). Hypnosis for rehabilitation after stroke: Six case studies. *Contemporary Hypnosis*, *23*(4), 173–180. 10.1002/ch.319

Dickinson, P., & Looper, K. J. (2012). Psychogenic nonepileptic seizures: A current overview. *Epilepsia*, *53*(10), 1679–1689. 10.1111/j.1528-1167.2012.03606.x

Donaldson, I., Marsden, D. C., Schneider, S. A., & Bhatia, K. P. (2012). *Marsden's book of movement disorders* (1st ed.). Oxford University Press.

Elkins, G. R. (Ed.). (2016). *Handbook of medical and psychological hypnosis: Foundations, applications, and professional issues* (1st ed.). Springer Publishing Company.
Evatt, M. I., Freeman, A., & Factor, S. (2011). Adult-onset dystonia. In W. J. Weiner, E. Tolosa, M. J. Aminoff, F. Boller, & D. F. Swaab (Eds.), *Hyperkinetic movement disorders (Handbook of clinical neurology, Volume # 100; 3rd series)* (1st ed., Vol. 100, pp. 481–512). Elsevier.
Ewin, D. M., & Elmer, B. N. (2006). *Ideomotor signals for rapid hypnoanalysis: A how-to manual.* Charles C Thomas Publisher.
Flamand-Roze, C., Célestin-Lhopiteau, I., & Roze, E. (2016). Hypnosis and movement disorders: State of the art and perspectives. *Revue Neurologique*, *172*(8–9), 530–536. 10.1016/j.neurol.2016.07.008
Jacobson, A. M., Hackett, T. P., & Surman, O. S. (1973). Raynaud phenomenon: Treatment with hypnotic and operant technique. *The Journal of the American Medical Association (JAMA)*, *225*(7), 739–740. 10.1001/jama.225.7.739
Jankovic, J., Tsui, J., & Bergeron, C. (2007). Prevalence of cervical dystonia and spasmodic torticollis in the United States general population. *Parkinsonism & Related Disorders*, *13*(7), 411–416. 10.1016/j.parkreldis.2007.02.005
Jensen, M. P., Barber, J., Romano, J. M., Molton, I. R., Raichle, K. A., Osborne, T. L., Engel, J. M., Stoelb, B. L., Kraft, G. H., & Patterson, D. R. (2009). A comparison of Self-Hypnosis versus progressive muscle relaxation in patients with multiple sclerosis and chronic pain. *International Journal of Clinical and Experimental Hypnosis*, *57*(2), 198–221. 10.1080/00207140802665476
Jensen, M. P., Ehde, D. M., Gertz, K. J., Stoelb, B. L., Dillworth, T. M., Hirsh, A. T., Molton, I. R., & Kraft, G. H. (2011). Effects of self-hypnosis training and cognitive restructuring on daily pain intensity and catastrophizing in individuals with multiple sclerosis and chronic pain. *International Journal of Clinical and Experimental Hypnosis*, *59*(1), 45–63. 10.1080/00207144.2011.522892
Johnson, A. (2016). Raynaud's syndrome. In G. R. Elkins (Ed.), *Handbook of medical and psychological hypnosis: Foundations, applications, and professional issues* (1st ed., pp. 391–398). Springer Publishing Company.
Kohen, D., & Kaiser, P. (2014). Clinical hypnosis with children and adolescents – What? Why? How?: Origins, applications, and efficacy. *Children*, *1*(2), 74–98. 10.3390/children1020074
Kurlan, R. M. (2014). Treatment of Tourette syndrome. *Neurotherapeutics*, *11*(1), 161–165. 10.1007/s13311-013-0215-4
Kuyk, J., Jacobs, L. D., Aldenkamp, A. P., Meinardi, H., Spinhoven, P., & Van Dyck, R. (1995). Pseudo-epileptic seizures: Hypnosis as a diagnostic tool. *Seizure –European Journal of Epilepsy*, *4*(2), 123–128. 10.1016/s1059-1311(95)80091-3
Lindeløv, J. K., Overgaard, R., & Overgaard, M. (2017). Improving working memory performance in brain-injured patients using hypnotic suggestion. *Brain*, *140*(4), 1100–1106. 10.1093/brain/awx001
Lisak R., Truong D., Carroll W., & Bhidayasiri R. (2016). *International neurology.* Stati Uniti: Wiley-Blackwell.
Lublin, F. D., Reingold, S. C., & National Multiple Sclerosis Society (USA) Advisory Committee on Clinical Trials of New Agents in Multiple Sclerosis. (1996). Defining the clinical course of multiple sclerosis: Results of an international survey. *Neurology*, *46*(4), 907–911. 10.1212/WNL.46.4.907
Martínez-Taboas, A. (2002). The role of hypnosis in the detection of psychogenic seizures. *American Journal of Clinical Hypnosis*, *45*(1), 11–20. 10.1080/00029157.2002.10403493
Moene, F. C., Spinhoven, P., Hoogduin, K., & Van Dyck, R. (2003). A randomized controlled clinical trial of a hypnosis-based treatment for patients with conversion disorder, motor type. *International Journal of Clinical and Experimental Hypnosis*, *51*(1), 29–50. 10.1076/iceh.51.1.29.14067
Mozzoni, M. (2018). Ipnosi e parkinson. *Ipnosi*, *n*(1), 41–50. 10.3280/ipn2018-001003
Müller, K., Bacht, K., Schramm, S., & Seitz, R. J. (2012). The facilitating effect of clinical hypnosis on motor imagery: An fMRI study. *Behavioural Brain Research*, *231*(1), 164–169. 10.1016/j.bbr.2012.03.013
Olson, S. (2004). Making sense of Tourette's. *Science*, *305*(5689), 1390–1392. 10.1126/science.305.5689.1390
Peckham, E. L., & Hallett, M. (2009). Psychogenic movement disorders. *Neurologic Clinics*, *27*(3), 801–819. 10.1016/j.ncl.2009.04.008

Robertson, M. M. (2000). Tourette syndrome, associated conditions and the complexities of treatment. *Brain*, *123*(3), 425–462. 10.1093/brain/123.3.425

Rosati, G. (2001). The prevalence of multiple sclerosis in the world: An update. *Neurological Sciences*, *22*(2), 117–139. 10.1007/s100720170011

Schlesinger, I., Benyakov, O., Erikh, I., Suraiya, S., & Schiller, Y. (2009). Parkinson's disease tremor is diminished with relaxation guided imagery. *Movement Disorders*, *24*(14), 2059–2062. 10.1002/mds.22671

Senders, A., Wahbeh, H., Spain, R., & Shinto, L. (2012). Mind-body medicine for multiple sclerosis: A systematic review. *Autoimmune Diseases*, *2012*, 1–12. 10.1155/2012/567324

Shenefelt, P. D. (2003). Biofeedback, cognitive-behavioral methods, and hypnosis in dermatology: Is it all in your mind? *Dermatologic Therapy*, *16*(2), 114–122. 10.1046/j.1529-8019.2003.01620.x

Singer, H. S. (2005). Tourette's syndrome: From behaviour to biology. *The Lancet Neurology*, *4*(3), 149–159. 10.1016/S1474-4422(05)01012-4

Singer, H. S., & Walkup, J. T. (1991). Tourette syndrome and other tic disorders: Diagnosis, pathophysiology, and treatment. *Medicine*, *70*(1), 15–32. 10.1097/00005792-199101000-00002

The Epidemiological Study of Dystonia in Europe (ESDE) Collaborative Group. (2000). A prevalence study of primary dystonia in eight European countries. *Journal of Neurology*, *247*(10), 787–792. 10.1007/s004150070094

Vacherot, F., Vaugoyeau, M., Mallau, S., Soulayrol, S., Assaiante, C., & Azulay, J. (2007). Postural control and sensory integration in cervical dystonia. *Clinical Neurophysiology*, *118*(5), 1019–1027. 10.1016/j.clinph.2007.01.013

Waddy, H. M., Fletcher, N. A., Harding, A. E., & Marsden, C. D. (1991). A genetic study of idiopathic focal dystonias. *Annals of Neurology*, *29*(3), 320–324. 10.1002/ana.410290315

Wahbeh, H., Elsas, S. M., & Oken, B. S. (2008). Mind-body interventions: Applications in neurology. *Neurology*, *70*(24), 2321–2328. 10.1212/01.wnl.0000314667.16386.5e

Wigley, F. M., & Flavahan, N. A. (2016). Raynaud's phenomenon. *The New England Journal of Medicine*, *375*(6), 556–565. 10.1056/nejmra1507638

Wilkinson, I., & Lennox, G. (2005). *Essential neurology* (4th ed.). Wiley-Blackwell.

Witt, K., Kalbe, E., Erasmi, R., Ebersbach, G. (2017). Nichtmedikamentöse Therapieverfahren beim Morbus Parkinson [Nonpharmacological treatment procedures for Parkinson's disease]. Nervenarzt, *88*(4), 383–390. German. 10.1007/s00115-017-0298-y. PMID: 28251243.

41
HYPNOSIS FOR SKIN DISORDERS

Philip D. Shenefelt

Retired Professor, Dermatology and Cutaneous Surgery, University of South Florida, Tampa, FL, USA

The skin and the nervous system develop side by side together in the growing fetus in the ectoderm layer. The skin and nervous system remain strongly interconnected and continue to influence each other significantly throughout life, providing a natural link by which hypnosis can affect skin disorders. Stress, negative feelings, and undesirable behaviors such as scratching or picking or noncompliance with prescribed treatments can adversely affect many skin disorders. For most patients, having a serious or cosmetically disfiguring skin disorder can negatively affect the psyche. Hypnosis can help patients deal with the emotional and physical effects that the skin disease or disorder has on their lives. Some patients are overly fearful of minor surgical skin procedures, and hypnosis can be used to reduce procedure anxiety. Many inflammatory skin disorders can be improved through hypnotic suggestions, and some skin conditions such as viral warts can resolve via suggestions influencing the immune response to the virus. Recognizing natural shifts of patients briefly into trance during office visits allows the practitioner to intersperse appropriate suggestions during hypnomoments without further need to take time to induce trance (Shenefelt, 2019). For cases involving skin disorders unexpectedly resistant to ordinary suggestion, the effective use of medical psychosomatic hypnoanalysis may produce desired results (Shenefelt, 2007). If still resistant, spiritual or religious areas can be evaluated with further hypnoanalysis (Shenefelt & Shenefelt, 2014).

Medical Hypnotherapy for Treating Specific Skin Disorders

Most reported evidence on the effectiveness of hypnosis for specific dermatologic conditions was until recently based on one or a few uncontrolled case examples (Shenefelt, 2000). The trend toward controlled trials has produced more reliable information (Kaschel et al., 1991), although randomized controlled trial results are still not available for most skin disorders. See Table 41.1.

The extent to which the various skin disorders are subject to mental influence was examined by Dr Griesemer (1978), a dermatologist and psychiatrist. See Table 41.2.

Acne tends to flare with stress in many individuals. Relaxation through teaching self-hypnosis can help reregulate the autonomic nervous system and decrease stress hormones.

DOI: 10.4324/9781003449126-55

Table 41.1 Skin Disorders Responsive to Hypnosis

Randomized Control Trials (representing strong evidence of effectiveness)
- Hypnotic relaxation and anxiety reduction during dermatologic procedures
- Verruca vulgaris
- Psoriasis

Nonrandomized Control Trials
- Atopic dermatitis

Case Series
- Alopecia areata
- Urticaria

Single or Few Case Reports (representing weak evidence of effectiveness)
- Acne excoriée
- Congenital ichthyosiform erythroderma
- Dyshidrotic dermatitis
- Erythema nodosum
- Erythromelalgia
- Furuncles
- Glossodynia
- Herpes simplex
- Hyperhidrosis
- Ichthyosis vulgaris
- Lichen planus
- Neurodermatitis
- Nummular dermatitis
- Post-herpetic neuralgia
- Pruritus
- Rosacea
- Trichotillomania
- Vitiligo

Table 41.2 Skin Disorders Rank Ordered as Being Triggered by Psychological Factors

Diagnosis	*% Triggered*	*Time elapsed*
Hyperhidrosis	100.0	seconds
Lichen simplex chronicus	98.5	days–2 weeks
Neurotic excoriations	97.5	seconds
Alopecia areata	96.4	2 weeks
Warts, multiple and spreading	94.9	days
Rosacea	94.1	2 days
Pruritus	85.7	seconds
Lichen planus	81.8	day–2 weeks
Dyshidrotic hand dermatitis	75.8	2 days
Atopic dermatitis	70.2	seconds
Factitial dermatosis	69.2	seconds
Urticaria	68.1	minutes
Psoriasis	62.3	day–2 weeks
Traumatic dermatitis	55.6	seconds
Dermatitis not otherwise specified	55.6	days
Acne vulgaris	55.3	2 days
Telogen effluvium	54.7	2–3 weeks
Nummular dermatitis	51.8	days

(*Continued*)

Table 41.2 (Continued)

Diagnosis	*% Triggered*	*Time elapsed*
Seborrheic dermatitis	40.6	day–2 weeks
Herpes simplex/zoster	35.7	days
Vitiligo	33.3	2–3 weeks
Pyoderma/bacterial infect	29.1	days
Nail dystrophy	28.5	2–3 weeks
Cysts	27.0	2–3 weeks
Warts, single/multiple	17.4	days
Contact dermatitis	15.3	2 days
Fungal infections	8.7	day–2 weeks
Basal cell carcinoma	0	n/a
Keratoses	0	n/a
Nevi	0	n/a

Note: Modified from *Hypnosis in Dermatology* by Shenefelt, 2000, p. 394. Copyright 2000 Shenefelt.

Picking performed with *acne excoriée* also intensifies with stress. Posthypnotic suggestion was successful in reducing or stopping the picking associated with acne excoriée in two reported cases (Hollander, 1959). One patient was instructed to remember the word "scar" whenever she wanted to pick her face and to refrain from picking by saying "scar" instead. The author has had similar success in one case and also reminded the patient in trance that perfect is less beautiful than natural is (Shenefelt, 2004). Hypnosis may be an appropriate treatment for the picking habit aspect of acne excoriée in conjunction with standard treatments for the acne itself.

Alopecia areata commonly flares with stress in most individuals. In a small clinical trial of medical hypnotherapy with five patients having extensive alopecia areata, only one patient showed significant increase in hair growth. Hypnosis did improve stress and psychological parameters in these five patients, although three patients had only slight increase in hair growth and one had no change (Harrison & Stepanek, 1991). In a larger clinical trial (Willemsen et al., 2006), all 21 patients with severe alopecia areata had improvement of anxiety and depression with hypnotherapy. Nine patients had total regrowth of scalp hair, and another three patients had better than 75% regrowth. Hypnosis is appropriate as a supportive treatment for the psychological impact of having alopecia areata and may sometimes have a positive effect on the condition itself. Hypnosis may be used adjunctively with other treatments such as Janus kinase (JAK) inhibitors that modulate the immune system by inhibiting one or more of the Janus kinase family of enzymes, interfering with the JAK-STAT signaling pathway in lymphocytes. This often permits hair regrowth.

Stress can exacerbate *atopic dermatitis*. A number of case reports describe improvement of atopic dermatitis in both children and adults as a result of hypnotherapy (Twerski & Naar, 1974). In a nonrandomized controlled clinical trial, Stewart and Thomas (1995) treated 18 adults with extensive atopic dermatitis who had been resistant to conventional treatment with hypnotherapy that included relaxation, stress management, direct suggestion for non-scratching behavior, direct suggestion for skin comfort and coolness, ego strengthening, posthypnotic suggestions, and instruction in self-hypnosis. The results were statistically significant ($p < 0.01$) for reductions in itch, scratching, sleep disturbance, and tension. Topical corticosteroid use decreased by 40% at 4 weeks, 50% at 8 weeks, and

60% at 16 weeks. For atopic dermatitis, hypnosis can be a very useful therapy that can decrease the needed number of other treatments.

Clearing of *congenital ichthyosiform erythroderma* of Brocq in a 16-year-old boy was reported following direct suggestion for clearing under hypnosis (Mason, 1952). Mason mistakenly thought that the boy had warts and strongly believed in the efficacy of hypnosis. Similar though less spectacular results were confirmed with two sisters aged eight and six (Wink, 1961), with a 20-year-old woman (Schneck, 1966), and with 34-year-old father and his four-year-old son (Kidd, 1966). Based on these case reports, hypnosis may be potentially very useful as a therapy in addition to emollients.

Stress is a common trigger factor for *dyshidrotic dermatitis*, to the point where some individuals can use the flaring of their dyshidrotic dermatitis as a barometer of their stress levels. Reduction in severity of dyshidrotic dermatitis has been reported while using hypnosis as a treatment (Tobia, 1982).

The author reported a case of *erythema nodosum* which had failed to resolve with medical treatment for nine years but which resolved following psychosomatic hypnoanalysis (Shenefelt, 2007).

There is one case report of successful treatment of *erythromelalgia* in an 18-year-old woman using hypnosis alone followed by self-hypnosis (Chakravarty et al., 1992). Permanent resolution occurred.

A 33-year-old man with a negative self-image and recurrent multiple Staphylococcus aureus containing *furuncles* occurring since age 17 had been unresponsive to multiple treatment modalities. Hypnosis and self-hypnosis with imagined sensations of warmth, cold, tingling, and heaviness brought about dramatic improvement over five weeks with full resolution of the recurrent furuncles (Jabush, 1969). The patient also had substantial mental attitude improvement. Conventional antibiotic therapy is the first line of treatment for furuncles, but in unusually resistant cases with significant psychosomatic overlay, use of hypnosis may help to end the chronic susceptibility to recurrent infection.

Oral pain such as *glossodynia* may respond well to hypnosis as a primary treatment if there is a significant psychological component (Golan, 1997). With organic disease, hypnosis may give temporary relief from pain.

Discomfort relief from *herpes simplex* through hypnotic suggestion is simpler than but similar to that for postherpetic neuralgia (see below). Reduction in the frequency of recurrences of herpes simplex following hypnosis has also been reported (Bertolino, 1983). In cases with an apparent emotional stress trigger factor, hypnotic suggestion may be useful as a therapy for reducing the frequency of recurrence.

Hypnosis or autogenic training may be useful as adjunctive therapy for *hyperhidrosis* (Hölzle, 1984). Suggestions for relaxation and thoughts of coolness may be helpful, Stress is a common trigger or exacerbator of hyperhidrosis.

A 33-year-old man with *ichthyosis vulgaris* which was better in summer and worse in winter began hypnotic suggestion therapy in the summer and was able to maintain the summer improvement throughout the fall, winter, and spring (Schneck, 1954).

Stress is a definite exacerbating factor in *lichen planus*. Pruritus and lesions of lichen planus may be reduced in selected cases using hypnosis (Scott, 1960; Tobia, 1982).

Some cases of *neurodermatitis* or psychogenic dermatitis have resolved and stayed resolved with up to four years of follow-up using hypnosis as an alternative therapy (Kline, 1953, Sacerdote, 1965; Collison, 1972; Lehman, 1978). Stress is a major factor in increasing scratching or picking of the skin in these patients.

Reduction of pruritus and resolution of lesions of *nummular dermatitis* has been reported with use of hypnotic suggestion (Scott, 1960; Tobia, 1982).

Pain from *herpes zoster* and *post-herpetic neuralgia* can be reduced by hypnosis (Scott, 1960; Tobia, 1982). Hypnosis may be useful as a therapy for postherpetic neuralgia. As an example, the author had one patient, a 70-year-old retired attorney who came to seek help through hypnosis out of desperation with a history of debilitating post-herpetic pain of six years duration. He had been an actively practicing trial lawyer in reasonably good health. At age 64, he developed acute herpes zoster on his left back, thigh, and leg primarily in the L4 dermatomal pattern associated with severe pain. After several weeks, the acute phase resolved, but severe post-herpetic neuralgia persisted. He retired early due to his difficulty concentrating while dealing with the pain. Various drug regimens had been ineffective in reducing the pain sufficiently, including acetaminophen, NSAIDS, oral cortisone, gabapentin and its derivatives, and morphine and its derivatives. Physical therapy methods, attempted nerve blocks, and regional infiltration with injected anesthetics had also failed to help sufficiently. He spent much time at home sitting and reading. When he attempted to play golf, one of his favorite pastimes, he usually quit after one or at most two holes. His assessed quality of life was poor due to the unrelenting pain.

He had no prior experience with hypnosis but was a highly motivated and intelligent person. After some discussion, and with informed consent, he experienced hypnosis using the Hypnotic Induction Profile (Spiegel & Spiegel, 2004) and he scored in the moderately hypnotizable range with no decrement. He did experience trance. He was taught in the alert state the various control imagery choices such as a discomfort versus comfort meter, a color indicator of discomfort versus comfort, applying a cooling lotion or cold pack, and glove anesthesia. He then again had trance induction using the Spiegel eyeroll method similar to that found in the Hypnotic Induction Profile (Spiegel & Spiegel, 2004) and deepened the trance with a ten-count descent on a path to a peaceful place he would rather be. After allowing him to enjoy the sights sounds, comfortable temperature, fragrances, and body positions of that place, it was suggested he experiment in turn with imagining a discomfort meter, imagining an increase and decrease in discomfort, and compare that with a color indicator of discomfort versus comfort and also had him imagine applying a cool pack or cooling lotion to the area and to note any changes in discomfort. After he re-alerted he was asked about his experiences. He had discovered that he could both increase and decrease discomfort using the meter or color scheme. Next, he was taught self-hypnosis using the Spiegel eyeroll induction, followed by self-deepening, going to a safe place, suggestions for changing discomfort toward comfort, and re-alerting himself. He was instructed to practice self-hypnosis daily and to give self-suggestions for comfort.

When the patient was seen two weeks later he was a transformed person. He had practiced self-hypnosis diligently and had regained a sense of control over his life. He reported that the pain intensity had not changed much, but it was no longer governing his life. He had been able to complete nine holes of golf without stopping except for brief self-hypnosis. He also was enjoying many other activities that he had previously given up doing. His interpersonal relationships had also improved. Now he felt like he was in control instead of letting the pain control him. He was very pleased and did not feel the need for further follow-up. His pain level was about the same, but he found he could lessen the pain for short periods using self-hypnosis, and his suffering had decreased dramatically. Having a sense of control over the pain freed him from letting the pain dominate him and run his life.

This case illustrates that hypnosis may not change the pain level much, depending on the source of the pain. Neuropathic pain such as from herpes zoster neuralgia often is difficult to alter in intensity except perhaps briefly. The hypnosis does not act much on the neuropathic source itself once established as a chronic post-inflammatory condition. By contrast, inflammatory pain may be more amenable to hypnosis because hypnosis can alter the inflammatory process inducing the pain. This patient experienced that he could modify the pain rather than feeling like the pain controlled him. He regained his sense of control and for him that made all the difference in his attitudes toward pain and life.

Pruritus typically increases with stress. Hypnosis can modify and lessen the intensity of pruritus (Scott, 1960). A man with chronic myelogenous leukemia had intractable pruritus that was much improved with hypnotic suggestion (Ament & Milgrom, 1967). Suggestions for cooling lotion or cool packs may be beneficial.

Stress is a common exacerbating factor in *psoriasis*. Hypnosis and suggestion have been demonstrated to have a positive effect on psoriasis (Kantor, 1990; Zachariae et al., 1996; Winchell & Watts, 1988). A 75% clearing of psoriasis was reported in one case using a hypnotic sensory-imagery technique (Kline, 1954). A case of extensive severe psoriasis of 20 years duration had marked improvement using sensory imagery to replicate the feelings in the patient's skin that he had experienced during sunbathing (Frankel & Misch, 1973). Another case of severe psoriasis of 20 years duration resolved fully with a hypnoanalytic technique (Waxman, 1973). Tausk and Whitmore (1999) performed a small randomized controlled trial using hypnosis as adjunctive therapy in psoriasis with significant improvement only in the highly hypnotizable subjects and not in the moderately hypnotizable subjects. Hypnosis can be quite useful as a therapy for resistant psoriasis, especially if there is a significant emotional factor triggering the psoriasis.

The vascular blush component of *rosacea* has been reported to improve in selected cases of resistant rosacea where hypnosis has been added (Scott, 1960; Tobia, 1982). Stress can increase blushing.

Several reports of successful adjunctive hypnotic treatment of *trichotillomania* have been published (Galski, 1981; Rowen, 1981; Barabasz, 1987). Stress is an exacerbating factor. Hypnosis may be a useful therapy for trichotillomania.

Two cases of *urticaria* with stress as a trigger factor responded to hypnotic suggestion in one study. An 11-year-old boy who had an urticarial reaction to chocolate could have the hives blocked by hypnotic suggestion so that hives appeared on one side of his face but not the other in response to hypnotic suggestion (Perloff & Spiegelman, 1973). In 15 patients with chronic urticaria of 7.8 years average duration, hypnosis with relaxation therapy resulted within 14 months in six patients being cleared and another eight patients improved, with decreased medication requirements reported by 80% of the subjects (Shertzer & Lookingbill, 1987).

Bloch (1927) and Sulzberger (Sulzberger & Wolf, 1934) reported on the efficacy of suggestion in treating *verruca vulgaris (warts)*. This has since been confirmed numerous times to a greater or lesser degree (Obermayer & Greenson, 1949; Ullman, 1959, Dudek, 1967; Sheehan, 1978) and failed to be confirmed in a few studies (Clarke, 1965; Stankler, 1967). A study that showed negative results was criticized for using a negative suggestion of not feeding the warts rather than a positive suggestion about having the warts resolve (Felt et al., 1998). Many reports confirm the efficacy of hypnosis in treating warts (McDowell, 1949; Ullman & Dudek, 1960; Vickers, 1961; Surman et al., 1972; Ewin, 1974; Clawson & Swade, 1975; Tasini & Hackett, 1977; Johnson & Barber, 1978;

Dreaper, 1978; Straatmeyer & Rhodes, 1983; Morris, 1985; Spanos et al., 1988; Noll, 1988; Spanos et al., 1990; Ewin, 1992; Noll, 1994). One study (Tenzel & Taylor, 1969) that tried to replicate the remarkable success reported in Lancet (Sinclair-Gieben & Chalmers, 1959) of using hypnotic suggestion to cause warts to disappear from one hand but not the other in persons with bilateral hand warts was unsuccessful. A well conducted randomized control study resulted in 53% of the experimental group having improvement of their warts three months after the first of five hypnotherapy sessions, while none of the control group had improvement (Surman et al., 1973). Genital warts in women have been demonstrated to be reduced or eliminated with hypnotic suggestions (Barabasz et al., 2010). Ewin (1992) reported a series of cases of warts resistant to ordinary hypnotic suggestions but with the addition of psychosomatic hypnoanalysis most of those cases of warts did resolve. Hypnosis has been proven to be successful as a therapy for warts.

Having *vitiligo* can be very stressful to some individuals, especially those with naturally dark skin tone. Vitiligo has improved using hypnotic suggestion as supportive therapy (Scott, 1960; Tobia, 1982), but it is unclear whether the recovery was simply spontaneous because spontaneous recovery is known to occur. Hypnosis may be appropriate as a supportive treatment for the psychological impact associated with having vitiligo.

Medical Hypnotherapy for Reducing Procedure Stress and Anxiety

Hypnosis can help reduce stress, anxiety, needle phobia, and pain during cutaneous surgery, as well as reduce postoperative discomfort and enhance postoperative healing. Fick et al. (1999) used self-guided imagery content during nonpharmacologic analgesia to help 56 nonselected patients referred for percutaneous interventional procedures in the radiology procedure suite. A standardized protocol and script were used to guide patients into a state of self-hypnotic relaxation followed by suggestion to go where they would rather be. All 56 patients developed an imaginary scenario. The imagery they chose was highly individualistic. They concluded that average patients can engage in imagery, but topics patients chose were highly individualistic, making recorded suggested scenarios or provider directed imagery likely to be less effective than self-directed imagery. The author has used this technique with good success in dermatology patients (Shenefelt, 2003, 2013).

Lang et al. (2000) conducted a larger randomized trial of adjunctive non-pharmacologic analgesia for invasive percutaneous vascular radiologic procedures consisting of three groups: standard care (control group), structured attention, and self-hypnotic relaxation. Pain increased linearly with time in the standard and the attention group, but remained flat in the hypnosis group. Anxiety decreased over time in all three groups, but more so with hypnosis. Conscious sedation drug use was significantly higher in the standard group than in the structured attention and self-hypnosis groups. The hemodynamic stability was significantly higher in the hypnosis group than in the attention and standard groups. Procedure times were significantly shorter in the hypnosis group than in the standard group, with the attention group intermediate. Cost analysis of this study (Lang & Rosen, 2002) showed that the cost associated with standard conscious sedation averaged $638 per case while the cost for sedation with adjunct hypnosis was $300 per case, making the latter considerably more cost-effective.

The author conducted a randomized control trial of hypnotically induced relaxation with self-guided imagery with 39 patients undergoing dermatologic surgery. They were randomly assigned to live induction, recorded induction, and control groups. The live induction group had significantly less anxiety by 20 minutes into the procedure than the controls, with the recorded induction group being close to the controls in response (Shenefelt, 2013).

A meta-analysis of hypnotically induced analgesia found that hypnosis can significantly relieve pain in patients with headache, burn injury, heart disease, cancer, dental problems, eczema (atopic dermatitis), and chronic back problems (Montgomery et al., 2000). For most purposes, light and medium trance is sufficient, but deep trance is required for hypnotic anesthesia for surgery (Barabasz & Watkins, 2005). Pain reduction mediated by hypnosis localized to the mid-anterior cingulate cortex in a study (Faymonville et al., 2000) using a positron emission tomography, suggesting that hypnotic effects with respect to pain regulation occur at least in part in the mid-anterior cingulate cortex.

In general, for hypnosis to be of benefit, patients must be mentally intact, not psychotic nor heavily intoxicated; be motivated, not resistant, and preferably medium or high hypnotizable as rated by the Hypnotic Induction Profile (Spiegel & Spiegel, 2004) or Stanford Hypnotic Susceptibility Scale and its variants. However, for self-guided imagery, a moderate or high degree of hypnotizability is not critical to success. Letting the patient choose his or her own self-guided imagery allows most individuals to reach a state of relaxation during procedures. Both the patient and the physician can benefit from a more pleasant experience attended by fewer complications during the procedure.

Psychosomatic Hypnoanalysis

Psychosomatic hypnoanalysis may help patients with skin disorders unresponsive to other simpler approaches. Using hypnoanalysis, results may also occur much more quickly than with standard psychoanalysis (Scott, 1960). Psychologists and psychiatrists have focused primarily on the mind and the emotions and have used hypnoanalysis to speed therapeutic results. Non-psychiatrist physicians and others have focused on the body and how the mind interacts with the body. To differentiate this from the type of hypnoanalysis used by psychologists and psychiatrists, the author has coined the term psychosomatic hypnoanalysis (Shenefelt, 2007; Shenefelt, 2018). This utilizes the somatic bridge starting with the bodily issue or complaint and using age regression back to the first time of occurrence or flaring and the associated negative experience or emotion that seemed to initiate or trigger it. Several key factors have been identified by Cheek and LeCron (1968) associated with psychosomatic issues. The author has slightly modified their naming to create a mnemonic. The key issues are *C*onflict, *O*rgan language, *M*otivation or secondary gain, *P*ast experiences or traumatic conditioning, *A*ctive identification, *S*uggestion, and *S*elf-punishment. The C.O.M.P.A.S.S. method of identifying seven trigger or exacerbating psychosomatic root causes is well described in Ewin and Eimer (2006). Ideomotor signaling is used for nonverbal communication (Ewin & Eimer, 2006; Shenefelt, 2011) Uncovering the initiating or trigger or exacerbating factors and neutralizing the associated negatively charged emotion often leads to the resolution of the psychosomatic aspects of the problem. Dr Ewin (1992) used psychosomatic hypnoanalysis on a series of 41 patients with recalcitrant warts that had failed to respond to ordinary hypnotic suggestion and had resolution in 33 of the 41 patients (Ewin, 1992). In these cases, a psychological blocking factor had inhibited the delayed cellular immune system from eliminating the warts until the negative emotional blockage was removed. One of the author's patients who had persistent erythema nodosum for nine years with no apparent physical trigger factors had resolution of the lesions after psychosomatic hypnoanalysis (Shenefelt, 2007). Another patient had resolution of resistant neurodermatitis on the face (Shenefelt, 2010). This C.O.M.P.A.S.S. method can be used for screening for psychosomatic factors. Although not empirically demonstrated, experience has taught that if all of the C.O.M.P.A.S.S. factors are negative, there is likely not a psychosomatic component to the disease process. If one or two factors are positive, appropriate neutralizing suggestions may be sufficient. If three or more factors are positive, referral to an appropriate psychologist or psychiatrist or other experienced mental health worker would be appropriate (Shenefelt, 2007). If the C.O.M.P.A.S.S. mnemonic is negative but the practitioner intuits that there may be something else to uncover, the P.O.I.N.T mnemonic may be added, representing *P*ast life experience ("real" or imagined), *O*ccult hex or curse, *I*ntruder spirit, *N*ocebo, or *T*rauma in their ancestral lineage (Shenefelt, 2012). What is important is what the person believes, whether "real" from an objective practitioner's standpoint or not.

Conclusions

The hypnotic use of trance often is capable of influencing amenable skin disorders in ways that are generally not feasible during ordinary conscious awareness. Direct suggestion, indirect suggestion, utilization of hypnomoments, and psychosomatic hypnoanalysis present useful tools that in selected cases can have significant effects on the skin disorders. For inflammatory conditions, suggestions such as imagining cooling sensations, imagining soothing lotion applications, imagining prior effective treatment results being used again, or imagining healthy skin before or after the onset of the condition can all be helpful. As Dr David Spiegel has said, "It is not all mind over matter, but mind matters" (Spiegel, 2001, p. 1768). As with most medical interventions, the results are variable, but hypnosis provides another available modality that currently is underutilized.

References

Ament, P., & Milgrom, H. (1967). Effects of suggestion on pruritus with cutaneous lesions in chronic myelogenous leukemia. *The Journal of the American Society of Psychosomatic Dentistry and Medicine*, *14*(4), 122–125. PMID: 5235108

Barabasz, A., Higley, L., Christensen, C., & Barabasz, M. (2010). Efficacy of hypnosis in the treatment of human papillomavirus (HPV) in women: Rural and urban samples. *International Journal of Clinical and Experimental Hypnosis*, *58*(1), 102–121. 10.1080/00207140903310899

Barabasz, A., & Watkins, J. G. (2005). *Hypnotherapeutic techniques* (2nd ed.). Brunner-Routledge.

Barabasz, M. (1987). Trichotillomania: A new treatment. *International Journal of Clinical and Experimental Hypnosis*, *35*(3), 146–154. 10.1080/00207148708416050

Bertolino, R. (1983). L'ipnosi in dermatologia [Hypnosis in dermatology]. *Minerva Medica*, *74*(51–52), 2969–2973. PMID: 6664593

Bloch, B. (1927). Über die Heilung der Warzen durch Suggestion. *Klinische Wochenschrift*, *6*, 2320–2325. 10.1007/bf01726552

Chakravarty, K., Pharoah, P. D., Scott, D. G., & Barker, S. (1992). Erythromelalgia – The role of hypnotherapy. *Postgraduate Medical Journal*, *68*(795), 44–46. 10.1136/pgmj.68.795.44

Cheek, D. B., & LeCron, L. M. (1968). *Clinical hypnotherapy*. Grune & Stratton.

Clarke, G. H. V. (1965). The charming of warts. *Journal of Investigative Dermatology*, *45*(1), 15–21. 10.1038/jid.1965.84

Clawson, T. A., & Swade, R. H. (1975). The hypnotic control of blood flow and pain: The cure of warts and the potential for the use of hypnosis in the treatment of cancer. *American Journal of Clinical Hypnosis*, *17*(3), 160–169. 10.1080/00029157.1975.10403735

Collison, D. R. (1972). Medical hypnotherapy. *Medical Journal of Australia*, *1*(13), 643–649. 10.5694/j.1326-5377.1972.tb46979.x

Dreaper, R. (1978). Recalcitrant warts on the hand cured by hypnosis. *The Practitioner*, *220*(1316), 305–310.

Dudek, S. Z. (1967). Suggestion and play therapy in the cure of warts in children: A pilot study. *Journal of Nervous and Mental Disease*, *145*(1), 37–42. 10.1097/00005053-196707000-00005

Ewin, D. M. (1974). Condyloma acuminatum: Successful treatment of four cases by hypnosis. *American Journal of Clinical Hypnosis*, *17*(2), 73–83. 10.1080/00029157.1974.10403717

Ewin, D. M. (1992). Hypnotherapy for warts (verruca vulgaris): 41 consecutive cases with 33 cures. *American Journal of Clinical Hypnosis*, *35*(1), 1–10. 10.1080/00029157.1992.10402977

Ewin, D. M., & Eimer, B. N. (2006). *Ideomotor signals for rapid hypnoanalysis: A how-to manual.* Charles C. Thomas Publisher.

Faymonville, M. E., Laureys, S., Degueldre, C., DelFiore, G., Luxen, A., Franck, G., Lamy, M., & Maquet, P. (2000). Neural mechanisms of antinociceptive effects of hypnosis. *Anesthesiology*, *92*(5), 1257–1267. 10.1097/00000542-200005000-00013

Felt, B. T., Hall, H., Olness, K., Schmidt, W., Kohen, D., Berman, B. D., Broffman, G., Coury, D., French, G., Dattner, A., & Young, M. H. (1998). Wart regression in children: Comparison of relaxation-imagery to topical treatment and equal time interventions. *American Journal of Clinical Hypnosis*, *41*(2), 130–137. 10.1080/00029157.1998.10404199

Fick, L. J., Lang, E. V., Logan, H. L., Lutgendorf, S., & Benotsch, E. G. (1999). Imagery content during nonpharmacologic analgesia in the procedure suite: Where your patients would rather be. *Academic Radiology*, *6*(8), 457–463. 10.1016/s1076-6332(99)80164-0

Frankel, F. H., & Misch, R. C. (1973). Hypnosis in a case of long-standing psoriasis in a person with character problems. *International Journal of Clinical and Experimental Hypnosis*, *21*(3), 121–130. 10.1080/00207147308409117

Galski, T. J. (1981). The adjunctive use of hypnosis in the treatment of trichotillomania: A case report. *American Journal of Clinical Hypnosis*, *23*(3), 198–201. 10.1080/00029157.1981.10403266

Golan, H. P. (1997). The use of hypnosis in the treatment of psychogenic oral pain. *American Journal of Clinical Hypnosis*, *40*(2), 89–96. 10.1080/00029157.1997.10403413

Griesemer, R. D. (1978). Emotionally triggered disease in a dermatologic practice. *Psychiatric Annals*, *8*(8), 49–56. 10.3928/0048-5713-19780801-08

Harrison, P. V., & Stepanek, P. (1991). Hypnotherapy for alopecia areata. *British Journal of Dermatology*, *124*(5), 509–510. 10.1111/j.1365-2133.1991.tb00644.x

Hollander, M. B. (1959). Excoriated acne controlled by post-hypnotic suggestion. *American Journal of Clinical Hypnosis*, *1*(3), 122–123. 10.1080/00029157.1959.10401777

Hölzle, E. (1984). Therapie der Hyperhidrosis [Treatment of hyperhidrosis]. *Der Hautarzt*, *35*(1), 7–15.

Jabush, M. (1969). A case of chronic recurring multiple boils treated with hypnotherapy. *Psychiatric Quarterly*, *43*(3), 448–455. 10.1007/bf01564260

Johnson, R. F., & Barber, T. X. (1978). Hypnosis, suggestions, and warts: An experimental investigation implicating the importance of "believed-in efficacy." *American Journal of Clinical Hypnosis*, *20*(3), 165–174. 10.1080/00029157.1978.10403925

Kantor, S. D. (1990). Stress and psoriasis. *Cutis*, *46*(4), 321–322.

Kaschel, R., Revenstorf, D., & Wörz, B. (1991). Hypnose und Haut: Trends und Perspecktiven. *Experimentelle Und Klinische Hypnose*, *7*(1), 65–82.

Kidd, C. B. (1966). Congenital ichthyosiform erythroderma treated by hypnosis. *British Journal of Dermatology*, *78*(2), 101–105. 10.1111/j.1365-2133.1966.tb12182.x

Kline, M. V. (1953). Delimited hypnotherapy: The acceptance of resistance in the treatment of a long standing neurodermatitis with a sensory-imagery technique. *Journal of Clinical and Experimental Hypnosis*, *1*(4), 18–22. 10.1080/00207145308410946

Kline, M. V. (1954). Psoriasis and hypnotherapy: A case report. *International Journal of Clinical and Experimental Hypnosis*, *2*(4), 318–322. 10.1080/00207145408410122

Lang, E. V., Benotsch, E. G., Fick, L. J., Lutgendorf, S., Berbaum, M. L., Berbaum, K. S., Logan, H., & Spiegel, D. (2000). Adjunctive non-pharmacological analgesia for invasive medical procedures: A randomised trial. *The Lancet*, *355*(9214), 1486–1490. 10.1016/s0140-6736(00)02162-0

Lang, E. V., & Rosen, M. P. (2002). Cost analysis of adjunct hypnosis with sedation during outpatient interventional radiologic procedures. *Radiology*, *222*(2), 375–382. 10.1148/radiol.2222010528

Lehman, R. E. (1978). Brief hypnotherapy of neurodermatitis: A case with four-year followup. *American Journal of Clinical Hypnosis*, *21*(1), 48–51. 10.1080/00029157.1978.10403957

Mason, A. A. (1952). Case of congenital ichthyosiform erythrodermia of Brocq treated by hypnosis. *British Medical Journal*, *2*(4781), 422–423. 10.1136/bmj.2.4781.422
McDowell, M. (1949). Juvenile warts removed with the use of hypnotic suggestion. *Bulletin of the Menninger Clinic*, *13*(4), 124–126.
Montgomery, G. H., DuHamel, K. N., & Redd, W. H. (2000). A meta-analysis of hypnotically induced analgesia: How effective is hypnosis? *International Journal of Clinical and Experimental Hypnosis*, *48*(2), 138–153. 10.1080/00207140008410045
Morris, B. A. (1985). Hypnotherapy of warts using the Simonton visualization technique: A case report. *American Journal of Clinical Hypnosis*, *27*(4), 237–240. 10.1080/00029157.1985.10402614
Noll, R. B. (1988). Hypnotherapy of a child with warts. *Journal of Developmental and Behavioral Pediatrics*, *9*(2), 89–91. 10.1097/00004703-198804000-00008
Noll, R. B. (1994). Hypnotherapy for warts in children and adolescents. *Journal of Developmental and Behavioral Pediatrics*, *15*(3), 170–173. 10.1097/00004703-199406000-00003
Obermayer, M. E., & Greenson, R. R. (1949). Treatment by suggestion of verrucae planae of the face. *Psychosomatic Medicine*, *11*(3), 163–164. 10.1097/00006842-194905000-00007
Perloff, M. M., & Spiegelman, J. (1973). Hypnosis in the treatment of a child's allergy to dogs. *American Journal of Clinical Hypnosis*, *15*(4), 269–272. 10.1080/00029157.1973.10402261
Rowen, R. (1981). Hypnotic age regression in the treatment of a self-destructive habit: Trichotillomania. *American Journal of Clinical Hypnosis*, *23*(3), 195–197. 10.1080/00029157.1981.10403265
Sacerdote, P. (1965). Hypnotherapy in neurodermatitis: A case report. *American Journal of Clinical Hypnosis*, *7*(3), 249–253. 10.1080/00029157.1965.10402426
Schneck, J. M. (1954). Ichthyosis treated with hypnosis. *Diseases of the Nervous System*, *15*(7), 211–214.
Schneck, J. M. (1966). Hypnotherapy for ichthyosis. *Psychosomatics*, *7*(4), 233–235. 10.1016/s0033-3182(66)72118-5
Scott, M. J. (1960). *Hypnosis in skin and allergic diseases*. Charles C. Thomas Publisher.
Sheehan, D. V. (1978). Influence of psychosocial factors on wart remission. *American Journal of Clinical Hypnosis*, *20*(3), 160. 10.1080/00029157.1978.10403924
Shenefelt, P. D. (2000). Hypnosis in dermatology. *Archives of Dermatology*, *136*(3), 393–399. 10.1001/archderm.136.3.393
Shenefelt, P. D. (2003). Hypnosis-facilitated relaxation using self-guided imagery during dermatologic procedures. *American Journal of Clinical Hypnosis*, *45*(3), 225–232. 10.1080/00029157.2003.10403528
Shenefelt, P. D. (2004). Using hypnosis to facilitate resolution of psychogenic excoriations in acne excoriée. *American Journal of Clinical Hypnosis*, *46*(3), 239–245. 10.1080/00029157.2004.10403603
Shenefelt, P. D. (2007). Psychocutaneous hypnoanalysis: Detection and deactivation of emotional and mental root factors in psychosomatic skin disorders. *American Journal of Clinical Hypnosis*, *50*(2), 131–136. 10.1080/00029157.2007.10401610
Shenefelt, P. D. (2010). Hypnoanalysis for dermatologic disorders. *Psychology Research and Behavior Management*, *2*(4), 439–445.
Shenefelt, P. D. (2011). Ideomotor signaling: from divining spiritual messages to discerning subconscious answers during hypnosis and hypnoanalysis, a historical perspective. *American Journal of Clinical Hypnosis*, *53*(3), 157–167. 10.1080/00029157.2011.10401754
Shenefelt, P. D. (2012). Hypnoanalysis for skin disorders. In L. V. Berhardt (Ed.), *Advances in medicine and biology* (Nova Medicine & Health, Vol. 190, pp. 163–175). Nova Science Publishers.
Shenefelt, P. D. (2013). Anxiety reduction using hypnotic induction and self-guided imagery for relaxation during dermatologic procedures. *International Journal of Clinical and Experimental Hypnosis*, *61*(3), 305–318. 10.1080/00207144.2013.784096
Shenefelt, P. D. (2018). Mindfulness-based cognitive hypnotherapy and skin disorders. *American Journal of Clinical Hypnosis*, *61*(1), 34–44. 10.1080/00029157.2017.1419457
Shenefelt, P. D. (2019). Inducing and utilizing hypnomoments in routine medical communications with patients. *Journal of Alternative Medicine Research*, *11*(1), 45–51.
Shenefelt, P. D., & Shenefelt, D. A. (2014). Spiritual and religious aspects of skin and skin disorders. *Psychology Research and Behavior Management*, *7*, 201–212. 10.2147/prbm.s65578
Shertzer, C. L., & Lookingbill, D. P. (1987). Effects of relaxation therapy and hypnotizability in chronic urticaria. *Archives of Dermatology*, *123*(7), 913–916. https://pubmed.ncbi.nlm.nih.gov/3300566/

Sinclair-Gieben, A. H., & Chalmers, D. (1959). Evaluation of treatment of warts by hypnosis. *The Lancet*, *2*(7101), 480–482. 10.1016/s0140-6736(59)90605-1

Spanos, N. P., Stenstrom, R., & Johnston, J. C. (1988). Hypnosis, placebo, and suggestion in the treatment of warts. *Psychosomatic Medicine*, *50*(3), 245–260. 10.1097/00006842-198805000-00003

Spanos, N. P., Williams, V., & Gwynn, M. I. (1990). Effects of hypnotic, placebo, and salicylic acid treatments on wart regression. *Psychosomatic Medicine*, *52*(1), 109–114. 10.1097/00006842-199001000-00009

Spiegel, D. (2001). Mind matters - Group therapy and survival in breast cancer. *The New England Journal of Medicine*, *345*(24), 1767–1768. 10.1056/nejm200112133452409

Spiegel, H., & Spiegel, D. (2004). *Trance and treatment: Clinical uses of hypnosis* (2nd ed.). American Psychiatric Association Publishing.

Stankler, L. (1967). A critical assessment of the cure of warts by suggestion. *The Practitioner*, *198*(187), 690–694. PMID: 6047163

Straatmeyer, A. J., & Rhodes, N. R. (1983). Condylomata acuminata: Results of treatment using hypnosis. *Journal of the American Academy of Dermatology*, *9*(3), 434–436. 10.1016/s0190-9622(83)70155-6

Stewart, A. C., & Thomas, S. E. (1995). Hypnotherapy as a treatment for atopic dermatitis in adults and children. *British Journal of Dermatology*, *132(5)*, 778–783. 10.1111/j.1365-2133.1995.tb00726.x

Sulzberger, M. B., & Wolf, J. (1934). The treatment of warts by suggestion. *Medical Record*, *140*, 552–556. https://psycnet.apa.org/record/1935-00691-001

Surman, O. S., Gottlieb, S. K., & Hackett, T. P. (1972). Hypnotic treatment of a child with warts. *American Journal of Clinical Hypnosis*, *15*(1), 12–14. 10.1080/00029157.1972.10402203

Surman, O. S., Gottlieb, S. K., Hackett, T. P., & Silverberg, E. L. (1973). Hypnosis in the treatment of warts. *Archives of General Psychiatry*, *28*(3), 439–441. 10.1001/archpsyc.1973.01750330111018

Tasini, M. F., & Hackett, T. P. (1977). Hypnosis in the treatment of warts in immunodeficient children. *American Journal of Clinical Hypnosis*, *19*(3), 152–154. 10.1080/00029157.1977.10403862

Tausk, F., & Whitmore, S. E. (1999). A pilot study of hypnosis in the treatment of patients with psoriasis. *Psychotherapy and Psychosomatics*, *68*(4), 221–225. 10.1159/000012336

Tenzel, J. H., & Taylor, R. L. (1969). An evaluation of hypnosis and suggestion as treatment for warts. *Psychosomatics: Journal of Consultation and Liaison Psychiatry*, *10*(4), 252–257. 10.1016/s0033-3182(69)71737-6

Tobia, L. (1982). L'ipnosi in dermatologia [Hypnosis in dermatology]. *Minerva Medica*, *73*(10), 531–537.

Twerski, A. J., & Naar, R. (1974). Hypnotherapy in a case of refractory dermatitis. *American Journal of Clinical Hypnosis*, *16*(3), 202–205. 10.1080/00029157.1974.10403677

Ullman, M. (1959). On the psyche and warts I.: Suggestion and warts: A review and comment. *Psychosomatic Medicine*, *21*, 473–488. PMID: 13840296

Ullman, M., & Dudek, S. (1960). On the psyche and warts II.: Hypnotic suggestion and warts. *Psychosomatic Medicine*, *22*, 68–76. 10.1097/00006842-196001000-00009

Vickers, C. F. H. (1961). Treatment of plantar warts in children. *British Medical Journal*, *2*(5254), 743–745. 10.1136/bmj.2.5254.743

Waxman, D. (1973). Behaviour therapy of psoriasis – A hypnoanalytic and counter-conditioning technique. *Postgraduate Medical Journal*, *49*(574), 591–595. 10.1136/pgmj.49.574.591

Willemsen, R., Vanderlinden, J., Deconinck, A., & Roseeuw, D. (2006). Hypnotherapeutic management of alopecia areata. *Journal of the American Academy of Dermatology*, *55*(2), 233–237. 10.1016/j.jaad.2005.09.025

Winchell, S. A., & Watts, R. A. (1988). Relaxation therapies in the treatment of psoriasis and possible pathophysiologic mechanisms. *Journal of the American Academy of Dermatology*, *18*(1 Pt 1), 101–104. 10.1016/s0190-9622(88)70015-8

Wink, C. A. S. (1961). Congenital ichthyosiform erythrodermia treated by hypnosis. *British Medical Journal*, *2*, 5254. 10.1136/bmj.2.5254.741

Zachariae, R., Øster, H., Bjerring, P., & Kragballe, K. (1996). Effects of psychologic intervention on psoriasis: A preliminary report. *Journal of the American Academy of Dermatology*, *34*(6), 1008–1015. 10.1016/s0190-9622(96)90280-7

42

HYPNOSIS IN GASTROENTEROLOGY

Peter J. Whorwell

WYTHENSHAWE HOSPITAL, UNIVERSITY OF MANCHESTER, MANCHESTER, UK

Disorders of Gut Brain Interaction

The functional gastrointestinal disorders are the commonest conditions seen by gastroenterologists and they are particularly difficult to manage. Extensive investigation always leads to negative results and treatment is notoriously unsatisfactory. The term "functional" is used to imply that they result from a disorder of function rather than structure but unfortunately in English, this term is often used to imply that the problem is all psychological. However, research over recent decades has shown that these conditions result from a whole variety of factors combining to cause symptoms. These include diet, disordered motility (gastrointestinal contractions), hypersensitivity of the gut, abnormal processing of pain inputs by the central nervous system, a disturbance of gut microbes (dysbiosis), and environmental influences. Psychological factors are also involved but are not the only trigger and this has led to the term "disorders of gut brain interaction" (DGBI) being introduced to replace the old terminology. It is traditional to divide these conditions into a number of named disorders such as irritable bowel syndrome (IBS), functional dyspepsia, and non-cardiac chest pain based on the pattern of symptoms and from where, in the gastrointestinal system, they are thought to originate. However, there is considerable overlap between these disorders and, for example, it is common for patients with IBS to complain of symptoms suggestive of functional dyspepsia, although the latter may be less severe. Consequently, it is tempting to speculate that all these conditions might just be differing expressions of a similar underlying disorder.

Irritable Bowel Syndrome

The commonest DGBI is IBS which affects up to 10% of the population and is characterized by abdominal pain, abdominal bloating or distension, and a disordered bowel habit. The bowel dysfunction can take the form of diarrhea, constipation, or an alternation between the two, with urgency or a feeling of incomplete emptying being relatively common. Sufferers also often experience a range of other "non-colonic" symptoms such as low backache, constant lethargy, nausea, chest pain, headaches, and urinary symptoms

DOI: 10.4324/9781003449126-56

suggestive of an irritable bladder (Whorwell et al., 1986). In the more severe cases, the women say that the pain can be as bad as that of childbirth and fecal incontinence is not unusual (Atarodi & Whorwell, 2014). Antispasmodic medication can help the pain and laxatives or antidiarrheals are used to control bowel function. However, even when these approaches are effective, they don't bring about long-lasting relief of symptoms. Antidepressants are frequently used based on the hypothesis that they might target both the central nervous system (brain) and the nerves in the gastrointestinal system (the enteric nervous system). Unfortunately, the majority of available medications only target single symptoms which results in patients having to take multiple medications in an attempt to control their problem. Despite all these approaches, many patients fail to make any progress and it has been shown that up to 38% of these individuals have contemplated suicide, not because they are depressed, but because they have difficulty in coping with the severity of their symptoms and the prospect of their symptoms not being improved in the future (Miller, 2004). Furthermore, the non-colonic symptoms of IBS seldom respond to conventional pharmaceutical treatment which is important as these symptoms can be just as intrusive as the gastrointestinal symptoms (Maxton, 1989).

Anxiety is a consistent feature in a large proportion of individuals with IBS and, therefore, it seems reasonable to propose that, because of its beneficial effects on anxiety, hypnotherapy might have a positive effect in IBS. Furthermore, for many years, there has been speculation that, with the aid of hypnosis, an individual might be able to influence certain physiological functions not normally considered to be under conscious control. In the field of gastroenterology, as far back as the 1970s (Stacher et al., 1975), there was some evidence that gastric acid secretion could be modulated using hypnosis and this was subsequently confirmed in a later study in 1989 (Klein & Spiegel, 1989). Consequently, we speculated that with the aid of hypnotherapy, patients might be able to learn how to control some of the physiological abnormalities associated with IBS and be able to take control of their illness rather than their illness controlling them. To test this hypothesis, we performed the first controlled trial of hypnotherapy in the field of gastroenterology and published our results in 1984 (Whorwell et al., 1984). Thirty patients with refractory IBS were randomized to receive seven sessions, on a one-to-one basis, of either what we called gut-directed hypnotherapy (GDH) or supportive therapy plus placebo medication. Both groups received a tutorial on the physiology of IBS and, in addition to standard hypnotic relaxation, participants in the active group were instructed how to control gut function and relieve spasm first, by using visualization (controlling the flow of the gut as a river) and second, by placing a hand on their abdomen and feeling warmth radiating into the gut and soothing it. At the end of the study, the hypnotherapy group was significantly improved compared to the controls. A link to our hypnosis protocol is available in the supporting information section at the end of one of our 2019 reviews (Vasant & Whorwell, 2019).

These encouraging results led us to introduce GDH into our routine service for the management of patients with severe refractory IBS. This has given us an opportunity to continue studying the phenomenon in terms of optimizing provision, predicting response to treatment, and better understanding the mechanisms involved in mediating its benefit.

In one of these studies, we compared the outcomes in 25 IBS patients who had been treated with hypnotherapy one year previously with 25 patients who had been on the waiting list for a similar length of time. The results were very similar to those reported in the 1984 trial but we also recorded some additional endpoints of interest, including non-colonic symptoms, quality of life, health seeking behavior, and employment (Houghton et al., 1996). Compared to controls, hypnotherapy patients showed a significant improvement in non-colonic symptoms and quality of life as well as a reduction in consultations with their general practitioner and less time of work because of their IBS. These results combined with the previous trial and a follow-up report (Whorwell et al., 1987) enabled us to obtain funding from the British National Health Service to establish a hypnotherapy unit for the treatment of IBS employing six non-medically qualified therapists. A condition for the continuation of funding was that we should confirm the previously reported effectiveness of hypnotherapy by submitting an audit of the first 250 patients treated by the unit and this was published in 2002 (Gonsalkorale et al., 2002). This study confirmed our previous efficacy data for IBS symptoms, non-colonic symptoms, and quality of life. New observations included a reduction in anxiety and depressions scores, a tendency for males to do less well, especially if they had diarrhea predominant IBS, and that all therapists achieved similar outcomes. A further audit of 1,000 consecutive patients was published in 2015 and, again, confirmed our previous results (Miller et al., 2015). In this audit, the overall response to treatment was 76% but females responded better (80%) than males (62%). There were no significant differences in the response rate between the different bowel habit subtypes and age had little effect although patients of a younger age experienced a greater reduction in their symptom severity score.

We have also assessed the long-term effects of hypnotherapy for IBS and shown that 83% of patients remain improved up to five years after treatment with 59% requiring no medication and 42% taking medication less often (Gonsalkorale et al., 2003). In addition, consultation behavior was reduced with both general practitioners and hospital consultants. Our results for the short- and long-term effects of hypnotherapy have been reproduced by others (Palsson, 2015; Peters et al., 2015; Lindfors et al., 2012) and its utility in children has also been extensively evaluated by Benninga's group in Amsterdam. They have shown that hypnotherapy is far superior to usual care in controlling pain and associated symptoms with an overall response rate of 85% compared to 25% in the control group (Vlieger et al., 2007) with the effects sustained for up to nearly five years (Vlieger et al., 2012). We have also published a small audit of hypnotherapy in 32 children showing very similar results (Vasant et al., 2021).

The effects of hypnotherapy have largely been evaluated in Caucasian populations although there is no obvious reason why it should not be similarly effective in other cultures. However, we thought it would be worth addressing this question and have recently shown that similar outcomes can be achieved in a British Asian population and, furthermore, the response is not affected by the ethnicity of the therapist (Sasegbon et al., 2022). One of the impediments to the uptake of hypnotherapy is the lack of suitably trained therapists who, when they are available, tend to be attached to a limited number of tertiary care centers. Consequently, patients often have to travel considerable distances to access treatment. We addressed this issue some years before the pandemic and showed that hypnotherapy via Skype was nearly as effective as face-to-face treatment (Hasan et al., 2019). This approach was adopted for all patients during the pandemic and we have shown that it was acceptable for the majority (Noble et al., 2022). Group hypnotherapy is another way of addressing the accessibility problem and has been shown to be effective (Flik et al., 2019) although the more severe cases seen in tertiary care may need the more individualized approach of one-to-one hypnotherapy. A number of digital applications of GDH are becoming available but the majority have not been submitted to critical evaluation and the response to treatment rate does appear to be substantially less than that seen with face to face or video GDH. This is presumably, at least in part, because the treatment has to be generic rather than tailored to the individual patient.

Functional Dyspepsia

Functional dyspepsia is another common DGBI affecting the top end of the gastrointestinal tract with the principal symptoms being upper abdominal pain, upper abdominal bloating, early satiety, nausea, vomiting, and feelings of fullness. The response to conventional medications is usually disappointing and in 2002 we reported the results of a trial of gut-focused hypnotherapy in this condition (Calvert et al., 2002). Patients were randomized to either GDH, supportive therapy plus placebo medication, or standard medical therapy for 16 weeks and re-assessed after 56 weeks. GDH was significantly superior to the other two treatments both in the short and long term with regard to symptom reduction, quality of life improvement, and medication reduction. As was observed for IBS, hypnotherapy also reduced consultation rates both with general practitioners and hospital consultants.

Non-Cardiac Chest Pain

As its name implies, patients with non-cardiac chest pain complain of chest pain that can be indistinguishable from angina even to the extent of radiation of the pain to the left arm. It is thought that the pain is due to a combination of abnormal contractions and increased sensitivity in the esophagus. Treatment is often unsatisfactory and patients frequently continue to worry about the possibility of heart problems, especially during bouts of severe pain. Not surprisingly sufferers often become regular attendees at accident and emergency departments. In 2006, we reported the outcome of a study comparing the effect of hypnotherapy or supportive treatment plus placebo medication in 28 patients with this condition (Jones et al., 2006). Participants randomized to the hypnotherapy group showed a significantly greater improvement in symptoms and quality of life than controls and this effect was sustained for at least two years. Interestingly, there was a tendency for patients to improve further during the follow-up period and we and others have previously reported this observation (Lindfors et al., 2012).

How Does Hypnotherapy Improve Symptoms in DGBIs?

In order to investigate how hypnotherapy may improve symptoms in patients with DGBIs, it is necessary to understand current thinking on the various factors that are likely to be involved in the pathogenesis of these conditions. These are best understood in IBS (Table 42.1) and separately or in combination are thought to lead to symptoms with some considered to be amenable to modulation by hypnosis.

Genetics, social learning, and diet: There is no doubt that DGBIs run in families and this could be because of genetic influences or learned behavior. Genetic studies in IBS have revealed some positive signals (Eijsbouts et al., 2021) but not enough to account for all of the observed familial clustering suggesting that other influences must also be important such as social learning and the environment. Many patients can be improved by dietary manipulation with the low fermentable oligosaccharide, disaccharide, monosaccharide, and polyol diet being particularly useful and having the best evidence (Gibson et al., 2022).

Table 42.1 Pathogenesis of IBS. Those Marked with * Have Been Shown to Be Amenable to Modification by Hypnotherapy

- Genetics, social learning, and diet
- Motility*
- Visceral hypersensitivity*
- Central processing*
- Bacterial imbalance (dysbiosis)
- Psychological factors*
- Inflammation

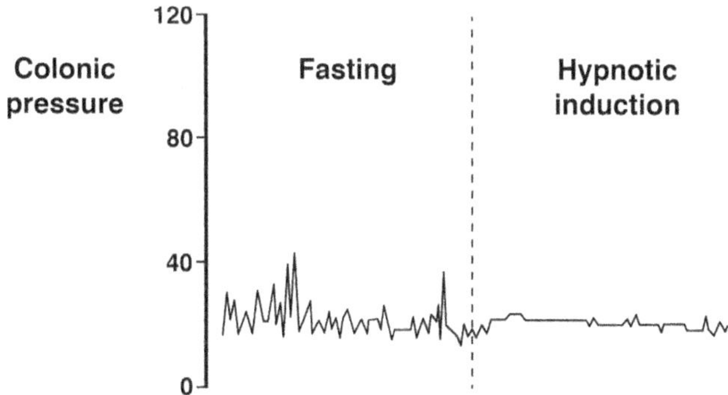

Figure 42.1 Reduction in colonic contractions following the induction of hypnosis. This figure was published in *The Lancet*, Volume 340, Whorwell et al., "Physiological effects of emotion: assessment via hypnosis", 69–72, Copyright Elsevier (1992).

Motility: It seems reasonable to assume that decreasing the strength of contractions of the circular smooth muscle of the gut might reduce the colicky pain associated with IBS and this is why antispasmodic medications are usually the first option for treating the abdominal pain associated with this condition. We speculated that hypnosis might have a similar effect and have shown (Figure 42.1) that it can reduce contractions in the sigmoid colon in volunteers at rest (Whorwell et al., 1992). In another study, it has been shown that hypnosis can accelerate gastric emptying in both healthy volunteers and patients with functional dyspepsia (Chiarioni et al., 2006).

Visceral hypersensitivity: Visceral hypersensitivity of the gastrointestinal tract is a consistent finding in many patients with IBS and may partly explain why the gut "over-reacts" to a variety of different to stimuli. One of the easiest ways to test for this abnormality is to slowly inflate a balloon in the rectum of an individual and record the pressure at which they feel pain. Patients with IBS feel pain at much lower pressures than healthy volunteers and this is called visceral hypersensitivity. We have used this technique to assess visceral sensation before and after a course of hypnotherapy (Lea et al., 2003; Prior et al., 1990) and found that those patients who were hypersensitive before treatment showed a significant shift toward more normal levels at the end of treatment (Figure 42.2).

Central processing (brain scanning): Since the advent of brain scanning techniques such as positron emission tomography (PET) and functional magnetic resonance imaging, these techniques have been applied to a whole range of scenarios and hypnosis is no exception with other chapters dealing with this in more detail. With regard to IBS, the findings are not always

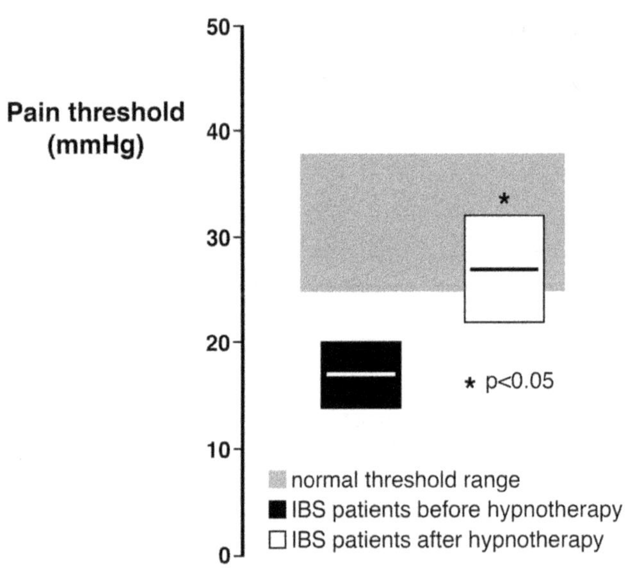

Figure 42.2 Improvement in colonic pain threshold following a course of hypnotherapy (adapted from Lea et al., "Gut-focused hypnotherapy normalizes disordered rectal sensitivity in patients with irritable bowel syndrome" (2003) 1;17(5):635–42, *Alimentary Pharmacology and Therapeutics*, © Wiley).

consistent, probably as a result of differences in the research paradigms, but it does seem that areas involved in the emotional response to painful stimuli from the gut are somewhat "overactive" and that this can be down regulated by hypnosis (Lowen et al., 2013; Mayer et al., 2019; Rainville et al., 1997). Furthermore, hypnosis seems to reduce abnormal functional connectivity in the brain which, in IBS, correlates with symptom reduction suggesting that hypnosis "modulates attention, perception and subjective awareness of aversive feelings by decoupling maladaptive classical conditioning to pain" (Simon et al., 2019 p. 478).

Bacterial imbalance (dysbiosis): The bacterial composition of the gut contents (the gut microbiome) is the subject of intense research in a whole variety of conditions and DGBIs are no exception. The microbiome in patients with IBS does not seem to be "normal" with the distribution and diversity of bacteria being less "healthy" than it should be (dysbiosis). This could be a reflection of abnormal motility leading to a degree of stagnation, but it is also of interest to note that a significant proportion of patients have been exposed to multiple antibiotics either resulting from the treatment of recurrent tonsillitis in childhood or severe acne in adolescence. There is now compelling evidence that the bacteria in the gut can affect the central nervous system and vice versa, so it would be of great interest to establish whether this interaction could be influenced by hypnosis. To date, there has only been one study assessing the microbiome before and after hypnotherapy which reported no significant changes (Peter et al., 2018). However, the study included all subtypes of IBS, and any changes confined to just one subtype might be overlooked by such an approach. Consequently, it might have been better to look at the effect of hypnosis on patients with a well-defined abnormality of their microbiome where change might be more easily detected. It is therefore probably fair to conclude that a possible effect on the microbiome has not yet been completely excluded.

Table 42.2 Anxiety and Depression Scores Before and After Hypnotherapy

	Pre-HT	*Post-HT*	*"p" value*
HAD "A" Score	11.1 ± 0.3	7.3 ± 0.3	$p < 0.001$
% anxious (score ≥9)	68.3	34.6	$p < 0.001$
HAD "D" Score	7.2 ± 0.3	4.1 ± 0.3	$p < 0.001$
% depressed (score ≥9)	36.1	14.6	$p < 0.001$

HAD scores expressed as mean ± S.E.M.
**post-HT versus pre-HT, paired "t" test.*

Psychological factors: Patients with IBS tend to be anxious and, although depression is less common than anxiety, it can be a problem in the more severe cases. There is still some debate about how much of the anxiety and depression could be the result of having a condition, which can lead to such a range of severe and intrusive symptoms, rather than the cause. However, there is evidence from genetic studies that patients with IBS have some loci associated with mood and anxiety disorders (Eijsbouts, et al., 2021). IBS patients are often not taken seriously by healthcare providers, so there must be a "non specific" beneficial effect from suddenly having an intensive course of treatment on a regular basis by someone who takes an interest in their illness and its care. However, in all of our studies over the years, we have consistently shown a reduction in anxiety and depression scores using the Hospital Anxiety and Depression Scale (HAD) (Table 42.2). In addition, we have shown that the negative cognitions associated with IBS can be improved following a course of hypnotherapy (Toner et al., 1998). It could be argued that a treatment such as hypnotherapy might be associated with a considerable amount of expectation which could contribute to the therapeutic effect. In a study on how patients perceive hypnotherapy, we looked at expectation and it did not seem to influence outcome (Donnet et al., 2022) although further investigation specifically addressing expectation is needed.

Inflammation: There is evidence that some patients with IBS have low-grade inflammation in their gastrointestinal tract but the changes can be subtle and therefore looking for the effect of hypnotherapy could be challenging. However, the inflammatory changes in inflammatory bowel disease (IBD) are much better characterized and the effect of hypnotherapy in these disorders is discussed later.

In summary, it can be seen from the above discussion that hypnosis has the potential to influence at least half of the factors (Table 42.1) involved in the pathogenesis of DGBIs.

Inflammatory Bowel Disease

Crohn's disease and ulcerative colitis, collectively known as IBD, are chronic conditions where the exact cause remains unknown although they have a definite genetic component and there is a disturbance of control of the inflammatory cascade. Ulcerative colitis only affects the colon, whereas Crohn's disease can affect any part of the gastrointestinal tract although it most commonly affects the last part of the small bowel or the colon or both. The typical symptoms of ulcerative colitis are diarrhea, rectal bleeding, and abdominal discomfort whereas Crohn's disease tends to cause more pain with a variable bowel habit and less bleeding. Despite being thought of as different, but closely related diseases, the medical treatment is quite similar in both and usually involves suppression of inflammation and the immune system. When in remission, patients with both of these conditions can develop the symptoms of IBS (Isgar et al., 1983; Meng et al., 2013). There is no doubt that psychological factors and stress can exacerbate the symptoms of IBD, so it is somewhat surprising that in contrast to IBS, there has been so little research on the effect of hypnotherapy in these conditions. This is probably because the treatment approach of modulating the immune and inflammatory response is relatively effective and therefore the drivers for exploring additional approaches are less than in IBS where conventional treatments are far less effective. Furthermore, the pathogenesis of IBD is far better understood than in IBS, making the investment in and development of new medications by pharmaceutical companies much more likely to be successful than in IBS. Nevertheless, a significant proportion of IBD patients either fail to respond or are intolerant of conventional medication and therefore the possible role of hypnotherapy deserves far more attention.

Hypnotherapy in IBD: In 2007, Keefer and Keshavarzian reported that hypnotherapy improved the quality of life of eight patients with inactive IBD, four with Crohn's disease, and four with ulcerative colitis (Keefer & Keshavarzian, 2007). The following year we reported that hypnotherapy was effective in reducing symptoms and improving quality of life in 15 patients with severe active IBD, 12 with ulcerative colitis, and 3 with Crohn's disease (Miller & Whorwell, 2008). Despite these two encouraging reports nearly 15 years ago, there have only been a couple of case reports and only two controlled trials, one in adults with ulcerative colitis (Keefer et al., 2013) and the other in children with Crohn's disease (Lee et al., 2021). In the first study, compared to controls, hypnotherapy significantly prolonged the length of remission in patients with ulcerative colitis. In the other trial, compared to controls, hypnotherapy improved symptoms in children with Crohn's disease as well as a series of other outcomes. Perhaps rather surprisingly, a study investigating the effect of hypnotherapy on IBS symptoms in IBD, which are quite common especially when IBD patients are in remission, did not find benefit over standard medical therapy (Hoekman et al., 2021). However, despite this disappointing outcome in terms of IBS relief, these results suggest that hypnotherapy is directly affecting the pathogenesis of IBD in some way, rather than just relieving an associated IBS which could have been an alternative explanation of why hypnotherapy seems to improve IBD.

Interestingly, a study of the possible mechanism by which hypnotherapy could be modifying IBD revealed that, compared to controls, hypnotherapy resulted in a significant reduction in some components of the systemic and mucosal inflammatory response in patients with active ulcerative colitis (Mawdsley et al., 2008). All these findings have led to calls for more research on what appears to be a neglected possible treatment option for IBD which has a near perfect safety profile especially when compared to some of the more potent pharmacological options available for IBD.

Duodenal Ulcer

Before the discovery of the association between *Helicobacter pylori* and duodenal ulceration, this condition was challenging to manage with gastric acid reduction being the main target of treatment. When that failed, patients were often subjected to surgery such as partial gastrectomy, vagotomy, and pyloroplasty or highly selective vagotomy with these operations often causing long-term side effects. We speculated that hypnotherapy might have therapeutic potential especially as duodenal ulcer was associated with stress and there was evidence that hypnosis might reduce gastric acid production (Stacher, et al., 1975). In a controlled trial published in 1988, we compared the relapse rate over one year following ulcer healing with ranitidine in patients randomized to be treated with either GDH or control treatment. The relapse rate was only 53% in the hypnotherapy group compared to 100% in controls (Colgan et al., 1988). However, the uptake of hypnotherapy following this study was not good as many patients preferred to take ranitidine long term rather than spending seven weeks learning how to use hypnotherapy to control their condition. Furthermore, once the dramatic effect of *H. pylori* eradication on eliminating duodenal ulcer disease completely was demonstrated, hypnotherapy for this condition became obsolescent.

Esophageal Disorders

Reflux esophagitis leads to the symptom of "heartburn" and is an extremely common condition. The first line management of this problem is the use of medications to suppress the production of acid such as the histamine type 2 receptor blockers or the proton pump inhibitors. However, some patients don't respond suggesting that hypersensitivity of the esophagus, rather than inflammation or exposure to excessive amounts of acid, may be more of a problem. In this group of patients, hypnotherapy may have a role (Luo & Keefer, 2022; Riehl et al., 2015) and there is some preliminary evidence to support this opinion (Hurtte et al., 2022; Riehl et al., 2016). Similarly, hypnotherapy may have a role in globus pharyngeus which is a disorder where the patient feels they have a lump or a foreign body in their throat (Kiebles et al., 2010; Riehl, et al., 2015).

Conclusions

The DGBIs are notoriously challenging to treat but there seems little doubt that hypnotherapy can significantly improve the symptoms and quality of life of sufferers. The best evidence is in IBS followed by functional dyspepsia and non-cardiac chest pain. Hypnotherapy should be regarded as part of a treatment package consisting of education, dietary manipulation, and "as necessary" medication rather than being a "stand alone" approach to managing these conditions. It is particularly interesting to note that hypnotherapy relieves a wide range of symptoms associated with IBS which is in contrast to medications which often only target one symptom such as pain or bowel function. Furthermore, it often relieves the non-colonic symptoms which seldom improve with pharmacological approaches. With regard to bowel habit, diarrhea responds better than constipation, although it is perfectly acceptable for patients to use anti-diarrheals or laxatives if necessary, and for the more severe forms of constipation may need to take laxatives on a continuous basis. The exact number of sessions required to achieve an optimum outcome varies from patient to patient but we allow a maximum of 12, although we have shown that in a large proportion of patients, six sessions can be as effective as 12 (Hasan, 2021). We and others have reported that it is not uncommon for patients to continue improving after a course of hypnotherapy has been completed. We have also noticed that patients with very mild symptoms do not necessarily do so well with hypnotherapy presumably because the motivation for embarking on a time consuming, relatively labor intensive form of treatment is not strong in an individual who experiences only mild symptoms relatively infrequently. It seems unlikely that we will ever be able to accurately predict who will respond to hypnotherapy but it would be useful if we could identify patients who are more likely to do well. We have undertaken some studies to address this question and have shown that patients who have a clear mental image of their condition (Carruthers et al., 2009, 2010c) and who chose a positive color to describe their mood on the Manchester Colour Wheel (Carruthers et al., 2010a, 2010b) are more likely to respond to treatment. Interestingly, high hypnotizability measured indirectly on the Tellegen Absorption Scale did not seem to be associated with a better response to GDH (Miller et al., 2015).

It seems that, at last, it is being accepted that the interaction between the mind and the health of the rest of the body is a critically important target for therapeutic interventions. Hopefully, in the field of gastroenterology, this will encourage studies to confirm all the preliminary data suggesting that hypnotherapy has great potential in a wide range of conditions.

References

Atarodi, S. R. S., & Whorwell, P. J. (2014). Faecal incontinence – The hidden scourge of irritable syndrome: A cross sectional study. *BMJ Open Gastroenterology*, *1*, 1–6. doi: 10.1136/bmjgast-2014-000002

Calvert, E. L., Houghton, L. A., Cooper, P., Morris, J., & Whorwell, P. J. (2002). Long-term improvement in functional dyspepsia using hypnotherapy. *Gastroenterology*, *123*(6), 1778–1785.

Carruthers, H. R., Miller, V., Morris, J., Evans, R., Tarrier, N., & Whorwell, P. J. (2009). Using art to help understand the imagery of irritable bowel syndrome and its response to hypnotherapy. *International Journal of Clinical and Experimental Hypnosis*, *57*(2), 162–173. doi: 908917198 [pii] 10.1080/00207140802665401

Carruthers, H. R., Morris, J., Tarrier, N., & Whorwell, P. J. (2010a). The Manchester Color Wheel: development of a novel way of identifying color choice and its validation in healthy, anxious and depressed individuals. *BMC Medical Research Methodology*, *10*, 12. doi: 1471-2288-10-12 [pii] 10.1186/1471-2288-10-12

Carruthers, H. R., Morris, J., Tarrier, N., & Whorwell, P. J. (2010b). Mood color choice helps to predict response to hypnotherapy in patients with irritable bowel syndrome. *BMC Complementary and Alternate Medicine*, *10*(1), 75. doi: 1472-6882-10-75 [pii] 10.1186/1472-6882-10-75

Carruthers, H. R., Morris, J., Tarrier, N., & Whorwell, P. J. (2010c). Reactivity to images in health and irritable bowel syndrome. *Alimentary Pharmacology & Therapeutics*, *31*(1), 131–142.

Chiarioni, G., Vantini, I., De Iorio, F., & Benini, L. (2006). Prokinetic effect of gut-oriented hypnosis on gastric emptying. *Alimentary Pharmacology & Therapeutics*, *23*(8), 1241–1249.

Colgan, S. M., Faragher, E. B., & Whorwell, P. J. (1988). Controlled trial of hypnotherapy in relapse prevention of duodenal ulceration. *Lancet*, *1*(8598), 1299–1300.

Donnet, A. S., Hasan, S. S., & Whorwell, P. J. (2022). Hypnotherapy for irritable bowel syndrome: Patient expectations and perceptions. *Therapeutic Advances in Gastroenterology*, *15*, 17562848221074208. doi: 10.1177/17562848221074208

Eijsbouts, C., Zheng, T., Kennedy, N. A., Bonfiglio, F., Anderson, C. A., Moutsianas, L., ... Parkes, M. (2021). Genome-wide analysis of 53,400 people with irritable bowel syndrome highlights shared genetic pathways with mood and anxiety disorders. *Nature Genetics*, *53*(11), 1543–1552. doi: 10.1038/s41588-021-00950-8

Flik, C. E., Laan, W., Zuithoff, N. P. A., van Rood, Y. R., Smout, A., Weusten, B., ... de Wit, N. J. (2019). Efficacy of individual and group hypnotherapy in irritable bowel syndrome (IMAGINE): A multicentre randomised controlled trial. *Lancet Gastroenterology and Hepatology*, *4*(1), 20–31. doi: S2468-1253(18)30310-8 [pii]

Gibson, P. R., Halmos, E. P., So, D., Yao, C. K., Varney, J. E., & Muir, J. G. (2022). Diet as a therapeutic tool in chronic gastrointestinal disorders: Lessons from the FODMAP journey. *Journal of Gastroenterology and Hepatology*, *37*(4), 644–652. doi: 10.1111/jgh.15772

Gonsalkorale, W. M., Houghton, L. A., & Whorwell, P. J. (2002). Hypnotherapy in irritable bowel syndrome: A large-scale audit of a clinical service with examination of factors influencing responsiveness. *American Journal of Gastroenterology*, *97*(4), 954–961.

Gonsalkorale, W. M., Miller, V., Afzal, A., & Whorwell, P. J. (2003). Long term benefits of hypnotherapy for irritable bowel syndrome. *Gut, 52*(11), 1623–1629.

Hasan, S. S., Pearson, J. S., Morris, J., & Whorwell, P. J. (2019). SKYPE HYPNOTHERAPY FOR IRRITABLE BOWEL SYNDROME: Effectiveness and comparison with face-to-face treatment. *International Journal of Clinical and Experimental Hypnosis, 67*(1), 69–80. doi: 10.1080/00207144.2019.1553766

Hasan, S. S., Whorwell, P. J., Miller, V., Morris, J., & Vasant, D. H. (2021). Six versus twelve sessions of gut-focused hypnotherapy for irritable bowel syndrome: A randomized trial. *Gastroenterology*. doi: S0016-5085(21)00463-7 [pii] 10.1053/j.gastro.2021.02.058

Hoekman, D. R., Vlieger, A. M., Stokkers, P. C., Mahhmod, N., Rietdijk, S., de Boer, N. K., & Benninga, M. A. (2021). Hypnotherapy for irritable bowel syndrome-type symptoms in patients with quiescent inflammatory bowel disease: A randomized, controlled trial. *Journal of Crohn's and Colitis, 15*(7), 1106–1113. doi: 10.1093/ecco-jcc/jjaa241

Houghton, L. A., Heyman, D. J., & Whorwell, P. J. (1996). Symptomatology, quality of life and economic features of irritable bowel syndrome – The effect of hypnotherapy. *Alimentary Pharmacology & Therapeutics, 10*(1), 91–95.

Hurtte, E., Rogers, B. D., Richards, C., & Gyawali, C. P. (2022). The clinical value of psychogastroenterological interventions for functional esophageal symptoms. *Neurogastroenterology & Motility, 34*(6), e14315. doi: 10.1111/nmo.14315

Isgar, B., Harman, M., Kaye, M. D., & Whorwell, P. J. (1983). Symptoms of irritable bowel syndrome in ulcerative colitis in remission. *Gut, 24*(3), 190–192. doi: 10.1136/gut.24.3.190

Jones, H., Cooper, P., Miller, V., Brooks, N., & Whorwell, P. J. (2006). Treatment of non-cardiac chest pain: A controlled trial of hypnotherapy. *Gut, 55*(10), 1403–1408.

Keefer, L., & Keshavarzian, A. (2007). Feasibility and acceptability of gut-directed hypnosis on inflammatory bowel disease: A brief communication. *International Journal of Clinical and Experimental Hypnosis, 55*(4), 457–466. doi: 10.1080/00207140701506565

Keefer, L., Taft, T. H., Kiebles, J. L., Martinovich, Z., Barrett, T. A., & Palsson, O. S. (2013). Gut-directed hypnotherapy significantly augments clinical remission in quiescent ulcerative colitis. *Alimentary Pharmacology & Therapeutics, 38*(7), 761–771. doi: 10.1111/apt.12449

Kiebles, J. L., Kwiatek, M. A., Pandolfino, J. E., Kahrilas, P. J., & Keefer, L. (2010). Do patients with globus sensation respond to hypnotically assisted relaxation therapy? A case series report. *Diseases of the Esophagus, 23*(7), 545–553. doi: 10.1111/j.1442-2050.2010.01064.x

Klein, K. B., & Spiegel, D. (1989). Modulation of gastric acid secretion by hypnosis. *Gastroenterology, 96*(6), 1383–1387.

Lea, R., Houghton, L. A., Calvert, E. L., Larder, S., Gonsalkorale, W. M., Whelan, V., ... Whorwell, P. J. (2003). Gut-focused hypnotherapy normalizes disordered rectal sensitivity in patients with irritable bowel syndrome. *Alimentary Pharmacology & Therapeutics, 17*(5), 635–642.

Lee, A., Moulton, D., McKernan, L., Russell, A., Slaughter, J. C., Acra, S., & Walker, L. (2021). Clinical hypnosis in pediatric Crohn's disease: A randomized controlled pilot study. *Journal of Pediatric Gastroenterology and Nutrition, 72*(3), e63–e70. doi: 10.1097/MPG.0000000000002980

Lindfors, P., Unge, P., Nyhlin, H., Ljotsson, B., Bjornsson, E. S., Abrahamsson, H., & Simren, M. (2012). Long-term effects of hypnotherapy in patients with refractory irritable bowel syndrome. *Scandinavian Journal of Gastroenterology, 47*(4), 414–420. doi: 10.3109/00365521.2012.658858

Lowen, M. B., Mayer, E. A., Sjoberg, M., Tillisch, K., Naliboff, B., Labus, J., ... Walter, S. A. (2013). Effect of hypnotherapy and educational intervention on brain response to visceral stimulus in the irritable bowel syndrome. *Alimentary Pharmacology & Therapeutics, 37*(12), 1184–1197. doi: 10.1111/apt.12319

Luo, Y., & Keefer, L. (2022). The clinical value of brain-gut behavioral therapies for functional esophageal disorders and symptoms. *Neurogastroenterology & Motility, 34*(6), e14373. doi: 10.1111/nmo.14373

Mawdsley, J. E., Jenkins, D. G., Macey, M. G., Langmead, L., & Rampton, D. S. (2008). The effect of hypnosis on systemic and rectal mucosal measures of inflammation in ulcerative colitis. *American Journal of Gastroenterology, 103*(6), 1460–1469. doi: 10.1111/j.1572-0241.2008.01845.x

Maxton, D. G., Morris, J. A., & Whorwell, P. J. (1989). Ranking of symptoms by patients with the irritable bowel syndrome. *BMJ, 299*(6708), 1138.

Mayer, E. A., Labus, J., Aziz, Q., Tracey, I., Kilpatrick, L., Elsenbruch, S., & Borsook, D. (2019). Role of brain imaging in disorders of brain-gut interaction: A Rome Working Team Report. *Gut, 68*(9), 1701–1715. doi: 10.1136/gutjnl-2019-318308

Meng, J., Agrawal, A., & Whorwell, P. J. (2013). Refractory inflammatory bowel disease-could it be an irritable bowel? *Nature Reviews Gastroenterology & Hepatology, 10*(1), 58–61. doi: 10.1038/nrgastro.2012.173

Miller, V., Carruthers, H. R., Morris, J., Hasan, S. S., Archbold, S., & Whorwell, P. J. (2015). Hypnotherapy for irritable bowel syndrome: An audit of one thousand adult patients. *Alimentary Pharmacology Therapeutics, 41*(9), 844–855. doi: 10.1111/apt.13145

Miller, V., Hopkins, L., & Whorwell, P. J. (2004). Suicidal ideation in patients with irritable bowel syndrome. *Clinical Gastroenterology and Hepatology, 2*(12), 1064–1068.

Miller, V., & Whorwell, P. J. (2008). Treatment of inflammatory bowel disease: A role for hypnotherapy. *International Journal of Clinical and Experimental Hypnosis, 56*, 1–12.

Noble, H., Hasan, S. S., Simpson, V., Whorwell, P. J., & Vasant, D. H. (2022). Patient satisfaction after remotely delivered gut-directed hypnotherapy for irritable bowel syndrome during the COVID-19 era: Implications for future practice. *BMJ Open Gastroenterology, 9*(1). doi: 10.1136/bmjgast-2022-001039

Palsson, O. S. (2015). Hypnosis treatment of gastrointestinal disorders: A comprehensive review of the empirical evidence. *American Journal of Clinical Hypnosis, 58*(2), 134–158. doi: 10.1080/00029157.2015.1039114

Peter, J., Fournier, C., Keip, B., Rittershaus, N., Stephanou-Rieser, N., Durdevic, M., ... Moser, G. (2018). Intestinal microbiome in irritable bowel syndrome before and after gut-directed hypnotherapy. *International Journal of Molecular Sciences, 19*(11). doi: 10.3390/ijms19113619

Peters, S. L., Muir, J. G., & Gibson, P. R. (2015). Review article: Gut-directed hypnotherapy in the management of irritable bowel syndrome and inflammatory bowel disease. *Alimentary Pharmacology & Therapeutics, 41*(11), 1104–1115. doi: 10.1111/apt.13202

Prior, A., Colgan, S. M., & Whorwell, P. J. (1990). Changes in rectal sensitivity after hypnotherapy in patients with irritable bowel syndrome. *Gut, 31*(8), 896–898.

Rainville, P., Duncan, G. H., Price, D. D., Carrier, B., & Bushnell, M. C. (1997). Pain affect encoded in human anterior cingulate but not somatosensory cortex. *Science, 277*(5328), 968–971.

Riehl, M. E., Kinsinger, S., Kahrilas, P. J., Pandolfino, J. E., & Keefer, L. (2015). Role of a health psychologist in the management of functional esophageal complaints. *Diseases of the Esophagus, 28*(5), 428–436. doi: 10.1111/dote.12219

Riehl, M. E., Pandolfino, J. E., Palsson, O. S., & Keefer, L. (2016). Feasibility and acceptability of esophageal-directed hypnotherapy for functional heartburn. *Diseases of the Esophagus, 29*(5), 490–496. doi: 10.1111/dote.12353

Sasegbon, A., Hasan, S. S., Whorwell, P. J., & Vasant, D. H. (2022). Experience and clinical efficacy of gut-directed hypnotherapy in an Asian population with refractory irritable bowel syndrome. *JGH Open, 6*(7), 447–453. doi: 10.1002/jgh3.12770

Simon, R. A., Engstrom, M., Icenhour, A., Lowen, M., Strom, M., Tillisch, K., ... Walter, S. (2019). On functional connectivity and symptom relief after gut-directed hypnotherapy in irritable bowel syndrome: A preliminary study. *Journal of Neurogastroenterology and Motility, 25*(3), 478–479. doi: 10.5056/jnm19069

Stacher, G., Berner, P., Naske, R., Schuster, P., Bauer, P., Starker, H., & Schulze, D. (1975). Effect of hypnotic suggestion of relaxation on basal and betazole-stimulated gastric acid secretion. *Gastroenterology, 68*(4 Pt 1), 656–661.

Toner, B. B., Stuckless, N., Ali, A., Downie, F., Emmott, S., & Akman, D. (1998). The development of a cognitive scale for functional bowel disorders. *Psychosomatic Medicine, 60*(4), 492–497.

Vasant, D. H., Hasan, S. S., Cruickshanks, P., & Whorwell, P. J. (2021). Gut-focused hypnotherapy for children and adolescents with irritable bowel syndrome. *Frontline Gastroenterology, 12*(7), 570–577. doi: 10.1136/flgastro-2020-101679

Vasant, D. H., & Whorwell, P. J. (2019). Gut-focused hypnotherapy for functional gastrointestinal disorders: Evidence-base, practical aspects, and the Manchester Protocol. *Neurogastroenterology & Motility, 31*(8), e13573. doi: 10.1111/nmo.13573

Vlieger, A. M., Menko-Frankenhuis, C., Wolfkamp, S. C., Tromp, E., & Benninga, M. A. (2007). Hypnotherapy for children with functional abdominal pain or irritable bowel syndrome: A randomized controlled trial. *Gastroenterology*, *133*(5), 1430–1436.

Vlieger, A. M., Rutten, J. M., Govers, A. M., Frankenhuis, C., & Benninga, M. A. (2012). Long-term follow-up of gut-directed hypnotherapy vs. standard care in children with functional abdominal pain or irritable bowel syndrome. *American Journal of Gastroenterology*, *107*(4), 627–631. doi: 10.1038/ajg.2011.487

Whorwell, P. J., Houghton, L. A., Taylor, E. E., & Maxton, D. G. (1992). Physiological effects of emotion: Assessment via hypnosis. *Lancet*, *340*(8811), 69–72.

Whorwell, P. J., McCallum, M., Creed, F. H., & Roberts, C. T. (1986). Non-colonic features of irritable bowel syndrome. *Gut*, *27*(1), 37–40.

Whorwell, P. J., Prior, A., & Colgan, S. M. (1987). Hypnotherapy in severe irritable bowel syndrome: Further experience. *Gut*, *28*(4), 423–425.

Whorwell, P. J., Prior, A., & Faragher, E. B. (1984). Controlled trial of hypnotherapy in the treatment of severe refractory irritable-bowel syndrome. *Lancet*, *2*(8414), 1232–1234.

43
HYPNOSIS AND CHRONIC PAIN MANAGEMENT

Mark P. Jensen

DEPARTMENT OF REHABILITATION MEDICINE, UNIVERSITY OF WASHINGTON, SEATTLE, WA, USA

Introduction

Pain is critical to our survival. It is an experience we create when we conclude that the body is at imminent risk for harm. As such, we can take steps to protect ourselves from harm before any damage actually occurs. Nociceptors distributed throughout the body, and in particular near the surface of the skin, start to fire in response to heat before that heat produces damage, allowing us the opportunity to remove ourselves from the heat source. A healthy person can and does experience pain regularly.

However, in the case of chronic pain – generally defined as ongoing pain that has occurred for three months or more -- the experience of pain is often less than useful. It can result in needless suffering and contribute to other long-term health conditions including insomnia and disability. Chronic pain is also by its very definition refractory to many treatments; yet this does not stop people with chronic pain from seeking out and ultimately obtaining treatments, even when those treatments themselves result in even more pain and disability.

Hypnosis treatment – including teaching people with chronic pain self-hypnosis – is a viable alternative to pharmacological and invasive biomedical treatments. In fact, given its proven efficacy and positive side effect profile, it should be the first treatment offered to individuals with chronic pain. This chapter summarizes the key information needed to provide effective hypnosis treatment for chronic pain. It begins with a discussion of three key research findings that inform the use of clinical hypnosis: (1) that treatment outcome is variable; (2) that hypnosis treatment has two primary benefits, so both should be targeted for treatment; (3) that hypnosis treatment has many benefits in addition to pain reduction; and (4) using hypnosis to change pain-related thoughts appears to have greater benefit than using hypnosis to change pain intensity or quality. The chapter then presents a detailed and specific treatment protocol (with proven efficacy based on decades of research) for using hypnosis to treat chronic pain in adults.

Four Key Research Findings

Hypnosis Treatment for Chronic Pain Is Effective, But Outcomes Vary

Among the many psychological treatments for pain, those that incorporate hypnosis may be the most effective (Jensen et al., 2020; Montgomery et al., 2000; Patterson, 2010;

DOI: 10.4324/9781003449126-57

Williams et al., 2022). However, not everyone benefits in the same way after receiving hypnosis treatment. If the *only* treatment outcome of interest to the patient is a marked reduction in daily pain intensity, many patients who receive hypnosis treatment – which for the patients I have worked with includes learning self-hypnosis skills – will be disappointed. For example, in our studies, among individuals with chronic pain associated with spinal cord injury – a population whose pain is particularly refractory to all available treatments – the treatment response rate ranges from 22% to 27%, using a pain reduction amount of 30% or more as indicating treatment response (Jensen et al., 2005, 2009a). We have also found that the response rates of individuals with multiple sclerosis and chronic pain are higher – 33% to 47% range (Jensen et al., 2005, 2009b). People with chronic pain associated with amputation have even higher response rates – 60% (Jensen et al., 2005). That said, of those who are able to experience meaningful pain reductions in pain intensity with hypnosis treatment, most are able to maintain those benefits for at least a year following treatment (Jensen et al., 2008). In short, while many individuals with chronic pain have a good chance of obtaining significant and meaningful pain reductions with hypnosis treatment, for most if not all chronic pain conditions, there will be individuals who do not respond to this treatment with clinically meaningful reductions in daily pain. Nonetheless, hypnosis treatment often provides other significant benefits for these individuals.

Self-Hypnosis Training Has Two Primary Beneficial Effects on Pain Intensity

Given our findings that not all people who receive hypnosis treatment for chronic pain report clinically meaningful reductions pain intensity, we were somewhat surprised to learn in follow-up interviews that only 3% of individuals reported "no benefit" to hypnosis treatment (Jensen et al., 2006). Perhaps related to this, the vast majority of patients who receive self-hypnosis training – 80–85% – continue to practice self-hypnosis following treatment (Jensen et al., 2009a, b).

To investigate this apparent contradiction, we asked individuals who have received hypnosis treatment to describe the effects of that treatment and their ongoing self-hypnosis practice. First, we learned that many experienced an *immediate* reduction in pain that often lasted for hours following self-hypnosis (Jensen et al., 2009a, b). Thus, many use self-hypnosis as a coping response to experience immediate but short-term reductions in pain.

Based on these findings, we have concluded that self-hypnosis training for chronic pain has *two* effects on pain intensity. First, hypnotic treatment can have a substantial effect on the way that people with chronic pain process sensory information on a daily basis, effects that result in substantial and clinically meaningful reductions in pain intensity that are durable and may require little additional effort on the part of the patient. This benefit is not experienced by everyone and appears to vary as a function of pain condition. Second, training in self-hypnosis teaches patients a skill that they can use whenever they choose to experience an immediate reduction in pain that can last for several hours – much like they might use a medication (but one with few negative side effects, as discussed in the next section). This short-term beneficial effect on pain intensity is consistent with evidence showing that the immediate effects of hypnosis on *current pain* can be very large (see Jensen et al., 2009b).

Hypnosis Treatment Has Many More Benefits Than Just Pain Reduction

During and after hypnosis treatment, many of the participants in our research studies – including many of those who did not report clinically meaningful reductions in daily chronic pain intensity – spontaneously reported a very high degree of treatment satisfaction. To understand what might have contributed to this, we asked the study participants about both the positive and negative effects of hypnosis treatment (Jensen et al., 2006).

We found that the ratio of positive to negative benefits (32/3) was extremely high. Moreover, the three "negative" effects about the treatment were in fact not that negative. One was that the treatment "... didn't work," another was that the treatment was less effective than was hoped, and the third was that the treatment benefits did not last as long as the person hoped it would. Moreover, despite the fact that the focus of the hypnotic suggestions was pain reduction, only nine of the treatment benefits identified were pain-related. The three most common pain-related benefits were pain reduction, an increased sense of control over pain, and a sense of having a new option or tool for pain management.

Perhaps most interestingly, the majority of the benefits identified were not pain related. These benefits included a feeling of increased energy, increased self-awareness, improved sleep, and lowered blood pressure.

Focusing Hypnosis Treatment on Pain-Related Thoughts May Be More Effective Than Focusing on Pain Reduction

Among the most interesting – and clinically useful – finding from our research is that hypnotic suggestions that focus on changing maladaptive pain-related beliefs to more neutral or adaptive ones appear to be more effective for reducing pain than suggestions that focus on pain reduction. The initial hints suggesting this finding came from a pilot study, in which we examined the effects of using hypnosis to alter pain-related thoughts (referred to in our work as hypnotic cognitive therapy; see Jensen et al., 2011). The inspiration for this study came from a systematic review conducted by Irving Kirsch and colleagues (1995), in which they concluded that the benefits of hypnosis combined with cognitive behavioral therapy treatments are substantially greater than cognitive behavioral therapy alone (Kirsch et al., 1995). This finding was subsequently replicated in a more recent meta-analysis (Ramondo et al., 2021).

In our preliminary pilot study, we found that using hypnosis to suggest changes in pain-related maladaptive beliefs (such as "It is never going to get better," and "My life is ruined because of pain") to more adaptive ones (such as "I can learn strategies to feel better," and "It is always possible to live a meaningful life consistent with my values") was not only associated with larger reductions in pain intensity than an intervention that used traditional cognitive therapy approaches to change pain-related beliefs but also substantially more effective than using hypnosis to suggest reductions in pain intensity. The relative benefit of hypnotic cognitive therapy over both hypnosis focused on pain reduction and traditional cognitive therapy was replicated in a subsequent fully powered clinical trial (Jensen et al., 2020).

Clinical Implications

The clinical implications of the four key findings from our research program are clear. First, clinicians and patients can hope for substantial decreases in daily characteristic pain intensity with treatment – indeed, substantial subsets of patients can achieve this – but not everyone experiences this. However, even without this benefit, the great majority of patients who learn self-hypnosis can use it to experience immediate pain relief that can last for hours. This gives them an important tool that can increase self-efficacy and hope. To ensure that patients benefit from both the possible durable and likely immediate reductions in pain, self-hypnosis training (in particular, post-hypnotic suggestions, see below) should target both benefits. The finding that patients usually experience improvements across multiple quality of life domains with hypnosis treatment also gives patients hope that even if or when they do not experience large pain reductions, they can experience improvements in other aspects of their lives. In fact, in my experience, the patient who obtains no benefits from learning self-hypnosis is extremely rare. This finding can be used to give patients hope early in treatment, and also seed curiosity regarding the specific benefits that they will find with treatment (see treatment protocols, below). The finding also emphasizes the importance of targeting hypnosis treatment to address the multiple factors impacted by pain, including sleep quality, depression, anxiety, and activity restrictions. Finally, the finding that hypnosis treatment targeting changes in pain-related beliefs results in larger improvements than hypnosis treatment targeting pain reductions means that clinicians should ensure that they evaluate patients' thoughts about pain and use hypnosis to address any maladaptive thoughts that are present.

Self-Hypnosis Training for Chronic Pain

The hypnotic treatment recommendations described in the remainder of this chapter are based on the findings from a long-standing and ongoing research program on the development and evaluation of hypnotic treatments for chronic pain (Jensen & Barber, 2000; Jensen et al., 2005, 2008, 2009a, b, 2011, 2020; Williams et al., 2022). Here the essential parts of the intervention will be reported, even more information is available from a published therapist manual (Jensen, 2011).

Overall Session Structure

Each session usually begins with a check in with the patient to discuss progress made with home practice, review overall treatment goals, and establish the goals for the current session, including the sensory, cognitive, emotional, and behavioral responses that will be targeted during the hypnosis session. The specific words that will be used during the hypnosis session can be identified prior to the hypnosis session using open questions and reflections (see Jensen, 2019).

This is usually followed by the hypnosis portion of the session (usually about 20–30 minutes), leaving enough time de-brief the patient and discuss goals for the week (Jensen, 2011). Many of the treatment benefits begin to emerge following just two to four sessions, and some patients achieve substantial benefits by the fourth session. For these patients, additional sessions may not be required. Others may feel that they are just getting started and could benefit from an additional four sessions. It is the rare patient that requires more than eight sessions of hypnosis treatment for pain management.

Because the model of hypnosis treatment presented here is a model of self-hypnosis training – that is, hypnosis as something that patients learn to do and use for themselves, rather than something that is done *to* patients – between-session practice is critical. Thus, an audio recording is made of each hypnosis session, and provided to the patient in his or her preferred form (e.g., as a CD or audio file). Patients are asked to listen to the recording at least once/day. They are also asked to practice self-hypnosis on their own for 2–3 minutes or longer as they wish at least three to five times daily.

Each session begins with a specific cue or anchor that, over time, can be used to initiate self-hypnosis followed by self-suggestions (given to oneself as either words or images; for example, an image of a future self who has achieved a specific goal). A favorite cue I use is to invite the patient to take a deep breath and hold it for several seconds. Others can include touching or rubbing the thumb and forefinger of one hand together, or even allowing a specific image to come to mind.

The scripts presented here should be considered as at most a starting point or as "ideas to be considered." They should not be administered (or read to) patients exactly as written without consideration of the patient's specific needs and treatment goals.

Inductions

I often start treatment with a relaxation induction for a number of reasons. First, almost everyone has had at least some experience at some point in their lives with feeling relaxed. It is therefore an experience that resonates with many – although clearly not all – individuals. As a result, it is often relatively easy for many individuals to feel relaxed following this induction. This success can build confidence that the approach is "working" and promote self-efficacy.

In addition, the experience of relaxation is inconsistent with pain. Thus, even in the presence of severe pain, suggestions for feeling relaxed can disrupt a patterned response, which then disrupts pain intensity and pain-related suffering. As a result, many patients report some pain relief and greater control over pain during the induction itself. This can help to create and build positive outcome expectancies very early. Finally, teaching patients to be able to feel relaxed (which is almost always experienced as pleasant) can help patients learn that the presence of pain does not necessarily have to be associated with negative affect. This is a critical truth that can be associated with significant improvements once it is clearly understood by a patient.

Although rare, some patients find the experience of relaxation uncomfortable. For some, this is psychological discomfort associated with a sense of losing control. Others describe a physical sensation of "falling" when they feel relaxed, which can be distressing. Still others have reported an increase in spasms and/or pain with relaxation suggestions – perhaps due to a decrease in activity in areas of the brain that are needed and being used for sensory and/or spasm suppression. To help decrease the chances that the patient would feel like he or she is "falling" with relaxation suggestions, and to encourage a mindset associated with feeling "supported" by the clinician, the reader will see in the script that follows wording that refers to experiencing the "strong support" of the chair. In any case, however, in the rare instance that a patient finds suggestions for relaxation uncomfortable, simply use other inductions. The most important thing, of course, is that the patient be able to focus his or her mind increasingly on the clinical suggestions that are offered following the induction.

Another favorite induction which I almost always use along with the relaxation induction is a favorite place induction. Prior to using this induction, it is a good idea to tell the patient that the session will include an invitation for them to experience themselves in a place where they feel comfortable and at ease – a "favorite place." They can be invited to select a place that they can very clearly imagine in detail.

As a final note, for readers who have experience inviting their patients to imagine going to a favorite place, you can pause and consider where it is your patients usually choose to go. You are likely to identify a beach as the most common, and a mountain or forest as the second most common. This choice is consistent with research that demonstrates that two colors are analgesic in humans and animals: blue and green (Khanna et al., 2019; Martin et al., 2021a, 2021b).

> What follows are examples of text outtakes from a typical relaxation and favorite place induction used in my clinical work and our research program.[1]
>
> Okay ... just settle back. ... And allow the eyes to close. ...
>
> Now ... I'm going to talk to you for a while. ... All you have to do is listen to what I'm saying, and allow yourself to have as pleasant an experience as you know how. ... Go ahead and adjust yourself to the most comfortable position you can. ...
>
> Go ahead and draw a deep, satisfying breath into your belly ... and gently hold the breath for as long as it feels comfortable ... and now ... let it go. ...
>
> And now, allow the whole body to relax. ... Maybe noticing that the top of your head is feeling more relaxed and comfortable. ... Letting that relaxation and comfort spread down into your forehead, your eyes, into your jaw, down the neck, deep, relaxing, and comfortably heavy. ... Letting your neck go, into your shoulders, deep, warm, and heavy.
>
> Down into the right arm, the right hand. ... And now ... the left arm ... and the left hand. More deeply relaxed. And now that relaxation spreads down into the chest, ... breathing even more deeply, slowly, and completely ... down into the right thigh, right calf, the right foot. Into the left thigh, left calf, the left foot. The entire body now very, very relaxed. Deep, comfortable, relaxation, not a care in the world. It may even be the sense of lightness and drifting. ...
>
> And now you find yourself in your favorite place. It can be whatever you want, as long as it is comfortable ... Notice what you are able to see in front of you, really notice what you can see. ... And now notice what you are able to hear. ... Notice what you are able to feel, perhaps a light breeze on your face, ... and the temperature is just right. ... And if you can see the sky ... you might notice how very BLUE it is ... And if you can see trees or plants or both ... you might notice the many pleasant greens ... light greens ... dark greens. ... And aware that when you are in your favorite place, your mind can serve you in wonderful ways, and allow you to have profound experiences that serve your ability to achieve your goals that are most important to you.

Clinical Suggestions

Following the induction, the clinician then makes the suggestions that are consistent with the patient's needs and treatment goals. Of course, the clinical suggestions offered to any one patient will depend entirely on their treatment goals. For individuals with chronic pain, treatment goals could and often do include improved sleep, increased activity, diet management, and becoming a non-smoker, among many others. Ideas for suggestions to address these issues as well as number of other pain-related issues are presented in various books and textbooks (Hammond, 1990; Patterson, 2010), including the book that is also based on our clinical research program (Jensen, 2011). Here, I present outtakes presenting the key ideas from clinical suggestions that I have found to be particularly helpful. They include suggestions for (1) a decreased awareness of uncomfortable suggestions, (2) an increased understanding that pain is not necessarily an indication of harm, (3) an increase in reassuring pain-related thoughts, and (4) age progression for comfort and confidence.

DECREASED AWARENESS OF UNCOMFORTABLE SENSATIONS

You can notice that something very interesting is happening. ..., that as your comfort grows ... any other feelings or sensations just seem to be drifting farther and farther away. ... Perhaps like leaves on a stream. ... I don't know what color they are, or what the image is ... but you do see them. ... You can see details, watching as the image changes. Perhaps floating slowly, drifting down the stream. ... Or you might see those feelings or sensations as the embers of a fire slowly burning out ... the colors of the embers slowly dimming, becoming cooler and more comfortable. ... Leaves floating down a stream or embers becoming cool and comfortable. ... Either way, the image is getting smaller and smaller ... less and less

And now, maybe you can take these images of any feelings or sensations that are diminishing and see them going into a strong insulated box that has a secure lid. ... And you can see yourself shutting the lid and securing it ... Muffling the sensations ... and then putting this box into a second very secure box and shutting the lid of the second box. ... And then, I wonder how you are going to find that the box is moving far, far away? ...

And with those sensations so far away, it is even easier to feel the comfort of every breath.

INCREASED UNDERSTANDING THAT PAIN IS NOT NECESSARILY AN INDICATION OF HARM

Now I would like you to think about your brain, and how it works. Wouldn't it be interesting, if you could come up with a model for how your brain works. Some people might see this in terms of switches that turn on and off. ...

And we know that the brain is also designed to respond to warning signals ... signals telling us about a possible threat. In this way, the brain and body can take really good care of us.

As useful as it can be to have warning signals when there is real danger, sometimes our brains become confused and give off warning signals when we are not in danger. The alarm turns on when there is no fire. ... What can we do when our brains are telling us that there is something wrong when we are really fine? ...

So, it is very useful for our brains to be able to detect which signals are real threats and which ones are not. For the sensations that are no longer threatening, it becomes very useful for us to learn how to dim those signals. ...

We might do this by picturing in our minds that we have a dimmer switch. When we turn it down ... from maybe a 5 to a 3 ... or a 2 ... the noise and sense of threat become less.

Perhaps you can look into your own brain now and see how you might dim those signals. ...

INCREASE IN REASSURING PAIN-RELATED THOUGHTS

Perhaps you might wonder how the things you learn and practice somehow happen to become automatic. ... Helpful thoughts about pain that once took some practice to learn and now just seem natural and effortless because you have thought about them enough. ... Isn't it interesting that helpful thoughts about your body, your sensations and your coping can grow to occur naturally ... almost without any effort at all.

With the mind drifting now, ... go ahead and notice if there might be even other thoughts that are helpful and reassuring. Maybe thoughts like "This too shall pass." ... Or "Deep inside, my body will know how to help me feel more comfortable." ...

And as long as the thought or thoughts are helpful, allow them to sink deep into your unconscious ... become an idea that you embrace ... deep down in your bones. ... An idea, a thought that can be available to you when you need it, a reassuring thought ... bringing you comfort ...

AGE PROGRESSION FOR COMFORT AND CONFIDENCE

And as you might be continuing to experience yourself in today's favorite place, perhaps noticing, again, what you see around you. ... You are now moving forward in time and are able to see clear images of yourself in the future

You can see a future version of yourself ... maybe a few weeks or few months older ... You can see that you are feeling better than you do now ... You have met some important goal or goals. ... Perhaps you are stronger in some ways. ... Perhaps more comfortable and confident. ... Perhaps you can see this person walking towards you ... or maybe standing or sitting with you. ... Yes, it is you, but it is you in the future.

Notice what you see in your future self. How you look. ... How wonderful you feel. And you can tell ... just by looking, that you are doing better. ... Perhaps you are stronger ... perhaps more fit. ...

And now ... you can experience yourself as becoming that future self. Experience your present self and future self becoming one. And you can feel the greater comfort, the greater confidence ... experience yourself as having made real progress. ... So nice to feel better.

And now, allowing yourself to come back into your current self. ... The future and present now blended into one ... anything that you discovered or found helpful now has become part of you. Perhaps a way of thinking ... a way of feeling ... greater confidence ... greater hope ... perhaps a sense of hopeful excitement ... all this and anything else that is helpful is a part of your current self, now.

Post-Hypnotic Suggestions

The goals of the post-hypnotic suggestions are to teach the participant how to use the hypnotic skills on his or her own, and to make any beneficial changes permanent, consistent with our findings that hypnosis can have two categories of benefits, discussed earlier in this chapter. The general idea is to suggest (1) that the experience of analgesia, relaxation, and comfort will stay with the patient and linger beyond the session, lasting for "... hours, days, weeks, and years ..."; (2) that the more the patient practices, by listening to a recording of the session and also by using the cue to enter a hypnotic state and re-experience the comfort of hypnosis without the recording, the more effective and long lasting the suggestions will be; and (3) that the participant will be able to enter this relaxed and absorbed state using a specific cue more easily with time and practice, and can do so any time he or she wishes to experience comfort. The post-hypnotic suggestions are also designed to increase the patient's confidence in using these skills and a sense of control over pain and its impact.

> And now we have reached the time to extend what has been most useful to you in this session into the rest of your day, and your daily life. ...
>
> Any time you want to feel more comfortable, to allow yourself to again experience the benefits of today's session, ... all you ever have to do ... is to take a very deep, very satisfying breath, and hold it, hold it for a moment, ... and then let it go. And any of the comfortable feelings and benefits, any helpful responses that you have created for yourself in this session will come washing over you ... naturally, easily, and automatically. ...
>
> And the more you practice, however you find yourself doing it ... listening to the recordings ... or practicing on your own several times every day ... the easier it will be for your mind to use these skills, automatically, so that you can create comfort and relaxation, and an inner strength, whenever you need it. And the benefits you create for yourself ... these benefits can linger and last beyond the sessions ... for minutes ... hours ... days ... and years. Becoming a permanent part of your comfort ... These benefits will last for as long as they continue to be helpful.

Re-Orienting

The goal of re-orienting is to bring patient out of hypnosis, while also maximizing the chances that he or she will bring any benefits of the sessions, including any feelings of calmness and relaxation into their day.

> Now, ... getting ready to return. You are looking at the number 10 in front of you. And in a moment, I am going to start counting with you as we move back up into a state of alertness, from 10 to 1. With each number I count you will feel more alert, awake, and refreshed. No hurry, we have plenty of time, you do not need to come back to a full state of alertness until you are ready. When we reach one at the top, your eyes will remain closed for a little longer ... and will only open when your mind finds that you are feeling alert and finished with this part

De-Briefing

The goals of the de-briefing session include (1) ensuring that the patient is actually alert and not just sitting, compliantly with his or her eyes open and (2) understanding how the patient responded to the induction and the suggestions, in order to inform what changes, if any, should be made in these for the next session. If, after conversing with the patient, it appears that he or she is not yet completely alert, you might give him or her some time to re-orient on his or her own. Or, if needed, you might provide additional suggestions for being alert.

Then discuss with the patient how they are feeling right now and their experience during the hypnosis session. Modifications in the hypnosis suggestions may be made based on the information obtained from this discussion (e.g., if a participant states that a suggestion was not helpful or did not like it, that suggestion should be dropped or reworded; if the participant describes a specific suggestion or image that was particularly helpful, that suggestion or image might be emphasized in the next session). Also, of course, this is a good time to address any questions or concerns about the hypnosis session or hypnosis in general, as appropriate.

Summary and Conclusions

Hypnosis and hypnotic interventions can, and often should, be a part of chronic pain treatment. The use of hypnosis for pain management should be informed by the findings from research. Four key findings include: (1) that treatment outcome is variable, (2) that hypnosis treatment has two primary benefits so both should be targeted for treatment, (3) that hypnosis treatment has many benefits in addition to pain reduction, and (4) using hypnosis to change pain-related thoughts appears to have greater benefit than using hypnosis to change pain intensity or quality. Clinicians should therefore not be surprised to see what each patient responds to hypnosis treatment in a unique way. Some, in fact, might respond better to alternative approaches such as those that teach mindfulness or cognitive restructuring skills (Jensen et al., 2020; Williams et al., 2022). Few, if any, patients should be offered or provided only hypnosis. When using hypnosis, post-hypnotic suggestion should ideally include those that suggest durable changes in how the brain processes sensory input and in the use of hypnosis as a practical daily skill. Hypnotic suggestions should focus on more than just pain reduction, and should also include suggestions for changing alarming and less useful pain-related thoughts to more reassuring ones that contribute to confidence and comfort.

The chapter contained the text based on scripts used in our clinical trials that have demonstrated the efficacy of hypnosis, and that therefore have evidence supporting their utility. The scripts presented here should not be read verbatim to patients, but should serve as inspiration for ideas for suggestions that can be tailored to each patient's needs and goals.

Disclosures

Mark P. Jensen is the author of two books (*Hypnosis for chronic pain management: Therapist guide* and *Hypnosis for chronic pain management: Workbook)*, is the editor of five others (*The art and practice of hypnotic induction: Favorite methods of master clinicians*, *Hypnotic techniques for chronic pain management: Favorite methods of master clinicians*, *Hypnosis for acute and procedural pain management: Favorite methods of master clinicians; Handbook of hypnotic techniques, Vol. 1: Favorite methods of master clinicians;* and *Handbook of hypnotic techniques, Vol. 1: Favorite methods of master clinicians*) and facilitates workshops related to the topic of this paper. He receives royalties for book sales and sometimes receive financial remuneration for facilitating workshops on the topic of this paper.

Acknowledgments

Preparation of this chapter was supported by grants from the National Institutes of Health (R01HD070973 and R01AT0008336). The author would like to thank the many scientists and clinicians who have contributed to the development and evaluation of treatment protocol described in this chapter, including Joseph Barber, Tiara Dillworth, Dawn Ehde, Marisol Hanley, Adam Hirsh, M. Elena Mendoza, Ivan Molton, Travis Osborne, Katherine Raichle, Joan Romano, Brenda Stoelb, and Gabriel Tan, and in particular David R. Patterson. The author would also like to thank Lisa C. Murphy for her helpful comments and suggestions on an earlier version of this chapter.

Note

1 All of the portions from hypnosis scripts presented here are copyrighted by the University of Washington and printed with permission. Readers can write the author to obtain the full scripts used in clinical trials.

References

Hammond, D. C. (1990). *Handbook of hypnotic suggestions and metaphors*. New York, NY: Norton and Company.

Jensen, M. P. (2011). *Hypnosis for chronic pain management: Therapist guide*. New York, NY: Oxford University Press.

Jensen, M. P. (2019). Using hypnotic reflective listening for identify effective suggestions for behavior change. In M. P. Jensen (Ed.), *Handbook of hypnotic techniques, Vol 1: Favorite methods of master clinicians* (pp. 140–170). Kirkland, WA: Denny Creek Press.

Jensen, M. P., & Barber, J. (2000). Hypnotic analgesia of spinal cord injury pain. *Australian Journal of Clinical and Experimental Hypnosis*, *28*, 150–168.

Jensen, M. P., Barber, J., Hanley, M. A., Engel, J. M., Romano, J. M., Cardenas, D. D., Kraft, G. H., Hoffman, A. J., & Patterson, D. R. (2008). Long-term outcome of hypnotic-analgesia treatment for chronic pain in persons with disabilities. *International Journal of Clinical and Experimental Hypnosis*, *56*(2), 156–169. 10.1080/00207140701849486

Jensen, M. P., Barber, J., Romano, J. M., Hanley, M. A., Raichle, K. A., Molton, I. R., Engel, J. M., Osborne, T. L., Stoelb, B. L., Cardenas, D. D., & Patterson, D. R. (2009a). Effects of self-hypnosis training and EMG biofeedback relaxation training on chronic pain in persons with spinal-cord injury. *International Journal of Clinical and Experimental Hypnosis*, *57*(3), 239–268. 10.1080/00207140902881007

Jensen, M. P., Barber, J., Romano, J. M., Molton, I. R., Raichle, K. A., Osborne, T. L., Engel, J. M., Stoelb, B. L., Kraft, G. H., & Patterson, D. R. (2009b). A comparison of self-hypnosis versus progressive muscle relaxation in patients with multiple sclerosis and chronic pain. *International Journal of Clinical and Experimental Hypnosis*, *57*, 198–221. 10.1080/00207140802665476

Jensen, M. P., Ehde, D. M., Gertz, K. J., Stoelb, B. L., Dillworth, T. M., Hirsh, A. T., Molton, I. R., & Kraft, G. H. (2011). Effects of self-hypnosis training and cognitive restructuring on daily pain intensity and catastrophizing in individuals with multiple sclerosis and chronic pain. *International Journal of Clinical and Experimental Hypnosis*, *59*(1), 45–63. 10.1080/00207144.2011.522892

Jensen, M. P., Hanley, M. A., Engel, J. M., Romano, J. M., Barber, J., Cardenas, D. D., Kraft, G. H., Hoffman, A. J., & Patterson, D. R. (2005). Hypnotic analgesia for chronic pain in persons with disabilities: A case series. *International Journal of Clinical and Experimental Hypnosis*, *53*(2), 198–228. 10.1080/00207140590927545

Jensen, M. P., McArthur, K. D., Barber, J., Hanley, M. A., Engel, J. M., Romano, J. M., Cardenas, D. D., Kraft, G. H., Hoffman, A. J., & Patterson, D. R. (2006). Satisfaction with, and the beneficial side effects of, hypnotic analgesia. *International Journal of Clinical and Experimental Hypnosis*, *54*(4), 432–447. 10.1080/00207140600856798

Jensen, M. P., Mendoza, M. E., Ehde, D. M., Patterson, D. R., Molton, I. R., Dillworth, T. M., Gertz, K. J., Chan, J., Hakimian, S., Battalio, S. L., & Ciol, M. A. (2020). Effects of hypnosis, cognitive therapy, hypnotic cognitive therapy, and pain education in adults with chronic pain: A randomized clinical trial. *Pain*, *161*(10), 2284–2298. 10.1097/j.pain.0000000000001943

Khanna, R., Patwardhan, A., Yang, X., Li, W., Cai, S., Ji, Y., Chew, L. A., Dorame, A., Bellampalli, S. S., Schmoll. R. W., Gordon, J., Moutal, A., Vanderah, T. W., Porreca, F., & Ibrahim, M. M. (2019). Development and characterization of an injury-free model of functional pain in rats by exposure to red light. *Journal of Pain*, *20*(11), 1293–1306. 10.1016/j.jpain.2019.04.008

Kirsch, I., Montgomery, G., & Sapirstein, G. (1995). Hypnosis as an adjunct to cognitive-behavioral psychotherapy: A meta-analysis. *Journal of Consulting and Clinical Psychology*, *63*(2), 214–220. 10.1037/0022-006x.63.2.214

Martin, L. F., Moutal, A., Cheng, K., Washington, S. M., Calligaro, H., Goel, V., Kranz, T., Largent-Milnes, T. M., Khanna, R., Patwardhan, A., & Ibrahim, M. M. (2021a). Green light antinociceptive and reversal of thermal and mechanical hypersensitivity effects rely on endogenous opioid system stimulation. *Journal of Pain*, *22*(12), 1646–1656. 10.1016/j.jpain.2021.05.006

Martin, L. F., Porreca, F., Mata, E. I., Salloum, M., Goel, V., Gunnala, P., Gillgore, W. D. S., Jain, S., Jones-MacFarland, F. N., Khanna. R., Patwardhan. A., & Ibrahim, M. M. (2021b). Green light exposure improves pain and quality of life in fibromyalgia patients: A preliminary one-way crossover clinical trial. *Pain Medicine*, *22*(1), 118–130. 10.1093/pm/pnaa329

Montgomery, G. H., Duhamel, K. N., & Redd, W. H. (2000). A meta-analysis of hypnotically induced analgesia: How effective is hypnosis? *International Journal of Clinical and Experimental Hypnosis*, *48*(2), 138–153. 10.1080/00207140008410045

Patterson, D. R. (2010). *Clinical hypnosis for pain control.* Washington, DC: American Psychological Association.

Ramondo, N., Gignac, G. E., Pestell, C. F., & Byrne, S. M. (2021). Clinical hypnosis as an adjunct to cognitive behavior therapy: An updated meta-analysis. *International Journal of Clinical and Experimental Hypnosis*, *69*(2), 169–202. 10.1080/00207144.2021.1877549

Williams, R. M., Day, M. A., Ehde, D. M., Turner, A. P., Ciol, M. A., Gertz, K. J., Patterson, D., Hakimian, S., Suri, P., & Jensen, M. P. (2022). Effects of hypnosis vs mindfulness meditation vs education on chronic pain intensity and secondary outcomes in veterans: A randomized clinical trial. *Pain*, *163*(10), 1905–1918. 10.1097/j.pain.0000000000002586

44
HYPNOSIS AND FIBROMYALGIA SYNDROME

Winfried Häuser[1] *and Giuseppe De Benedittis*[2]
[1]Technical University Munich, Germany; [2]University of Milano, Italy

Introduction and Definition

A feature of general pain in muscles and tendons (fibromyalgia) has been earlier described by the Greek physician Theophrastus (from 372 BC to 287 BC) (Higgs, 2018). The physician Guillaume de Baillou (1734) published the very first medical description of a fibromyalgia syndrome (FMS)-like muscular pain in 1592. At the end of the 19th century, the first pathophysiological and psychological approaches emerged with the concepts of fibrositis and psychosomatic rheumatism. The controversies on the definition and classification of FMS are not finished yet. "Fibromyalgia" was listed in the International Classification of Diseases (ICD) of the World Health Organization since 1994 in the chapter of the diseases of the musculoskeletal system and connective tissue as a rheumatic disease. Several psychosocial health care professionals avoid the diagnostic label "fibromyalgia" and prefer diagnostic labels such as "somatoform pain disorder" or "somatic symptom disorder". It is important to note that not all patients with fibromyalgia meet the criteria of somatoform pain disorder (Häuser & Henningsen, 2014) or of a somatic symptom disorder (Häuser et al., 2020).

A working group of the International Association of the Study of Pain succeeded to classify FMS as a pain disorder. In the most recent version of the ICD (ICD-11) (Nicholas et al., 2019), FMS is listed in the chapter "Symptoms, signs or clinical findings, not elsewhere classified", as an inclusion term under Chronic primary pain > Chronic widespread pain (CWP). FMS is a form of CWP which is defined as pain in at least four of five body regions (in at least three or four body quadrants), and is associated with sleep disorders, cognitive dysfunction, and somatic symptoms. The symptoms have been present at a similar level for at least three months and are not better accounted for by another diagnosis (Nicholas et al., 2019). However, a pain-centered view on the polysymptomatic clinical picture of patients diagnosed with FMS is too narrow (Häuser et al., 2019).

Epidemiology

The population prevalence in the general population is approximately 2% (Häuser et al., 2015). The prevalence increases with age. However, children and adolescents can be

DOI: 10.4324/9781003449126-58

affected by FMS. In clinical settings, FMS is more frequently diagnosed in women with a gender ration of 8 to 10:1. It is likely underdiagnosed in men (Häuser et al., 2015).

Clinical Symptoms and Signs

The main symptoms of FMS (required for diagnosis) are CWP in muscles and tendons, unrefreshed sleep, and cognitive problems such as concentrations problems and memory problems. Nearly all patients report other somatic symptoms of the gastrointestinal, urogenital, and cardiovascular tract. Many patients meet the criteria of so-called functional syndromes such as irritable bowel syndrome, functional dyspepsia, or painful bladder syndrome. Most patients report other psychological symptoms, especially of anxiety and depression. About 60–80% meet the criteria of a mental disorder (anxiety and/or depressive disorder) (Häuser et al., 2015). Tenderness of muscles and tendons at palpation is a typical sign of FMS. Based on the amount of somatic and psychological symptom load and associated disability in daily functioning, slight, moderate, and severe forms of FMS can be differentiated. The severity of FMS is determined by somatic and psychiatric comorbidities (Häuser et al., 2015).

Diagnostic Criteria

There is no gold standard for the clinical diagnosis. Different diagnostic criteria have been published over the years. Since 2010, the modified American College of Rheumatology diagnostic criteria of 2011 (Wolfe et al., 2011) and 2016 criteria (Wolfe et al., 2016) have been used in clinical studies.

According to clinical guidelines on the management of FMS, the diagnosis is established as follows:

a Full medical history taking to capture the three main symptoms
b Complete physical examination to assess signs of diseases which might cause or contribute to muscle pain and fatigue
c Basic laboratory tests to screen for other disease leading to widespread pain and fatigue.

In younger persons with no relevant somatic comorbidity, the diagnosis is easy. The diagnosis is more difficult in older people with multiple somatic comorbidities. There can be a combination of osteoarthritis or inflammatory rheumatic disease pain with FMS (Häuser et al., 2017).

Etiology and Pathophysiology

A model of interacting biological and psychosocial variables in the predisposition, triggering, and development of the chronicity of fibromyalgia symptoms has been suggested (Üçeyler et al., 2017). Inflammatory rheumatoid arthritis, depression, genetics, obesity combined with physical inactivity, physical and sexual abuse in childhood, and sleep problems predict future development of FMS. Psychosocial stress (e.g., working place and family conflicts) and physical stress (e.g., infections, surgery, accidents) might trigger the onset of CWP and fatigue. Depression and post-traumatic stress disorder worsen fibromyalgia symptoms (Üçeyler et al. 2017).

Several factors are associated with the pathophysiology of FMS. The functional changes include alteration of sensory processing in the brain (so-called central sensitization), reduced reactivity of the hypothalamus-pituitary-adrenal axis to stress, increased pro-inflammatory and reduced anti-inflammatory cytokine profiles (produced by cells involved in inflammation), disturbances in neurotransmitters such as dopamine and serotonin, and small nerve fiber pathology (Üçeyler et al., 2017).

Traumatic Life Events, PTSD, and FMS

Ortiz (2019) investigated physical abuse during childhood in 111 women with FMS compared with those without a history of childhood abuse. The study demonstrated a clinically modest, yet statistically significant, association with increased tenderness as measured by pain pressure thresholds and tender points, showing that experience of child abuse is associated with FMS symptom severity.

Häuser et al. (2013) evaluated the incidence of PTSD in a population of 395 consecutive FMS patients. Results showed 45.3% of FMS patients presented with PTSD symptoms and signs as compared with 3% only in the healthy controls. In more than 2/3 of the cases, adverse events antedated the onset of FMS; in less than 1/3 of the cases, these events followed the onset of FMS, with adverse events occurring in the same year of FMS in 4% of the cases.

A recent study by Nardi et al. (2020) confirmed the high prevalence of PTSD in FMS patients estimated at approximately 56%. Some FMS patients seem to have a dysregulation of the stress response capacity, with endocrine and sympathetic hyporeactivity (Üçeyler et al., 2017). FMS patients may have an increased hyperalgesic response different from the healthy control group. The FMS patients might have a distinctive hypothalamic–pituitary–adrenocortical dysfunction pattern that is different from other psychiatric disorders and control subjects (López-López et al., 2021).

A common hypothesis states that trauma and major life stressful events are not likely to cause FMS or PTSD but, in genetically susceptible people, early life events, besides acute or prolonged traumatic stress in adulthood, may affect the brain modulatory circuitries of both pain and emotions responsible for the enhanced pain responses and co-occurring symptoms that are reported by patients with FMS and PTSD (Häuser et al., 2013).

Nociplastic pain is the semantic term suggested by the international community of pain researchers to describe a third category of pain that is mechanistically distinct from nociceptive pain, which is caused by ongoing inflammation and damage of tissues, and neuropathic pain, which is caused by nerve damage. The mechanisms that underlie this type of pain are not entirely understood, but it is thought that augmented CNS pain and sensory processing and altered pain modulation play prominent roles. FMS is regarded to be a prototype of a pain condition with predominant nociplastic pain mechanisms (Fitzcharles et al., 2021). There is some evidence from basic research findings that traumatic stress can lead by glia activation to slight neuroinflammation and can thus contribute to central hypersensitivity (Nijs et al., 2017).

Treatment

General Principles of Treatment

These include education, pharmacological treatment, physical exercise, and psychological treatments, mainly cognitive-behavioral including acceptance-based therapies (Macfarlane et al., 2017). A tailored approach adapted to the severity of the main disabling symptoms and of disability and to comorbidities of patients has been recommended (Häuser et al., 2018; Macfarlane et al., 2017). Multimodal and multidisciplinary approaches for severe forms of FMS have been widely advocated (De Benedittis, 2016; De Benedittis, 2018; Macfarlane et al., 2017; Petzke et al., 2017).

The Importance of Psychological Therapies

Because of the importance of psychological factors in most (not all) FMS-patients, psychological therapies should be offered to the majority of patients. The German guideline recommends psychological therapies for these clinical constellations (Köllner et al., 2017):

- Maladaptive disease management (e.g., catastrophizing, inappropriate physical avoidance behavior, or dysfunctional perseverance) and/or
- Relevant modulation of the symptoms due to stress of daily life and/or interpersonal problems and/or
- Comorbid mental disorders.

The Importance of Hypnosis in FMS Guidelines

Hypnosis/guided imagery has received a weak recommendation by the German and Israeli guidelines, but not by the Canadian guidelines (Ablin et al., 2013). The European League Against Rheumatism gave a weak recommendation (Macfarlane, 2017). The strength of recommendation is based on the balance between desirable and undesirable effects, confidence in the magnitude of effects, and resource use. A strong recommendation implies that, if presented with the evidence, all or almost all informed persons would make the recommendation for or against the therapy, while a weak recommendation would imply that most people would, although a substantial minority would not.

The Role of Hypnosis in FMS

Current State of Evidence-Based Medicine

Hypnosis used alone, as well as in combination with other treatments, has been shown to be effective in the control of chronic pain of various origins (De Benedittis, 2016; De Benedittis, 2018; Miró et al., 2016; Milling et al., 2021).

Zech et al. (2017) reported a systematic review aimed at evaluating the efficacy, acceptability, and safety of guided imagery/hypnosis (GI/H) for fibromyalgia. Randomized controlled trials (RCTs) comparing GI/H with controls were analyzed. Primary outcomes were ≥50% pain relief, ≥20% improvement of health-related quality of life, psychological distress, disability, acceptability, and safety at end of therapy and three-month follow-up. Seven RCTs with 387 subjects were included into a comparison of GI/H versus controls. There was a clinically relevant benefit of GI/H compared to controls on ≥50% pain relief and psychological distress at the end of therapy. Acceptability at the end of treatment for GI/H was not significantly different from the control. Two RCTs with 95 subjects were included in the comparison of hypnosis combined with cognitive behavioral therapy (CBT) versus CBT alone. Combined therapy was superior to CBT alone in reducing psychological distress at the end of therapy. No study reported on safety. The methodological quality of most studies was poor as some details required for calculation of the risk of bias and treatment quality scores were not reported.

Recently, Aravena et al. (2020) evaluated the effectiveness of audio-recorded hypnosis in ameliorating fibromyalgia symptoms in 95 FMS patients. Both groups maintained their standard pharmacological treatment and continued their usual physical or psychological activities. The experimental group received an audio-recorded hypnosis intervention in the first session; subsequently, they received another audio hypnosis session to use for daily practice for a month. They found that the self-administered audio-recorded hypnotic intervention significantly decreased the intensity and interference of pain and fatigue, as well as the depressive symptomatology, providing an effective, practical, and economical alternative for reducing fibromyalgia-related symptoms.

Hypnosis and Hypnotherapy for FMS

Hypnosis for FMS can be used as symptom-oriented hypnosis aiming to reduce symptoms (pain, fatigue, sleep problems, anxiety, depression) and as hypnotherapy aiming to resolve emotional conflicts and/or unresolved traumata associated with FMS. The variety of hypnosis and hypnotherapy is reflected by the methods of the studies included in the systematic review of Zech et al. (2017): Two studies offered individually tailored (Ericksonian) and one study used a traditional approach with a standardized protocol. Two studies used non-pain-related (e.g., relaxation, ego-strengthening, feelings of security, improvement of sleep, stress management) and pain-related (e.g., pain control, pain acceptance) suggestions. One study focused on the solution of intrapsychic (emotional) conflicts.

Audio files with symptom-oriented hypnosis can be used by patients for daily practice. Some fee paying and not scientifically tested audio files with hypnosis for FMS are available. Hypnosis via audio files can be combined with aerobic exercise or movement therapies (e.g., Yoga, Tai-Chi) into a self-management program. Self-management of patients is strongly recommended by FMS guidelines (Macfarlane et. al, 2017; Petzke et al., 2017).

Hypnotherapy can be combined with other psychotherapeutic methods, e.g., acceptance-based CBTs to improve coping with pain or with CBTs or psychodynamic therapies in the therapy of comorbid mental disorders such as depressive disorder or PTSD.

Clinical Illustrations

Here are some suggestions from the audio file, *Healing Room*, of one of the authors (Häuser, 2003):

> (After induction and deepening of the hypnotic state): "You now open another door. You have now arrived in your actual healing room. A pleasant temperature immediately surrounds you. You feel a pleasant temperature enveloping you and further loosening your muscles and tendons. If you wish, you can also hear pleasant sounds that touch your ears only lightly and gently, only gentle soothing sounds soothing … . only hear what does good … . If it stimulates you pleasantly, you can feel a delicate pleasant fragrance in the nose, you can smell it now. There are scents that trigger a feeling of well-being … .

In this room is everything you need now. In this room there is also a special tub, where you can lie down and a resting bed, where you can rest after a pleasant bath. You will first look around the room with pleasure and let the temperature, the sounds and the smells gently caress you … .

Now you can go to the tub, which is already filled with a pleasant temperature water. Perhaps, in addition to the pleasant temperature, which you will first feel on your ankles and legs when you get into the tub now, you will notice a pleasant scent of an essence rising from the water. It smells so good. You now sit down in the tub and feel how pleasantly the water now surrounds your pelvis. You let yourself slide a little further into the tub and feel the water on your back, shoulders and neck. The water loosens and cleanses, everything falls away from you that you want to let go of…. This is a good thing.

You don't have to do anything, you don't have to perform anything, you don't have to think anything, you can just feel good. It's okay to allow yourself and your muscles and internal organs this rest and recovery so that their muscles and tendons loosen up and feel smooth".

Hypnotherapy Protocol for Fibromyalgia Patients

FMS patients usually receive one weekly hypnotic session for the first three months, with two monthly sessions for the next three months; about 14 sessions in all. Patients are instructed to practice self-hypnosis twice daily (approximately 20 minutes per session).

As far as hypnotic procedures are concerned, following standard trance induction by eye fixation, deepening of hypnosis is achieved with suggestions for multisensory imagery and progressive relaxation. Subsequently, indirect (Ericksonian) suggestions are given as target suggestions for cognitive modulation of pain in an individualized form. These include (De Benedittis, 2016): (1) dissociation ("Pain does not belong to you"); (2) imagining swimming in a magic swimming pool; (3) respiratory pacing (slow breathing, shown to be effective in reducing pain); (4) age progression (projecting to a pain-free future); and (5) partial posthypnotic amnesia for the pain experience.

Some other, rather innovative hypnotherapeutic methods have been used in selected cases. Algovisual synaesthesia (De Benedittis, 2001) has been successfully applied to patients with FMS. The rationale is to cognitively modulate pain by multisensory cross talk. In one case, the patient with FMS was asked, during trance, to associate her pain experience with a color. The starting color was pink. Subsequently, the patient was asked to associate another color with the experience of well-being. In this case, the ending color was a white, marble color. In the following hypnotic session, suggestions were given to trance-form the starting pink-rose color into the ending white-marble color, thereby resulting in significant pain relief without even mentioning the term pain. In another case, a patient was asked to trance-form the starting deep-blue color, associated with pain, into the ending sky-blue color, associated with the sense of well-being, resulting in significant pain relief.

Finally, in selected cases of highly hypnotizable subjects with a clear history of abuse and PTSD, hypnoanalytical treatment has been successful. Unconscious trauma and conflicts were unveiled by age regression and worked through. This eventually led to (almost complete) symptom resolution.

Case Example

The patient was a 48-year-old woman who presented with a complaint of widespread, severe, disabling pain lasting for 15 years. The pain, described as burning, and pins and pricks, increased substantially in the last four years.

On examination, she showed abnormal myofascial tenderness conforming to the distribution outlined in the 1990 American College of Rheumatology criteria for the diagnosis of FMS.

The patient had received multiple pharmacological treatments over many years and was currently taking nonsteroidal anti-inflammatory drugs which were ineffective.

Imaging studies of the spine and brain showed no structural pathology and neurophysiologic investigations, including needle EMG, did not show any evidence of radiculopathy, compressive mononeuropathy, or myopathic conditions. Her Visual Analog Scale scored 9/10. She also complained of chronic fatigue syndrome, cognitive impairment (fibrofog), and reported sleep problems that she attributed to her pain. Psychopathological patterns (MMPI) revealed high scores on Hypochondriasis and Depression scales. The WHOQOL-100 questionnaire of the HRQoL (Health-Related Quality of Life) showed very poor self-evaluation.

Relevant history. Her father died when she was 17 years old. Her brother died at the age of 3. When she was born a few months later, she received the name of her dead brother. After school, she became sales director in a women's fashion store, but became unable to work because of her painful disease. She described her life as emotionally poor with very few affective relationships. The patient reported multiple adverse life events in terms of active, physical, and emotional abuse at the age of 19, 36, and 41 years old, respectively.

A multimodal approach, including combined hypnosis + self-hypnosis + drug treatment (i.e., amitriptyline, 100 mg/day), was adopted. The patient received one weekly hypnotic session + self-hypnosis twice/day (20 minutes). Hypnotic approach was used to cognitively modulate pain and to address and work-through traumatic memories.

In the short run, hypnosis + self-hypnosis acted synergistically with medications. In the long run, the patient developed and enhanced hypnotic skills and pain self-control, while progressively tapering off medications.

Hypnotic strategies included cautious exploration of traumatic memories by age regression, followed by abreaction and carefully controlled flow of the material into awareness. This process was associated with a great deal of emotional relief. The end-result of the hypnotherapeutic treatment was the emergence of a new identity of the self.

Long-term clinical results (at one-year follow-up) showed 90% pain relief, significant reduction of hyperpathia and chronic fatigue, reduction of medication, and remarkable improvement of the Quality of Life.

Safety Profile and Contraindications

The safety profile of hypnotic treatment for FMS is excellent, with the absence of significant side effects. There are no absolute or relative contraindications, but it should be taken into consideration that very often these are "difficult" and demanding patients, for whom hypnotic treatment requires specific skills and prolonged time (De Benedittis, 2018).

Future Orientation

Gut-directed hypnosis (standardized protocol with disease-specific suggestions, high-quality-controlled studies, recommendations by evidence-based guidelines of medical associations) (Vasant & Whorwell, 2019) shows the way to improve the role of hypnosis in the management of FMS. The recommendations of a task force of six major hypnosis organizations for establishing efficacy standards for clinical hypnosis should be followed (Kekecs et al., 2022).

Implications for Training and Professional Development

Curricula (training programs) for pain psychotherapists should include hypnosis for acute and chronic pain in general and for defined diseases such as FMS in particular.

References

Ablin, J., Fitzcharles, M.-A., Buskila, D., Shir, Y., Sommer, C., & Häuser, W. (2013). Treatment of fibromyalgia syndrome: Recommendations of recent evidence-based interdisciplinary guidelines with special emphasis on complementary and alternative therapies. *Evidence-Based Complementary and Alternative Medicine: ECAM, 2013*, 485272. 10.1155/2013/485272

Aravena, V., García, F. E., Téllez, A., & Arias, P. R. (2020). Hypnotic intervention in people with fibromyalgia: A randomized controlled trial. *American Journal of Clinical Hypnosis*, *63*(1), 49–61. 10.1080/00029157.2020.1742088

Baillou, G. (1734). *Opera omnia medica*. Angelum Jeremiam.

De Benedittis, G. (2001). The revolving doors of pain: Hypnotic synesthesia for modulation of the pain experience. In C. Loriedo & B. Peter (Eds.), *The new hypnosis – The utilization of personal resources in Ericksonian practice and training (Proceedings of the 3rd European Congress of Ericksonian Hypnosis and Psychotherapy, 1998 in Venice, Italy* (Hypnosis international monographs (HIM) (Vol. 5., pp. 33–48). M.E.G. Stiftung.

De Benedittis, G. (2016). Hypnosis and fibromyalgia. In G. R. Elkins (Ed.), *Handbook of medical and psychological hypnosis: Foundations, applications, and professional issues* (1st ed., pp. 235–244). Springer Publishing Company.

De Benedittis, G. (2018). Hypnotherapy for fibromyalgia. In M. P. Jensen (Ed.) *Hypnotic techniques for chronic pain management: Favorite methods of master clinicians* (pp. 54–75). Denny Creek Press.

Fitzcharles, M. A., Cohen, S. P., Clauw, D. J., Littlejohn, G., Usui, C., & Häuser, W. (2021). Nociplastic pain: Towards an understanding of prevalent pain conditions. *The Lancet*, *397*(10289), 2098–2110. 10.1016/s0140-6736(21)00392-5

Häuser, W. (2003). *Fibromyalgia. Active pain control*. Hypnos Publishers.

Häuser, W., Galek, A., Erbslöh-Möller, B., Köllner, V., Kühn-Becker, H., Langhorst, J., Petermann, F., Prothmann, U., Winkelmann, A., Schmutzer, G., Brähler, E., & Glaesmer, H. (2013). Posttraumatic stress disorder in fibromyalgia syndrome: Prevalence, temporal relationship between posttraumatic stress and fibromyalgia symptoms, and impact on clinical outcome. *Pain*, *154*(8), 1216–1223. 10.1016/j.pain.2013.03.034

Häuser, W., & Henningsen, P. (2014). Fibromyalgia syndrome: A somatoform disorder? *European Journal of Pain*, *18*(8), 1052–1059. 10.1002/j.1532-2149.2014.00453.x

Häuser, W., Ablin, J., Fitzcharles, M.-A., Littlejohn, G., Luciano, J. V., Usui, C., & Walitt, B. (2015). Fibromyalgia. *Nature Reviews Disease Primers*, *1*(1), 15022. 10.1038/nrdp.2015.22

Häuser, W., Ablin, J., Perrot, S., & Fitzcharles, M. A. (2017). Management of fibromyalgia: Practical guides from recent evidence-based guidelines. *Polish Archives of Internal Medicine*, *127*(1), 47–56. 10.20452/pamw.3877

Häuser, W., Perrot, S., Clauw, D. J., & Fitzcharles, M. A. (2018). Unravelling fibromyalgia – Steps toward individualized management. *Journal of Pain*, *19*(2), 125–134. 10.1016/j.jpain.2017.08.009

Häuser, W., Clauw, D., & Fitzcharles, M. A. (2019). Fibromyalgia as a chronic primary pain syndrome: Issues to discuss. *Pain*, *160*(11), 2651–2652. 10.1097/j.pain.0000000000001686

Häuser, W., Hausteiner-Wiehle, C., Henningsen, P., Brähler, E., Schmalbach, B., & Wolfe, F. (2020). Prevalence and overlap of somatic symptom disorder, bodily distress syndrome and fibromyalgia syndrome in the German general population: A cross sectional study. *Journal of Psychosomatic Research*, *133*, 110111. 10.1016/j.jpsychores.2020.110111

Higgs, J. B. (2018). Fibromyalgia in primary care. *Primary Care: Clinics in Office Practice*, *45*(2), 325–341. 10.1016/j.pop.2018.02.008

Kekecs, Z., Moss, D., Elkins, G., De Benedittis, G., Palsson, O. S., Shenefelt, P. D., Terhune, D. B., Varga, K., & Whorwell, P. J. (2022). Guidelines for the assessment of efficacy of clinical hypnosis applications. *International Journal of Clinical and Experimental Hypnosis*, *70*(2), 104–122. 10.1080/00207144.2022.2049446

Köllner, V., Bernardy, K., Greiner, W., Krumbein, L., Lucius, H., Offenbächer, M., Sarholz, M., Settan, M., & Häuser, W. (2017). Psychotherapie und psychologische Verfahren beim Fibromyalgiesyndrom [Psychotherapy and psychological procedures for fibromyalgia syndrome: Updated guidelines 2017 and overview of systematic review articles]. *Der Schmerz*, *31*(3), 266–273. 10.1007/s00482-017-0204-3

López-López, A., Matías-Pompa, B., Fernández-Carnero, J., Gil-Martínez, A., Alonso-Fernández, M., Alonso Pérez, J. L., & González Gutierrez, J. L. (2021). Blunted pain modulation response to induced stress in women with fibromyalgia with and without posttraumatic stress disorder comorbidity: New evidence of hypo-reactivity to stress in fibromyalgia? *Behavioral Medicine*, *47*(4), 311–323. 10.1080/08964289.2020.1758611

Macfarlane, G. J., Kronisch, C., Dean, L. E., Atzeni, F., Häuser, W., Fluß, E., Choy, E., Kosek, E., Amris, K., Branco, J., Dincer, F., Leino-Arjas, P., Longley, K., McCarthy, G. M., Makri, S., Perrot, S., Sarzi-Puttini, P., Taylor, A., & Jones, G. T. (2017). EULAR revised recommendations for the management of fibromyalgia. *Annals of the Rheumatic Diseases*, *76*(2), 318–328. 10.1136/annrheumdis-2016-209724

Milling, L. S., Valentine, K. E., LoStimolo, L. M., Nett, A. M., & McCarley, H. S. (2021). Hypnosis and the alleviation of clinical pain: A comprehensive meta-analysis. *International Journal of Clinical and Experimental Hypnosis*, *69*(3), 297–322. 10.1080/00207144.2021.1920330

Miró, J., Castarlenas, E., De La Vega, R., Roy, R., Solé, E., Tomé-Pires, C., & Jensen, M. (2016). Psychological neuromodulatory treatments for young people with chronic pain. *Children*, *3*(4), 41. 10.3390/children3040041

Nardi, A. E., Karam, E. G., & Carta, M. G. (2020). Fibromyalgia patients should always be screened for post-traumatic stress disorder. *Expert Review of Neurotherapeutics*, *20*(9), 891–893. 10.1080/14737175.2020.1794824

Nicholas, M., Vlaeyen, J. W. S., Rief, W., Barke, A., Aziz, Q., Benoliel, R., Cohen, M., Evers, S., Giamberardino, M. A., Göbel, A., Korwisi, B., Perrot, S., Svensson, P., Wang, S. J., Treede, R. D. (2019). The IASP Taskforce for the Classification of Chronic Pain. The IASP classification of chronic pain for ICD-11: Chronic primary pain. *Pain*, *160*(1), 28–37. 10.1097/j.pain.0000000000001390

Nijs, J., Loggia, M. L., Polli, A., Moens, M., Huysmans, E., Goudman, L., Meeus, M., Vanderweeën, L., Ickmans, K., & Clauw, D. (2017). Sleep disturbances and severe stress as glial activators: Key targets for treating central sensitization in chronic pain patients? *Expert Opinion on Therapeutic Targets*, *21*(8), 817–826. 10.1080/14728222.2017.1353603

Ortiz, R., Ballard, E. D., Machado-Vieira, R., Saligan, L. N., & Walitt, B. (2019). Quantifying the influence of child abuse history on the cardinal symptoms of fibromyalgia. *Clinical and Experimental Rheumatology*, *34*(2 Suppl 96), S59–S66.

Petzke, F., Brückle, W., Eidmann, U., Heldmann, P., Köllner, V., Kühn, T., Kühn-Becker, H., Strunk-Richter, M., Schiltenwolf, M., Settan, M., Von Wachter, M., Weigl, M., & Häuser, W. (2017). Allgemeine Behandlungsgrundsätze, Versorgungskoordination und Patientenschulung beim Fibromyalgiesyndrom [General treatment principles, coordination of care and patient education in fibromyalgia syndrome: Updated guidelines 2017 and overview of systematic review articles]. *Der Schmerz*, *31*(3), 246–254. 10.1007/s00482-017-0201-6

Üçeyler, N., Burgmer, M., Friedel, E., Greiner, W., Petzke, F., Sarholz, M., Schiltenwolf, M., Winkelmann, A., Sommer, C., & Häuser, W. (2017). Ätiologie und Pathophysiologie des

Fibromyalgiesyndroms [Etiology and pathophysiology of fibromyalgia syndrome: Updated guidelines 2017; Overview of systematic review articles and overview of studies on small fibre neuropathy in FMS subgroups]. *Der Schmerz*, *31*(3), 239–245. 10.1007/s00482-017-0202-5

Vasant, D. H., & Whorwell, P. J. (2019). Gut-focused hypnotherapy for functional gastrointestinal disorders: Evidence-base, practical aspects, and the Manchester Protocol. *Neurogastroenterology & Motility*, *31*(8), e13573. 10.1111/nmo.13573

Wolfe, F., Clauw, D. J., Fitzcharles, M. A., Goldenberg, D. L., Häuser, W., Katz, R. S., Mease, P., Russell, A. S., Russell, I. J., & Winfield, J. B. (2011). Fibromyalgia criteria and severity scales for clinical and epidemiological studies: A modification of the ACR preliminary diagnostic criteria for fibromyalgia. *Journal of Rheumatology*, *38*(6), 1113–1122. 10.3899/jrheum.100594

Wolfe, F., Clauw, D. J., Fitzcharles, M. A., Goldenberg, D. L., Häuser, W., Katz, R. L., Mease, P. J., Russell, A. S., Russell, I. J., & Walitt, B. (2016). 2016 Revisions to the 2010/2011 fibromyalgia diagnostic criteria. *Seminars in Arthritis and Rheumatism*, *46*(3), 319–329. 10.1016/j.semarthrit.2016.08.012

Zech, N., Hansen, E., Bernardy, K., & Häuser, W. (2017). Efficacy, acceptability and safety of guided imagery/hypnosis in fibromyalgia – A systematic review and meta-analysis of randomized controlled trials. *European Journal of Pain*, *21*(2), 217–227. 10.1002/ejp.933

45

A SUGGESTIVE PRESENCE DURING LABOR AND BIRTH

Sándor Bálint[1], *Balázs Bálint*[1], *Katalin H. Kondor*[1], *and Katalin Varga*[2,3]

[1]Gólyafészek Birthcenter, Budapest, Hungary; [2]Institute of Psychology, ELTE Eötvös Loránd University, Budapest, Hungary; [3]Hungarian Association of Hypnosis

You are a woman ... . You are a woman, like so many in the world.
Your task now is to have children ...
And you are perfect, you can do it, that is your special ability on Earth ...
Now you are the most important in the world ...
You send the message from the ancestors to the future ...,
now you are the most important ...

Sándor Bálint

Introduction

Hypnosis is used during the birth preparation process, facilitating the mother's attachment to the baby. It empowers women by means of self-affirmation and visualization, decreasing anxiety and allowing the mother to gain control. Formal hypnosis can effectively be used in cases of hyperemesis gravidum (McCormack, 2010), preventing preterm labor (Reinhard et al., 2009; Shah et al., 2011), and supporting external cephalic version procedure (Reinhard et al., 2012). Various techniques can be used for pain management, including hypnoanesthesia (Azizmohammadi & Azizmohammadi, 2019; Beebe, 2014; Catsaros & Wendland, 2020; Cyna et al., 2004). Its use can potentially reduce the need for synthetic oxytocin (Cyna et al., 2006) and potentially reduce complications (Catsaros & Wendland, 2020). Self-hypnosis can be used for emotional management and to reduce the fear of childbirth (Babbar & Oyarzabal, 2021; Finlayson et al., 2015) or the risk of developing post-partum depression (Guse et al., 2006). Various neonatal outcomes have proven to benefit from hypnosis (Khadem Rezaiyan et al., 2018).

In this chapter, we propose a "suggestive presence" model of hypnotic suggestions to assist labor and birth. We provide examples of the opportunities for therapeutic suggestion that affect the mother throughout pregnancy and during childbirth. Based on the authors' experience, we find that these openings for therapeutic suggestion are practical opportunities for clinicians to facilitate both the mother's and newborn baby's well-being.

 DOI: 10.4324/9781003449126-59

The authors, comprising two doctors, a midwife, and a psychologist, who have approximately 138 years of combined field experience in assisting birthing experiences, determined that the "suggestive presence" model may be the best approach to facilitate the natural labor and delivery processes. The main roles and responsibilities adopted by the professionals who use this approach worldwide are to support and facilitate the *naturally occurring* pain relief and to monitor emotion-regulating changes in the state of consciousness that occur during labor and birth. This allows the neurochemical mechanisms (e.g., central oxytocin, endorphins, and epinephrine) that have been evolving over millions of years, to be most beneficial (Buckley, 2015; Uvnäs-Moberg et al., 2020).

To this end, we prioritize (1) providing a suitably relaxing physical environment, (2) minimizing communication between those present at the birth, (3) ensuring that the mother's and baby's rest time is undisturbed during the intervals between contractions, and (4) focusing on the suggestive duration of the communication involved in the process, rather than on long, sophisticated suggestions. In other words, we pay critical attention to what we would usually say and do. For professionals, it is essential to:

1 **Recognize the altered state of consciousness or non-ordinary mental processing** (Facco et al., 2021; Farthing, 1992; Vaitl et al., 2005). Just as in many other situations, clinical observation shows that a woman enters a spontaneous trance, altered state of consciousness, state during pregnancy, labor, and delivery, and potentially in the post-partum period (Bierman, 1989; Orne, 1959). Thus, formal hypnosis induction is not needed, as the effect of suggestion is exerted without it. The spontaneous trance commonly involves changes in concentration, memory, perception, reality-orientation, emotional expression, time, and body sense (Ludwig, 1969). In these circumstances, according to the classical suggestive effect the suggestions are followed involuntarily (Weitzenhoffer, 1989). Instead of the "dominant" mode of consciousness (where logic, voluntary control, instructions, serial processing, rational judgments, and analytical thinking prevail), the characteristics of "alternative" mode are present: intuition, automaticity, holism, and modeling (Uneståhl, 1981). Several circumstances increase the likelihood of this trance state starting with the gynecological examination, when a sacred part of the body, that is usually hidden during most medical examinations, is brought to the fore (Hilden et al, 2003). Pregnancy and childbirth are emotional events in a woman's life and that of her family. The process, although physiologically natural, also involves significant physical changes. These are accompanied by the considerable physical demands of childbirth, sleep deprivation, and, in most cases, a strange and unfamiliar environment.

2 **To know how the altered mind works in the altered state of consciousness.** There are many phenomena of the trance state that can be frightening to the uninformed. However, trance can be useful in promoting a positive birth experience. These include diminished voluntary muscle activity, lethargy, muscle relaxation, changes in breathing patterns, catalepsy, amnesia, analgesia, anesthesia, feeling of detachment, selective awareness, dissociation, altered time perception (e.g., time distortion), and heightened susceptibility to suggestions without critical evaluation (i.e., trance logic) (Rossi & Cheek, 1988).

3 **Be familiar with the rules of suggestion formation** (Varga, 2013). Recent neuropsychological research shows the impact of negative suggestion on bodily functions. It is noteworthy that pain and pain-related words can activate the pain neuromatrix, emphasizing that our words may do harm (Corsi et al., 2019; Zech et al., 2019).

4 **Be able to build up and maintain an appropriate rapport** with the mother and her attendants, creating an atmosphere of trust that is a prerequisite for the natural neurochemical birthing process (Varga, 2022).
5 **Be self-aware of one's own involvement**, emotional vulnerability, and how this can be inadvertently and even negatively expressed. For example, during perinatal care, the care provider who is legally responsible for the care does everything possible to detect risks and reduce complications. In this way, the mother's and even father's attention is constantly drawn to the possible problems throughout pregnancy and during childbirth. If the personnel, such as the midwife, obstetrician, nurse, or family doctor, involved in the care, is inattentive to the way in which each communication is made, the mother's and father's stress level is likely to increase.

It has been elucidated that the suggestive or unconscious use of suggestion in care can have an impact on the fetus's development (fetal programming, see e.g., Stevenson et al., 2020). Thus, when communicating necessary information to – or in the presence of – the mother, attention to the prosody (volume, cadence, tone of voice, inflection) or the "music" of our language is imperative. The mother's perception of the communication affects her stress level. The maternal stress level will have an impact on the maturation of the fetal endocrine, immune, and nervous systems. These effects, in turn, may influence their regulatory processes even into adulthood (Coe & Lubach, 2008).

Supporting the *natural* childbirth process is important for many reasons. Pharmacological interventions (inducing or speeding up the birth or for pain management) prescribing the mother's body position, restricting her movements or voice, separating mother and baby right after the birth are all possible ways of diverting the process from its natural course. In the authors' opinion, it is likely that the technical obstetric practices of recent decades are among the many other causes that have led to infertility, affecting more than 70 million women globally. Currently, the use of hypnosis as a possible solution to infertility is gaining increasing interest (Casareno, 2016; James, 2009). Similarly, the inhibition of the unfolding of natural psycho-affective processes may be associated with post-partum depression, which has a prevalence of 10–40%, depending on definition and criteria (Bai et al., 2021). Hypnosis is also increasingly used in its treatment (Beevi et al., 2019; Sado et al., 2012; Yexley, 2007).

We are of the opinion that it is preferable to use hypno-suggestive techniques in the first place for *prevention*, thus mitigating side effects later.

Pregnancy

During pregnancy, sensitivity to suggestion increases. The trained obstetrician/midwife/nurse can utilize the natural "trance"/readiness of the woman to accept positive, helpful suggestions, making the interaction more effective. It is easier for the midwife or obstetric nurse to tune into the patient, empathizing with their concerns. The providers can even use the increased sensitivity to reassure the mother.

Also, during pregnancy, a woman experiences numerous bodily changes and undergoes a psychological maturation process. The developmental transition from young lady to woman and then to mother does not always take place until childbirth. These questions indicate the woman's uncertainty about her ability to cope. Notice the supportive, informative response of Doctor B, versus Doctor A:

Patient: Will I have enough milk, doctor? My mum said she had small breasts and was unable to breastfeed me ...

A. Doctor: Oh, you will see when the time comes ...

B. Doctor: There is no correlation between breast size and the amount of milk produced. Ninety-eight percent of women can breastfeed, only some of them have an anatomical problem. If nature has given you a child, it gives you milk. (The doctor provides positive factual information, that corrects grandmother's negative suggestion, skillfully providing encouragement and connecting the success of breastfeeding to pregnancy.)

Taking this into consideration, it makes sense to continuously communicate throughout the pregnancy. The findings should always be assessed; however, it is also important to confirm good results and, in the case of any discrepancies, to refer to the subsequent follow-up test as a safety factor: "Let's see how the hematoma is absorbed in two weeks' time." The suggestion also articulates the expected change (absorption), while making it clear that a control is needed. This brings the focus from "danger" to maternal competence and the naturalness of the birth. Studies have confirmed this assumption and daily practical experience shows that the positive suggestion of the doctor, whether expressed in words or deeds, has a strong and positive impact on the mother and thus during birth (Bálint et al., 2021; Martis et al., 2017).

Negative Suggestions

During pregnancy, women receive negative suggestion from many sources including friends, media, and medical personnel.

The following are a few common negative suggestions:

1 Childbirth is a painful process and there are no exceptions.
2 Childbirth is suffering, and a person that is suffering needs assistance.
3 Women want children but are afraid of giving birth.
4 Doctor: The woman's pelvis is below normal size ...
5 Physician: The cardiotocography curve looks good, nothing looks out of the ordinary, but the tests need to be repeated ...
6 Nurse: Ma'am the findings are fine, but you look very calm and this is concerning ...

The ultrasound examination results may increase the concern of mother already worried about her baby. A few examples of (otherwise professionally correct) ultrasound findings:

1 the fetus is alive but the gestational sac is small
2 a tiny bit more amniotic fluid
3 the placenta is calcified
4 the umbilical cord is nuchal
5 the placenta is low laying

These (and similar alarming formulations) are worth "interpreting," putting them into an appropriate positive suggestive framework, as average non-professional person may easily misinterpret them.

Messages from acquaintances or the internet:

During pregnancy, it is typical for mothers who are informed by acquaintances, relatives, or even by the social media posts, to be terrified of an upcoming examination because they have read or heard negative experiences. It takes major effort for the caregiver to help the mother accept that she is *another* person, unique, who is likely to react differently in such and such situation. And miraculously, this often happens!

Positive Suggestion

To counteract the countless negative suggestion heard for decades, let us repeatedly and with conviction convey the positive ones!

A woman's body is perfect and knows everything.

"*Just as your body is able to accept the baby and give it everything it needs to grow, so too your body is able to birth the baby.*" Here it is important to pay attention to the circumstances of conception, as the meaning is different if the baby was conceived with ease or with difficulty.

At each appointment (check-up, visit), the assessment of the tests according to the protocol for antenatal care should be included. It is very important to report back as many results as possible, that is, good results, for example:

These results are perfect; they indicate that everything is fine!

When there is a slight discrepancy in the lab result, but it is acceptable in pregnancy:

This value is indeed different compared to the lab limits, which are the average values for humans, in pregnancy this value is excellent, it indicates that everything is fine, the baby is feeling well, the mother's body is giving the baby everything it needs.

However, if the results reveal that supplements, such as iron, are indeed needed, we can convey it in the following manner:

This value is below the acceptable level for pregnancy, and that's fine, because it indicates that the mother's body is giving the baby everything that is needed. And we can supplement so that we have enough to feed both the mother and the baby.

It is also good for the professional to be aware of their self-suggestions, and *reframe* them (in italics) if necessary:

My oath is to always help in every situation. / *Sometimes it is better not to intervene.*

Childbirth hurts, so I must use the quickest and best method. / *What I see is not suffering. It is an unusually energetic process.*

Childbirth is a dangerous process, so I must prevent trouble. / *Birth and delivery are natural processes.*

The safety of the mother and her baby is ensured by constant monitoring. / *Safety lies in the wisdom of nature. Observing the face, voice and movements of the mother will guide what is needed for safety*

Loss

People who have experienced previous perinatal loss may be even more anxious than usual about interpreting natural signs. Again, notice the supportive, positive, and informative response from Doctor B:

Patient: *I have constant abdominal cramps, doctor. I have feelings like when I lost my baby... I get very scared. And then I have to sit down...*
A. Doctor: *It's nothing...*
B. Doctor: *You feel this tension all the time... ? Probably at night too...*
Patient: *No, not at night, and I did not have to take any antispasmodics.*
Doctor: *Great! The sensation you are experiencing could merely be the relaxation and tightening of your uterus.* (The doctor asks the woman to lie on the examination table. When the abdominal wall is examined externally, the uterus is completely soft and a good fetal heartbeat can be heard with the small ultrasound machine). *Now your uterus is relaxed. Let's see how your uterus behaves when it is stimulated.* (The doctor taps the abdominal wall very lightly with his fingertips. The uterus contracts in response to the stimulus and relaxes after a few seconds). *And soon the sensation of tensing appears...*
Patient: *Yes, that's it! That's what I feel!*
Doctor: *The uterus is a constantly growing organ. It contracts whenever it is stimulated. Just like a snail pulls in its horns when it is stimulated. This phenomenon is completely natural. The fact that your body is aware of this sensation is a good sign, which means you can sit down and relax.*

If the findings confirm a definitive undesirable condition (e.g., the fetus is not alive, or it has clearly suffered some kind of damage), the doctor must console the woman who might be in a state of shock or despair. This is not always easy.

The psychotherapeutic technique of crisis intervention is often confused with trivializing the event. It is a way of comforting a crying woman:

Doctor A.
- Do not cry, do not cry... Calm down... You'll have another baby ...

And they tell you statistics about the percentage of mothers who will have a baby ...

Doctor B.
Empathy, listening, offering assistance, may be provided by leaning in a little closer:
- Express your emotions, cry as long as you need to. The pain has to be released. You lost your baby. Now is the moment to say goodbye. Letting go of your baby is not an easy process and may take some time, but when the time comes you will be able to make peace with this situation, and as soon as your body says yes and opens up, you will feel it. You will not be alone on this healing journey: your partner, your family, and I will help you every step of the way, in every way we can.

As a way forward in the case of miscarriage, we can also point out that, although the miscarriage itself is not really a pleasure, we learn a lot about what works well for the two of you.

> *There are ovaries that are definitely functioning, there are mature eggs, there are permeable fallopian tubes, and there is a uterus that is capable of receiving them, and on the paternal side, there are definitely sperm that are capable of fertilization. These tests have practically been done by nature.*

These suggestions are always made according to the reactions of the woman and her partner (looks, gestures, facial expressions), pacing how much she/he takes in.

Delivery

In studies conducted by Michel Odent (Davies & Borland, 2015; Odent, 2012, 2017), it was found that pain during childbirth can be reduced or even eliminated if the woman gives birth in an environment free of strong stimuli such as noise, speech, and bright lights. According to Odent (2012, 2017), this environment allows for suppression of cortical function of the cerebrum, the woman is not thinking rationally, her inhibitions are removed, she feels safe, she directs her attention inward toward her body, and the primal reflexes take over. This is regulated by a combination of hormones and the fetus is born with the help of the "ejection reflex" (Davies & Borland, 2015; Odent, 2012, 2017).

Simkin in her model "Road Map of Labor" provides a great summary of how to recognize the coping style of a woman in labor (Simkin & Ancheta, 2011).

1 If a laboring woman is focused inwards on her body and is not distracted by the outside world, she will find her own rhythm. The natural state of arousal and pain during contractions can be greatly reduced by listening to rhythmic movement and sounds.
2 When a laboring mother demonstrates the following behaviors, it could be a sign of emotional dystocia: being excessively alert, asking a lot of questions, reacting violently to even the slightest contractions, nervousness, and/or distrust. In such cases, the laboring baby needs more help. Simkin (Simkin & Ancheta, 2011) recommends the use of the technique known as the three Rs (relaxation, rhythm, and ritual), which can help the mother achieve a sense of introversion, a feeling of security in a familiar (because repetitive) situation and the possibility of relaxation.

The following negative suggestions are also common during the birthing period:

> "Do not strain!"
> "Do not close your legs!"
> "If you do not push properly, you will never give birth!"

Instead, positive suggestions can be used to support the natural birthing process, in the mother's inwardly turning state, in which she is particularly susceptible to suggestion.

Below, we review the most important suggestion principles and rules, with an example, to illustrate their essence. Detailed explanations of the methods and further examples can be found elsewhere (Hammond, 1990; Varga, 2015).

1 Positivity – *"Let go... , relax... , release..."*
2 Repetition – *virtually any important message can and should be repeated as often as possible, either literally or in terms of content.*
3 Involuntariness – *"This is the time of rest, baby rests, mum rests... just let yourself relax."*
4 Motivation – *"As the head gets ahead, you feel more and more how you can help it..."*
5 Future orientation – *"It is birth day today! A year from now, there will be a candle on the cake..."*
6 Rhythm and pauses – we sit and do nothing, because everything is fine...
7 Doing, not trying – *"Let your body work! You can do it!"*
8 The illusion of alternatives – *"It is worth experiencing whether standing or squatting feels better..."*
9 Timing – *"Gradually the tension will go away..."*
10 Utilization – *"Big sigh at the end of the contraction, and as you exhale, your belly and your body relax..."*
11 Pacing-leading – *"Yes, it is very tight now... very uncomfortable... On the next contraction, it's worth pushing hard to get through this..."*
12 Reframing – *"Frequent contractions are a good sign, as they are an indication that your baby will be born sooner..."*

The way the midwife greets the woman expecting a breech baby can go a long way in alleviating negative expectations of such a birth:

> *Ma'am! I'm glad you came in. Your delivery is going well. I have spoken to your doctor, and I am very happy that you have decided to have your baby vaginally. Many people consider this a dangerous route for a breech position; however, we believe otherwise. Your doctor has delivered many babies with pelvic thrust and knows exactly what to do under these circumstances. And your baby knows as well...*

In the final stages of labor, it is often the case that when the baby's head presses against the perineum, the squeeze causes feces and urine to be passed. This often triggers social inhibition (it is not right, it is not appropriate) and the birth, which was going well up to that point, stops. Assistance and positive reassurance should immediately be given:

> *This is absolutely normal, these are natural human things, and this is not alien to us...*
> *This happens often.*
> *I can see the baby's head now, and soon you can hold it in your arms...*

There are situations during the course of a birth, when progress slows down. Sometimes the pushing-out period is prolonged, the uterine activity is slow, the mother is tired, and the fetus is showing signs of wanting to be born.

> Doctor A.
> *Ma'am, push because the baby is not feeling well. Everything depends on you! If you do not push properly, the baby will suffer!* No *and no, that's nothing! Now I'm have to use the vacuum to get the baby out!*

Doctor B.

You did a great job, but I can see you're a little tired. Your baby is anxious to meet you. I can see her head now. Let's help her together. Concentrate, and when the push comes, push, and I'll help you from underneath with a little suction. That way, in a few minutes, you'll be able to put your arms around her...

Involvement of a Professional

During the birth, the "birth couple" is more sensitive to the staffs' movement in the delivery room, and there is constant metacommunication monitoring on their part. Therefore, in addition to obstetric expertise, the ability of the doctor and midwife to control their own behavior and emotions is imperative.

The health professionals must learn to recognize that, although they do not know what to do yet, they are still considering various options, and their body is already giving them signals: dry mouth, change in tone of voice, blinking, heaving shoulders, uncontrolled muscle twitching. Inappropriate movements (running in and out of the delivery room) and uttering inappropriate sentences are very characteristic of staff and confusing or frightening to the birthing couple.

The doctor or midwife often projects their own anxiety, that may even reach the level of a reprimand: "*What an irresponsible person, why should such a person have a child...*" Of course, these are extreme examples, but the phrases have been uttered.

Fortunately, when the doctor notices the increase in tension and the metacommunication error in time and explains the steps to be taken in relation to the obstetric phenomenon everyone calms.

After Delivery

Examples of negative suggestions:

"You cannot breastfeed with small breasts, I couldn't either..."
"Stop breastfeeding because your teeth will become brittle."
"If you conceive while breastfeeding, stop because it will harm the new baby."

Examples of positive suggestions:

People who have not yet given birth and are not on birth control are mostly aware of hormonal changes in their bodies. They may also have uncomfortable breast sensations (e.g., tightness, tenderness). They seek medical help for the complaint. If there are no abnormalities on examination, this sentence may be uttered:

"Madam, your body is working perfectly and when the time comes, you will have just enough milk..."

Summary

Bohren and colleagues (2015) reviewed 65 publications from 34 countries. They looked at communication errors made by staff in maternity wards. The order of errors was as follows: physical, sexual, and verbal abuse. The latter were characterized by the frequent use of harsh, mocking, threatening, shouting, intimidating, humiliating, and insulting words. This tone was mostly preceded by an unfriendly reception and bad rapport. Disrespectful and unfriendly greetings were followed by unsupportive, judgmental, and impolite behavior. It was found that if there was a lack of attention and information (what is happening, what is expected, and what interventions are needed), fear and anxiety increased during the birth (i.e., the technical care was useless if there was no emotional support). It is therefore no coincidence that women who give birth consider it important to have helpers (husbands, partners, partners, or doulas) present during the birth, but in this case, the helpers are there to protect rather than to share in the fulfilling experience of the birth (Bohren et al., 2015).

When a woman who gives birth feels safe, she is able to relax, to direct her attention inward, to disconnect from the outside world, and to allow her body to function in a state of altered consciousness, in its own rhythm and in hormonal harmony (oxytocin, endorphin, and adrenaline).

According to Simkin and Ancheta (2011), this happens:

1 When the woman in labor receives the appropriate attention and respect,
2 When she can remain active and mobile,
3 If she can maintain her upright position,
4 If her pain is adequately managed,
5 If a caring partner is present.

Childbirth is a natural process and intervention is only necessary when it is needed. But *being present* is always important. Accompanying a birth, or a stage of it, consists of nothing more than the presence of the attendants (doctor, midwife, doula, father, etc.). Although they do not assist in the actual birthing process, it is important that they are with the mother to convey the suggestion that everything is fine because there is no need to intervene.

Starting during pregnancy, it is worth emphasizing through positive suggestion that it is not a task to be learned, but about experiencing the body's good and pleasant sensations in the present, because:

> *When you go into labor, your body will know what to do, be proud of this wonderful knowledge, you will not be alone, you will have helpers, accept that it is a woman's job.*

In a study conducted by Graziottin (2010), the doctor–patient relationship was investigated by means of the placebo-nocebo effect, using neurobiological and brain imaging tools. He found that the favorable and unfavorable reactions elicited in the patient by the doctor's behavior, that is, the use of all his communication channels, act through the same system (dopamine-serotonin opiate and adrenergic) but in opposite ways. Namely, the placebo (I will help) and nocebo (I will harm) effects cannot be separated (Graziottin, 2010).

Failure to recognize or incorrectly manage the natural trance state associated with childbirth can have a number of negative consequences. Physiological processes are reversed when a woman is overcome by fear and anxiety (Uvnäs-Moberg et al., 2005). This physical and mental state is closely related to any traumas suffered in the past, the memory, or even the reliving of the memory which may intrude on the birth process.

In obstetrical and midwifery practice, all channels of communication are important. An altered state of consciousness makes the natural course of childbirth more vulnerable if the mother is subjected to negative suggestion or if the process turns into a negative trance. However, it is precisely this that gives us the opportunity to support her through appropriate communication. The use of all types of suggestion, or a combination of them, improves obstetric outcomes (Bálint, 2014).

These unconventional processes do not leave the professional untouched. In order to release their own tensions, they can use self-awareness (Who am I? Where do I belong? Where are my limits? Do I need to know everything? etc.). Relaxation training is also useful.

Case Vignette

The description of the situation will be followed by *analysis, comments, and applied techniques.*

I (KK, midwife) once arrived at the delivery room for night duty. The doctor on duty, my daytime colleague, and the cleaning lady were sitting in the midwife's chair like a beaten army. Finally, I had arrived, they said, I should do something with the laboring mother in the delivery room because they had tried everything.

The exhaustion and unimaginativeness of colleagues can add weight to an already heavy situation. The "invitation" is public, so the effectiveness of the current intervention will be too.

These circumstances may be inspiring for some (while others may be rather off-putting).

The mother was standing in the shower next to the delivery room, and kept screaming that she could not take it anymore.

The signs of negative trance were obvious. The typical reaction to this usually: Do not waste your energy shouting! You will be exhausted!

She was young, 21 years old, carrying her first baby. Such young mothers are rare nowadays. She had several piercings and tattoos on her body. Her partner was in the shower with her, but she was obviously desperate. I got the impression that this baby was not planned, and their relationship was not that long ago.

Based on the description, the midwife's first impression of the woman or couple was not very positive. Moreover, it seems that she could not find a real partner in the father at that moment.

She was fighting the contractions with all her strength, trying to escape the situation. She had been in labor and in the delivery room since the morning, her cervix was dilated around three fingers (6 cm).

The mother did not accept the situation, she avoided it. The process, which lasted for hours, produced hardly any results in dilation.

I introduced myself, and the next moment, a strong contraction made her whole body tense up, and I watched a contraction with yelling.

The introduction is a key factor for the acceptance of the raport.

The midwife is initially a passive observer of the situation.

I complimented her on how well she was doing. At the next contraction, I encouraged her to make an even stronger and more powerful sound. "Let the whole delivery room know when her uterus was working and when her baby was moving out."

The key to the solution is not to 'dissuade' the woman from shouting, but to accept and even reinforce it (paradoxical suggestion, the first element of 'pacing').

Unlike before, the woman giving birth hears regarding her shouting a different meaning (reframing): it is a sign, a message of the natural process of childbirth, and within it, the work of the uterus. It links this to the expected goal: the coming of the baby (positivity, future orientation).

We did this through several contractions, and then I asked her to notice when her tummy was soft, when her uterus was resting, so that she could rest too.

The rhythmical functioning of the uterus is brought into focus. This is done by anticipating the possibility of "rest" (motivation), since a mother who has been in labor since the morning is obviously extremely exhausted.

I asked her to signal this to me by inhaling very slowly and exhaling even slower.

The midwife asks for a signal (reinforcement of the **rapport***) and gives a task that physiologically supports the* **goal** *to be achieved – relaxation, reduction of agitation (i.e., slow breathing).*

In the beginning, she could not relax between contractions, she would scream the usual "I cannot take it anymore" at the top of her lungs. I asked her to watch when the contractions came because I needed to know when they occurred, I needed her to help me. "You are only allowed to shout during contractions, at that time as much as you can."

Despite the apparent failure – that is, not being able to relax – the strategy continued.

In Hungarian, a contraction is called pain. I wanted her to shout, but not use the word for contraction. I was using the permission to shout as repeated **pacing**, but now I was **leading** her experience.

For another 15 minutes I had to dictate the rhythm of "Now we take rest, now we shout," and then the shouting was gradually replaced by slow exhalation and then involuntary pressure.

*By "dictating" along the established rapport, the midwife takes control: the "pacing-leading" elements come into play here. The plural first person (we) formulation of "resting, shouting" already reflects the joint activity (***rapport** *maintenance, cooperation).*

Her body was no longer tense. Two hours later, she gave birth to her son without a sound.

The practitioner does not expect immediate quick results (principle of successive approximation), slow breathing, relaxation, and attunement to the natural rhythm of the birth are slowly introduced.

Conclusion

In our experience, there is increased responsiveness to suggestion during pregnancy, labor, birth, and the postpartum period. It is amazing how finely tuned the physiological, endocrine, psychological, affective, and social processes are in the mother and the baby. Each knows their part in the activity of birthing. The suggestive presence of a professional is a major contribution to support the unfolding natural processes.

References

Azizmohammadi, S., & Azizmohammadi, S. (2019). Hypnotherapy in management of delivery pain: A review. *European Journal of Translational Myology*, *29*(3), 210–217. 10.4081/ejtm.2019.8365

Babbar, S., & Oyarzabal, A. J. (2021). The application of hypnosis in obstetrics. *Clinical Obstetrics and Gynecology*, *64*(3), 635–647. 10.1097/grf.0000000000000635

Bai, X., Song, Z., Zhou, Y., Wang, X., Wang, Y., & Zhang, D. (2021). Bibliometrics and visual analysis of the research status and trends of postpartum depression from 2000 to 2020. *Frontiers in Psychology*, 12, 665181. 10.3389/fpsyg.2021.665181

Bálint, B. (2014). *A szülés körüli és alatti szuggesztiók, ezek háttere és eredménye a mindennapi gyakorlatban. {The background and outcome of suggestions around and during childbirth in everyday practice}* [Presentation]. XXIII National Scientific Assembly of the Hungarian Psychological Society, 15-17 May 2014, Târgu Mures, Romania.

Bálint, S., Bálint, B., H. Kondor, K. (2021). Szuggesztív kommunikáció a szülészetbenn. {The use of suggestions in obstetrics}. In. Varga, K. (ed), *A szülési Fájdalom kezelése.* {The management of obstetric pain.} (pp. 311–336). Budapest: Medicina.

Beebe, K. R. (2014). Hypnotherapy for labor and birth. *Nursing for Women's Health*, *18*(1), 48–59. 10.1111/1751-486x.12093

Beevi, Z., Low, W. Y., & Hassan, J. (2019). The effectiveness of hypnosis intervention in alleviating postpartum psychological symptoms. *American Journal of Clinical Hypnosis*, *61*(4), 409–425. 10.1080/00029157.2018.1538870

Bierman, S. F. (1989). Hypnosis in the emergency department. *American Journal of Emergency Medicine*, 7(2), 238–242. 10.1016/0735-6757(89)90145-9

Bohren, M. A., Vogel, J. P., Hunter, E. C., Lutsiv, O., Makh, S. K., Souza, J. P., Aguiar, C., Coneglian, F. S., Diniz, A. L. A., Tunçalp, Ö., Javadi, D., Oladapo, O. T., Khosla, R., Hindin, M. J., & Gülmezoglu, A. M. (2015). The mistreatment of women during childbirth in health facilities globally: A mixed-methods systematic review. *PLoS Medicine*, *12*(6), e1001847. 10.1371/journal.pmed.1001847

Buckley, S. J. (2015). Executive summary of hormonal physiology of childbearing: Evidence and implications for women, babies, and maternity care. *Journal of Perinatal Education*, *24*(3), 145–153. 10.1891/1058-1243.24.3.145

Casareno, G. E. (2016). *Using hypnosis to enhance fertility for women experiencing infertility* [A graduate project submitted in partial fulfillment of the requirements for the degree of Master of Science in Counseling, Marriage and Family Therapy]. Northridge: California State University; Retrieved April 3, 2023, from https://dspace.calstate.edu/bitstream/handle/10211.3/185996/Casareno-Gianina-thesis-2017.pdf?sequence=1

Catsaros, S., & Wendland, J. (2020). Hypnosis-based interventions during pregnancy and childbirth and their impact on women's childbirth experience: A systematic review. *Midwifery*, *84*, 102666. 10.1016/j.midw.2020.102666

Coe, C. L., & Lubach, G. R. (2008). Fetal programming: Prenatal origins of health and illness. *Current Directions in Psychological Science*, *17*(1), 36–41. 10.1111/j.1467-8721.2008.00544.x
Corsi, N., Andani, M. E., Sometti, D., Tinazzi, M., & Fiorio, M. (2019). When words hurt: Verbal suggestion prevails over conditioning in inducing the motor nocebo effect. *European Journal of Neuroscience*, *50*(8), 3311–3326. 10.1111/ejn.14489
Cyna, A. M., Andrew, M. I., & McAuliffe, G. L. (2006). Antenatal self-hypnosis for labour and childbirth: A pilot study. *Anaesthesia and Intensive Care*, *34*(4), 464–469. 10.1177/0310057x0603400402
Cyna, A. M., McAuliffe, G. L., & Andrew, M. I. (2004). Hypnosis for pain relief in labour and childbirth: A systematic review. *British Journal of Anaesthesia*, *93*(4), 505–511. 10.1093/bja/aeh225
Davies, M., & Borland, S. (2015, July 2). *Dr Michel Odent reveals secret to quick painless childbirth*. Mail Online. Retrieved April 3, 2023, from https://www.dailymail.co.uk/health/article-3147111/The-secret-quick-painless-childbirth-Just-don-t-think-ban-partner-room-leading-doctor-claims.html
Facco, E., Fracas, F., & Tressoldi, P. (2021). Moving beyond the concept of altered state of consciousness: The Non-Ordinary Mental Expressions (NOMEs). *Advances in Social Sciences Research Journal*, *8*(3), 615–631. 10.14738/assrj.83.9935
Farthing, G. W. (1992). *The psychology of consciousness*. Prentice Hall.
Finlayson, K., Downe, S., Hinder, S., Carr, H., Spiby, H., & Whorwell, P. J. (2015). Unexpected consequences: Women's experiences of a self-hypnosis intervention to help with pain relief during labour. *BMC Pregnancy and Childbirth*, *15*(1), 229 (2015). 10.1186/s12884-015-0659-0
Graziottin, A. (2010). Doctor/patient relationship: The neglected power of placebo-nocebo effect: Abstracts of XVI international congress of ISPOG, Venezia, Italy, October 28–30, 2010. *Journal of Psychosomatic Obstetrics & Gynecology*, *31*(sup1), 27. 10.3109/0167482x.2010.536387
Guse, T., Wissing, M., & Hartman, W. (2006). The effect of a prenatal hypnotherapeutic programme on postnatal maternal psychological well-being. *Journal of Reproductive and Infant Psychology*, *24*(2), 163–177. 10.1080/02646830600644070
Hammond, D. C. (1990). *Handbook of hypnotic suggestions and metaphors*. W. W. Norton & Company.
Hilden, M., Sidenius, K., Langhoff-Roos, J., Wijma, B., & Schei, B. (2003). Women's experiences of the gynecologic examination: Factors associated with discomfort. *Acta Obstetricia Et Gynecologica Scandinavica*, *82*(11), 1030–1036. 10.1034/j.1600-0412.2003.00253.x
James, U. (2009). Practical uses of clinical hypnosis in enhancing fertility, healthy pregnancy and childbirth. *Complementary Therapies in Clinical Practice*, *15*(4), 239–241. 10.1016/j.ctcp.2009.09.005
Khadem Rezaiyan, M., Saeidi, R., Ghazanfarpour, M., Mashhadi, M. E., & Najafi, M. N. (2018). Relationship between hypnosis for pain management in labor and adverse neonatal outcomes: A systematic review. *Iranian Journal of Neonatology IJN*, *9*(3), 70–75. 10.22038/ijn.2018.30047.1407
Ludwig, A. M. (1969). Altered states of consciousness. In C. T. Tart (Ed.), *Altered states of consciousness: A book of readings* (1st ed., pp. 9–22). John Wiley & Sons.
Martis, R., Emilia, O., Nurdiati, D. S., & Brown, J. (2017). Intermittent auscultation (IA) of fetal heart rate in labour for fetal well-being. *The Cochrane Database of Systematic Reviews*, *2017*(2). 10.1002/14651858.cd008680.pub2
McCormack, D. (2010). Hypnosis for hyperemesis gravidarum. *Journal of Obstetrics and Gynaecology*, *30*(7), 647–653. 10.3109/01443615.2010.509825
Odent, M. (2012). The function of joy in pregnancy [E-book]. In N. Halsede (Ed.), *Birth wisdom from Michel Odent; a collection of articles from Midwifery Today magazine (Chapter 8)*. Midwifery Today, Inc.
Odent, M. (2017). *The birth of Homo, the marine chimpanzee: When the tool becomes the master* (1st ed.). Pinter & Martin.
Orne, M. T. (1959). The nature of hypnosis: Artifact and essence. *Journal of Abnormal Psychology*, *58*(3), 277–299. 10.1037/h0046128
Reinhard, J., Heinrich, T. H., Reitter, A., Herrmann, E., Smart, W., & Louwen, F. (2012). Clinical hypnosis before external cephalic version. *American Journal of Clinical Hypnosis*, *55*(2), 184–192. 10.1080/00029157.2012.665399

Reinhard, J., Huesken-Janßen, H., Hatzmann, H., & Schiermeier, S. (2009). Preterm labour and clinical hypnosis. *Contemporary Hypnosis*, *26*(4), 187–193. 10.1002/ch.387

Rossi, E. L., & Cheek, D. B. (1988). *Mind-body therapy: Methods of ideodynamic healing in hypnosis* (1st ed.). W. W. Norton & Company.

Sado, M., Ota, E., Stickley, A., & Mori, R. (2012). Hypnosis during pregnancy, childbirth, and the postnatal period for preventing postnatal depression. *The Cochrane Database of Systematic Reviews*, *6*(CD009062). 10.1002/14651858.cd009062.pub2

Shah, M. C., Thakkar, S. H., & Vyas, R. B. (2011). Hypnosis in pregnancy with intrauterine growth restriction and oligohydramnios: An innovative approach. *American Journal of Clinical Hypnosis*, *54*(2), 116–123. 10.1080/00029157.2011.580438

Simkin, P., & Ancheta, R. (2011). *The labor progress handbook: Early interventions to prevent and treat dystocia* (3rd ed.). Wiley-Blackwell.

Stevenson, K., Lillycrop, K. A., & Silver, M. J. (2020). Fetal programming and epigenetics. *Current Opinion in Endocrine and Metabolic Research*, *13*, 1–6. 10.1016/j.coemr.2020.07.005

Uneståhl, L.-E. (1981). *Inner mental training*. Sweden: Veje Publishing.

Uvnäs-Moberg, K., Arn, I., & Magnusson, D. (2005). The psychobiology of emotion: The role of the oxytocinergic system. *International Journal of Behavioral Medicine*, *12*(2), 59–65. 10.1207/s15327558ijbm1202_3

Uvnäs-Moberg, K., Ekström-Bergström, A., Buckley, S., Massarotti, C., Pajalic, Z., Luegmair, K., Kotlowska, A., Lengler, L., Olza, I., Grylka-Baeschlin, S., Leahy-Warren, P., Hadjigeorgiu, E., Villarmea, S., & Dencker, A. (2020). Maternal plasma levels of oxytocin during breastfeeding: A systematic review. *PLoS One*, *15*(8), e0235806. 10.1371/journal.pone.0235806

Vaitl, D., Birbaumer, N., Gruzelier, J., Jamieson, G. A., Kotchoubey, B., Kübler, A., Lehmann, D., Miltner, W. H. R., Ott, U., Pütz, P., Sammer, G., Strauch, I., Strehl, U., Wackermann, J., & Weiss, T. (2005). Psychobiology of altered states of consciousness. *Psychological Bulletin*, *131*(1), 98–127. 10.1037/0033-2909.131.1.98

Varga, K. (2013). Suggestive techniques connected to medical interventions. *Interventional Medicine and Applied Science*, *5*(3), 95–100. 10.1556/IMAS.5.2013.3.1

Varga, K. (2015). *Communication strategies in medical settings: Challenging situations and practical solutions. Consciousness and human systems*, Vol. 3. Peter Lang Group. 10.3726/978-3-653-05313-5

Varga, K. (2022). Communication with people in altered states of consciousness: Techniques of rapport management. In A. G. Gómez, & A. Carrara (Eds.), *Decoding consciousness: Bioethical perspectives on consciousness and on its altered states* (1st ed., pp. 53–71).

Weitzenhoffer, A. M. (1989). *The practice of hypnotism* (1st ed., Vols. 1–2). Wiley Interscience Publication, John Wiley and Sons.

Yexley, M. J. (2007). Treating postpartum depression with hypnosis: Addressing specific symptoms presented by the client. *American Journal of Clinical Hypnosis*, *49*(3), 219–223. 10.1080/00029157.2007.10401584

Zech, N., Seemann, M., Grzesiek, M., Breu, A., Seyfried, T. F., & Hansen, E. (2019). Nocebo effects on muscular performance: An experimental study about clinical situations. *Frontiers in Pharmacology*, *10*. 10.3389/fphar.2019.00219

Critical Care

46

HYPNOSIS IN SURGERY

The Social-Psycho-Biological Model of Surgical Hypnosis

Edit Jakubovits

Faculty of Humanities, Institute of Psychology, Károli Gáspár University of the Reformed Church in Hungary, Budapest, Hungary

Background

I used to work as an anesthesiologist. During my 15 years of medical practice, I have successfully used hypnosis during numerous operations. Over time, I have found that the technique of suggestion without formal hypnosis is also useful, not only during surgery but also before. I began to pay attention to my words and then to my behavior to see what messages they might be conveying. With my psychologist colleagues, we carried out tests and statistical analyses that confirmed, in accordance with the international literature, that hypnosis not only reduced pain but also stabilized physiological variables, improved doctor–patient cooperation, and reduced drug consumption. The use of suggestion was also reassuring for me, and the interesting images and experiences I received from patients added color to the routine. The wisdom of the unconscious has always fascinated me, strengthening my faith. I am now a psychotherapist in private practice preparing patients for surgery and teaching at university.

Theoretical Framework

The demand for surgical care is going to increase in the future, as modern surgical procedures allow interventions on patients with increasingly poor health (Cutti et al., 2020). The topic of surgical hypnosis may therefore become increasingly important, as surgical hypnosis does not require any equipment, only human communication, and has no proven side effects in the operating room (Facco, 2016). Surgical hypnosis can be used not only for pain relief and anxiety reduction but also to counteract the effects of negative spontaneous suggestion (Enqvist et al., 1997; Hansen & Zech, 2019), and to harness the potential of positive physiological and psychological changes which can reduce treatment time, costs, and mortality (Defechereux et al., 1999; Disbrow et al., 1993; Esdaile, 1851; Facco, 2016; Meurisse et al., 1999; Montgomery et al., 2002; Schnur et al., 2008; Wobst, 2007; Zeng et al., 2022) both in adults and in children (Calipel et al., 2005). Hypnosis is a non-pharmacological procedure that is usually used as an adjuvant treatment (Montgomery et al., 2002), rather than as a stand-alone treatment (Facco et al., 2021; Hansen et al., 2013), both under regional

DOI: 10.4324/9781003449126-61

anesthesia, and narcosis, both in major and minor surgery, and invasive maneuvers (Facco, 2016; Schnur et al., 2008). Hypnosis supports the patient to remain conscious while still meeting surgical expectations, so sometimes it can also replace narcosis. This makes cooperation easier (Faymonville et al., 1999; Hansen et al., 2013; Meurisse et al., 1999). The effect is stronger when hypnosis was delivered with a "live" administration method as compared to audio recording (Schnur et al., 2008).

On both a physical and psychological level, invasive interventions during anesthesia involve the deep human relationship. I would like to show that hypnosis is more than just an inexpensive, "attractive technique" for pain and anxiety relief, and to add a new aspect to the rich body of knowledge that exists.

Introduction

In this I will first present some of the surgical uses of hypnosis that do not deal with pain and blood loss, because this is discussed in another chapter, see also in this volume. In the second part, I would like to draw attention to specific surgical conditions that deepen the change in state of consciousness. A socio-psycho-biological model of hypnosis (Bányai, 1998; Varga, 2021) may explain the powerful effects of hypnotic suggestion in the operating room, as the surgical setting may revive the patients' physiological and emotional patterns of early childhood experiences, so hypnosis can be an important tool not only for physical but also for mental healing for clinicians to utilize during invasive procedures.

The Biological Effects of Mental Stress

Traditional Literature Review

The risk of surgical mortality has been reduced by a number of factors over the centuries (Cutti et al., 2020); yet to this day, in addition to the physical difficulties of surgery, the most unpleasant experience for many patients is the anxiety before surgery (Eberhart et al., 2020). In a vascular surgery population, patients were more fearful of anesthesia before more difficult surgeries if anesthesia was used and if they did not know the anesthesiologist personally (Jovanovic et al., 2022). Anxiety is associated with greater changes in heart rate and blood pressure before surgery, higher likelihood of experiencing headache, vomiting, pain, problem behavior, prolonged wound healing, long-term persistence of symptoms, dissatisfaction after surgery, and even increased mortality (Kiecolt-Glaser et al., 1998; Montgomery & Bovbjerg, 2004; Székely et al., 2007; Takagi et al., 2017). The role of social support in reducing preoperative anxiety to increase feelings of safety was highlighted by many (e.g., 95% of patients requiring a preoperative talk with an anesthetist; Eberhart et al., 2020; Jovanovic et al., 2022; Mavridou et al., 2013). The sense of safety is associated with a shift in sympathetic autonomic nervous function towards parasympathetic control, changes in stress mediators, and circulatory balance. The anti-anxiety effect of hypnosis has been shown to result in favorable physiological, immunological, and hormonal changes in healthy subjects, in the operating room, and in the postoperative period (DeBenedittis et al., 1994; Gruzelier, 2002; Kiecolt-Glaser et al., 1998; Montgomery & Bovbjerg, 2004; Zachariae et al., 1991).

Postoperative nausea and vomiting (PONV) are the most common accompanying adverse events at the end of anesthesia, and in the days after surgery. In addition to individual characteristics (age, gender, weight, sensitivity), PONV is associated with anesthetic, surgical, and postoperative care factors, which may be exacerbated by anxiety (Enqvist et al., 1997; Ghosh et al., 2020). This is not only uncomfortable for the patient but can also be dangerous, for example, if stomach acid leaks into the lungs or there is increased pressure in the eye or nervous system, this can jeopardize the success of surgery in these areas (Hansen et al., 2013; Lewenstein et al., 1981). Several studies have shown a beneficial effect of hypnosis on postoperative nausea (Defechereux et al., 1999; Enqvist et al., 1997; Evans & Richardson, 1988). Therapeutic suggestion given under general anesthesia halved the incidence of PONV in a group of patients at high risk of nausea ($N = 345$) in a double-blind, multicenter, randomized controlled trial (Nowak et al., 2022).

Hemodynamic stability also occurs with a reduction in anxiety, although other processes (drug effects, the disease itself, body position, blood loss, fluid replacement) during surgery play a role in this, and it is therefore difficult to separate. Nevertheless, some studies have described more stable blood pressure and more rhythmic cardiac function in hypnotic intervention groups (Defechereux et al., 1999). Direct suggestion has an effect on the vascular status, as evidenced by the change in hemorrhagic phenomena (Meurisse et al., 1999; Szeverényi et al., 2016).

In our prospective, randomized, controlled clinical pilot study of elective abdominal surgery, patients were divided into three groups: standard treatment ($N = 17$), music during surgery ($N = 15$), and pre-, and intraoperative live, personalized suggestion ($N = 15$) (Jakubovits et al., 2011). During surgery, 93% of patients had a rapid and spontaneous recovery of bradycardia while receiving the "Heart beats more and more calmly ..." suggestion. The suggestion group had a significantly higher incidence of heart rate reduction exceeding the pre-anesthetic value by 30%. Compared to controls on the day of surgery and in the following days, patients who received suggestion had significantly fewer complaints, their appetite returned sooner, and their stools settled more quickly during their hospital stay, and the suggestion group needed fewer painkillers. On the day of discharge, 13–15% of patients in the control groups rated their own recovery as worse than expected, compared with none in the suggestion group. Significantly more patients in the suggestion group (57%) than in the control group (13%) felt that their recovery was better than expected. There was no difference between groups for the length of hospital stay.

In our other study of cataract surgery, we compared data from a usual care control group ($N = 50$) and a suggestion group ($N = 34$) who listened to a standard preoperative suggestion audio recording at home (Kekecs et al., 2014). During surgery, we observed significantly calmer feelings and greater cooperativeness in the suggestion group versus control group. The groups did not differ in terms of preoperative sleep quality, subjective well-being before and after surgery, and heart rate during surgery. In the rest of the chapter, quotations in italics are taken from our research, from personal sources, or from the literature.

The Mental Effects of Mental Stress

The efficacy of hypnosis in the operating room is enhanced by the fact that high levels of stress lead to a hypnotic type of information processing, a spontaneous trance state (Bejenke, 2011; Cheek, 1962; Enqvist et al., 1997; Varga et al., 1995). The spontaneous trance state is here defined as a change of state of consciousness that occurs intentionally, without formal induction (Varga, 2011). Emotional functioning takes priority over learned behaviors. There is increased sensitivity to social exclusion and peer support as seen, for example, in patients reporting:"*It had been raining and they were all in coats and I was in my nightie. I was pushed to one side of the room and I just sat there and felt very nervous and really very vulnerable.*" "*One thing that really, really helped, there was another lady on the ward ... and we got on like a house on fire. I was talking to her the evening before the operation, all the same sort of anxieties ... everything that I'd worried about she'd got exactly the same ... and that really helped. In fact she was one of the best things about the whole thing, I can honestly say*" (Carr et al., 2006, p. 347).

At the most intense stage of the traumatic experience, in life-threatening situations, many people experience emotional paralysis, temporarily alienated from reality and from their own self. A defense mechanism against traumatic threats is dissociation. Dissociation is also an intrinsic pattern of the hypnotic experience (Spiegel, 2006; Spiegel & Cardeña, 1991). The dopaminergic anterior attentional system is activated and creates a state of narrowed attention well known in hypnosis (Spiegel & Cardeña, 1991). Oxytocin levels are increased under stress and enhance social connectivity and the reception of hypnotic suggestion (Bryant & Hung, 2013; Janeček & Dabrowska, 2019). The evolutionary background to this may be that, in the absence of social support, when life is threatened, the shutdown of emotions is necessary to maintain heightened vigilance. Thinking and value judgments are also pushed temporarily into the background. This leaves more strength and time to carry out the behavior needed to survive. Seeking social support helps us to more easily follow involuntarily the person we think has the solution. This means that the suggestibility increases. But this "other" can also be our own inner intuitive wisdom.

I would like to illustrate this process with the experience of a midwife who, while giving birth, realized that her baby was in danger of dying: "*I was looking at myself from somewhere outside. I even remember looking at my face ... I was breathing at a nice slow pace as I dictated to myself from the outside ... the heartbeat still hadn't settled. Desperation was growing in my mind, but I was only looking outside at my other self-dictating the breath. The fetal heartbeat became slower than my pulse. I wanted to scream, to panic. I stood next to my body and dictated the breath. It felt like floating. To this day I don't know how I managed to do that. My little boy needed me. I was life to him. They took me to the operating room. He was born a beautiful, healthy, lively newborn. In extreme situations, I can still see myself being there to dictate what to do and not let my inner self panic*" (detail of a personal letter). In this case, a life-threatening situation resulted in a spontaneous hallucinatory perception of social support. During hypnosis, however, conscious social support occurs in which participants pay intense attention to each other, as the mother in the story does to her fetus.

The Complex Effects of Socio-Psycho-Biological Stress

Social Relationship Aspects

In Éva Bányai's socio-psycho-biological model, the word "social" has been brought to the front (Bányai, 1998). That is, she regards social relationships as the primary mechanism of action that causes emotional, behavioral, and physiological changes. Social relations play a role in the regulation of tension, the selection of important stimuli, and the modulation of physiological rhythms (Schore, 2021; Varga, 2021). "Self in context" theories suggest that by giving an adaptive personal meaning to events, our organism (whole body) can prepare for similar situations, which can be reinterpreted through new experiences. Meaning and reinterpretation occur in the neural structures that have been described in hypnosis (ventromedial prefrontal cortex and default-mode network) (Demertzi et al., 2011; Koban et al., 2021). The phenomenon of synchrony and the hormone/neurotransmitter oxytocin are considered important in early infant development as well as in hypnosis (Bryant & Hung, 2013; Varga, 2021). Both concepts have to do with the intense social relationship in which the caregiver is a stimulus-based regulator. This intense social relationship can also be experienced in hypnosis. "Labelling a social situation as 'hypnosis' allows participants to engage in an intense interpersonal relationship without undue risk to themselves or others, as they can leave the situation at any moment of the interaction. Thus, in a controlled situation, new cognitive and emotional – possibly corrective – experiences can emerge. By helping two individuals to enter into a close relationship in which mutual attunement and meaningful cognitive experiences are generated, hypnosis can broaden the horizons of both participants in the interaction" (Bányai, 1998, p. 60). Love, relationship difficulties, motherhood are some examples of situations in which we enter into intense social situations in adulthood where we can gain new experiences, sometimes in a protected situation, sometimes not. Nor do we make healing the goal of relationships. But surgery is similar to hypnosis. We call "surgery" a consciously created, therapeutic, protected, intense, and short-term interpersonal relationship in which the participants are mutually immersed. "Surgery is a strange profession. During surgery, I think, there is a narrowed state of consciousness that allows one to focus only and exclusively on what one is doing," says Ferenc Perner (surgeon) (Kondor, 2007, p. 21). Because of the invasive physical intervention and other special circumstances, the patient easily recalls the early caregivers who were important to him. During preoperative preparation, hypnosis provides a context to re-evaluate early traumatic experiences. The body is thus prepared for surgery at an optimal level. In an unprepared patient, surgery can trigger a high level of separation anxiety due to childhood memories. Due to the memories, the autonomic nervous system effects already set a vegetative pattern characteristic of existential anxiety (Koban et al., 2021; Sterling, 2012). However, the danger perceived by the patient is greater than what is surgically justified. Excessive anticipatory autonomic preparation for perceived danger stresses the body. The time to return to optimal homeostatic levels is also prolonged as the body has less power to recover. For a prepared patient, the same surgery is an intervention to improve health. The patient is well informed, has sufficient resources, and can adapt flexibly. He recovers relatively quickly and can return to work quickly.

I would like to provide some personal testimonies to support what I have described. The first example is that of a stressed ophthalmology patient. She was verbally abused by people around her in childhood, which she could not defend herself against. This caused anxiety, which she must have known well from childhood. Her face was already covered when she heard the comment that her eyelashes were falling out. "*Why do you say that, I have enough tension, I don't need this. I still get nervous just thinking about it. I felt like I was under-informed.*" The hypnotically prepared patient experienced something different: "*When they put me on the table, everything was natural, I didn't feel any excitement. In hindsight I thought it was the effect of the recording I had listened to before.*"

Psychobiological Aspects

Donald Houge (Houge, 2002) has grouped his hypnotic strategies used in the operating room along Ronald Shor's dimensions (Shor, 1962): (1) acceptance of analgesic suggestion (role taking as motivated participation in the hypnotic relationship); (2) spontaneous trance (weakening of general reality orientation); (3) archaic involvement as interpersonal relations in the operating theater (archaic object relations and referential relations to the hypnotist and the involvement of the core of the personality in the process). Continuing Houge's line of thought, we will now consider the characteristics of the operating theater trance state, specifically along the lines of the stressors that occur in the operating theater.

Acceptance of Analgesic Suggestion

When cognitive processes are inhibited by stress, it is difficult to make decisions, and it is easier to accept suggestions. Sentences of the unprepared patient are: "*I couldn't deal with what someone was saying in the background, would the operation be cancelled for that? Confusion in listening. Leave me alone in this vulnerable situation*!" What a patient said to me from the operating theater: "*Even when numbly spread out, every human word and touch reached me, offering me precious straws in the loneliness of fear and uncertainty…*"

Spontaneous Surgery Trance

The surgical procedure is a physical intrusion with the patient in an unnatural, restrained body position. In animal experiments, when animals are restrained in unusual positions from which they cannot escape, a freezing reaction occurs. They are in a state known as "tonic immobilization." Some of the animals become completely relaxed and exhibit physiological and postural signs typical of death. In vertebrates, for example, defecation, urination, eyes open wide while the tongue hangs out, pulse decreases, and respiration become shallow in this state. Despite appearing dead and unresponsive, the animals are aware of their surroundings and are internally active (Humphreys & Ruxton, 2018) as they prepare for the possibility of escape. In patients, the unusually narrow table, supine, prostrate posture may evoke this ancient defensive response. The condition is similar to relaxation hypnosis in that the person under hypnosis also appears to be asleep. Victor Rausch (1980), who successfully performed self-hypnosis during his own abdominal surgery, reports on his "lethargic" state: "*My eyes were open and according to the operating team there was no visible tensing of the muscles, no change in breathing, no flinching of the eyelids and no change in facial expression. I was intently staring at the nurse to my immediate right and she later commented that I turned a funny colour as if I were dead*" (Rausch, 1980, p. 126).

Archaic Involvement as Interpersonal Relations

The patient on the operating table sees the world from the perspective of the infant. The caregiver is sometimes seen, sometimes unexpectedly disappears. The table on which she/he lies moves in different directions until she/he is placed in the optimal position. This may include rocking like that of the baby in the womb, in a cradle, or in a pram. The tubes of an infusion or the respirator feed the body in a similar way to an umbilical cord. Feelings of indifference, exclusion, loneliness or caring physical touch may be familiar at a visceral level, even if there is no conscious memory of it. "*It was bad that no one spoke to me, they were just testing my vein, I couldn't see anything. I felt like I was just a body*" (unprepared patient). "*It was good to have my hand held in the operating theater and reassured, it was part of the miracle that happened to me*" (prepared patient).

The surgical mask makes the gaze the primary channel of communication, and the mask also distorts the voice. The lack of other facial information increases the patient's loneliness. In animals, the freezing response has been induced by the presentation of frightening eyes (Gallup et al., 1971). In hypnosis, eye fixation, developed by Braid, is still widely used for hypnosis induction (Braid, 1853). He explained the hypnotic effect of eye fixation by focusing attention. According to him, intense concentration causes the respiration to slow down and the nervous system to become fatigued in a state of oxygen deprivation. However, modern scientific studies suggest that sustained eye contact can generate a positively charged force field, which is explained by neural intersubjective synchronization (Schore, 2021). This promotes the maturation of brain areas involved in the analysis of stimulus input during the infant's early developmental stages (Feldman, 2015). When using hypnotic suggestion, one can consciously pay attention to the benefits of sustained eye contact, as Victor Rausch (1980) describes the initial stages of his surgery: "*I dissociated very effectively, but almost instantly realized that if I dissociated completely, I could not control my reflexes. ... I again turned to the operating room nurse ... and looked at her. As soon as I had eye contact with her, I again felt the same kind of flowing sensation I had experienced when the initial incision was made. ... I could mentally direct the flowing sensation to any area and achieve complete control... I suddenly felt strong and knew that the procedure would be absolutely successful*" (Rausch, 1980, p. 127) This example shows that although the infantile vegetative pattern can be reactivated, the adult is not a helpless infant, but can consciously use his memories and experiences for his own purposes. Perhaps fetuses are not entirely helpless either, as they can elicit physiological responses from their mothers, just as anesthetized patients can elicit actions from an anesthetist.

Therapeutic Relevance

The most important contraindication to hypnosis is the patient's and the team's aversion to it (Meurisse et al., 1999), but consciously used suggestive communication works in this cases too. Drugs and equipment should always be on standby in the operating room, where the patient's well-being is the most important thing, not the success of hypnosis. The adverse effects are failure of suggestion (Bejenke, 2011) which hypnosis training and self-awareness can avoid or correct. It is useful and facilitates hypnosis if all team members agree and cooperate (Meurisse et al., 1999), because of the social involvement and synchronization (Bányai, 1998; Varga, 2021), suggestion can affect all participants of the surgery.

The operating theater is a special social space where early infantile attachment patterns, behavioral, stimulus regulation processes, and their physiological effects may be continuously revived. Those who have the means are able to consciously steer the force field of the relationship in a positive direction (Rausch, 1980; Schore, 2021), so that the patient can move out of a victim role to become an active participant in their own healing team (Bejenke, 2011). This requires a more vigorous and conscious attention to the patient, to oneself, and to the relationship than usual. Not just in the context of formal hypnosis, not just for pain relief, but perhaps always.

Future Orientation

In planning for the future, the brain compares past experiences with the present. In this way, it is able to prepare in advance for anticipated stressful situations (Koban et al., 2021;

Sterling, 2012). The hypnotist, through a conscious interpersonal relationship, can help the patient to re-evaluate the intrapersonal relations of his past and to use his resources in a more economical, adaptive, and responsible way in the future. In planning for an energy-economic future, it is useful to integrate the healing power of ancient hypnosis in human relationships with the safe, surgical techniques of today.

References

Bányai, É. I. (1998). The interactive nature of hypnosis: Research evidence for a social-psychobiological model. *Contemporary Hypnosis*, *15*(1), 52–63. 10.1002/ch.116

Bejenke, C. (2011). The widespread use of suggestive communication in clinical practice: One practitioner's observations, lessons and practice over 35 years. In *Beyond the words: Communication and suggestion in medical practice* (pp. 107–123). Nova Sciences Publishers, Inc.

Braid, J. (1853). Hypnotic therapeutics, illustrated by cases. *Monthly Journal of Medical Science*, *8*(43), 14–47.

Bryant, R. A., & Hung, L. (2013). Oxytocin enhances social persuasion during hypnosis. *PLoS One*, *8*(4), e60711. 10.1371/journal.pone.0060711

Calipel, S., Lucas-Polomeni, M.-M., Wodey, E., & Ecoffey, C. (2005). Premedication in children: Hypnosis versus midazolam. *Paediatric Anaesthesia*, *15*(4), 275–281. 10.1111/j.1460-9592.2004.01514.x

Carr, E., Brockbank, K., Allen, S., & Strike, P. (2006). Patterns and frequency of anxiety in women undergoing gynaecological surgery. *Journal of Clinical Nursing*, *15*(3), 341–352. 10.1111/j.1365-2702.2006.01285.x

Cheek, D. B. (1962). Importance of recognizing that surgical patients behave as though hypnotized. *American Journal of Clinical Hypnosis*, *4*, 227–236. 10.1080/00029157.1962.10401905

Cutti, S., Klersy, C., Favalli, V., Cobianchi, L., Muzzi, A., Rettani, M., Tavazzi, G., Delmonte, M. P., Peloso, A., Arbustini, E., & Marena, C. (2020). A multidimensional approach of surgical mortality assessment and stratification (Smatt Score). *Scientific Reports*, *10*(1), 10964. 10.1038/s41598-020-67164-6

DeBenedittis, G., Cigada, M., Bianchi, A., Signorini, M. G., & Cerutti, S. (1994). Autonomic changes during hypnosis: A heart rate variability power spectrum analysis as a marker of sympatho-vagal balance. *International Journal of Clinical and Experimental Hypnosis*, *42*(2), 140–152. 10.1080/00207149408409347

Defechereux, T., Meurisse, M., Hamoir, E., Gollogly, L., Joris, J., & Faymonville, M. E. (1999). Hypnoanesthesia for endocrine cervical surgery: A statement of practice. *Journal of Alternative and Complementary Medicine (New York, N.Y.)*, *5*(6), 509–520. 10.1089/acm.1999.5.509

Demertzi, A., Soddu, A., Faymonville, M.-E., Bahri, M. A., Gosseries, O., Vanhaudenhuyse, A., Phillips, C., Maquet, P., Noirhomme, Q., Luxen, A., & Laureys, S. (2011). Hypnotic modulation of resting state fMRI default mode and extrinsic network connectivity. *Progress in Brain Research*, *193*, 309–322. 10.1016/B978-0-444-53839-0.00020-X

Disbrow, E. A., Bennett, H. L., & Owings, J. T. (1993). Effect of preoperative suggestion on post-operative gastrointestinal motility. *The Western Journal of Medicine*, *158*(5), 488–492.

Eberhart, L., Aust, H., Schuster, M., Sturm, T., Gehling, M., Euteneuer, F., & Rüsch, D. (2020). Preoperative anxiety in adults—A cross-sectional study on specific fears and risk factors. *BMC Psychiatry*, *20*(1), 140. 10.1186/s12888-020-02552-w

Enqvist, B., Björklund, C., Engman, M., & Jakobsson, J. (1997). Preoperative hypnosis reduces postoperative vomiting after surgery of the breasts. A prospective, randomized and blinded study. *Acta Anaesthesiologica Scandinavica*, *41*(8), 1028–1032. 10.1111/j.1399-6576.1997.tb04831.x

Esdaile, J. (1851). *Mesmerism in India, and its practical application in surgery and medicine*. Silas Andrus and Son.

Evans, C., & Richardson, P. H. (1988). Improved recovery and reduced postoperative stay after therapeutic suggestions during general anaesthesia. *Lancet (London, England)*, 2(8609), 491–493. 10.1016/s0140-6736(88)90131-6

Facco, E. (2016). Hypnosis and anesthesia: Back to the future. *Minerva Anestesiologica*, *82*(12), 1343–1356.
Facco, E., Bacci, C., & Zanette, G. (2021). Hypnosis as sole anesthesia for oral surgery: The egg of Columbus. *Journal of the American Dental Association (1939)*, *152*(9), 756–762. 10.1016/j.adaj.2021.04.017
Faymonville, M. E., Meurisse, M., & Fissette, J. (1999). Hypnosedation: A valuable alternative to traditional anaesthetic techniques. *Acta Chirurgica Belgica*, *99*(4), 141–146. 10.1080/00015458.1999.12098466
Feldman, R. (2015). Sensitive periods in human social development: New insights from research on oxytocin, synchrony, and high-risk parenting. *Development and Psychopathology*, *27*(2), 369–395. 10.1017/S0954579415000048
Gallup, G. G., Nash, R. F., & Ellison, A. L. (1971). Tonic immobility as a reaction to predation: Artificial eyes as a fear stimulus for chickens. *Psychonomic Science*, *23*(1), 79–80. 10.3758/BF03336016
Ghosh, S., Rai, K. K., Shivakumar, H. R., Upasi, A. P., Naik, V. G., & Bharat, A. (2020). Incidence and risk factors for postoperative nausea and vomiting in orthognathic surgery: A 10-year retrospective study. *Journal of the Korean Association of Oral and Maxillofacial Surgeons*, *46*(2), 116–124. 10.5125/jkaoms.2020.46.2.116
Gruzelier, J. H. (2002). A review of the impact of hypnosis, relaxation, guided imagery and individual differences on aspects of immunity and health. *Stress*, *5*(2), 147–163. 10.1080/10253890290027877
Hansen, E., Seemann, M., Zech, N., Doenitz, C., Luerding, R., & Brawanski, A. (2013). Awake craniotomies without any sedation: The awake-awake-awake technique. *Acta Neurochirurgica*, *155*(8), 1417–1424. 10.1007/s00701-013-1801-2
Hansen, E., & Zech, N. (2019). Nocebo effects and negative suggestions in daily clinical practice—Forms, impact and approaches to avoid them. *Frontiers in Pharmacology*, *10*, 77. 10.3389/fphar.2019.00077
Houge, D. R. (2002). A model for the application of hypnotic techniques in surgery. In *Hypnosis international monographs, No. 6* (pp. 185–190). MEG Stiftung.
Humphreys, R. K., & Ruxton, G. D. (2018). A review of thanatosis (death feigning) as an anti-predator behaviour. *Behavioral Ecology and Sociobiology*, *72*(2), 22. 10.1007/s00265-017-2436-8
Jakubovits, E., Janecskó, M., Varga, K., Diószeghy, C., & Pénzes, I. (2011). The Efficacy of pre-operative psychological preparation and positive suggestions during general anaesthetic. In the perioperative period. In *Beyond the words: Communication and suggestion in medical practice* (pp. 293–306). Nova Sciences Publishers, Inc.
Janeček, M., & Dabrowska, J. (2019). Oxytocin facilitates adaptive fear and attenuates anxiety responses in animal models and human studies—Potential interaction with the corticotropin releasing factor (CRF) system in the bed nucleus of the stria terminalis (BNST). *Cell and Tissue Research*, *375*(1), 143–172. 10.1007/s00441-018-2889-8
Jovanovic, K., Kalezic, N., Sipetic Grujicic, S., Zivaljevic, V., Jovanovic, M., Savic, M., Trailovic, R., Vjestica Mrdak, M., Novovic, M., Marinkovic, J., Kukic, B., Dimkic Tomic, T., Cvetkovic, S., & Davidovic, L. (2022). Patients' fears and perceptions associated with anesthesia. *Medicina (Kaunas, Lithuania)*, *58*(11), 1577. 10.3390/medicina58111577
Kekecs, Z., Jakubovits, E., Varga, K., & Gombos, K. (2014). Effects of patient education and therapeutic suggestions on cataract surgery patients: A randomized controlled clinical trial. *Patient Education and Counseling*, *94*(1), 116–122. 10.1016/j.pec.2013.09.019
Kiecolt-Glaser, J. K., Page, G. G., Marucha, P. T., MacCallum, R. C., & Glaser, R. (1998). Psychological influences on surgical recovery. Perspectives from psychoneuroimmunology. *The American Psychologist*, *53*(11), 1209–1218. 10.1037//0003-066x.53.11.1209
Koban, L., Gianaros, P. J., Kober, H., & Wager, T. D. (2021). The self in context: Brain systems linking mental and physical health. *Nature Reviews. Neuroscience*, *22*(5), 309–322. 10.1038/s41583-021-00446-8
Kondor, K. (2007). *Titoknyitogató—Perner Ferenc.* Semmelweis Kiadó és Multimédia Stúdió.
Lewenstein, L. N., Iwamoto, K., & Schwartz, H. (1981). Hypnosis in high risk ophthalmic surgery. *Ophthalmic Surgery*, *12*(1), 39–41.
Mavridou, P., Dimitriou, V., Manataki, A., Arnaoutoglou, E., & Papadopoulos, G. (2013). Patient's anxiety and fear of anesthesia: Effect of gender, age, education, and previous experience of anesthesia. A survey of 400 patients. *Journal of Anesthesia*, *27*(1), 104–108. 10.1007/s00540-012-1460-0

Meurisse, M., Defechereux, T., Hamoir, E., Maweja, S., Marchettini, P., Gollogly, L., Degauque, C., Joris, J., & Faymonville, M. E. (1999). Hypnosis with conscious sedation instead of general anaesthesia? Applications in cervical endocrine surgery. *Acta Chirurgica Belgica*, *99*(4), 151–158.

Montgomery, G. H., & Bovbjerg, D. H. (2004). Presurgery distress and specific response expectancies predict postsurgery outcomes in surgery patients confronting breast cancer. *Health Psychology: Official Journal of the Division of Health Psychology, American Psychological Association*, *23*(4), 381–387. 10.1037/0278-6133.23.4.381

Montgomery, G. H., David, D., Winkel, G., Silverstein, J. H., & Bovbjerg, D. H. (2002). The effectiveness of adjunctive hypnosis with surgical patients: A meta-analysis. *Anesthesia and Analgesia*, *94*(6), 1639–1645, table of contents. 10.1097/00000539-200206000-00052

Nowak, H., Wolf, A., Rahmel, T., Oprea, G., Grause, L., Moeller, M., Gyarmati, K., Mittler, C., Zagler, A., Lutz, K., Loeser, J., Saller, T., Tryba, M., Adamzik, M., Hansen, E., & Zech, N. (2022). Therapeutic suggestions during general anesthesia reduce postoperative nausea and vomiting in high-risk patients—A post hoc analysis of a randomized controlled trial. *Frontiers in Psychology*, *13*, 898326. 10.3389/fpsyg.2022.898326

Rausch, V. (1980). Cholecystectomy with self-hypnosis. *American Journal of Clinical Hypnosis*, *22*(3), 124–129. 10.1080/00029157.1980.10403216

Schnur, J. B., Kafer, I., Marcus, C., & Montgomery, G. H. (2008). Hypnosis to manage distress related to medical procedures: A meta-analysis. *Contemporary Hypnosis: The Journal of the British Society of Experimental and Clinical Hypnosis*, *25*(3–4), 114–128. 10.1002/ch.364

Schore, A. N. (2021). The interpersonal neurobiology of intersubjectivity. *Frontiers in Psychology*, *12*, 648616. 10.3389/fpsyg.2021.648616

Shor, R. E. (1962). Three dimensions of hypnotic depth. *International Journal of Clinical and Experimental Hypnosis*, *10*, 23–38. 10.1080/00207146208415862

Spiegel, D. (2006). Recognizing traumatic dissociation. *American Journal of Psychiatry*, *163*(4), 566–568. 10.1176/ajp.2006.163.4.566

Spiegel, D., & Cardeña, E. (1991). Disintegrated experience: The dissociative disorders revisited. *Journal of Abnormal Psychology*, *100*(3), 366–378. 10.1037//0021-843x.100.3.366

Sterling, P. (2012). Allostasis: A model of predictive regulation. *Physiology & Behavior*, *106*(1), 5–15. 10.1016/j.physbeh.2011.06.004

Székely, A., Balog, P., Benkö, E., Breuer, T., Székely, J., Kertai, M. D., Horkay, F., Kopp, M. S., & Thayer, J. F. (2007). Anxiety predicts mortality and morbidity after coronary artery and valve surgery—A 4-year follow-up study. *Psychosomatic Medicine*, *69*(7), 625–631. 10.1097/PSY.0b013e31814b8c0f

Szeverényi, C., Csernátony, Z., Balogh, Á., Simon, T., & Varga, K. (2016). Effects of positive suggestions on the need for red blood cell transfusion in orthopedic surgery. *International Journal of Clinical and Experimental Hypnosis*, *64*(4), 404–418. 10.1080/00207144.2016.1209041

Takagi, H., Ando, T., Umemoto, T., & ALICE (All-Literature Investigation of Cardiovascular Evidence) Group. (2017). Perioperative depression or anxiety and postoperative mortality in cardiac surgery: A systematic review and meta-analysis. *Heart and Vessels*, *32*(12), 1458–1468. 10.1007/s00380-017-1022-3

Varga, K. (2011). Possibilities of suggestive communication. In *Beyond the words. Communication and suggestion in medical practice* (pp. 3–17). Nova Sciences Publishers, Inc.

Varga, K. (2021). Possible mechanisms of hypnosis from an interactional perspective. *Brain Sciences*, *11*(7), 903. 10.3390/brainsci11070903

Varga K., Jakubovits E., & Janecskó M. (1995). A tudatállapot általános anesztézia alatt. *Magyar Pszichológiai Szemle*, *51*(35), 58–82.

Wobst, A. H. K. (2007). Hypnosis and surgery: Past, present, and future. *Anesthesia and Analgesia*, *104*(5), 1199–1208. 10.1213/01.ane.0000260616.49050.6d

Zachariae, R., Bjerring, P., Zachariae, C., Arendt-Nielsen, L., Nielsen, T., Eldrup, E., Larsen, C. S., & Gotliebsen, K. (1991). Monocyte chemotactic activity in sera after hypnotically induced emotional states. *Scandinavian Journal of Immunology*, *34*(1), 71–79. 10.1111/j.1365-3083.1991.tb01522.x

Zeng, J., Wang, L., Cai, Q., Wu, J., & Zhou, C. (2022). Effect of hypnosis before general anesthesia on postoperative outcomes in patients undergoing minor surgery for breast cancer: A systematic review and meta-analysis. *Gland Surgery*, *11*(3), 588–598. 10.21037/gs-22-114

47

PERIOPERATIVE MEDICAL INTERVENTIONS AND DEVICES

Kristóf Perczel

BETHESDA CHILDREN'S HOSPITAL, BUDAPEST, HUNGARY; HUNGARIAN ASSOCIATION OF HYPNOSIS, BUDAPEST, HUNGARY

Outline

In this chapter, I will explore the theoretical framework underlying the assumption that there is an altered state of consciousness in the acute medical and perioperative setting. After summarizing the evidence available in the literature, I will move on to clinical applications: first I present the lucid approach of Christel Bejenke (1996), then add some additional applications that I have found useful. I conclude with some suggestions for further research and training.

The author is an anesthesiologist and hypnotherapist with a special interest in pain management, who has been using therapeutic suggestions for ten years now to complement his medical work.

Theoretical Framework

The perioperative situation elicits an altered state of consciousness, just like any highly stressful, threatening, and extreme situation (Field, 1992). "Tart (1975) argued that our normal, alert waking state of consciousness is maintained by certain *stabilizing conditions*, including a sufficient level of physiological arousal, a changing array of external stimuli, and an attitude of maintaining attention to them so that we can make appropriate decisions and responses consistent with our motives. In order to produce an altered state of consciousness we must first disrupt or *destabilize* the normal state" (Farthing, 1992, p. 213, emphasis in original). The perioperative condition, acute medical, and surgical situations are rife with such destabilizing factors.

Physiological *arousal* can be extremely elevated in the case of severe homeostatic derangements (such as trauma, sepsis, or any other acute life-threatening condition) and, to a lesser degree, by the fight or flight response of an anxious and fearful patient preparing for an elective procedure. Arousal can also be greatly reduced by sedative and anesthetic drugs, or pathological processes interfering with normal central nervous system functioning. The *level of external stimulation* can also vary greatly. At one extreme, there can be severe overstimulation with practically incomprehensible quantities of medical

DOI: 10.4324/9781003449126-62

information or, in case of an emergency, the cacophony of device alarms and noisy teamwork. At another extreme, there are the hours and days spent waiting in hallways and wards, which in certain special cases (e.g., isolation for infection control purposes or prolonged intensive care) can approach the conditions of sensory-deprivation experiments.

An altered state of consciousness can be characterized by changes in many dimensions of the subjective experience. These include attention, perception, imagery, time experience, memory, higher-level thought processes, meaning of experience, self-control, suggestibility, and sense of personal identity (Farthing, 1992, p. 208). Many of these changes are readily identifiable in the perioperative patient. *Attention* can be markedly focused on some aspect of the patient's condition or the procedure, making it difficult to develop a well-rounded and realistic understanding of one's condition. This highly focused attention leads to diminished responsiveness to other stimulation, which can range from subtle difficulties to process new information to the severe inability to interact with other people. Changes in *perception* partially stem from the focused state of attention but are also aggravated by the frightened person's pessimistic interpretation of any communication with multiple possible meanings.

The *decreased ability to recall information* compounds the alterations of higher-level thought processes leading to difficulties in problem solving and decision making (Farthing, 1992, p. 209). Changes in *self-control* are evident in the case of the raging patient, but probably of greater clinical importance in the ubiquitous form of lethargy and the inability to initiate action.

The changes typical of altered states of consciousness foster a shift in information processing: logical and rational modes of understanding fade away and the world becomes primarily understood in a way similar to that of small children. Communication is often understood verbatim, complex concepts can be grasped only through images and metaphors. The ability to rationally weigh and contrast information is reduced or lost, contradicting details are easily accepted as valid.

Becoming highly dependent on the figures of authority for guidance under such circumstances arises from the inability to cope with the threatening situation alone. This reliance is further intensified by psychological regression, which is "the process of returning to an earlier, more primitive level of adaptation in response to stress that taxes mature coping abilities" (Corradi, 1983, p. 353). One form of such earlier level of adaptation is the child's complete dependence on the parents who are perceived as omnipotent and all-knowing.

The increased responsiveness to suggestions can be explained by the interplay of all the aforementioned factors. "Patients become very susceptible to the signs which can help them interpret the uncontrollable situation in which they find themselves" (Varga, 2013, p. 97). *Suggestions*, according to Barber (1996) are "an invitation to an experience" (p. 7). A more specific definition could be that suggestions are "verbal and nonverbal messages that the receiver involuntarily accepts and follows. Not only our spoken or written words but the environment, objects, and nonverbal messages (eye contact, sighs, and touches) can have suggestive effects" (Varga, 2013, p. 95).

This hypersuggestibility may render the patient defenseless against all the negative suggestions he encounters. Communication with negative suggestive effects is copious in medical settings, partly as an effort to be "true" to the patient. "Physicians and nurses often use relatively harsh words to describe invasive procedures in an attempt to prepare, and possibly calm and reassure the patient in advance of what may be an uncomfortable procedure" (Varelmann et al., 2010, p. 869). This observation can easily be generalized to discussions about medication side-effects and most other aspects of patient care as well.

The result of the spontaneously occurring altered state of consciousness, the consequential hypersuggestibility, and the myriad of well-meant negative suggestive effects create a state which we can call a *negative trance*. A very exciting parallel to this state – characterized above and familiar from the clinic everyday – is given by Ziss (2020) from the differing context of anticipatory trauma at a community level:

> When an extreme situation occurs, the SoA [sense of agency] mostly decreases ... Anxiety and fear can create borders and shrink the space around the community, both mentally and physically (Ahmed, 2004). Feeling like a victim or a passive subject can cause involuntary actions, contradictory behavior and beliefs, loss of a sense of time, dissociative processes, and other cognitive-affective signs of an altered state of consciousness (Ludwig, 1966), where all these ... work toward stronger feelings of victimhood and passivity. A symmetrical process can happen with the feeling of heroism, activity or even omnipotence. This is the process of the polarization of the SoA ... in the state of trance the SoA is more fictile. (p. 2)

Understanding the impact of our communication (which will be the goal of the proximate literature review) opens up a world of possibilities to utilize language in a way that protects, comforts, orientates, and even inspires our patients. To connect in a way that turns the spontaneous negative trance, via conscious and professional communication, into a positive one.

Hypnosis is a method that utilizes various induction techniques to increase suggestibility and then seeks to foster change via delivering therapeutic suggestions (for elaboration on the possible definitions of hypnosis we refer to the relevant chapters of this volume). In the perioperative and acute medical setting, such hypersuggestibility is typical, so any communication following the rules of suggestion can be considered to have the potential to induce hypnotic phenomena.

The Importance of Appropriate Communication in Light of the Literature

This issue at hand is not new by far. As early as 1964, Egbert demonstrated that a pre- and postoperative visit by the anesthesiologist, involving only education and instructions about pain, was sufficient to halve narcotic needs after major intraabdominal surgery. He concluded that an important factor at work was probably the relationship: "The anesthetist who understands his patient and who believes that each patient is "his" patient ceases to be merely a clever technician in the operating room" (Egbert et al., 1964, p. 827).

The term *placebo* is used to denote the non-specific effects of a treatment, or the "complex psychosocial context surrounding the patient, which constitutes the ritual of the therapeutic act" (Benedetti, 2012, p. 98). A study conducted by Amanzio et al. (2001) showed that the effect of well-established opioid and non-opioid analgesics could be diminished by up to 50% if given as a "hidden injection", which is a striking indication of the *magnitude* of influence that the psychosocial context has on drug effects.

The *nocebo* effect of well-meant negative wording is well documented for both local anesthetic injections (Varelmann et al., 2010) and peripheral venous cannulation (Dutt-Gupta et al., 2007). A study by Wang et al. (2008) demonstrated that when negative wording was used to communicate with postoperative patients, their morphine requirement increased by up to 60%.

There are a multitude of articles and studies indicating the beneficial effects of therapeutic suggestions in the perioperative and acute medical setting. I refer to the seminal work of pioneers such as Christel J. Bejenke (1996), Katalin Bloch-Szentágothai (1991), David B. Cheek (1969), Dabney M. Ewin (1983), Leora Kuttner (2012), and Katalin Varga (2011, 2015). More recent studies have shown that using therapeutic suggestions without a formal hypnosis induction could shorten mechanical ventilation time in critically ill patients (Szilágyi et al., 2014), decrease intraoperative blood loss in hip and knee arthroplasty patients (Szeverényi et al., 2016), and soothe anxiety during cataract surgery (Kekecs et al., 2014). For a summary of the literature, I refer you to the review by Kekecs and Varga (2013), and Kekecs et al. (2014) alongside the relevant chapters of this volume.

Suggestions given to patients under general anesthesia are an especially interesting application of the technique. Although the evidence that seemingly unconscious anesthetized patients maintain auditory contact with the environment is contradictory (see Tzovara et al., 2015 and Trustmanz et al., 1977), a recently published study by Nowak et al. (2020) found significantly diminished postoperative analgesic needs in patients who were given positive suggestions, while under general anesthesia. The fact that such an effect could be demonstrated in a multicenter randomized trial provides very strong evidence for the clinical relevance of this phenomenon and vindicates further research to clarify the factors at work.

Hypnotic interventions have proven to be beneficial for surgical patients in a multitude of ways, as summarized in a meta-analysis by Montgomery et al. (2002). Since in the perioperative setting, an altered state of consciousness and hypersuggestibility is present, it can be difficult to draw the line between hypnosis and suggestive communication. This leads me to believe that findings from studies of hypnotic interventions in perioperative patients can also be relevant to the usage of therapeutic suggestions, even if no formal induction procedure is realized.

Hypnosedation, a term coined by Marie-Elisabeth Faymonville, refers to the combination of conscious analgosedation, local anesthesia, and hypnosis (Meurisse et al., 1999, p. 151). The combination of these techniques – in contrast to pure hypnoanalgesia – allows for a quick induction of good operating conditions without any prior hypnotic practice and independence from the patient's level of hypnotic susceptibility. Faymonville and her team (Meurisse et al., 1999) reported their experience with over 2,000 cases of plastic and endocrine cervical surgery with hypnosedation. The results showed significantly less postoperative pain, higher patient satisfaction, shorter hospital stay, and an astonishing 21 days earlier return to previous functional state, compared to general anesthesia (Meurisse et al., 1999). It is difficult to estimate the human and financial gain if such results – when replicable in a multicentered setting – could inform widespread practice. For a rigorous analysis of time- and cost-effectiveness of adequate perioperative communication and hypnosis, see also Lang et al. (2000) and Lang and Rosen (2002).

In the section on our theoretical framework, I outlined a *deductive* argument for the application of therapeutic suggestions in the acute medical setting. I believe that the literature summarized here complements this, by constituting a solid *inductive* argument for the implementation of suggestive techniques in perioperative and acute medical situations.

Clinical Application

It is difficult to see what one could add to the existing rich literature and practice of suggestive communication, since engaging reports from clinicians with great experience are abundant. Choosing to reframe this difficulty of relevant contribution as freedom to put forth what I find personally meaningful and relevant, I decide to present the lucid approach of Christel Bejenke (1996), and then share a few examples of clinically challenging situations where I have found suggestive communication helpful. Great care is taken to cite any known source of phrases and techniques that I present as part of my work, but due to the organic nature in which one's tone and clinical work develops such reconstruction may not always be possible.

Christel Bejenke's Approach

Bejenke (1996) puts forward a framework for managing perioperative negative trance states via "INFORMATION, INSTRUCTION, SUGGESTIONS (with or without hypnosis) and *the implicit message of commitment and caring*" (p. 211, emphasis in original).

Giving *information* in a language and at a pace that the patient can understand is highly empowering. The health literacy of patients is often overrated by medical caregivers, so care should be taken to explain underlying anatomical and physiological basics in simple language to most patients. Recording what is said at the physician's office for later review can help the patient overcome the difficulty to recall information and minimize repeat visits.

A direct consequence of understanding is the possibility to make choices either relevant to patient care (e.g., regional anesthesia or a patient-controlled analgesia pump for post-operative pain control) or as a therapeutic double-bind (e.g., "On which finger would you like me to place the pulse oximeter?"). Choices bring about a sense of control and agency that directly counter feelings of helplessness and passivity.

> Well intended admonitions from nurses or physicians to "just relax" are *not* helpful, instead confirming to the patient his or her inability to do so. This only further amplifies a sense of helplessness. It can, however, be very helpful to show a patient *how* to relax.
>
> *(Bejenke, 1996, p. 223, emphasis in original)*

Effective *instructions* empower patients, strengthening their sense of control and agency. Such instructions given in advance of surgery can be to learn abdominal breathing before a thoracic procedure (or thoracic breathing before an abdominal one), or to learn to relax muscles around the surgical area. Patients already connected to a monitor can be shown how they can influence the various readings, grasping attention by the obvious changes in heart rate brought about by a Valsalva's maneuver (where a forced expiratory effort against a closed glottis causes an elevation of heart rate) and then by progressive relaxation. Another creative method recommended by Bejenke (1996) is to show patients – when breathing through the mask of the anesthesia machine – how they can influence the displayed capnogram by the depth of the breath they take. This not only turns potentially threatening pieces of equipment into intelligible devices they can explore but also sets the scene for a gradual inward shift of attention.

> Independence and self-sufficiency can be supported by reinforcing the patient's characteristic skills and by designing suggestions to be self-perpetuating. *Self-perpetuation* is achieved by linking suggestions to cues that can be expected to recur automatically or repeatedly for extended periods of time ... [such as] breathing, rhythmic beeping of monitors ... ringing of telephones, nurses or visitors walking into the room. (ibid., p. 225, emphasis in original)

An exceptionally important aspect is to protect patients from the unintended negative suggestions they encounter which can be very effectively done by reminding them that

> ... there are ever so many sounds and conversations in the operating room, and you might find it very *reassuring* to hear the hustle and bustle that goes on, which lets you know that everything that is happening in that room happens only for *your* benefit ... to make everything safe. It all might sound to you like just a babbling brook ... or gentle raindrops ... with no meaning other than that you can feel peaceful, comfortable and relaxed ... And you don't even need to bother to pay attention to any of them, unless you are addressed by name. (ibid., p. 227, emphasis in original)

Notice that once again an inward shift of attention is elicited and that the auditory channel is emphasized, being the "most persistent mode of perception, even under profound sedation and anesthesia" (ibid., p. 225).

This framework can be applied to many medical devices, recognizing that by providing information, giving instructions, and adding goal-directed suggestions, we can help the patient recognize them for what they truly are: allies toward recovery. "[Chest tubes] help drain away fluid and air ... and allow your lungs to work in a healthier way as they are healing ... Each time you hear the gurgling sound in the suction apparatus ... you can know that it protects you" (ibid., p. 231).

Bladder catheters can be irritating, but if we tell our patients that they "can be so relieved ... because it means, that [they] don't even have to think about finding a bathroom ... [they can just] let all those muscles down there know that they can just relax, and let go" (ibid., p. 231).

The awareness of nasogastric tubes "lets you know that your operation is safely finished. And you can be so relieved. It means that [your stomach] is being given the best chance to rest and heal quickly ... because the stomach juices that might be irritating to the healing tissues are being siphoned away" (ibid., p.232).

Endotracheal tubes and ventilators can be recontextualized to provide the sense of safety since they are a sign that "healing has already begun ... As you know, this sophisticated machine *helps* you, so that you don't even need to do the work of breathing ... So when you hear the huffing and puffing of the machine, and feel your chest rise and fall ... you can just settle back and relax and let that machine do the work for you" (p. 233, emphasis in original).

Clinical Examples from Practice

Neuraxial techniques form an integral part of obstetric anesthetic practice. Although these procedures brought a breakthrough in the safety and efficacy of obstetric pain management, most women are more apprehensive about these procedures than any other part of their labor experience. In my experience, a combination of information, instruction, suggestion, and distraction has been found to be profoundly helpful for the mothers-to-be. After rapport is established and the routine assessment completed, the subject is positioned sitting on the surgical table. She is told that:

> I would like to show you how to position yourself so that together we can achieve this nice numbness quickly and comfortably, so that you can hold [baby XY] in your hands very soon now. Just take a deep breath and then let it all out, to help let go of any unnecessary tension and make you feel more and more comfortable. *[The anesthesiologist here can benefit greatly from his legitimate use of touch, by lightly pressing down on the patient's shoulders at the end of exhalation. He further adjusts the patient's posture for optimal position.]* Now you will feel the coolness of the antiseptic at your back as I prep the skin, which helps you to be so safe in this regard as well. Now I would like to ask you to focus on your toes and feet. I will be giving the anesthetic here at your back, but what matters is what you feel in your toes. Please let me know when you start to feel a nice, warm, tingling sensation. It could be in your left big toe, or in the second toe on your right foot, maybe in the other sole, I'm not sure, but you do know. I am giving the medicine now, and you're helping me greatly by letting me know as soon as you start feeling anything interesting in your feet.

The usual response of the women is to start reporting nice sensations from their feet even before any medication has been injected and the overwhelming majority doesn't even notice the sting of the needle. Before one urgent cesarean section, the surgeon scrubbing remarked that listening to these words kind of made him also want a spinal anesthetic, a comment that I consider a compliment of a lifetime.

The perioperative situation is often perceived as threatening and uncontrollable, so suggestions building on personal strengths can be very effective tools. These suggestions not only reconnect the patient with a resourceful state in their lives but also imply attention and foster dignity stemming from being noticed as a person. One colleague referred to the activity of eliciting personal resources as "pearl-diving", pointing out both the effort and the great reward implied (E. Jakubovits, personal communication, 2014). This technique can be utilized to enhance the placebo effect of analgesics, as in the case of the nine-year-old girl screaming from unbearable pain after minor surgery:

> Katie, I have brought you now an even stronger medicine, you will be surprised by how strong it is. I know you are in a lot of pain now, and this pain will go on for some time, before it starts to subside. And with time it will start to get better and better. Let's do this together: I'll give the medicine and you blow the little painkiller dwarves to where it is sensitive. *[The intravenous analgesic is given.]* Breathe in ... .and out. You are a big schoolgirl now in third grade, so you know what the double of any number is. So as you inhale to a count of two, you will know to exhale to a count of four. Inhale... one ... two, and let it out one... two ... three ... four. That's it. And now if you inhale to a count of three, you can blow the little midgets for a full count of six. That's it, very good. The worst is over now, you will get better and better. It might still be sensitive, but you can just let the feelings change, it might feel like it's pulling, or like small kittens scratching.

Katie was greatly relieved in a few minutes by the synergy of pharmacology, suggestions, and the sense of support and accompaniment. I also felt greatly rewarded when Katie's cries of despair turned into an enthusiastic account of her kittens at home.

Such mobilization of personal resources can be very helpful in soothing anxiety in adults too as seen in the following example.

Case Vignette 1

Peter was a middle-aged man with a hyperactive gag reflex, who came to ask for general anesthesia to cope with the necessary dental interventions to manage his accumulating oral hygiene problems. After the first interview, he was offered the possibility to experience the procedure under hypnosis and dental local anesthesia. When asked about his favorite activities, he enthusiastically told us about his competency as a rally driver. The sense of control and strength he experienced while racing on the road could be mobilized and transferred into the dental chair. The conscientious driver's care for his vehicle lent itself easily as a metaphor for the dental care he needed. His desire to impress his girlfriend could be used as a goal toward which he was driving through the procedure as well. He endured a 30-minute procedure without gagging and the need for any sedatives. Even though in this case a formal induction was used to deepen the trance in order to help him overcome his unnecessary gagging, I believe that the same suggestions would have been immensely helpful as "waking suggestions" too.

Case Vignette 2

John was a man in his eighties, who needed postoperative intensive care after an extensive intraabdominal surgery because of a malignant colon tumor. After extubation, he needed additional, intermittent non-invasive respiratory support in the intensive care unit (ICU). The daytime passed uneventfully, but in the evenings, he experienced severe agitation and confusion requiring heavy sedation, which led to prolonged somnolence constraining him to further days in the ICU. During a lucid daytime period, I found the time to sit with him, seeking resources he could build upon in the evenings he found so terrifying. He articulated a love for fishing, so I gave the following suggestions:

> And you know, when you are fishing on those banks you love so much, you just sit and wait. You can't make the fish come by yelling or running around, every skillful angler knows that isn't the way it is done. You do the preparation and then just sit around waiting for nature to do its job. Isn't it interesting that you can do the most by not doing too much, just relaxing and patiently waiting? Now your healing is also like that, you can just lie here, let the machine do its job and help you, and let the healing forces of your body do their job to help you be back by the river you love so much. With every relaxed and deep breath that you take with the help of the machine you are making a step towards that river, to being back there fishing again.

In the evening time, when he started to show the first signs of becoming agitated – and the physician on duty was piled under work – he could be comforted with a short reminder of his goal to be back fishing and only a mild sleeping pill.

Patients preparing for surgery mandated by a malignant disease have to cope with many forms of grief: there can be a realistic chance of limited life expectancy, limitations brought about by the severe side effects of chemotherapy, and the consequences of a radical surgical approach. The possibility to express this grief can be very beneficial for these patients in the midst of a health care system and society who expects them to be "tough". Bejenke (1996) emphasizes the importance of mourning the organ to be removed and I too have found it to be immensely helpful as a part of the preoperative anesthetic visit.

> Many patients find it very helpful to spend some time, maybe in the evening before surgery, to say goodbye to their part which will be removed. You have to say goodbye to a part of you, which has been with you since the day you were born, but now, for some reason, it has to go, so that you can live on. This can be very difficult. So be free to take your time, think about all that you have been through together, as if talking to a friend, sum up all that you are grateful for, you can thank your [organ] for helping you through so many years in so many ways. Some find it helpful to imagine what it looks like, or even to start a conversation [organ], so that when the time comes you are ready to let go. By doing this you are contributing greatly to your healing and recovery.

We believe that this short invitation not only gives the patient a meaningful activity for the long hours of waiting but also validates their negative feelings and allows them to start working through them toward recovery.

Conclusion and Closing Remarks

This chapter shows the theoretical foundations and the scientific evidence indicating the existence of an altered state of consciousness in the perioperative setting and the consequential therapeutic possibilities offered by hypersuggestibility. I have described an established model of effective communication in such a state, along the lines of Christel Bejenke's work (Bejenke, 1996), adding some techniques that I have found effective in similar situations. These techniques are viewed as theoretically sound and corroborated by ample scientific evidence and the experience of countless devoted professionals.

The question remains why such a method is not more widespread in the medical community? How can one explain the striking divide between everyday medical communication and a suggestively mindful and theoretically sound one? I suggest that research directed toward answering this question should be a priority for the community of professionals invested in hypnosis and suggestive communication. Meanwhile, awaiting the results of such an inquiry, I propose training in the usage of therapeutic suggestions for medical professionals *separate* from training in hypnosis. The complex technical and legal aspects of using formal hypnosis demand strict training curricula and entry criteria, which create a high threshold for entry. In contrast, the science of effective communication via suggestions can be mastered much quicker, and their usage in an already given, informal trance can be legally more relaxed, so such a training can be made available to a wider public. An inspiring model could be the highly successful psychological support based on positive suggestions training in Hungary (Varga, 2013).

The effective usage of therapeutic suggestions rests not only on sound technical knowledge but also on the capacity of the professional to contain the patient's experience and emotions. The power of such an encounter can not only provide us with deeply satisfying experiences but also has the potential to burden us significantly. Such an intense relationship does not self-evidently form a part of how biomedical professionals conceive their roles in patient care. Research exploring how such a connection is perceived by health care professionals and how it relates to long-term well-being and burnout could reveal deeper aspects of the acceptance and dissemination of this highly effective therapeutic tool.

References

Amanzio, M., Pollo, A., Maggi, G., & Benedetti, F. (2001). Response variability to analgesics: A role for non-specific activation of endogenous opioids. *Pain*, *90*(3), 205–215. 10.1016/s0304-3959(00)00486-3

Ahmed, S. (2004). The affective politics of fear. In S. Ahmed (Ed.), *The cultural politics of emotion* (pp. 62–81). Edinburgh University Press.

Barber, J. (1996). *Hypnosis and suggestion in the treatment of pain: A clinical guide* (1st ed.). W. W. Norton & Co.

Bejenke, C. J. (1996). Painful medical procedures. In J. Barber (Ed.), *Hypnosis and suggestion in the treatment of pain: A clinical guide* (1st ed., pp. 209–266). W. W. Norton & Co.

Benedetti, F. (2012). Placebo-induced improvements: How therapeutic rituals affect the patient's brain. *Journal of Acupuncture and Meridian Studies*, *5*(3), 97–103. 10.1016/j.jams.2012.03.001

Bloch-Szentágothai, K. (1991). Hypnose und Regionalanasthesie beim Kind. *Hypnose Bulletin*, *16*.

Cheek, D. B. (1969). Communication with the critically ill. *American Journal of Clinical Hypnosis*, *12*(2), 75–85. 10.1080/00029157.1969.10734309

Corradi, R. B. (1983). Psychological regression with illness. *Psychosomatics*, *24*(4), 353–362. 10.1016/s0033-3182(83)73214-7

Dutt-Gupta, J., Bown, T., & Cyna, A. M. (2007). Effect of communication on pain during intravenous cannulation: A randomized controlled trial. *British Journal of Anaesthesia*, *99*(6), 871–875. 10.1093/bja/aem308

Egbert, L. D., Battit, G. E., Welch, C. E., & Bartlett, M. K. (1964). Reduction of postoperative pain by encouragement and instruction of patients: A study of doctor-patient rapport. *The New England Journal of Medicine*, *270*(16), 825–827. 10.1056/nejm196404162701606

Ewin, D. M. (1983). Emergency room hypnosis for the burned patient. *American Journal of Clinical Hypnosis*, *26*(1), 5–8. 10.1080/00029157.1983.10404130

Farthing, G. W. (1992). *The psychology of consciousness*. Prentice Hall.

Field, N. (1992). The therapeutic function of altered states. *Journal of Analytical Psychology*, *37*(2), 211–234. 10.1111/j.1465-5922.1992.00211.x

Kekecs, Z., Jakubovits, E., Varga, K., & Gombos, K. (2014). Effects of patient education and therapeutic suggestions on cataract surgery patients: A randomized controlled clinical trial. *Patient Education and Counseling*, *94*(1), 116–122. 10.1016/j.pec.2013.09.019

Kekecs, Z., Nagy, T., & Varga, K. (2014). The effectiveness of suggestive techniques in reducing postoperative side effects: A meta-analysis of randomized controlled trials. *Anesthesia & Analgesia*, *119*(6), 1407–1419. 10.1213/ane.0000000000000466

Kekecs, Z., & Varga, K. (2013). Positive suggestion techniques in somatic medicine: A review of the empirical studies. *Interventional Medicine and Applied Science*, *5*(3), 101–111. 10.1556/imas.5.2013.3.2

Kuttner, L. (2012). Pediatric hypnosis: pre-, peri-, and post-anesthesia. *Paediatric Anaesthesia*, *22*(6), 573–577. 10.1111/j.1460-9592.2012.03860.x

Lang, E. V., Benotsch, E. G., Fick, L. J., Lutgendorf, S., Berbaum, M. L., Berbaum, K. S., Logan, H., & Spiegel, D. (2000). Adjunctive non-pharmacological analgesia for invasive medical procedures: A randomised trial. *The Lancet*, *355*(9214), 1486–1490. 10.1016/s0140-6736(00)02162-0

Lang, E. V., & Rosen, M. P. (2002). Cost analysis of adjunct hypnosis with sedation during outpatient interventional radiologic procedures. *Radiology*, *222*(2), 375–382. 10.1148/radiol.2222010528

Ludwig, A. M. (1996). *Altered states of consciousness*. In Trat T. C. (Ed.), Altered states of consciousness (pp. 11-24). Doubleday.

Meurisse, M., Defechereux, T., Hamoir, E., Maweja, S., Marchettini, P., Gollogly, L., Degauque, C., Joris, J., & Faymonville, M. E. (1999). Hypnosis with conscious sedation instead of general anaesthesia? Applications in cervical endocrine surgery. *Acta Chirurgica Belgica*, *99*(4), 151–158. 10.1080/00015458.1999.12098468

Montgomery, G. H., David, D., Winkel, G., Silverstein, J. H., & Bovbjerg, D. H. (2002). The effectiveness of adjunctive hypnosis with surgical patients: A meta-analysis. *Anesthesia & Analgesia*, *94*(6), 1639–1645. 10.1097/00000539-200206000-00052

Nowak, H., Zech, N., Asmussen, S., Rahmel, T., Tryba, M., Oprea, G., Grause, L. W., Schork, K., Moeller, M., Loeser, J., Gyarmati, K., Mittler, C., Saller, T., Zagler, A., Lutz, K. A., Adamzik, M., & Hansen, E. (2020). Effect of therapeutic suggestions during general anaesthesia on post-operative pain and opioid use: Multicentre randomised controlled trial. *British Medical Journal*, *371*(8273:m4284), 510–511. 10.1136/bmj.m4284

Szeverényi, C., Csernátony, Z., Balogh, Á., Simon, T., & Varga, K. (2016). Effects of positive suggestions on the need for red blood cell transfusion in orthopedic surgery. *International Journal of Clinical and Experimental Hypnosis*, *64*(4), 404–418. 10.1080/00207144.2016.1209041

Szilágyi, A. K., Diószeghy, C., Fritúz, G., Gál, J., & Varga, K. (2014). Shortening the length of stay and mechanical ventilation time by using positive suggestions via MP3 players for ventilated patients. *Interventional Medicine and Applied Science*, *6*(1), 3–15. 10.1556/imas.6.2014.1.1

Trustmanz, R., Dubovsky, S., & Titley, R. (1977). Auditory perception during general anesthesia-myth or fact? *International Journal of Clinical and Experimental Hypnosis*, *25*(2), 88–105. 10.1080/00207147708415969

Tzovara, A., Simonin, A., Oddo, M., Rossetti, A. O., & De Lucia, M. (2015). Neural detection of complex sound sequences in the absence of consciousness. *Brain*, *138*(5), 1160–1166. 10.1093/brain/awv041

Varelmann, D., Pancaro, C., Cappiello, E., & Camann, W. (2010). Nocebo-induced hyperalgesia during local anesthetic injection. *Anesthesia & Analgesia*, *110*(3), 868–870. 10.1213/ane.0b013e3181cc5727

Varga, K. (Ed.). (2011). *Beyond the words: Communication and suggestion in medical practice*. Nova Science Publishers.

Varga, K. (2013). Suggestive techniques connected to medical interventions. *Interventional Medicine and Applied Science*, *5*(3), 95–100. 10.1556/imas.5.2013.3.1

Varga, K. (2015). *Communication strategies in medical settings: Challenging situations and practical solutions*. PL Academic Research.

Wang, F., Shen, X., Xu, S., Liu, Y., Ma, L., Zhao, Q., Fu, D., Pan, Q., Feng, S., & Li, X. (2008). Negative words on surgical wards result in therapeutic failure of patient-controlled analgesia and further release of cortisol after abdominal surgeries. *Minerva Anestesiologica*, *74*(7–8), 353–365.

Ziss, M. (2020). Pre-trauma growth under terror threat: Suggestive communication method in anticipatory trauma. *International Journal of Clinical and Experimental Hypnosis*, *68*(4), 475–482. 10.1080/00207144.2020.1799712

48

BLEEDING, HEMOSTASIS

Suggestive Techniques

Csenge Szeverényi

Department of Orthopedic Surgery, University of Debrecen, Debrecen, Hungary

Every year, 310 million major operations are performed worldwide, 40–50 million in the US, and 20 million in Europe (Dobson, 2020). This stunning number has been rising steadily since 2004 (Weiser et al., 2015), making the quality of patient care and ensuring the most effective recovery more and more important. Stress around surgeries results in activation of the body's sympathetic discharge (Desborough, 2000). The sympathetic response is a highly complex physiological phenomenon, all the components of which are still unknown, but changes in hemodynamic parameters may also occur to maintain hemostasis and ensure survival (Giannoudis et al., 2006).

Hemostasis, Bleeding, Coagulation

Hemostasis in the body is such a mechanism that ensures that blood retains its fluid state within the vessels but creates a local blood clot as it leaves them. It has three phases: vascular reaction, platelet reaction, and coagulation. During the vascular reaction, the smooth muscle of the damaged vessel segment contracts, and the vessel lumen narrows to minimize blood loss. During the platelet reaction, platelets attach to the collagen fibers of the damaged vascular segment and accumulate. Meanwhile, the proteolytic chain reaction of coagulation factors leads to the formation of fibrin, which forms a mesh. Formed elements are also incorporated into the fibrin mesh, which creates the red thrombus. After the vascular injury heals, the clot that has formed dissolves over a few days, a process called fibrinolysis. In this case, tissue plasminogen activator (tPA) converts the plasminogen into plasmin, which dissolves the fibrin (Fonyó, 1999).

Disruption of hemostasis may be associated with increased tendency to bleeding (e.g., hemophilia A, B, C) or to thrombosis (Fonyó, 1999).

Factors Affecting Bleeding during Surgery

The amount of bleeding during surgery is significantly affected by the surgical technique. The aim is to work quickly and atraumatically. Patient positioning, use of electrocautery, tourniquets, vasoconstrictors, and topical or systemic (e.g., tranexamic acid) drugs are

 DOI: 10.4324/9781003449126-63

important. There have been several studies showing that tranexamic acid reduces the amount of transfusion for large joint replacement, but it is not available everywhere and it may increase the risk of thromboembolic complications (Charoencholvanich, 2011; de Jonge, 2012; Lee et al., 2013; Yang et al., 2012).

During anesthesia, controlled low blood pressure usually helps to reduce bleeding accompanied by appropriate infusion and, if necessary, targeted factor replacement. However, bleeding often increases when the blood pressure temporarily increases. The patient's body temperature is ideally normothermic, which is achieved at an ambient temperature of 21 degrees Celsius. Low hemoglobin levels and acidosis may result in increased bleeding (Kozek-Langenecker et al., 2017; Shander et al., 2012; Spahn & Goodnough, 2013).

Consequences of Perioperative Bleeding, Transfusion

Though pain and anxiety are two of the most common problems around major surgeries for patients, but blood loss can also have a significant impact on patient recovery. Perioperative bleeding of varying severity is very common in cardiac surgery, which has been shown to increase thromboembolic complications, the number of surgical re-explorations, and infection rates. These also lead to an increase in mortality (Buccheri et al., 2019; Ranucci et al., 2013). Postoperative bleeding during tonsillectomies increases the number of second surgeries (Albright et al., 2020).

If blood loss has reached a certain level, red blood cell transfusion should be given. Although nowadays transfusion is considered safe, it is not a risk-free intervention. Transfusion may be associated with immediate (hemolysis, thrombolysis, fever, anaphylaxis, lung injury) and delayed (hemolysis, purpura, graft versus host disease) immunological and non-immunological (hemolysis, sepsis, infections, circulatory overload, coagulopathy, air embolism) reactions (Baróti-Tóth et al, 2016; Daurat & Renaudier, 2012). Several studies have demonstrated that patients undergoing hip and knee replacement surgery have an increased incidence of complications (dislocation, infection, wound healing disorder, urinary tract infection, pneumonia, deep vein thrombosis, myocardial infarction) and increased length of hospital stay in case of receiving transfusions compared to patients not receiving them (Abbas et al., 2012; Innerhofer et al., 2005; Jonas et al., 2013). Similar complications have been found in patients requiring transfusion after surgery for hip fracture (Carson et al., 1999).

In addition, the preparation and administration of transfusions is a burden on healthcare staff, and blood products also represent a significant cost burden for institutions.

In view of the above, it is understandable that reducing the need for transfusions is a priority for these operations.

The Relationship between Bleeding and Mental State

A review of the literature shows that there is a correlation between patients' mental state and bleeding. Either physical or mental stress can lead to an imbalance of hemostasis, which can be associated with hypercoagulability, i.e., a tendency toward thrombosis, and increased fibrinolysis, i.e., increased tendency to bleeding (Hoirisch-Clapauch, 2018). Anxiety increases the levels of several clotting factors and platelet aggregability in the body. These are predisposing factors for the development of thrombosis. At the same time, tPA is released from the cells at higher levels, resulting in increased fibrinolysis. If the balance between the prothrombotic state and increased fibrinolysis is tipped in favor of fibrinolysis, the tendency to bleeding is increased. Such a phenomenon can also occur when stress causes epistaxis (Seidel et al., 2017), hypermenorrhea (Thomas, 2011), or when the number of bleeding episodes in hemophiliac patients increases (Fung, 1983; Hoirisch-Clapauch, 2018).

Based on the above, it is obvious that in addition to mechanical and pharmacological hemostatic treatments, there is a third potential option to reduce blood loss during surgery: the use of psychological methods such as relaxation, suggestion, and hypnosis, which can effectively complement medical interventions.

Brief Review of Literature – Psychological Techniques to Reduce Blood Loss

A review of the literature reveals studies in which hypnosis and therapeutic suggestions have been used to control bleeding, although the number of such studies is not yet large.

Enqvist (1995) used hypnosis before and during surgery in patients undergoing maxillofacial surgery in general anesthesia. The hypnosis was played from a tape recorder. The 17 minutes of audio material started with hypnosis induction, followed by direct and indirect suggestion and metaphors to promote healing and reduce bleeding. Suggestions for maintaining low blood pressure were also used. 60 patients were included in the control group and 60 in the hypnosis group. The hypnosis patients were divided into three groups: (1) hypnosis was given only preoperatively, (2) hypnosis was given pre- and intraoperatively, and (3) hypnosis was used only in the intraoperative period. In all three groups, a reduction in blood loss was found compared to the control group. The biggest reduction was in the group who listened to hypnosis before surgery. Hypnotisability showed no correlation with the amount of blood loss (Enqvist & Bystedt, 1995).

Hart investigated the effect of tape-recorded hypnosis applied preoperatively on blood loss reduction in 40 patients undergoing cardiopulmonary bypass surgery (Hart, 1980). The study found that patients required significantly fewer transfusions in the postoperative period.

In our own study, hip and knee replacement surgery patients received preoperative (in person) and intraoperative (audiotaped) therapeutic suggestions, aimed at improving recovery and reducing the need for transfusion. Compared to the control group (50 patients), the percentage of patients in the suggestion group (45 patients) who did not need transfusion was significantly higher (Szeverényi et al., 2016).

Bensen (1971) used personal suggestions in the immediate postoperative period in 100 patients undergoing small surgical procedures. Bleeding was 90% controlled in the suggestion group (Bensen, 1971).

Bennett et al. (1986) used suggestive techniques without hypnosis in patients undergoing spinal surgery, with which they could reduce the estimated blood loss during surgery (Bennett et al., 1986).

Lucas (1975) has used hypnosis successfully in oral surgery for hemophilia patients for decades. Among other things, the suggestions aimed to reduce saliva production and pain in addition to reduce bleeding. Regarding the control of capillary bleeding, he used the image of severe cold, contraction of blood vessels, and numbness of the surgical site (Lucas, 1975).

Opposing the above results, Rapkin et al. (1991) were unable to achieve a reduction in bleeding with preoperative hypnosis at head and neck surgery (Rapkin et al., 1991). Similarly bleeding control could not be achieved by Ross (1981), who used hypnosis to reduce bleeding and oedema in 18 patients undergoing oral surgery (Ross, 1981). In a study by Hopkins et al. (1991), they investigated under laboratory conditions whether bleeding from skin pouches caused by a device called Surgicut could be reduced by hypnotic suggestions. The hypnosis used failed to reduce the bleeding time in the involved 32 subjects (Hopkins et al., 1991). Peimani et al. (2017) showed that hypnosis did not significantly change the hemorrhage volume 24 and 48 hours after tooth extraction in 16 patients (Peimani et al., 2017). Efsun Ozgunay et al. (2019) investigated the effects of preoperative hypnosis on hemorrhage in open septorhinoplasty. The authors found no difference in intraoperative bleeding between the control (11 patients) and suggestion (11 patients) groups (Efsun Ozgunay et al., 2019).

In the literature, we can also find reports where the hypnosis used was not to reduce bleeding around operations, but to change vascular diameters. This technique could also be used to reduce blood loss in certain cases. Klapow et al. (1996) presented the case of a male patient with Bürger's disease (severe lower limb arteriosclerosis), where the threat of amputation was avoided by hypnotic suggestions aiming the increase of circulation. The study also showed a measurable change in lower limb temperature and a significant reduction in pain (Klapow et al., 1996). Badiul et al. (2019) used 50–60 minutes of hypnosis in 18 patients undergoing plastic surgery to achieve a detectable improvement in blood flow of the transplanted perforator flap (perforator flap is a skin flap having a supplying vessel coming from deeper structures; it is used to reconstruct a part of the body) (Badiul et al., 2019). Reinhard et al. (2009) found cardiotocography-detectable improvement in the circulation of the umbilical artery during hypnosis in six pregnant women (Reinhard et al., 2009). Zachariae et al. (1994) were able to influence skin blood flow with hypnotic suggestions in ten highly hypnotizable erythematous (red inflammatory skin reaction) patients (Zachariae et al., 1994).

Mechanism of Action of the Interventions

The pathophysiological mechanism underlying the reduced blood loss induced by suggestions is not clearly understood. Several possibilities have been proposed as explanations. One possibility is that the interventions put patients in a more relaxed state, which in itself may directly help to maintain hemostasis balance (Hoirisch-Clapauch S, 2018). A more balanced mental state may also have made patients' blood pressure lower and less volatile, which may also help reduce blood loss (Solovey & Milechnin, 1958). A third option is to directly change the vessels diameters (Badiul et al., 2019; Klapow et al., 1996; Reinhard et al., 2009; Zachariae et al., 1994).

It is known that hypnosis can effectively modulate the autonomic nervous system activity, which modulates the arterial vasoconstriction and the blood pressure as well (De Benedittis et al., 1994). This also means that these three hypothetical "attack points" (anxiety relief – blood pressure reduction – vessel diameter reduction) may be correlated. Only a few studies in the literature have investigated simultaneously the changes in both the amount of blood loss and the patient's blood pressure under hypnosis (Enqvist et al., 1995; Hart, 1980). Enqvist et al. (1995) used targeted therapeutic suggestions to reduce blood loss and blood pressure, while Hart used relaxation techniques under hypnosis (Enqvist et al., 1995; Hart, 1980). Surprisingly, no clear correlation between patients' blood pressure and blood loss was found in either study. However, these studies also have their limitations; they worked with relatively small numbers of cases and did not record mean blood pressure, so further, better designed studies are needed to explore the relationships and effects.

Suggestion Techniques with or without Hypnosis

In the literature review above, we found many examples of hypnosis being used well around surgery, but there are also examples of therapeutic suggestions being used by researchers without formal hypnosis induction. In the latter case, we hypothesize that in the hospital setting, in the stressful situation of surgery, patients' mental states spontaneously shift to a state where they become more receptive to suggestions (Varga, 2017). This can be well exploited in clinical practice for the use of therapeutic suggestions.

When we want to use suggestions to reduce blood loss, we can give direct suggestions, but considering the possible mechanisms of action mentioned above, we can also use suggestions aiding to relax the patients. To increase effectiveness, the method of repetition may also be useful.

Below are examples of suggestion already used to reduce bleeding:

> *...Your body knows that you are undergoing a sterile, clean procedure, of which you are prepared for, of which you can safely undergo ... There is no need for bleeding, nor inflammation ... No need for bleeding, nor inflammation ... Your blood circulation and the tightness of your muscles is precisely matched to help the surgery progress and to help your recovery ... Your body will only let that amount of blood to the surgical site which provide just enough nourishment and oxygen to the tissues. This is enough to create a healthy, well-closed, nice surface ... The rest of the blood flows to other parts of the body ... The rest of the blood flows to other parts of the body ... During the operation, just enough blood is supplied to the tissues. Your body knows this all by itself, which gives you peace of mind....*
>
> *(Szeverényi, 2020, pp. 33–34)*

The effectiveness of the suggestions is increased if we do not expect the patients to be voluntary, i.e. if we do not ask them to tighten his veins to lose less blood, but if we draw attention to the spontaneous, natural process that occurs involuntarily (Varga, 2017).

> *As well as being able to digest or breathe, your body knows how to let the right amount of blood to the surgical site to nourish the tissues and create well-healed, fused surfaces ....*
>
> *(Szeverényi, 2020, p. 29)*

Confusion techniques can also be used:

> *You may notice a particular sensation when the blood stops flowing to that area, or you may simply be aware that you can stop the bleeding without being quite sure how you know it.*
>
> *(Godot, 2016, p. 67)*

Dünzl (2011) listed several suggestion possibilities in his publication:

Your arm is getting number and number. Bleeding ***is going to stop.***

I am going to clean the wound. A little bleeding would be very helpful. And soon as the wound is clean you can stop the bleeding and healing will begin. Very good.

That's a really healthy, red blood you have. And now, you know you were bleeding enough that your wound was cleansed. You can begin to stop bleeding while I put the bandage on your arm. OK?

(Dünzl, 2011, p. 213)

Guided imagery can be used as well, for example, pictures of turning off or opening water taps:

You can start and stop bleeding by imagining turning a faucet for warm water on and off. See the faucet, feel the faucet in your hand. Switch it off, now! – tighter. Well done.

I'd like you to imagine workers in your blood vessels sealing the leaking spot. Your blood pressure is being stabilized. And I would recommend thinking about these images on the way to the hospital....

(Dünzl, 2011, p. 213)

The more acute and dramatic the situation, the more serious the threat, the more likely the patient is to respond to a direct suggestion:

Stop bleeding! Now!

(Dünzl, 2011, p. 213)

Indirect suggestion can also be used, where we then make the patient an active participant, giving the patient a sense of control:

When the bleeding stops soon on your arm/jaw, please place the ice on your elbow/face etc.

(Dünzl, 2011, p. 213)

Rossi and Cheek (1994) have successfully used suggestions in the field of obstetrics:

If you want to see your child stop the bleeding NOW.

(Rossi & Cheek, 1994, p. 191)

A nice example of the yes-set can be seen in the following suggestion:

I imagine the injury must be very painful and you may have been frightened by this cut. You're bleeding a lot. And it may bleed even more - yet it will stop - now!

(Dünzl, 2011, p. 213)

It can also help to use existing memories, for example, if you are bleeding, to imagine what it was like to dip your hands or feet in icy water (Trenkle, 2011).

Clinical Usage

According to the literature and case reports, suggestions, whether used under hypnosis or without hypnosis induction, can help patients to heal and reduce blood loss. In clinical practice, we find that the role of suggestive communication is significantly underestimated, from the perspective of surgeons, anesthetists, and other health professionals. Of course, suggestive techniques are primarily a complement to, and not a substitute for, professional medical care, but they can aid patients' recovery.

Audio materials can be listened to before, during, and after planned surgery. For the more common types of surgery, these can be pre-recorded, but they can also be personalized for one certain intervention. Varga (2019) provides an excellent guide on how to create a personalized suggestion soundtrack when preparing for surgery (Varga, 2019). Where possible, personal presence can make hypnotic suggestions even more effective. In some cases, the two methods (face-to-face interview + audio material) can be combined. The effectiveness is likely to be increased if the intervention can be repeated. Our previous meta-analysis pointed out that psychological interventions are more effective for acute surgeries than for planned surgeries, i.e., they should be used when we feel we do not have the time or when unexpected situations mean that we do not have the standardized tools available (Szeverényi et al., 2018). Though with proper organization and preparation, this problem could be solved in most circumstances. For example, any healthcare professional can learn to use suggestive communication. The use of suggestions becomes automatic after a more conscious period of time, the terms and techniques used become part of the daily routine, so they can be easily used in emergency situations as well as without hypnosis induction (Dünzl, 2011; Tanenbaum, 2005). Suggestions were also used with good results in emergency situations by EMS (emergency medical services) personnel, who had to recite a pre-rehearsed text to each patient (Dünzl, 2011). Learning suggestion techniques also help to avoid the unintentional use of negative suggestions around patients.

Research Goals and Difficulties

Reports and meta-analyses in the literature suggest that the effectiveness of hypnosis and suggestion techniques around surgery, for example in reducing bleeding, is important and worth investigating in better designed clinical trials.

Our own practice and experience have shown us that it is very difficult to measure the amount of blood loss directly, since during the operations some of the blood flows onto the textiles, some of it is soaked up with wipes, and the rest is collected in a tank with the help of a suction system. Neither the amount of blood on the textiles nor the blood in the wipes can be measured well, nor is the secretion in the container pure blood since the surgical site is sometimes washed with physiological saline or disinfectant solution. The measurement inaccuracies make it easier and more accurate to record the number of red blood cell transfusions required during the operation rather than the blood loss, but this is an indirect parameter, and its value may be influenced by other factors (e.g., who indicated the transfusion).

It would also be interesting to explore the mechanism of action of suggestions, to record the mean blood pressure during surgeries and compare this with the blood loss, or to find a correlation between some parameters of hemostasis (e.g., tPA) and hypnosis.

Based on the studies so far, we do not know clearly whether the effect of the suggestions is actually due to the suggestions, or to the patient more relaxed state, or perhaps just due to the extra care they receive. It may also be worth investigating whether preoperative or intraoperative suggestions are more effective.

The accuracy of studies is increased if the participating patients' hypnotizability/suggestibility is measured before the study, if hypnosis is performed under standardized conditions, e.g., by playing an audio recording.

Double (triple) blind design is important for good quality research. This is usually not feasible in the operating theater due to the nature of the intervention, but it is worth striving for it.

References

Abbas, K., Murtaza, G., Umer, M., Rashid, H., & Qadir, I. (2012). Complications of total hip replacement. *Journal of the College of Physicians and Surgeons Pakistan: JCPSP*, *22*(9), 575–578.

Albright, J. T., Duncan, N. O., Smerica, A. M., & Edmonds, J. L. (2020). Intra-capsular complete tonsillectomy, a modification of surgical technique to eliminate delayed post-operative bleeding. *International Journal of Pediatric Otorhinolaryngology*, *128*, 109703. 10.1016/j.ijporl.2019.109703

Badiul, P. O., Sliesarenko, S. V., Saliaiev, M. G., & Kriachkova, L. V. (2019). Hypnosis influence on the perfusion in perforator flaps in early postoperative period. *Plastic and Reconstructive Surgery – Global Open*, *7*(11), e2491. 10.1097/gox.0000000000002491.

Baróti-Tóth, K. C. Z., Hoffer, I., Jenei, B., Szekeres, V., Vörös, K. (2016). *Transzfúziós szabályzat.*

Bennett, H. L., Benson, D. R., & Kuiken, D. A. (1986). Preoperative instructions for decreased bleeding during spine surgery. *Anesthesiology*, *65*(Supplement 3A), A245.

Bensen, V. B. (1971). One hundred cases of post-anesthetic suggestion in the recovery room. *American Journal of Clinical Hypnosis*, *14*(1), 9–15. 10.1080/00029157.1971.10402137

Buccheri, S., Capodanno, D., James, S., & Angiolillo, D. J. (2019). Bleeding after antiplatelet therapy for the treatment of acute coronary syndromes: A review of the evidence and evolving paradigms. *Expert Opinion on Drug Safety*, *18*(12), 1171–1189. 10.1080/14740338.2019.1680637

Carson, J., Altman, D., Duff, A., Noveck, H., Weinstein, M., Sonnenberg, F., Hudson, J., & Provenzano, G. (1999). Risk of bacterial infection associated with allogeneic blood transfusion among patients undergoing hip fracture repair. *Transfusion*, *39*(7), 694–700. 10.1046/j.1537-2995.1999.39070694.x

Charoencholvanich, K., & Siriwattanasakul, P. (2011). Tranexamic acid reduces blood loss and blood transfusion after TKA: A prospective randomized controlled trial. *Clinical Orthopaedics and Related Research*, *469*(10), 2874–2880. 10.1007/s11999-011-1874-2

Daurat, G., & Renaudier, P. (2012). Risques spécifiques de la transfusion en médecine [Specific hazards of transfusion in medical units]. *Transfusion Clinique Et Biologique*, *19*(4–5), 206–211. 10.1016/j.tracli.2012.07.002

De Benedittis, G., Cigada, M., Bianchi, A., Signorini, M. G., & Cerutti, S. (1994). Autonomic changes during hypnosis: A heart rate variability power spectrum analysis as a marker of sympatho-vagal balance. *International Journal of Clinical and Experimental Hypnosis*, *42*(2), 140–152. 10.1080/00207149408409347

de Jonge, T. (2012). Pharmacological reduction of bleeding during hip endoprosthetic replacement, *Orvosi Hetilap*, *153*(41), 1607–1612. 10.1556/oh.2012.29455

Desborough, J. (2000). The stress response to trauma and surgery. *British Journal of Anaesthesia*, *85*(1), 109–117. 10.1093/bja/85.1.109

Dobson, G. P. (2020). Trauma of major surgery: A global problem that is not going away. *International Journal of Surgery*, *81*, 47–54. 10.1016/j.ijsu.2020.07.017

Dünzl, G. (2011). Suggestive communication in somatic medical emergencies. In K. Varga (Ed.), *Beyond the words: Communication and suggestion in medical practice* (1st ed., pp. 209–222). Nova Science Publishers.

Efsun Ozgunay, S., Ozmen, S., Karasu, D., Yilmaz, C., & Taymur, I. (2019). The Effect of hypnosis on intraoperative hemorrhage and postoperative pain in rhinoplasty. *International Journal of Clinical and Experimental Hypnosis*, *67*(3), 262–277. 10.1080/00207144.2019.1612670

Enqvist, B., Konow, L. V., & Bystedt, H. (1995). Pre- and perioperative suggestion in maxillofacial surgery: Effects on blood loss and recovery. *International Journal of Clinical and Experimental Hypnosis*, *43*(3), 284–294. 10.1080/00207149508409971

Fonyó, A. (1999). *Az orvosi élettan tankönyve. [Textbook of medical physiology.]* Medicina Könyvkiadó Rt.

Fung, E. H., & Lazar, B. S. (1983). Hypnosis as an adjunct in the treatment of von Willebrand's disease. *International Journal of Clinical and Experimental Hypnosis*, *31*(4), 256–265. 10.1080/00207148308406621

Giannoudis, P. V., Dinopoulos, H., Chalidis, B., & Hall, G. M. (2006). Surgical stress response. *Injury*, *37*, S3–S9. 10.1016/s0020-1383(07)70005-0

Godot, D. (2016). Formulating hypnotic suggestions. In R. Elkins (Ed.), *Handbook of medical and psychological hypnosis: Foundations, applications, and professional issues* (1st ed., pp. 57–68). Springer Publishing Company.

Hart, R. R. (1980). The influence of a taped hypnotic induction treatment procedure on the recovery of surgery patients. *International Journal of Clinical and Experimental Hypnosis*, *28*(4), 324–332. 10.1080/00207148008409861

Hoirisch-Clapauch, S. (2018). Anxiety-related bleeding and thrombosis. *Seminars in Thrombosis and Hemostasis*, *44*(07), 656–661. 10.1055/s-0038-1639501

Hopkins, M. B., Jordan, J. M., & Lundy, R. M. (1991). The effects of hypnosis and of imagery on bleeding time. *International Journal of Clinical and Experimental Hypnosis*, *39*(3), 134–139. 10. 1080/00207149108409629

Innerhofer, P., Klingler, A., Klimmer, C., Fries, D., & Nussbaumer, W. (2005). Risk for postoperative infection after transfusion of white blood cell-filtered allogeneic or autologous blood components in orthopedic patients undergoing primary arthroplasty. *Transfusion*, *45*(1), 103–110. 10.1111/j.1537-2995.2005.04149.x

Jonas, S. C., Smith, H. K., Blair, P. S., Dacombe, P., & Weale, A. E. (2013). Factors influencing length of stay following primary total knee replacement in a UK specialist orthopaedic centre. *The Knee*, *20*(5), 310–315. 10.1016/j.knee.2012.07.010

Klapow, J. C., Patterson, D. R., & Edwards, W. T. (1996). Hypnosis as an adjunct to medical care in the management of Burger's disease: A case report. *American Journal of Clinical Hypnosis*, *38*(4), 271–276. 10.1080/00029157.1996.10403351

Kozek-Langenecker, S. A., Ahmed, A. B., Afshari, A., Albaladejo, P., Aldecoa, C., Barauskas, G., De Robertis, E., Faraoni, D., Filipescu, D. C., Fries, D., Haas, T., Jacob, M., Lancé, M. D., Pitarch, J. V., Mallett, S., Meier, J., Molnar, Z. L., Rahe-Meyer, N., Samama, C. M., …Zacharowski, K. (2017). Management of severe perioperative bleeding. *European Journal of Anaesthesiology*, *34*(6), 332–395. 10.1097/eja.0000000000000630

Lee, S. H., Cho, K. Y., Khurana, S., & Kim, K. I. (2013). Less blood loss under concomitant administration of tranexamic acid and indirect factor Xa inhibitor following total knee arthroplasty: A prospective randomized controlled trial. *Knee Surgery, Sports Traumatology, Arthroscopy*, *21*(11), 2611–2617. 10.1007/s00167-012-2213-1

Lucas, O. N. (1975). The use of hypnosis in hemophilia dental care. *Annals of the New York Academy of Sciences*, *240*, 263–266. 10.1111/j.1749-6632.1975.tb53358.x

Peimani, A., Irannezhad, M., & Ahmadi, A. M. (2017). Comparing the effect of hypnosis and local anesthesia injection on induction of local anesthesia, anxiety, hemorrhage and pain control during tooth extraction. *Journal of Research in Medical and Dental Science*, *5*(4), 44–49. http://eprints.rums.ac.ir/4337/

Ranucci, M., Baryshnikova, E., Castelvecchio, S., & Pelissero, G. (2013). Major bleeding, transfusions, and anemia: The deadly triad of cardiac surgery. *Annals of Thoracic Surgery*, *96*(2), 478–485. 10.1016/j.athoracsur.2013.03.015

Rapkin, D. A., Straubing, M., & Holroyd, J. C. (1991). Guided imagery, hypnosis and recovery from head and neck cancer surgery: An exploratory study. *International Journal of Clinical and Experimental Hypnosis*, *39*(4), 215–226. 10.1080/00207149108409637

Reinhard, J., Hüsken-Janßen, H., Hatzmann, H., & Schiermeier, S. (2009). Veränderung des Gefäßwiderstands der Arteria umbilicalis, der fetalen Bewegung und der Herzzeitvariation durch Hypnose – Erste Ergebnisse. [Changes in resistance of the umbilical artery, foetal movements and short time variation through clinical hypnosis – Preliminary results] *Zeitschrift Für Geburtshilfe Und Neonatologie, 213*(01), 23–26. 10.1055/s-0028-1128127

Ross, D. (1981). *The use of hypnosis in the control of surgical bleeding and postoperative edema* [Doctoral Dissertation]. The Fielding Institute ProQuest Dissertations Publishing, 1981. 8221800.

Rossi, E. L., & Cheek, D. B. (1994). *Mind-body therapy: Methods of ideodynamic healing in hypnosis.* W. W. Norton.

Seidel, D., Jacob, L., Kostev, K., & Sesterhenn, A. (2017). Risk factors for epistaxis in patients followed in general practices in Germany. *Rhinology Journal, 55*(4), 312–318. 10.4193/rhin17.105

Shander, A., Van Aken, H., Colomina, M., Gombotz, H., Hofmann, A., Krauspe, R., Lasocki, S., Richards, T., Slappendel, R., & Spahn, D. (2012). Patient blood management in Europe. *British Journal of Anaesthesia, 109*(1), 55–68. 10.1093/bja/aes139

Solovey, G., & Milechnin, A. (1958). Some points regarding hypnosis in dentistry. *American Journal of Clinical Hypnosis, 1*(2), 59–77. 10.1080/00029157.1958.10734337

Spahn, D. R., & Goodnough, L. T. (2013). Alternatives to blood transfusion. *The Lancet, 381*(9880), 1855–1865. 10.1016/s0140-6736(13)60808-9

Szeverényi, C., Csernátony, Z., Balogh, G., & Varga, K. (2013). Examples of positive suggestions given to patients undergoing orthopaedic surgeries. *Interventional Medicine and Applied Science, 5*(3), 112–115. 10.1556/imas.5.2013.3.3

Szeverényi, C. (2020). *Pszichoterápiás módszerek alkalmazásának lehetőségei ortopédiai, traumatológiai műtétek során (Possible use psychotherapeutic methods during orthopaedic and traumatological operations)* [PhD dissertation]. Hungary: Univesity of Debrecen.

Szeverényi, C., Csernátony, Z., Balogh, G., Simon, T., & Varga, K. (2016). Effects of positive suggestions on the need for red blood cell transfusion in orthopedic surgery. *International Journal of Clinical and Experimental Hypnosis, 64*(4), 404–418. 10.1080/00207144.2016.1209041

Szeverényi, C., Kekecs, Z., Johnson, A., Elkins, G., Csernatony, Z., & Varga, K. (2018). The use of adjunct psychosocial interventions can decrease postoperative pain and improve the quality of clinical care in orthopedic surgery: A systematic review and meta-analysis of randomized controlled trials. *Journal of Pain, 19*(11), 1231–1252. 10.1016/j.jpain.2018.05.006

Tanenbaum, B. (2005). Ericksoni technikák vészhelyzetekben: Fájdalomkontroll. [Ericksonian techniques in emergencies: Pain control.]. In K. Varga (Ed.), *Szuggesztív kommunikáció a szomatikus orvoslásban [Positive suggestion techniques in somatic medicine]* (pp. 107–116). Országos Addiktológiai Intézet.

Thomas, M. C. (2011). Treatment options for dysfunctional uterine bleeding. *The Nurse Practitioner, 36*(8), 14–20. 10.1097/01.npr.0000399716.79607.39

Trenkle, B. (2011). Being a patient and utilizing and experiencing hypnosis and self-hypnosis during medical procedures. In K. Varga (Ed.), *Beyond the words: Communication and suggestion in medical practice* (1st ed., pp. 351–362). Nova Science Publishers.

Varga, K. (2019). Suggestive techniques for the management of postoperative pain. In M. Jensen (Ed.), *Hypnosis for acute and procedural pain management: Favorite methods of master clinicians* (pp. 26–47). Denny Creek Press.

Varga, K. (2017). Suggestive techniques without inductions for medical interventions. In M. Jensen (Ed.), *The art and practice of hypnotic induction: Favorite methods of master clinicians* (pp. 114–135). Denny Creek Press.

Weiser, T. G., Haynes, A. B., Molina, G., Lipsitz, S. R., Esquivel, M. M., Uribe-Leitz, T., Fu, R., Azad, T., Chao, T. E., Berry, W. R., & Gawande, A. A. (2015). Estimate of the global volume of surgery in 2012: An assessment supporting improved health outcomes. *The Lancet, 385*, S11. 10.1016/s0140-6736(15)60806-6

Yang, Z. G., Chen, W. P., & Wu, L. D. (2012). Effectiveness and safety of tranexamic acid in reducing blood loss in total knee arthroplasty. *The Journal of Bone and Joint Surgery, 94*(13), 1153–1159. 10.2106/jbjs.k.00873

Zachariae, R., Oster, H., & Bjerring, P. (1994). Effects of hypnotic suggestions on ultraviolet B radiation-induced erythema and skin blood flow. *Photodermatology, Photoimmunology and Photomedicine, 10*(4), 154–160.

49

EPILEPSY, STROKE AND PSYCHOSES AFTER TRAUMATIC BRAIN INJURY

Susanna Carolusson

PRIVATE PRACTICE GÖTEBORG, SWEDEN

In my profession as a hypnosis-competent psychologist and psychotherapist, I have been consulted to treat various psycho-neuro-somatic problems. Among those were patients with traumatic brain injuries (TBI), and epileptic seizures of known or unknown origin. Regarding evidence, I found a few case studies of hypnosis. These factors and a request for my hypnotic competence inspired me to learn more.

During three partly overlapping periods, I treated hundreds of patients with epilepsy, stroke and/or TBI. The first period started in 1980. A woman in her forties, with a 12-year history of severe epilepsy, unfortunate side effects from heavy medication and an imminent disability retirement, consulted me for hypnosis. After 12 sessions of hypnotherapy, she had developed a capacity to control and postpone her seizures. The predicted disability retirement did not occur. Her doctor, professor Olle Hambert, chief neurologist at Sahlgrenska University Hospital and well known in Sweden for his expertise on epilepsy, continued to refer patients with epilepsy to me during the following ten years, until his retirement.

The second period with brain injured patients started after my adult son's bicycle accident. To enhance his survival options, damaged left hemisphere tissue was surgically removed. The remaining brain was severely affected. I found myself treating my own son, motivated to be in tune and creative to an extent I hardly would have managed with someone less close. When my first book on this subject was published, I was frequently invited to teach and supervise rehab staff and personal assistants, with a focus on how to deal with aphasia, cognitive losses, loss of self-esteem, post-traumatic stress disorder and psychotic reactions. And finally, a third ten-year period suddenly presented itself in 2005, with several stroke patients being referred to me.

A few years after his TBI, my son developed psychotic episodes. My psychodynamic competence, and my experience with psychotic patients, provided me with the necessary skills to help him out of these psychotic states. This experience resulted in a second book on TBI (Carolusson, 2012).

 DOI: 10.4324/9781003449126-64

Epilepsy: Prevalence, Traditional Treatments and Their Limitations

According to the World Health Organization (WHO), globally an estimated 5 million people are diagnosed with epilepsy each year, with the estimated prevalence of active epilepsy in the general population ranging from 4 to 10 per 1000. Traditional treatment is the use of anti-seizure medicines. For those who do not respond to medicine, surgery may be an option (World Health Organization, 2023).

However, medication has its limitations. According to my clinical experience, confirmed by the neurologist Hambert, patients with major seizures have limited help from medication or suffer side effects of such severity that their quality of life is decreased. Reported side effects are weakening of skeletal bone structure, severe dermatitis, aggressive mood swings, confusion, apathy and inability to concentrate or initiate actions (Hambert, personal communication, 1985–1990).

Epilepsy and Rational for Hypnosis

Betts (2003) reported a pilot study, in which a combination of hypnosis, massage and aromatherapy had the best effect, compared to each treatment separately: "a mixture of aromatherapy, massage and simple hypnosis seems the most long-lasting in effect" (Betts, 2003, p. 537). In this study, "simple hypnosis" is defined as merely inducing a hypnotic state, but without any targeted suggestions. I believe that this explains the limited effect of hypnosis alone. However, as Betts (1992) discusses, the mere induction of the hypnotic state is well indicated for stress management. Since stress triggers seizures, hypnosis has a place as a preventive treatment (Betts, 1992).

Stroke: Prevalence, Traditional Treatments and Their Limitations

The prevalence of stroke is as high as 101 million (GBD 2019 Stroke Collaborators, 2021). In 2020, 13.7 million people suffered stroke annually (Markus et al., 2020).

Traditional treatments are physio-, logo- and occupational therapies. The treatment goal is rehabilitation, aimed at retrieving as much as possible of lost functions. Most stroke patients suffer from left hemispheric injury. In modern cultures, skills attributed to that hemisphere are indispensable for an independent life. Lesions affect verbal communication, logic, reason and the complex skills of putting data together into serial patterns or activities. Reading, writing, using a cell phone or computer, planning, organizing, cooking, dressing, brushing teeth and even the simple act of eating a meal involve serial organizational cognition and behavior.

Traditional treatments rarely deal with emotional and relational consequences such as confused identity, amnesia, loss of self-esteem and human dignity. These consequences inhibit the patients' curiosity and joy, thus decreasing the motivation to learn new skills or how to compensate for lost functions.

The need to treat emotional consequences is illustrated by neurologist Jill Taylor (2008). After her own stroke, she experienced a need to feel loved, not as the one she used to be, but as the one she was going to be. Her loss of left hemispheric functions made her incapable of linear thinking, and she needed to learn everything from scratch. She needed to meet people who had patience and a peaceful mind. Taylor (2008) used gestalt therapy in her search for a narrative to remember what exactly happened when she had her stroke.

She also practiced meditation and massage, thus utilizing the beneficial effects of the right hemisphere's dominance after her stroke, which resulted in an enhanced body awareness and a spiritual sense of meaning (Taylor, 2008).

Stroke and Rational for Hypnosis

A study of six people was designed utilizing hypnosis to help stroke patients regain motor activity. Hypnotic suggestions were made to "feel" an activity as they had before the stroke and to imagine muscular movements. It was hypothesized that this would stimulate neuromuscular connections. After hypnosis, they observed qualitative improvements in motor function, increased grip strength and reduced spasticity of the paretic limb. Subjects reported an improved outlook, increased motivation, greater awareness of and decreased effort to perform motor tasks (Diamond et al., 2006).

An experience of the use of night dreams in stroke rehabilitation was published by an expert on hypnosis (Rossi, 2005). Before his own stroke, Rossi (2004) published an epigenetic model of hypnotic healing, which gives us well-founded theories for understanding the efficacy of hypnosis in neurological rehabilitation. The essence of his model for stroke rehabilitation is the activation of memory traces. Hypnotherapy can evoke a "creative replay of activity-dependent gene expression, protein synthesis, and brain plasticity" (Rossi, 2005, p. 5).

Stroke patients often have aphasia, problems with abstract thinking and other complications as a result of left hemispheric injury. In clinical hypnosis, stroke patients are guided to focus on internal autonomic processes that are more connected to the right hemisphere such as breathing. For the same reason as Taylor (2008) recommends massage, I recommend hypnotic suggestions to stimulate kinesthetic perception and somatic awareness, with the aim of regenerating neuro-physiological connections and functionality, concurrent with Rossi's theory (Rossi, 2005). Hypnosis can also be used to lift amnesia and to discover new existential meaning. My clinical experience of hypnotic communication in a case with left hemispheric injury is illustrated in detail elsewhere (Carolusson, 2010, 2011).

Psychosis Following Traumatic Brain Injury: Prevalence, Traditional Treatments and Their Limitations

The diagnosis of psychosis following traumatic brain injury (PFTBI) is the presence of psychotic positive symptoms after an externally caused brain injury. Symptoms occur during the period of post-traumatic amnesia, in association with post-traumatic epilepsy, TBI-related mood disorders and/or as a chronic, schizophrenia-like syndrome.

Epidemiologic data are mixed and contradictory. Some claim that psychosis is a rare, but serious complication of TBI (McAllister & Ferrell, 2002). In 2003, Arciniegas wrote "Psychosis is a relatively infrequent but potentially serious and debilitating consequence of traumatic brain injury" (Arciniegas et al., 2003, p. 328). In a meta-analysis from 2011, the estimated risk of schizophrenia after TBI was 60% higher than for the general population (Molloy et al., 2011). Gurin and Arciniegas (2019) hypothesized an underdiagnosing of psychoses after TBI, because of a latency period of five years or more after the trauma, before psychosis was diagnosed. In Sweden, I have observed that neurologists regard psychotic symptoms as organically caused cognitive dysfunctions and rarely diagnose them as PFTBI.

The traditional treatment is medication (Fujii & Ahmed, 2002; McAllister & Ferrell, 2002). Lauterbach et al. (2015) pointed out that cognitive dysfunction is a problem for most patients, but medication has poor efficacy and behavioral side effects.

The poor efficacy and the negative side effects with pharmacological treatment of psychosis in general, not merely after TBI, are well documented by Whitaker (2010). He summarizes longitudinal studies, reporting a correlation between nonmedical psychosocial treatment and a decrease of psychotic symptoms, while those who were medicated had more lasting psychotic symptoms. Whitaker (2010) supports his drug skepticism with reference to MRI studies: the more medication, the more decrease of gray matter. He claims a causal correlation between neuroleptic blocking of basal ganglia activity and a deterioration of the prefrontal cortex (Whitaker, 2010).

I have seen indications that TBI patients who suffer psychosis regress to primitive functionality that may be considered as a defensive/protective avoidance of psychological insights and grief (Carolusson, 2012).

PFTBI and Rationales for Hypnosis

Patients suffering from TBI are rarely referred to psychotherapy, and even less so, if they have developed psychotic episodes. In discussions with neurologists and neuropsychologists, I have met a skepticism to hypnosis, in particular to trauma-oriented psychotherapy. Supportive coaching is sometimes considered, given it does not evoke emotional reactions.

However, patients with acquired left hemispheric injuries suffer not only from organic but also from emotional trauma. With faulty vocabulary and no narrative for the trauma, the trauma memories present themselves in right hemispheric psychotic language, that is, irrational, nonserial, illogical and symbolic. Hypnotherapists' familiarity with such language, known as "trance logic", gives them a privileged competence in the attempts to understand how to communicate with these patients. The skill to interpret trance logic is also needed, when patients during the process of gaining some insight in their trauma and its consequences temporarily relapse into psychosis, as an escape from an intimidating reality. How to deal with that from a hypnotic approach is described in my second book (Carolusson, 2012).

Measuring Outcome and Perspectives on Evidence

Treatment procedures are influenced by the explicit and implicit assumptions of what is a successful outcome, revealed in how outcome is measured. Traditionally, measurement instruments assess degree of symptoms before and after treatment. In TBI treatment, traditional measurements focus on functional improvement. Accordingly, treatment procedures focus on functional rehabilitation. However, given the unpredictability of these patients' prognosis, a long-term goal for optimal restoration of psychological, neurological and social resources moves via a labyrinth of progress, setbacks, impasses and unforeseen complications. In case of permanently lost functions, a goal can be to grieve and compensate for the losses, and to find new meaning of life. How to measure that?

Another complication is that in research study designs, treatment outcome and follow-ups are usually measured within planned intervals, but TBI patients rarely present stable recovery over time. When assessed, they may be in a temporary regression or progression which may confuse a traditional "outcome-measurer".

Outcome measure is also problematic with respect to amnesia and denial. TBI patients often have amnesia for their trauma. Besides hippocampal injury as a cause, a psychogenic denial is likely. Denial preserves self-esteem as it used to be. This is particularly obvious during the first years after trauma. Eventually, life itself confronts the bereaved with their limitations. During such periods, the patients need support to deal with setbacks, grief and lost self-esteem, to find a new meaning of life and accept the slower than expected progress.

Total acceptance of lost skills, or "insight", is rarely possible nor recommended. Most patients need hope for functional improvement. Fortunately, evidence of neuroplasticity supports a professional attitude of optimism (Khan et al., 2017; Patel, 2022). Rossi's early publications on how to influence neuronal circuits with hypnosis (Rossi, 2004; Rossi, 2005) support the clinical practice of hypnotic interventions to assist patients in their search for healing resources. For some patients, this is a condition for their motivation to engage in daily rehabilitation.

My hope is that we abandon the classical division between insight-oriented and future-oriented treatment. A certain insight is needed for motivation, because if psychological denial and amnesia are massive, they decrease motivation, causing a belief that the executive disabilities are nothing but parenthetic contextual nuisances.

Treatment needs to include awareness of the injury and its consequences, combined with curiosity and joy, affects that nourish self-esteem and motivation.

The emotional reactions that accompany insight are rarely addressed or measured in traditional treatment after TBI. Staff may mistake grief for depression and initiate medication. But if we clarify depressive symptoms as repressed grief, the patients are relieved that their dysphoria can be understood as a normal reaction to enormous loss. Regarding psychotic symptoms, I address them as symptoms to be decoded. This approach of finding a meaning fosters motivation, but it also prevents chronic depression. I use hypnosis as an adjunct to find resources from subconscious levels to deal with the emotional reactions.

Conclusively, in traditional measurement of outcome, "negative" emotional reactions may be mistaken as a lack of improvement. The treatment process and outcome measurements need to include not only functional improvements but also insight, the capacity and quality of life.

Outcome Measurement with Relevance for Relational Hypnosis

I suggest frequently interspersed assessments of patients' insight regarding injured functions, as a natural part of the treatment. I may ask: "How does your injury affect your everyday living, practically and in your relations?" I also suggest to patients to evaluate the therapist's capacity to evoke and use their unique resources for healing. I do that by observing the patients' reactions to my interventions and encourage them to give feedback to me regarding what works and what doesn't work, in their own opinion. When applicable, I invite next of kin to assess to what degree patients generalize therapeutic progress to everyday life.

Conclusively, since the effects of brain injuries are individually different, prognosis, treatment content and procedures have to be unique and individualized. Therefore, case studies and case publications will be more inspirational for future clinical development than statistically presented generalizations from such work.

Indications and Definition of Hypnosis in Treatment of Epilepsy, Stroke and PFTBI

There is a paucity of research on applied hypnosis for patients with brain injuries. Although some authors claim that hypnosis is contraindicated for psychoses or schizophrenia (Spiegel & Spiegel, 2004; Spiegel et al., 1982), my own and other colleagues' clinical and experimental evidence indicate that hypnosis can be constructively utilized (Baker, 1983; Brown & Fromm, 1986; Gafner & Young, 1998; Hodge, 1988; Murray-Jobsis, 1993; Pyun, 2013; Scagnelli, 1976). I consider psychosis to be a state of unwanted trance, and skilled hypnotherapists to have the competence to deal with trance states, whether they are wanted or not. Hypnotherapists understand the trance logic and therefore have the assets to help stabilize these patients (Carolusson, 2012). Baker (1981) illustrates in detail how to constructively utilize the psychotics' hypnotic state and seamlessly guide them into safe communication (Baker, 1981). However, I would only recommend hypnosis to be used with psychotic patients, given the therapist is experienced both with such patients and as a hypnotherapist.

Most patients with a brain injury need the hypnotic procedures to be individualized. If a patient resists hypnosis, it usually means the hypnotist has yet to find their unique way to enter, utilize and leave the state of trance. The question is not about "if" hypnosis, but "how". A hypnotherapist can be too authoritative and directive, or too vague and indirect. Patients with a history of being violated may be unwilling to submit to direct suggestions. On the other hand, patients with aphasia might feel stupid and overwhelmed when offered multiple choices as often is the case in "indirect" approaches.

My approach does not follow any manualized procedure. Just like a neurosurgeon proceeds differently with each patient, guided by the individual unique brain in the moment of the surgery, I will, in the moment of hypnotizing, use the individual patient's feedback to guide me to the next step, moment by moment.

Definitions of Hypnosis

For most patients in a medical context, the 2015 APA definition is applicable. It defines hypnosis in a way that includes different theoretical orientations: "A state of consciousness involving focused attention, and reduced peripheral awareness characterized by an enhanced capacity for response to suggestion" (Elkins et al., 2015, p. 6). This definition covers direct, indirect, hetero- and self-hypnosis. I use the concept "trance" as equivalent to the hypnotic state, as defined above, and I use the concept "hypnosis" for the clinical context, in which the induction of trance is followed by individually created suggestions, concurrent with the treatment contract.

A definition of hypnosis in clinical work needs to also include therapist factors such as the competence to adapt to patients' individual cognitive and communicative style and resources. Patients with trauma-related amnesia may have acquired a negative association to the trance state. In traumatic situations, fear activates the fight or flight response, but if flight is not an option, the victim escapes mentally by a phenomenon called dissociation, also experienced as a kind of trance. This defense mechanism isolates from the memory, threatening perceptions of the traumatic situation, in particular horror. Therefore, amnesia indicates that the trauma might have been experienced as life-threatening and a dissociative barrier has been created to escape from terror.

Hypnotherapists need to make the state of trance safe. Brain injured patients need safety and clarity in a reliable, predictable relationship that can protect them from re-traumatization, while simultaneously resolving the amnestic barrier, when possible.

Finally, to define clinical hypnosis, some relational aspects need specific attention.

Clinical Hypnosis Is Affect-Dependent and Relational

In their article, Hope and Sugarman (2015) explain the efficacy of individualized hypnotic interventions: "the most effective clinicians (...) can, however, provide a safe and supportive containment of change within the confines of a therapeutic relationship" (Hope & Sugarman, 2015, p. 218). I agree.

Clinical Hypnosis Is Induced with Simple Vocabulary, Safe Voice and Slow Tempo

With brain injuries, information processing may be difficult. Some cannot comprehend abstract or complex verbal instructions, nor respond verbally. Nonverbal or simple-language inductions enhance motivation and the sense of being competent. Slow and easy inductions with attention on one sense at a time engage right hemispheric functions and subconscious "knowledge", without cognitive effort. Johnson and Korn (1986) described a patient with TBI who improve surprisingly well. Anxiety and depression were relieved with the use of hypnosis and the imagination of a safe place, while playing the piano. In 1992, Spellacy wrote: "Unfortunately, it is not uncommon even for rehabilitation personnel to speak rapidly with a high-level vocabulary when speaking to persons with brain injury. The injured person feels overwhelmed and embarrassed by poor comprehension (...) In hypnotherapy this is less likely to occur" (Spellacy, 1992, p. 38).

Clinical Hypnosis Evokes Positive Affect

Patients with epilepsy, stroke or TBI often suffer from negative emotional connotations to their symptoms. Nathanson (2009) explains how hypnosis can help in general, and I find it applicable to these patients. "How people think about or understand anything is controlled by the affect with which it has become linked. Cognitions locked to unpleasant emotions can be disturbingly resistant to change until trance work alters the affective environment of the participant" (Nathanson, 2009, p. 319).

According to Nathanson (2009), the basic affect *interest-excitement* is more accessible in hypnosis than in the normal alert state. This affect opens the mind for more acceptance of losses and changes. It also facilitates a reframing of shame to more constructive feelings. Since hypnotherapists often are in a "working trance", i.e., the state clinicians enter when deeply focused on attunement with patients' intrapsychic and somatic experience, the therapists' own *interest-excitement* in the attempt to understand is an attitude which influences the patients' affects and healing capacities (Nathanson, 2009).

Clinical Hypnosis for Dealing with Repressed Feelings

After a brain injury or stroke, the identity is destabilized. That can cause grief, guilt or shame. In traditional rehabilitation, such feelings are rarely addressed. If not encouraged to express and share, patients deny negative emotions. Some exhibit a positive facade and deny their emotions. Symptoms of such internal conflict can be nightmares, seizures, dysregulated anger or psychotic reactions. With hypnosis we evoke, accept and contain repressed feelings and use them as resources. Grief, guilt or shame is included in the treatment as resources for healing.

Applied Hypnosis: PFTBI

As I have discussed in detail (Carolusson, 2012), psychosis occurs when cognitive coping mechanisms and higher levels of defense mechanisms are absent. In psychosis, right hemispheric and subcortical primitive survival functions are activated, causing a polarized categorization of self and others, e.g., "me good, you bad" and persecutory avoidance; or the opposite; "me bad, you good". Both states can lead to violently provocative behavior. I have observed that contextual triggers precipitate psychotic episodes, such as being reminded of lost competencies in a vulnerable situation, where self-esteem is absent. TBI patients who experience such emotional pain and shame have not only organic but also psychological reasons to become psychotic (Carolusson, 2012).

A psychological containment of trauma-related affect can stop psychotic symptoms to such a degree that medication can be dramatically reduced. During a psychotic period, medication is necessary for sleep and to reduce excessive anxiety. In agreement with neurologists, I have found barbiturates effective for muscular relaxation, and an antipsychotic type of sleeping pill during the initial and acute days of psychosis, and directly after, when the patient is vulnerable and prone to relapse. This very limited medication needs to be combined with supportive and clarifying psychotherapy throughout the psychotic period.

A therapeutic goal is to help patients accept reality and gain self-esteem. To get there, we need to first meet the patients where they are. You can never lead psychotic persons anywhere, until you have acknowledged and understood their present experience. As Nathanson (2009) has described, hypnotherapists easily enter a working trance, which evokes their right hemispheric functionality, facilitate their creativity and an understanding of the symbolic language of psychosis.

I do that by entering a therapeutic trance myself, then I imagine the patient's inner world and verbalize that experience to my patient. In the psychotic state, they expect me to read their mind anyway. If my interpretation is correct, the patient easily accepts it. If not, they look at me with a skeptical eye.

By understanding the patients' experiences, interpreting the meaning of the symbols and hallucinations, we strengthen their self-understanding and self-respect. Such interventions are labeled "ego strengthening" (Phillips & Frederick, 1992; Torem, 1990). The hypnotic language is validating, and the focus is on idiosyncratic resources. How to do this is illustrated in detail in my second book (Carolusson, 2012).

Applied Hypnosis: Epilepsy

Epilepsy, like psychosis, is a state of intensive and increased speed in the central nervous system (CNS). Antiepileptics, just as antipsychotic drugs, have the function of slowing down the cerebral activity. Hypnosis serves the same purpose. In hypnotic inductions we guide patients to focus attention, and then we suggest imagery to calm down the seizure-triggering brain activity. There are as many variations of imagery as there are patients; therefore, we adapt imagery to idiosyncratic sense modalities and preferences.

I have found two treatment approaches effective. One is suggestive hypnosis for seizure control, the second is hypnosis for exploring, interpreting, reframing emotional triggers, within a scope of tolerance. The first approach teaches patients self-hypnosis for stopping, postponing or reducing the intensity of seizures. How to create a metaphor and visualization of over-active brain circuits and how to calm them down are described in detail in a chapter on rehabilitation after brain injury (Carolusson, 2011). The second approach deals with seizures that are triggered by trauma reminders or flashbacks. When seizures start with a scream of terror, it may indicate a flashback. Hypnosis can be applied to manage flashbacks and trauma. My verbatim report on how that can be done is described elsewhere (Carolusson, 2010).

Applied Hypnosis: Stroke

Inspired by Dr Taylor's personal experience of stroke (Taylor, 2008) and my clinical experience, I will specify three main goals for hypnosis after stroke: (1) finding a narrative for the time of the stroke, (2) finding ways to regain or compensate for lost functions, (3) finding new meanings of life by validating and using the best functioning hemisphere, often the right. Trance engages right hemispheric functions, so hypnotic language and hypnotic imagery are easily accessible.

Many stroke patients suffer from aphasia, with difficulty to understand or express verbal language. Nonverbal techniques can be used as hypnotic inductions as well as in trance work. Hypnotist and patient can both draw pictures, the hypnotist can use relaxing body touch, if it's comfortable for the patient. For patients who have some intact understanding of vocabulary, the hypnotic language is perfect: slow, concrete, melodic and simple. When sentences are spoken in a melodic fashion, the right hemisphere's musical functions assist the understanding of words. I have also observed that stroke patients who have studied a second language sometimes have easier access to that vocabulary.

In hypnosis, we do not need verbal responses. We can invite patients to respond with ideomotor signaling, gestures or drawing. One of the most detailed manuals on how to do that was created by Ewin and Eimer (2006).

Case: Barney

After three months of stroke rehabilitation, Barney, a 40-year-old engineer, was referred to me by his neurologist. Ten sessions of therapy were offered, paid by his employment insurance.

Barney was now back home with his wife, trying to adapt their relation to his functional losses. He was also scheduled for regular two-hour visits at work, as a middle manager, but with no pressure to produce. His superior was very supportive.

Barney's motivation was two-fold: (1) he had a strong wish to regain his previous capacity of being a skilled professional. (2) He suffered from amnesia around the time of his stroke and wanted to find out exactly what had happened. We agreed to use explorative (bottom-up) hypnosis for both themes. As a home assignment he listened once a day to my audio file *Healing Imagery* (Carolusson, 1999).

My intake interview revealed a socially capable, psychologically mature man with no relational issues. I responded to his wish to regain occupational capacity, with humility and respect for an unknown future, conveying my belief that his subconscious mind had information about his resources for an optimal rehabilitation. I induced a trance state, with focus on his exhalations. I addressed his subconscious mind, "that knows more than your conscious mind about how to recover and how it can assist this healing. Is that OK?" Barney nodded. "And you, the conscious part of Barney, you just relax, trusting and allowing the subconscious mind to present in its own way what you need to know".

Regarding what resources to discover or skills to regain, I was nondirective. My reason for not specifying the content of such imagery is based on the empirical evidence that future improvements are quite unpredictable. I espouse an attitude of not knowing, for professional and ethical reasons. Nevertheless, my verbalizations aimed to evoke all available resources.

Barney told me: "I see my garden. It has nothing to do with my work". I responded: "Maybe it has. Your wise mind knows. Just look at the garden as it appears. Do you notice anything in particular?" "Yes, I see a snail. Should I remove it?"

"This snail is here for a reason. It has something to tell you. Look at it and place yourself in a convenient communication distance to this snail". (Pause) "Now ask the snail what it has to show you or tell you". Then I added, with interest, joy and curiosity in my voice: "Now, dear snail, tell Barney your secret, a secret that will help him!"

With a surprised look on his face, Barney suddenly opened his eyes. He responded: "The snail said: *Be patient, move slowly, you need lots of rest. Spend time with me in the garden*".

When he was alerted from the trance state, we discussed this message and its implications for his rehabilitation. Barney concluded that he had spent too much time at work. He had pretended to understand things he used to know, but the level was, sadly enough, too advanced for his actual cognitive capacity.

Barney's second wish was to resolve his amnesia. I asked him about all the details before and immediately after the amnestic period. He had been abroad on a business conference in a hotel. He remembered leaving his colleagues after dinner, walking upstairs, passing a corridor and then entering his room. From there he had amnesia. Barney's next conscious memory was lying in a hospital bed, with a nurse by his side, telling him he had had a stroke and would soon be sent home to Sweden.

Again, I used the suggestion of subconscious knowledge beyond awareness. Amnesia after brain injury may be associated to a near death experience, and memory reconstruction can be retraumatizing. Hence, I offered some extra safety in my suggestions. After induction and deepening his trance, I suggested Barney to go double as deep as in the previous hypnosis. Down there, he would be able to speak and tell me again everything he experienced that night.

Barney reported being there again, doing his bathroom rituals and then going to bed, falling asleep. I said: "So, now you are sleeping. In sleep you may not know that time passes ... Just let me know when anything happens". After a minute Barney said: "I'm waking up. I feel strange, something is very wrong. I'm afraid. I leave my bed and walk out, into the corridor. Must have air! Can't breathe, am dizzy! Back to my room. I call the room service, something is wrong. I lift the receiver; my voice sounds weird. I fall on the floor ... hear a voice ... Someone lifts me, I am carried ... They are talking to me". Barney continued the story, and I wrote down every word.

After hypnosis, I read my notes aloud. Barney felt relieved and satisfied to have a narrative with a "before, during, and after" the stroke. A year later, in a follow-up, Barney told me he had yet to find an occupational level that matched his reduced capacity, he was still happily married and life had a new and more spiritual meaning.

References

Arciniegas, D. B., Harris, S. N., & Brousseau, K. M. (2003). Psychosis following traumatic brain injury. *International Review of Psychiatry*, *15*(4), 328–340. 10.1080/09540260310001606719
Baker, E. L. (1981). An hypnotherapeutic approach to enhance object relatedness in psychotic patients. *International Journal of Clinical and Experimental Hypnosis*, *29*(2), 136–147. 10.1080/00207148108409154
Baker, E. L. (1983). The use of hypnotic techniques with psychotics. *American Journal of Clinical Hypnosis*, *25*(4), 283–288. 10.1080/00029157.1983.10404117
Betts, T. (1992). Epilepsy and stress. *British Medical Journal*, *305*(6850), 378–379. 10.1136/bmj.305.6850.378
Betts, T. (2003). Use of aromatherapy (with or without hypnosis) in the treatment of intractable epilepsy: A two-year follow-up study. *Seizure – European Journal of Epilepsy*, *12*(8), 534–538. 10.1016/s1059-1311(03)00161-4
Brown, D. P., & Fromm, E. (1986). *Hypnotherapy and hypnoanalysis* (1st ed.). Routledge.
Carolusson, S. (1999). *Susanna Carolusson - Audio files: Audiofile #6 – A healing imagery*. Susanna Carolusson. Retrieved March 23, 2023, from https://www.carolussons.se/english.htm#:~:text=6.%20A%20healing%20imagery
Carolusson, S. (2010). *There is someone in there: Confidence and conscience after acquired brain injury*. Recito: Alom Editores.
Carolusson, S. (2011). Brain trauma and hypnotic communication; Tobias and family love. In K. Varga (Ed.), *Beyond the words: Communication and suggestion in medical practice* (1st ed., pp. 363–387). Nova Science Publishers.
Carolusson, S. (2012). *Brain trauma, psychosis and a meaningful life: Being present*. Recito.
Diamond, S. G., Davis, O. C., Schaechter, J. D., & Howe, R. D. (2006). Hypnosis for rehabilitation after stroke: Six case studies. *Contemporary Hypnosis*, *23*(4), 173–180. 10.1002/ch.319
Elkins, G. R., Barabasz, A. F., Council, J. R., & Spiegel, D. (2015). Advancing research and practice: The revised APA Division 30 definition of hypnosis. *International Journal of Clinical and Experimental Hypnosis*, *63*(1), 1–9. 10.1080/00207144.2014.961870
Ewin, D. M., & Eimer, B. N. (2006). *Ideomotor signals for rapid hypnoanalysis: A how-to manual*. Charles C. Thomas Publisher.
Fujii, D., & Ahmed, I. (2002). Psychotic disorder following traumatic brain injury: A conceptual framework. *Cognitive Neuropsychiatry*, *7*(1), 41–62. 10.1080/135468000143000131
Gafner, G., & Young, C. (1998). Hypnosis as an adjuvant treatment in chronic paranoid schizophrenia. *Contemporary Hypnosis*, *15*(4), 223–226. 10.1002/ch.139
GBD 2019 Stroke Collaborators (2021). Global, regional, and national burden of stroke and its risk factors, 1990–2019: A systematic analysis for the Global Burden of Disease study 2019. *Lancet Neurology*, *20*(10), 795–820. 10.1016/s1474-4422(21)00252-0
Gurin, L., & Arciniegas, D. B. (2019). Psychotic disorders. In J. M. Silver, T. W. McAllister, & D. B. Arciniegas (Eds.), *Textbook of traumatic brain injury* (pp. 413–430). American Psychiatric Publications.
Hodge, J. R. (1988). Can hypnosis help psychosis? *American Journal of Clinical Hypnosis*, *30*(4), 248–256. 10.1080/00029157.1988.10402747
Hope, A. E., & Sugarman, L. I. (2015). Orienting hypnosis. *American Journal of Clinical Hypnosis*, *57*(3), 212–229. 10.1080/00029157.2014.976787
Johnson, K., & Korn, E. (1986). Hypnosis and imagery in the rehabilitation of a brain-damaged patient. *Hypnos*, *XIII*(3), 134–137.
Khan, F., Amatya, B., Galea, M. P., Gonzenbach, R., & Kesselring, J. (2017). Neurorehabilitation: Applied neuroplasticity. *Journal of Neurology*, *264*(3), 603–615. 10.1007/s00415-016-8307-9
Lauterbach, M. D., Notarangelo, P. L., Nichols, S. J., Lane, K. S., & Koliatsos, V. E. (2015). Diagnostic and treatment challenges in traumatic brain injury patients with severe neuropsychiatric symptoms: Insights into psychiatric practice. *Neuropsychiatric Disease and Treatment*, *2015*(11), 1601–1607. 10.2147/ndt.s80457
Markus, H. S., Brainin, M., & Fisher, M. (2020). Tracking the global burden of stoke and dementia: World Stroke Day 2020. *International Journal of Stroke*, *15*(8), 817–818. 10.1177/1747493020959186

McAllister, T. W., & Ferrell, R. B. (2002). Evaluation and treatment of psychosis after traumatic brain injury. *NeuroRehabilitation*, *17*(4), 357–368. 10.3233/nre-2002-17409
Molloy, C., Conroy, R. M., Cotter, D. R., & Cannon, M. (2011). Is traumatic brain injury a risk factor for schizophrenia? A meta-analysis of case-controlled population-based studies. *Schizophrenia Bulletin*, *37*(6), 1104–1110. 10.1093/schbul/sbr091
Murray-Jobsis, J. (1993). The borderline patient and the psychotic patient. In J. W. Rhue, S. J. Lynn, & I. Kirsch (Eds.), *Handbook of clinical hypnosis* (pp. 425–451). American Psychological Association.
Nathanson, D. L. (2009). Affect and hypnosis: On paying friendly attention to disturbing thoughts. *International Journal of Clinical and Experimental Hypnosis*, *57*(4), 319–342. 10.1080/00207140903098361
Patel, B. (2022). The brain-environment relationship: Part II. *ECO Journal of Environmental Health Association of Québec*. Retrieved March 21, 2023, from https://aseq-ehaq.ca/wp-content/uploads/2022/03/4.-Brain-2_April-EN.pdf
Phillips, M., & Frederick, C. (1992). The use of hypnotic age progressions as prognostic, ego-strengthening, and integrating techniques. *American Journal of Clinical Hypnosis*, *35*(2), 99–108. 10.1080/00029157.1992.10402992
Pyun, Y. D. (2013). The effective use of hypnosis in schizophrenia: Structure and strategy. *International Journal of Clinical and Experimental Hypnosis*, *61*(4), 388–400. 10.1080/00207144.2013.815059
Rossi, E. L. (2004). *A discourse with our genes: The psychosocial and cultural genomics of therapeutic hypnosis and psychotherapy*. Editris.
Rossi, E. L. (2005). The memory trace reactivation and reconstruction theory of therapeutic hypnosis: The creative replaying of gene expression and brain plasticity in stroke rehabilitation. *Hypnos*, *XXXII*(1), 5–16.
Scagnelli, J. (1976). Hypnotherapy with schizophrenic and borderline patients: Summary of therapy with eight patients. *American Journal of Clinical Hypnosis*, *19*(1), 33–38. 10.1080/00029157.1976.10403829
Spellacy, F. (1992). Hypnotherapy following traumatic brain injuries. *Hypnos*, *XIX* (1), 34–39.
Spiegel, D., Detrick, D., & Frischholz, E. (1982). Hypnotizability and psychopathology. *American Journal of Psychiatry*, *139*(4), 431–437. 10.1176/ajp.139.4.431
Spiegel, H., & Spiegel, D. (2004). *Trance and treatment: Clinical uses of hypnosis* (2nd ed.). American Psychiatric Publications.
Taylor, J. B. (2008). *My stroke of insight: A brain scientist's personal journey*. Penguin Books.
Torem, M. S. (1990). Ego-strengthening. In D. C. Hammond (Ed.), *Handbook of hypnotic suggestions and metaphors* (1st ed., pp. 110–112). W. W. Norton & Company.
World Health Organization (2023, February 9). *Epilepsy*. Retrieved March 21, 2023, from https://www.who.int/news-room/fact-sheets/detail/epilepsy
Whitaker, R. (2010). *Anatomy of an epidemic: Magic bullets, psychiatric drugs, and the astonishing rise of mental illness in America*. Crown Publishing.

50

HYPNOSIS IN THE INTENSIVE CARE UNIT

Utilization of the Superorganismic Connection State

Adrienn Kelemen-Szilágyi

Doctoral School of Psychology, ELTE Eötvös Loránd University, Budapest, Hungary

Introduction

I think of the intensive care unit (ICU) as a magnifying glass which shows our real needs. The know-how to handle critically ill patients has furnished me with a lot of practical knowledge, courage, and self-confidence and given me a compass in psychotherapeutic and hospital work and everyday life.

You may wonder about what a psychologist – even if it's a hypnotherapist – can do in the ICU, where vital parameters are the highest priority: breath, circulation, and brain functions. For many years, psychologists only mapped the iatrogenic effects of being in the ICU (Ely et al., 2004; Huang et al., 2015; Jackson et al., 2007; Kamdar et al., 2012; Weinhouse et al., 2009) and some elaborate interventions aiming to alleviate the fear, anxiety, and nightmares after being in an ICU and to prevent PTSD (Berg et al., 2006; Berger et al., 2010; Chien et al., 2006; Chlan, 1998; Fleischer et al., 2014; Garrouste-Orgeas et al., 2012; Hatch et al., 2011; Jaber et al., 2007; Novoa & Ballesteros de Valderrama, 2006; Peris et al., 2011).

In 2006, our team was the first in the world to run a randomized controlled trial (RCT) meeting the following three criteria at the same time: (1) the empirical impact assessment of a psychological intervention at the ICU (2) used with critically ill patients at the same time as their intensive therapy (and not after), and (3) aimed to have an impact not (just) on subjective but on the objective data of the physiological care such as drug consumption, length of mechanical ventilation, and length of care (Varga et al., 2007). In our RCT, mechanically ventilated patients received psychological support based on positive suggestions following the rules of hypnotic communication, irrespective of their state of health and their state of consciousness. Patients receiving care from the same person at least 50% of their time in ICU (K. Szilágyi et al., 2007) or having a standard hypnotic text via earphones (K. Szilágyi et al., 2014) had 20% (i.e., two days) faster recovery (K. Szilágyi et al., 2014) among other benefits (Schlanger et al., 2013).

I believe that the relationship potentiated the power of suggestions. We know from Harlow and Harlow's research (1962) that without maternal warmth and security, the baby monkeys showed severe developmental delays, and some simply stopped eating and

DOI: 10.4324/9781003449126-65

died. Spitz (1945) observed that after the Second World War, about half of the orphans who had no fixed attachment figure for the first six months of their lives died despite adequate physical care. This showed that warmth, love, and security are essential for life. If we can have a positive impact on the somatic state of a critically ill patient by adding these psychological factors, it shows that psychological needs are also vital and essential. By ignoring that basic human need, we unnecessarily add at least 20% healing time to critically ill patients (K. Szilágyi, 2011).

We used hypnotic communication strategies to incorporate the psychological component of healing. I will outline how a network is put together, the pathways in and between our consciousnesses, that allows hypnosis (and suggestive techniques) to be effective in life-threatening situations. Indeed, it is the method by which it can be truly effective. And the so-called superorganismic connection state (SCS) provides the playing field for this, which is created along our evolutionary needs and the way our brains function as a result. I will exemplify this approach with case-vignettes.

The Evolutionary Roots and the ICU

According to Csányi (1993, 2002, 2003), relationship has evolutionarily roots.

He theorizes that the purpose of evolution is better survival. Just as cooperating *cells* provide an organ with higher functioning than the same quantity of unorganized cells would have, well-organized *organs* yield a well-functioning organism. A solitarily wild animal needs to perceive and understand the signs of the physical environment. A social animal needs information coming from peers. The human way to surpass other species was to live in a group. When the members of the group are connected to each other through sensitively attuned cooperation, the group becomes a "superorganism". The "connective tissue" of this superorganism is in our minds due to human-specific attributes. These attributes are: having common ideas, belief systems, rules, fidelity, and indoctrination – that means following values and beliefs without questioning them. Socialization means that the member of the group acquires these rules by living in the group. A well-organized group of humans by socialization is the superorganism of its members, a survival machine, able to sustain a well-organized life around us (electricity, schools, water supply, etc.). The link between our brains is the "connective tissue" of a very effective superorganism, a community. To strengthen this superorganism, we have many sophisticated synchronizing mechanisms shown in several MRI studies (Kulcsár, 2005; Singer et al., 2004; Sanfey et al., 2003; Winston et al., 2002). This synchronized link is woven by common actions, like singing, dancing, chatting, telling stories, gossiping, doing sports together, cheering for a team, and being together in altered states of consciousness. Hypnosis can be viewed as a guided synchronizing mechanism consciously going for a common goal.

Further, devaluation and aversion of the outgroup, of outsiders, reinforces the sense of community, the sense of belonging to our community. Considering the outgroup as a mortal danger helps our beliefs, rules, and doctrines to stay more intact. This is why it's still so easy to provoke xenophobia (Csányi, 1993, 2002, 2003).

In the ICU, employing this evolutionary perspective, the staff is a hostile outgroup, representing mortal danger for the patients who are alone, vulnerable, and far from their primary group. The patients do not know the rules to live safely in this strange community and this threatening situation.

Stress-Response

Kulcsár (2005) describes the effects of stress-response triggered in the central nervous system (CNS) of everybody experiencing positive or negative stress. Due to stress, the hippocampus underperforms, while the amygdala is overactive. This change in the CNS produces an explicit emotional openness. This is manifested in the following ways. The social urges, emotional sensitivity, and suggestibility increase with stress. We behave less logically, and "decide" with our emotions, what is dangerous or safe (Ewin, 2011). For example, ventilated patients experience the tube in their throat as dangerous, and not the action, which is dangerous, when they try to rip it out. The other explicit change is that stress negatively affects the brain's "who system" (Georgieff & Jeannerod, 1998). This is the system that helps to distinguish "me" from "not me". When I refer to "not me", I use the word *Other*. When stress affects "who-system", it means it impairs the separation of self and non-self and intensifies the need to belong, and makes self-boundaries more permeable emotionally and physically. For example, when I was giving birth and the doctor asked me not to squeeze his shoulder, I couldn't tell or feel which was his shoulder and which was my arm, so I couldn't even loosen my grip. You may recognize this pattern as characteristic of the altered state of consciousness (ASC). In this emotional state, the social-visceral-emotional mirror system circulates information in every direction and between the bodies and minds of people in interaction. This creates the possibility that the emotional state of the *Other* directly influences our bodily state and that social influences may take hold at a visceral level (Gallese et al., 2004; Rizzolatti et al., 1996; Rosenthal, 2002; Rosenthal & Jacobson, 1968). We may take on others' fears, pain, and negative affect, but we may also absorb others' positive, supportive feelings. It depends on the attitude of the *Others* if this state goes in a positive or a negative direction (Uchino et al., 1996).

The Superorganismic Connection State

Evolution didn't push us to "lose our minds" in a dangerous situation but rather to create a condition where re-socialization is allowed when it's needed. Stable socialization gives the superorganism the strength to protect its members and increase its chances of survival. However, when we fall out of our original community or fall in love (when we enter into a new, strong bond), it is essential to be able to leave our original socialization, because survival is aided by adapting to new circumstances. Group loyalty and indoctrination protect the stability of the superorganism when we take collective action with our original community. However, at the gateway to a new community, it is essential to be able to override this indoctrination and acquire new knowledge, new habits, rules, and roles. The change triggered by the stress response in the CNS like change in the functioning of the hippocampus, the amygdala, the "Who system", and the social-visceral-emotional mirror system causes a particular mental state to occur. This special, ASC allows for a new community of people from different socializations who are placed in a common situation (in our case, caregivers and patients) to unite. This mental state creates the conditions for a new "connective tissue" to form between the brains and minds of these different people. This new community, this new superorganism, is better able to adapt to the demands of new circumstances, promoting a better chance of survival. Therefore, it is worthwhile and evolutionarily advantageous to leave our original stable socialization.

I have titled this special, permeable, and customizable mental state triggered by stress in the CNS that promotes a better chance of survival by enabling new connectivity, the SCS.

Those who are in the stronger group, those who are less vulnerable, can determine whether the situation moves in a positive or negative direction. In the relationship between healthcare staff and patients, the stronger, less vulnerable is always the staff. Patients are frequently afraid of caregivers until they have cues to feel the staff's support and goodwill. In the absence of this, they can build up a negative picture of the mosaic of stimuli that affect them, because it's evolutionarily more adaptive to perceive danger in unfamiliar situations (Ewin, 2011).

To move in a positive direction, the staff must include patients in the medical community, give them the feeling of being hosted, and help them understand they are the center, the very purpose of this community. In this way, patients can feel accepted, have status, tasks, warmth, and security in their new community, where cooperation with the ICU team is safe and indispensable.

It is therefore worthwhile for the staff to be aware of this and to know techniques and tools to take control of the situation and then even caregivers become the beneficiaries of the SCS. This is why it is beneficial if not only the "extra person", i.e., the psychologist, is responsible for the hypnotic work, but that the staff also has basic hypnotic knowledge. It is also in the staff's interest to make the patient feel supported, because if there are hostile feelings toward the patient or from the patient, this emotion will reverberate between them harming both parties physically and psychologically. It is not the patient's poor condition that negatively affects the staff. If the patient is unwell but feels a sense of help and compassion, feelings of camaraderie, gratitude, and belonging will flow toward the staff and even the staff will gain a protective factor through compassion. Patient support also has a positive impact on the supporter, both physically and psychologically (Kulcsár, 2005; Vargay et al., 2019), but only if it does not involve excessive sacrifice (Kulcsár, 2005).

The healing factor provided by the group, in this case, the medical staff, is the expected protection and good intention toward its members. Understanding the SCS makes the protection and care more explicit and makes them resilient against burdens. Staff can provide this healing relationship for the patients, as was the case in our study.

Caregiver in Trouble

Stressful places and situations put participants in the SCS. The person in the most stressful situation is both the most vulnerable and the most flexible and needs the appropriate presence of the *Other* (Kulcsár, 2005). Staff who are well used to traumatic sights, at a different level than the patient, are also in the SCS. They also need a sense of security to perform well under duress. Patient cooperation can make the workplace less stressful. Perceived organizational support increases job satisfaction (Cropanzano et al., 1997), commitment, and sacrificial behaviors (Organ & Ryan, 1995). Perceived social support from military leadership was associated with fewer PTSD symptoms and in its absence, there is a higher risk of suicidal ideation (Kelley et al., 2019) and burnout (Maslach et al., 2016). If healthcare personnel are under too much physical and psychological strain, without mental and physical protection and appreciation, they may rightly feel that "I am not important to my group". The feeling of "not having the same ideas" can be traumatic, leading to moral distress and demoralization. This can occur with unclear protocol or guidance in end-of-life care, when it's not clear that staff are extending life or prolonging dying, when they don't have control over whether they participate or not, leading to a loss of a common belief system. It's easy to find themselves in a situation where they witness or commit an atrocity, or where they can't help or can't handle a situation, because there is an asset shortage on the ward. They may feel guilty, instead of feeling like a heroic healer. Then the trauma affecting the staff is not vicarious, but an individual's primal trauma. It manifests as healthcare staff's PTSD symptoms such as disturbing memories, nightmares, feeling that the events are inexplicable and/or incommunicable, and avoidance of the topic of death and dying. If the burden, tasks, workload, or support, eligibility, and connectivity is not suitable for one cell of the superorganism (e.g., by putting a heavier burden on one cell/one member while providing less support), this will lead to mental problems. These may be psychosomatic symptoms, anxiety, mood disorders, lack of motivation, burnout, PTSD, and substance (ab)use, and sometimes even the helper syndrome (Schmidbauer, 1977) in which compulsive helping maintains dependency of the helped person. Not surprisingly patients can show the same symptoms.

We can prevent these symptoms by providing the optimum to the "cells". For the patients, the staff can provide the supportive community. For the staff, it can be a case discussion group, a bereavement group, and abreaction sessions after a difficult ICU situation. A recovering patient returning to the ICU or writing a short thank you note with a photo can also remind staff that this is a battle worth fighting.

Self-Connection

Patients will take on staff's feelings and if they cannot perceive the staff as trustworthy, they will go into a "fight or flight" coping mode. In this case, the staff's priority is to regulate their own feelings. Staff must accept they are influenced by the events around them and need to find their balance.

I realized the importance of that when I trained intensivist doctors to be able to calm down patients needing non-invasive ventilation to avoid mechanical ventilation, which would lead to longer and more burdensome care. Doctors were asked to list the physical symptoms of respiratory failure that patients can experience. They included difficulty to breathe and speak, pressure in the chest, a pounding heartbeat, cold sweaty palms, weakness in the legs. And of course, anxiety. I explained that the patients experience discomfort globally. We can develop trust and cooperation by drawing their attention to some of the details that they are certainly experiencing, but are not in their conscious awareness. The patients will be surprised and satisfied that we know what is happening to them and they will believe we know how they'll get better. This is called pacing the treatment.

During the theoretical part of the training, doctors seemed to understand everything. But when they practiced the new behavior with a patient role-played by a colleague, they returned to their former, bad communication habits. At that moment, I realized that we need to understand what doctors need to be relaxed and comfortable in a medically stressful situation, and only then will they be able to help patients feel comfortable. It is the same synchronicity and connection as in hypnosis, where before touching or speaking to the subject – in a psychotherapeutic or medical setting – hypnotists have to put away their problems, fears, and disbeliefs if they don't want their bad feelings to harm the patient (Bányai, 1998; Ewin, 2011).

So, I asked the internists what they experienced when they tried to put the mask on the face of the resistant patient. They reported pressure in the chest, a pounding heartbeat, cold sweaty palms, weakness in the legs, and of course, anxiety, the same symptoms of respiratory failure they had previously listed. At that moment, they understood that to provide the patients with a trusting balance they have to first calm down themselves. It helps if they recall a previous success or colleagues who exemplify this indispensable skill. They have realized that they have the tools that have already helped them to overcome difficult situations and that even simple things can make a difference. A deep breath or thinking of something peaceful can also lead them to their positive SCS, which can ease finding the connecting path to the patients and lead them to their new team to fulfill this healing project together.

Hypnosis in the Superorganismic Connection State

We have to keep in mind that the SCS's pivotal role is to provide a framework for all parties involved to "merge" and work together for one common goal, for one common project as one team. This process is for a limited period: the healing of the patient. This team unity is completed when this project is done, and everyone returns to their previous roles. For the patient, this process lasts until their time in the ICU is ended. As for the staff, they have to check out of this team every day at the end of their workload and check in again the next day. This is how the deep connection between caregiver and patient in this period of healing makes the ICU a safe workplace for the staff and patients as well.

To be in SCS is both to be in an emotionally vulnerable mental state and to have the opportunity to develop trust in caregivers. Patients are then able and willing to "re-socialize", i.e., to learn new rules and new habits. This state is reached when leaving the old community is more conducive to survival than clinging to the old one.

The pacing-leading hypnosis technique ensures a smooth transition and continuity between the patient's new and old communities. This can be achieved simply by helping the patients feel that staff knows what they are feeling.

For example, when patients are suffocating, naming the symptoms that they are experiencing but are not aware of (palpitations, cold sweats, etc.) or expressing our empathy by saying, "I can imagine how difficult this must be for you" – conveys that staff are thinking the same way they are. Knowing how to consciously engage with the critically ill patient's experience in SCS will gain the patient's trust and willingness to re-socialize and cooperate. It can facilitate recovery for both patient and caregiver. This protective connection can overwrite the power of the healthcare hierarchy from which Bejenke (1996) derives the power of suggestion. With the pacing-leading technique, the psychologist gives the patient a sense of familiarity, which gives the patient the confidence to tune into a new, trusted, strong, supportive group in the middle of the alien minds.

Rapport by Gaining the Patient's Perspective

To build the relationship, the rapport, healthcare providers can tune into the current physical, emotional, or cognitive experience of the patients, and then lead them to the desired state. The aim is to ensure continuity between the existing "socialization" and the new relationship to be acquired. Observing patients' environment, imagining what it is to be them in the critical care setting, and how the overall situation might impact their physical, cognitive, and mental state enable staff to communicate with therapeutic suggestions.

For example, to a shouting patient in respiratory failure:

(loudly): - *That's it! Can you shout louder? Because it's an important signal to me when you have enough air left and when you absolutely need help.*

Swearing:

- *Yes! Can you say something stronger? Very good, let it out! By releasing your tension you'll be relaxed, and when you are relaxed, you'll be able to follow my requests much more easily so I can help you breathe easier.*

I focus on self-related information and reframe it to promote cooperation and their inner resources. For example, when patients' hands are secured to the bed, I explain, lying in a semi-sleeping state is currently the most effective way to help them recover. With their hands secured, they don't have to pay attention to their involuntary gestures. This allows all the medical equipment to stay in place and do its best work for them while they help their recovery by resting comfortably. This will reduce stress by raising the level of information, control, and sense of security of the patients (Levine et al., 1978).

The "ICU mental state" ceases when the patient leaves the ward (Ewin, 2011). It may be the responsibility of the staff during the patient's stay in the ICU to set the emotional/sensational homeostasis that is most appropriate for the patient's recovery. It's evolutionarily adaptive to detect negative signals (danger) earlier than positive ones because it can save our life if we react in time. So, we can be quite sure in the patient's focus there will be some negative aspect of the situation. By pacing these negative aspects, we can lead them to the positive aspects of the situation that have not yet been realized.

A young colleague was unable to provide a positive statement to a patient just one step away from recovery, because he always refused it, saying that here it was like being in an inquisition. I counseled her to tell the patient:'I've been thinking how hard it must be for you to spend your days in the ICU, being in a weak state and experiencing pain and discomfort every day. I've realized, how difficult it is for you to notice what a great job your body has done with the help of the doctors, and how little the recovery period remains for you! The patient looked at the colleague with surprise. "Are you working in that ward?" From then he started to cooperate with the staff, and when the young colleague visited him, he no longer needed the positive reframing of the situation but increased his self-power by telling her stories about his family (showing his supportive background).

In this example, the patient has independently extended the rapport to the whole ward. But sometimes we have to encourage this extension.

Once during a training lunch break one of my colleagues had an epileptic seizure, and was choking on food in her throat. I held her and removed the obstacle from her throat while telling her in a positive manner what was happening. When she alerted from the seizure, she snarled offensively at her friends until I reassured her that they were okay. When the paramedics arrived, she tried to bite and kick them until

I reassured her that paramedics were there to help, she was safe and could cooperate. I then remembered to highlight the people the paramedics were going to take her to, as they were also worth cooperating with, they are "with us".

Explaining the superorganismic theoretical framework, I can tell that while I was the least known person to her, our relationship became higher ranking in the hierarchy of previous friendships, or the authority of the healthcare staff because this relationship was born in the SCS. That's why it was possible to hand over the rapport and that's why she needed me to approve these subsequent relationships.

Sometimes symptoms that disturb or block recovery such as nightmares and inexplicable symptoms that don't fit in the process of recovery disappear, when the patients understand that the goal of their hospital stay is to cure them with teamwork. And in this team, it isn't only the security and good intention they receive from the medical team, but they are VIPs, and are at the very center of the team, having tasks, a role, and a position.

With this theoretical framework, the symptom can be reframed by saying that the symptom is a well-intentioned part of him that wants to help him in something or protect him against something. *The symptom is a friend, that wants to alert you that your house is on fire and it will bang on your door louder and louder if you don't listen to it.* In that hypnotic framework, you can realize that your panic just wants you to let you feel your emotions. No longer surprising when a patient "sees" earlier during hypnosis her actual abdominal abscess (Kelemen-Szilágyi, 2019) or his intestinal perforation (K. Szilágyi et al., 2014) or a pregnant woman the malformation of her fetus. These are "seen" before the medical tests are performed and confirm what the patient knows about their body. Subconsciously, we are aware of everything that is happening inside us, and if we pay attention to what's going on inside us, it can sometimes help to control it a bit more easily.

Providing basic information about the treatment helps the patient to cope with the frightening unknown, because the lack of information increases the fear, the pain, and the negative alteration of the mind.

An old man arriving at the ICU to drain his chest with a large needle became psychotic in 2 minutes because doctors didn't wait a few minutes for the calming explanation about the intervention waiting for him.

But if we provide a helping hand, both literally and metaphorically, they will catch it and use it to build a secure basis even in hard circumstances.

I was asked to hold the hand or restrain the hand of a patient when 4–5 people on the staff were providing him care. We couldn't see or hear each other. When he tightened his body, I squeezed his hand tightly, and after I relaxed my grip, I waited for his hand to relax. And *to anchor this desired state I tapped a simple rhythm on his palm. And in the middle of the health care chaos, I realized he was calmly tapping the same rhythm in my palm.*

Patients in the ICU are very open to relationships where their perceived "savior" arrives. If they receive anything small that helps them to get better, from someone who they can trust, they will use it for their own good, and amplify it. Patients understand the logic of using their own inner resources quite quickly because they feel it can save or just ease their life. They are grateful for the information that they don't have to monitor every stimulus around them. They can save their energy by concentrating only on their new task in the new situation in their new community – surrendering to recovery. For example:

A lady remembered that she could survive the one-month-long ICU care because I was her non-stop guardian angel for a month while we only met 3 or 4 times. Did she hallucinate my presence? Maybe. Her mind helped her to survive and come back to a normal state of mind when the danger had passed.

And:

Once I told a patient that while we're concerned with his recovery in the ICU, he can switch to another channel of his brain and immerse himself in whatever he wants. After 2 weeks of mechanical ventilation the patient – surprised and satisfied – explained to me that he'd experienced he was fly-fishing in Switzerland in these two weeks. So, he immediately understood how to get the remote control of his brain.

Would it be more adaptive to register reality by a normal state of mind? Or even sleeping unconsciously? Yes, sometimes hallucination and daydreaming can be very harmful when it's without any helpful basis as in the following example:

A 75-year-old factory worker became catatonic on the ward. When I realized that he had defended himself against the tremendous amount of unknown and frightening stimuli experienced in the ward, I did a dehypnosis, and explained the situation, the new rules, and isolated him from the ward by a curtain, and offered him the possibility to connect to us in his own rhythm. Then half an hour was enough for him to come back to a normal state of mind. He told me, that until this moment he spent his ICU stay (more than two weeks) in horrifying nightmares and hallucinations.

He was already near the end of his life, but it was a massive difference to pass away with dignity and without nightmares ... .

It's very dangerous in the ICU when patients feel left out of every group and lose the motivation to cooperate. Inclusion can be regained by helping them to find their own purpose and showing how our team can help them in achieve it, even if the expected lifetime is short.

An elderly woman thought her family didn't care about her. She was angry with them and wanted to die. She said her relatives didn't deserve her. I answered in this case she certainly doesn't deserve to suffer because of them. But she persisted in her desire to die. I reminded her that without the tracheal tube even dying is more comfortable. It was an undeniable fact. From that moment she started to cooperate and recovered nicely. Once the staff alerted me that this lady was just lying with closed eyes. But it wasn't resistance. She told me enthusiastically she was on a big field with plenty of flowers and playing with children. It gave her peace and calm. So, she just filled herself with a gift from her brain. She told me, the day before she dreamed of being in a cemetery. It rained and her skin was cold. But that image wasn't good. She preferred the image with the flowers. At that moment her willingness to live was without question. So, she stayed alive and left the hospital.

Do you wonder if we can induce psychosis on the ward? As shown, it's possible. Fear, pain, the lack of information about the situation, the flooding of unknown stimuli, and the lack of a peaceful frame can lead to psychosis.

Once a woman arrived at the ward after surgery. She was so confused and resistant that doctors called a psychiatrist and asked me to see her. I paced her resistance and called her attention to the fact that she could use the force, and strength, of her resistance for her recovery. Once the rapport was established, she remembered when the healing mud of the Dead Sea healed her warts when she was lying on the Dead Sea beach exactly in the same position as she was lying in the hospital bed. I left her to recover from this healing mud on the beach and I went to see another patient. In a few minutes, the psychiatrist arrived and started the Mini Mental Test (MMT). MMT begins with questions like "What day is it? What time is it? Where you are now?" This is exactly the information patients expect from staff or anyone when they regain consciousness. I think that it is a professional mistake to use MMT to assess the cognitive status of patients in intensive care. Would the patient say she was at Dead Sea beach as I left her there? Then she might not avoid the antipsychotic medication ... I waited for the answer with bated breath. The lady answered as clearly as could be: "I am in the ICU of this hospital after my surgery.

In the ICU, it's not just the drug-induced mental state that we have to consider. *Others* can affect the mental state of patients in both positive and negative ways. The "human-induced peaceful state" leads to benign mental states, as we have seen in the case of this lady.

Closing Remarks

At the Mayo Clinic ICU, our method has been established (Karnatovskaia et al., 2021a; Karnatovskaia et al., 2021b). In Hungary, Varga (Varga & Diószeghy, 2003; Varga, 2015) created training to master the use of positive suggestions for psychologists and healthcare staff (doctors, nurses, midwives, physiotherapists, etc.). These trainees have integrated this hypnotic approach into a wide range of somatic medicine (László et al., 2014). During COVID, we provided this healing relationship via suggestive posters and standard hypnotic sound clips to staff as well as to relatives and patients, and in supervision for psychologists and some intensivists (Kelemen-Szilágyi, 2019). We hope that this method will one day become part of primary care in somatic medicine for the benefit of all involved.

References

Bányai, É. I. (1998). The interactive nature of hypnosis: Research evidence for a social-psychobiological model. *Contemporary Hypnosis*, *15*(1), 52–63. 10.1002/ch.116

Bejenke, C. J. (1996). Painful medical procedures. In J. Barber (Ed.), *Hypnosis and suggestion in the treatment of pain: A clinical guide* (1st ed., pp. 209–266). W. W. Norton & Company.

Berger, M. M., Davadant, M., Marin, C., Wasserfallen, J.-B., Pinget, C., Maravic, P., Koch, N., Raffoul, W., & Chioléro, R. L. (2010). Impact of a pain protocol including hypnosis in major burns. *Burns: Journal of the International Society for Burn Injuries*, *36*(5), 639–646. 10.1016/j.burns.2009.08.009

Berg, A., Fleischer, S., Koller, M., & Neubert, T. R. (2006). Preoperative information for ICU patients to reduce anxiety during and after the ICU-stay: Protocol of a randomized controlled trial [NCT00151554]. *BMC Nursing*, *5*(4). 10.1186/1472-6955-5-4

Chien, W.-T., Chiu, Y. L., Lam, L.-W., & Ip, W.-Y. (2006). Effects of a needs-based education programme for family carers with a relative in an intensive care unit: A quasi-experimental study. *International Journal of Nursing Studies*, *43*(1), 39–50. 10.1016/j.ijnurstu.2005.01.006

Chlan, L. (1998). Effectiveness of a music therapy intervention on relaxation and anxiety for patients receiving ventilatory assistance. *Heart & Lung: The Journal of Critical Care*, *27*(3), 169–176. 10.1016/s0147-9563(98)90004-8

Cropanzano, R., Howes, J. C., Grandey, A. A., & Toth, P. (1997). The relationship of organizational politics and support to work behaviors, attitudes and stress. *Journal Of Organizational Behavior*, 18(2), 159–180. DOI: 10.1002/(SICI)1099-1379(199703)18:2<159::AID-JOB795>3.0.CO;2-D

Csányi, V. (1993). Human evolution: Emergence of the group-self. *Behavioral and Brain Sciences*, *16*(4), 755–756. 10.1017/s0140525x00032738

Csányi, V. (2002). Single-person group and globalisation. *The Hungarian Quarterly*, *43*(167), 3–18. Retrieved April 4, 2023, from http://real-j.mtak.hu/12051/1/HungarianQuarterly_167_2002.pdf

Csányi, V. (2003). Reconstruction of the major factors in the evolution of human behavior. *Praehistoria*, *4–5*, 1–12. Retrieved April 4, 2023, from http://etologia.elte.hu/file/publikaciok/2003/CsanyiV_Prehistoria_human-complex.pdf

Ely, E. W., Shintani, A., Truman, B., Speroff, T., Gordon, S. M., Harrell, F. E., Inouye, S. K., Bernard, G. R., & Dittus, R. S. (2004). Delirium as a predictor of mortality in mechanically ventilated patients in the intensive care unit. *Journal of American Medical Association (JAMA)*, *291*(14), 1753–1762. 10.1001/jama.291.14.1753

Ewin, D. M. (2011). The laws of hypnotic suggestion. In K. Varga (Ed.), *Beyond the words: Communication and suggestion in medical practice* (1st ed., pp. 75–82). Nova Science Publishers.

Fleischer, S., Berg, A., Behrens, J., Kuss, O., Becker, R., Horbach, A., & Neubert, T. R. (2014). Does an additional structured information program during the intensive care unit stay reduce anxiety in ICU patients?: A multicenter randomized controlled trial. *BMC Anesthesiology*, *14*(48). 10.1186/1471-2253-14-48

Gallese, V., Keysers, C., & Rizzolatti, G. (2004). A unifying view of the basis of social cognition. *Trends in Cognitive Sciences*, *8*(9), 396–403. 10.1016/j.tics.2004.07.002

Garrouste-Orgeas, M., Coquet, I., Périer, A., Timsit, J.-F., Pochard, F., Lancrin, F., Philippart, F., Vesin, A., Bruel, C., Blel, Y., Angeli, S., Cousin, N., Carlet, J., & Misset, B. (2012). Impact of an intensive care unit diary on psychological distress in patients and relatives. *Critical Care Medicine*, *40*(7), 2033–2040. 10.1097/ccm.0b013e31824e1b43

Georgieff, N., & Jeannerod, M. (1998). Beyond consciousness of external reality: A "who" system for consciousness of action and self-consciousness. *Consciousness and Cognition*, 7(3), 465–477. 10.1006/ccog.1998.0367

Harlow, H. F., & Harlow, M. K. (1962). Social deprivation in monkeys. *Scientific American*, *207*(5), 136–146. 10.1038/scientificamerican1162-136

Hatch, R., McKechnie, S., & Griffiths, J. R. (2011). Psychological intervention to prevent ICU-related PTSD: Who, when and for how long? *Critical Care*, *15*(2), 141. 10.1186/cc10054

Huang, H.-W., Zheng, B.-L., Jiang, L., Lin, Z.-T., Zhang, G.-B., Shen, L., & Xi, X.-M. (2015). Effect of oral melatonin and wearing earplugs and eye masks on nocturnal sleep in healthy subjects in a simulated intensive care unit environment: Which might be a more promising strategy for ICU sleep deprivation? *Critical Care*, *19*(1), 124. 10.1186/s13054-015-0842-8

Jaber, S., Bahloul, H., Guétin, S., Chanques, G., Sebbane, M., & Eledjam, J.-J. (2007). Effets de la musicothérapie en réanimation hors sédation chez des patients en cours de sevrage ventilatoire versus des patients non ventilés [Effects of music therapy in intensive care unit without sedation in weaning patients versus non-ventilated patients]. *Annales Francaises D' Anesthesie et de Reanimation*, *26*(1), 30–38. 10.1016/j.annfar.2006.09.002

Jackson, J. C., Hart, R. P., Gordon, S. M., Hopkins, R. O., Girard, T. D., & Ely, E. W. (2007). Post-traumatic stress disorder and post-traumatic stress symptoms following critical illness in medical intensive care unit patients: Assessing the magnitude of the problem. *Critical Care*, *11*(1), R27. 10.1186/cc5707

Kamdar, B. B., Needham, D. M., & Collop, N. A. (2012). Sleep deprivation in critical illness: Its role in physical and psychological recovery. *Journal of Intensive Care Medicine*, *27*(2), 97–111. 10.1177/0885066610394322

Karnatovskaia, L. V., Varga, K., Niven, A. S., Schulte, P. J., Mujic, M., Gajic, O., Bauer, B. A., Clark, M. M., Benzo, R. P., & Philbrick, K. L. (2021a). A pilot study of trained ICU doulas providing early psychological support to critically ill patients. *Critical Care*, *25*(1), 446. 10.1186/s13054-021-03856-3

Karnatovskaia, L. V., Schultz, J., Niven, A. S., Steele, A. J., Baker, B. A., Philbrick, K. L., Del Valle, K. T., Johnson, K. R., Gajic, O., & Varga, K. (2021b). System of psychological support based on positive suggestions to the critically ill using ICU doulas. *Critical Care Explorations*, *3*(4), e0403. 10.1097/cce.0000000000000403

Kelemen-Szilágyi, A. (2019). Léna. In A. Zseni (Ed.), *Hipnózis a gyakorlatban 4. Testünk bajai [Hypnosis in practice 4. The troubles of our body]* (1st ed., pp. 48–68). Animula Kiadó.

Kelley, M. L., Bravo, A. J., Davies, R. L., Hamrick, H. C., Vinci, C., & Redman, J. C. (2019). Moral injury and suicidality among combat-wounded veterans: The moderating effects of social connectedness and self-compassion. *Psychological Trauma: Theory, Research, Practice and Policy*, *11*(6), 621. 10.1037/tra0000447

Kulcsár, Z. s. (2005). A társas interakciók pszichológiai hatásai és agyi mechanizmusai. Egy hipotézis körvonalai. Társas támogatás [Psychological effects and brain mechanisms of social interactions. Outline of a hypothesis. Peer support]. In Z. s. Kulcsár (Ed.), *Teher alatt ... Pozitív traumafeldolgozás és poszttraumás személyiségfejlődés [Under pressure ... Positive trauma processing and posttraumatic personality development]* (1st ed., pp. 315–393). Trefort Kiadó.

László, Z. s., Papi, R., & Szilágyi, A. K. (2014). *Pozitív szuggesztiókon alapuló pszichoterápiás munka egy kritikus állapotú Chron-beteg férfi pácienssel az intenzív osztályon – Esetismertetés [Psychotherapeutic work based on positive suggestion in the intensive care unit with a critically ill a male patient with Chron's disease – case report]* [Presentation]. XXIII National Scientific Assembly of the Hungarian Psychological Society, May 15–17, 2014, Târgu Mures, Romania.

Levine, S., Weinberg, J., & Ursin, H. (1978). Definition of the coping process and statement of the problem. In H. Ursin, E. Baade, & S. Levine (Eds.), *Psychobiology of stress: A study of coping men* (pp. 3–22). Academic Press.

Maslach, C., Jackson, S. E., & Leiter, M. P. (2016). *Maslach burnout inventory: Manual* (4th ed.). Mind Garden.

Novoa, M., & Ballesteros de Valderrama, B. P. (2006). The role of the psychologist in an intensive care unit. *Universitas Psychologica*, *5*(3), 599–612. Retrieved April 4, 2023, from https://www.redalyc.org/pdf/647/64750314.pdf

Organ, D. W., & Ryan, K. (1995). A meta-analytic review of attitudinal and dispositional predictors of organizational citizenship behavior. *Personnel Psychology*, *48*(4), 775–802. 10.1111/j.1744-6570.1995.tb01781.x

Peris, A., Bonizzoli, M., Iozzelli, D., Migliaccio, M. L., Zagli, G., Bacchereti, A., Debolini, M., Vannini, E., Solaro, M., Balzi, I., Bendoni, E., Bacchi, I., Trevisan, M., Giovannini, V., & Belloni, L. (2011). Early intra-intensive care unit psychological intervention promotes recovery from post traumatic stress disorders, anxiety and depression symptoms in critically ill patients. *Critical Care*, *15*(1), R41. 10.1186/cc10003

Rizzolatti, G., Fadiga, L., Gallese, V., & Fogassi, L. (1996). Premotor cortex and the recognition of motor actions. *Brain Research: Cognitive Brain Research*, *3*(2), 131–141. 10.1016/0926-6410(95)00038-0

Rosenthal, R. (2002). Covert communication in classrooms, clinics, courtrooms, and cubicles. *American Psychologist*, *57*(11), 839–849. 10.1037/0003-066x.57.11.839

Rosenthal, R., & Jacobson, L. (1968). *Pygmalion in the classroom: Teacher expectation and pupil's intellectual development.* Crown House Publishing.

Sanfey, A. G., Rilling, J. K., Aronson, J. A., Nystrom, L. E., & Cohen, J. D. (2003). The neural basis of economic decision-making in the Ultimatum Game. *Science*, *300*(5626), 1755–1758. 10.1126/science.1082976

Schlanger, J., Fritúz, G., & Varga, K. (2013). Therapeutic suggestion helps to cut back on drug intake for mechanically ventilated patients in intensive care unit. *Interventional Medicine and Applied Science*, *5*(4), 145–152. 10.1556/imas.5.2013.4.1

Schmidbauer, W. (1977). *Die hilflosen Helfer: Über die seelische Problematik der helfenden Berufe [The helpless helpers: On the mental problems of the helping professions]*. Rowohlt.

Singer, T., Kiebel, S. J., Winston, J. S., Dolan, R. J., & Frith, C. D. (2004). Brain responses to the acquired moral status of faces. *Neuron*, *41*(4), 653–662. 10.1016/s0896-6273(04)00014-5

Spitz, R. A. (1945). Hospitalism: An inquiry into the genesis of psychiatric conditions in early childhood. *The Psychoanalytic Study of the Child*, *1*(1), 53–74. 10.1080/00797308.1945.11823126

K. Szilágyi, A., Diószeghy, C. s., Benczúr, L., & Varga, K. (2007). Effectiveness of psychological support based on positive suggestion with the ventilated patient. *European Journal of Mental Health*, 2(2), 149–170. 10.1556/ejmh.2.2007.2.2

K. Szilágyi, A. (2011). Suggestive communication in the intensive care unit. In K. Varga (Ed.), *Beyond the words: Communication and suggestion in medical practice* (1st ed., pp. 223–237). Nova Science Publishers.

K. Szilágyi, A., Diószeghy, C. s., Fritúz, G., Gál, J., & Varga, K. (2014). Shortening the length of stay and mechanical ventilation time by using positive suggestions via MP3 players for ventilated patients. *Interventional Medicine and Applied Science*, *6*(1), 3–15. 10.1556/imas.6.2014.1.1

K. Szilágyi, A., László, Z. s., Diószeghy, C. s., & Varga, K. (2014). Healing effects of positive suggestions with ventilated patients [Paper presented]. In 13th Congress of European Society of Hypnosis, October 21–25, 2014, Sorrento, Italy.

Uchino, B. N., Cacioppo, J. T., & Kiecolt-Glaser, J. K. (1996). The relationship between social support and physiological processes: A review with emphasis on underlying mechanisms and implications for health. *Psychological Bulletin*, *119*(3), 488–531. 10.1037/0033-2909.119.3.488

Varga, K., & Diószeghy, Cs. (2003). The use of hypnotic communication and hypnotic suggestions in the intensive care unit. *Hypnos*, *30*(1), 16–26.

Varga, K., Diószeghy, C. s., & Fritúz, G. (2007). Suggestive communication with the ventilated patient. *European Journal of Mental Health (EJMH)*, *2*(2), 137–147. 10.1556/ejmh.2.2007.2.1

Varga, K. (2015). *Communication strategies in medical settings: Challenging situations and practical solutions: Vol. Consciousness and Human Systems, Volume 3*. Peter Lang Group. 10.3726/978-3-653-05313-5

Vargay, A., Józsa, E., Pájer, A., & Bányai, É. (2019). The characteristics and changes of psychological immune competence of breast cancer patients receiving hypnosis, music or special attention. *Mentálhigiéné és Pszichoszomatika*, *20*(2), 139–158. 10.1556/0406.20.2019.009

Weinhouse, G. L., Schwab, R. J., Watson, P. L., Patil, N., Vaccaro, B., Pandharipande, P., & Ely, E. W. (2009). Bench-to-bedside review: Delirium in ICU patients – Importance of sleep deprivation. *Critical Care*, *13*(6), 234. 10.1186/cc8131

Winston, J. S., Strange, B. A., O'Doherty, J., & Dolan, R. J. (2002). Automatic and intentional brain responses during evaluation of trustworthiness of faces. *Nature Neuroscience*, *5*(3), 277–283. 10.1038/nn816

51
CLINICAL HYPNOSIS IN PALLIATIVE CARE

Maria Paola Brugnoli
Department of Philosophy and Neurobioethics, Pontifical Athenaeum Regina Apostolorum, Roma, Italy

Introduction: Psychophysiology, Perspectives, and Applications of Clinical Hypnosis in Palliative Care

Even if some diseases are not curable, symptoms are. The saying, "When nothing remains to be done, everything remains to be done" is fundamental to palliative care. Palliative care focuses on physically and psychologically distressing symptom relief, including pain, anxiety, shortness of breath, fatigue, constipation, nausea, loss of appetite, difficulty sleeping, and depression. The goal is to improve quality of life for both the patient and their family. One commonly accepted early definition of palliative developed by the World Health Organization (WHO) was: "Palliative care is the active total care of patients whose disease is not responsive to curative treatment." Subsequently, in 1990, WHO broadened its definition to emphasize the control of pain and attention to psychological, social, and spiritual elements of care. The goal of Clinical Hypnosis in Palliative Care is this global approach aimed at the best quality of life for patients and their families (WHO Expert Committee on Cancer Pain Relief and Active Supportive Care & World Health Organization, 1990).

One commonly accepted early definition of palliative developed by the WHO begins: "Palliative care is the active total care of patients whose disease is not responsive to curative treatment." Subsequently, in 1990, WHO suggested a more global approach by stating: "… control of pain, of other symptoms, and of psychological, social and spiritual problems is paramount." The goal of Clinical Hypnosis in Palliative Care is to achieve this global approach aimed at the best quality of life for patients and their families (WHO Expert Committee on Cancer Pain Relief and Active Supportive Care & World Health Organization, 1990).

Clinical hypnosis and self-hypnosis in palliative care is that state of inner concentration, which means presence of mind and attentiveness to the present (Landry et al., 2018). It is used to relieve pain and distressing symptoms associated with cancer and severe chronic diseases (Brugnoli, 2014a; Handel, 2001). Hypnosis has documented efficacy in severe chronic diseases, in a variety of conditions such as mental health disorders, psychosomatic symptoms, pain reduction, anxiety, nausea, vomiting, and other distressing symptoms

DOI: 10.4324/9781003449126-66

(Elkins et al., 2007; Lankton, 2013; Moss, 2018; Satsangi & Brugnoli, 2018). Clinical hypnosis research bridges phenomenology and neuroscience (Landry et al., 2018; Raz., 2005, 2011). Most researchers leverage bottom-up suppression to unlock the underlying mechanisms of unconscious processing. However, a top-down approach – for example via hypnotic suggestion – paves the road to experimental innovation and complementary data that afford new scientific insights concerning attention and the unconscious mind (Landry et al., 2018). The following neurophysiological features of clinical hypnosis are very important in palliative care: Hypnosis can: (1) selectively target and modify perception of sensory events (Landry et al., 2018), (2) induce experiences of modified or cross-modal sensations (i.e., interactions of the sense, such as synesthesia; Anbar & Linden, 2010; Barber et al., 1974), and (3) temporarily abolish co-occurrences of secondary sensory experiences in synesthetes (Terhune et al., 2016).

We can use these effects of hypnosis on perceptions to modulate acute and chronic pain, and to reduce anxiety, depression, and the distressing physical and psychological symptoms (Brugnoli, 1974a, 1974b, 2014a, 2014b, 2016; Brugnoli et al., 2018; De Benedittis, 1979a, 1979b; Ewin, 1978; Erickson et al., 1976; Jensen & Patterson, 2008; Néron & Stephenson, 2007; Vannoni & Brugnoli, 1971). Hypnosis is emerging as a valuable tool for investigating the default mode network (DMN) of brain regions that show increased activity at rest (Deeley et al., 2012). DMN activity correlates with a wide range of internally directed conscious activity and cognitive processes, including mind-wandering, self-oriented thinking, moral reasoning, and episodic memory (Landry & Raz, 2015). These studies illustrate how influencing the experiential state of the subject can enrich and even guide not only the investigation of brain networks but also their psychological and clinical correlates when using hypnosis in palliative care (Brugnoli et al., 2016; Landry et al., 2018).

Clinical Hypnosis and the Challenge of Its Therapeutic Relevance in Palliative Medicine

The WHO (World Health Organization, 2002, 2018a, 2018b, 2021) established a revised definition of palliative care for adults and children:

> Palliative care is an approach that improves the quality of life of patients and their families facing the problems associated with life-threatening illness, through the prevention and relief of suffering by means of early identification and impeccable assessment and treatment of pain and other problems, physical, psychosocial and spiritual. (p. 3)

Palliative care entails multidimensional assessment and interventions that improve the quality of life and provide assistance to individuals and families from different cultures, as they approach the end of life. The complexity of medical therapies includes the allocation of individual, family, and societal resources, and the recognition of changing goals of care. This concerns individuals' deepest and most dearly held fears, values, beliefs, and hope (Frankl, 1988; Gawande, 2017). Addressing end-of-life issues requires skilled, insightful, interdisciplinary care. Palliative care is based on the needs of the patient, not on the patient's prognosis (Bruera et al., 1991). It is appropriate at any age and at any stage in a severe disease and it can be provided along with curative treatment. Palliative care is increasingly used with people who have cancer, cardiac disease, chronic obstructive pulmonary disease, kidney failure, HIV/AIDS, and progressive neurodegenerative conditions. Pediatric palliative care has rapidly grown in response to the need for services geared specifically for children with severe illness (Friedrichsdorf & Kohen, 2018; Kuttner & Friedrichsdorf, 2013).

Clinical hypnosis has different modalities of complementary therapy in the various medical and psychological treatments. In palliative care, both medical and psychological hypnotic approaches are essential. We view hypnosis as a therapeutic relationship with the patient, in a dynamic and collaborative process (Varga, 2013, 2021). When using hypnosis, one person (the subject) is guided by another (the hypnotist) to respond to suggestions for changes in subjective experience, alterations in perception, sensation, emotion, thought, or behavior. Persons can also learn self-hypnosis, which is the act of administering hypnotic procedures on one's own (Brugnoli et al., 2018; see chapter on self-hypnosis). Therapeutic hypnosis can have profound effects on the most common symptoms addressed in palliative care. So it emerges as a realistic and sometimes primary treatment option (Casiglia et al., 2020; Squintani et al., 2018).

The two primary clinical effects of hypnosis treatment on symptoms are as follows: (1) the reductions in daily background pain, anxiety, and distressing symptoms intensity (Jensen & Patterson, 2008); and (2) an increased ability to use self-hypnosis to reduce the symptoms (Brugnoli & Brugnoli, 2016; Brugnoli et al., 2018; Ewin, 1978).

Specifically, clinicians treating patients in palliative care with clinical hypnosis should include suggestions that impact the distressing symptom's relief; apply hypnotic techniques that impact all of the neurophysiological processes that may underlie a patient's pain; train patients in the use of self-hypnosis to achieve immediate pain and symptoms' relief; and provide audio recordings of treatment sessions to enhance treatment effects (Brugnoli, et al., 2016; Brugnoli et al., 2018; Hammond, 2010; Handel & Néron, 2017).

The Goals of Clinical Hypnosis in Palliative Care

The goal of palliative care is to improve the quality of life for both the patient and the family. Patient-centered care is central to treatment (World Health Organization, 2018a, 2018b, 2019) Clinical hypnosis, remarkably, can accomplish all the following components of palliative care, which WHO (World Health Organization, 2018a, 2018b, 2019) emphasizes as essential.

1 Provide relief from pain and other distressing symptoms.
2 Affirm life and dying as a normal process.
3 Intend neither to hasten or postpone death.
4 Integrate the psychological and spiritual aspects of patient care.
5 Offer a support system to help patients live as actively as possible until death.
6 Offer a support system to help the family cope during the patients' illness and in their own bereavement.
7 Use a team approach to address the needs of patients and their families, including bereavement counseling, if indicated.
8 Enhance quality of life, and also positively influence the course of illness.
9 Begin early in the course of illness, in conjunction with other therapies that are intended to prolong life, such as chemotherapy or radiation therapy, and include those investigations needed to better understand and manage distressing clinical complications.

The goals of clinical hypnosis in palliative care and the WHO guidelines for Palliative Care (World Health Organization, 2018a, 2018b, 2019) are the same.

To Provide Relief from Pain, Anxiety, and Other Distressing Symptoms

We do not perceive pain and suffering as separate entities. The physical, anatomic, and neurochemical expression of pain is treated with physical therapy, medicine, nerve block, electric stimulators, and surgery. Clinical hypnosis is a complementary therapy for pain relief (Brugnoli, 2014a, 2016, 2018; Jensen & Patterson, 2008). Hypnosis is used for both chronic and acute pain conditions with promising results:

a hypnotic analgesia in palliation consistently results in greater decreases in a variety of pain outcomes compared to no treatment/standard care (Brugnoli et al., 2018);
b hypnosis frequently out-performs non-hypnotic interventions (e.g., education, supportive therapy) in terms of reductions in pain-related outcomes (Brugnoli, 2014a);
c hypnosis performs similar to treatments that contain hypnotic elements (such as progressive muscle relaxation) but is not surpassed in efficacy by these alternative treatments (Squintani et al., 2018).

Studies using laser-evoked potentials, functional MRI, and positron emission tomography (PET) have revealed that a number of brain structures involved in the perception of pain, e.g., somatosensory cortex, anterior cingulate cortex, and the insula, are demonstrably affected through hypnotic suggestion (Rainville et al., 1997; Raz, 2011; Squintani et al., 2018).

Fear of suffering is significant in people with chronic illnesses and at end of life. Fear is ameliorated with self-control and efficacy. Table 51.1 lists the many psychological complications.

Hypnosis provides a means for self-control. Patterson and Jensen (2003) and Willmarth (2017) supported the use of hypnosis for both acute and chronic pain conditions. "Total pain" is the summation of the patient's physical, psychological, social, and spiritual pain.

Table 51.1 Clinical and Psychological Complications in Palliative Care Pain

Reluctance to report pain
Suffering may be perceived as the "*conditio sine qua non*" for serious diseases or death
Fear of increasing functional deficits
Concerns with cognitive function
High number of cognitively impaired
Fear of the unknown in children
Fear of hastening death in the frail elderly
Anxiety
More depression and desperation
Decreased socialization
Sleep disturbances
Social suffering
Communication barrier due to sensory or cognitive impairment
Communication barrier due to anxiety and depression.
Nausea and vomiting
Other physical distressing symptoms
Spiritual suffering

This notion is fundamental to the assessment and diagnosis of pain and suffering (Saunders, 1996). Treating the patient's total pain is imperative, especially at the end of life (Kuebler et al., 2007). Although hundreds of valid creative suggestions and metaphors for pain control have been presented in the scientific literature, for palliative care we highlight the recommendations of Hilgard and Hilgard (1994). They propose three general classes of (total) pain management approaches with clinical hypnosis. These are (1) direct suggestion of symptom reduction, (2) alteration of the experience of symptom, and (3) redirection of attention.

In palliative care, anxiety is addressed as a special form of mind/body problem involving deep interaction between mental and physical distress. Untreated anxiety can often lead to a depressive syndrome. Hypnosis and self-hypnosis training represent rapid, cost-effective, and safe additions to medication for the treatment of anxiety-related conditions (Handel, & Néron, 2017; Moss, 2018). Cognitive hypnotherapy (CH) can be effectively applied to the treatment of anxiety disorders and depression (Alladin, 2018). Rapid and sustained relief of severe anxiety is necessary to achieve comfort at the end of life. Skillful use of psychological therapies such as clinical hypnosis with breathing exercises and meditation led to control of anxiety (Agarwal et al., 2018; Casula, 2018). Insomnia, excessive sleeping, fatigue, loss of energy, or aches, pains, or digestive problems that are resistant to treatment may also be present (NIH, 2004; National Institute of Mental Health [NIMH], 2012). While apparently not painful for the patient, the association of the symptom with impending death can create fear and uncertainty for those at the bedside (Rodin et al., 2009). Nonpharmacological strategies such as hypnosis and progressive relaxation are highlighted for managing medical and anesthesiologic procedures, common chemotherapy, symptoms adverse effects (Kekecs & Varga, 2013), and psychosomatic symptoms (Satsangi & Brugnoli, 2018). Both research and clinical experience highlight the potential value of hypnosis in the management of anticipatory nausea and vomiting in chemotherapy (Marchioro et al., 2000).

Palliative Care Affirms Life and Regards Dying as a Normal Process

Clinical hypnosis significantly integrates the pharmacological and psychological care of dying patients. In fact, we help the patient and his family live with less stress in the last hours of life. The empathic relationship we create can better help the patient and the therapist in his important pathway: "clinical hypnosis affirms life and regards dying as a normal process" (Brugnoli, 2014a). Current literature reflects numerous studies suggesting that psychological, social, and/or spiritual dimensions influence positive patient health outcomes and affects overall quality of life (Puchalski, 2007). Caring for a person during the last few weeks and days of life can be traumatic and demanding. At this time, both the patient and the family need to feel that they are not alone and have some control during this journey.

Palliative Care Intends Neither to Hasten or Postpone Death

Palliative care and clinical hypnosis intend neither to hasten or postpone death. This means that clinical hypnosis respects the bioethical principles of medicine and the dignity of the patient.

Clinical hypnosis is a therapeutic approach that respects life and death (Gómez et al., 2021). Practicing clinical hypnosis, we are responsible for working not only according to rules and laws but also in an ethical manner of person-centered therapy. Life is unconditionally meaningful, no matter what happens. It follows that an (ultimate) meaning exists even when one cannot find a meaning in a life-situation (Frankl, 1988).

Palliative Care Integrates the Psychological and Spiritual Aspects of Patient Care

Psychological and spiritual aspects of hypnotic care combine effective medical treatment with compassionate relationships. This establishes a secure "inner space" in which the process of a patient's healing may take place over time (Agarwal et al., 2018; Brugnoli, 2009). The psychological and socio-spiritual component of suffering involves the patient's (a) non-acceptance, (b) fear of the unknown and anxiety, (c) pessimistic evaluation of the meaning of pain and depression, (d) feeling of no time limit to suffering, and (e) often self-destructive feelings of guilt and resentment (Saunders, 1996). These emotions and imaginings are quite amenable to hypnotherapy. When inner suffering is reduced, physical and psychological pain tends to become tolerable or may even disappear (Alladin, 2018; Brugnoli et al., 2018). The patient can experience feelings of deepest peace (Agarwal et al., 2018).

Religion and spirituality, which are multidimensional concepts, have positive effects on psychological and spiritual health. Viktor Frankl (1988) wrote that he needed to find meaning in his life so that he could sustain his life physically, psychologically, and spiritually. In other words, when an individual understands meaning in life, especially at the end of life, these three dimensions will be in a healthy interaction. Clinical hypnosis can be a life transforming change process, for the psycho-social and spiritual healing of the patients. In this context, we may consider clinical hypnosis as a "short psychotherapy" for a transformative psycho-social spiritual learning of better ways to live.

Palliative Care Offers a Support System to Help Patients Live as Actively as Possible Until Death

Hypnosis helps the patient to maximize the benefits of therapies and to live as well as possible with a better quality of life. We can consider clinical hypnosis a modified state of consciousness for the physical, mental, social, and spiritual processes of recovery, repair, renewal, and transformation (Brugnoli et al., 2016). In psychosocial oncology, paths of both psychotherapy with hypnosis (Alladin, 2018) and art therapy through hypnosis (Brugnoli & Brugnoli, 2016, 2019) can help the patient to live as gladly as possible until death.

Palliative Care Offers a Support System to Help the Family Cope during the Patient's Illness and in Their Own Bereavement

Clinical hypnosis in palliative care assesses the care needs of each patient and their families across the domains of physical, psychological, social, spiritual, and information needs. Hypnotherapy can reduce anxiety, not only for the patients but also for the family (Agarwal et al., 2018). The therapists in the palliative care team construct the communication with the family so that confidentiality and dignity for the patient's last stage of life are maintained (Beauchamp & Childress, 2001). Empathic communication with patients and family deals with ethical questions regarding two fundamental aspects of palliative: to explain the pathway of a good death and to resolve the conflicting needs of patient vis-à-vis family (NIH, 2004).

Palliative Care Uses a Team Approach to Address the Needs of Patients and their Families, Including Bereavement Counseling, If Indicated

Teamwork is an indispensable component of palliative care. A functional narrative analysis reveals the fundamental themes: many different ways to communicate with the patient, the voice of the lifeworld, and the bereavement counseling (NIH, 2004). Hypnotherapy in palliative care can be a method of communication and psychotherapy used to create unconscious change in the patient and family, in the form of new responses, thoughts, attitudes, behaviors, or feelings (Alladin, 2018). Losing a loved one is one of life's greatest stressors. Prolonged grief disorder is associated with higher risk for depression, posttraumatic stress disorder, and suicidal ideation and behaviors (Alladin, 2018; Handel & Néron, 2017; Néron & Stephenson, 2007). Hypnotic communication is a way to handle the different states of mind in bereavement counseling. Non-clinical studies raise the possibility to consider hypnosis as a potential corrective/reparative possibility in cases of persons with unfavorable experiences in the childhood (e.g., having non-attentive parents) (Költő et al., 2019; Varga, 2013, 2021).

Palliative Care Will Enhance Quality of Life, and May Also Positively Influence the Course of Illness

Even when we cannot cure the illness, we can give the patients a better quality of life (Saunders, 1996). It is normal for patients at the end of life to worry and grieve the loss of their health. Alladin (2018) investigated the effectiveness of CH, combined with cognitive-behavioral therapy, on depression in palliative care. His study represents a controlled comparison of hypnotherapy with a well-established psychotherapy for depression. The treatment of anxiety and depression in terminally ill patients can optimize their physical comfort at the end of life and provide them the opportunity to confront and prepare for death. Hypnosis may also positively influence the course of illness, from the psychological, social, and spiritual point of view.

Palliative Care Is Applicable Early in the Course of Illness, in Conjunction with Other Therapies That Are Intended to Prolong Life, Such as Chemotherapy or Radiation Therapy, and Includes Those Investigations Needed to Better Understand and Manage Distressing Clinical Complications

Clinical hypnosis is applicable early in the course of illness (Handel & Néron, 2017; Marcus et al., 2003; Néron & Stephenson, 2007). Clinical hypnosis, in conjunction with other therapies, can cure the total pain and suffering. The advantages of clinical hypnosis in palliative care include:

- Simplicity, as complementary analgesic and symptom relief;
- Applicability early in the course of illness as an adjunct in conjunction with other therapies;
- Flexibility for a large variety of pain and symptoms situations;
- Safety from side effects;
- A multimodal approach on suffering relief and total suffering (Brugnoli, 2014a).

Brief Introduction to Clinical Hypnosis in Palliative Care for Children

Palliative care for children is closely related field to adult palliative care. The following principles apply to pediatric chronic disorders (American Academy of Pediatrics Committee on Pediatric Emergency Medicine, 1995; World Health Organization, 1998)

- Palliative care for children is the active total care of the child's body, mind, and spirit, and also involves giving support to the family;
- It begins when illness is diagnosed and continues regardless of whether or not a child receives treatment directed at the disease;
- Health providers must evaluate and alleviate a child's physical, psychological, and social distress;
- Effective palliative care requires a broad multidisciplinary approach that includes the family and makes use of available community resources: it can be successfully implemented even if resources are limited;
- It can be provided in tertiary care facilities, in community health centers, and even in children's homes (Friedrichsdorf & Zeltzer, 2012; Gardner, 1976).

Integration of palliative care into the routine care of children, adolescents, and young adults with cancer and severe chronic diseases has resulted in enhanced outcomes in patients and their families. Family-centered communication helps a dialog between children, families, and therapists with a goal of effective and empathic pediatric health care (Kuttner & Friedrichsdorf, 2013; Wolfe et al., 2008).

Psychosocial care of children and families is a key element of palliative care in pediatric oncology patients. Recent clinical guidelines for the psychological approach (Ferrell et al., 2018) and suggestions of care for psychosocial palliative care (Kuttner & Friedrichsdorf, 2013) have emphasized the importance of routine psychosocial assessments for patients and their family members, and the importance of an interdisciplinary palliative care team (Wolfe et al., 2008; Culbert et al., 2012).

Hypnosis for pediatric patients experiencing a life-limiting disease not only provides an integral part of advanced pain and symptom management but also supports children dealing with loss and anticipatory loss, sustains and enhances hope, and helps children and adolescents live fully, making every moment count, until death (Friedrichsdorf & Kohen, 2018; Kohen & Olness, 2011; Kuttner & Friedrichsdorf, 2013). Advanced effective treatment and prevention of symptoms in palliative care requires employing "multi-modal" therapies, commonly including pharmacology, rehabilitation, procedural intervention, psychology, psychosocial, spiritual therapies, and clinical hypnosis (Liossi et al., 2009; Sugarman & Wester, 2014).

When a child with a serious illness learns hypnosis early during treatment, either as self-hypnosis or during psychotherapy, it becomes part of the supportive therapeutic scaffold, which the child leans on and builds upon to deal with life and death concerns. Hypnosis helps to evoke experiences within the child's imagination that diminish the fear of death and ease their present experience (Kuttner & Friedrichsdorf, 2013; Kohen & Olness, 2011). The words of the dying child Mattie Stepanek (1990–2004) were: "Palliative care no longer means helping children die well, it means helping children and their families to live well, and then, when the time is certain, to help them die gently" (Stepanek, n.d.).

Conclusions: Future Orientation for Professional Development of Clinical Hypnosis as an Integrative Therapy in Palliative Care

The goal of integration of hypnosis in palliative care is to optimize patient access to supportive care, and ultimately, to improve the quality of life of patients, family, therapists, and caregivers. In 2021, the WHO outlined some essential components needed to provide optimal palliative care with an integrated, person-centered approach (World Health Organization, 2021).

Clinical hypnosis in palliative care is appropriate for all the patients with advanced incurable disease, and not only those in the last weeks/months of life. It should be fully integrated with diagnosis and treatment. The development of guidelines for the use of clinical hypnosis as an adjunctive therapy is important because they will ensure that evidence-based methodology is used to establish national consensus protocols of hypnosis (Kekecs et al., 2022). Further studies are needed to explore whether the observed benefits are a direct result of the hypnotherapy, and how the intervention could most advantage the therapy of these patients. Given the tremendous heterogeneity in healthcare systems, patient population, resource availability, clinician training, and attitudes and beliefs toward palliative care worldwide, it is important to emphasize that no one model of palliative care will offer the final solution for all.

Clinical hypnosis in palliative care is best introduced early in the disease trajectory. Pharmacologic and non-pharmacological therapies are combined into an integrative framework of medical, psychological, and cognitive functions. Clinical hypnosis considers roles of bottom-up and top-down processes involved in threat-evaluation, orienting, and inhibitory control in the different manifestations of the psychosomatic symptoms (Satsangi & Brugnoli, 2018).

The importance of psycho-social and spiritual care with hypnosis has increased in recent years (Agarwal et al., 2018; Brugnoli, 2009). Clinical hypnosis is a psychological and psychotherapeutic approach to be considered in psychosocial oncology for adults and children (Alladin, 2018; Brugnoli, 2018; Handel., 2001; Handel & Néron, 2017; Kuttner & Friedrichsdorf, 2013; Marcus et al., 2003; Moss, 2018). Integrating clinical hypnosis into palliative care is both necessary and achievable. They share fundamental goals, as described earlier.

In conclusion, clinical hypnosis is a clinical and psychological person-centered therapy: "... A meaning centered psychotherapy views even man's orientation toward ultimate meaning as a human phenomenon rather than anything divine ... . We must remain aware of this fact as long as absolute truth is not accessible to us" (Frankl, 1988, p. 9). Today, more than ever, we must also remember the importance of palliative care in particular social contexts: the palliative care needs of people affected by natural hazards, political, or ethnic conflict, wars, epidemics of life-threatening infections, and other humanitarian crises (World Health Organization, 2012). Through clinical hypnosis, communication, and empathy at the end of life, we can be close to the sick person and his or her family ... as if we were observing together the blue reflections of the sky ... in the light of early morning dew drops ... and together smiling at the immense mystery of life.

References

Agarwal, S., Kumar, V., Agarwal, S., Brugnoli, M. P., & Agarwal, A. (2018). Meditational spiritual intercession and recovery from disease in palliative care: A literature review. *Annals of Palliative Medicine*, 7(1), 41–62. 10.21037/apm.2017.08.08

Alladin, A. (2018). Cognitive hypnotherapy for psychological management of depression in palliative care. *Annals of Palliative Medicine*, *7*(1), 112–124. 10.21037/apm.2017.08.15

American Academy of Pediatrics Committee on Pediatric Emergency Medicine. (1995). Guidelines for pediatric emergency care facilities. *Pediatrics*, *96*(3), 526–537. 10.1542/peds.96.3.526

Anbar, R. D., & Linden, J. H. (2010). Understanding dissociation and insight in the treatment of shortness of breath with hypnosis: A case study. *American Journal of Clinical Hypnosis*, *52*(4), 263–273. 10.1080/00029157.2010.10401731

Barber, T. X., Spanos, N. P., & Chaves, J. F. (1974). *Hypnosis, imagination, and human potentialities* (1st ed.). Pergamon Press.

Beauchamp, T. L., & Childress, J. F. (2001). *Principles of biomedical ethics* (5th ed.). Oxford University Press.

Bruera, E., Kuehn, N., Miller, M. J., Selmser, P., & Macmillan, K. (1991). The Edmonton Symptom Assessment System (ESAS): A simple method for the assessment of palliative care patients. *Journal of Palliative Care*, *7*(2), 6–9. 10.1177/082585979100700202

Brugnoli, A. (1974a). Tecniche di terapia ipnotica del dolore [Hypnotic therapeutic methods for pain]. *Minerva Medica*, *65*(47), 2637–2641.

Brugnoli, A. (1974b). Ipnoterapia del dolore [Hypnotherapy of pain]. *Minerva Medica*, *65*(63), 3288–3295.

Brugnoli, M. P. (2009). *Clinical hypnosis, spirituality and palliation. The way of inner peace*. Delmiglio Editore.

Brugnoli, M. P. (2014a). *Clinical hypnosis in pain therapy and palliative care: A handbook of techniques for improving the patient's physical and psychological well-being*. Charles C Thomas Publisher, Ltd.

Brugnoli, M. P. (2014b). Clinical hypnosis and relaxation in surgery room, critical care and emergency, for pain and anxiety relief. *Journal of Anesthesia & Critical Care: Open Access*, *1*(3). 10.15406/jaccoa.2014.01.00018

Brugnoli, M. P. (2016). Clinical hypnosis for palliative care in severe chronic diseases: A review and the procedures for relieving physical, psychological and spiritual symptoms. *Annals of Palliative Medicine*, *5*(4), 280–297. 10.21037/apm.2016.09.04

Brugnoli, M. P. (2018). Clinical hypnosis in palliative care: Neural correlates, clinical, psychological and spiritual therapies. *Annals of Palliative Medicine*, *7*(1), 3–6. 10.21037/apm.2017.09.11

Brugnoli, M. P., Brugnoli, A., & Recchia, L. (2016). *A new classification of the modified states of consciousness*. LAP Lambert Academic Publishing.

Brugnoli, M. P., & Brugnoli, M. (2016). *Art, mindfulness and self-hypnosis in psychosocial oncology: The way of inner consciousness*. Officina Grafica.

Brugnoli, M. P., & Brugnoli, M. (2019). *Art and meditation for the peace of heart*. Youcanprint Publisher.

Brugnoli, M. P., Pesce, G., Pasin, E., Basile, M. S., Tamburin, S., & Polati, E. (2018). The role of clinical hypnosis and self-hypnosis to relief pain and anxiety in severe chronic diseases in palliative care: A 2-year long-term follow-up of treatment in a nonrandomized clinical trial. *Annals of Palliative Medicine*, *7*(1), 17–31. 10.21037/apm.2017.10.03

Casiglia, E., Finatti, F., Tikhonoff, V., Stabile, M. R., Mitolo, M., Albertini, F., Gasparotti, F., Facco, E., Lapenta, A. M., & Venneri, A. (2020). Mechanisms of hypnotic analgesia explained by functional magnetic resonance (fMRI). *International Journal of Clinical and Experimental Hypnosis*, *68*(1), 1–15. 10.1080/00207144.2020.1685331

Casula, C. (2018). Clinical hypnosis, mindfulness and spirituality in palliative care. *Annals of Palliative Medicine*, *7*(1), 32–40. 10.21037/apm.2017.07.07

Culbert, T., Friedrichsdorf, S., & Kuttner, L. (2012). Mind/body skills for children in pain. In H. Breivik, W. Campbell, & W. Nicholas (Eds.), *Clinical pain management: Practice and procedures* (2nd ed., pp. 478–495). Hodder Arnold.

De Benedittis, G. (1979a). A new strategy for chronic pain control: The multi-modal approach. Preliminary results (Part I). *Journal of Neurosurgical Sciences*, *23*(3), PMID: 43360. https://pubmed.ncbi.nlm.nih.gov/43360/

De Benedittis, G. (1979b). A new strategy for chronic pain control: the multi-modal approach. Preliminary results (Part II). *Journal of Neurosurgical Sciences*, *23*(3), PMID: 529002. https://pubmed.ncbi.nlm.nih.gov/529002/

Deeley, Q., Oakley, D. A., Toone, B., Giampietro, V., Brammer, M., Williams, S., & Halligan, P. W. (2012). Modulating the default mode network using hypnosis. *International Journal of Clinical and Experimental Hypnosis*, *60*(2), 206–228. 10.1080/00207144.2012.648070

Elkins, G. R., Jensen, M. P., & Patterson, D. A. (2007). Hypnotherapy for the management of chronic pain. *International Journal of Clinical and Experimental Hypnosis*, *55*(3), 275–287. 10.1080/00207140701338621

Erickson, M. H., Rossi, E. L., & Rossi, S. I. (1976). *Hypnotic realities: The induction of clinical hypnosis and indirect forms of suggestion*. Irvington Publishers.

Ewin, D. M. (1978). Relieving suffering – and pain – with hypnosis. *Geriatrics*, *33*(6), 87.

Ferrell, B., Twaddle, M., Melnick, A., & Meier, D. E. (2018). National Consensus Project Clinical Practice Guidelines for Quality Palliative Care (NCP Guidelines): 4th edition. *Journal of Palliative Medicine*, *21*(12), 1684–1689. 10.1089/jpm.2018.0431

Frankl, V. E. (1988). *The will to meaning: Foundations and applications of logotherapy*. Meridian.

Friedrichsdorf, S. J., & Kohen, D. P. (2018). Integration of hypnosis into pediatric palliative care. *Annals of Palliative Medicine*, *7*(1), 136–150. 10.21037/apm.2017.05.02

Friedrichsdorf, S. J., & Zeltzer, L. (2012). Palliative care for children with advanced cancer. In S. Kreitler, M. W. Ben-Arush, & A. Martin (Eds.), *Pediatric psycho-oncology: Psychosocial aspects and clinical interventions* (2nd ed., pp. 160–174). Wiley-Blackwell.

Gómez, A. G., Brugnoli, M. P., & Carrara, A. (Eds.). (2021). *Bioethics and consciousness*. Cambridge Scholars Publishing.

Gardner, G. G. (1976). Childhood, death, and human dignity: Hypnotherapy for David. *International Journal of Clinical and Experimental Hypnosis*, *24*(2), 122–139. 10.1080/00207147608405603

Gawande, A. (2017). *Being mortal: Illness, medicine and what matters in the end*. Metropolitan.

Hammond, D. C. (2010). Hypnosis in the treatment of anxiety- and stress-related disorders. *Expert Review of Neurotherapeutics*, *10*(2), 263–273. 10.1586/ern.09.140

Handel, D. L. (2001). Complementary therapies for cancer patients: What works, what doesn't, and how to know the difference. *Texas Medicine*, *97*(2), 68–73.

Handel, D. L., & Néron, S. (2017). Cancer palliation: Layered hypnotic approaches mending symptoms, minding hope, and meaning. *American Journal of Clinical Hypnosis*, *60*(1). 10.1080/00029157.2017.1299678

Hilgard, E. R., & Hilgard, J. R. (1994). *Hypnosis in the relief of pain*. Routledge.

Jensen, M. P., & Patterson, D. R. (2008). Hypnosis and the relief of pain and pain disorders. In M. R. Nash & A. J. Barnier (Eds.), *The Oxford handbook of hypnosis: Theory, research, and practice* (pp. 503–533). Oxford University Press.

Kekecs, Z., Moss, D., Elkins, G., De Benedittis, G., Palsson, O. S., Shenefelt, P. D., Terhune, D. B., Varga, K., & Whorwell, P. J. (2022). Guidelines for the assessment of efficacy of clinical hypnosis applications. *International Journal of Clinical and Experimental Hypnosis*, *70*(2), 104–122. 10.1080/00207144.2022.2049446

Kekecs, Z., & Varga, K. (2013). Positive suggestion techniques in somatic medicine: A review of the empirical studies. *Interventional Medicine and Applied Science*, *5*(3), 101–111. 10.1556/imas.5.2013.3.2

Kohen, D. P., & Olness, K. (2011). *Hypnosis and hypnotherapy with children* (4th ed.). Taylor & Francis.

Költő, A., Józsa, E., & Bányai, É. I. (2019). Recalled parental rearing style and dimensions of hypnotic response. *International Journal of Clinical and Experimental Hypnosis*, *67*(2), 157–191. 10.1080/00207144.2019.1580968

Kuebler, K. K., Heidrich, D. E., & Esper, P. (2007). *Palliative and end-of-life care: Clinical practice guidelines* (2nd ed.). Saunders Elsevier.

Kuttner, L., & Friedrichsdorf, S. J. (2013). Hypnosis and palliative care. In L. I. Sugarman & W. C. Wester (Eds.), *Therapeutic hypnosis with children and adolescents* (2nd ed., pp. 491–509). Crown House Publishing.

Landry, M., & Raz, A. (2015). Hypnosis and imaging of the living human brain. *American Journal of Clinical Hypnosis*, *57*(3), 285–313. 10.1080/00029157.2014.978496

Landry, M., Stendel, M., Landry, M., & Raz, A. (2018). Hypnosis in palliative care: From clinical insights to the science of self-regulation. *Annals of Palliative Medicine*, *7*(1), 125–135. 10.21037/apm.2017.12.05

Lankton, S. (2013). Special issue on placebo, hypnosis, and antidepressants. *American Journal of Clinical Hypnosis*, *55*(3), 207–208. 10.1080/00029157.2013.741024

Liossi, C., White, P. D., & Hatira, P. (2009). A randomized clinical trial of a brief hypnosis intervention to control venepuncture-related pain of paediatric cancer patients. *Pain*, *142*(3), 255–263. 10.1016/j.pain.2009.01.017

Marchioro, G., Azzarello, G., Viviani, F., Barbato, F., Pavanetto, M., Rosetti, F., Pappagallo, G. L., & Vinante, O. (2000). Hypnosis in the treatment of anticipatory nausea and vomiting in patients receiving cancer chemotherapy. *Oncology*, *59*(2), 100–104. 10.1159/000012144

Marcus, J., Elkins, G. R., & Mott, F. L. (2003). The integration of hypnosis into a model of palliative care. *Integrative Cancer Therapies*, 2(4), 365–370. 10.1177/1534735403259065

Moss, D. (2018). I hurt so: Hypnotic interventions and palliative care for traumatic brain injury. *Annals of Palliative Medicine*, *7*(1), 151–158. 10.21037/apm.2017.08.16

Néron, S., & Stephenson, R. (2007). Effectiveness of hypnotherapy with cancer patients' trajectory: Emesis, acute pain, and analgesia and anxiolysis in procedures. *International Journal of Clinical and Experimental Hypnosis*, *55*(3), 336–354. 10.1080/00207140701338647

NIH. (2004). NIH State-of-the-Science conference statement on improving end-of-life care. *NIH Consensus and State-of-the-Science Statements*, *21*(3), PMID: 17308546. https://pubmed.ncbi.nlm.nih.gov/17308546/

National Institute of Mental Health [NIMH]. (2012). *Depression*. National Institute of Mental Health (NIMH). Retrieved March 12, 2023, from https://www.nimh.nih.gov/health/topics/depression

Patterson, D. R., & Jensen, M. P. (2003). Hypnosis and clinical pain. *Psychological Bulletin*, *129*(4), 495–521. 10.1037/0033-2909.129.4.495

Puchalski, C. M. (2007). Spirituality and the care of patients at the end-of-life: An essential component of care. *Omega – Journal of Death and Dying*, *56*(1), 33–46. 10.2190/om.56.1.d

Rainville, P., Duncan, G. E., Price, D. L., Carrier, B., & Bushnell, M. C. (1997). Pain affect encoded in human anterior cingulate but not somatosensory cortex. *Science*, *277*(5328), 968–971. 10.1126/science.277.5328.968.

Raz, A. (2005). Attention and hypnosis: Neural substrates and genetic associations of two converging processes. *International Journal of Clinical and Experimental Hypnosis*, *53*(3), 237–258. 10.1080/00207140590961295

Raz, A. (2011). Hypnosis: a twilight zone of the top-down variety: Few have never heard of hypnosis but most know little about the potential of this mind-body regulation technique for advancing science. *Trends in Cognitive Sciences*, *15*(12), 555–557. 10.1016/j.tics.2011.10.002

Rodin, G., Lo, C., Mikulincer, M., Donner, A., Gagliese, L., & Zimmermann, C. (2009). Pathways to distress: The multiple determinants of depression, hopelessness, and the desire for hastened death in metastatic cancer patients. *Social Science & Medicine*, *68*(3), 562–569. 10.1016/j.socscimed.2008.10.037

Satsangi, A. K., & Brugnoli, M. P. (2018). Anxiety and psychosomatic symptoms in palliative care: From neuro-psychobiological response to stress, to symptoms' management with clinical hypnosis and meditative states. *Annals of Palliative Medicine*, *7*(1), 75–111. 10.21037/apm.2017.07.01

Saunders, C. (1996). Into the valley of the shadow of death: A personal therapeutic journey. *British Medical Journal (BMJ)*, *313*(7072), 1599–1601. http://hdl.handle.net/10822/898833

Squintani, G., Brugnoli, M. P., Pasin, E., Segatti, A., Concon, E., Polati, E., Bonetti, B., & Matinella, A. (2018). Changes in laser-evoked potentials during hypnotic analgesia for chronic pain: A pilot study. *Annals of Palliative Medicine*, *7*(1), 7–16. 10.21037/apm.2017.10.04

Stepanek, M. (n.d.). *Matttie Stepanek's definition of palliative care*. What Is Paediatric Palliative Care | Paedspal Paediatric Palliative Care. Retrieved March 13, 2023, from https://paedspal.org.za/about-us/what-is-paediatric-palliative-care

Sugarman, L. I., & Wester, W. (2014). *Therapeutic hypnosis with children and adolescents* (2nd ed.). Crown House Publishing.

Terhune, D. B., Polito, V., Barnier, A. J., & Woody, E. Z. (2016). Variations in the sense of agency during hypnotic responding: Insights from latent profile analysis. *Psychology of Consciousness: Theory, Research, and Practice*, *3*(4), 293–302. 10.1037/cns0000107

Vannoni, S., & Brugnoli, A. (1971). L'ipnoterapia in ortopedia e traumatologia [Hypnotherapy in orthopedics and traumatology]. *Minerva Ortopedica*, *22*(3), 77–83, PMID: 5579742.

Varga, K. (2013). Suggestive techniques connected to medical interventions. *Interventional Medicine and Applied Science*, *5*(3), 95–100. 10.1556/imas.5.2013.3.1

Varga, K. (2021). Possible mechanisms of hypnosis from an interactional perspective. *Brain Sciences*, *11*(7), 903. 10.3390/brainsci11070903

WHO Expert Committee on Cancer Pain Relief and Active Supportive Care & World Health Organization. (1990). *Cancer pain relief and palliative care: Report of a WHO expert committee [meeting held in Geneva from 3 to 10 July 1989]: World Health Organization Technical Report Series; No: 804*. Retrieved March 13, 2023, from https://apps.who.int/iris/handle/10665/39524

World Health Organization. (1998). *Cancer pain relief and palliative care in children*. Retrieved March 13, 2023, from https://apps.who.int/iris/handle/10665/42001

World Health Organization (2002). *Community participation in local health and sustainable development: Approaches and techniques*. Retrieved March 13, 2023, from https://apps.who.int/iris/handle/10665/107341

World Health Organization. (2012 [updated 2019]). *Palliative care*. Retrieved March 13, 2023, from https://www.who.int/health-topics/palliative-care

World Health Organization. (2018a). *Integrating palliative care and symptom relief into primary health care: A WHO guide for planners, implementers and managers*. Retrieved March 13, 2023, from https://apps.who.int/iris/handle/10665/274559

World Health Organization. (2018b). *Integrating palliative care and symptom relief into responses to humanitarian emergencies and crises: A WHO guide*. Retrieved March 13, 2023, from https://apps.who.int/iris/handle/10665/274565

World Health Organization. (2019). *WHO definition of palliative care*. Royal Commission Into Aged Care Quality and Safety. Retrieved March 13, 2023, from https://agedcare.royalcommission.gov.au/system/files/2020-06/LCM.9999.0001.0009.pdf

World Health Organization. (2021). *Assessing the development of palliative care worldwide: a set of actionable indicators*. Retrieved March 13, 2023, from https://www.who.int/publications/i/item/9789240033351

Willmarth, E. K. (2017). Clinical hypnosis in pain therapy and palliative care: A handbook of techniques for improving the patient's physical and psychological well-being by Brugnoli, Maria Paola: Book reviews. *American Journal of Clinical Hypnosis*, *59*(Issue 3: Exploring, Evolving, and Refining Hypnosis Education), 318–320. 10.1080/00029157.2016.1169719

Wolfe, J., Hammel, J. F., Edwards, K. E., Duncan, J., Comeau, M., Breyer, J., Aldridge, S. A., Grier, H. E., Berde, C., Dussel, V., & Weeks, J. C. (2008). Easing of suffering in children with cancer at the end of life: Is care changing? *Journal of Clinical Oncology*, *26*(10), 1717–1723. 10.1200/jco.2007.14.0277

SECTION IV

Frontiers of Hypnosis

Hypnosis and Society

52

EFFORTS, PITFALLS, AND CRITERIA TO BUILD A BRIDGE BETWEEN HYPNOSIS AND MEDICINE

Ernil Hansen

DEPARTMENT OF ANESTHESIOLOGY, UNIVERSITY HOSPITAL REGENSBURG, GERMANY

My Background

I am a scientist and anesthesiologist with a training in hypnosis strongly influenced by Milton Erickson. For me, hypnosis is a skill that perpetuates and influences trance in order to access unconscious resources and use them to induce beneficial psychological and physiological changes by suggestions. In this chapter, I am using the term "hypnotherapy" for psychotherapy using hypnosis to distinguish applications in psychologic and psychiatric indications from use in somatic medicine.

Working in acute medicine, I am inspired by the realization that patients in these situations are already in a natural trance state that can be used without formal trance induction and no need for artificial deepening. This is a situation quite different from experimental hypnosis, hypnotherapy, or the treatment of chronic diseases. It widens the application of hypnosis from a special treatment in some special patients by an external specialist to a better treatment of all patients. The hypnotic interventions then can be named "Therapeutic Communication" and the word "Hypnosis" – disturbing for many patients and medical colleagues – need not be carried in front as a flag.

Hypnosis and suggestions provide a model to explain a wide variety of beneficial as well as harmful effects in medicine. It can supplement the widely used model of placebo and nocebo effects that originate from one's own experiential learning (conditioning), from suggestions given that induce expectations, and from observational learning (co-patients, relatives, friends, media; Manaï et al., 2019). My main interest and work are to support research in hypnosis and its publication and to help integration of hypnosis into medicine by teaching students (mandatory courses for medical and for dental students at the University of Regensburg), young doctors, and other health care personnel.

Introduction

This is not a chapter about visions of the potential of hypnosis to increase general health and wellness in the future, but about our current need for desirable improvements in health

DOI: 10.4324/9781003449126-69

care in the prevailing health care system that is the practice of medicine. Acknowledging the rules in this system opens a realistic and practical way to re-integrate hypnosis into medicine for the benefit of patients. Instead of designing a future time, where hypnosis and meditation and mindfulness and mind-body techniques have brought health and well-being to everyone, this chapter gives practical advice for the incorporation of hypnosis into the practice of medicine making it available for patients here and now.

Hypnosis holds the potential to make important contributions to four major challenges in medicine:

1 Understanding, recognition, avoidance, and neutralization of widespread harmful effects such as nocebo effects and negative suggestions;
2 Accompanying and supporting medical treatments, especially in acute medical situations and interventions;
3 Induction of changes in physiology, namely involuntary body functions;
4 More effective therapeutic communication and relationship.

Since this hypnosis has not yet been sufficiently re-integrated in medicine it is necessary to ask, how can its potential be fulfilled?

Above all, hypnosis can bring medicine closer to a fundamentally different view of patients, illness, and healing, as well as to the role of the therapist. Here and in the following, "therapist" includes both psychotherapists and physicians, since the common principles of their attitude and practice of whatever therapy are addressed. The medical doctor tends to look primarily at the "illness" from an objective observer position and to overlook the patient's "being ill" as subjective (Ebell, 2018). Their way of thinking is predominantly "interventional," i.e., every identified problem is followed by an intervention. Modern hypnotherapy has largely left this view and use of tools behind. Milton Erickson described hypnosis as a relational interaction (Flemons, 2020).

In medicine, the misconception is still widespread that the doctor–patient interaction is relationally neutral. The doctor obtains information about symptoms and reports and derives from them a diagnosis and a therapy, which is then communicated to the patient. From the therapeutic treatment, strictly therapy-specific effects and side effects follow (A in Figure 52.1). This traditional medical theory of practice ignores the relational dynamics and phenomena that influence symptoms and their treatment (Lang et al., 2005; Cyna & Lang, 2010). Asking, "Do you have pain?" can induce or intensify pain, depending on the

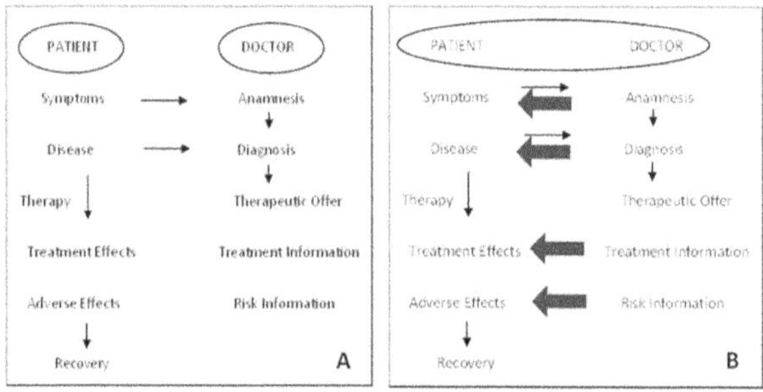

Figure 52.1 Doctor–patient relationship. A. Classic model, where disease and therapy have fixed, predetermined effects. B. Interaction model, where communication about disease and therapy add to and shape the effects.

context and relationships involved. With the pronouncement of the diagnosis, the therapist can shape the disease and its further course. "You are a high-risk patient!" pigeonholes a patient and can affect their health status for years (Lown, 1999). In giving the treatment and risk information, the therapist unknowingly contributes to a considerable extent to the success of therapy as well as the incidence and severity of side effects. Figure 52.1 graphically compares and contrasts the classical and this interactive model of doctor–patient relationship. Disease and therapy are not objective variables that only have an effect in a way that is determined by themselves, but are co-determined to a large extent by the doctor, the patient, and their interaction (Hansen & Zech, 2019). Only the realization of one's own participation and role in what is happening enables effective intervention. Here hypnosis can open a new perspective because it has long recognized the influential power of the therapist and therapeutic relationship.

Moreover, recognition and prevention of avoidable additional burdens such as nocebo effects and negative suggestions are essential prior to any treatment or positive communication. Evolution values negative effects as more influential than positive ones. Half the battle for better communication is won with their avoidance. Working with hypnosis provides valuable knowledge about the recognition and treatment of negative influences in both the medical (Häuser et al., 2016) and the hypnotic treatment context (Hassan and Scheflin, in this volume).

Building Bridges – How Can Hypnosis (Re-)enter Medicine?

Many hypnotherapists and even professional hypnosis societies are quite happy with the situation of hypnosis in medicine; physicians participate in hypnosis congresses and trainings, some hypnotherapists are consulted to prepare patients for operations, every now and then a hypnotherapist is invited to give a lecture to students or doctors. However, the full potential of hypnosis in medicine is far from being realized. Whether hypnosis has ultimately arrived within the practices of medicine and dentistry can be assessed on the basis of a few parameters that are also the goals for reintegration (Table 52.1). Those most optimistic about clinical hypnosis would confess that we still have a long way to go. Contrasting the limited acceptance with the tremendous potential and value of hypnosis in medicine compels the motivation and the energy necessary to work toward the goal of a full integration according to the criteria listed in Table 52.1.

Full integration is when the idea of hypnosis can be spread within medical science and the health care system itself instead of during occasional efforts from an outside consultant.

Table 52.1 Criteria and Goals for the Integration of Hypnosis in Medicine

Hypnosis in
Medical curriculum (compulsory courses)
Medical education and specialization
Medical training and refresher courses
Medical textbooks
Medical scientific journals (searchability, availability, review)
Medical congresses
Treatment guidelines (indication, legal certainty, reimbursement)
University (chair of hypnosis)

For hypnosis and hypnotherapy, such a condition would be the result of both greater acceptance and wider application. When, for example, hypnotherapy is not listed in the treatment guidelines for a disease, it is rarely requested or applied by the attending physician. But it can find its way into the guidelines when Guideline Commissions have been convinced by rigorously derived evidence of effectiveness. That scientifically derived evidence is only now increasing.

Need for Hypnosis

There is a great need for hypnosis in modern medicine that stems from a number of unsolved challenges and limited points of view. These deficiencies include neglect of the therapeutic relationship; the limitations of a monistic problem-oriented approach; the passivity prescribed to the patient; the neglect of natural changes in states of consciousness (trance); an underdeveloped practice of self-care in the part of both clinicians and patients; and more (see Table 52.2). There is less need for hypnosis expertise in addressing well-mastered conditions such as acute pain, surgery, fighting infections, or tumor therapy, and especially not for evidence-based therapies (Table 52.3). Nevertheless, hypnosis also can add benefit in medical treatment of those conditions, when applied supplementarily and not as the first-line treatment or replacement. Hypnosis can be a powerful adjunct to treating chronic pain as well as health challenges that are not well-addressed by conventional biomedicine such as stress, fear, loneliness, alienation, dependency, and helplessness. These conditions, with their roles in chronic disease, can be best addressed with therapeutic hypnosis.

To my knowledge, there is no country in which hypnosis is found in treatment guidelines as a primary or sole treatment in somatic medicine. Hypnosis as an "alternative" method of treatment such as "hypnosis instead of anesthesia" does not find acceptance among conventionally trained doctors and dentists. Instead, it promotes their resistance and a lack of understanding. However, these are the persons that decide whether hypnosis is included in the mandatory textbooks and treatment guidelines for medical care; then hypnosis can be very attractive as an "adjuvant," "complementary," and "supportive" strategy.

Hypnosis is particularly helpful and supportive in overcoming previously insufficiently solved problems like anxiety or depressive reactions. Every excellently trained dentist can feel helpless in the face of a patient who does not open his mouth. Every anesthetist is at the

Table 52.2 Knowledge and Experiences That Hypnosis Can Offer Medicine

- The special state of consciousness, "trance"
- The nature, effects, and applications of suggestions
- Change of psychological phenomena and states (fear, stress, state of mind)
- Influencing involuntary bodily functions
- Solution orientation instead of pure problem orientation
- Focusing on the patient and his or her illness instead of symptoms and disease
- Therapeutic communication with hypno-strategies (mirroring, utilization, etc.)
- Therapeutic relationship with the patient through rapport and resonance
- Guidance for resource activation and self-help (self-hypnosis)
- Experience of self-efficacy instead of prescribed passivity
- Self-care of the therapist

Table 52.3 What Is Needed and What Is Not to Get Hypnosis Back to Medicine

	Positive Approach, Needed	*Negative Approach, Not Useful*
Adaptation to the need	Complementary	"Alternative," "Hypnosis instead of ... "
	Use of natural trance	Trance induction without necessity
	Applicability to many/all patients	Exclusive (patient and therapist)
	Therapist's communication skills	Specific psychotherapy
	Stimulation to self-activity	Healer dependency
	Self-hypnosis (active, self-effective)	Passive consumption (CDs)
Compatibility	Stay in your competence	Negative suggestion "Hypnosis" (manipulative, authoritarian, esoteric)
	Limitation of colorfulness	
	Therapeutic communication	Guru
Science	Measurements of effects	Only qualitative
	Objective parameters when possible	Only subjective parameters
	Studies	Only stories and case reports
	Sufficient group size (multicenter)	Small test group
Evidence	Evidence-based	Eminence-based
	Publish in recognized scientific journals	Only books
	Discuss (scientific congresses)	Only in own workshops
	Review and meta-analysis of data	Reviews of views
	Define treatment guidelines	Arbitrary techniques ("in my experience")

mercy of a screaming child. In these conditions, clinicians can neither apply nor derive satisfaction from their professional competence.

In medicine, the need for the application of hypnotic tools and principles is wide. It differs from and reaches beyond psychotherapy. In the latter case, an expert treats selected patient with defined complaints and pathological conditions by use of a special treatment. In somatic medicine, all patients, irrespective of their specific medical problem, must endure stress, a difficult and poor condition, pain, anxiety, and perceived life threat. This situation is often precisely conditioned or reinforced by the very persons who actually want to help (Lang et al., 2005). For this reason, all health care providers can be more effective when they have knowledge of hypnosis and therapeutic communication and use it with all patients and in all situations.

An especially important and helpful contribution to medicine is the understanding of trance as a state of consciousness different from the everyday functional mode (Faymonville et al., 2006; Demertzi et al., 2011; Bicego et al., 2022). In trance, critical and conscious mind processes are bypassed and access is allowed to non-conscious inner resources and less voluntary body functions. Trance is not limited to the practice of hypnotherapy ("hypnotic trance") or dependent on a hypnotic induction. A "common everyday trance" occurs spontaneously and repeatedly all day after 90 minutes of intellectual activity, for about 20 minutes in a natural ultradian rhythm (Rossi, 1991; Rossi et al., 2008). Also, and especially important in medicine, trance often includes dissociation. It is an automatic emergency response (Jacobs, 1991; Acosta & Prager, 2014).

Accordingly, in acute conditions such as emergency medicine, surgery, anesthesia, or intensive care, the situation is quite different from psychotherapy or the treatment of chronic diseases: most often the patient already is in trance ("natural trance") as a natural dissociative distress response to pain, anxiety, helplessness, and the feeling of existential threat. David Cheek (1962) titled his critical paper "Importance of recognizing that surgical patients behave as though hypnotized" (p. 227). This means that techniques for trance induction and deepening are far less important, both in clinical work and hypnosis training. Instead, trance phenomena can be recognized in and by the patient, and trance depth can be regulated by the patients according to their need (Barber, 1991; Erickson, 2009).

Hardly any method can compensate for the lack and gaps in training and experience of communication skills in medicine better than skills in hypnosis. What is offered in medical school and medical training with regard to communication is largely limited to conducting conversations to take medical histories, communicating therapeutic options, explaining risks for legally valid informed consent, exchanging information for error avoidance, and patient-centered client counseling. These represent very important competencies, but are different from a "therapeutic communication" and the "therapeutic relationship" that affects the patient and their health as do drugs or surgery (Table 52.2). Experience with hypnosis can provide insight into a patient's non-ordinary state of consciousness (trance), an understanding of the nature and effect of suggestion, and a recognition of the importance of rapport and resonance (Hansen et al., 2023). With regard to the medical interview and risk information for informed consent, for instance, the longer the time duration between patient interview for obtaining informed consent and receiving risk information and the operation date, the less the anxiety and susceptibility to negative suggestion, an inverse correlation. Zech et al. (2020) found that the increase in anxiety with approaching surgery correlated with the reduction in muscle strength after risk information. With an understanding of the nature and effects of suggestions, alternative formulation of risk information verifiably can avoid weakening and traumatization of the patient (Zech et al., 2019; Zech et al., 2022). The skills to utilize rapport and resonance can be added to necessary screening with risk lists in order to individualize patient interviews.

Hypnosis, especially self-hypnosis, encourages active involvement and self-efficacy. Rarely can a therapy allow a patient to experience so much active contribution. The passivity that is almost typically prescribed in medicine ("Let us do it. Just hold still!") is one of the worst negative suggestions with deleterious effects on homeostasis and the immune system (Hansen & Zech, 2019). With hypnotic suggestions and simple application of hypnotic principles (e.g., a suggestion to dissociate to a safe place), the patient can learn to continue to apply these effective measures and to develop them further individually. When patients are thus challenged and guided to become a partner in their own recovery, they can experience an appreciation of their abilities and resources that enable them to endure and bring about incredible changes and achievements within and beyond the therapeutic relationship.

While posters on the ceiling during anesthesia induction are helpful to encourage dissociation to a "safe place" (Hansen & Bejenke, 2010), video clips are not. These, instead of active imagination, just provide distraction, which has been shown to be far less effective than hypnosis (Faymonville et al., 1995; Lang et al., 2000; Zech et al., 2017). With adequate guidance, patients can master the challenge of even their own brain surgery while awake without sedation (Hansen et al., 2013; Zech et al., 2018). Their active involvement can build their self-confidence for any subsequent chemotherapy and radiation treatment.

Similarly, guided imagery or application of virtual reality is significantly less effective than what a patient can do for themselves when properly stimulated and guided. With "virtual reality hypnosis" a most important basis of hypnosis, the human relationship, is missed (Erickson, 2009; Flemons, 2020; Rousseaux et al., 2020).

Finally, medical practitioners can learn and practice self-care from psychotherapy. Several studies show that treatment quality and efficacy are lower in stressed physicians, e.g., lower performance and survival in resuscitation (Hunziker et al., 2012). And that self-care improves doctor's performance and patient's outcome (West et al., 2016). Accordingly, part of clinicians' obligations to their patients is to look after themselves. The same hypnotic techniques that can so effectively reduce tension and stress in the patient can be used for self-care of the health care providers, especially in acute situations. For example, during stressful hospital rounds, they can use progressive muscle relaxation by clenching and unclenching their fist in the pocket of their doctor's coat. Before a difficult procedure, they can breathe in strengthening together with the oxygen and breathe out anxiety and uncertainty together with the used air. They can remember words and images of strength, get support from imagined helper animals or other inner resources, and so much more (see also Criswell in this volume).

Compatibility – "Hypnosis" as a Negative Suggestion

The "alternative-ness" with which hypnosis is sometimes offered both attracts some doctors looking for new methods and repels many others. Those "others" often include decision-makers and opinion-leaders who are needed for integration of hypnosis into clinical practice and guidelines. Perception of hypnosis is strongly shaped, mischaracterized, and sensationalized by the media. A negative image can originate from the connection with stage-hypnosis, miracle healers, authoritarian guru-like manipulators, reactions of unwillingness and dependency, and symbols such as an electric magic ball or magic spirals like the eyes of snake "Kaa" in the movie *Jungle Book* (Reitherman, 1967). Advertisement for "hypnosis for erotic wellness, penis enlargement, reincarnation" can be found abundantly on the internet. It seems incumbent upon hypnosis societies to take responsibility, as a joint effort, in order to carefully research and correct the media.

Nevertheless, there is just as much need for bringing medicine to hypnosis. Without the connection to the findings, procedures, and explanatory models of medicine, and without understanding and taking into account the physical and somatic aspects of illnesses, one cannot do justice to the complexity of problems of a patient and of possible solutions.

Science and Evidence

One of the main reasons for the ignorance and lack of acceptance of hypnosis is the shortage of a rigorous clinical research to generate an evidence base. Scientific evidence is the basis for contemporary medical decision-making, both with regard to therapies offered and their reimbursement. One can argue about the advantages and disadvantages of the principle of evidence-based medicine, but hardly about the need for criteria to determine beneficial interventions and limit costs. The availability of unproven therapy options impedes the further development of treatments by critical and competitive examination. Health care resources are limited. With increasing costs for more sophisticated and effective medical therapies such as immunomodulatory tumor therapy, health insurances will have to cut their benefits or increase premiums. On the other hand, as patients have to spend more money on supplemental insurance (e.g., for dental implants, hearing aids, glasses, and new therapeutic options) and as they get older and sicker, they will be less willing or able to pay for treatments on their own, even when apparently beneficial. Evolution of health care requires us to offer only the most effective, evidence-based treatments. While for some time there was doubt that rules for randomized controlled trials (RCT) could be applied in psychotherapy because of subjective effects and the essential role of the therapist, methods have been developed and feasibility has been demonstrated (Leichsenring, 2004; Falkenström et al., 2013). The research methods of Jensen, Benedetti, De Benedittis, and many others represented in this volume demonstrate that rigorous hypnosis and hypnosis-related research can now be accomplished.

"Evidence" also results from case reports on therapy effects, and from experimental research (e.g., biochemical, physiological, radiological), but primarily from scientific clinical studies. Their quality is given by the study design, for which there are now established and approved recommendations and standards (e.g., CONSORT checklist) including the preparation and registration of a study plan with a case number calculation, the definition of a primary and secondary outcome parameters, and the vote of an ethics committee. RCTs are now considered the gold standard, and found feasible also for studies in hypnosis and hypnotherapy. Scientific investigations are always accompanied by controls that limit translation to real-world clinical settings. This is the problem of ecological validity. The knowledge gained from such research becomes more precise when as many factors as possible are kept constant, and focus is limited to one or a few variables. Anecdotal clinical evidence about such imprecise variables such as "health" does not allow conclusions to be drawn about the contribution of individual factors that could define a well-founded indication and likely outcome for a specific intervention. Therefore, rather physiological parameters, biobehavioral correlates, and gene expression (Rossi, 2009) should be included in research on hypnosis effects.

Measuring

The basis of scientific evidence is measurement and objectification. The therapist's idea and impression that a certain intervention is good for the patient must be verified. Even the patient's subjective feeling about what is good for him is not sufficient, despite the power of belief. In the past, for example, all patients with disc surgery felt that bed rest was good for them. In the meantime, it has been shown that early mobilization leads more quickly and safely to freedom from pain and the ability to move, and thus to recovery. Subjective scales are dominant in psychotherapy research and continue to be widespread in medicine such as the numerical or visual "pain scale." On the other hand, it is becoming increasingly clear that these impressions by patients are multifactorial and that they are strongly influenced by context, previous experiences (conditioning), and expectations (nocebo effect). Hence, results are significantly dependent on the choice of words in the query. This query determines not only the measurement result (e.g., NRS score) but also the actual symptom (Hansen & Zech, 2019). In a study on pain after cesarean section, a comfort scale instead of a pain scale resulted not only in less pain and less need for analgesics but also in fewer women that reported the sensation as "unpleasant" or as "tissue damage" instead of "healing and recovery," with potential long-term effects on the relationship between mother and child (Chooi et al., 2013).

In studies on the effect of verbal and non-verbal suggestions from the medical environment, objective parameters can be used instead of subjective assessments by patients and therapists. In recent studies, maximum arm muscle strength during abduction, a parameter from physiology, was measured by dynamometry in response to different suggestions from everyday clinical practice (Zech et al., 2019; Zech et al., 2020). All tested suggestions resulted in significant reduction in muscle strength, a weakening. This example shows that the quality of a suggestion is not only to be assumed or felt, but can be objectively measured. By using a uniform and quantitative parameter, different suggestions can be tested for their negative or positive effect and compared. The impact of words such as "pain" or "nauseous" thereby can be weighed, while usually incomparable, since the first is tested for its effect on pain and the second for its effect on nausea. Even the impact of verbal and non-verbal suggestions can be compared, e.g., "words that hurt" and watching the ceiling during a transport in a hospital. A transportation in strict supine position is often unnecessary, disturbing, and "weakening," as is the common overhead view of the anesthetist before induction of anesthesia (standing at the head end of the operating table and thereby making biological face recognition impossible, a situation standard all over the world). Very often the negative factors are small but numerous. During a hospital stay, they may sum up to overall anxiety, and their combination effect can be evaluated with this scientific approach.

In this study, alternative versions of the suggestions were tested as well, and they were able to avoid the disempowerment of the patient and to neutralize a prior corresponding negative suggestion. Likewise, combinations of negative or positive suggestions can be tested and analyzed to see if they are non-additive, additive, or potentiating. This is just an example of how a physiological parameter can provide an easy, quick, and comprehensible tool to traceably evaluate alternative formulations, examine communication factors, and improve therapeutic communication in a reproducible scientific way (Hansen & Zech, 2019).

This approach has impact on concrete, pressing clinical issues. For instance, how to fulfill the obligation for extensive risk information to obtain informed consent. An ethical dilemma exists, since medical practitioners are committed to the Hippocratic principle of not doing harm ("primum nihil nocere," nonmaleficence), but they do ("nocebo" = I will harm). The harmful effects of informed consent are now recognized and several proposals for a less traumatizing informative interview have been made, including some from psychotherapists (Manai et al., 2019, Evers et al., 2021). However, only few have been tested for efficacy and verification, and of those some led to inconclusive or only weak results (Barnes et al., 2019). Even the most intriguing ideas need to be verified. The evaluation of effects of risk information on arm muscle strength shows a significant reduction that is avoided when presented together with benefits of the respective therapy (Zech et al., 2019; Zech et al., 2022).

Evaluation

The results of studies can be evaluated following defined standards such as the "CONSORT statement" (Schulz et al., 2010). Statistical and clinical significance, correlations between parameters, and effect sizes of interventions are calculated. No longer is a search in the study data for any significant result acceptable. The controlled analysis of predefined outcome parameters is required. The number of cases is of crucial importance.

Small studies tend to overestimate effects, so it makes sense to combine them to multicenter studies. A meta-analysis of studies on the clinical effects of hypnotic suggestions given during general anesthesia (Rosendahl et al., 2016), for instance, showed no effect on postoperative pain and only little impact on the use of analgesics, while a recent multicenter study on 385 patients revealed strong and significant reductions of pain scores and total amount of analgesics (Nowak et al., 2020), as well as of postoperative nausea and vomiting and need for antiemetics (Nowak et al., 2022). Acceptance and significance increase when a number of cases common in medicine research is reached.

Publishing

Publication of research in peer-reviewed, scientific journals increases perception, dissemination, and replication. Peer review also provides a valuable check, discussion, and usually improvement of data interpretation. There is an exchange with the knowledge, experiences, and findings of others. This enables a better assessment of one's own approaches and views, a more reliable view of the essential findings, and ultimately better treatment of patients than simply relying only on one's own insights and skills. In contrast to books and book chapters, study results in scientific journals are easy to find (via keywords in literature search portals such as PubMed) and available (increasingly online and free of charge). The aim is to publish in a reputable and widely used journal.

Most peer-reviewed professional hypnosis journals are unavailable in university clinics and libraries. The articles are rarely read by medical doctors. The importance and dissemination of the peer-reviewed professional journals are measured by the impact factor (IF). It reflects how many colleagues read that journal, a given article, and cite those publications (i.e., rate them as important and disseminate them). If an article, like the one on intraoperative hypnotic suggestions already mentioned (Nowak et al., 2020), is published in the *British Medical Journal* with an IF of 96, instead of in the *American Journal of Clinical Hypnosis* or the *International Journal of Clinical and Experimental Hypnosis* with IFs of 0.7 and 2.0 respectively, it reaches not only a larger number of readers but also a more diverse population of medical specialists who rarely ever think about hypnosis. Many important studies on the clinical application of hypnosis are lost in low-rated or specialized journals. Books and DVDs, such as those on display at hypnosis congresses, can reach doctors who have found their way to hypnosis through an interest in unusual and fringe areas. But they rarely reach the direction- and application-determining authorities and opinion leaders. At the time of this writing, in the most widely read medical journals —*The Lancet, the Journal of the American Medical Association,* and the *New England Journal of Medicine*—very few papers on hypnosis have been published since 2000 aside the one (Lang et al., 2000) mentioned. For this to change, users of medical hypnosis will need to put more energy and commitment into publication of peer-reviewed papers in mainstream journals than books.

Meta-Analyses

The published studies on a topic can then be found, analyzed, and summarized. Even if different measurement parameters are used, a joint effect size can be calculated. A large number of studied cases allows subgroup analyses. However, the quality of the meta-analysis is limited by the quality of the included studies, which today can be determined and presented in a standardized and comprehensible way (Murad et al., 2014). A meta-analysis can be created from as few as three studies with 20 patients each, but its significance and acceptance will be very limited. Therefore, in a systematic review of the effectiveness of hypnosis in medicine (Häuser et al., 2016), the criterion used was that the included meta-analyses each had to cover at least 400 patients in order to make it suitable and acceptable for medical conditions. The current status of evidence for hypnotherapy in medicine is limited and not much better in psychotherapy. The mentioned review found only five meta-analyses that met the condition. Three showed low to moderate evidence for medical interventions. One demonstrated good evidence for irritable bowel syndrome. The Cochrane meta-analysis on hypnosis in labor and childbirth did not yield proof of efficacy. Whereas a later repetition demonstrated reduction in drug use, there was no reduction in the rate of epidural anesthesia, spontaneous births, and many other items (Madden et al. 2016). No meta-analyses for dental or other interventional procedures were found. Meanwhile, a meta-analysis has been published supporting evidence for minimal invasive procedures under local anesthesia showing small effects on procedure time and pain (Noergaard et al., 2019). The Cochrane Library (www.cochrane.org) of systematic reviews and trials for evidence-based medicine lists the evidence for hypnosis in labor, surgery, headache, spinal cord injury, multiple sclerosis, cancer pain, dentistry, and pediatric chronic pain or abdominal and non-specific chest pain or needle placement as "lacking, insufficient, uncertain, or low to very low" and state "little confidence in the reported effect estimates." All meta-analyses of interventions with hypnosis criticize the lack of studies and the low quality of the few available.

Studies and meta-analyses are finally presented, discussed, and evaluated at congresses of the various medical societies. This is where the perception and acceptance of a therapeutic procedure emerge, which can then find its way into teaching (textbooks and student curriculum), into the training regulations for doctors, and into treatment guidelines via committees and commissions. Such authoritative acceptance increases the likelihood of hypnosis being used, reimbursed by insurance companies, and supported as legitimate in legal disputes. The basis for legal actions in medicine is the "state of scientific knowledge," which is currently derived from literature reviews, the knowledge and opinion of medical experts, and, above all, from practical guidelines with indication of the degree of evidence. In a lawsuit of a patient that suffered a heart attack during dental treatment, for instance, the dentist has weak arguments if quoting the patient's fear or allergies as the reason he used hypnosis instead of local anesthesia. The judge will ask for the "state of the art" that is given by reviews and guidelines and will not allow meanwhile unjustified reference to high allergy rates in former times. Accordingly, scientific evidence is necessary for several reasons (Table 52.4).

Why does this chapter call for more use of hypnosis in medicine? Because our experience is that hypnosis works and helps in many applications. Experience and confidence are not enough to reintegrate hypnosis into medicine, but evidence can. The existing studies do not reflect the actual potential of hypnosis, and the gathering of evidence has to be more rigorous.

Table 52.4 Advantages of Evidence-Based Approach to Hypnosis

- Hypothesis testing
- Therapy improvement
- Dissemination and acceptance
- Cost coverage
- Legal certainty

Teaching Hypnosis in Medicine

As great as the benefit to physicians and the potential to learn from psychotherapists may be, still it is important and helpful to involve physicians in the education and training of physicians in hypnosis. The proposal of hypnotic strategies in medicine is of limited use, if the course instructor has never been present at a medical emergency, has never delivered care within an intensive care unit, and is not familiar with the legal requirements for medico-surgical informed consent. Physicians in the hypnosis courses should be recognized, supported, and guided to become part of hypnosis training. For effective application of hypnosis and hypnotic communication in the clinical environment and well-functioning teamwork, invitations for training and co-operation must be made also to other members of health care such as nurses, physiotherapists, and paramedics. The course content should be directed to teach communication skills and beneficial dealing with people in trance within common medical contexts (Jacobs, 1991; Varga et al., 2011; Cyna et al., 2023).

The primary aim of medical hypnosis training and education is not to generate more psychotherapists but to improve physicians' care, competence, and clinical outcomes. Serious damage has occurred when "hypnodoctors," "hypnodentists," and "hypnonurses" used their "hypnotraining" for therapy with PTSD patients, practicing outside of their area of competence and training. What is learned should be used to recognize and avoid negative suggestions and to use the increased suggestibility of the patient for the benefits of positive suggestions. Furthermore, the primary objective of the training in hypnosis techniques is not to substitute or interfere but to support and enhance the necessary medical treatment.

References

Acosta, J., & Prager, J. S. (2014). *The worst is over: What to say when every moment counts – Verbal first aid to calm, relieve pain, promote healing, and save lives.* 2nd ed. CreateSpace Independent Publishing Platform.

Barber, J. (1991). The locksmith model. In S. J. Lynn & J. W. Rhue (Eds.), *Theories of hypnosis: Current models and perspectives* (pp. 241–274). New York: Guilford Press.

Barnes, K., Faasse, K., Geers, A. L., Helfer, S. G., Sharpe, L., Colloca, L., et al. (2019). Can positive framing reduce nocebo side effects? Current evidence and recommendation for future research. *Frontiers in Pharmacology, 10*, 167. doi: 10.3389/fphar.2019.00167.

Bicego, A., Rousseaux F., Faymonville, M. E., Nyssen, A. S., & Vanhaudenhuyse, A. (2022). Neurophysiology of hypnosis in chronic pain: A review of recent literature. *American Journal of Clinical Hypnosis, 64*(1), 62–80.

Cheek, D. B. (1962). Importance of recognizing that surgical patients behave as though hypnotized. *American Journal of Clinical Hypnosis, 4*, 227–236. doi: 10.1080/00029157.1962.10401905.

Chooi, C. S., White, A. M., Tan, S. G., Dowling, K., & Cyna, A. M. (2013). Pain vs comfort scores after Caesarean section: A randomized trial. *British Journal of Anaesthesia, 110*(5), 780–787. doi: 10.1093/bja/aes517.

Cyna, A. M., & Lang, E. V. (2010). How words hurt. In A. M. Cyna, M. I. Andrew, S. G. M. Tan, A. F. Smith (Eds.), *Handbook of communication in anaesthesia and critical care.* Oxford: Oxford University Press, pp. 30–37.

Cyna, A. M., Andrew, M. I., Tan, S. G. M., & Smith, A. F. (Eds.) (2023). *Handbook of communication in anaesthesia and critical care.* 2nd ed. Oxford: Oxford University Press.

Demertzi, A., Soddu, A., Faymonville, M. E., Bahri, M. A., Gosseries, O., Vanhaudenhuyse, A., et al (2011). Hypnotic modulation of resting state fMRI default mode and extrinsic network connectivity. *Progress in Brain Research, 193*, 309–322.

Ebell, H. J. (2018). Resonance based medicine: A systems perspective for managing chronic pain. In M. P. Jensen (Ed.), *Hypnotic techniques for chronic pain management: Favorite methods of master clinicians*. Washington: Denny Creek Press.

Erickson, M. H. (2009). Naturalistic techniques of hypnosis. 1958. *American Journal of Clinical Hypnosis*, *51*(4), 333–340. doi: 10.1080/00029157.2009.

Evers, A. W. M., Colloca, L., Blease, C., Gaab, J., Jensen, K. B., Atlas, L. Y., Beedie, C. J., Benedetti, F., Bingel, U., Büchel, C., Bussemaker, J., Colagiuri, B., Crum, A. J., Finniss, G., Consortium of Placebo Experts, et al. (2021). What should clinicians tell patients about placebo and nocebo effects? Practical considerations based on expert consensus. *Psychotherapy and Psychosomatics*, *90*(1), 49–56. doi: 10.1159/000510738.

Falkenström, F., Markowitz, J. C., Jonker, H., Philips, B., & Holmqvist, R. (2013). Can psychotherapists function as their own controls? Meta-analysis of the crossed therapist design in comparative psychotherapy trials. *Journal of Clinical Psychiatry*, *74*(5), 482–491. doi:10.4088/JCP.12r07848.

Faymonville, M. E., Fissette, J., Mambourg, P. H., Roediger, L., Joris, J., & Lamy, M. (1995). Hypnosis as adjunct therapy in conscious sedation for plastic surgery. *Regional Anesthesia*, *20*(2), 145–151.

Faymonville, M. E., Boly, M., & Laureys, S. (2006). Functional neuroanatomy of the hypnotic state. *Journal of Physiology-Paris*, *99*(4-6), 463–469.

Flemons, D. (2020). Toward a relational theory of hypnosis. *American Journal of Clinical Hypnosis*, *62*(4), 344–363. doi: 10.1080/00029157.2019.1666700.

Häuser, W., Hagl, M., Schmierer, A., & Hansen, E. (2016). The efficacy, safety and applications of medical hypnosis. *Deutsches Ärzteblatt International*, *113*(17), 289–296. doi: 10.3238/arztebl.2016.0289.

Hansen, E., & Bejenke, C. (2010) Negative and positive suggestions in anaesthesia: Improved communication with anxious surgical patients. *Der Anaesthesist*, *59*(3), 199–209. German. doi: 10.1007/s00101-010-1679-9.

Hansen, E., Seemann, M., Zech, N., Doenitz, C., Luerding, R., & Brawanski, A. (2013). Awake craniotomies without any sedation: The awake-awake-awake technique. *Acta Neurochirurgica*, *155*(8), 1417–1424. doi: 10.1007/s00701-013-1801-2.

Hansen, E., & Zech, N. (2019). Nocebo effects and negative suggestions in daily clinical practice – Forms, impact and approaches to avoid them. *Frontiers in Pharmacology*, *10*, 77. doi: 10.3389/fphar.2019.00077.

Hansen, E., Faymonville, M. E., Bejenke, C. J., & Vanhaudenhuyse, A. (2023). Hypnotic techniques. In A. Cyna, M. I. Andrew, S. G. M. Tan, & A. F. Smith (Eds.), *Handbook of communicationin anaesthesia and critical care*. 2nd ed. Oxford: Oxford University Press, chap. 20 (in press).

Hunziker, S., Semmer, N. K., Tschan, F., Schuetz, P., Mueller, B., & Marsch, S. (2012). Dynamics and association of different acute stress markers with performance during a simulated resuscitation. *Resuscitation*, *83*(5), 572–578. doi: 10.1016/j.resuscitation.2011.11.013.

Jacobs, D. T. (1991). *Patient communication for first responders and EMS personnel*. Englewood Cliffs: Brady.

Lang, E. V., Benotsch, E. G., Fick, L. J., Lutgendorf, S., Berbaum, M. L., Berbaum, K. S., Logan, H., & Spiegel, D. (2000) Adjunctive non-pharmacological analgesia for invasive medical procedures: A randomised trial. *Lancet*, *355*(9214), 1486–1490. doi: 10.1016/S0140-6736(00)02162-0.

Lang, E. V., Hatsiopoulou, O., Koch, T., Berbaum, K., Lutgendorf, S., Kettenmann, E., Logan, H., & Kaptchuk, T. J. (2005). Can words hurt? Patient-provider interactions during invasive procedures. *Pain*, *114*(1–2), 303–309. doi: 10.1016/j.pain.2004.12.028.

Leichsenring, F. (2004). Randomized controlled versus naturalistic studies: A new research agenda. *Bulletin of the Menninger Clinic*, *68*(2), 137–151. doi: 10.1521/bumc.68.2.137.35952.

Lown, B. (1999). *The lost art of healing*. New York: Balantine Books.

Madden, K., Middleton, P., Cyna, A. M., Matthewson, M., & Jones, L. (2016). Hypnosis for pain management during labour and childbirth. *Cochrane Database Syst Rev*, *2016*(5), CD009356. doi: 10.1002/14651858.

Manaï, M., van Middendorp, H., Veldhuijzen, D. S., Huizinga, T. W. J., & Evers, A. W. M. (2019). How to prevent, minimize, or extinguish nocebo effects in pain: A narrative review on mechanisms, predictors, and interventions. *Pain Reports*, *4*(3), e699. doi: 10.1097/PR9.0000000000000699.

Murad, M. H., Montori, V. M., Ioannidis, J. P., Jaeschke, R., Devereaux, P. J., Prasad, K., Neumann, I., Carrasco-Labra, A., Agoritsas, T., Hatala, R., et al. (2014). How to read a systematic review and meta-analysis and apply the results to patient care: Users' guides to the medical literature. *Journal of the American Medical Association*, *312*(2), 171–179. doi: 10.1001/jama.2014.5559.

Noergaard, M. W., Håkonsen, S. J., Bjerrum, M., & Pedersen, P. U. (2019) The effectiveness of hypnotic analgesia in the management of procedural pain in minimally invasive procedures: A systematic review and meta-analysis. *Journal of Clinical Nursing*, *28*(23-24), 4207–4224. doi: 10.1111/jocn.15025.

Nowak, H., Zech, N., Asmussen, S., Rahmel, T., Tryba, M., Oprea, G., Grause, L., Schork, K., Moeller, M., Loeser, J., Gyarmati, K., Mittler, C., et al. (2020). Effect of therapeutic suggestions during general anaesthesia on postoperative pain and opioid use – Multicentre randomised controlled trial. *British Medical Journal*, *371*, m4284. doi: 10.1136/bmj.m4284.

Nowak, H., Wolf, A., Rahmel, T., Oprea, G., Grause, L., Moeller, M., Gyarmati, K., Mittler, C., Zagler, A., Lutz, K., Loeser, J., Saller, T., et al. (2022). Therapeutic suggestions during general anesthesia reduce postoperative nausea and vomiting in high-risk patients – A post-hoc analysis of a randomized controlled trial. *Front Psychol*, *13*, 898326. doi: 10.3389/fpsyg.2022.898326.

Reiherman, W. (Director). (1967). The Jungle Book [Film]. Walt Disney Productions

Rosendahl, J., Koranyi, S., Jacob, D., Zech, N., & Hansen, E. (2016). Efficacy of therapeutic suggestions under general anesthesia: A systematic review and meta-analysis of randomised controlled trials. *BioMed Central Anesthesiology*, *16*, 125. doi 10.1186/s12871-016-0292-0.

Rossi, E. (1991). *The 20-minute break*. Kirkwood: Tarcher Press.

Rossi, E., Erickson-Klein, R., & Rossi, K. (2008). Novel activity-dependent approaches to hypnosis and psychotherapy: The general waking trance. *American Journal of Clinical Hypnosis*, *51*(2), 185–200. doi: 10.1080/00029157.2008.10401664.

Rossi, E. L. (2009). The psychosocial genomics of therapeutic hypnosis, psychotherapy, and rehabilitation. *American Journal of Clinical Hypnosis*, *51*(3), 281–298. doi: 10.1080/00029157.2009.10401678.

Rousseaux, F., Bicego, A., Ledoux, D., Massion, P., Nyssen, A. S., Faymonville, M. E., Laureys, S., & Vanhaudenhuyse, A. (2020). Hypnosis associated with 3D immersive virtual reality technology in the management of pain: A review of the literature. *Journal of Pain Research*, *13*, 1129–1138. doi: 10.2147/JPR.S231737.

Schulz, K. F., Altman, D. G., Moher, D., CONSORT Group. (2010). CONSORT 2010 Statement: Updated guidelines for reporting parallel group randomised trials. *BMC Med*, *8*, 18. doi: 10.1186/1741-7015-8-18.

Varga, K. (2011). *Beyond the words: Communication and suggestion in medical practice*. New York: Nova Science Publishers.

West, C. P., Dyrbye, L. N., Erwin, P. J., & Shanafelt, T. D. (2016). Interventions to prevent and reduce physician burnout: A systematic review and meta-analysis. *Lancet*, *388*(10057), 2272–2281. doi: 10.1016/S0140-6736(16)31279-X.

Zech, N., Hansen, E., Bernardy, K., & Häuser, W. (2017). Efficacy, acceptability and safety of guided imagery/hypnosis in fibromyalgia – A systematic review and meta-analysis of randomized controlled trials. *European Journal of Pain*, *21*, 217–227. doi: 10.1002/ejp.933.

Zech, N., Seemann, M., Seyfried, T. F., Lange, M., Schlaier, J., & Hansen, E. (2018). Deep brain stimulation surgery without sedation. *Stereotactic and Functional Neurosurgery*, *96*(6), 370–378. doi: 10.1159/000494803.

Zech, N., Seemann, M., Grzesiek, M., Breu, A., Seyfried, T. F., & Hansen, E. (2019). Nocebo effects on muscular performance – An experimental study about clinical situations. *Frontiers in Pharmacology*, *10*, 219. doi: 10.3389/fphar.2019.00219.

Zech, N., Schrödinger, M., Seemann, M., Zeman, F., Seyfried, T. F., & Hansen, E. (2020). Time dependent negative effects of verbal and nonverbal suggestions in surgical patients – A study on arm muscle strength. *Frontiers in Psychology*, *11*, 16932020. doi: 10.3389/fpsyg.2020.0169.

Zech, N., Schrödinger, M., & Hansen, E. (2022). Avoidance of nocebo effects by coincident explanation of treatment benefits during the medical interview for informed consent – Evidence from dynamometry. *Frontiers in Psychology*, *13*, 923044. doi: 10.3389/fpsyg.2022.923044.

53

UNDERSTANDING THE DARK SIDE OF HYPNOSIS AS A FORM OF UNDUE INFLUENCE EXERTED IN AUTHORITARIAN CULTS AND ONLINE CONTEXTS

Implications for Practice, Policy, and Education

Steven A. Hassan[1] *and Alan W. Scheflin*[2,*]

[1]Freedom of Mind Resource Center; [2]Professor Emeritus, Santa Clara University School of Law

Typically, human predators (Atack, 2021) and authoritarian cult leaders pursue power, money, and sex (Fromm, 1964). We explore case examples of cult leaders who display traits of narcissism and psychopathology, unlicensed uses of hypnosis, and exploitative companies—in other words, a different arena from communities of ethically bound healthcare clinicians. This nefarious arena is one in which playbooks demand obedience and dependence of members and supplant ethical codes. Hypnosis is used with ignorance or indifference to scientific rigor. Consequently, it can be used to do great harm: to defraud and enslave people.

Protecting the Field, Supporting the Individual

The damage caused by hypnosis in cults and online spaces is not limited to their impact on individuals. Most alarmingly, unregulated uses of hypnosis pose a threat to the benefits of the therapeutic application of hypnosis. The unethical use of hypnosis—the systematic exploitation of human vulnerabilities—is the opposite of the instruction to "do no harm," respected by every ethical clinician.

The healthcare field would benefit from perceiving unethical forms of hypnosis as a subset of undue influence—in which individuals downplay their own interests in service of a dominant other (Hassan & Shah, 2019). These clinicians need to know the impact of exploitative practices that affect the status of their profession and how their clients may have been previously affected by these practices.

[*] He died (august 27, 2023) during the publication process of this article.

DOI: 10.4324/9781003449126-70

Hassan postulates that there is a strong possibility of harm from exposure to hypnotic techniques because the public cannot discern due (or proper) influence from undue influence. This discernment is vital given the many lay hypnotists with credentials and expertise below or without professional standards. As of this writing, only Israel (State of Israel, 1984) has legislated the need for a license to practice hypnosis.

The dark use of hypnosis can covertly affect our daily lives in many different areas, including religious groups, political ideologies, and digital media. The forms of influence range from doomsday cults to addictive social media platforms. The harm of the latter is bolstered because many countries lack data privacy legislation and platform regulation. Indeed, artificial intelligence harnesses personalized data to manipulate, exploit, and indoctrinate users. Collected data are used to expose users to addictive advertising, affirming prejudices, and shaping views.

The public is subjected to an inaccurate understanding of hypnosis. As unethical hypnosis spreads, a distrustful public is directed toward pharmaceutical remedies or unnecessary medical procedures for help. Pharmaceutical companies that profit from this dynamic may support the unchecked spread of unethical uses and the ensuing damage done to the reputation of ethical hypnosis. This chapter is a start in addressing this unfortunate reality by shining a light on this dangerous abuse of human rights. We support promoting the positive, beneficial use of hypnosis, including better achievement of personal goals (for instance, in sports or for better sleep), pain control, improvement of many health issues, and as an aid in therapy.

A Definition of Hypnosis

We focus on hypnosis as conversational and naturalistic, rooted in Milton Erickson's approach that uses language and nonverbal communication to induce suggestibility and responsiveness (Erickson, 2008). Elkins et al. (2015) echo this definition, calling hypnosis: "a state of consciousness involving focused attention and reduced peripheral awareness characterized by an enhanced capacity for response to suggestion" (p. 6).

The Dual Identity Model

Because hypnosis involves concentrating attention and the reduction of external perception, hypnosis involves dissociation (Spiegel, 1991). Destructive cults program a "cult self" (formed in the leader's or ideology's image) that negates a person's conscious and critical thinking, feelings, and abilities to make their own choices (West & Martin, 1994). As the basis for clinical work and research, Hassan (1998, 2015) calls this the "dual identity model." This is akin to what the DSM-5-TR recognizes as a dissociative disorder (American Psychiatric Association, 2022, section 330).

The following case study detailing Hassan's identity in the Moon organization highlights this concept of dissociative disorder. Hassan (2000) hypothesizes that his cult identity was created by utilizing child ego states he outgrew as he matured. However, our embodied minds (Sugarman, 2021) are layered and adapt to our environmental context. Watkins and Watkins' (1997) concept of ego states is helpful for understanding this dual identity model.

It is important to realize that we tend to meta-comment internally about our ongoing experiences. Hassan posits that an external voice takes over the meta-commentator position when one is in a hypnotic trance; the external voice is accepted as the internal voice. The "cult self" is programmed to suppress the organic, "authentic" self. This hypothesis aligns with

Jaynes' and Kuistjen's bicameral mind models of hypnosis (see Sugarman, 2021). Cult leaders and members use hypnotic techniques to program this internalized (cult) voice. Hypnosis can lead to the belief that a cult leader is divine, superior to all humans, and deserving of all sacrifices (financial, sexual, etc.). The cult self is programmed to believe that the authentic self is a dangerous internal enemy to be silenced at all costs. This dismantles self-efficacy because cult influence suppresses but does not erase the unique, authentic self. Clinicians educated about how to conduct appropriate counseling for victims of undue influence can help people to reach their potential as they rebuild themselves (Hassan, 2022a).

A Foundational Case Study of Cult Recruitment and Maintenance

We begin with Hassan's story of recruitment into the Moon organization and membership for over two years, from 1974, when he underwent a radical personality change, such that he was trained to die or kill on command. Unlike regulated ethical military recruitment, Hassan was deceived and indoctrinated when joining the Moon organization. He received no compensation or ability to exit with honor and was not bound by any formal ethical code—a fact further complicated by the group's lack of healthy checks and balances. Finally, he was given no indication that such a warrior-like orientation would be imposed on him.

In retrospect, Hassan learned that hypnosis was used on him and by him on others. Hassan experienced how cult doctrine and policies can shape an individual to act according to the cult's goals. These experiences were instrumental in his personal and professional quest to understand how clinical hypnosis can be abused for undue influence. His work since his deprogramming has attuned him to undue influence as exerted by authoritarian cults and unregulated individuals and companies.

Although Hassan did not experience training that was explicitly named hypnosis, he was urged to copy Moon and other leaders—to model himself upon them: to think, feel, and act as they did. He spent substantial time around cult elders who had likewise absorbed the imitative methodology of hypnosis.

Hassan was deprogrammed in 1976 but did not study hypnosis formally until 1980. This study filled a significant gap in his understanding of his experiences with destructive cults. He went on to learn hypnosis from the Erickson Foundation, the American Society of Clinical Hypnosis, and the International Society of Hypnosis programs, providing a valuable and evolving understanding of this work.

Hypnosis in the Moon Organization Cult

Hassan's first exposure to induction-style hypnosis came four years after leaving when he experienced a workshop on Neuro-Linguistic Programming (NLP). He realized he had been trained to use naturalistic, conversational hypnosis with members, including audible prayers to recruit and indoctrinate obedience. He had learned to repeat language and communication to elicit altered states. He had used single binds, prompting members to consider two realities at once. For example, "Sure, this could all be made up, but what if it isn't? Let us pray. Oh, Heavenly Father, please help John's heart and mind to the truth! Don't let him fall under Satan's spell. Help him make the right choice."

These audible prayers, which conditioned people into suggestible states, lasted from a few minutes to several hours. They were often performed in a group setting. So, the prayer's content was internalized without content evaluation. Hassan also modulated how he spoke (i.e., prosody), for instance, whispering to draw a person into listening more carefully. This was followed by a loud, emotionally charged voice to emphasize intensity. He used other techniques when speaking one-on-one. For example, he learned explicitly to focus on an imaginary point that converged three inches into the skull when looking into another's eyes. Hassan believes this created not only eye fixation but also a sense of superior authority.

Mystical manipulation (Lifton, 1961) was often used to create the illusion of being psychic or influenced by spiritual forces. Information gathered surreptitiously was used to create awe and surrender through manipulated experiences. This technique of thought reform (Lifton, 1961) is incredibly potent in religious cults.

Recruitment, Despite Hesitations

Hassan grew up in a conservative Jewish household in Queens, New York. He was the youngest of three and had a solid education. He loved to read books, write poetry, play basketball, and travel. He had a relatively healthy childhood. His social network was supportive. Nevertheless, within two weeks, he came to believe that Sun Myung Moon was the "Messiah" and that both WWIII and Armageddon were imminent. How?

At age 19, while in college and vulnerable after his girlfriend ended their relationship, he was approached by three women recruiters who flirted with him. They seemed to want to know everything about him. Hassan was invited to dinner and then asked to attend a lecture. Years later, he realized that the experience was filled with hypnotic patterning. While Hassan had no desire to join any group or drop out of college, a sequence of events led him to wonder if there was some "higher" force at work (Hassan, 1988, 2015,2018, 2022).

The cult members were happy and confident. The "humanitarian mission" they described elicited his curiosity and motivation to make a positive difference in the world. Perhaps Hassan's religious values played a role. He was raised to believe in the Judaic notion of a future Messiah to bring world peace and "Tikkun Olam"—repairing the world. The Moonies seemed to have the same goal.

Membership and Maintenance

These factors all influenced Hassan. He was soon moved to leadership positions in the US, gaining access to Sun Myung Moon and the workings of cult leadership. Hassan strove to be the best he could be within the formulations of the cult. This meant total surrender to Moon and the group. Hassan was trained to automatically practice "thought-stopping": chanting internally to suppress doubts.

Hassan became convinced of the infallibility of the group's doctrine, interpreting critical thoughts as Satan testing him. He believed he was building the "Garden of Eden" on Earth. He could not imagine living a happy, fulfilled existence outside of the cult.

Extensive and deceptive propaganda supported these instilled phobias and thought control practices. Hassan worked 18–21 hours a day, seven days a week, without compensation. He recruited and indoctrinated others to join and bring more money and influence to Moon.

Eventually, sleep deprivation and poor health led to a traumatic motor vehicle crash. He was hospitalized for two weeks away from the cult's influence. Hassan experienced compassionate interaction with clinicians, adequate sleep, and improved nutrition there. Without constant reinforcement, his original, authentic self began to resurface. He reached out to his sister, and this led to a deprogramming intervention. Among other strategies, his father asked him to consider how he would feel if his own son left college, became estranged from his family, and joined a controversial group. This led Hassan to agree to meet with former Moonies in an effort to convince his family that he was not brainwashed, was not in a cult, and was thinking for himself. He has been a researcher and activist ever since.

The Dark Side of Hypnosis in Cults

Many destructive cults have risen to prominence: the Charles Manson "Family" (Manson attributed his power over his followers to his Scientology counseling [Emmons, 1986]), the Symbionese Liberation Army (SLA), Jim Jones's People's Temple, David Koresh's Branch Davidians, Luc Jouret's Order of the Solar Temple, Marshall Applewhite and Bonnie Nettles' Heaven's Gate, Shoko Asahara's Aum Shinrikyo, Yogi Bhajan's 3HO cult, and the Bhagwan Shree Rajneesh (Osho) cult (Hassan, 2020a). There are hundreds more destructive cults.

Destructive cults take many forms, including religious, therapy, large-group awareness training, political, and commercial (both human trafficking and multi-level marketing). In an abusive relationship, one person can coercively control another, sometimes reaching the level of a one-on-one cult. We acknowledge that aspects and variations of control can be justified such as a teacher "demanding" a certain level of effort or a parent "controlling" screen time. We bring more nuance to this discussion in our concluding section on models of Undue Influence, notably the Influence Continuum (Hassan, 1988, 2015, 2018, 2022).

These cults all use hypnotic techniques to exert undue influence. More of these techniques have been popularized by Scientology than by any other group. It is worth diving deep into Scientology's founder L. Ron Hubbard's relationship to hypnosis. Hubbard is one of the few cult leaders who studied hypnosis (Atack, 1995, 2014). Since it was first incorporated in 1953 by Hubbard, Scientology has exerted a tremendous influence on the practices of hundreds of destructive cults (Atack, personal communication, December 24, 2022).

The Role of Hypnosis in the Life of Ron Hubbard

In his article "Never Believe a Hypnotist," scholar and former member of Scientology Jon Atack (1995, 2014) examines Hubbard's relationship to hypnosis. He provides a revelatory perspective into Hubbard's unethical use of hypnosis, his contradictory statements, and his overall fascination with the topic. We cite Atack's research throughout this section because of his unique access to sources, his experiences within Scientology, and his focus on hypnosis in Hubbard's life.

Despite Scientology's protestations to the contrary, Hubbard was already interested in hypnosis by the age of 16 years. Later, he credited it with shaping his initial book *Dianetics: The Modern Science of Mental Health* (Hubbard, 1950). Hubbard also recommended books on hypnosis, including the work of Estabrooks (Estabrooks, 1943, as cited in Atack, 2014, p. 39), the *Twenty-Five Lessons in Hypnosis* (Young, 1944), and his averred favorite text, *Hypnotism Comes of Age* (Wolfe & Rosenthal, 1948).

On hypnosis, Hubbard "was initially outspoken on the subject" (HCO Technical Bulletin, 1956, as cited in Atack, 2014, p. 2). Atack writes, "Hubbard was versed in various approaches to hypnotism" (p. 6). Hubbard said he used amnesia, amnestic trances, deep trance, and light trance. He candidly recalls using hypnosis with one individual to change his identity:

> I threw him into a deep trance and gave him the full routine. I gave him the suggestion ... wiped the whole experience out of his mind, wiped out the experience of his coming to tell me that he wanted it done ... woke up this patient, and had a psychotic on my hands. (Volume 1 of Research and Discovery Series, 1950, as cited in Atack, 2014, p. 9)

Hubbard used both nitrous oxide and amphetamines with hypnosis. He was relentless in admitting dark uses of hypnotism: As Atack writes, "Hubbard asserted that it was possible using drugs and hypnotism to 'drive somebody insane by accident ... [or], we could bring about, in the awakened subject, a semblance to every insanity'" (Hubbard, 1950 as cited in Atack, 2014, p. 15).

Hubbard's claims about the power of his hypnotic practices provide evidence of his malignant narcissism. "He even wrote a manual on brain-washing ... and in a letter offered to sell his 'brain-washing' techniques to the FBI. He was also to claim, 'we can brainwash faster than the Russians. 20 secs to total amnesia" (HCO Technical Bulletin, 1956, as cited in Atack, 2014, p. 2).

A Window into Prevalent Cult Practices

Hubbard's understanding of an authority's role in heightening suggestibility was foretold how cults would later use hypnosis. For example, he describes a concept called "altitude teaching." This technique involves claiming to be an authority on an esoteric and inscrutable subject and actively wielding that influence over someone:

> In altitude teaching, somebody is a "great authority." He is probably teaching some subject that is far more complex than it should be. He has become defensive down through the years, and this is a sort of protective coating that he puts up, along with the idea that the subject will always be a little better known by him than by anybody else and that there are things to know in this subject which he really wouldn't let anybody else in on. This is altitude instruction. (Education and Dianetics, 1950, as cited in Atack, 2014, p. 23)

Elsewhere, Hubbard explained, "Any time anybody gets enough altitude he can be called a hypnotic operator, and what he says *will* act as hypnotic suggestion. Hypnotism is a difference in levels of altitude" (Education and Dianetics, 1950, cited in Atack, 2014, p. 20).

Unraveling Jargon: Dianetics, Auditors, and Hypnosis

Hubbard originally called his technique Dianetics (Hubbard, 1950), though Atack argues that Hubbard plagiarized Freud and others. Later, he would incorporate Dianetics into his Scientology as a part of a larger agenda of creating dependency and obedience in followers. Scientology added a wide range of hypnotic techniques to the light trance or "reverie" advocated in his original 1950 text, *Dianetics: The Modern Science of Mental Health* (Atack, personal communication, November 28, 2022).

Hubbard claimed Scientology was an extension of Dianetics after selling all rights to the latter subject in 1952 (Atack, 1990, 2018). Much of the language of Dianetics was absorbed into Scientology. For instance, counselors were renamed "auditors," and the hypnotic aspect of the mind was renamed the "reactive mind." At the time of publication, every counseling or "auditing" session is recorded and often filmed, filling stacks of folders full of notes with followers' intimate details. Former members have been documented as being hesitant to criticize Scientology because they are well aware of this fact. Indeed, Scientology has used supposedly confidential details to harass critics in smear campaigns, blackmail, or subtle manipulation (Atack, 1990, 2018).[1]

Hubbard writes that the auditor "must be prepared to use hypnotism, he must know how it works, what he should do to make it function, how to regress a person in hypnotism and so on" (Volume 1 of Research and Discovery Series, 1950, as cited in Atack, 2014). Aside from the pernicious use of session notes, there is a further problem with Scientology auditors: they lack adequate training in hypnosis. Atack says they "share an ignorance of hypnotism with the general populace and simply parrot Hubbard's calming assurance that 'auditing is not a form of hypnosis' or that 'auditing removes hypnosis'" (p. 40).

A Legacy Practice: Scientology Training Routines

Among the techniques avidly adopted by other manipulative groups are Scientology's Training Routines ("T.R.s"). T.R.s employ various hypnotic methods to put the subject into an altered state. Individuals sit across from a coach, first with their eyes closed ("OT-TR0"). They then stare into each other's eyes fixedly for "some hours," according to Hubbard's directions (TR-0). The "coach" has already learned to enter a passive trance and models trance for the "student." Each step can only be passed with the coach's assent.

Students believe they are learning to communicate more effectively, but T.R.s ultimately aim to cultivate the Scientologist identity and altered perception of reality. With further practice, drivers of undue influence accumulate, and suggestibility heightens. This makes it easier for behavior, interpretation of information, thoughts, and emotions to be shaped (Atack et al., 2015, J. Atack, personal communication, November 28, 2022).

After Hubbard: Hypnosis Used for Undue Influence in Other Cults

Overriding one's self-generated voice to replace it an externally generated cult voice creates susceptibility to an authoritarian cult's influence. This cements involvement and adherence to cult doctrines. If the natural self is subordinated to the cult self, the individual is primed for all kinds of abuse. Abuse, however, is not limited to this form of undue influence.

The NXIVM Cult of Keith Raniere

In 1998, Keith Raniere collaborated with Nancy Salzman (who was trained in NLP) to found NXIVM, known for its "Executive Success Programs." According to former insiders (Edmonson, 2019), Raniere used his studies of Scientology and NLP (Grinder et al., 1979), a model based on Milton Erickson's work. This cult followed in the footsteps of other personal development "coaching" cults (Hassan, 2019, 2021).

Hypnosis was central to Raniere's cult control. Some participants claimed they had no memory of meetings that dragged on for hours, pointing toward the use of amnestic trances (Noujaim, 2020). The cult later used sub-groups to exert more influence on followers; these groups masqueraded as female empowerment but were eventually shown to employ many abusive practices, including 500-calorie diets and the physical branding of women members.

Members learned dependence and obedience to the cult and ultimately to Raniere or "Vanguard," as followers were told to call him. In 2020, Raniere was convicted and sentenced to jail for 120 years for trafficking and racketeering (Department of Justice, 2020).

The Rajneesh Movement

Bhagwan Shree Rajneesh reportedly used hypnosis as early as age six. One member of his inner circle, Erin Robbins (one of his many lovers), who was directed to be sterilized at age 25, said it was well known that Rajneesh hypnotized everyone in his community (Ames & Edmondson, 2022). Rajneesh gave talks about hypnosis (Osho World, 2022). He used typical hypnotic techniques such as voice modulation, staring, linguistic binds, and embedded commands; during this time, he claimed to be Jesus, Buddha, and a "perfect master."

Yogi Bhajan and 3HO

Yogi Bhajan was taught NLP in the early 1980s by a high-ranking disciple. Bhajan amassed a fortune by recruiting and indoctrinating bright, talented westerners. Bhajan used hypnotic methods to control, indoctrinate, and abuse his followers. He claimed to be a kundalini master. He also called himself a Sikh, though he is not accepted by that community (Dyson, 2019; Hassan, 2020c; Singh, 2012).

Solo Sex Predators

Cult leaders are often sexual predators who prey on their flock. Attorney Michael Fine is a distinct case in this section. He was not a cult leader but a divorce attorney who hypnotized female clients to engage in sexual encounters (confirmed by police video and court records). At least 25 women came forward after one court case against him ended (Hassan, 2016).

An investigation began when one of his clients went to the police, and they wired her with a hidden microphone to record his use of hypnosis. Fine was charged with multiple counts of kidnaping with sexual motivation and agreed to a plea deal of 12 years in prison.

Fine had earlier made several appearances in judge Lisa Swenski's court. In law school, Swenski was covertly hypnotized and raped by her male roommate. Informed and sensitized by her subsequent study of hypnosis, Swenski was unnerved by Fine's behavior in trying to use hypnotic manipulation on her and recused herself from his cases. She provides training in covert hypnosis for law enforcement and forensic experts and is committed to helping dispel the common myths held by many professionals about the power of covert hypnosis and undue influence.

Hypnosis Misuse Online

As with cults, there are no licensing requirements for people who use hypnotic techniques who are not healthcare professionals. In fact, hypnosis and NLP are used, and no international regulations exist to protect consumers. Meta (Facebook), Instagram, Twitter, and TikTok are massive networks that influence human behavior for both good and ill. These platforms have been used to influence elections, as described in several documentaries, including The Great Hack (2019) (Seadle, 2020). Foreign governments and other bad actors use troll farms and artificial intelligence to radicalize many people worldwide. These effects spilled into the world, for instance, on January 6, 2021, a violent insurrection intended to prevent the peaceful transfer of presidential power at the U.S. Capitol.

Academic studies support intuitive claims that users of online media experience the dissociative phenomena of time distortion and increased vulnerability to suggestion (Marci, 2022; Turel & Cavagnaro, 2019). Documentaries (e.g., *The Social Dilemma*; Orlowski, 2020) build arguments using evidence from social media officials to show that platforms are engineered to encourage screen addiction.

Online influence goes beyond the individual wasting time, getting lost in predatory ads, or clicking away on the path to radicalization. Cults use online scenarios to assist in recruitment. Unlike the pre-internet world, cults no longer need remote locations to create isolation. Powerful computers that communicate directly with our unconscious processes can create isolation through ads and algorithms (Marci, 2022).

So long as individuals are connected by a device, the desired environment can be created. An American teenager can be recruited by ISIS or a white supremacy cult or be radicalized into violence (Hassan et al., 2022a). Individuals attracted to a video game or dating app can be led to a chat room by a recruiter, then into a financially destructive multi-level marketing group.

As in cults, social media companies proactively keep users hooked. Algorithms detect reduced activity and then dole out notifications to pull users back. Apps will show images of those the user will ostensibly be "leaving" to disincentivize them from deleting the app (Harris, 2021). Similar to Hassan's phobias as a member of the Moon organization, leaving social media can feel like abandoning friends, a supportive network, one's sense of routine and stability, and ultimately the direct influence of the cult leader (Marci, 2022). Finally, some online cults resort to blackmail, public criticism, threats of litigation, and more (Berman, 2020).

A Preview of Future Online Threats

Social media platforms gather users' data. With artificial intelligence, they can tune into users' preferences and shape beliefs covertly. NetCitizens always remain steps behind research devoted to predicting and controlling human behavior. Immersive virtual realities can be more influential than a hypnotist. They directly substitute dissociative "realities."

ASMR as Hypnosis

Autonomous sensory meridian response (ASMR) has been described as the "experience [of] a tingling, static-like sensation across the scalp, back of the neck and at times further areas in response to specific triggering audio and visual stimuli" (Barratt & Davis, 2015, p. 1). We see ASMR as a hypnotic technique capable of producing the narrowing effect of hypnosis on a mass scale: producing trance, raising suggestibility, and leading the listener to home on embedded messages and ideologies. Not surprisingly, some online cults use ASMR as a core component of their recruitment and membership maintenance.

The online group "Bambi Sleep," which describes itself as "Deep Bimbo Erotic Hypnosis," is one such cult. Their YouTube videos frequently feature what could be described as a whispery, cacophonous, immersive song-like soundscape laden with messages and stories (Sleep, 2019).

Hypnosis and Sex

Reddit forums such as r/EroticHypnosis were created in 2011. Its users often post hypnotic videos, including guides. Other websites, such as Breakthrough Addiction Recovery (2022), tout hypnotic devices such as NLP and its ability to re-program the brain to cure addictions to love or sex. Others citing NLP, such as *SoSuave*, to discuss the merits of using NLP to secure sexual encounters (Marlimus, 2005).

Hypnoporn experienced a boom following the COVID-19 pandemic, with sophisticated online videos on sites including PornHub.com using hypnotic methods to induce individuals to transition to the opposite sex or identify as having a different sexual orientation. Variations of hypnoporn include "femdom hypnosis," which uses hypnosis to "guid [e] someone into an altered state of conscious, a flow state, to create heightened states of arousal and pleasure and relaxation" (Ekemezie, 2022).

Future Uncertainties

Digital technologies now under development offer both transformational benefits and potential for harm. If we understand how digital contexts create this harm, we can make informed guesses about how they will play out as new technologies and media become more prevalent.

The Search for a Legal Remedy

In the 1970s, the rise and global spread of cults and their techniques of mental enslavement became public knowledge and a matter of substantial public concern. While most researchers focused on the cults themselves, Scheflin, then President of the International Cultic Studies Association (ICSA), wanted to find ways for victims who escaped cult control to find legal redress. At that time, courts were disinclined to grant any relief. The most frequently used idea in courts was that cult victims had been "brainwashed" or subjected to "mind control." However, judges did not respond favorably because no legal construct was available that would support awarding damages. Moreover, judges did not tend to believe that "brainwashing" was anything more than a public relations label.

In one sense, the courts were correct. "Brainwashing" was a term attributed to Edward Hunter, a government propaganda specialist, who in the late 1950s was tasked with countering the bad publicity for the US generated during the Korean War. In the late 1950s, Hunter was tasked with countering the bad publicity for the US generated during the Korean War. This was when captured American soldiers were put on television to claim they had committed war crimes (Hunter, 1951). He found a unique way to say, "they are not true." Hunter claimed that "the soldiers were brainwashed," and thus "brainwashing" became the generic label for all efforts to claim that people's minds could more easily be manipulated than we would want to believe. *The Manchurian Candidate* idea (Condon, 1959) is perhaps the most significant testament to Hunter's achievement.

Unfortunately, the courts dismissed the basic idea of mental manipulation by focusing merely on the label "brainwashing." There exists a sizeable literature on the feasibility of mind manipulation. The American Psychiatric Association's DSM-III (p. 260), DSM-IV (p. 331), and DSM-5-TR (see section 330) all recognize "brainwashing" as a form of mental enslavement (3rd ed.; DSM-III; American Psychiatric Association, 1980; 4th ed.; DSM-IV; American Psychiatric, Association 1994; 5th ed.; DSM-5-TR; American Psychiatric Association, 2022).

Scheflin suggested that a more traditional legal theory was needed because judges could not see beyond the "brainwashing" label. He chose "undue influence," a concept recognized by British and American courts for centuries. However, undue influence generally dealt with providing a remedy for *financial* exploitation. It did not involve *psychological* harm, which raised important questions concerning freedom of the mind. Indeed, Sloman and Fernbach (2018) convincingly argue that people are necessarily dependent on others, which makes them especially vulnerable to trusting untrustworthy sources, as they argue in their book *The Knowledge Illusion.*

Two essential tasks remained: first to overcome the fundamental judicial reluctance to intervene in an area involving private thoughts, and second, how to use the existing legal notion of undue influence to show judges and juries a way to demonstrate how manipulators could overcome the will of their victims to the point where legal redress was essential.

Scheflin called the first problem *The Myth of the Unmalleable Mind* (Atack, 2021), a common belief that each of us is in complete control of what we think. As the U.S. Supreme Court has said: "Our whole constitutional heritage rebels at the thought of giving government the power to control men's minds" (Stanley v. Georgia, 1969). It is one thing for the law to protect a person's finances, but it is another thing to ask courts to step into the private arena of private thought.

The Myth of the Unmalleable Mind challenges courts to understand mental processes. It is no surprise courts have been hesitant to do so. The faith in our independence leads us to conclude that either (1) mind control does not exist, or, if it does, (2) we can easily spot it and will not fall prey to it. To protect our minds effectively, we must be familiar with the tactics and techniques others may use to penetrate our natural defenses. One may see a punch coming but not a carefully crafted lie or manipulation strategy.

Because the mind is indeed malleable, the law should consider those who, for their gain, take unfair advantage of other's vulnerability. With the framework of undue influence as a passport into the judicial arena, Hassan and Scheflin have constructed a three-part presentation to explain *Undue Influence* to judges and jurors via expert witnesses and lawyers.

Three Frameworks for Understanding Undue Influence

When people interact, they naturally influence one another. When the influence is not helpful, it may become unethical. As mentioned, British common law has long recognized "undue influence" as a remedy that provides monetary compensation for individuals harmed by an influence beyond what the law tolerates as legitimate communication.

But finding the point at which an influence becomes "undue" is no easy task. It is essentially the law being used to say, "you cannot treat another person that way, and having done so, you must pay that person damages for the harm you have caused." Undue influence has been a "slippery slope," incapable of precise delineation. A U.S. Supreme Court Justice once said regarding an obscenity case that he "couldn't define it, but he will know it when he sees it" (Lattman, 2007). The same holds for undue influence.

The Influence Continuum

Hassan developed what he calls the Influence Continuum (Hassan, 2018, 2022), a visualization of the spectrum of influence to help judges and others assess when influence has become "undue." On the ethical, healthy side (the left side of the Figure 53.1 graphic), there is respect for the individual's sense of self, autonomy, conscience, and informed consent, including an "internal locus of control." Qualities like creativity, compassion, and love are respected and even encouraged. If a person wishes to exit a relationship or involvement in a group, the decision is respected.

On the unethical, unhealthy side of the Continuum (the right side), there is a dissociated "cloned" self, created in the image of the cult leader or rigid ideology. The subject operates out of fear, hate, dependency, dogma, and blind obedience. Indeed, a person is programmed with fears and phobias that make it difficult to imagine ever exiting the group without drastic consequences. The cloned (or cult) self has an external locus of control.

A robust model—the BITE Model of Authoritarian Control—lists many specific factors categorized into four overlapping categories. The more of these factors exist, the stronger the undue influence. Research is being undertaken to use a quantitative study (Hassan, 2020b) to develop a model which weighs each factor. This study could demonstrate how deleterious the influence is from predators or predatory organizations.

The graphic below (Figure 53.1) offers criteria to ascertain important values applied to leadership and an organization's health.

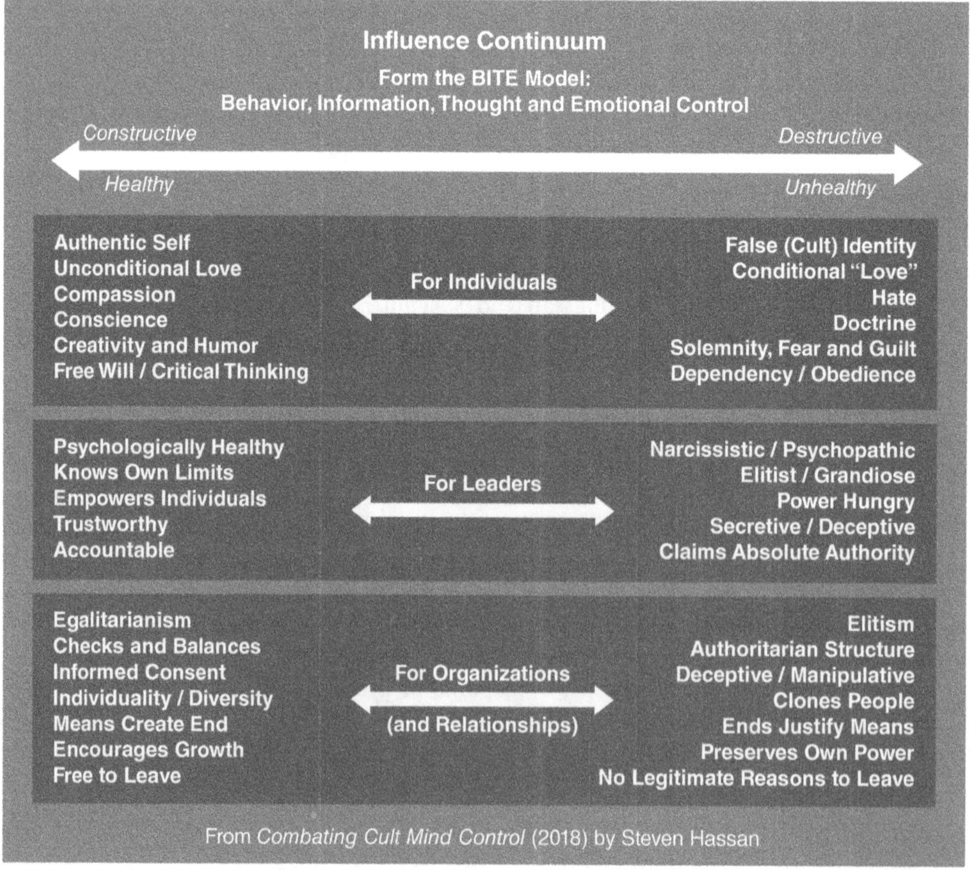

Figure 53.1 The Influence Continuum.

Hassan (2018, 2022). *Influence Continuum* [Image]. Freedom of Mind Resource Center. https://freedomofmind.com/cult-mind-control/influence-continuum/

The BITE Model of Authoritarian Control

Answering the question of when an influence becomes "undue" demands an examination of the biopsychosocial factors surrounding communication (Hassan, S. 2022b). Experts will often testify in court about the nature of the environment as well as communications between the parties. In these situations, they will explain the science of the impact and consequences these communications can have.

To assist in this process, Hassan created the BITE Model of Authoritarian Control (Hassan, 1988, 2015, 2020) building upon Leon Festinger's work (Festinger, 1957). While the Influence Continuum sorts influences on a spectrum from healthy to unhealthy, the BITE Model acknowledges four overlapping, interactive forms of influence. Authoritarian Control can be identified by examining these components, explained in the following four paragraphs.

Behavior Control refers to control of sleep, including sleep deprivation and interference with natural circadian rhythms; overly long indoctrination sessions and rituals; control of diet, dress, financial dependence, isolation from outside communication; and rigid rules and regulations. These controls are often accompanied by a host of different punishments to enforce obedience.

Information Control starts with deceptive recruitment, often by lying, withholding vital information, or distorting information to make it more acceptable. It then moves to control a person's time through manipulation. It is referred to elsewhere as "gatekeeping" (Lewin, 1943).

Thought Control is a crucial component that instills a rigid, dichotomous, us versus them, good versus evil ideology. It internalizes the cult's belief system.

Emotion Control aims to make the person feel special, chosen, and part of an elite group while using various guilt and fear techniques to motivate, indoctrinate, and control that person. It includes flattery and denigration. Phobia indoctrination is the universal mind control technique that creates invisible psychological prison bars.

The most extreme form of undue influence creates a dissociative identity in the mold of the cult leader and ideology. There are many specific recognizable criteria in each of these four components; the more these individual factors are identified, the more influential the Influence will be on the Continuum. This provides a structure within a framework and gives clarity by articulating easily understandable dimensions. Using this framework, experts can structure their testimony and help juries to understand how science contributes to deciding whether an influence is reasonable or undue. The updated list of the four factors of Authoritarian Control can be found online at https://freedomofmind.com/cult-mind-control/bite-model/.

The Social Influence Model

The final model is the Social Influence Model (SIM) (Scheflin, 2015; revised in Atack, 2021), or SIM. The Influence Continuum delineates the dangers of influence, and the BITE Model structures the data obtained from experts. The SIM, however, is designed to use these insights to present coherent arguments to the judge and jury. It visually directs jurors and others to reach a moral conclusion based on the facts of a given case.

The SIM is a visual representation of the "Six Servants" from Kipling's (1902) poem. It allows the jury to look at (1) the leading players in the case, with their strengths and weaknesses, (2) how and why they interacted with each other, and (3) what happened to each after their encounter. The idea is to take the science and the facts and tell a visual story regarding a human interaction that has led the parties to court. Lawyers can create a slide or poster so the judge and jurors can see the whole case structure. At the same time, they can also see how to organize the evidence presented (Scheflin, 2015; revised in Atack, 2021). Clearly, in the world of persuasion, the eye is more powerful than the ear. When jurors can visualize something, it is more vivid and real to them.

The SIM confronts the myth that we are built to resist situational forces head-on. It allows us to understand how influence is exerted by considering the following aspects: who (i.e., influencer); why (i.e., influencer's motive); what and how (i.e., influencer's methods); where and when (i.e., circumstances); who (i.e., influencee's receptivity/vulnerability); and what (i.e., consequences).

At the time of this writing, the undue influence concept has already attracted the attention of courts and legislatures in many countries. As such, the problem of mental manipulation is increasingly in the media (Wood, 2022). Beyond human trafficking laws in existence worldwide (Office for Victims of Crime, n.d.), https://www.legislation.gov.uk/ukpga/2015/2/contents/enacted specific laws targeting "Coercive Control" (U.K. Criminal Justice Act, amended 2015; The Crown Prosecution Service, 2017; Luck, 2021; Rose, 2022; Sundaram, 2022), and "Predatory Alienation" (Laisure, 2021; LegiScan, 2017) have been debated or enacted in several countries. Lawyers working on human trafficking cases also use Influence Models to obtain justice for physically and mentally enslaved clients. Legislators and judges are more aware than ever that there is a need for legal protection for freedom of the mind.

The Question of Whether the Law Protects Freedom of the Mind

Ironically, the U.S. Constitution's First Amendment protects freedom of speech, but not freedom of thought/mentation. Indeed, what we think must be more important than what we say. The First Amendment would be hollow if it merely protected the right to be a marionette expressing the thoughts implanted by others. The Universal Declaration of Human Rights (1948) states in Article 18 that "everyone has the right to freedom of thought [and] conscience." This protection is essential. Chief Justice Earl Warren, writing in the U.S. Miranda v. Arizona (1966) case requiring police officers to read criminal suspects' rights before being questioned, made such a point. He wrote that "the interrogation environment is created for no other purpose than to subjugate the individual to the will of his examiner."

It is sad but true that the world is not unlike a police interrogation room, except that, in some ways, it is worse. At least the interrogation room setting warns that what we say and think will be scrutinized and influenced. Social media gives the world no such warning. This chapter has demonstrated that malevolent influencers do not wear badges or uniforms. Worse yet, they disguise their true intent behind an invisible wall of misrepresentations and prevarications. Nor have they sworn a professional oath to act in the best interests of the clients they aim to fleece or control.

Conclusion

This chapter focuses on the abuse of hypnosis by unethical influencers. We have exposed the world of non-licensed people who use hypnosis, bound solely to their own personal moral codes if they have any morality beyond their self-interest. What they do with hypnosis reflects adversely on healthcare clinicians using hypnosis to heal. In short, when the *image* of hypnosis is abused, all healers are harmed, as are their patients. The good name of hypnosis is essential to the work of its ethical practitioners can do. Considering the influences we have discussed, the law should pay more attention to current threats to our mental integrity (Hassan et al., 2022a; Hassan et al., 2022b; Hassan et al., 2022c; Scheflin, 1983).

Indeed, although the 17th century has been called the "Age of Enlightenment," the 18th century the "Age of Reason," the 19th century the "Age of Progress," and the 20th century the "Age of Anxiety" (Coleman, 1980), we propose the 21st century as the *Age of Influence.*

With the internet, social media, and other forms of media reaching mass markets worldwide, the need to protect the right to think, free from fraud and covert manipulation, is greater than ever. To uphold humanity's *Freedom of Mind,* it is necessary for us to teach and practice ethical influence, as well as to criminalize authoritarian mind control. Human rights demand that we respect and defend the sovereignty of our minds. The tools now exist to guide us. It is time we make better use of them.We have no known conflict of interest to disclose.

Note

1 See, for instance, the Hartwell case (Atack, 1990, 2018).

References

Ames, A. & Edmondson, S. (Hosts). (2022, April). Surviving wild wild country: Erin Robbins speaks out on Osho horrors. [Audio Podcast Episode] In *A Little Bit Culty.* Citizens of Sound. https://open.spotify.com/episode/2hJoK9coCkXB0n3jrNrJwD?si=8459d6fa0a3b405d

American Psychiatric Association. (1980). *Diagnostic and statistical manual of mental disorders* (3rd ed.)

American Psychiatric Association. (1994). *Diagnostic and statistical manual of mental disorders* (4th ed.)

American Psychiatric Association. (2022). *Diagnostic and statistical manual of mental disorders: DSM-5-TR.*

Atack, J. (1990). *A piece of blue sky: Scientology, dianetics and L. Ron Hubbard exposed.* Carol Publishing Group.

Atack, J. (1995). Never believe a hypnotist. Unpublished manuscript.

Atack, J. (2014). Never believe a hypnotist. Unpublished manuscript.

Atack, J. (2018). *Let's sell these people a piece of blue sky: Hubbard, dianetics and scientology.* Trentvalley Limited.

Atack, J. (2021). *Opening our minds: Avoiding abusive relationships and authoritarian groups.* Trentvalley Ltd. (Personal communication, November 28, 2022).

Atack, J., Hassan, S., & Szurko, C. (2015, June 24). *The hypnotic and social influence techniques of Scientology deconstructed.* [Conference presentation]. Getting Clear; A Conference[jl1] [SH2] on Scientology. Toronto, Ontario, Canada, http://gettingclear.co/schedule.html

Barratt, E. L., & Davis, N. J. (2015). Autonomous Sensory Meridian Response (ASMR): A flow-like mental state. *PeerJ, 3,* e851.

Berman, S. (2020, March 12). Accused cult leader threatened ex members after VICE investigation. *Vice.*

Breakthrough Addiction Recovery. (2022). Using neuro-linguistic programming (NLP) to manage sex and love addictions. https://breakthroughaddictionrecovery.net/using-neuro-linguistic-programming-nlp-to-manage-sex-and-love-addictions/

Coleman, J. S. (1980). The structure of society and the nature of social research. *Knowledge, 1,* 333–350.

Condon, R. (1959). *The Manchurian candidate*. Mc-Graw Hill.
The Crown Prosecution Service. (2017, June 30). Controlling or coercive behaviour in an intimate or family relationship. National Police Chiefs' Council. https://www.cps.gov.uk/
Department of Justice (2020). https://www.justice.gov/usao-edny/pr/nxivm-leader-keith-raniere-sentenced-120-years-prison-racketeering-and-sex-trafficking
Dyson, P. S. (2019). *Premka: White bird in a golden cage: My life with Yogi Bhajan*. Eyes Wide Publishing.
Edmonson, S. & Gasbarre, K. (2019) *Scarred: The true story of how I escaped NXIVM the cult that bound my life*. Chronicle Books
Erickson, M. H. (2008). *The collected works of Milton H. Erickson*. Milton H. Erickson Foundation.
Ekemezie, C. (2022, September 26). FEMDOM hypnotists are getting tired of the kink shaming. *The Daily Beast*. https://www.thedailybeast.com/femdom-hypnotists-are-getting-tired-of-the-kink-shaming
Elkins, G. R., Barabasz, A. F., Council, J. R., & Spiegel, D. (2015). Advancing research and practice: The revised APA Division 30 definition of hypnosis. *American Journal of Clinical Hypnosis*, *57*(4), 378–385. 10.1080/00029157.2015.1011465
Emmons, N. (1986). *Manson in his own words as told to Nuel Emmons*. Grove Press.
Festinger, L. (1957). *A theory of cognitive dissonance*. Stanford University Press.
Fromm, E. (1964). *The heart of man*. Harper and Row Publishers.
Grinder, J., Bandler, R., & Andreas, S. (1979). *Frogs into princes: Neuro linguistic programming*. Real People Press.
Harris, T. H. (Host). (2021, April). Can your reality turn on a word? – With Anthony Jacquin [Audio Podcast Episode] In *Your undivided attention*. TED. https://open.spotify.com/show/4KI3PtZaWJbAWK89vgttoU?si=db68b1f072074d23&nd=1
Hassan, S. (1988, 2015, 2018, 2022). *Combating cult mind control: The# 1 best-selling guide to protection, rescue, and recovery from destructive cults*. Freedom of Mind Press.
Hassan, S. A. (2016). *Unethical use of covert hypnosis to rape*. Freedom of Mind Resource Center. https://freedomofmind.com/unethical-use-of-covert-hypnosis-to-rape/
Hassan, S. A., & Shah, M. J. (2019). The anatomy of undue influence used by terrorist cults and traffickers to induce helplessness and trauma, so creating false identities. *Ethics, Medicine and Public Health*, *8*, 97–107. 10.1016/j.jemep.2019.03.002
Hassan, S. (2000). *Releasing the bonds: Empowering people to think for themselves*. Freedom of Mind Press.
Hassan, S. (2020a). *The cult of Trump: A leading cult expert explains how the president uses mind control*. Free Press.
Hassan, S. A. (2020b). *The BITE model of authoritarian control: Undue influence, thought reform, brainwashing, mind control, trafficking and the law* (Doctoral dissertation, Fielding Graduate University). 10.13140/RG.2.2.12755.60965
Hassan, S. (2020c, April 18). *Former 3HO Official Pamela Dyson discusses Yogi Bhajan's use of sex, money and power to deceive and control*. Freedom of Mind Resource Center. https://freedomofmind.com/former-3ho-official-pamela-dyson-discusses-yogi-bhajans-use-of-sex-money-and-power-to-deceive-and-control/
Hassan, S. (2021, February 14). *Keith Raniere and NXIVM on trial: Mind control and manipulation*. Freedom of Mind Resource Center. https://freedomofmind.com/keith-raniere-and-nxivm-on-trial-mind-control-and-manipulation/
Hassan, S. (2022a) Understanding cults: A foundational course for clinicians https://freedomofmind.com/understanding-cults-a-foundational-course-for-clinicians/
Hassan, S. (2022b, January 27). *A paradigm shift for health: A biopsychosocial model of hypnosis*. Freedom of Mind Resource Center. https://freedomofmind.com/ethical-hypnosis/
Hassan, S., Caven-Atack, J., Shah, M., & Malhotra, S. (2022a). Chapter 19: Lone-actor terrorism: Understanding online indoctrination. In J. Holzer, A. Dew, P. Recupero, P. Gill, and J. Wyman (Eds.), *Lone-actor terrorism: An integrated framework*. Oxford University Press. 10.1093/med/9780190929794.001.0001
Hassan, S., Gutheil, T., & Shah, M. (2022b, February). Putting the new framework into practice. *Psychiatric Times*. https://www.psychiatrictimes.com/view/putting-the-new-framework-into-practice
Hassan, S., Gutheil, T., & Shah, M. (2022c, February). A new framework: Exploring efficacy. *Psychiatric Times*. https://www.psychiatrictimes.com/view/putting-the-new-framework-into-practice

Hassan, S., Gutheil, T., & Shah, M. (2022d, February). Responding to authoritarian cults and extreme exploitations: A new framework to evaluate undue influence. *Psychiatric Times*. https://www.psychiatrictimes.com/view/putting-the-new-framework-into-practice

Hubbard, L. R. (1950). *Dianetics: The modern science of mental health*. Hermitage House.

Hunter, E. (1951). *Brain-washing in red China: The calculated destruction of men's minds*. Vanguard Press.

Kipling, R. (1902). *The elephant's child, just so stories*. Tauchintz.

Laisure, R. (2021). Preventing predatory alienation by high-control groups: The application of human trafficking laws to groups popularly known as cults, and proposed changes to laws regarding federal immigration, state child marriage, and undue influence. *International Journal of Coercion, Abuse, and Manipulation*, *1*(2). 10.54208/0002/004

Lattman, P. (2007, September 27). The origins of Justice Stewart's "I know it when I see it." *Wall Street Journal*.

Lewin, K. (1943). Forces behind food habits and methods of change. National Academies Press.

LegiScan. (2017, May 8). New Jersey Senate Bill 2562. LegiScan. https://legiscan.com/NJ/text/S2562/2016

Lifton, R. J. (1961). *Thought reform and the psychology of totalism: A study of "brainwashing" in China*. W. W. Norton & Company.

Luck, S. (2021, December 7). *Coercive control, the silent partner of domestic violence, instils fear, helplessness in victims*. CBC. https://www.cbc.ca/news/canada/nova-scotia/relationships-domestic-violence-control-1.6271236

Marlimus (2005, July 5). *Discussion post asking if somebody could explain NLP*. SoSuave. Retrieved November 20, 2022, from https://www.sosuave.net/forum/threads/could-somebody-explain-nlp.79287/

Marci, C. D. (2022). *Rewired: Protecting your brain in the digital age*. Harvard University Press.

Miranda v. Arizona (1966). 384 U.S. 436.

Noujaim (2020). Director (n.d.). HBO Documentary Series "The Vow" Taking an Inside Look at the NXIVM Organization.

Office for Victims of Crime. (n.d.). Human trafficking task force e-guide: Strengthening collaborative responses. https://www.ovcttac.gov/taskforceguide/eguide/1-understanding-human-trafficking/resources-14-human-trafficking-laws/

Orlowski, J. (Director). (2020). *The social dilemma* [Film]. Exposure Labs; Argent Pictures; The Space Program.

Osho World. (2022, February 6). *The secret of hypnosis*. Osho World. https://oshoworld.com/the-secret-of-hypnosis/

Rose, T. (2022, November 16). NSW passes law to make coercive control a stand-alone offence in an Australian first. *The Guardian*. https://www.theguardian.com/australia-news/2022/nov/16/nsw-passes-law-to-make-coercive-control-a-stand-alone-offence-in-an-australian-first

Scheflin, A. W. (1983). Freedom of the mind as an international human rights issue. *Human Rights Law Journal*, *3*, 1–64.

Scheflin, A. W. (2015). Supporting human rights by testifying against human wrongs. *International Journal of Cultic Studies*, *6*, 69–82.

Seadle, M. (2020). The great hack (documentary film). Produced and directed by Karim Amer and Jehane Noujaim. Netflix, 2019. 1 hour 54 minutes. *Journal of the Association for Information Science and Technology*, *71*(12), 1507–1511.

Singh, G. (2012). *Confessions of an American Sikh: Locked up in India, corrupt cops & my escape from a "New Age" tantric yoga cult!* CreateSpace Independent Publishing Platform.

Sleep, B. (2019, December 31). *Bambi sleep –Bambi mental makeover –03 automatic airhead* [Video file]. YouTube. https://www.youtube.com/watch?v=IL_9muYLk20

Sloman, S., & Fernbach, P. (2018). *The knowledge illusion: Why we never think alone*. Penguin.

Spiegel, D. A. (1991). Neurophysiological correlates of hypnosis and dissociation. *Journal of Neuropsychiatry and Clinical Neurosciences*.

State of Israel: Ministry of Health (1984). *A word from the chairperson*. State of Israel. https://www.health.gov.il/English/MinistryUnits/HealthDivision/MedicalAdministration/hypnosis/Pages/default.aspx

Stanley v. Georgia (1969). 394 U.S. 557, 565.

Sugarman, L. I. (2021). Leaving hypnosis behind? *American Journal of Clinical Hypnosis*, *64*(2), 139–156. 10.1080/00029157.2021.1935686

Sundaram, V. (2022, November 16). *How California's coercive control law could help women manipulated by partners*. San Francisco Public Press. https://www.sfpublicpress.org/how-californias-coercive-control-law-could-help-women-manipulated-by-partners/

Turel, O., & R Cavagnaro, D. (2019). Effect of abstinence from social media on time perception: Differences between low-and at-risk for social media "addiction" groups. *Psychiatric Quarterly*, *90*(1), 217–227. 10.1007/s11126-018-9614-3

The Great Hack (2019). Netflix https://www.youtube.com/watch?v=CAMoPbj3jQE

Universal Declaration on Human Rights, 1948 Rights, U. O. (1948). Universal Declaration of Human Rights. United Nations. https://www.un.org/en/universal-declaration-human-rights/

Watkins, J. G., & Watkins, H. H. (1997). *Ego states: Theory and therapy*. W. W. Norton & Company.

West, L. J., & Martin, P. R. (1994). Pseudo-identity and the treatment of personality change in victims of captivity and cult. In J. L. Stephen & J. W. Rhue (Eds.), *Dissociation: Clinical and theoretical perspectives*. (pp. 268–288). Guilford Press.

Wolfe & Rosenthal (1948). *Hypnotism comes of age*. The Bobbs-Merrill Company.

Wood, D. (2022, October 26). This is why only a handful of coercive control relationship cases go to court. *Yahoo!Finance*. https://uk.finance.yahoo.com/news/why-only-handful-coercive-control-140700977.html

Young, L. E. (1944). *25 Lessons in Hypnotism*. Padell Book Co.

54
THE IMAGE OF HYPNOSIS
Public Perception of the Negative Aspects of Trance

Alan W. Scheflin[1,*] *and Steven A. Hassan*[2]

[1]Professor Emeritus, Santa Clara University School of Law California, USA; [2]Freedom of Mind Resource Center, Newton, MA, USA

The Image of Hypnosis: Public Perception of the Negative Aspects of Trance

Hypnosis is a centuries-old therapeutic technique that has provided much-needed relief for people suffering from a wide variety of physical and mental ailments. It requires no pills, prescriptions, needles, or other paraphernalia. In the hands of licensed professionals, countless numbers of people around the globe have had their lives vastly improved by exposure to this life-affirming and enriching procedure.

But there is another perception of hypnosis that is far more problematic. In the public mind, hypnosis often means something far less appealing. When asked, people tend to view hypnosis with some suspicion, and that is no surprise. Images of hypnotic subjects acting like barnyard animals or fools are the legacy of the stage hypnotists who employ it for demeaning entertainment purposes. Even worse, social media has distorted the concept of hypnosis into an increasingly bizarre myriad of schemes shaped solely by the profit motive and megalomania of the individual huckster.

Perhaps most serious and frightening of all, the public has a more sinister view of hypnotized subjects as individuals who have lost their own free will and now act as mind-controlled automatons doing the bidding of their malevolent masters. Images of Svengali, Rasputin, and the Manchurian Candidate permeate this darker vision of hypnosis. The perception that hypnosis is a method of mind control allowing someone else to manipulate another person's thoughts and behavior is, with good reason, a truly terrifying idea. In the chilling science fiction movie *Invasion of the Body Snatchers* (Siegel, 1956), aliens arrive on Earth, surreptitiously capture people, replicate their bodies, but completely program and control their minds. Thus, "Uncle Fred" looks and acts just like himself, but he does the bidding of his captors. It is this perception of hypnosis that is the most unnerving of all – that a person seems to be himself, yet he is not.

In this chapter, we examine hypnosis' "dark side," with its exotic, mysterious, mystical powers, involving the ability to alter how people ordinarily think and act. Still, it is

* He passed away August, 2023 while chapter was in press.

DOI: 10.4324/9781003449126-71

important to focus on image, as his perception receives constant reinforcement from stories in the media involving sex, mind control, and loss of individual identity. These images hold our attention and trigger our fears. News of the beneficial aspects of hypnosis' use receive little comparable attention. Hypnosis is neutral. The intent of its user is decisive.

Licensed professionals have contributed, wittingly and unwittingly, to the controversial and often unflattering ways in which hypnosis is perceived by the general public. We will present examples of this about which the reader can study further. The issues we address are controversial and contentious, so it is not surprising that the hypnosis community has long been divided about them.

The Methodological Dilemma

"Mind control" is at the core of the public's concerns and fears. Free will, autonomy, and voluntary control are core to the human experience; their loss should frighten anyone (Hassan, 2020). Can hypnosis obliterate a person's voluntary control to the point that the unwitting subject becomes a puppet of the hypnotist's desires?

There are many obstacles to answering this question. The central problem is proving that hypnosis caused a person to engage in antisocial or criminal conduct against that person's will or moral code. We call this the "Methodological Dilemma." The difficulty is that there is no definitive way to prove or disprove causation for several reasons. First, it is unethical and illegal to test the hypothesis, at least as far as criminal conduct or one's personal moral code. Second, no method of testing is completely valid. If the subject violates the law or a personal moral code after a hypnotic interaction, hypnosis is not necessarily the cause. Third, there is disagreement about whether the hypnotized subject retains some element of voluntary control. Fourth, there is controversy within the hypnosis community about how to define "hypnosis."

Laboratory Experiments

In the laboratory, researchers have reported success in inducing hypnotized subjects to throw what they have been told is acid into someone else's face; shoot or stab friends or relatives; put their hands in a box containing poisonous snakes; steal money or property; rip or destroy bibles; and commit apparently self-injurious or criminal acts (Temple, 1989). Critics of such experiments have rejected them on the grounds that subjects were aware or had reason to believe that precautions had been taken to avoid harm. As Moll (1889) has noted, "these laboratory experiments prove nothing, because some trace of consciousness always remains to tell the subject he is playing a comedy ..." (p. 338).

Barber (1961) has written that by telling a person that he or she will be hypnotized, the hypnotist is actually informing the subject "[t]hat he is not only permitted but also expected to carry out [a] performance which he would otherwise inhibit." Indeed, even using the word "hypnosis" "may also contain a concomitant message [that the subject] "advocate(s) control of his behavior [and] the hypnotist is responsible for the consequences" (p. 111). Decades earlier, Bramwell had written that: "If a subject believed that hypnosis was a condition of helpless automatism and that the operator could make him do whatever he liked, harm might result, not through the operator's power, but in consequence of the subject's self-suggestions" (Bramwell, 1903, p. 425).

Furthermore, it is argued that subjects do not necessarily behave in the laboratory the same way they would in social situations. Orne has argued that hypnosis is a superfluous label to explain a subject's compliant behavior. Increased suggestibility, a core concept of hypnosis, "may be viewed as an increase in motivation to conform to the wishes of the hypnotist and not as some mysterious state in and of itself" (Orne, 1959, p. 277). Thus, in the laboratory, the charade of a hypnotic state is merely enhanced motivation to obey the requests made by the hypnotist. The same results can be achieved without prior induction of a hypnotic state. Orne (1960) has explained:

> Volunteer subjects are often motivated to tolerate dangerous and stressful situations for the sake of advancing scientific knowledge. [...] Moreover, the laboratory hypnotist is generally known by the subject to be a reputable investigator who will undoubtedly ensure the safety of all involved despite the appearance of the situation. [...] In our opinion, no situation which is perceived by the subject to be a scientific experiment can validly test the question of the possibility of hypnotically inducing antisocial behavior.
>
> *(Orne, 1960, p. 133)*

To the extent that the subject has "an intense interpersonal relationship [...] with the hypnotist" (Orne, 1960, p. 133), hypnosis cannot be the cause of the antisocial conduct.

By contrast, West and Deckert (1965) have described several cases persuading them that a hypnotist can, in effect, induce antisocial conduct without a prior intimate relationship. This view finds support in secret U.S. government Central Intelligence Agency (CIA) documents that we shall discuss later. West worked for the CIA and was involved in covert hypnosis experiments and activities. Furthermore, as we shall see shortly, for the last 100 years, the possibility of mind control has been birthed, nurtured, and fueled by hypnosis researchers.

Actual Court Cases

To overcome the "demand characteristics" of the laboratory environment, researchers have turned to actual court cases to determine whether the hypnotic inducement of crime is possible.

The Bombard Trial

In 1889, Mr Gouffe was found murdered. Prosecutors accused Gabrielle Bompard, a 22-year-old prostitute, of using herself as bait so that her lover, Michel Eyraud, could rob and kill him. At trial, Bombard accused Eyraud of hypnotizing her into unconscious criminality. She said he reduced her to an automaton devoid of free will. Eyraud responded by claiming that he himself was captivated by love and unable to resist her romantic dominance.

This drama played out in a Paris courtroom where experts from the two leading hypnosis centers in France offered conflicting testimony about hypnosis and criminality. Experts from the Nancy School in Strasbourg concluded that Bompard was highly suggestible and was probably unduly influenced by Eyraud. Jules Liégeois provided expert testimony that hypnosis could undermine the will and morality of almost any subject. He argued that Bompard had been rendered unconscious by Eyraud and therefore was neither morally nor legally culpable.

On the other hand, experts from the Salpêtrière School in Paris, led by Charcot, acknowledged that hypnosis could induce conduct for which there was no conscious awareness or memory, but they argued that some element within the subject's consciousness remained to resist commands that were repugnant to their own moral center. To argue that, the Nancy position would eliminate all legal culpability.

The jury favored the Salpêtrière approach, and Eyraud was guillotined after the guilty verdict. Bompard was sentenced to 20 years in prison. She received early parole in 1903, and Liégeois reportedly got the opportunity to hypnotize her one last time and watch her relive the murder. More than a century after the *Bompard* case, the hypnosis community remains as divided as were the two French schools of thought (as cited in Laurence & Perry, 1988).

The Manchurian Candidate

A recent article in *The Guardian* (Hassenger, 2022) is titled "The Manchurian candidate at 60: does the paranoid thriller still resonate?" The author comments that "the plot is (probably?) preposterous: a group of captured U.S. Korean war soldiers is brainwashed into serving as sleeper agents for a consortium of communist forces so that seeming military hero Raymond Shaw ... will assassinate a presidential candidate." As you read this next section, ask yourself whether the plot is as preposterous as the author suggests.

As we shall see, the "Manchurian Candidate" concept was essentially created by licensed hypnosis professionals and has been sustained by them for more than a century. Although Richard Condon's book *The Manchurian Candidate* (1959) was a work of fiction, it was inspired by several significant social factors.

First, during the 1930s, as Joseph Stalin consolidated his power as the ruler of the Soviet Union, he ordered the arrest of his powerful political enemies and put these men in the courtroom to plead for their lives. But they did not do so. Instead, they confessed to a litany of crimes they could not possibly have committed and begged to be punished. The men appeared quite normal and there was no clear sign of torture. How could such strong and independent men lose their character and integrity? (Conquest, 1968; Vaksberg, 1990). These widely publicized and terrifying political trials were the inspiration for two of the most acclaimed novels published in the twentieth century: Arthur Koestler's *Darkness at Noon* (1940) and George Orwell's 1984 (1949).

Second, the idea of "mind control" was becoming a matter of public interest, with books such as *The Hidden Persuaders* (Packard, 1957) revealing how advertisers were influencing the public's thinking outside of its conscious awareness. In the U.S. culture of the 1950s, social conformity became a prime virtue, and obedience was good manners. The arrival of the 1960s gave rise to its polar opposite – the eruption of unbridled liberty, individuality, and the desire to be free from external control.

Third, Edward Hunter's best-selling book *Brain-Washing in Red China: The Calculated Destruction of Men's Minds* (1951) inspired the Manchurian Candidate idea. Hunter, who worked for the CIA in 1958, provided the following explanation to Congress for the mind control research being conducted in the USSR: "War has changed its form. The Communists have discovered that a man killed by a bullet is useless. He can dig no coal. They have discovered that a demolished city is useless. Its mills produce no cloth. The objective of Communist warfare is to capture intact the minds of the people and their possessions so that they can be put to use. This is the modern conception of slavery, that puts all others in the kindergarten age" (Committee on Un-American Activities, 1958; Hunter, 1958).

Fourth, Condon researched hypnosis and social conformity, and he mentions several studies in the hypnosis and psychology literature supporting the possibility of a person being programmed to be an unconscious spy or killer (Brenman, 1942; Wells, 1941). Condon's evil hypnotist, Yen Lo, explains: "I am sure that all of you have heard that old wives' tale ... which is concerned with the belief that no hypnotized subject may be forced to do that which is repellant to his moral nature, whatever that is, or to his own best interests. That is nonsense, of course" (Condon, 1959, p. 40).

Estabrooks and Dissociation

This fascinating and frightening idea of hypnotic mind control actually has more historical depth than one might otherwise think. Morton Prince's classic *The Dissociation of a Personality* (1906) raised the possibility that a single individual may possess several independent personalities who might not be aware of each other. This possibility intrigued and influenced psychologist George H. Estabrooks enough to make him imagine creating hypnotically controlled couriers and assassins.

The modern story begins with Dr George H. Estabrooks in the early 1920s working at Harvard University's Prince Laboratory. Estabrooks reasoned that if multiple personalities could be *cured* by hypnosis, they could also be *created* by hypnosis. With two distinct personalities, and one not aware of the other, a "double agent" could be fashioned. In this scenario, it would be possible to create a perfect spy, and it would be possible to create a perfect messenger/courier or assassin. Imagine scenarios in which a citizen or member of the military of one country was induced, through hypnosis performed without their knowledge and permission to (1) be an unwitting courier of information with a second, hidden persona (see Bain, 1976); (2) perform acts of sabotage against one's own country; (3) when triggered by a code phrase, carry out a planned assignation followed by complete amnesia for the act (e.g., *The Manchurian Candidate*).

Estabrooks spent his life exploring whether these scenarios were fact or fiction. One issue he faced was the question of whether a person who has been hypnotized would act contrary to his or her own moral codes. Writing in 1928, Estabrooks admitted that "my views are here somewhat different than those of most psychologists. [...] In fact, I believe the hypnotist's power to be unlimited – or rather to be limited only by his intelligence and his scruples" (Estabrooks, 1928, p. 340).

During the 1920s, Estabrooks researched using hypnosis to override individual subjects' will (Estabrooks, 1929). In his early writing, he bragged about the manipulative powers of hypnosis (Scheflin, 1982). In the 1920s, he was unsuccessful in his attempts to interest military and intelligence personnel in the government. There is evidence of this effort in the Colgate University Archive files of Estabrooks's work, where bibliography of his writings includes his statement that after 1930, "I became involved in the military applications of hypnotism and spent my efforts in the field where publication was frowned on" (Estabrooks, 1951, 1962; Estabrooks & Gross, 1961).

Indeed, throughout his life, Estabrooks became a crusader for the idea that hypnotic couriers were essential to the military (Estabrooks, 1955). In correspondence with the

Central Intelligence Agency (Estabrooks, 1957), the Federal Bureau of Investigation (Estabrooks, 1939a & b; 1940a & b; The Black Vault, 2022), the Army (Estabrooks, 1935), the Navy (Estabrooks, n.d.), and the Royal Canadian Mounted Police (Bronskill, 1997; Estabrooks, 1940, 1940), he urged that his ideas be put into practice.

Estabrooks (1957) publicly advocated creating hypnotically programmed couriers and assassins in his book *Hypnotism.* Two years later, he co-authored *Death in the Mind* (Lockridge & Estabrooks, 1945), a novel in which he portrayed Allied officers committing treasonous acts for no apparent reason. The hero discovers that the Nazis have captured these men and converted them into hypnotically programmed double agents. Before long the tables are turned, and the Allies start sending double agents against the Nazis. While the public thought this was scary fiction, Estabrooks hinted otherwise in the 1957 revision of his book *Hypnotism,* suggesting that hypnotically controlled double agents were legitimate possibilities.

Estabrooks went further in an interview with the *Providence, Rhode Island Evening Bulletin* in May 1968 (Blake, 1968). Confessing to having been a consultant for the FBI, the Army, and the CIA, Estabrooks stated that the possibility of hypnotic spies "is not science fiction. [...] This has and is being done. I have done it." He explained that the key to creating an effective spy or assassin "rests in splitting a man's personality or creating a multi-personality, with the aid of hypnotism." Three years later, writing in *Science Digest*, he provided details of some of his efforts (Estabrooks, 1971). Many of the scenarios he described were quite complex, involving intricate programming and reprogramming requiring several months of effort.

In the 1940s, the Office of Strategic Services (the predecessor to the CIA), the CIA, the FBI, the Air Force, the Army, and the Navy all explored the feasibility of hypnotically controlled individuals for use in covert operations, which tested the limits of mind and behavior control techniques. Top Secret CIA programs entitled Project BLUEBIRD, Project ARTICHOKE, and MKULTRA involved countless experiments in the laboratory and public, testing the limits of hypnotic control (Scheflin & Opton, 1978). Estabrooks's work figured prominently in these covert activities (Bowart, 1978; Marks, 1979; Scheflin, 1993; Scheflin & Opton, 1978). Indeed, many of the twentieth century's most prominent scholars and leaders in the hypnosis community were involved in this covert research.

By the 1940s, Project ARTICHOKE assembled an impressive array of hypnosis researchers and interrogation specialists to help answer the following question: "Can we get control of an individual to the point where he will do our bidding against his will and even against such fundamental laws of nature such [sic] as self-preservation?" (Memorandum, 1952). "Hypnotism has been reported to have been used in some cases by the Soviets as an adjunct to interrogation [… .] It would be possible for a skilled Soviet operator to lower a prisoner's resistance to questioning and yet leave him with no specific recollection of having been interrogated. [...] it would be possible to brief a prisoner or other individual, subsequently dispatch him on a mission and successfully debrief him on his return without his recollection of the whole proceeding" (Memorandum, 1951).

It is important to observe that none of Estabrooks's writings describe in detail the procedures he used, and he, himself, indicated that his views were at variance with the opinions of many of his hypnosis colleagues. On the other hand, it would have been counterproductive to reveal such information to the public. Estabrooks neither claimed nor intended to produce a clinical dissociative disorder, though it could be argued that the phenomena he claims to have induced may have met clinical criteria. His goal was practical, not theoretical. Would it be possible to seal off a portion of a person's identity/memory such that only the programmer would be aware of its existence? Moreover, would the amnesia barrier between the two personalities withstand both passage of time and the use of torture?

In the Soviet Union, A. R. Luria's (1932) work on techniques for creating artificial affective complexes provided a possible explanation. In the United States, Milton Erickson and Lawrence Kubie (1939) noted the link between Luria's work and dissociative states in their publication regarding communications with an unsuspected dual personality. They suggested the possibility of one individual having multiple personalities.

Building on this idea, Major Harry C. Leavitt (1947) of the U.S. Army Medical Corps. explored the idea of creating a series of "secondary personalities" whose existence was unknown to the host personality. These ideas paralleled those of Estabrooks's more sinister pursuits.

The idea of creating hypnotically controlled individuals is as old as hypnosis itself since dissociation is an essential hypnotic phenomenon. The public will still fear that hypnosis is a dangerous form of mind control, and professionals will continue to reassure them publicly that it is not. It seems a stubborn methodological fact that, in order to make such a determination, hypnotists must act in a criminal and unethical manner. This debate will likely continue because the Methodological Dilemma virtually assures that opinion is not likely to be overridden by facts. Moreover, the public's appetite for stories of hypnotic mind control is bound to persist.

Forensic Hypnosis

The California Supreme Court in *People v. Ebanks* (1896) wrote with elegant simplicity: "American law does not recognize hypnotism." Events in the new century were emblematic of a great change underway. Indeed, as the Supreme Court of Kentucky pointed out a century later: "Perhaps no issue in the law of evidence has been more hotly debated over the past twenty-five years than the admissibility of testimony by a witness who has been previously subjected to hypnotism" (Roark v. Commonwealth, 2002).

There is a difference between legal cases that involve hypnosis as part of a crime and legal cases that involve hypnosis used to refresh recollections of a crime. The former cases test the power of hypnosis to override a person's will. In contrast, the latter cases involve hypnosis to obtain an accurate memory from a witness, victim, or the accused defendant. In short, the former cases involve the *commission* of a crime, while the latter involves searching for a *solution* to a crime.

In this section, we address the issue of whether the law should permit hypnotically refreshed recollections to be admissible in court. This discussion is especially significant in that, beginning in the 1960s and 1970s when the issue arose in a significant way, hypnosis, in essence, turned on itself.

One of the major factors leading to the use of hypnosis as a memory refresher was the outrage in the 1920s and thereafter to harsh U.S. police interrogation methods, including beatings with rubber hoses, sustained deprivation of food and beverage, around-the-clock questioning of suspects and witnesses, physical abuse, and threats of severe violence. Courts eventually shut down these barbaric practices, necessitating more humane methods of solving crimes. The famous case of Miranda v. Arizona (1966) documents just how cruel and brutal these practices were and why confessions obtained by using such methods could not be considered reliable. The now famous "*Miranda* warning" requires U.S. police to inform criminal suspects that they have the right to remain silent and that anything they say will be used against them.

Hypnosis came of age in the post-World War II era. The 1950s saw the rise of the acceptance of hypnosis as a valid therapeutic procedure, and it received professional recognition from the British Medical Association (British Medical Journal, 1955), the Canadian Medical Association (1958), and the American Medical Association (Council on Mental Health, 1958).

Lay hypnotists had been advising U.S. police departments about the virtues of hypnosis for several decades (Arons, 1967). Many police departments invited individuals to be trained in hypnosis to teach untrained individuals in a variety of hypnotic techniques.

In the United States, from the 1800s to 1968, only 44 cases involving hypnosis reached appellate courts. By contrast, since 1968, more than 500 cases have been decided by appellate judges (Scheflin & Shapiro, 1989).

The first case in the United States that permitted the introduction of hypnotically refreshed testimony was Harding v. State (1968). A rape victim was hypnotized, and she recollected facts she had not previously reported. The court concluded that hypnotically refreshed recollection was admissible evidence. Any challenge to its credibility could be raised at the trial. From 1968 to 1978, courts generally followed this "open admissibility" rule.

There were no guidelines that had to be followed in conducting the hypnosis session, and the hypnotist did not need to possess any professional credentials. For example, the Wyoming Supreme Court had no difficulty admitting the testimony of a "hypnotist" who was a maintenance man at the local Pacific Power and Light Company. His training consisted of a "32-hour home course" (Haselhuhn v. State, 1986). Three years earlier, two judges in a dissenting opinion found a unique way to criticize the lack of any reasonable standards: "There is a man in Oakland, California, who is the dean and lone 'professor' at 'Croaker College.' For the sum of $150 each, this man trains frogs to jump. (Many graduates, after receiving their degrees, go on to compete in the famous jumping contest of Calaveras County.) As part of his rigorous training curriculum, the 'professor' claims that he hypnotizes the frogs; while they are in their hypnotic trance, he plays an attitude-improvement tape to them. Under our present standards, the dean of 'Croaker College,' would be over-qualified as hypnotist" (Gee v. State, 1983). The Calaveras County, California "jumping frog contest" first began in 1928 and has continued ever since.

In one case, told to Scheflin by a law enforcement officer (personal communication), the police hypnotist placed the witness in a trance and asked for a description of his assailant. The witness said he could not describe the man's face because it was hidden by a mask. The police hypnotist responded: "Under hypnosis, you can actually lift the mask and see his face." The witness then proceeded to give a description of what his assaulter looked like. There can be no justification for admitting such testimony in a trial.

To remedy the problem of using unqualified hypnotists, some licensed professionals established police training units to improve the quality of the instruction (Reiser, 1980). However, the hypnotists they trained were not licensed professionals.

In 2020, the *Dallas Morning News* published the results of an extensive investigation conducted into the use of police hypnotists in Texas. This state has the deepest commitment to their involvement in hypnosis in memory recollection (Boucher & McGaughy, 2020). The

Dallas Morning News reporters interviewed police hypnotist Stephen Hatchel who explained that he used progressive relaxation to ease tension in the subject's muscles and open the subject's mind to the concept of hypnosis:

> In videos of some sessions ... hypnotists used the same method before instructing witnesses to imagine standing atop a staircase. As they walk down the steps in their minds, they are supposed to go deeper and deeper into a trance. At the bottom, they are told they see a door ... . A sign on or above that door reads 'Memory Room.' Upon entering, they are told to sit in front of a television. The hypnotist directs them to watch their memories on the screen ... . Hatchel told Barbre [the victim of a physical assault] that hypnosis would help her recall anything from her life as far back as birth. He believed she could review events as though they were a movie, with the ability to rewind, fast forward, and pause at a specific spot.

Barbre said that it was too dark to see the face of the man in her room looking out the window, so Hatchel told her to rewind the memory back to the point where she first realized someone was in the room. Barbre complied and provided identifying characteristics. Hatchel suggested: "Is the light shining on his face?" Barbre responded, "Yes." She was then told that from now on, she would remember the attack better every time she recalled it.

The *Dallas Morning News* investigation reported that prosecutors sent at least 54 people to prison in cases that involved a hypnosis session since the mid-1970s. Courts reversed the convictions of five of these men based at least in part on the use of hypnosis in their cases. Four remained on death row, and 11 were executed. It also noted that record-keeping in these cases was shoddy and that hundreds of cases of police questioning with hypnosis are no longer available for study.

The story is a devastating indictment of unbridled abuse of hypnosis in the absence of legitimate restraints. Almost immediately after this devastating report, the Texas Rangers announced that they were ending their 40-year use of hypnosis (Oli, 2021), and the Texas legislature thereafter considered a bill to prohibit hypnotically refreshed recollection in court (McGaughy, 2021).

As the number of these police-hypnosis cases escalated around the country, many licensed professionals began to sound the alarm. Led by Martin H. Orne, a psychiatrist with a specialty in hypnosis, courts were urged to require some guidelines before any hypnotically refreshed testimony could be introduced into evidence. Orne was torn between his dislike of nonprofessionals utilizing hypnosis and by his appreciation of professionals who conducted hypnosis sessions under strict guidelines crafted to reduce potential contamination of memory.

Guidelines were soon drafted, some of them by Orne himself, and adopted by courts as a requirement for the admission of hypnotically refreshed testimony (Orne, 1979). The intent was to eliminate the "open admissibility" rule and remove lay and police hypnotists from any involvement in the solution of crimes. In general, these are the Guidelines:

1. Competence: The hypnosis session should be conducted by a licensed psychiatrist or psychologist trained in the use of hypnosis.
2. Neutrality: The professional conducting the hypnosis session should be independent of, and not regularly employed by, the prosecutor, investigator, or defense.

3 Documentation: Any information provided to the hypnotist by the prosecution, law enforcement personnel, or the defense prior to the hypnosis session must be in written form or recorded.
4 Pre-hypnotic Narrative: Before the induction of hypnosis, the hypnotist should obtain from the subject a fully detailed description of the facts as the subject remembers them.
5 Documentation: All contact between the hypnotist and the subject should be recorded so that there is no undue suggestion or non-verbal communication contaminating the subject's memory. Videotaping is strongly encouraged.
6 Avoidance of Suggestion: Only the hypnotist and the subject should be present during any phase of the hypnosis session, including the prehypnotic testing and posthypnotic interview.

At that point, it appeared that using guidelines would solve all the problems. Only licensed professionals with hypnosis credentials could question a witness. Their entire encounter would be filmed for a review allowing experts on both sides to evaluate the hypnosis interaction.

Of course, the "guidelines" approach, even in the hands of licensed professionals, can be misused. For example, in Wisconsin in 2001, Evan Zimmerman was charged with the murder of a young woman he used to date. The only piece of evidence tying him to the crime was the testimony of Brice Rene, who was driving his car at 5:30 am and saw a van that he thought looked like Zimmerman's van and he thought he saw a young woman in the passenger's seat. It wasn't much, but it was all the police had. A licensed psychologist, who worked with the police for almost three decades using hypnosis with witnesses, conducted a session with Rene. Wisconsin at the time had nine guidelines that must be followed. The hypnotist violated almost all of them, including being told by the police what they wanted Rene to say and failing to videotape his encounters with the police and with Rene.

Not surprisingly, Zimmerman was found guilty and sentenced to life imprisonment. The Wisconsin Innocence Project retained Scheflin, who explained the guidelines violations and why each violation tainted the hypnosis session. After completing his testimony, Scheflin returned to his seat and looked at Zimmerman, who was crying, but he mouthed the words "Thank you" just as the judge announced that the hypnotist was a personal friend. On appeal, Zimmerman's conviction was reversed. He was tried again, but the prosecution gave up after three weeks. And the case ended with Zimmerman in limbo because the prosecution still thought he was guilty but could not prove it (Boodell & DuBow, 2006).

By the late 1970s, Orne had changed his mind. He concluded that hypnotically refreshed recollection should *never* be used in court. Others also reached similar conclusions, including Dr Bernard Diamond, a psychiatrist who had previously hypnotized Sirhan Sirhan (see Jackman, 2021 for more on Sirhan Sirhan), though his work on that case came under immediate attack by Dr Eduard Simson-Kallas, the chief prison psychologist who spent considerable time with Sirhan (Diamond, 1969; Scheflin, 1982). It also was questioned by Daniel Brown and Scheflin, who acted as experts in the attempt to secure a retrial for Sirhan based on newly discovered data, including the 80 hours of hypnosis and additional questioning of Sirhan by Brown. Not surprisingly, a California federal district court rejected the idea of the possibility of a person being programmed to kill because others in the hypnosis community, who were not named, did not believe this was possible (Sirhan v. Galaza, 2015).

Diamond wrote an influential law review article in which he urged courts not to allow any hypnotically refreshed recollection to be admitted into evidence (Diamond, 1980). This "*per se* inadmissibility rule" position had the effect of splitting the profession into two warring camps. In order to maintain his new view that hypnotically refreshed recollection should never be admissible in court, Orne had to attack hypnosis directly, and he encouraged others to do so as well. This new position had a devastating impact. In the minds of judges, hypnosis became a pariah and was shunned by many courts of law across the country and abroad. His vehemence also split the hypnosis field itself, with proponents and opponents attacking each other, often in the public press. Because the topic was intriguing and timely, newspapers, magazines, and other media outlets ran a barrage of stories detrimental to hypnosis. Hypnosis had become its own worst enemy.

Scheflin pointed out that Orne's *per se* exclusion rule led to absurd conclusions:

> According to the Karlin and Orne position supporting the *per se* exclusion rule for hypnotized witnesses, a person who has been lobotomized can testify in court, a person who has received massive electroshock treatments can testify in court, a person who has taken enormous dosages of mind-altering psychiatric drugs or psychedelics can testify in court, a person who has suffered substantial organic brain damage can testify in court; but a person who had been competently hypnotized by an experienced licensed professional who carefully followed strict guidelines to avoid undue suggestions, cannot testify in court.
>
> *(Scheflin, 1997, p. 26)*

Furthermore, Scheflin posed the following hypothetical in a conversation with Orne:

> Suppose a therapist hypnotized a patient and then had sex with her. Under the *per se* exclusion rule, all her memories would be post-hypnotic, and she would not be able to testify about them. This would, in effect, constitute a license to rape.

Orne conceded that perhaps an exception would be necessary. However, what if a victim of a crime later used a hypnosis-based relaxation tape and remembered some events of the crime afterward? And what if a therapist used hypnosis or guided imagery to help relax an agitated crime victim and asked him to talk about the crime if he wanted to do so?

The original rule of open admissibility and the *per se* exclusion rule arguably share the same problem. Both are too extreme. Admitting everything or admitting nothing hardly serves the interest of justice. The "Guidelines" approach (Kihlstrom, & Frankel, 2000) by contrast found strong support among hypnosis specialists, initially including Orne, and did not lead to unfavorable media stories about hypnosis. Furthermore, we are left with the intriguing and frightening question of whether licensed professionals using hypnosis with patients must give them a warning that any memories, whatever they might be, that result from the induction of hypnosis might ultimately disqualify that patient from obtaining a legal remedy.

The impact of Orne's change of mind, and the increasing number of media stories about the dangers of hypnosis to refresh recollection, eventually resulted in a significant number of state courts rejecting hypnosis outright. Federal courts and agencies generally continue to follow the "guidelines" approach. Many crimes that might not otherwise have been solved have resulted in convictions or led to evidence that might not have otherwise been discovered.

Unfortunately, but not coincidentally, the Orne-Diamond approach arose at a time when there was an increasing number of news stories about child sexual abuse and the defensive response that has come to be called "the false memory" and/or "repressed memory" movements. These discussions, which continue to be volatile even today, added additional negative impressions of hypnosis in the *clinical* setting.

Clinicians must ask themselves: if hypnosis always contaminates memories, especially involving traumatic events, should patients be told about this beforehand, as in an informed consent statement? Would the use of hypnosis under these circumstances constitute the destruction of evidence? The interested reader can find a lively four-paper debate on some of these topics between Scheflin and Karlin & Orne in the *Cultic Studies Journal* (Karlin & Orne, 1996; Karlin & Orne, 1997; Scheflin, 1996; Scheflin, 1997).

The Image of Hypnosis: The International Dimension

The story begins in the 1970s, with the increasing public awareness of child sexual abuse. Sensitive topics involving children and sex were not matters of public discussion before then because of their delicacy and the unwillingness of the public to acknowledge the existence of such private and offensive matters. What broke the ice was the increasingly frequent reports of child sexual abuse at the hands of the clergy – the shocking reports cascaded in the press from across the globe. And then a second wave hit, this time accusing not the clergy but the parents of young children who began reporting their memories of unwanted sexual molestations. Two classes of defendants, clergy and parents, found themselves in courtrooms addressing accusations of the most heinous sins and crimes. Two primary defenses emerged – the children's memories were "false," or if the memories of the abuse had been "repressed," they were inaccurate because "repressed memory" is not a valid concept.

Orne and other memory researchers entered the legal arena to testify that memory was highly fallible and that "repressed memory" was not real; it was mostly the figment of the imagination of the therapists who treated the alleged victims. An avalanche of scientific papers accompanied a cascade of stories in the media, essentially blaming therapists for misusing hypnosis to cue children to relate "memories" of having been sexually abused. The battle pitted academic researchers with scientific data against clinical therapists using "improper" techniques regarding memory retrieval. Hypnosis and other "suggestive" therapies became the problem. This changed the target from the alleged molester to the incompetent healer. The real victims, the children, got lost in the scuffle (Brown et al., 1998).

The false memory/repressed memory attacks reverberated around the world to the glee of the media. Discussions shifted from the reality of sexual abuse to the threat to patients from unskilled clinicians. Just when it looked like matters could not get worse, they did. Added to this toxic stew was the rise of the "satanic ritual abuse" movement, which further encouraged the media's appetite for sensational stories. Hypnosis practitioners found themselves immersed in controversies having nothing to do with how they helped patients. Indeed, many lawyers, like hungry wolves, stalked the therapy community, especially targeting mental health professionals using hypnosis. The news media around the globe had a feeding frenzy reporting these sensationalized cases. Indeed, we are aware of many instances where the media stories were actually encouraged or written by opponents of hypnosis involving memory. The result was bad press for hypnosis before the trial even began.

One final point is worth raising. Clinicians obtain malpractice insurance to protect them in lawsuits. In very many cases involving hypnotherapy, insurance companies representing the therapists decided to settle these cases rather than fight them, often against the will of the insured therapist. Thus, clinicians were denied their rights, and they got tarnished without ever having the option to protect their actions and reputations in a court of law. Even worse, and against the advice of many of us, by settling, the insurers actually inspired more lawyers to file suit for the quick money that was available. And many of these cases also were settled against the expressed wishes of the insured therapist.

Conclusion

Our focus has been on how the *image* of hypnosis has been detrimental to the professional *practice* of hypnosis. Sadly, the image problem worsens as hypnosis falls into the hands of lay exploiters, not healthcare clinicians. For them, the negative image and mystery of hypnosis is the candle that attracts their followers to the flame.

Despite the problems addressed here, it appears that hypnosis is more robust than ever in the healing arts (Sugarman et al., 2020). We applaud this fact. Further, we acknowledge the positive impacts of hypnosis in the past and look forward to a future both in which the *image* of hypnosis is improved and in which the *use* is directed toward positive ends.

We envision a future where hypnosis is used not for mind control, but for pain control; for recovering from unethical mind control; for performing better in sports; for boosting creativity; for improving sleep quality; for activating the immune system; and for improving well-being.

We desire a future in which hypnosis is used properly in a forensic setting, especially as we acknowledge that hypnosis can certainly be used as a tool to understand if someone was unethically influenced. These kinds of usages are critical in individual legal cases and the setting of influential, fair, and sensible legal precedents.

This process of forensic hypnosis, however, can be conducted in an unethical way, involving the planting of ideas into another's mind. At the same time, it can be used ethically by supporting individuals in opening their minds to access memories. Not only do we stand by the ethical use of this kind of forensic hypnosis, but we also believe that this ethical use will flourish when the negative image of hypnosis is confronted.

We have no known conflict of interest to disclose.

References

Arons, H. (1967). *Hypnosis in criminal investigation*. Power Publishers, Inc.

Bain, D. (1976). *The control of Candy Jones*. Playboy Press.

Barber, T. X. (1961). Antisocial and criminal acts induced by hypnosis. *Archives of General Psychiatry*, *5*(Issue), 301–312.

Blake, A. F. (1968, May 13). To 'sleep:' Perchance to kill. *Evening Bulletin*.

Boodell & DuBow. (Executive Producers). (2006). Facing life: The retrial of Evan Zimmerman. [T.V. series]. A & E Home Video; A & E Network.

Boucher, D. & McGaughy, L. (April 12, 2020). The memory room: Does hypnosis really uncover the truth? *The Dallas Morning News*.

Bowart, W. H. (1978). *Operation mind control*. Dell.

Bramwell, J. M. (1903). *Hypnotism: Its history, practice and theory*. London: Grant Richards. 10. 1037/10668-000

British Medical Journal. (1955, April 23). Supplementary annual report of council, 1954–5. Supplement, 190–193.
Brenman, M. (1942). Experiments in the hypnotic production of anti-social and self-injurious behavior. *Psychiatry: Journal for the Study of Interpersonal Processes*, *5*, 49–61.
Bronskill, J. (1997, December 28). Manchurian candidates of our own: When RCMP flirted with brainwashing. *The Ottawa Citizen.*
Brown, D., Scheflin A. W., & Hammond, D. C. (1998). *Memory, trauma treatment, and the law.* W. W. Norton and Company.
Canadian Medical Association Journal. (1958). Miscellany: Hypnotism and medicine. *78*, 367–368.
Committee on Un-American Activities. (1958). *Communist psychological warfare (brainwashing): Consultation with Edward Hunter.*
Condon, R. (1959). *The Manchurian candidate.* Mc-Graw Hill.
Conquest, R. (1968). *The great terror: Stalin's purge of the thirties.* Random House.
Council on Mental Health, American Medical Association (AMA). (1958). Medical use of hypnosis. *Journal of the American Medical Association*, *168*, 186–189.
Diamond, B. (1969, September). Psychiatrist Bernard L. Diamond tells of the bizarre paranoia he found in Sirhan B. Sirhan: A conversation with T. George Harris. *Psychology Today*, *3* (4), 48–56.
Diamond, B. L. (1980). Inherent problems in the use of pretrial hypnosis on a prospective hypnosis. *California Law Review*, *68*(2), 313–349. 10.2307/3479989
Erickson, M. H., & Kubie, L. S. (1939). The permanent relief of an obsessional phobia by means of communications with an unsuspected dual personality. *The Psychoanalytic Quarterly*, *8*(4), 471–509. 10.1080/21674086.1939.11925402
Estabrooks, G. H. (1928). Facts about hypnotism. *Scientific American*, *4*, 340–341. 10.1038/scientificamerican0428-340
Estabrooks, G. H. (1929). Mysterious mesmerism. *North American Review*, *8*(4), 435–443.
Estabrooks, G. H. (May 8, 1935). [Estabrooks to Navy, 1935 May 8] Retrieved from George H. Estabrooks papers (A1026). Colgate University Libraries.
Estabrooks, G. H. (April 20, 1939a). [Estabrooks to Hoover, 1939 April 20] Retrieved from George H. Estabrooks papers (A1026). Colgate University Libraries.
Estabrooks, G. H. (June 19, 1939b). [Estabrooks to Hoover, 1939 June 19] Retrieved from George H. Estabrooks papers (A1026). Colgate University Libraries.
Estabrooks, G. H. (October 25, 1940a). [Estabrooks to Hoover, 1940 October 25] Retrieved from George H. Estabrooks papers (A1026). Colgate University Libraries.
Estabrooks, G. H. (October 7, 1940b). [Estabrooks to Bavin, 1940 October 7] Retrieved from George H. Estabrooks papers (A1026). Colgate University Libraries.
Estabrooks, G. H. (1957). *Hypnotism.* Dutton & Co., Inc.
Estabrooks, G. H. (1951). The possible anti-social use of hypnotism. *Personality*, *1*, 294–299.
Estabrooks, G. H. (1955). The possible antisocial use of hypnotism. *British Journal of Medical Hypnotism*, *6*(4), 2–7.
Estabrooks, G. H. (March 20, 1957). [To Morse Allen from Estabrooks, 1957 February 6] Retrieved from George H. Estabrooks papers (A1026). Colgate University Libraries.
Estabrooks, G. H. & Gross, N. E. (1961). *The future of the human mind.* Dutton & Co.
Estabrooks, G. H. (1962). The social implications of hypnosis. In G. H. Estabrooks (Ed.). *Hypnosis: Current problems.* Harper & Row.
Estabrooks, G. H. (May 7, 1935). [Estabrooks to Navy, 1935 May 7] Retrieved from George H. Estabrooks papers (A1026). Colgate University Libraries.
Estabrooks, G. H. (1971). Hypnosis comes of age. *Science Digest, volume number* (issue number), pp. 44–50.
Gee v. State, 662 P.2d 103 (1983).
Harding v. State (1968), 5 Md. App. 230, 246 A.2d 302, *cert. denied, Harding v. Maryland*, 395 U.S. 949 (1969).
Haselhuhn v. State, 727 P.2d 280 (1986), *cert. denied, Haselhuhn v. Wyoming*, 497 U.S. 1098 (1987).
Hassan, S. A. (2020). *The BITE model of authoritarian control: Undue influence, thought reform, brainwashing, mind control, trafficking and the law* (Doctoral dissertation, Fielding Graduate University). 10.13140/RG.2.2.12755.60965

Hassenger, J. (2022, October 24). The Manchurian candidate at 60: Does the paranoid thriller still resonate? *The Guardian*. https://www.theguardian.com/film/2022/oct/24/the-manchurian-candidate-john-frankenheimer-thriller-1962.
Hunter, E. (1951). *Brain-washing in red China: The calculated destruction of men's minds*. Vanguard Press.
Hunter, E. (1958). *Communist psychological warfare (brainwashing)*. Congressional Testimony.
Jackman, T. (2021, August 25). Sirhan Sirhan, convicted of Robert F. Kennedy assassination, seeks parole with no opposition from prosecutors. *The Washington Post*.
Karlin, R. A., & Orne, M. T. (1996). Commentary on Borawick v. Shay: Hypnosis, social influence, incestuous child abuse, and satanic ritual abuse: The iatrogenic creation of horrific memories for the remote past. *Cultic Studies Journal*, *13*(1), 42–94.
Karlin, R. A., & Orne, M. T. (1997). Hypnosis and the iatrogenic creation of memory: On the need for a per se exclusion of testimony based on hypnotically influenced recall. *Cultic Studies Journal*, *14*(2), 172–206.
Kihlstrom, J. F., & Frankel, F. H. (2000). In memoriam: Martin T. Orne, 1927–2000. *International Journal of Clinical and Experimental Hypnosis*, *48*, 355–360.
Koestler, A. (1940). *Darkness at noon*. Macmillan.
Laurence, J. R., & Perry, C. (1988). *Hypnosis, will, and memory: A psycho-legal history*. Guilford Press.
Leavitt, M. H. C. (1947). A case of hypnotically produced secondary and tertiary personalities. *Psychoanalytic Review*, *34*(3), 274–295.
Lockridge, R., & Estabrooks, G. H. (1945). *Death in the mind*. E. P. Dutton, Incorporated.
Luria, A. R. (1932). *The nature of human conflicts*. Liveright.
Marks, J. (1979). *The search for the "Manchurian Candidate:" the CIA and mind control*. Times Books.
McGaughy, L. (2021, June 24). Texas gov. Greg Abbott vetoes bill to ban testimony based on hypnosis. *The Dallas Morning News*.
Memorandum (January 25, 1952).
Memorandum (February 10, 1951). Defense against Soviet medical interrogation and espionage techniques.
Miranda v. Arizona (1966). 384 U.S. 486.
Moll, A. (1889). *Hypnotism*. Walter Scott Publishing Co.
Oli, S. (2021, March 18). After 40 years in the Texas Rangers are no longer using hypnosis. *National Post*.
Orne, M. T. (1959). The nature of hypnosis: Artifact and essence. *Journal of Abnormal and Social Psychology*, *58*(3), 277–299. 10.1037/h0046128
Orne, M. T. (1960). A book review of Reiter, P.J. M.D., Antisocial or criminal acts and hypnosis: A case study. *International Journal of Clinical and Experimental Hypnosis*, 8, 131–134.
Orne, M. T. (1979). The use and misuse of hypnosis in court. *International Journal of Clinical and Experimental Hypnosis*, 27(4), 311–341. 10.1080/00207147908407571
Orwell, G. (1949). *1984*. Secker & Warburg.
Packard, V. (1957). *The hidden persuaders*. McKay Co.
People v. Ebanks, 117 Cal. 652, 49 P. 1049 (1897).
Prince, M. (1906). *Dissociation of a personality*. Longman.
Reiser, M. (1980). *Handbook of investigative hypnosis*. Law Enforcement Hypnosis Institute.
Roark v. Commonwealth, 90 S.W.3d 24 (Ky. 2002).
Scheflin, A. W. (1982). Freedom of the mind as an international human rights issue. *Human Rights Law Journal*, *3*(1–4), 1–64.
Scheflin, A. W., & Opton, Jr., E. M. (1978). *The mind manipulators*. Paddington Press.
Scheflin, A. W., & Shapiro, J. L. (1989). *Trance on trial*. Guilford Press.
Scheflin, A. W. (1993). The use of medicine and psychiatry to commit human rights violations: The mind control experiments. In P. Mahoney & K. Mahoney (Ed.), *Human rights in the twenty-first century: A global challenge*, pp. 831–843. Brill-Nijhoff.
Scheflin, A. W. (1996). Commentary on Borawick v. Shay: The fate of hypnotically retrieved memories. *Cultic Studies Journal*, *13*(1), 26–41.

Scheflin, A. W. (1997). False memory and Buridan's ass: A response to Karlin and Orne, *Cultic Studies Journal*, *14*(2), 207–289.
Siegel, D. (Director). (1956). *Invasion of the body snatchers.* [Film]. Walter Wanger Productions.
Sirhan v. Galaza, 76 F. Supp. 3d 1073 (C.D. Cal. 2015).
Sugarman, L. I., Linden, J. H., & Brooks, L. W. (2020). *Changing minds with clinical hypnosis: Narratives and discourse for a new health care paradigm.* Routledge.
Temple, R. (1989). *Open to suggestion: The uses and abuses of hypnosis.* The Aquarian Press.
The Black Vault (2022) Freedom of Information Act correspondence between George H. Estabrooks and J. Edgar Hoover. https://documents.theblackvault.com/documents/fbifiles/scientists/georgeestabrooks-fbi2.pdf
Vaksberg, A. (1990). *The Prosecutor and the prey: Vyshinsky and the 1930s, Moscow Show Trials.* Weidenfeld and Nicolson.
Wells, W. R. (1941). Experiments in the hypnotic production of crime. *Journal of Psychology*, *11*(1), 63–102.
West, L. J., & Deckert, G. H. (1965). Dangers of hypnosis. *Journal of the American Medical Association*, *192*(1), 9–12. 10.1001/jama.1965.03080140015003

Professional Development

55

HOW TO ENCOURAGE SELF-CARE IN HELPING PROFESSIONALS THROUGH PROCESS-ORIENTED HYPNOSIS

Shawn R. Criswell

Kaiser Permanente Northwest, Keizer, OR, USA

Introduction

Many helping professionals, such as clinicians and teachers, gain deep satisfaction from their contributions to the well-being of others. However, neglect of essential self-care skills and practices by professionals inevitably erodes their own health. Self-care and caring for others seem to be competing needs with no one-size-fits-all formula for finding the balance between them.

As a mental health therapist, I typically see helping professionals when they are weeks, months, or even years into negative consequences from their neglected self-care: burnout, depression, anxiety, relationship problems, and harmful habits. Often clients[1] are not aware that self-care neglect contributes so significantly to their problems. Ironically, and quite humanly, my helping professional clients, even with their expert level of knowledge about self-care, can fail to heed their own advice. With so much of their attention focused on caring for others, they may not notice the early signs that indicate a need to better address their self-care.

The core of this chapter is a description of how to use Yapko's Process-Oriented Hypnosis (2016, 2019, 2021) to encourage self-care in helping professionals. The tools, concepts, and case examples are designed to provide enough detail to be of practical use for experienced clinicians.

Leading up to the clinical application section of the chapter is a definition of "hypnosis" and an overview of the hypnosis literature that is focused on self-care for helping professionals. A brief description of what inspired my interest in both Process-Oriented Hypnosis and self-care for helping professionals provides insight into the clinical orientation and personal experiences that informed the how-to clinical guide. The chapter concludes with an exploration of the future of self-care for helping professionals and the role of Process-Oriented Hypnosis in the overall future of hypnosis.

Due to the broad applicability of wellness topics such as self-care, there may be personal benefit to anyone who reads the chapter. Allowing a part of yourself to consider beneficial adjustments to your own self-care as you read can add value to your experience.

DOI: 10.4324/9781003449126-73

Definitions and Framework

Despite the recognized efficacy of therapeutic hypnosis, there remains no consensual definition of it. Jensen et al. (2015) separate "hypnosis" from "hypnotic responding." When defining hypnosis, Hope and Sugarman (2015) limited the term to describe the intentional interactive process – not its effects – and the word "trance" to describe the target of that process.

When a clinician intentionally applies certain communication skill sets (i.e., the process of hypnosis), it tends to allow clients/patients to deliberately, yet more automatically, access and change their physiology, emotions, beliefs, and perceptions – a whole range of at least partly nonconscious processes. Mind/body capacities and resources within clients exist independently from the process of hypnosis. When I refer to "hypnosis," I am referring to the process that I am applying to evoke, build, and beneficially direct innate client resources and capacities.

When I use the word "resource," I do not speak of preidentified and specific items within a client to mine and exploit. It is not that you might not want to target a specific resource to harness on behalf of the client. It is more about orienting yourself and your client to expansive possibilities within them and their relationships. "Hypnosis" without a capacity to interact with "resources" within clients would be meaningless. The English-language idiom "squeezing blood from a turnip" comes to mind. Words themselves are simply tools to provide a bridge of communication so that an exchange of the concepts underlying those words can occur. Client "resources" are those unique, vast, multilayered, and complex networks of possibilities within clients. The "resources" also encompass client relationships to people and to other elements of the world. Some of the "resources" are familiar to the client and some are, yet, unknown. Other "resources" have not been perceived yet as a "resource." The client without the benefit of a fuller perspective may only have had awareness for the negative aspects. Perhaps the client had only used the "resource" in contexts in which the "resource" was inappropriate. The analogy that brings the concept of "resources" to life for clients will necessarily flow from client interests and experiences. A nature lover may relate to the concept of an old growth forest with its beautiful and complex ecosystem extending both above and below the surface of the ground. A diver may relate descriptions of an ocean reef. A gamer could prefer reference to how, in questing video games, the characters bring and discover a range of items, talents, and companions. An animal lover may relate more to an interchange about their relationship with their pet and the rich nuances of the shared connection. A client "resource" is what is activated and engaged with in the process of "hypnosis."

Process-Oriented Hypnosis aims hypnosis strategically. It helps clients to more clearly define and then achieve their goals. Rather than trying to create a specific predetermined, clinician-selected result, Process-Oriented Hypnosis uses hypnosis to focus client attention, resources, and abilities on activating beneficial changes in the direction of their goals. Consideration of context rather than only suggesting a global use of a skill is fundamental to this approach. Any given action or perception can be adaptive in one context and problematic in another. Taking a brief break during a lengthy surgical procedure can enhance both self-care and the outcome of the operation. During that same procedure, the surgeon ought not to divert their attention from the patient at a critical moment. That could result in the death of the patient. While most context-by-context discriminations are not so immediately dangerous, they can still be crucial in determining outcomes. The patterns in which clients think and act also contribute to the creation and maintenance of problems. The surgeon tends to lose focus as they approach critical steps well into long procedures. When these patterns are adaptively changed, the problems often disappear or become irrelevant. The surgeon recognizes this pattern and takes intentional breaks in anticipation instead of reaction.

Using hypnosis opens the possibility of discovering and building a range of abilities – both conscious and nonconscious – within the client. Aiming those resources strategically increases the likelihood of lasting change around the client goal.

Hypnosis for Self-Care: General Background

For well over 100 years, hypnosis has been used in psychological and medical care. Part of the ongoing relevance of hypnosis may rest on its potential to enhance health and well-being. One key element of ongoing well-being, regardless of a person's state of health, is self-care.

Within the peer-reviewed, English-language hypnosis literature, there are articles in which self-care and/or enhancing well-being is a primary focus (Elkins et al., 2018; Guse, 2014; Ruysschaert, 2014). Self-care is also a component in dozens of hypnotically based treatments for individuals dealing with the consequences of challenges ranging from perceived stress, to depression, to PTSD, to cancer, to pain.

Highlighting how this chapter's topic has received little attention, only two relatively recent articles specifically address the use of hypnosis for helping professionals to enhance their self-care.

Ruysschaert (2009), a Belgian psychiatrist, exclusively focused on the use of hypnosis for self-care for caregivers. She provided an overview of the risk factors faced by health care professionals including burnout and compassion fatigue. She also discussed positive treatment targets such as resilience, engagement, and compassion satisfaction. The bulk of the article outlined hypnotic strategies to address caring for the self, setting boundaries, increasing inner strength, and connection to positive feelings and habits at work.

Carolusson (2014) described her successful use of hypnosis to help clients with burnout. Of the two case intervention examples she presented, one involved a helping professional. She described an important focus of her work with 50 clients with burnout to be on "the balance between achievement and rest and also between outward and inward focus of attention" (p. 72).

The literature, though limited, reports good results using hypnosis to increase well-being in helping professionals. The need for increased resources to promote well-being for helping professionals is evident. The United States Surgeon General issued an advisory to sound an alarm about the level of burnout and resignations in many helping professionals (HHS.gov, May 23, 2022).

Hypnosis for Self-Care: Personal Background

In my work setting at a health care organization, I had been witnessing the magnitude of the suffering in helping professionals, both colleagues and clients, during the first years of the COVID-19 pandemic. However, I also knew how to use Process-Oriented Hypnosis to enhance self-care in ways that were making a positive difference for helping professionals. This chapter was inspired by seeing a need and having a resource that could help.

My own hypnosis journey started with those same circumstances. As an undergraduate, I volunteered at a crisis line, a woman's shelter, and a group home for children who had been badly abused. The training that was provided did not always help enough. In my search for creative approaches, I found and read books about Ericksonian hypnosis including ones by Haley (1973), Erickson et al. (1976), Zeig (1980), and Lankton and Lankton (1983). Intrigued, I sought training and personal hypnosis to explore the methods further. The personal and professional payoff was profound, enriching both my therapeutic relationships and the benefits to those in my care. This inspired me to continue my study. I took classes and read materials from a variety of hypnosis experts. My early training, after graduate school, was primarily with Stephen Gilligan. He taught me how to first access and embody my own resources before actively engaging in the provision of care to others. Lusijah Marx, another Ericksonian hypnosis mentor, provided individual guidance that helped me further personalize my own methods of self- and other-care.

The most galvanizing experience that I had related to hypnosis was years into using hypnosis professionally. In a class I was taking with Michael Yapko, he demonstrated his use of Process-Oriented Hypnosis with a woman who was experiencing depression as a result of interpersonal issues. The positive transformation that the woman went through was apparent. Prior to the demonstration, Yapko had explained how he was going to use Process-Oriented Hypnosis to help the woman with her presenting complaints. After the demonstration, he gave a detailed description of what he did. He did not stop there, he showed us how we could, regardless of the specifics of the presenting concerns and the particulars of the person we were working with, yet with all those details in mind, create similarly powerful results. While the content of the demonstration was fascinating on many levels, it was this combination of showing and telling, demonstrating and explaining that stood out for me. That this combination of science and art was done on a parallel level with both the audience and the demonstration partner only made it more impressive and compelling. I obtained every recording I could find where Yapko demonstrated his style of hypnosis. Again and again, he was able to use his method to help his demonstration partners create rapid, yet lasting change related to a variety of complex problems. My clinical approach to encouraging self-care in helping professionals that I present in this chapter is directly based on Yapko's work (2016, 2019, 2021).

Phenomenology and Therapeutic Relevance

Some of the most significant issues that helping professionals face with self-care involve nonconscious processes. When they are immersed in the other-oriented flow of their work, professionals are often not consciously aware of personal needs or wants. Even when helping professionals briefly notice a cue indicating a want, a need, or that they are approaching their limit, they may push it aside as only of secondary importance relative to their role as a helper. This dedicated and self-sacrificing behavior is often modeled by faculty as a virtue during the training of helping professionals. As a result, type of pattern can become so habitual and automatic that the person even forgets that there is a series of potentially important decisions being made, and needs are accumulating. They may not know that they are forfeiting something essential to their own well-being. Perhaps the concept self-care seems so familiar that the helping professional underestimates its value in their life.

The therapeutic task then becomes creating ways to support helping professionals in developing not only sustainable, deliberate habits of self-care but also ways to notice and respond to cues about their evolving needs, limits, and desires. Encouraging self-care for helping professionals involves both individualized self-care habits and a connection to an attitude of self-protection that includes noticing and proactively responding to cues signaling risk and opportunities to flourish.

New Applications – How to Do a Process-Oriented Hypnosis Session to Encourage Self-Care

Each Process-Oriented Hypnosis interaction involves more than formal hypnosis. If a client has not presented a specific, solvable goal, one can postulate a goal that may be relevant to their concerns. A client may come to therapy because they used to love their job and now dread going to work. They may not be able to provide much detail about what contributes to the global situation that they are labeling "dread about going to work." If they want to change their "dread," it would be reasonable to consider setting a goal related to building skills for proactively and effectively shifting their mood states.

A key element of any therapeutic encounter is the accurate identification of specific patterns that maintain and/or create client problems and subsequently can keep them from achieving their goals. One also strives to determine what skills and resources they will need to use to meet their goals. This is more targeted than a general goal, such as client empowerment, that may be in the background of every session.

I follow a generic structure that naturally includes the key elements of any hypnosis session (e.g., induction, deepening). However, the actual time spent on each element of a session can vary dramatically and is influenced by verbal and nonverbal feedback received from the client. When using hypnosis, some clients can focus quickly and only need a short transition time (i.e., induction) before actively working on their goals. Other clients need a lengthy buildup of momentum and focus before they are ready to directly work on the primary goal. Readiness and responsiveness can often be implied from nonverbal cues (e.g., changes in breath rate and muscle tone, body movements including facial expressions). The clinician can also use verbal check ins and/or ideomotor signaling.

When designing a hypnosis session, I use a relatively complex set of evaluations to determine client and problem characteristics. These characteristics inform many of the details of the session – the tailoring. For example, if a client has a short attention span or starts to fall asleep, that is likely to influence how interactive the session is. If a client is very guarded, I usually spend more time building responsiveness before launching into more sensitive topics (i.e., lengthening response sets and starting with themes that are more acceptable). I tailor sessions according to what seems to be working to achieve the client goal. To make sure that what I am doing is both generally and specifically helpful, I check in verbally during my hypnosis sessions to provide more clarity about clients' internal experiences. I also encourage clients to audio record at least the more formal hypnosis portion of the session for later use. We discuss guidelines for how to best use the audio recordings.

There are four core self-care skills (see Table 55.1). A client does not necessarily have to consciously understand all the core self-care skills to benefit from this approach. However, for a clinician to apply the concepts, they will need to be able to not only understand each of the core skills but also spot the myriad ways that skill deficits or neglect of their importance to a healthy self-care process can manifest. These core skills may appear deceptively simple yet each one could easily be the topic for an entire book. Rather than

Table 55.1 Core Self-Care Skills for Helping Professionals (Based on Yapko, 2016)

1 Know your limits, needs, and wants. (Have self-awareness about your limits, needs, and wants. Know what it takes for you to flourish, now and in the future. To be helpful, the awareness must be detailed enough to allow a specific action plan to be created, and then adapted as things change.)
2 Respect your limits, needs, and wants. (Realize that your needs and wants are important enough to actively prioritize. It isn't enough to think about self-care – even when something competes for attention, you must act on your own behalf through doing self-care.)
3 Enforce your limits and needs. (Actively set boundaries with yourself and others. As a helping professional, it is often your responsibility to help. Helping yourself enables you to better help others. You will need to regulate relationships according to many factors, including your own limits, needs, and wants. Boundaries are a way of enforcing and clarifying.)
4 Adjust your limits as needed in response to internal and external feedback. (Cultivate a culture of feedback within your relationships. Sometimes others may be in a better position than you are to notice your limits, needs, and wants. Take the time to notice and respond to your internal feedback – physical, emotional, and mental signals – when they first appear.)

prescribe an exact solution for a client's problem, the therapeutic goal is to identify the skill(s) that seems to be most central to the client's goals and teach them or associate them to new, effective behaviors. This is done within a hypnotic context through the use of compassionately provocative and helpfully instructive content. The process-oriented aspects of the session will relate to the overarching patterns that are central to the problems and the solutions. Metaphorically, it might be framed as teaching how to fish rather than just offering a fish.

Clinical Illustrations: Examples of Process-Oriented Hypnosis Sessions to Encourage Self-Care

The basic outline of what I do to encourage self-care in helping professionals is relatively concise (see Tables 55.1 and 55.2). The messages that are being conveyed in this process-oriented core, if accepted and utilized, can be enough to both resolve the current concerns and prevent future issues. However, simply giving the messages, even within a hypnotic context, is usually not enough. The bulk of the content and much of the artistry of the session involve adding details that are intended to evoke meaningful responses. Personalized details can help build the intensity of responsiveness related to the process-oriented themes. Metaphors and word choices that are based on client interests and experiences increase the probability of the client understanding, accepting, and then incorporating suggested possibilities.

There are also times when adding content-oriented portions to the session can enhance the treatment result. In each of the two clinical examples that follow, I work with the specific symptom that the clients bring to the session. This content-oriented work is nested within the process-oriented work. The process-oriented portions provide generally useful attentional, decision-making, and behavioral shifts around the processes that were necessary elements for the specific symptoms to emerge. The content-oriented aspect of the session uses the context of hypnosis to experience the transformation of the specific symptom.

Table 55.2 Essential Elements of a Session That Features Process-Oriented Hypnosis

1 Build rapport through
   a articulating an understanding of the goal for the session and
   b creating a relationship environment that is respectful and supportive while also therapeutically provocative.
2 Gather information about interests, strengths, life experiences, and values that can be used to create metaphors and choose words that are engaging and intuitively understood.
3 Postulate specific core self-care skill(s) that are being neglected or applied problematically.
4 Direct the client's conscious and nonconscious attention toward process themes that may benefit them.
   (I ask clients discrimination questions about how they make certain decisions, come to specific conclusions, or direct their attention and/or actions. This process helps check my postulation about their core self-care skill issue(s). I can tell that I have a topic area of value when they indicate through, for example, a long pause, saying "I don't know," or giving an inadequate answer. At this point, they often understand how it could be important to have a good answer to my question. This active search, consciously and nonconsciously, is the core of one of the major benefits of Process-Oriented Hypnosis – aimed skill and resources acquisition.)
5 Encourage productive mindsets – positive, yet realistic expectancy (linking it to their active participation and highlighting changes already happening in the session); curiosity and openness; self-compassion and/or sense of humor; flexibility and exploration; and an orientation to growth and willingness to experiment.
6 Use hypnosis formally in the following ways:
   a to explore their options – potentially including the approach they are using and alternatives that may be available.
   b to connect them with their strengths and resources.
   c to encourage context appropriate decision-making – now that they have clarity that they are making a choice and have options.
   d to build motivation, expertise, and realistic confidence through imaginal practice of skills and enjoyment of future successes – including successes with navigating possible challenges.
   e to increase comfort with and connection to potentially useful words, phrases, and concepts (Some people who use hypnosis call these techniques anchoring and seeding.)
   f to link the resources and skills and hypnotic experiences to the contexts where they could be most useful (i.e., post-hypnotic suggestions).
7 Create and/or collaborate on an action plan.
8 Follow-up (This may include another session or emails. This can be prearranged or more spontaneous. Follow-up is both an opportunity to refine skills and reinforce positive change.).

I have provided an example of each of two common themes: (1) ignoring internal cues (feedback) that indicate a need for a change in self-care in response life changes; and (2) automatically responding to the needs of others without first assessing, and then appropriately prioritizing, self-care needs. The first theme primarily involves the fourth skill from the core self-care skills. The second theme involves elements of each of the four skills. The foundational intervention in each case is drawing the client's attention to the neglected yet essential skills. Once the client's attention is aimed toward the skill(s), engaging in more formal hypnosis unlocks a powerful combination of conscious and nonconscious resources that build new possibilities.

In the following examples, I provide partial transcripts. Spoken content is italicized. I use bolded words to indicate words and phrases that I emphasized vocally during the sessions. The transcript dialog is interspersed with non-italicized descriptions and explanations. While it can be helpful to see examples of wording, the transcript portions are short in acknowledgment that each person applying hypnosis may use their own style to expand the specific content.

Even a Well-Balanced Life Requires Rebalancing at Times: The Case of Sam

Sam is a psychologist who is single and in his 30s. His work is divided between his private practice and teaching at one of the local universities. Early in his career, he realized the importance of self-care and had built an impressive self-care plan. His regular program included running five days a week, a daily meditation practice, healthy eating, and an active social life. Then, unfortunately, the COVID-19 pandemic occurred. There were new technologies and procedures he had to learn, and his workload increased substantially. Clients and students needed more from him than ever before, and he wanted to be there for them. They told him what a difference he was making in their lives. The positive feedback was gratifying for him. Despite his success within his work settings and his ongoing dedication to his self-care plan, he began to experience a surge of panic attacks and dread about going to work. At first it only affected him on Sundays, but eventually it was with him every day.

Presession Postulation to Test

Sam's initial request for treatment provided enough data to indicate the self-care issues that may need more attention. Our interview also gave me plenty of information about his interests and strengths.

Sam has done a great job with formulating and then prioritizing his self-care. He also seems to be effective in his work. His skills include impulse control, foresight, frustration tolerance, and social skills – including the ability to effectively set boundaries with himself and others. There are plenty of strengths and interests to draw on. Once he knows where to focus his energies, he can stick with a plan.

He already seemed to have a series of positive coping strategies that could help transform discomfort—running, socializing, noticing positive feedback at work, and the ability to shift attention intentionally. I wanted to explore whether and how he used awareness of his discomfort to help him understand and respond to his changing needs and limits. As the demands had increased in both of his work settings, his only adjustment had been to work harder. It had been a crisis. It was not pathological to want help in any way that he could. However, his physiology and his emotions were providing feedback that he had exceeded his limits. It was time to consider whether to adjust based on those internal cues (i.e., the fourth core self-care skill, see Table 55.1).

My session with Sam started with a brief discussion of his goal to build momentum, positive expectation, and rapport. Several of the initial essential elements of a session (see Table 55.2) were well under way within minutes.

The following transcript illustrates directing the client's attention to process themes.

Therapist: *What happens when you just sit with the panic and notice what is happening?*

Sam: *I don't.* For the first time when he is speaking, he pauses for several seconds. His breathing slows and his eye defocus. *I guess I always try to change it. Hmm.*

Therapist: Pausing to allow the curiosity to build. Sam's rigid and nonconscious response of automatically seeking to transform discomfort without first considering the possible value was his primary process-oriented theme.

Transition to Formal Hypnosis

Therapist: *Would you be okay with doing a brief focusing activity to get some more information?*

Sam: *Sure.*

Therapist: *I am going to guide you through some steps that may allow you to experience and then learn more about your panic.* I begin to slow my breathing and my pace of speaking. I insert slight pauses and allow my body to be more still, closing my eyes briefly. *So that it can help you have more control over your life again ...* His eyes close.

The hypnosis session provided a series of experiences, including stories based on his interests, that shifted Sam's relationship to his former feelings of "panic" and "overwhelm." The final verbal check-in with him suggested the potential value of a condensed content rich experience that would associate his previously troubling symptoms to calm curiosity followed by adjustments to self-care. I often include post-hypnotic suggestions throughout the session and always include suggestions for how to extend the benefits of the sessions to the contexts where they could be useful. Typically, I reiterate and consolidate the key suggestions at the end of the formal hypnotic portion of the session.

Post-Hypnotic Suggestions Given to Sam

Therapist: *You can continue to breathe ... to experience that calm ... that calm that you also experience with your meditation ... that you can experience throughout the day... now ... and in the future ... it could be that your body signals are like reminders ... reminders to create a plan ... a realistic plan for how to adjust your schedule ... your work ... to be more realistic for your current situation ... And as you breathe ... now and later ... perhaps you can imagine the freedom ... after the work ... of recalibrating your work day ... your work tasks ... in ways that invite and bring more of what you love ...*long pause *And each time your body signals you... panic ... and each time your emotions signal you... overwhelmed ... dread ... you might be surprised and even pleased ... very pleased ... to discover yourself responding in pleasant new ways ... a smile* commenting on his smile ... *an internal thank you* associating internal experiencing with something of potential value ... *as you use the signals to adjust in little ways ... or big ways ... to meet your needs ... your wants ...* long pause ... *again and again... now ... later today... tomorrow ... next week ... always* associating changes to a variety of times ... *exploring, experimenting ... settling into a plan that works for now* reinforcing the need to adapt over time ... *outside ... inside* reinforcing both external and internal attention ... *confident in your ability to respond ... doing ... on the way to being ... more and more comfortable ... living a life you can really enjoy ... and value ... that's right* responding to another smile.

Developing an Action Plan

We spent the rest of the session, at his request, problem solving how to adjust his workload. We set up a template schedule that included time for addressing his basic needs and integrating his self-care plans. As he struggled to fit his work responsibilities and personal needs and wants into the limited slots of time, he realized how many changes he would need to make to create a more balanced life.

Follow-Up to Sam's Session

At his follow-up session three weeks later, Sam had exciting news to report. Ever since the initial session, he sometimes had stress signals but no further panic attacks. Whenever he felt dread or overwhelm, he simply used the awareness as a cue to decide whether to adjust something in his day or in his life. This transformation of how Sam interpreted and then responded to his emotions and sensations was the process-oriented target of his treatment.

There were details that helped Sam refine his self-care habits. He found that referring to his calendar and using electronic reminders several times during the day helped him maintain his personal boundaries. When he did not use his reminders for reflective down time, he found himself pushing to get one more thing done or connecting socially by responding to a personal or professional communication. He set aside weekly and quarterly reflection times to proactively decide about how many and what types of clients and classes to take on.

During our second and final session, we used hypnosis to reinforce successes over the last weeks and explore how to extend the skills and enjoy the rewards of using his calendar and reminders to help guide his decision-making. Sam was encouraged to continue cultivating and using his internal and external resources recognition of situational cues to adapt.

Through periodic emails over the next several months, Sam let me know that he was earning less money due to reducing his workload but that he was happier than he had been in a long time.

Deciding Whether and How to Respond to Others' Needs and Requests: The Case of Juliana

Prior to my initial visit with Juliana, I had received the following email from her:

> This last year has been a stressful one. I am a physician so the pandemic itself and all the work stresses and changes have been one factor. My parents' and siblings' ill health has been another. And finally, my wife has been upset with how much time I have been putting in at work and with my family. She strongly suggested that I come to therapy. I want my marriage to be good, but I also need to work and help my family. I have a hypnosis app that helps me go to sleep at night. I heard that you use hypnosis.

Presession Postulation to Test

Juliana appeared to have strong values in many areas – job, family, and marriage. Her training as a physician and the culture in her workplace encouraged dissociating from personal needs during her workday to allow focus on patient needs. I suspected that this habit of automatically focusing on doing what she can to respond to the needs of others was interfering with the awareness that she could benefit from stepping back to assess her situation from a broader perspective. Though she probably understood the concept of limits, I wondered whether she was experientially connected to how limits – especially related to time and energy – dictated the need to be selective rather than reflexive in her decision-making about how to spend her time and energy.

When I signed onto the virtual session, Juliana and her wife Amy were playing with their cat, Tiger. I was able to have a brief interview with all of them to gather information about experiences that could form a basis for potentially meaningful metaphors and to develop rapport with both Juliana and Amy while building a momentum for and expectation of positive change.

Directing the Client's Attention to Process Themes

After brief exchanges with Juliana and Amy, I asked a question that Juliana's response confirmed was pivotal to how she was contributing to the problems she was experiencing. This became the central process-oriented theme of her treatment with me. The transcript follows:

Therapist: *How do you decide whether and how to respond to the needs or requests of others?*

Juliana: After a several second pause ... *I guess I don't. If it seems important and it seems like I can or should do it, I do it ... It isn't working out very well for my marriage though.*

Juliana's response highlights the rigidity and automaticity of her pattern of setting boundaries, especially with her family.

Therapist: *Well, I think we have a focus for our session. Amy, will you be willing to help Juliana with an action plan that we will be coming up with in the session? It might involve saying "yes" to helping her family. It would be a different kind of helping though, helping that leaves you and Juliana more freedom and more fun.*

Amy: *That sounds interesting.*

Therapist: *Juliana, do you want to continue the session with all of us together or would you like to do the hypnosis portion with just the two of us?*

Juliana: *Let's have it be just us.*

Therapist smiling and laughing and waving goodbye as Tiger and Amy leave: *Amy, look at that, she is already setting boundaries!*

Transition to Formal Hypnosis

Therapist: *Is there anything else you want to talk about before we start with hypnosis? We will have time to check in during and afterwards.*

Juliana: *No, I am ready.*

Therapist: *Is there anything you need to do to limit interruptions or make your body more comfortable? Do you need to shut any doors, turn off a phone, or take a bathroom break?*

Seeding the idea of stepping back to assess the situation relative to the goal, then actively taking care of her body and doing her part to put up boundaries to protect the time.

Juliana shakes her head "no."

You already know how to focus inside ... like when you use your hypnosis app ... or practice yoga ... you use your breath to center ... body relaxed ... face relaxed ... mind slow and easy.

If you **choose** to, you can continue to use your breath now ... to keep you where you want most to be ... in a special kind of flow that has a familiar feel. That's right.

You can **gently guide** your attention in ways that are pleasant, productive. You may hear sounds on the outside ... the world is going about its usual business as it does ... you can allow those sounds to fade, to grow more and more distant. Pleasantly distant. Nothing you need to respond to ... unless it makes sense to.

As you continue to settle ... to center ... you may be aware of thoughts or feelings or feelings about thoughts or thoughts about feelings ... you can let those go ... if you want to ... drifting or directing ...**directing your attention** toward your main intention ... or perhaps enjoying the moment ... doing nothing at all ... on purpose ... I used a conversational induction that utilized her prior successes with altering her internal experience in pleasant ways. I chose and emphasized words that seeded a variety of core self-care skills: multidimensional self-awareness, empowerment (some people call this ego-strengthening), prioritizing based on thoughtful consideration, adapting based on her needs/wants, and increased comfort with boundary setting.

I did not include the transcript section where I first began to push at increasing her awareness of the extent to which she seemed relatively unaware of the signs that she had exceeded her limits. I provided several metaphors about others going beyond reasonable limits. My hope was that telling stories that were playful and involved cats would help Juliana engage more easily while still getting the point. The transcript resumes after this series of metaphors and immediately after I have requested that she verbally report what she was aware of.

Juliana: *It is getting easier at work, but it is really hard to say "no" when my family needs something ... I feel relaxed.*

Therapist: *Isn't it nice to feel relaxed ... You can feel relaxed and consider complicated things ... at the same time ... a breath ... that's right. Choosing whether and how to respond to the needs of others can be uncomfortable* ***at first*** *... it can be more comfortable when you consider,* ***it isn't necessarily about whether the need or request is met, it is perhaps more about who meets it.***

At work, you often see patients leaving from seeing other providers ... all kinds of providers ... your clinic is full of caring competent people ... and wouldn't it be uncomfortable ... really uncomfortable ... if you were feeling guilty about not having met all of those needs and requests of everyone ... the billing needs, the pharmacy needs, the medical assistant needs, the social worker needs, you get the idea ...

You recently got someone to take notes for you at work, a scribe. At first it was awkward, uncomfortable. Some of your patients complained initially ... which made it even more difficult emotionally, ***at first****. You found yourself in the interesting position of justifying it to them. And then agreeing with what you said ... adapting how you care ... distancing from their initial discomfort ... more and more certain of the value ... to make space for what is* *essential in those relationships ... The medical record is a need, of course. It must be done. The negotiable part is who does it. And* ***isn't it nice to be able to be present for what is most important, most enjoyable*** *with your patients. Now that they are all used to it, they appreciate the benefits too ... even if some of them would never admit it ...*

Juliana already had experience increasing her ease and familiarity with boundary setting in one context (work). I enhanced her association to both her positive feelings about her growth and the details of steps that she had taken. The process-oriented issue stopping her from effective boundary setting with her family involved her reflexive, rather than carefully considered, responses.

And isn't it interesting where you are now ... in your process compared to where you were at the beginning of the session ... when you first emailed ... you know where to ***focus your problem solving ...***

I wonder how it will feel when you see the look in Amy's eyes as you are setting limits in new ways ... what will she say and do ... how will you celebrate together ... and how you can feel the ***pride in setting just the right limits for the situation ... So many positive possibilities.***

Post-Hypnotic Suggestions

Each time that you notice a need or get a request ... you can pause ... carefully consider how or if ***you*** *meeting that need or request fits into what is most important: for you, for your marriage, and for them. This process can get more and more automatic as you practice.*

And each time that you see a speed limit sign, I wonder how much more you can consider the value of all kinds of limits ... situation by situation ... and what respecting those limits allow ... in your marriage and in your life ... and that is certainly worth protecting.

Action Plan

Juliana and I collaborated on a plan for her, with Amy's help, to create a document for each family member that she is currently helping. It would list at least 20 possible resources and ideas, that did not directly involve her, that could meet the needs of the family member. We discussed the medical social worker on her work team as a resource for additional ideas. We agreed to schedule a follow-up session after she was able to work on the action plan and listen to her recording of the hypnosis session a few more times.

Follow-Up

The next session, two months and a few brief email exchanges later, I again met with the couple together. In the interim, they had created a resource list and a plan. They were also using their shared electronic calendar to schedule in more fun time as a couple and a monthly fun-focused extended family event.

Once Juliana realized that she was reflexively responding to needs and requests that could, and perhaps sometimes should, be met by others, she was able to allocate her finite resources differently. When Amy realized that Juliana was protecting their time together and taking better care of herself, she was able to enthusiastically participate in plans to meet Juliana's family's needs.

Over a six-month post-treatment period, a few emails were exchanged reinforcing and refining mindsets and practices and celebrating the successful changes.

Juliana and Sam shared a strong value for helping others – and, with the help of Process-Oriented Hypnosis, developed new ways to also value themselves in contexts where they had previously, beyond their conscious awareness, neglected self-care.

Implications for Training and Professional Development and Future Orientation

The well-being of helping professionals requires more than personal efforts. The various contexts where helping professionals work and are educated should support well-being through prioritizing ongoing training in and dedicating adequate resources for self-care. Changes could include appropriate workloads, scheduling flexibility, and enough resources to meet helping professionals' personal and family needs. Culturally based stigma within professional and educational settings against both self-care and seeking assistance can create internalized reluctance to do either. As strengths-based, empowering approaches such as Process-Oriented Hypnosis have gained in popularity, helping professionals may be more responsive to engaging a range of opportunities to getting training and care around developing their self-care.

Changes, predictable and unpredictable, will continue to shape the ways that hypnosis and self-care are practiced. Technological advances have allowed us to expand where and how clinical care is provided. The COVID-19 pandemic necessitated an increase in virtually provided care. Its popularity among both clinicians and people seeking their care has remained high.

Clinicians now have increased access to training, consultation, and collaboration from professionals across the globe as more professionals were forced and/or inspired to use virtual platforms. The comparative affordability and convenience of these options have already increased the number of clinicians who are trained in Process-Oriented Hypnosis.

Subjective reports and now even some empirical research attests to the efficacy of virtual interactions that are both synchronous (i.e., live) and asynchronous (i.e., materials that are produced for general audiences and/or specific individuals that may include written messages and documents, images, videos, and/or audio recordings stored and then accessed later). Apps and websites can provide portals for synchronous care as well as access to a range of asynchronous resources. Though versions of synchronous and asynchronous virtual care and training have been with us for a while (e.g., phone calls, written materials, and audio recordings of hypnosis sessions), the current level of proliferation is remarkable and seems likely to continue to expand in both clinical and educational contexts.

As technology evolves, it will provide more tools and resources. As our knowledge about how to access and develop innate human potential expands, it can allow us to use hypnosis with increased precision and power. However, no matter how much we know or how many technological advances we have, we will face the need to make choices. Some of those choices will be made consciously. Some of those choices will be made nonconsciously. Whether it involves a helping professional making choices about balancing their care of others with their self-care, or a clinician choosing how to focus their care, choices are the foundation from which the future rises. One reason that Process-Oriented Hypnosis is so central to the future of clinical hypnosis is its focus on enhancing the quality of decision-making. Much of the recent progress in health and care can be attributed to enhancing our abilities to include and prioritize different contexts, e.g., from prolonging life to improving its quality (see Gawande, 2014). Choosing well, context by context, among all the possibilities, will determine how we promote the well-being of ourselves in the service of others.

Note

1 Since this chapter focuses on enhancing the self-care of helping professionals, the term "client" will be used primarily to refer to helping professionals. While these same skills can help the clients/students/patients in the care of these helping professionals, in this chapter "client" does *not* refer to the people in the helping professional's care.

References

Carolusson, S. (2014). Burnout syndrome and analytical hypnosis. *Archives of Psychiatry and Psychotherapy*, 2, 71–84.

Elkins, G. R., Roberts, R. L., & Simicich, L. (2018). Mindful self-hypnosis for self-care: An integrative model and illustrative case example. *The American Journal of Clinical Hypnosis*, *61*(1), 45–56. 10.1080/00029157.2018.1456896

Erickson, M. H., Rossi, E. L., & Rossi, S. I. (1976). *Hypnotic realities: The induction of clinical hypnosis and forms of indirect suggestion*. Irvington.

Gawande, A. (2014). *Being mortal: Medicine and what matters in the end*. New York, NY: Metropolitan Books, Henry Holt and Company.

Guse, T. (2014). Increasing psychological well-being through hypnosis. In Fava, G., and Ruini, C. (Eds.), *Increasing psychological well-being in clinical and educational settings. Cross-cultural advancements in positive psychology, vol 8*. Dordrecht: Springer. 10.1007/978-94-017-8669-0_6

Haley, J. (1973). *Uncommon therapy: The psychiatric techniques of Milton H. Erickson, M.D.* W. W. Norton.

Hope, A. E., & Sugarman, L. I. (2015). Orienting hypnosis. *The American Journal of Clinical Hypnosis*, *57*(3), 212–229. 10.1080/00029157.2014.976787

Jensen, M. P., Adachi, T., Tomé-Pires, C., Lee, J., Osman, Z. J., & Miró, J. (2015). Mechanisms of hypnosis: Toward the development of a biopsychosocial model. *International Journal of Clinical and Experimental Hypnosis*, *63*(1), 34–75. 10.1080/00207144.2014.961875

Lankton, S. R., & Lankton C. H. (1983). *Theanswer within: A clinical framework of Ericksonian hypnotherapy* (1st ed.). Routledge. 10.4324/9781315803937

Ruysschaert, N. (2009). (Self) hypnosis in the prevention of burnout and compassion fatigue for caregivers: Theory and induction. *Contemporary Hypnosis*, 26, 159–172. 10.1002/ch.382

Ruysschaert, N. (2014). The use of hypnosis in therapy to increase happiness. *American Journal of Clinical Hypnosis*, *56*(3), 269–284, 10.1080/00029157.2013.846845

Yapko, M. D. (2021). *Process-oriented hypnosis: Focusing on the forest, not the trees*. New York, NY: W. W. Norton.

Yapko, M. D. (2019). *Trancework: An introduction to the practice of clinical hypnosis* (5th ed). New York, NY: Routledge.

Yapko, M. D. (2016). *The discriminating therapist: Asking "how" questions, making distinctions, and finding direction in therapy*. Fallbrook, CA: Yapko.

Zeig, J. K. (Ed.). (1980). *Teaching seminar with Milton H. Erickson* (1st ed.). Routledge. 10.4324/9780203776117

56

MINDFULNESS MEDITATION AND HYPNOSIS IN CLINICAL PRACTICE

An Integrated Approach

Akira Otani

PRIVATE PRACTICE

Mindfulness meditation (hereafter, the terms *mindfulness* and *meditation* are used interchangeably unless otherwise noted) has come of age. Long considered esoteric and even cult-like Eastern quackery, Buddhist meditation has recently transformed into one of healthcare's most popular, science-based complementary and integrative health methods. According to Centers for Disease Control and Prevention (CDC) statistics, approximately 36 million adult Americans, that is 14.2 percent of the U.S. population, used mindfulness in 2017 (U.S. Department of Health and Human Services, 2018). Worldwide, 275 million people, roughly 3.4 percent of the global population, are estimated to meditate (Kane, 2022). Mindfulness is now a Western phenomenon and a billion-dollar business (LaRosa, 2019).

It is no surprise that a growing number of healthcare providers, including hypnosis-informed clinicians, showed interest in incorporating mindfulness into their practice (e.g., Alladin, 2014; Elkins, 2020; Lynn et al., 2006; Otani, 2003, 2016; Slonena & Elkins, 2021). Combining hypnosis and mindfulness makes good sense because they utilize attention skills, yet each offers additional clinical perspectives and techniques.

Specifically, integrating mindfulness meditation with hypnosis has three advantages. First, hypnosis and mindfulness utilize attentional mechanisms to evoke various cognitive, somatic, and neurophysiological phenomena germane to clinical applications. Clinicians familiar with hypnotic techniques can quickly expand their skill repertoire using the knowledge and training in clinical hypnosis.

Second, like hypnotherapy, mindfulness may be applied with or without the healthcare provider (i.e., guided versus solo practice). This commonality notwithstanding, because mindfulness evolved from the Buddhist meditation framework (see "What Is Mindfulness Meditation?" below), it encourages the client's regular self-practice. This promotes the client's self-management and raises self-efficacy.

Finally, hypnosis and mindfulness meditation can enhance understanding of the fundamental nature of each practice. Studies have begun unraveling similarities and differences in brain mechanisms and cognitive functions between hypnosis and mindfulness (see "Hypnosis vs. Mindfulness Meditation: Commonalities and Differences" below). Nevertheless, there is

DOI: 10.4324/9781003449126-74

much more to be accomplished. For example, ancient Buddhist meditation texts describe the eight sequential stages of consciousness as meditation deepens. The first four stages allegedly accompany pleasant thoughts, feelings, and eventually one-pointed concentration. Following these stages, the next four "formless" states called "infinite space," "infinite spaciousness," "nothingness," and "neither perception nor non-perception" emerge. These highly concentrated mental states are considered to be the precursors to enlightenment (see Cousins, 2022, for a detailed review). Nothing in the current hypnosis literature describes anything resembling these esoteric conscious states (e.g., Pekala et al., 2010; Shore, 1962). Once understood scientifically, these and other topics in Buddhist meditation texts will enhance the knowledge of hypnosis and its clinical applications.

Conversely, the scientific paradigm and applications adopted in developing various hypnotizability scales will be an excellent model to guide future mindfulness research. No reliable and valid instruments currently exist to measure the individual's capacity and competence to engage in mindfulness. Establishing the norm and identifying characteristics of individuals in various mindful capacities will advance the scientific understanding of mindfulness meditation.

In summation, the cross-fertilization of knowledge and research methodology of hypnosis and mindfulness will advance both disciplines.

What Is Hypnosis?

Defining hypnosis[1] has been historically challenging because competing theories (e.g., neo-dissociation, socio-cognitive, psychoanalytic, role enactment, Ericksonian) present different, sometimes opposing, views regarding its nature, mechanism, and process (see Lynn et al., 2015 for a review). As a result, an effort was made to achieve a consensus by describing hypnosis in a "theoretically neutral" manner (Rhodes et al., 2022). One example is "a state of consciousness involving focused attention and reduced peripheral awareness characterized by an enhanced capacity for response to suggestion" (Elkins et al., 2015, p. 6). Note that this definition avoids jargons such as "unconscious," "altered states," and "trance," which led to controversies in the past. Instead, it explains hypnosis by its commonly acceptable characteristics, i.e., "focused attention," "reduced peripheral awareness," and "response to suggestion." The first two terms also apply to mindfulness meditation (see "What Is Mindfulness Meditation?").

Among the factors that make hypnosis viable as a clinical tool, the most vital is the hypnotist–subject relationship. Hypnosis typically occurs in an interpersonal context, i.e., hetero-hypnosis. The healthcare provider and the client engage in dialogs in which the former communicates empathy, respect, and therapeutic suggestions to the latter to achieve desired therapeutic goals. The therapeutic relationship is the key.

Woody and Sadler (2022) contended insightfully that "the interpersonal aspects of hypnosis may be of considerable, relatively broad social importance. They also lend support to the idea that the qualities of the hypnotist and the characteristics of the hypnotist-subject interaction may be of greater significance than has been typical in most hypnosis research" (p. 175). The provider must remember to establish a solid, secure relationship with the client in hypnotic work.

The phenomenology of hypnosis is diverse and well-documented (Rhodes et al., 2022). Many hypnotic phenomena also appear in mindfulness meditation, particularly in the focused attention type relative to the open monitor type (see "The Types of Mindfulness

Meditation" for the distinction of mindfulness in the next section). For instance, absorption, reduced volitional control, alterations in self-awareness, changes in the sense of time, diminished sense of agency, and suspension of the rational thinking process emerge in both practices (De Benedittis, 2015; Kasos et al., 2022).

Finally, suggestions are the primary mechanism underlying hypnotic induction and treatment. Studies comparing the relative efficacy of hypnosis and relaxation in pain reduction demonstrate that hypnotic suggestion, not relaxation, reduces pain (Castel et al., 2007; Sebastiani et al., 2007). Furthermore, the different types of suggestion activate distinct regions of the brain. For instance, the suggestions that target pain intensity reduction (e.g., "The pain eases and fades away") reveal activation in the somatosensory area. In contrast, hypnotic directives to suggest emotional distancing from the pain unpleasantness (e.g., "The sensation will not bother you") activate the anterior cingulate cortex (ACC) (Hofbauer et al., 2001; Rainville et al., 1997, 1999). The relative impact of these hypnotic suggestions, one aiming at the sensory-discriminative domain and the other at the motivational-affective component of the pain experience, advocates the importance of goal-specific formulation of hypnotic suggestions (De Benedittis, 2021).

Individually tailored and carefully worded suggestions are, in short, the heart of hypnosis and hypnotherapy.

What Is Mindfulness Meditation?

Mindfulness, as mentioned earlier, has its roots in Buddhism, especially the Theravāda tradition that maintains the rites and rituals in the original form as practiced in the days of the Buddha (463–383 BCE). According to Buddhist theology, meditation, or Right Mindfulness (*samma sati*), is one of the eight "noble paths" to enlightenment. Its goal is to "see things as they are" by way of direct, dispassionate observation of four essential tenets of reality: (1) the breath and body, (2) the feelings,[2] (3) the mental factors, and (4) the laws of nature. The original instructions of the first tenet, i.e., awareness of the breath and body, are as follows:

> Breathing in long, he knows 'I breathe in long,' breathing out long, he knows 'I breathe out long.' Breathing in short, he knows 'I breathe in short,' breathing out short, he knows, 'I breathe out short.'
> He trains thus: 'I shall breathe in experiencing the whole body,' he trains thus: 'I shall breathe out experiencing the whole body.' He trains thus: 'I shall breathe in calming the bodily formation,' he trains thus: 'I shall breathe out calming the bodily formation.'
>
> *(Anālayo, 2004, p. 140)*

Note that the described process consists of two stages: first, the observation of the breath per se (i.e., long versus short inhalation and exhalation), followed by the awareness of the whole body and relaxation (i.e., experiencing the entire body and calming of the bodily formation) *using* the breath. The practitioner repeats this format with the subsequent "feelings," "the mental factors," and "the laws of nature" until he/she can consistently maintain breath awareness in all activities. This is Right Mindfulness.

The concept of "seeing things as they are" has been adapted in contemporary mindfulness practice as *decentering*. It refers to a metacognitive process of "stepping outside the automated mode of perceptual processing and attending to the minute details of mental activity that might otherwise escape awareness" (Bishop et al., 2004, p. 235). Simply put, it is an awareness that *thoughts do not correspond to physical reality*. A famous phrase, "Do not believe everything you think," underscores this idea (Buggy, undated). Its mastery allows the practitioner to detach the self from perturbing cognitions.

Types of Mindfulness Meditation

There are two types of practice in contemporary mindfulness: Open Monitor (OM, or *vipassanā*) and Focused Attention (FA, or *śamatha*). OM consists in "paying attention in a particular way; on purpose, in the present moment, nonjudgmentally" (Kabat-Zinn, 1995, p. 4). In OM, the practitioner observes thoughts, feelings, sensations, and any ongoing experience with openness and receptivity. Indian philosopher Jiddu Krishnamurti called it "choiceless awareness" (Krishnamurti, 2000). Most mindfulness-based therapies currently practiced, e.g., Mindfulness-Based Stress Reduction, Mindfulness-Based Cognitive Therapy, Dialectical Behavior Therapy (Linehan, 2020), and Acceptance and Commitment Therapy (Hayes, 2016), utilize the OM method.

The other method, FA, differs from OM in that it focuses attention on selected objects, e.g., breath, sound, color, scenery, sensation, image, and person. The methodology resembles hypnosis. The best-known FA-based mindfulness is the body scan. Jon Kabat-Zinn introduced it as "body sweeping," a procedure adopted by an ancient Buddhist meditation to promote body awareness (Kabat-Zinn, 1982). It resembles progressive muscle relaxation but differs from it because of its emphasis on focused observation, not deliberate tensing and relaxation, of body parts. Body scan has been compared to hypnosis, particularly Autogenic Training (Schultz & Luthe, 1959), without active body imagery or the "aims to alter body sensations" (Dreeben et al., 2013, p. 396). The similarity with hypnosis is unequivocal.

The technical distinction between OM and FA aside, the demarcation between them is less evident in practice. Many OM practitioners, for instance, use the breath as an anchor (i.e., focal point) during continuous observation of internal- and external-experience. In so doing, momentary absorption states (*khanika samadhi*) occur (Sparby, 2019). This phenomenon is comparable to "everyday trance" in hypnosis, advocated by Milton Erickson (Erickson & Rossi, 1981). Similarly, FA meditators notice and "let go" of any awareness that falls outside the object of concentration until absorption emerges. OM and FA are better viewed as a continuum on which the open-ended attention lies on one end and the mental concentration on the other.[3] The meditator's task is to stay attentive to where the awareness falls at a given moment, depending on OM or FA. This conceptualization allows the healthcare provider to easily integrate hypnosis and mindfulness in clinical work and switch from mindfulness to hypnosis during sessions (see *Basic Techniques of Mindfulness Meditation* below).

Hypnosis Versus Mindfulness Meditation: Commonalities and Differences

So how do hypnosis and mindfulness compare with one another? There has been a growing interest among researchers and practitioners to integrate mindfulness into hypnosis (e.g., Brown, 2006; De Benedittis, 2015, 2021; Elkins, 2020; Holroyd, 2003; Lynn et al., 2006; Otani, 2003, 2016, 2020; Pekala & Creegan, 2020; Wickramasekera, 2020; Yapko, 2011). Recent studies have focused on plausible brain regions and neurophysiological functions commonly shared by and unique to the two respective approaches. The interested reader is referred to excellent resources by Amir Raz and his colleagues (Lifshitz & Raz, 2012; Lynn et al., 2012; Penazzi & De Pisapia, 2022; Raz & Lifshitz, 2016; Semmens-Wheeler & Dienes, 2012).

A thorough review of the similarities and differences is beyond the scope of this chapter (see Chapter 11, "Neural Correlates of Hypnosis," for details). However, a few summary remarks are in order. Given the complexity inherent in hypnosis and mindfulness meditation, respectively, the following is an abridged account of the reported commonalities and differences between the two:

- Therapeutic hypnosis is used solely as a clinical tool, whereas mindfulness may be applied as either a clinical skill or practiced as a religious/spiritual ritual (Otani, 2016);
- Suggestion is the central operative mechanism in hypnosis, while self-observation is the primary method in mindfulness;
- Aside from expectation in both, dissociation is a primary explanatory construct in hypnosis, whereas in mindfulness, decentering (i.e., viewing thoughts and feelings as simply mental phenomena, not the actuality. See p. 5) is a central concept (Kirsch, 2001; Spiegel, 1991; Vancappel et al., 2021);
- According to meta-analytic studies to date, the overall efficacy of clinical hypnosis appears to be medium to high (e.g., IBS, pain, anxiety) (Schaefer et al., 2014; Thompson et al., 2019; Valentine et al., 2019), whereas that of mindfulness to be low to medium (e.g., insomnia, pain, anxiety) (Eberth & Sedlmeier, 2012; Hilton et al., 2017; Ren et al., 2018);
- Higher quality research, i.e., randomized controlled trials, is needed in both hypnosis and mindfulness to assess their clinical efficacy (Goyal et al., 2014; Thompson et al., 2019);
- Existing neuroscientific studies suggest that both hypnosis and mindfulness involve the default mode network and ACC (McGeown et al., 2009). While ACC is decoupled from the prefrontal cortex in hypnosis (Egner et al., 2005), their association is strengthened in mindfulness (Lynn et al., 2012);
- In general, the prefrontal cortex (PFC) is involved in both hypnosis and meditation. However, its activation level is increased in hypnosis but is decreased in mindfulness (Raz & Lifshitz, 2016).
- The general PFC function pattern appears in pain management as well, which indicates hypnotic suggestion enhances cognitive reappraisal to achieve the goal, whereas mindfulness accomplishes pain reduction by attention withdrawal;
- The functional connectivity between the dorsal anterior cingulate cortex and the dorsolateral prefrontal cortex (DLPFC) increases in hypnosis. In contrast, it decreases in mindfulness (Raz & Lifshitz, 2016). This indicates that the DLPFC is engaged in hypnosis due to suggestion but not in mindfulness (Del Casale et al., 2015);
- The generalized reality orientation lowers in hypnosis (Shor, 1959), whereas it is heightened in OM mindfulness (Tang et al., 2015);
- Neuroplastic changes have been observed in long-term meditators (Guidotti et al., 2021), but they have yet to be confirmed in highly hypnotizable practitioners (Spina et al., 2020);
- Absorption occurs in both hypnosis and mindfulness meditation. However, its phenomenology and quality vary depending on various factors (e.g., hypnotizability, types of mindfulness, expertise level), and finally,

- Hypnosis reflects primarily the Western European cultural, social, and medical values given its historical origin with Franz Anton Mesmer in the 18th century. In contrast, mindfulness meditation has historical, methodological, and soteriological roots in Asia, particularly in ancient Indian Buddhism (De Benedittis, 2015).

Based on this summary, one may reasonably conclude that hypnosis and mindfulness meditation are distinct yet share certain commonalities. As Penazzi and De Pisapia (2022) observed in their review of the two modalities, "[T]he large number of meditative practices and the many possible hypnotic inductions open to a combinatorial explosion of interesting experimental contrasts, many of which have not been yet performed" (p. 5). Future research will shed light on the shared and disparate properties of hypnosis and mindfulness meditation.

Hypnosis and Mindfulness: An Integrative Approach

The Buddhist concept of Right Mindfulness (*samma sati*) has been reformulated into a clinically and user-friendly format as contemporary mindfulness. One method is *Touch-and-Return* which comprises OM and FA (Otani, 2016). The practitioner continually monitors the here-and-now awareness (sight, sound, smell, taste, touch, and cognition) (i.e., Touch [OM]) with the alternating observation of the breath as an anchor (i.e., Return [FA]). It follows the principle of "noticing the body, feelings, thoughts, and the laws of nature with the breath" delineated in the Buddhist text.

Although it sounds simple, a few practitioners find Touch-and-Return challenging, at least initially, because of mind wandering, a common phenomenon humorously named the "monkey mind" or "untamed horse" (Gimian, 2016). Fortunately, it becomes easier over time as the practitioner learns to "let go" of distraction without attending to its content (i.e., decentering).

Touch-and-Return Protocol for Mindfulness

Here is the standard Touch-and-Return protocol for mindfulness meditation (modified from Otani, 2020). It consists of six steps: (1) Introductory verbal set, (2) External/internal awareness, (3) Breath awareness, (4) Repeat, (5) Finish, and (6) Post-session assessment. The length of practice depends on the client's needs and comfort. Italicized remarks indicate the clinician's statements.

Step 1 Introductory verbal set

Goal: Explain the overall process of Touch-and-Return to the client.

Touch-and-Return is a simple technique to learn mindfulness. It is to help you become aware of things. I will guide you step-by-step to become aware of things around you, in your body, mind, and breath. You can stay quiet while practicing. You may keep your eyes open, closed, half-open, closed sometime, and open sometime ... it does not matter. Let me know when you are ready.

Step 2 External/internal awareness (Touch)

Goal: Guide the client's awareness of the immediate experience, starting with surrounding prompts (e.g., sound, sight, smell), gradually moving toward bodily sensations, and finally, cognitive activities.

Notice what is around you. Any sound, view, smell ... whatever catches your attention, you openly monitor that ... it's very simple. Do this for a while (wait 10–15 seconds).

Now, what do you notice in your body? Any sensation, tension, movement, warmth ... Whatever they are, acknowledge them as you did with the awareness of things around you (wait 10–15 seconds).

And what about your mind? What is on your mind? Whatever you become aware of, just note it. If you notice your mind noticing the things around you or body sensations at the same time, acknowledge it. It is very simple (wait 10–15 seconds).

If you become aware of several things at the same time or if the mind wanders from time to time, that's no problem. Just notice them as they are.

Step 3 Breath awareness (Return)

Goal: Facilitate the awareness of the breath without altering the pace.

Whenever you feel ready, bring your attention to your breath. Make sure NOT to change the pace or depth or the breathing. Feel your natural breaths. That's right (wait a few seconds).

Step 4 Repeat (2) and (3) (Touch-and-Return)

Goal: Alternate between external/internal awareness and breath observation.

After you observe the breath, notice the things around you, body sensations, and mental activity. Then return to the breath. Become aware of your experience, then go back to the breath. If you become aware of other things together with the breath, let it be and attend to the breath. Repeat this process comfortably (wait 1 minute or longer).

Step 5 Finish

Goal: Complete Touch-and-Return mindfully.

When you feel ready to complete this exercise, tell yourself you will finish now. Then take a nice slow breath. When it is done, you may open your eyes (if the client had the eyes closed). This completes mindfulness for now.

Step 6 Post-session assessment

Goal: Review the client's experience with Touch-and-Return, e.g., comfort level, ease, difficulty, positive and negative reactions, and general and specific comments.

People have different experiences with Touch-and-Return, positive, negative, and neutral. What was your experience? Especially things you found helpful and not so beneficial. Feel free to share with me whatever you find during the practice. We will incorporate your feedback in future practice.

Although most clients find the experience with Touch-and-Return calming and pleasant, some may complain about "not being able to follow the directions well" due to mind wandering. Others may express anxiety analogous to relaxation-induced anxiety observed in relaxation training (Heide & Borkovec, 1983). A few report physical discomfort (e.g., muscle tension, pain, itching) or emotional distress (e.g., unpleasant memory recall, unexpected emotion) during practice. Clients with chronic pain, for example, may fall in the first category, while trauma survivors represent the second. To safeguard the client's well-being, the healthcare provider and the client should thoroughly discuss difficulties and make necessary adjustments (e.g., using an external object for an anchor instead of the breath, avoiding mindfulness in favor of hypnosis).

Nevertheless, adverse reactions during mindfulness practice, in general, are not uncommon. Recent studies (Britton et al., 2021; Kaufmann et al., 2021; Lindahl et al., 2017; Taylor et al., 2022) show that many practitioners have experienced adverse effects during practice, some even lasting afterward. One silver lining is a study by Ruth Bare and her colleagues, who found that 90 percent of practitioners find the unpleasant reactions associated with mindfulness practice "not bothersome" (Baer et al., 2021). Only 10 percent require adequate care to restore somatic comfort and a sense of safety to avoid lingering complications. For this reason, the adverse effects of mindfulness remain a severe issue and must be monitored carefully.

As for the potential risks associated with hypnosis, a recent meta-analytic study revealed an overall rate of 0.47% of adverse events, mainly anxiety-related symptoms (e.g., disturbing images, nightmares, dizziness). No "serious" effects were attributable to hypnosis (Bollinger, 2018). These findings corroborate Lynn et al.'s (1996) earlier conclusion that "there is no reason to believe that hypnosis poses special or unique risks to participants. Indeed, well-controlled experimental studies suggest that hypnotized participants are not at particular risk" (p. 16). Thus, it is safe to conclude that hypnosis is safer than mindfulness.

This being said, the clinician must always ensure the safety of the client when hypnosis and mindfulness are implemented.

Touch-and-Return Protocol for Hypnosis Induction

Extended focus on the breath alone may be adopted for clients who constantly shift attention between awareness and the breath. This adjustment will help facilitate absorption and can induce hypnosis. Conversely, clients with difficulty entering hypnosis can engage in mindfulness meditation by Touch-and-Return. This flexibility is an advantage of this method. A case study using hypnosis and mindfulness by Touch-and-Return is available in Otani (2016), as well as the case illustration in this chapter.

To use Touch-and-Return for hypnosis induction, the clinician may substitute the following modified protocol in Step 4. Steps 1 through 3, 5, and 6 remain the same.

Step 4 (**modified**): Intensify focused attention and absorption.

Goal: Provide directives to concentrate on internal cues to induce hypnosis.

As you continue paying attention to your breath, (pause) are you aware that your out-breath is slightly warmer than the in-breath? (pause) What about the length of your in- and out-breaths? Are they even … or uneven? (pause) Is one longer than the other? (pause) Some people realize the air in one nostril feels smoother than the other … what about yours? (pause) As you continue discovering these fascinating facts about your breath, let your mind and body relax. Let the breath continue doing its own thing. You can just monitor the process from a safe, secure place. Enjoy going deeper into this special place.

The clinician monitors the client closely, paces response, and manages the tempo and tone of voice to ensure hypnotic emergence. It is no different from regular hypnotic induction using observation and pacing.

In summation, Touch-and-Return allows both mindfulness mediation and hypnotic induction depending on its application. The choice is determined by the client's preference or capacity for either skill.

The Importance of Therapeutic Alliance in Mindfulness and Hypnosis

Touch-and-Return is a versatile protocol for mindfulness meditation and hypnosis induction (Brito, 2014). This advantage notwithstanding, the practitioner must remember that the *therapeutic alliance* between clinician and client is quintessential in successful hypnotic induction and intervention (see "What Is Hypnosis?"). In mindfulness, the healthcare provider shows *non-judgmental acceptance of clients* and *openness to experience* to maintain a positive alliance with the client (Razzaque et al., 2015). These two characteristics parallel Carl Rogers' well-known therapist conditions, i.e., unconditional positive regard for clients and congruence (Rogers, 1957).

Research suggests that "mindful clinicians," those practicing mindfulness meditation for up to 10 hours per week, are viewed more favorably by clients as exhibiting more warmth, acceptance, and genuineness (Greason & Welfare, 2013). Some theorists even contend that mindfulness cultivates personal "presence," i.e., personal qualities such as equanimity, empathy, and interpersonal attunement. Such clinicians can "focus on the internal state of another individual with kindness and compassion" (Parker et al., 2015, p. 225). Simply put, a solid interpersonal relationship is crucial for mindfulness meditation to be effective as a therapeutic tool.

Concerning hypnosis, it remains unclear if repeated personal hypnotic experiences will enhance the clinician's ability to relate to clients better. Nevertheless, good rapport-building is indispensable in hypnotic work. Spiegel and Spiegel (2008) argued this point: "The good hypnotist can create an appropriate atmosphere in which the patient may explore his or her trance capacity ... the respectful demeanor appropriate to any clinical setting provides the best atmosphere for hypnosis" (pp. 16–17).

Milton Erickson also gave a similar rationale:

> Now in hypnotizing the psychiatric patient I think one of the important things to do first is to establish an excellent conscious rapport. Let him know that you are interested in him and his problems, and definitely interested in using hypnosis if in your judgment you think it will help.
>
> *(Erickson & Rossi, 1981, p. 5)*

He demonstrated this principle when he decided to work with a terminally ill client, "Joe," whom he *reluctantly* accepted. Wrote Erickson:

> Despite the author's unfavorable view of possibilities, there was one thing of which he could be confident. He could keep his doubts to himself and he could let Joe know by manner, tone of voice, by everything, said that the author was genuinely interested in him, was genuinely desirous of helping him. If even that little could be communicated to Joe, it should be of some comfort, however small, to Joe and to the family members and to the nurses within listening distance in the side room.
>
> *(Emphasis added. Erickson, 1966, p. 203)*

In clinical work, whether hypnosis or mindfulness, the healthcare provider must establish a quality rapport with the client. Otherwise, as the Zen saying goes, "a right tool in the wrong hand becomes a wrong tool" applies to mindful mediation and hypnosis practices.

A Case Illustration

In the last section of this chapter, a case illustrating the applications of mindfulness meditation and hypnosis is provided for a client with chronic trigeminal neuralgia and depression. It should be of interest to the reader to appreciate the nuance of Touch-and-Return in clinical work.

Basic Information about the Client

The client, Mrs JMN,[4] is a 70-year-old retired lawyer happily married with two adult sons. Her contented life halted five years ago when she began having frequent headaches, vision and hearing problems, and limb weakness. Upon consulting a neurologist at a major research hospital, she was diagnosed with a benign meningioma. A team of experienced neurosurgeons operated on her and removed all tumors successfully. Thirty-five-day radiation treatment followed the surgery. Not able to drive herself, she had arranged rides for all sessions and completed the rigorous regimen without missing a day. She was pleased with the "outstanding medical treatment" that she had received.

To her dismay, unfortunately, a few weeks after the treatment, she began experiencing headaches on the left side of her scalp, where the tumors had been excised. The neurologist determined it as postsurgical trigeminal neuralgia.[5] He prescribed several analgesic medications, but they were not effective. Botox injections and sphenopalatine ganglion (SPG) block, a local anesthetic in the nasal spray format, were added. This regiment "helped some," but the pain persisted. Over time, she became depressed, feeling helpless over her condition and predicament. At this time, she sought psychological help from the author.

During the initial assessment session, Mrs JMN detailed her medical history. While listening to her narrative, the author conveyed empathy and willingness to do anything to help her manage pain and suffering. The client appreciated these words very much. She indicated that the trigeminal pain was limited to the left side of her face from above the ear down to the chin. Ironically, this area was paralyzed and numb due to the surgery, except for the pain.

The overall intensity of the pain was moderate, ranging between 4 and 5 out of a maximum of 10. What was unnerving to her were sudden, paroxysmal "sharp shooting pains" typical of this condition. They would happen several times a day without warning. The residual pain would last up to 20 minutes. Although SPG blocks reduced the intensity and frequency of the attacks, she began ruminating about "future attacks." The preoccupation triggered a depressive outlook on the future and caused depressive affect.

Disappointed with the medical treatment for maxillofacial pain and distress, Mrs JMN expressed interest in the "mind-body" approach, especially hypnosis and mindfulness meditation. Subsequent sessions, therefore, focused on psychoeducation about hypnosis and mindfulness, the intricate relationship between self-talk and physiological response, plausible roles of attention in pain management, and the positive impact of social support and fun activities. The client was fascinated by the information while admitting that she all but "gave up" her social life because of her hectic schedule with medical appointments.

Despite her emotional distress, the client expressed interest in resuming gardening, particularly growing daffodils, for competition. It had been her long-time hobby, and she had won several awards. Mrs JMN regretted not being able to do it since the onset of her illness and wished to resume it. She also conveyed that listening to music and reading had always been enjoyable. The author noted this information and welcomed her interest in resuming fun activities.

Intervention

In the following session, Mrs JMN stated that she had enjoyed the initial session and was looking forward to pursuing the mind-body interventions. Mindfulness meditation was introduced as an attention- and awareness-based approach using the breath. The author explained the presumed neurophysiology of mindfulness meditation using a brain scan photo on the iPad. She then practiced Touch-and-Return with the author's guidance. It lasted no more than 10 minutes in total.

Mrs JMN found the mindfulness exercise relaxing. She acknowledged her mind wandering and had to remind herself to "return" to her breath. The "monkey mind" became most noticeable when she became aware of the numbness and pain on the left side of her face. When the author asked if she was willing to practice it at home, she answered affirmatively and decided to do it for five minutes daily.

When she returned the following week, Mrs JMN reported that she could not do Touch-and-Return at home. The partial paralysis of the face was "too uncomfortable" when shifting her attention to her breath. This "monkey mind" predominated in her mind. As a result, she would stay with immediate awareness. Her difficulty was accepted as valid, and it was decided that hypnotherapy was more appropriate than mindfulness.[6] It is the "utilization approach" advocated by Milton Erickson (Erickson, 1959).

According to Erickson, hypnotic induction and efficacy can be enhanced by "(utilizing) the patient's unique repertory of response potentials to achieve therapeutic goals that might have been otherwise beyond reach" (Erickson & Rossi, 1981, p. 5). In Mrs JMN's situation, it meant accepting her mind wandering ("monkey mind") associated with Touch-and-Return and encouraging instead hypnotic responses by using these spontaneously occurring images.

To accomplish this goal, she was encouraged to *focus on the images without returning to the breath* (i.e., modified Step 4). She had done this at home, and the protocol worked well. While observing and pacing her nonverbal responses, the author emphasized relaxation, selective attention, absorption, involuntariness, and detachment from reality, all typical hypnotic phenomena. Suggestions for physical and mental comfort were repeated intermittently. The session lasted about 25 minutes. Despite no direct suggestion for pain control, the intervention produced significant pain reduction. When she came out of her hypnosis, Mrs JMN exclaimed in a surprised tone, "There is no pain!" She could hardly believe the outcome. She was most eager to practice it at home and requested that future sessions be recorded for home practice. The author gladly agreed to it.

The modified version of Touch-and-Return was utilized in subsequent sessions. She would be mindful of external and internal stimuli (Step 2) and, instead of breath awareness (Step 3), would continue noticing the images for absorption to occur. Her hobbies and favorite activities, i.e., gardening, music listening, and reading, were incorporated to facilitate hypnosis induction. For example,

> *You enjoy gardening. You're good at it because you pay attention to details. You check the temperature, ground condition, and moisture in the soil to ensure everything is right. Daffodil bulbs find it easy to relax ... and the roots go deeper to ensure it is safe and secure.*

The reader will note the direct (e.g., "pay attention to details," "make sure everything is right") and indirect (e.g., "Daffodil bulbs find it easy to relax," "the roots go deeper to assure it is safe and secure") suggestions in this quote. Mrs JMN found these words comforting and allowed her to relax quickly.

For pain management, here is an example of the suggestions:

> *As you let your mind wander, it allows you to move away from the pain. Any discomfort, sharp, dull, quick, or long, will go away ... fade away ... and a sense of peace and comfort will fill your mind and body (pause) (intensity reduction). Continue immersing yourself in calming and cozy images. That makes you feel so comfortable that no pain will bother you (affect modulation). It is delightful to know you can do this.*

These suggestions were repeated during several sessions and were recorded every week. Mrs JMN listened to them at home for daily pain management.

Outcome

Hypnotherapy using the modified Touch-and-Return protocol proved to be beneficial for Mrs JMN. Although she kept experiencing mild chronic pain in the facial region, she "did not mind" it as before, allowing her to focus on fun activities, i.e., music appreciation and books on tape. During the COVID lockdown, she started growing daffodils again on the back porch of her house. It allowed her to go outside for 15–20 minutes daily. Although her social contact was limited due to COVID lockdowns, she maintained online communication with family and friends, lifting her mood gradually.

As for the paroxysmal sharp shooting pains, SPG blocks and hypnotherapy using Touch-and-Return helped to reduce the frequency and intensity, but her negative rumination continued. To ameliorate this problem, mindfulness-based thought-stopping was introduced (Otani, in press). She understood that the sharp pains triggered her preoccupation afterward. This tendency was explained to her as the "mental movie trailers" enticing her to watch the "lengthy feature horror film" depicting her endless misery. As such, she needed to avoid them by switching her attention away from them as soon as they occurred. This metaphor and intervention made good sense to her. After a few weeks of practice, she was able to circumvent rumination. It was not always easy, especially after intense pain, but the situation improved.

She continues therapy with the author after two and a half years. Mild chronic and sharp intermittent pains persist. Nevertheless, she acknowledges the positive impact of Touch-and-Return hypnosis on her, especially her improved quality of life. She also expresses calmness during and after the sessions. Alternatively, in the mindfulness framework, she has understood and accepted the concept, "Pain is inevitable; suffering is optional."

Conclusion

Hypnosis and mindfulness meditation are two accepted mind-body approaches in medicine and psychology. They share commonalities and complement each other despite the differences in history, theory, neural correlates, and technique. Healthcare providers familiar with hypnosis will find it relatively easy to integrate mindfulness into practice. In so doing, Touch-and-Return will be a practical, versatile method. It is based on traditional Buddhist meditation and allows application in mindfulness practice and hypnosis.

Contrary to general belief, mindfulness meditation accompanies absorption (i.e., trance) even though its quality and duration vary depending on the OM or FA practice. The clinician needs to be aware of this fact and be flexible in responding to the client to maximize its therapeutic potential.

As true with hypnosis training, the clinician should be familiar with mindfulness experientially. What does it feel like to practice mindfulness by Touch-and-Return? How does the experience resemble or differ from that of hypnosis? These questions cannot be answered merely through knowledge acquisition but through personal experience. Therefore, the clinician's intimate knowledge and familiarity with mindfulness meditation are essential.

Finally, mindfulness meditation enhances the practitioner's emotion regulation and executive functioning (Leyland et al., 2019). Combined with hypnosis, these qualities will heighten the healthcare provider's efficacy. Integrating hypnosis and mindfulness will thus contribute to the client's well-being and, ultimately, the progress of hypnosis and mindfulness as healing science and art.

Notes

1 The term "hypnosis" in this chapter refers only to formal, therapeutic hypnosis unless specified.
2 The Pali term *vedanā* is generally translated as "feeling," but its nuance is closer to "feeling tone," i.e., pleasant, unpleasant, or neutral, in English. See Batchelor (2019).
3 An influential Thai meditation master Ajahn Chah explains this point as follows. "Meditation is like a single stick of wood. Insight (vipassana) (i.e., OM) is one end of the stick and serenity (samatha) (i.e., FA) the other. If we pick it up, does only one end come up or do both? When anyone picks up a stick both ends rise together. Which part then is vipassana, and which is samatha? Where does one end and the other begin? They are both the mind. As the mind becomes peaceful, initially the peace will arise from the serenity of samatha. We focus and unify the mind in states of meditative peace (samadhi)" (Chah, 2011, p. 460).
4 The author thanks the client for granting permission to describe her case. All identifiable information has been altered to guarantee her anonymity.
5 One of the editors, Dr De Benedittis, pointed out that the client might likely suffer from post-surgical headaches based on her favorable response to SPG blocks and the mindfulness-based hypnotic intervention. Trigeminal neuralgia is impervious to these treatments.
6 The relative efficacy of hypnosis and mindfulness meditation on pain management has yet to be established. Based on the review of available literature, Jensen and his colleagues concluded that "[T]he efficacy of hypnosis treatment for reducing chronic pain is supported by fairly consistent evidence." As for the impact of mindfulness, while noting the paucity of literature, they stated, "[T]he limited available evidence regarding efficacy is promising" (Jensen, Day, & Miró, 2014, p. 175).

References

Alladin, A. (2014). Mindfulness-based hypnosis: Blending science, beliefs, and wisdoms to catalyze healing. *American Journal of Clinical Hypnosis*, *56*, 285–302.
Analayo, B. (2004). *Sattipatthana: The direct path to realization.* Windhorse Publications.
Baer, R., Crane, C., Montero-Marin, J., Phillips, A., Taylor, L., Tickell, A., & Kuyken, W. (2021). Frequency of self-reported unpleasant events and harm in a mindfulness-based program in two general population samples. *Mindfulness*, *12*, 763–774.
Batchelor, M. (2019). Mindfulness theory: Feeling tones (vedanās) as a useful framework for research. *Current Opinion in Psychology*, *28*, 20–22.

Bishop, S. R., Lau, M., Shapiro, S., Carlson, L., Anderson, N. D., Carmody, J., Segal, Z. V., Abbey, S., Speca, M., Velting, D., & Devins, G. (2004). Mindfulness: A proposed operational definition. *Clinical Psychology: Science and Practice*, *11*, 230–241. 10.1093/clipsy/bph077.

Bollinger, J. W. (2018). The rate of adverse events related to hypnosis during clinical trials. *American Journal of Clinical Hypnosis*, *60*, 357–366.

Brito, G. (2014). Rethinking mindfulness in the therapeutic relationship. *Mindfulness*, *5*, 351–359.

Britton, W. B., Lindahl, J. R., Cooper, D. J., Canby, N. K., & Palitsky, R. (2021). Defining and measuring meditation-related adverse effects in mindfulness-based programs. *Clinical Psychological Science*, *9*, 1185–1204. 10.1177/2167702621996340.

Brown, D. P. (2006). *Pointing out the great way: The stages of meditation in the Mahamudra tradition*. Simon and Schuster.

Buggy, P. (Undated). Don't believe everything you think (suffering is optional). *Mindful Ambition*. https://mindfulambition.net/suffering-is-optional/

Casale, A. D., Stefano, F., Rapinesi, C., Serata, D., Caltagirone, S. S., Savoja, V., Piacentino, D., Callovini, G., Manfredi, G., Sani, G., Kotzalidis, G. D., & Girardi, P. (2015). Pain perception and hypnosis: Findings from recent functional neuroimaging studies. *International Journal of Clinical and Experimental Hypnosis*, *63*, 144–170. DOI: 10.1080/00207144.2015.1002371

Castel, A., Pérez, M., Sala, J., Padrol, A., & Rull, M. (2007). Effect of hypnotic suggestion on fibromyalgic pain: Comparison between hypnosis and relaxation. *European Journal of Pain*, *11*, 463–468.

Chah, A. (2011). *Collected teachings of Ajahn Chah*. Amaravati Buddhist Monastery.

Cousins, L. S. (2022). *Meditations of the Pali tradition: Illuminating Buddhist doctrine, history, and practice*. Shambhala Publications.

De Benedittis, G. (2015). Neural mechanisms of hypnosis and meditation. *Journal of Physiology-Paris*, *109*, 152–164. DOI:.1016/j.jphysparis.2015.11.001

De Benedittis, G. (2021). Neural mechanisms of hypnosis and meditation-induced analgesia: A narrative review. *International Journal of Clinical and Experimental Hypnosis*, *69*, 363–382. DOI: 10.1080/00207144.2021.1917294.

Dreeben, S. J., Mamberg, M. H., & Salmon, P. (2013). The MBSR body scan in clinical practice. *Mindfulness*, *4*, 394–401. DOI: 10.1007/s12671-013-0212-z

Eberth, J., & Sedlmeier, P. (2012). The effects of mindfulness meditation: A meta-analysis. *Mindfulness*, *3*, 174–189.

Egner, T., Jamieson, G., & Gruzelier, J. (2005). Hypnosis decouples cognitive control from conflict monitoring processes of the frontal lobe. *Neuroimage*, *27*, 969–978.

Elkins, G. R. (2020). Contemplative practices and hypnosis: Emerging perspectives and future directions. *International Journal of Clinical and Experimental Hypnosis*, *68*, 139–143.

Elkins, G. R., Barabasz, A. F., Council, J. R., & Spiegel, D. (2015). Advancing research and practice: The revised APA Division 30 definition of hypnosis. *International Journal of Clinical and Experimental Hypnosis*, *63*, 1–9.

Erickson M. D. (1959). Further clinical techniques of hypnosis: Utilization techniques. *American Journal of Clinical Hypnosis*, *2*, 3–21. DOI: 10.1080/00029157.1959.10401792

Erickson, M. H. (1966). The interspersal hypnotic technique for symptom correction and pain control. *American Journal of Clinical Hypnosis*, *8*, 198–209. DOI: 10.1080/00029157.1966.10402492

Erickson, M. H., & Rossi, E. L. (1981). *Experiencing hypnosis: Therapeutic approaches to altered states*. Irvington.

Gimian, C. R. (2016, August 24). What is monkey mind? Lion's roar. https://www.lionsroar.com/monkey-mind/

Goyal, M., Singh, S., Sibinga, E. M., Gould, N. F., Rowland-Seymour, A., Sharma, R., Berger, Z., Sleicher, D., Maron, D. D., Shihab, H. M., & Ranasinghe, P. D. (2014). Meditation programs for psychological stress and well-being: A systematic review and meta-analysis. *JAMA Internal Medicine*, *174*, 357–368.

Greason, P. B., & Welfare, L. E. (2013). The impact of mindfulness and meditation practice on client perceptions of common therapeutic factors. *Journal of Humanistic Counseling*, *52*, 235–253.

Guidotti, R., Del Gratta, C., Perrucci, M. G., Romani, G. L., & Raffone, A. (2021). Neuroplasticity within and between functional brain networks is based on long-term meditation in mental training. *Brain Sciences*, *11*, 1086–1192.

Hayes, S. C. (2016). *The ACT in context.* Routledge.
Heide, F. J., & Borkovec, T. D. (1983). Relaxation-induced anxiety: Paradoxical anxiety enhancement due to relaxation training. *Journal of Consulting and Clinical Psychology*, *51*, 171–182.
Hilton, L., Hempel, S., Ewing, B. A., Apaydin, E., Xenakis, L., Newberry, S., ... & Maglione, M. A. (2017). Mindfulness meditation for chronic pain: Systematic review and meta-analysis. *Annals of Behavioral Medicine*, *51*, 199–213.
Hofbauer, R. K., Rainville, P., Duncan, G. H., & Bushnell, M. C. (2001). Cortical representation of the sensory dimension of pain. *Journal of Neurophysiology*, *86*, 402–411.
Holroyd, J. (2003). The science of meditation and the state of hypnosis. *American Journal of Clinical Hypnosis*, *46*, 109–128.
Jensen, M. P., Day, M. A., & Miró, J. (2014). Neuromodulatory treatments for chronic pain: Efficacy and mechanisms. *Nature Reviews Neurology*, *10*, 167–178.
Kabat-Zinn, J. (1982). An outpatient program in behavioral medicine for chronic pain patients based on the practice of mindfulness meditation: Theoretical considerations and preliminary results. *General Hospital Psychiatry*, *4*, 33–47.
Kabat-Zinn, J. (1995). *Full catastrophe living: Using the wisdom of your body and mind to face stress, pain, and illness.* Bantam Dell.
Kabat-Zinn, J. (2003). Mindfulness-based stress reduction (MBSR). *Constructivism in the Human Sciences*, *8*, 73–107.
Kane, R. "How Many People Meditate In The World?" M_mindfulnessbox, April 22, 2022, https://mindfulnessbox.com/how-many-people-meditate-in-the-world/. (Accessed June 4, 2022).
Kasos, E., Kasos, K., Józsa, E., Varga, K., Bányai, E., Költő, A., & Szabó, A. (2022) Altered states of consciousness during exercise, active-alert hypnosis, and everyday waking state. *International Journal of Clinical and Experimental Hypnosis*, *70*, 300–313, DOI: 10.1080/00207144.2022.2093644
Kaufmann, M., Rosing, K., & Baumann, N. (2021). Being mindful does not always benefit everyone: Mindfulness-based practices may promote alienation among psychologically vulnerable people. *Cognition and Emotion*, *35*, 241–255.
Kirsch, I. (2001). The response set theory of hypnosis: Expectancy and physiology. *American Journal of Clinical Hypnosis*, *44*, 69–73.
Krishnamurti, J. (2000). *Choiceless awareness: A selection of passages for the study of the teachings of J. Krishnamurti.* Krishnamurti Foundation of America.
LaRosa, J. (2019, October 16). "$1.2 Billion U.S. Meditation Market Growing Strongly as It Becomes More Mainstream." Market Research Blog, October 16, 2019, https://blog.marketresearch.com/1.2-billion-u.s.-meditation-market-growing-strongly-as-it-becomes-more-mainstream. (Accessed June 3, 2022).
Leyland, A., Rowse, G., & Emerson, L. M. (2019). Experimental effects of mindfulness inductions on self-regulation: Systematic review and meta-analysis. *Emotion*, *19*, 108–125.
Lifshitz, M., & Raz, A. (2012). Hypnosis and meditation: Vehicles of attention and suggestion. *The Journal of Mind-Body Regulation*, *2*, 3–11.
Lindahl, J. R., Fisher, N. E., Cooper, D. J., Rosen, R. K., & Britton, W. B. (2017). The varieties of contemplative experience: A mixed-methods study of meditation-related challenges in Western Buddhists. *PLoS One*, *12*, e0176239.
Linehan, M. M. (2020). *Dialectical behavior therapy in clinical practice*. Guilford Publications.
Lynn, S., Malaktaris, A., Maxwell, R., Mellinger, D. I., & van der Kloet, D. (2012). Do hypnosis and mindfulness practices inhabit a common domain? Implications for research, clinical practice, and forensic science. *Journal of Mind-Body Regulation*, *2*, 12–26.
Lynn, S. J., Martin, D. J., & Frauman, D. C. (1996) Does hypnosis pose special risks for negative effects? A master class commentary, *International Journal of Clinical and Experimental Hypnosis*, *44*, 7-19. DOI: 10.1080/00207149608416064
Lynn, S. J., Surya Das, L., Hallquist, M. N., & Williams, J. C. (2006). Mindfulness, acceptance, and hypnosis: Cognitive and clinical perspectives. *International Journal of Clinical and Experimental Hypnosis*, *54*, 143–166.
Lynn, S. J., Green, J. P., Kirsch, I., Capafons, A., Lilienfeld, S. O., Laurence, J. R., & Montgomery, G. H. (2015). Grounding hypnosis in science: The "New" APA division 30 definition of hypnosis as a step backward. *American Journal of Clinical Hypnosis*, *57*, 390–401.

McGeown, W. J., Mazzoni, G., Venneri, A., & Kirsch, I. (2009). Hypnotic induction decreases anterior default mode activity. *Consciousness and Cognition*, *18*, 848–855.
Otani, A. (2023). Using Buddhist meditation-informed hypnotic techniques to manage rumination: Two case illustrations. *International Journal of Clinical and Experimental Hypnosis*, *71*, 48–62.
Otani, A. (2003). Eastern meditative techniques and hypnosis: A new synthesis. *American Journal of Clinical Hypnosis*, *46*, 97–108. DOI: 10.1080/00029157.2003.1040358.
Otani, A. (2016). Hypnosis and mindfulness: The Twain finally meet. *American Journal of Clinical Hypnosis*, *58*, 383–398. DOI: 10.1080/00029157.2015.1085364.
Otani, A. (2020). The mindfulness-based phase-oriented trauma therapy (MB-POTT): Hypnosis-informed mindfulness approach to trauma. *American Journal of Clinical Hypnosis*, *63*, 95–111. DOI: 10.1080/00029157.2020.1765726.
Parker, S. C., Nelson, B. W., Epel, E. S., & Siegel, D. J. (2015). The science of presence: No-self, self, and mindfulness in Buddhist thought and Western psychologies. In K. W. Brown, J. D. Creswell, & R. M. Ryan (Eds.) (2015). *Handbook of mindfulness: Theory, research, and practice* (pp. 225–244). Guilford.
Pekala, R. J., & Creegan, K. (2020). States of consciousness, the qEEG, and noetic snapshots of the brain/mind interface: A case study of hypnosis and sidhi meditation. *OBM Integrative and Complementary Medicine*, *5*, 1–35. DOI:10.21926/obm.icm.2002019.
Pekala, R. J., Kumar, V. K., Maurer, R., Elliott-Carter, N., Moon, E., & Mullen, K. (2010). Suggestibility, expectancy, trance state effects, and hypnotic depth: I. Implications for understanding hypnotism. *American Journal of Clinical Hypnosis*, *52*, 275–290.
Penazzi, G., & De Pisapia, N. (2022). Direct comparisons between hypnosis and meditation: A mini-review. *Frontiers in Psychology*, *13*, 958185. DOI: 10.3389/fpsyg.2022.958185.
Rainville, P., Duncan, G. H., Price, D. D., Carrier, B., & Bushnell, M. C. (1997). Pain affect encoded in human anterior cingulate but not somatosensory cortex. *Science*, *277*(5328), 968–971. DOI: 10.1126/science.277.5328.968.
Rainville, P., Carrier, B., Hofbauer, R. K., Bushnell, M. C., & Duncan, G. H. (1999). Dissociation of sensory and affective dimensions of pain using hypnotic modulation. *Pain*, *82*, 159–171.
Raz, A., & Lifshitz, M. (Eds.). (2016). *Hypnosis and meditation: Towards an integrative science of conscious planes*. Oxford University Press.
Razzaque, R., Okoro, E., & Wood, L. (2015). Mindfulness in clinician therapeutic relationships. *Mindfulness*, *6*, 170–174.
Ren, Z., Zhang, Y., & Jiang, G. (2018). Effectiveness of mindfulness meditation in intervention for anxiety: A meta-analysis. *Acta Psychologica Sinica*, *50*, 283–304.
Rhodes, J., Elkins, G., & Alldredge, C. (2022). Definition of hypnosis and hypnotherapy. In G. Elkins (Ed.), *Introduction to clinical hypnosis: The basics and beyond* (pp. 50–63). Waco, TX: Mountain Pine Publishing.
Rogers, C. R. (1957). The necessary and sufficient conditions of therapeutic personality change. *Journal of Consulting Psychology*, *21*, 95–103. 10.1037/h0045357.
Schaefert, R., Klose, P., Moser, G., & Häuser, W. (2014). Efficacy, tolerability, and safety of hypnosis in adult irritable bowel syndrome: Systematic review and meta-analysis. *Psychosomatic Medicine*, *76*, 389–398.
Schultz, J. H., & Luthe, W. (1959). *Autogenic training: A psychophysiologic approach to psychotherapy*. Grune & Stratton.
Sebastiani, L., D'Alessandro, L., Menicucci, D., Ghelarducci, B., & Santarcangelo, E. L. (2007). Role of relaxation and specific suggestions in hypnotic emotional numbing. *International Journal of Psychophysiology*, *63*, 125–132.
Semmens-Wheeler, R., & Dienes, Z. (2012). The contrasting role of higher-order awareness in hypnosis and meditation. *The Journal of Mind-Body Regulation*, 2, 43–57.
Shor, R. E. (1959). Hypnosis and the concept of the generalized reality-orientation. *American Journal of Psychotherapy*, *13*, 582.
Shor, R. E. (1962). Three dimensions of hypnotic depth. *International Journal of Clinical and Experimental Hypnosis*, *10*, 23–38.
Slonena, E. E., & Elkins, G. R. (2021). Effects of a brief mindful hypnosis intervention on stress reactivity: A randomized active control study. *International Journal of Clinical and Experimental Hypnosis*, *69*, 453–467.

Sparby, T. (2019). Phenomenology and contemplative universals: The meditative experience of dhyana, coalescence, or access concentration. *Journal of Consciousness Studies*, *26*, 130–156.

Spiegel, D. A. (1991). Neurophysiological correlates of hypnosis and dissociation. *Journal of Neuropsychiatry and Clinical Neurosciences*, *3*, 440–445.

Spiegel, E. B., Baker, E. L., Daitch, C., Diamond, M. J., & Phillips, M. (2019). Hypnosis and the therapeutic relationship: Relational factors of hypnosis in psychotherapy. *American Journal of Clinical Hypnosis*, *62*, 118–137. 10.1080/00029157.1966.10402492

Spiegel, H., & Spiegel, D. (2008). *Trance and treatment: Clinical uses of hypnosis*. American Psychiatric Pub.

Spina, V., Chisari, C., & Santarcangelo, E. L. (2020). High motor cortex excitability in highly hypnotizable individuals: A favorable factor for neuroplasticity? *Neuroscience*, *430*, 125–130.

Tang, Y. Y., Hölzel, B. K., & Posner, M. I. (2015). The neuroscience of mindfulness meditation. *Nature Reviews Neuroscience*, *16*, 213–225.

Taylor, G. B., Vasquez, T. S., Kastrinos, A., Fisher, C. L., Puig, A., & Bylund, C. L. (2022). The adverse effects of meditation-interventions and mind–body practices: A systematic review. *Mindfulness*, *13*, 1–18.

Thompson, T., Terhune, D. B., Oram, C., Sharangparni, J., Rouf, R., Solmi, M., Veronese, N., & Stubbs, B. (2019). The effectiveness of hypnosis for pain relief: A systematic review and meta-analysis of 85 controlled experimental trials. *Neuroscience & Biobehavioral Reviews*, *99*, 298–310.

U.S. Department of Health and Human Services (2018). Use of yoga, meditation, and chiropractors among U.S. adults aged 18 and over. [Online]. Available from: https://www.cdc.gov/nchs/data/databriefs/db325-h.pdf. (Accessed May 29. 2022).

Valentine, K. E., Milling, L. S., Clark, L. J., & Moriarty, C. L. (2019). The efficacy of hypnosis as a treatment for anxiety: A meta-analysis. *International Journal of Clinical and Experimental Hypnosis*, *67*, 336–363.

Vancappel, A., Guerin, L., Réveillère, C., & El-Hage, W. (2021). Disentangling the link between mindfulness and dissociation: The mediating role of attention and emotional acceptance. *European Journal of Trauma & Dissociation*, *5*, 100220. 10.1016/j.ejtd.2021.100220.

Wickramasekera, I. E. (2020). Hypnotic-like aspects of the Tibetan tradition of Dzogchen meditation. *International Journal of Clinical and Experimental Hypnosis*, *68*, 200–213.

Woody, E., & Sadler, P. (2022). Interpersonal aspects of hypnosis: Twisted pears and other forbidden fruit. *Psychology of Consciousness: Theory, Research, and Practice*, *9*, 172–186.

Yapko, M. D. (2011). *Mindfulness and hypnosis: The power of suggestion to transform experience*. W. W. Norton & Company.

57

ADVANCING EDUCATION IN CLINICAL HYPNOSIS

Donald Moss, Eric Willmarth, and David B. Reid

College of Integrative Medicine and Health Sciences, Saybrook University, Pasadena, CA, USA

Introduction

Clinical hypnosis is widely applied as an individualized, experiential, spontaneous therapeutic treatment intervention, eliciting a focused, yet receptive experience for a patient in the present moment (B. A. Erickson, 2017; Williamson, 2019; Yapko, 2012, 2021; Zeig, 2014). Ideally, hypnotic therapeutic experiences facilitate and enhance coping skills including flexibility in the management of behavior, cognition, and emotion. Seasoned trainers often encourage clinicians to utilize the patient's history, including seizing upon their words, personal stories, interests, and life experiences as pathways to promote a more flexible and adaptive way of living. Yet formal training in clinical hypnosis often over-emphasizes historical information, schools of theorizing about hypnosis, hypnosis research findings, and wordy definitions of hypnosis over clinical skills development.

The history of hypnosis can inform our understanding of hypnosis techniques and practice today. When practitioners are well-informed about recent research, neural correlates of hypnotic treatment, and evidence-based treatment protocols, they more readily accept the integration of hypnosis into their practice. Teaching and training in hypnosis occur within this tension between conveying relevant information about hypnosis and immersing the trainee in hypnotic experiences. This chapter addresses hypnosis education and training and pursues a balance between recognizing a necessary core fund of knowledge and exposing the student to the living process of hypnotic experiencing.

By *hypnosis,* we refer here to a process of eliciting:

> A state of consciousness involving focused attention and reduced peripheral awareness, characterized by an enhanced capacity for response to suggestion.
>
> *(Elkins et al., 2015)*

This is the definition of hypnosis promulgated in 2014 by Division 30 of the American Psychological Association. Similarly, Milton Erickson provided a simple and practical definition of hypnosis in 1967 that is worth citing here:

DOI: 10.4324/9781003449126-75

> Hypnosis is essentially a communication of ideas and understandings to a patient in such a fashion that he will be most receptive to the presented ideas and thereby motivated to explore his own body potentials for the control of his psychological and physiological responses and behavior.
>
> *(Erickson, 1967, p. 83)*

The clinical process of eliciting this enhanced responsiveness creates the conditions for enhanced effectiveness of many forms of psychological and medical interventions.

Contributions of Leaders to Clinical Hypnosis Education and Training

Historically, it was Anton Mesmer who first recognized the need to educate others in his techniques of Animal Magnetism. In 1785, he established the Societies of Universal Harmony, first in Paris and then "component sections" throughout France. Each Society was limited to 50 members who were at least 25 years old, of "good morals," and who had "purity of view" (Tinterow, 1970, p. 80). Mesmer included in the Constitution of the Societies that he would hold the title of "Perpetual President," but by teaching others to teach, he set up a model that continues to be used to this day.

Worldwide, professional organizations and leaders in hypnosis research and practice have advanced and promoted clinical hypnosis training and education through establishing standards and publishing guidelines in peer-reviewed journals and textbooks.

In 1992, the American Society of Clinical Hypnosis (ASCH) established a Standards of Training and Certification Task Force, and in 1993 launched the ASCH Certification program, based on the Task Force's recommendations. In 1994, D. Corydon Hammond and Gary Elkins (1994) published the *Standards of Training in Clinical Hypnosis*, which provided detailed outlines and guidance for curriculum in both basic and intermediate hypnosis workshops, including time dedicated to each topic, in addition to requirements for obtaining ASCH Certification in Clinical Hypnosis and becoming an ASCH Approved Consultant in Clinical Hypnosis (Hammond & Elkins, 1994).

The proposed *Standards* are described in the introduction as flexible guidelines and not rigid curricula. However, the required content was so extensive that many introductory and intermediate workshops seemed somewhat shackled to the recitation of a great deal of information "about" hypnosis (i.e., history, definitions, theories, and common myths). The *Standards* also proposed extensive group practice, monitored by ASCH faculty, for eliciting and deepening hypnosis experiences, ensuring that all attendees would have opportunities to experience and facilitate the hypnosis process.

In 2005, ASCH revised the 1994 *Standards* and included updated resources and references in the Recommended Reading List (Hammond & Elkins, 2005). The introduction of this revised publication again reinforced that the Standards are intended to be flexible guidelines and not rigid curricula. The learning objectives for both basic and intermediate hypnosis workshops were essentially unchanged from the initial publication.

In 2019, ASCH released extensively updated *Standards of Training* for both basic and intermediate clinical hypnosis workshops (American Society of Clinical Hypnosis Education and Research Foundation, 2019). The updated *Standards* introduced new terminology, for example, shifting from a consideration of hypnotic "induction" to "elicitation" or "facilitation," from "deepening" to "intensification," and from "re-alerting" to "reorientation." The rationale for this modified terminology was primarily justified since older nomenclature lacked clarity and had accumulated "problematic associations." For instance, "induction" was recognized as a term that inaccurately reinforces the notion that clients are under the control of a clinician who "induces" a hypnotic experience (Reid, 2019). In addition, the updated *Standards* emphasize the *process* of hypnosis and minimized didactics on the knowledge of clinical hypnosis. The updated *Standards* also provided pragmatic guidance for introducing students to rapport and the hypnotic experience through small group practice.

In 2017, Laurence Sugarman served as guest editor for a special issue of the *American Journal of Clinical Hypnosis* (AJCH) dedicated to "Exploring, Evolving, and Refining Hypnosis Education." In his editorial for the special issue, Sugarman pointed out that only 3% (N = 14) of the papers published in the *International Journal of Clinical and Experimental Hypnosis* and the *American Journal of Clinical Hypnosis* between 1955 and 2002 addressed hypnosis education. He called for greater attention in the future to principles of education and training for clinical hypnosis (Sugarman, 2017, p. 231). A summary of the articles in that special issue serves to frame contemporary opinions and recommendations regarding training in clinical hypnosis.

Alter and Sugarman (2017) called for a reorienting in hypnosis education, a movement away from linear, diagnosis-based, and reductionist models to a more responsive, naturalistic, and disruptive approach. They proposed a skill set for training that emphasized systemic perturbation and reorientation, incorporating novelty and uncertainty in the training. A case narrative offered insight and guidance that supported their broad proposals. Alter and Sugarman argued that human beings possess adaptive resources and suggested that exposure to novel experiences – individualized to this person – provokes disorientation and an adaptive response.

Linden and Anbar (2017) suggested that training should shift its focus from "what to teach" and "who to teach" to a new focus on "how to teach." Their work drew on deliberations within a newer Task Force on Standards of Training in Clinical Hypnosis aimed at updating training and workshop curricula and approaches at that time (Linden et al., 2011). They also drew on pedagogical and andragogical principles for adult learning, including an emphasis on various teaching styles and learning styles. Linden and Anbar provided a detailed discussion of the process in ASCH training and advocated for an increased reliance on small group practice for learning skills as well as individualized consultation.

One issue that has served as the source of ongoing contention and contemplation over the years in the clinical hypnosis community involves the utilization and encouragement of scripts during training workshops. In response to this subject matter, Lankton (2017) highlighted the importance of recognizing and utilizing the individualized nature of the human person and human responsiveness during hypnosis. According to Lankton, prescribed scripts are useful for cooking meatloaf or assembling Ikea furniture but are not appropriate for clinical hypnosis. Dostoevsky (1994) would cheer Lankton's point, since he observed that the human being is not as predictable as a piano key. Lankton emphasized the importance of non-scripted interventions for both treatment of the client and the learning/training of the therapist. Lankton also opined that each hypnotic intervention should anticipate and contribute to the outcome of overall psychotherapy goals. The hypnotic process should, therefore, involve an interactive dialog, assisting the "next-step goals" of the therapy, and formulate suggestions and statements that support the next steps. Accordingly, training to support these non-linear processes should include approaches that assess the client's needs and resources and comprehension of the psychotherapeutic process supported by hypnotic suggestions.

Lindheim and Helgeland (2017) reported on their observations and data gathered from a hypnosis training program conducted annually in Norway since 2008. The training is framed with a biopsychosocial model and follows the guideline of Hammond (1996) that, "Almost as important as course content is the art of teaching and presenting ideas in a manner that is also hypnotic in that it both captivates our students and imparts practical skills that may be replicated outside the classroom" (p. 21). The authors emphasized that both understanding hypnosis as a concept and developing hypnotic skills require a personal experience of hypnosis. For this reason, they reinforced the value of hypnosis demonstrations and practical training.

Kohen et al. (2017) proposed a remodeling of curriculum and a refining of faculty development for training in pediatric hypnosis practice. The authors drew on their experience in pediatric hypnosis training through the National Pediatric Hypnosis Training Institute (NPHTI). NPHTI training emphasizes core social and adult learning principles, an experiential learning approach, as well as therapeutic principles borrowed from Milton Erickson (1958) and Michael Yapko (2012, 2016). NPHTI also includes group discussion and large group exercises to facilitate active processing and personal reflections about the participants' experiences in training (Kohen et al., 2017, p. 294). Video recordings of clinical hypnosis sessions also support the NPHTI teaching process.

Baker (2017) provides an integrative commentary on the five contributions to the AJCH special issue. Baker begins with an epigram attributed to Antoine de Saint-Exupery:

> If you want to build a ship, don't gather people to collect wood and don't assign tasks and work but rather teach them to yearn for the vastness of the sea.
>
> *(Saint-Exupery,* Citadelle, *1948)*

Baker lauded the congruence of many themes put forward in the special issue, including the emphasis on adaptability, creativity, uniqueness, and individualization in clinical hypnosis and in hypnosis training. He highlighted the relationship between how we conceptualize hypnosis, how we integrate it into practice, and how this shapes the educational model.

In summary, a number of leading figures in clinical hypnosis have advocated for a process of re-thinking approaches to hypnosis training and education. The emphasis has been on including the individualized, spontaneous, and non-linear process of hypnosis treatment into the training process. Specific recommendations include teaching that utilizes hypnotic principles and qualities of clinical hypnotic dialog, the importance of the ongoing context of clinical therapeutic work that is supported by hypnosis interventions, and inclusion of generous amounts of hypnosis demonstrations and guided practice in small groups.

Essential Competencies for Clinical Hypnosis

Clinicians and students seeking training in clinical hypnosis can benefit from learning a number of specific skills and competencies, reinforced by directly experiencing the hypnotic process. Essential competencies for clinical hypnosis can be identified as follows:

1 Establishing empathy and rapport.
2 Assessing the presenting problem, and screening for potentially serious medical or mental health problems that may require additional evaluation and treatment.
3 Exploring the patient's misconceptions and fears of hypnosis.

4 Discussing realistic expectations about the hypnotic treatment process and inviting openness to hypnosis.
5 Eliciting a hypnotic experience (hypnotic induction) and learning a variety of techniques to accomplish this.
6 Assisting patients to intensify the hypnotic experience (deepening, intensifying) and to re-alert.
7 Practicing utilization – that is perceiving elements in the patient's narrative that may serve as doors for further hypnotic experiencing.
8 Facilitating hypnotically assisted relaxation.
9 Explaining the continuum of hypnotic ability and identifying reliable tools for assessing hypnotic ability.
10 Mastering additional specific strategies for facilitating therapeutic work during hypnosis.
11 Introducing the concept of ego strengthening and practical strategies for accomplishing ego strengthening.
12 Introducing self-hypnosis strategies, techniques for guiding oneself to enter hypnosis, intensifying the experience, and using self-hypnosis for health and well-being.

Each of these 12 competencies will now be discussed in more detail.

Establishing Empathy and Rapport

Research on the "so-called" common factors in psychotherapy consistently demonstrates that regardless of the therapeutic technique or orientation, patients benefit more fully when they feel understood and supported by the therapist, when they believe the therapist is "present with them" (Moudatsou et al., 2020; Norcross & Lambert, 2018a, 2018b; Rogers, 1992; Spiegel & Baker, 2019). Empirical research consistently reveals that therapeutic response and patient satisfaction in both medical and mental health care are enhanced when patients perceive their medical practitioner as empathic. Riess (2010) concluded that "Evidence supports the physiological benefits of empathic relationships, including better immune function, shorter post-surgery hospital stays, fewer asthma attacks, stronger placebo response, and shorter duration of colds" (p. 1605).

One approach to addressing this need for empathy and rapport is the integration of ongoing mentoring into hypnosis training. The one-on-one relationship between the experienced mentor and the novice can mirror and teach the desired empathy and rapport of the therapeutic alliance.

Assessing the Presenting Problem

It is critical that the hypnotic practitioner engage in a thorough assessment process whenever a treatment process begins. Assessment is ever present, even in the brief and time urgent hypnotic interventions in many medical settings. A referral may be relatively clear on identifying an objective problem requiring intervention, yet the patient's own narrative frequently reveals much more than a diagnostic label or pain syndrome. Even a brief psychosocial/medical history may reveal significant life issues that frequently accompany or trigger both medical and mental health problems. One patient, referred for a major depressive episode upon his spouse's military deployment, commented that "every time I love someone, they leave me." A lifetime of separation and loss were re-experienced in this involuntary separation and occupied a central place in the therapeutic process.

Occasionally, an evaluation will reveal a sudden onset or abrupt change in physical symptoms in the absence of a systematic and comprehensive medical evaluation. Such circumstances warrant a referral for further medical evaluation. The present authors have identified patients with sudden onset of chest pain or limb pain where heart disease or undiagnosed cancer required immediate treatment. Absent careful evaluation, hypnosis may mask symptoms of a serious medical condition, particularly those associated with pain.

Exploring the Patient's Misconceptions of Hypnosis

Some patients express unfounded fears and maintain misconceptions about hypnosis. Unfortunately, the motion picture industry and social media continue to portray hypnosis as omnipotent and deceptive mind control. These are challenging treatment obstacles that should be addressed and mitigated. Discussion of the fears and misconceptions, and reassurance about the hypnotic process can be helpful in enhancing the patient's comfort with hypnosis.

Common fears about hypnosis include the loss of voluntary control, domination by the hypnotic practitioner, becoming stuck in a trance, and being belittled or made fun of (see Myerson, 2017; Yapko, 2012, pp. 21–45). In an effort to dispel common misconceptions associated with a loss of control during hypnosis, patients are often reassured that they can stop a hypnosis session at any time, "simply by opening your eyes" (Myerson, 2017, p. 31) and that the therapeutic goals for hypnotic sessions will be formulated by the patient.

Discussing Realistic Expectations about the Hypnotic Treatment Process

Positive expectancy about hypnosis is an important predictor of treatment outcome in hypnotherapy (Kirsch, 2018). Exploring the patient's current expectations about the likely outcome of hypnosis-based therapy can identify and confront any negative expectations and encourage more positive expectations. Occasionally, patients report unrealistically positive expectations. For example, some imagine that hypnosis will eliminate their craving for cigarettes without any need for further behavioral work or behavioral change on their part. Unrealistic expectations must be identified and addressed.

Patient education about hypnosis begins during the first session and continues throughout the therapeutic process. This includes addressing the fears and misconceptions cited above and providing information about the likely benefits for hypnosis-based therapy. For some patients, this means reviewing published research on positive outcomes using hypnosis for treating their disorder; for others, an anecdote about a recent patient with similar complaints who experienced relief through hypnosis will be more meaningful.

Eliciting a Hypnotic Experience (Hypnotic Induction)

One of the basic skills of hypnosis training involves introducing skills and strategies for inducing or eliciting a hypnotic experience. Students should master a variety of skills and approaches that elicit hypnotic experiences. Typical skills for training include the use of eye fixation, eye roll, images of descending a staircase, counting down, muscle relaxation, slow gentle breathing, arm heaviness and arm levitation exercises, and visualization of a comfortable, calm, and when appropriate, safe place.

Training should be structured to provide frequent and extended practice of elicitation skills, and trainees should be encouraged to introduce hypnotic elicitation as often as possible in clinical work, both for their patients' benefit and their own development and confidence in expanding hypnosis skills. Trainees should consider that an early experience of entering hypnosis, even a simple hypnotically assisted relaxation exercise, can dispel or minimize the patient's fears about hypnosis.

Assisting Patients to Intensify the Hypnotic Experience (Deepening, Intensifying), and to Re-Alert at the Close of the Session

Once the patient has entered a hypnotic state, the same strategies that elicit trance can also be used to intensify trance. Suggestions of calm soothing places, descending staircases, counting down, and somatic strategies such as muscle relaxation or paced breathing can facilitate greater intensity in the hypnotic experience.

Of equal importance, training should emphasize the importance of re-alerting the patient at the close of the hypnotic session. Patients may retain a somewhat disoriented or dissociative quality after intense hypnotic work. The trainee should learn specific strategies for assuring that the client is fully alert and oriented before leaving the session, in order to drive, navigate public transportation, and function effectively in everyday life (Howard, 2017).

Practicing Utilization

The principle of *utilization* is attributed to Milton Erickson, who often seized creatively on some image or expression from the patient that was strategically woven into the therapeutic process. Zeig (2014) promoted utilization as a foundational principle in hypnotic work. He observed that hypnotic influence on patients is greatest when founded on their own spontaneous images and experiences. In turn, Rossi took utilization further. He emphasized guiding patients and the patients' "inner minds" to utilize their own resources – their imagery, language, life experiences, and abilities – to resolve problems (Rossi, 1986, pp. 72–78).

Hypnotic training can introduce the concept and process of utilization for students and demonstrate the importance of listening to the patient's dialog and highlighting potential entry points for therapeutic utilization. Training should also include small group practice sessions dedicated to practicing utilization principles. Reviewing video recordings of therapeutic sessions illustrating both successful utilization and missed opportunities for utilization can also be helpful.

Facilitating Hypnotically Assisted Relaxation

One of the widest applications of hypnotic interventions is hypnotically assisted relaxation training (Elkins, 2014, 2017). Many patients show significant symptom reduction with relaxation, without sophisticated therapeutic work to resolve emotional issues. Research has documented the link between the human stress response and many medical and psychological symptoms (McEwen, 2017; Yaribeygi et al., 2017). Many relaxation-oriented therapies reduce the physiological and psychological effects of stress and produce reduction in clinical symptoms, including anxiety (Manzoni et al., 2008).

Elkins (2017) recommends introducing a relaxation-based hypnotic elicitation first and carrying out additional relaxation techniques and relaxation-oriented suggestions, when the patient is in a hypnotic state, for a deeper effect. Classical relaxation techniques can be implemented while the patient is in a hypnotic state. This includes progressive muscle relaxation (Jacobson, 1938), autogenic training (Linden, 2007; Schultz & Luthe, 1959), paced diaphragmatic breathing (Fried & Grimaldi, 1993), mindful acceptance (Kabat-Zinn, 2005), and imagery of a calm scene (Rossman, 2000). Lehrer and Woolfolk (2021) provide useful introductions and scripts for a variety of relaxation techniques.

Explaining the Continuum of Hypnotic Ability and Identifying Reliable Tools for Assessing Hypnotic Ability

Hypnotic susceptibility, suggestibility, and hypnotic ability are terms describing individual differences in human beings' level of responding to hypnotic suggestions. Hilgard described hypnotic ability as "an ability in which men differ, just as they differ in intelligence or athletic ability" (Hilgard,1965, p. 65). Hilgard showed that, like intelligence, hypnotic ability is normally distributed in the general population. Later, Piccione et al. (1989) showed that hypnotic ability is a relatively stable trait over a 25-year period, and Morgan (1973) documented the heritability of hypnosis through a twin study. In spite of the evidence that there are measurable differences in hypnotic responsiveness in the general population, few practitioners responding to a recent global survey rated hypnotizability as an important factor in producing effective treatment (Palsson et al., 2023). Furthermore, measures of hypnotizability are used primarily in empirical studies evaluating the efficacy of hypnosis.

Hypnosis training should acquaint students with common hypnotic experiences and variations in hypnotic ability, and introduce several measures of hypnotic susceptibility, including the Harvard Group Scale of Hypnotic Susceptibility (Shor and Orne, 1962), the Stanford Scale of Hypnotic Susceptibility (Weitzenhoffer & Hilgard, 1959, 1962), the Elkins Hypnotizability Scale (Elkins, 2014), and the Hypnotic Induction Profile (Spiegel, 1978). Students will also benefit from learning the signs of hypnotic engagement such as time distortion and a sense of involuntariness. Recognizing signs of depth provides clinical indications of the patient's state in the absence of formal assessment.

Mastering Additional Specific Strategies for Facilitating Therapeutic Work during Hypnosis

Once engaged in a hypnotic state, patients show a rich responsiveness to a variety of hypnotic interventions. Therapeutic work in hypnosis sessions can include desensitizing cues that previously triggered anxiety attacks or traumatic experiencing. Patients may revisit painful past experiences through age regression; the patients re-experience past trauma strengthened by hypnotic skills – experiencing the painful situation at a distance, through a window, on a video replay, and so on.

Hypnosis can be integrated with a variety of psychotherapeutic approaches, including cognitive behavioral therapy, acceptance and commitment therapy, dynamic psychotherapy, and ego state therapy. Similarly, hypnosis lends itself to integration in a variety of medical and dental settings, from facilitating wound closure to manage procedural pain (Chester et al., 2018; Jensen, 2019). The specific form of therapeutic work during hypnotic sessions will be shaped by the therapist's overall psychotherapeutic or clinical medical approach. Training can introduce a handful of examples of therapeutic work such as hypnosis in systematic desensitization, trauma resolution, cardiac rehabilitation, and habit control (e.g., smoking cessation, weight management).

Introducing the Concept of Ego Strengthening and Practical Strategies for Accomplishing Ego Strengthening

Ego strengthening began as a specific strategy for hypnotic interventions (Hartland, 1965, 1971; Stanton, 1979, 1989) and evolved into an attitude pervading psychotherapy and clinical hypnotic work (McNeal & Frederick, 1993; McNeal, 2020; Moss & Willmarth, 2017). Hartland introduced a specific and directive script with an emphasis on personal strengthening, clarity of thinking, relaxation, independence, and happiness, and documented that patients with moderate disorders showed significant improvement with this script and in some cases did not require more extensive therapy. The patients showed improvement in their overall coping and drew more effectively on internal resources. McNeal and Frederick introduced a variety of imagery strategies for enhancing self-soothing, self-love, and positive self-sentiments. Further, they proposed that ego-enhancing language, imagery, and suggestions should pervade all of hypnotic work, from the first contact throughout treatment, and form an element of every treatment plan. They also asserted that ego strengthening approaches in some sense blur the boundaries between hypnosis and psychotherapy.

Students in hypnosis training should be introduced to an ego strengthening attitude for clinical work, and master specific therapeutic interventions to induce ego strengthening. Such interventions may include guided imagery for self-acceptance and self-love, affirming language that counteracts negative self-talk, age regression to recapture forgotten strengths, and age progression to anticipate and imagine future wisdom and strengths (Frederick & McNeal, 1998; Torem, 1992).

Integrating both group and individual exercises in ego strengthening into training sessions provides the best introduction into the power of ego strengthening strategies.

Introducing Self-Hypnosis Strategies

Self-hypnosis practice provides a useful tool to extend and promote the effects of hetero-hypnotic sessions and provides long-term self-directed coping strategies for patients following the termination of treatment. Some individuals also use self-hypnosis as a form of self-help instead of seeing a professional, based on the many resources available through social media. Hammond (1992) published a manual for self-hypnosis and Elkins (2014, 2017) provided instructions and guidance for self-hypnosis in his publications on hypnotic relaxation therapy.

Training should provide clear guidance for teaching patients self-hypnosis. Elkins (2017) recommends introducing self-hypnosis after the patient becomes familiar with hypnotically assisted relaxation. He begins by providing patients with audio recordings of in-office hypnotic sessions and then proceeds to teach them how to initiate an independent hypnotic experience. Training should also include case narratives from the instructors' clinical use of self-hypnosis and small group time for trainees to practice introducing and teaching self-hypnosis to one other.

The Future

In several respects, the future of hypnosis practice is upon us. The final section of this chapter will address several aspects of hypnosis education and practice that are already emergent. This will include (a) the emergence of telemedicine and virtual hypnosis, (b) the emergence of both virtual and hybrid hypnosis education, (c) the emergence of digital resources and apps for hypnosis self-care, and (d) the expansion of hypnosis education and training to multiple disciplines treating diverse groups of medical and mental health patients within an integrative healthcare model.

Hypnosis and Telemedicine

As recently as 2017, in his chapter on ethics, Nagy (2017) discussed remote delivery of hypnosis largely through a series of well-justified cautionary statements, founded in clinical concerns, legal restrictions, and ethical principles. However, the Covid-19 pandemic created a brave new world in healthcare, forcing health professionals to advance remote medical and psychological assessment and treatment interventions. A recent global survey of 691 hypnosis practitioners in 31 countries found that 63.8% % of respondents were using video sessions to deliver hypnosis, and approximately one in five used it often, most of the time, or all of the time (Palsson et al., 2023). Among the respondents conducting virtual hypnotic sessions, 54% maintained that remote hypnosis was as effective as face-to-face hypnosis.

It is our personal experience, from conversations with many psychotherapists and hypnosis practitioners, that significant numbers of patients prefer the convenience of remote work and have been reluctant to resume in-office therapy. Some hybrid combination of face-to-face evaluation followed by remote hypnosis sessions and prescribed self-hypnosis practice may provide a happy medium.

Virtual and Hybrid Hypnosis Training and Education

Similarly, the leading clinical hypnosis organizations moved quickly, albeit reluctantly, into remote, virtual training. In the United States, the Society for Clinical and Experimental Hypnosis (SCEH) and the ASCH had previously conducted all basic, intermediate, and advanced training in person, yet both scheduled virtual training within the first year of the pandemic and of equal importance both accepted virtual training as a qualification for clinical certification. Universities such as Baylor University in Texas and Saybrook University in California moved rapidly into remote hypnosis training, with apparent success in terms of measurable student skills. Baylor also trained research staff virtually in clinical hypnosis, including the administration of the Elkins Hypnotizability Scale, and other hypnosis interventions. Then, virtual hypnosis was implemented with participants in an NIH-funded clinical study of interventions for hot flashes and sleep (G. Elkins, personal communication, 2022; E. Willmarth, personal communication, 2022).

At the time of this writing, as the Covid-19 pandemic of 2019–2023 is waning, face-to-face training is resuming again. However, the experience of the pandemic years has spurred increasing effectiveness in virtual training and virtual supervision of student-practitioners. In addition, an increasing number of trainees will be reluctant to undertake expensive travel when their experiences with virtual learning have proven effective. Various forms of hybrid education are likely to prevail: creative combinations of online asynchronous delivery of didactic information about hypnosis history, research findings, ethics, and similar topics, in combination with live virtual and/or face-to-face training in hypnosis techniques. With the availability of digital breakout rooms, virtual small group hypnosis practice and supervised individual hypnosis sessions are feasible.

Training organizations are reporting higher attendance and lower costs in providing virtual trainings. It is quite probable that a combination of remote and in-person training will prevail.

Digital Resources for Self-Hypnosis and Hypnosis-Guided Self-Care

Along with the emergence of virtual hypnosis treatment and virtual hypnosis training and education, we see an emergence of online resources and digital apps that offer an increasingly effective introduction to hypnosis. Clinical hypnosis education will do well to introduce and provide guidance on the use of digital resources.

If one searches the terms, "YouTube" and "Hypnosis," 3,370,000,000 items pop up. Consumers are finding and using online videos guiding them to learn self-hypnosis techniques, enhance their sleep, calm their anxiety, and enhance their sexual experiences. The challenge is not finding a site with hypnosis guidance; rather the challenge is in sorting through the plethora of hypnosis guidance, to identify the most effective and most credible. It is our hope that professional hypnosis organizations and medical institutions will utilize their websites to assist the general public in finding and utilizing the most credible online resources for self-help, including YouTube videos, podcasts, and other online materials. Meanwhile, user ratings are the only guide that the general public currently has in selecting online guidance.

Another emergent trend is the use of smart phone apps for learning in multiple areas. Again, the challenge is in sorting through the plethora of commercially available apps. Currently, a number of major leaders in professional hypnosis are releasing apps to assist self-help. David Spiegel of Stanford University has guided the development of the *Reveri* app, offering self-hypnosis guidance for better focus, relaxation, sleep, and health. Several leaders in hypnosis are partnering with MindsetHealth.com to create and promote apps, websites, and blogs providing hypnosis guidance (https://mindsethealth.com). Gary Elkins of Baylor University collaborated with MindsetHealth to create *Evia*, which provides mental imagery, guided relaxation, and self-hypnosis practices self-manage many of the problems of menopause, including hot flashes and night sweats. He also created *Finito* for smoking cessation. Simone Peters created *Nerva* with MindsetHealth, a hypnosis app to manage irritable bowel syndrome. Michael Yapko contributed several sessions for another MindsetHealth app called *Mindset: Hypnosis and Sleep*. MindsetHealth also provides a clinicians' portal that enables practitioners to use MindsetHealth apps as adjuncts to therapy and provides online processes for monitoring patients' use of apps.

The US Food and Drug Administration (FDA) has recognized the increasing consumer use of online resources. Terri Cornelison, assistant director for the health of women in the FDA's Center for Devices and Radiologic Health, commented that: "Consumers are increasingly using digital health technologies to inform their everyday health decisions ... "

(https://www.fda.gov/news-events/press-announcements/fda-allows-marketing-first-direct-consumer-app-contraceptive-use-prevent-pregnancy). Accordingly, the FDA has begun reviewing and approving mobile medical apps for consumer grade devices. For example, they have approved the Kardia Mobile app, produced by AliveCor, which records heart rhythms and detects atrial fibrillation. They also have approved the Nature Cycles app, which women can utilize for self-monitoring menstrual cycles to guide contraception. Longer term, FDA approvals may provide a means to assist consumers to sort through the plethora of digital apps and identify those with solid evidence-based support.

Inclusion of apps in applied behavioral health research will also provide a pathway of evidence-based support for specific consumer grade devices and apps. For example, Chung et al. (2021) conducted an entire research study on heart rate variability training for anxiety without any face-to-face contact, using a wearable device, a smart phone app, and telephone coaching. Even the pre- and post-anxiety and depression measures were administered through the app. The participants showed significant reductions in both anxiety and depression.

Future hypnosis education will need to include education on guiding patients on the use of digital resources, including online hypnosis training, smart phone apps, wearable monitors, and related technologies to remain relevant in the digital age. Integrating videos, apps, and similar technology into hypnosis treatment will extend the scope of treatment and provide support for the patient following discharge.

Concerns Regarding Future Developments

There remain many challenges. Digital teleconferencing platforms (e.g., ZOOM) typically display patients' head and shoulders, and the full body language and non-verbal synchrony between the therapist and patient are somewhat missing, although some therapists and patients report feeling significant attunement. The use of apps and videos also reduces the presence of rapport, empathy, and therapeutic relationship – the so-called common factors that play such a critical role in medical and psychological interventions. Embedding the use of apps and digital resources within an actual treatment process, with a therapist/practitioner, may optimize the impact of the digital resources while preserving the common factors critical for benefit.

New Professional Disciplines in Hypnosis Practice and Integrative Healthcare

In the United States, leading professional organizations for many years limited membership, hypnosis education, and certification to a narrow list of licensed health professionals. Consequently, the majority of members were physicians, doctoral level psychologists, social workers, and counselors. In addition, the majority of hypnosis practitioners worked in solo or group private practice settings.

Over the past decade, the restrictions have begun to lift, and the private practice model is no longer the only pathway for applying hypnosis. The SCEH, for example, has significantly opened its membership, hypnosis education, and certification processes for additional healthcare disciplines, including many non-doctoral-level practitioners. Currently, SCEH membership is open to:

> … physicians; dentists; doctoral level speech pathologists and pharmacists; doctoral level practitioners of Traditional Chinese Medicine (accredited by the Accreditation

> Commission for Acupuncture and Oriental Medicine); those with a master's or higher degree in psychology, marital/family therapy (or couples/family therapy), counseling, nursing, physicians assistants, social work (accredited by the Council on Social Work Education), health coaching, or physical and occupational therapy. Membership will also be available to those with a bachelor's or higher degree and licensure as nurses, dental hygienists, paramedics, midwives, or mental health counsellors/associates. (https://sceh.us/membership)

Expansion of professional organization membership and training to additional healthcare disciplines facilitates broader use of hypnosis and hypnosis-informed treatments within integrative healthcare settings, where allied professionals and paraprofessionals have significant patient contact. One of the markers of integrative healthcare is the concept of interprofessionalism, that is, the diverse professionals work on a *collaborative basis* in a single pediatric, family practice, or specialty medicine setting (Weeks, 2015, WHO, 2010). Decision making is carried out through communication across disciplines and engaging the patient integrally in the process. Educating multiple disciplines within integrative settings optimizes the impact of hypnosis for a broader group of patients.

SCEH educational programs and certification are open to most of the same professional groups, enabling a variety of health professionals throughout the world of integrative healthcare to learn and apply hypnosis and hypnosis-assisted interventions to a variety of patient groups with medical and emotional disorders.

Another example of emergent trends is Elvira Lang and her company, Comfort Talk™. Through Comfort Talk, Lang and her teams provide training for all disciplines including support staff personnel in hospitals in positive, hypnotically influenced language (Lang, 2012; Lang & Laser, 2011). One research report on MRI departments at three large academic medical centers, which implemented the Comfort Talk programs, showed that the training significantly reduced no show rates and incompletion rates for MRI services (Norbash et al., 2016). The study also reported improved patient compliance, with a reduction in motion artifacts, producing considerable cost savings.

Conclusion

Training and education in clinical hypnosis is critical for continued growth and development in hypnosis practice. North American professional hypnosis societies, especially the ASCH, SCEH, NPHTI, and the Milton H. Erickson Foundation provide regular training opportunities in clinical hypnosis, based on current standards of training. In recent years, critics have called for reorienting hypnosis education, and the perspectives of several authors on directions for a reorientation were included in a 2017 special issue of the *American Journal of Clinical Hypnosis.*

This chapter also reviewed the dramatic and essential increase in the use of virtual hypnosis treatment and hypnosis training since the onset of the Covid-19 pandemic. For the future, we are likely to see creative combinations of in-person evaluation, virtual treatment sessions, and digitally supported self-hypnosis practice, as well as hybrid combinations of in-person and virtual training. In addition, the future will include the use of hypnosis by many additional health professions within an integrative healthcare model.

The present chapter calls for a balance in training between a process-oriented immersion of trainees in hypnotic experiences and the review of minimal levels of hypnosis knowledge and theory. This chapter presented 12 competencies critical for hypnosis training and called for inclusion of an abundant amount of small group practice experiences during hypnosis training, to prevent training from deteriorating into an overemphasis on "knowledge about hypnosis." Inclusion of an abundance of hypnotic experiences in training workshops assures that trainees will come to "yearn for the vastness of the sea."We have no conflicts of interest to disclose.

References

Alter, D. S., & Sugarman, L. I. (2017). Reorienting hypnosis education. *American Journal of Clinical Hypnosis*, *59*(3), 235–259. http://dx.doi.org/10.1080/00029157.2016.1231657

American Society of Clinical Hypnosis Education and Research Foundation (2019). *Standards of training*, 2019.

Baker, E. L. (2017). Yearning for the vastness of the sea: Reflections and commentary on professional training in hypnosis. *American Journal of Clinical Hypnosis*, *59*, 311–315. 10.1080/00029157.2017.1247551

Chester, S. J., Tyack, Z., De Young, A., Kipping, B., Griffin, B., Stockton, K., Ware, R. S., Zhang, X., & Kimble, R. M. (2018). Efficacy of hypnosis on pain, wound-healing, anxiety, and stress in children with acute burn injuries: A randomized controlled trial. *Pain*, *159*(9), 1790–1801. 10.1097/j.pain.0000000000001276

Chung, A. H., Gevirtz, R. N., Gharbo, R. S., Thiam, M. A., & Ginsberg, J. P. (2021). Pilot study on reducing symptoms of anxiety with a heart rate variability biofeedback wearable and remote stress management coach. *Applied Psychophysiology and Biofeedback*, *46*(4), 347–358. 10.1007/s10484-021-09519-x

Dostoevsky, F. (1994). *Notes from underground.* (trans. by R. Pevear & L. Volokbosky). Vintage Classics.

Elkins, G. R. (2014). *Hypnotic relaxation therapy: Principles and applications.* Springer Publishing Company.

Elkins, G. R. (2017). Hypnotic relaxation therapy. In G. R. Elkins (Ed.), *Handbook of medical and psychological hypnosis* (pp. 83–97). Springer.

Elkins, G. R., Barabasz, A. F., Council, J. R., & Spiegel, D. (2015). Advancing research and practice: The revised APA Division 30 definition of hypnosis. *The International Journal of Clinical and Experimental Hypnosis*, *63*(1), 1–9. 10.1080/00207144.2014.961870

Erickson, B. A. (2017). Ericksonian hypnotherapy. In G. R. Elkins (Ed.), *Handbook of medical and psychological hypnosis: Foundations, medical, and psychological hypnosis* (pp. 119–131). Springer Publishing Company.

Erickson, M. H. (1967). An introduction to the study and application of hypnosis for pain control. In J. Lassner (Ed.), *Hypnosis and psychosomatic medicine* (pp. 83–90). Springer Verlag. 10.1007/978-3-642-87028-6_11

Erickson, M. H. (1958). Naturalistic techniques of hypnosis. *The American Journal of Clinical Hypnosis*, *1*(1), 3–8. 10.1080/00029157.1958.10401766

Frederick, C., & McNeal, S. A. (1998). *Inner strengths: Contemporary psychotherapy and hypnosis for ego strengthening.* Routledge.

Fried, R., & Grimaldi, J. (1993). *The psychology and physiology of breathing: In behavioral medicine, clinical psychology, and psychiatry.* Plenum Press. 10.1007/978-1-4899-1239-8

Hammond, D. C. (1992). *Manual for self-hypnosis.* American Society of Clinical Hypnosis.

Hammond, D. C., & Elkins, G. (1994). *Standards of training in clinical hypnosis.* ASCH Press.

Hammond, D. C. (1996). Experiential learning exercises in clinical hypnosis training. *American Journal of Clinical Hypnosis*, *39*(1), 21–36. 10.1080/00029157.1996.10403362

Hammond, D. C., & Elkins, G. (2005). *Standards of training in clinical hypnosis.* ASCH Education and Research Foundation.

Hartland, J. (1965). The value of "ego strengthening" procedures prior to direct symptom removal under hypnosis. *American Journal of Clinical Hypnosis*, *8*(2), 89–93. 10.1080/00029157.1965.10402470

Hartland, J. (1971). Further observations on the use of ego strengthening techniques. *American Journal of Clinical Hypnosis*, *14*(1), 1–8. 10.1080/00029157.1971.10402136

Hilgard, E. R. (1965). *Hypnotic susceptibility*. Harcourt Brace Jovanovich.

Howard, H. A. (2017). Promoting safety in hypnosis: A clinical instrument for the assessment of alertness. *American Journal of Clinical Hypnosis*, *59*(4), 344–362. 10.1080/00029157.2016.1203281

Jacobson, E. (1938). *Progressive relaxation*. University of Chicago Press.

Jensen, M. P. (Ed.) (2019). *Hypnosis for acute and procedural pain management*. Denny Creek Press.

Kabat-Zinn, J. (2005). *Wherever you go, there you are: Mindfulness meditation in everyday life (reprint edition)*. Hachette Books.

Kirsch, I. (2018). Response expectancy and the placebo effect. *International Review of Neurobiology*, *138*, 81–93. 10.1016/bs.irn.2018.01.003

Kohen, D. P., Kaiser, P., & Olness, K. (2017). State-of-the-art pediatric hypnosis training: Remodeling curriculum and refining faculty development. *American Journal of Clinical Hypnosis*, *59*(3), 292–310. 10.1080/00029157.2016.1233859

Lang, E. V. (2012). A better patient experience through better communication. *Journal of Radiology Nursing*, *31*(4), 114–119. 10.1016/j.jradnu.2012.08.001

Lang, E. V., & Laser, E. (2011). *Patient sedation without medication. Rapid rapport and quick hypnotic techniques: A resource guide for doctors, nurses, and technologists*. CreateSpace Independent Publishing Platform.

Lankton, S. R. (2017). Training in therapy—Induction without scripts. *American Journal of Clinical Hypnosis*, *59*(3), 276–281. 10.1080/00029157.2017.1247549

Lehrer, P. M., & Woolfolk, R. L. (Eds.). (2021). *Principles and practice of stress management* (4th edition). Guilford.

Linden, J. H., & Anbar, R. (2017). Hypnosis training and education: Distinctive features of training hypnosis educators. *American Journal of Clinical Hypnosis*, *59*(3), 260–275. 10.1080/00029157.2016.1225253

Linden, J., Hammond, D. C., Shapiro, M., Wark, D., & Zastrow, J. (Eds.). (2011). Standards of training in clinical hypnosis (unpublished manuscript). Committee Report submitted to Executive Committee of ASCH.

Linden, W. (2007). The autogenic training method of J. H. Schulz. In P. M. Lehrer, R. L. Woolfolk, & W. E. Sime (Eds.). *Principles and practice of stress management* (3rd ed., pp. 151–174). Guilford.

Lindheim, M. Ø., & Helgeland, H. (2017). Hypnosis training and education: Experiences with a Norwegian one-year education course in clinical hypnosis for children and adolescents. *American Journal of Clinical Hypnosis*, *59*(3), 282–291, 10.1080/00029157.2016.1230728

Manzoni, G. M., Pagnini, F., Castelnuovo, G., & Molinari, E. (2008). Relaxation training for anxiety: A ten-years systematic review with meta-analysis. *BMC Psychiatry*, 8(41). 10.1186/1471-244X-8-41

McEwen, B. S. (2017). Neurobiological and systemic effects of chronic stress. *Chronic Stress*, *1*, 1–11. 10.1177/2470547017692328

McNeal, S. (2020). Hypnotic ego strengthening: Where we've been and the road ahead. *American Journal of Clinical Hypnosis*, *62*(4), 392–408.

McNeal, S., & Frederick, C. (1993). Inner strength and other techniques for ego strengthening. *American Journal of Clinical Hypnosis*, *35*(3), 170–178. doi:10.1080/00029157.1993.10403001

Morgan, A. H. (1973). The heritability of hypnotic susceptibility in twins. *Journal of Abnormal Psychology*, *82*(1), 55–61.

Moudatsou, M., Stavropoulou, A., Philalithis, A., & Koukouli, S. (2020). The role of empathy in health and social care professionals. *Healthcare (Basel, Switzerland)*, *8*(1), 26. 10.3390/healthcare8010026

Moss, D., & Willmarth, E. (2017). Ego strengthening approaches in hypnotically assisted psychotherapy. In G. Elkins (Ed.), *Clinician's guide to medical and psychological hypnosis: Foundations, applications, and professional issues* (pp. 535–545). Springer.

Myerson, J. (2017). Presenting hypnosis to patients. In G. Elkins (Ed.), *Clinician's guide to medical and psychological hypnosis: Foundations, applications, and professional issues* (pp. 29–33). Springer.
Nagy, T. F. (2017). Ethics. In G. Elkins (Ed.), *Clinician's guide to medical and psychological hypnosis: Foundations, applications, and professional issues* (pp. 651–671). Springer.
Norbash, A., Yucel, K., Yuh, W., Doros, G., Ajam, A., Lang, E., Pauker, S., & Mayr, N. (2016). Effect of team training on improving MRI study completion rates and no-show rates. *Journal of Magnetic Resonance Imaging*, *44*(4), 1040–1047. 10.1002/jmri.25219
Norcross, J. C., & Lambert, M. J. (2018a). Psychotherapy relationships that work, III. *Psychotherapy*, *55*(4), 303–315.
Norcross, J. C., & Lambert, M. J. (2018b). Special issue: Evidence-based psychotherapy relationships III. *Psychotherapy*, *55*(4), 303–537.
Palsson, O., Kekecs, Z., De Benedettis, G., Moss, D., Elkins G., Terhune, D. B., Varga, K., Shenefelt, P. D., & Whorwell, P. J. (2023). Current practices, experiences, and views in clinical hypnosis: Findings of an international survey. *The International Journal of Clinical and Experimental Hypnosis*, *71*, 92–114.
Piccione, C., Hilgard, E. R., & Zimbardo, P. (1989). On the degree of stability of measured hypnotizability over a 25-year period. *Journal of Personality and Social Psychology*, *56*(2), 289–295. 10.1037/0022-3514.56.2.289
Reid, D. B. (2019). Hypnotic induction: Enhancing trance or mostly myth? In V. Kumar & S. R. Lankton (Eds.), *Hypnotic induction: Perspectives, strategies and concerns*. (pp. 6–16). Routledge, Taylor & Francis Group.
Riess, H. (2010). Empathy in medicine—A neurobiological perspective. *Journal of the American Medical Association*, *304*(14), 1604–1605. 10.1001/jama.2010.1455
Rogers, C. (1992). The necessary and sufficient conditions of therapeutic personality change. 1957. *Journal of Consulting and Clinical Psychology*, *60*(6), 827–832. 10.1037//0022-006x.60.6.827
Rossi, E. L. (1986). *The psychobiology of mind-body healing: New concepts of therapeutic hypnosis*. W. W. Norton.
Rossman, M. L. (2000). *Guided imagery for self-healing*. New World Library.
Schultz, J. H., & Luthe, W. (1959). *Autogenic training: A psychophysiological approach in psychotherapy*. Grune and Stratton.
Shor, R. E., & Orne, E. C. (1962). *Harvard Group Scale of Hypnotic Susceptibility. Form A*. Consulting Psychologists Press.
Spiegel, E., & Baker, E. (2019). Special issue: The generative presence of relatedness. *American Journal of Clinical Hypnosis*, *62*(1–2). 10.1080/00029157.2019.1609840
Spiegel, H. (1978). *Manual for the Hypnotic Induction Profile (1st ed.)*. Basic Books.
Stanton, H. E. (1979). Ego-enhancement through positive suggestion. *Australian Journal of Clinical Hypnosis*, *3*, 32–36.
Stanton, H. E. (1989). Ego-enhancement: A five step approach. *American Journal of Clinical Hypnosis*, *31*, 192–198.
Sugarman, L. I. (2017) Exploring, evolving, and refining hypnosis education. *American Journal of Clinical Hypnosis*, *59*(3), 231–232. 10.1080/00029157.2017.1247544
Tinterow, M. M. (1970) *Foundations of hypnosis: From Mesmer to Freud*. Charles C. Thomas.
Torem, M. S. (1992). Back from the future: A powerful age-progression technique. *American Journal of Clinical Hypnosis*, *35*(2), 81–88. 10.1080/00029157.1992.10402990
Weeks, J. (2015). What is the commitment to interprofessionalism in integrative health and medicine? *Global Advances in Health and Medicine*, *4*(3), 9–11. 10.7453/gahmj.2015.046
World Health Organization (2010). *Framework for action on interprofessional education and collaborative practice*. Geneva: Department of Human Resources for Health. Available at: https://apps.who.int/iris/bitstream/handle/10665/70185/WHO_HRH_HPN_10.3_eng.pdf;jsessionid=AF3022A6DB2F464B45B378D22826F537?sequence=1
Weitzenhoffer, A. M., & Hilgard, E. R. (1959). *Stanford Hypnotic Susceptibility Scale, Forms A and B*. Consulting Psychologists Press.
Weitzenhoffer, A. M., & Hilgard, E. R. (1962). *Stanford Hypnotic Susceptibility Scale, Form C*. Consulting Psychologists Press.
Williamson A. (2019). What is hypnosis and how might it work?. *Palliative Care*, *12*, 1178224219826581. 10.1177/1178224219826581

Yapko, M. D. (2012). *Trancework: An introduction to the practice of clinical hypnosis* (4th ed.). Routledge.

Yapko, M. D. (2016). *The discriminating therapist: Asking "how" questions, making distinctions, and finding direction in therapy*. Yapko Publications.

Yapko, M. D. (2021). *Process-oriented hypnosis: Focusing on the forest, not the trees*. W. W. Norton.

Yaribeygi, H., Panahi, Y., Sahraei, H., Johnston, T. P., & Sahebkar, A. (2017). The impact of stress on body function: A review. *EXCLI Journal*, *16*, 1057–1072. 10.17179/excli2017-480

Zeig, J. K. (2014). *The induction of hypnosis: An Ericksonian elicitation approach*. Milton H. Erickson Foundation.

58

A MODEL OF TRAINING IN CLINICAL HYPNOSIS GROUNDED IN INTERPERSONAL NEUROBIOLOGY

Reinhild Draeger-Muenke

PRIVATE PRACTICE, BALA CYNWYD, PA, USA

Traditional Training in Clinical Hypnosis

Since its inception, the standards of traditional training in clinical hypnosis focus on the dissemination of didactic, experiential, and practical information about hypnosis to healthcare professionals to further their competent elicitation of standard hypnotic protocols in their respective clinical settings (Elkins & Hammond, 1998; Linden & Anbar, 2017; Watkins, 1998).

However, many clinicians abandon hypnosis training after the introductory level, finding it procedurally and legally complicated, and emotionally risky. Modalities such as Mindfulness Meditation, Internal Family Systems, and Eye Movement Desensitization and Reprocessing (EMDR) promise easier access and faster proficiency. Meanwhile, clinicians are often left unaware that all of these treatment modalities utilize the human capacity for trance – the main focus of the field of clinical hypnosis. Cross-training in the competent recognition and utilization of trance in the process of healing could significantly enhance standard treatment in the major therapeutic modalities (Beere et al., 2001; Fine & Berkowitz, 2001; Gilligan, 2002; Otani, 2016; Sapp, 2016; Yapko, 2011).

In the author's experience, clinicians who do continue past the introductory training in clinical hypnosis acknowledge anxiety and self-doubt around "correctly" eliciting prescribed hypnotic phenomena, self-limiting their full utilization of hypnosis in their clinical work. Training situations these clinicians had experienced as evaluative and highly stressful led to their subsequent failure entrancements, preventing them from experiencing the satisfaction of facilitating trance collaboratively and with curiosity for their own patients.

After serving as chair and faculty for traditional training modules through the American Society of Clinical Hypnosis for a decade, the author was offered the opportunity by the International Society for the Study of Trauma and Dissociation (ISSTD) to develop a model of training in clinical hypnosis meeting the sought-after ASCH standards for certification, while addressing the particular needs of clinicians treating traumatized and dissociative patients.

DOI: 10.4324/9781003449126-76

Guided by the conceptualization of dissociation as an autohypnotic process (Craparo et al., 2019; Dell, 2017, 2019, 2021; Loewenstein, 1993; Putnam, 1989), clinical hypnosis as a skill set is uniquely equipped to teach mastery of problematic dissociation. Teaching clinical hypnosis in a trauma and dissociation informed way, less prescriptive and more person-centered, supports safety in learning and experiencing clinical hypnosis for the trainees as well as for their future traumatized patients. This model prioritizes individualized discovery of beneficial trance experiences throughout all components of the training. It allows for the trainees' growing competent engagement with hypnosis as a useful tool in their treatment of complex patients, supporting the clinician-trainees' sense of efficacy (Kumar et al., 2022; Sansbury et al., 2015). It appears to be equally beneficial for trainees from medical and mental health fields and underscores the necessity of training faculty from both fields to consider this model for their approach to training.

The following factors are associated with positive learning experiences that are conducive to the retention and dissemination of clinical hypnosis skills:

1 Honoring the trainees' competence as clinicians and their ability to learn new information through interactive teaching.
2 Consistently linking new and practice relevant clinical hypnosis knowledge and skills to the trainees' preexisting fund of clinical knowledge in their respective clinical specialties (e.g., medicine, physical therapy, dentistry, clinical psychology).
3 Appreciating and normalizing the process of learning to co-regulate conditioned fears of judgment when engaging in hypnotic experiences, and creating emotional safety through attunement and collaboration.

When we accept that learning and changing our minds is possible because of our neuroplasticity (Hawkins, 2021; Tovar-Moll & Lent, 2016; Voss et al., 2017), and when we claim that hypnosis facilitates neuroplasticity (Alter & Sugarman, 2017; Doidge, 2015; Nemeth et al., 2013; Spiegel & Baker, 2019), then the teaching of clinical hypnosis must become hypnotic in all its aspects. Content and process, teaching, learning, and experiencing the learned material need to complement each other, so that, for example, teaching the concept of attunement requires explicit and implicit attunement to the trainees and their varied responses and needs throughout the training.

As the author understands the teaching of hypnosis, it applies the principles of interpersonal neurobiology, respecting each trainee's Window of Tolerance (Siegel, 1999, 2012; Siegel et al., 2021), and encouraging the greater opening of their Window of Welcome (Peyton & Badenoch, 2017). Trainees are empowered to "own" their hypnotic abilities, as individual trance experiences create a felt knowledge of the phenomenon. Attending to the emotional and relational components of learning allows for a respectful and flexible individualized learning experience for clinicians with varied personal and professional backgrounds, incorporating newly learned hypnosis principles into their already existing clinical skill sets (Linden & Anbar, 2017). Trainees then can utilize this model with their future patients in a parallel process of collaborative pacing leading to the constructive utilization of clinical hypnosis.

Considerations for Adult Learners in Clinical Hypnosis

Learning, a life-long process, has been conceptualized as occurring in several domains: the domain of knowledge and cognition, of affective/attitudinal learning (readiness, motivation), and of psychomotor/behavioral skills (Bloom, 1956). Conditioning and motivation are also contributing factors in successful learning (Hilgard, 1962; Hilgard et al., n.d.). Newer models of learning have broadened the focus to include the role of attention and its (emotional) detractors (Jha, 2021), and the relational aspect of multi-layered communication for enhanced collaboration and joint problem-solving (Siegel, 2012). It makes sense then to let interpersonal neurobiology inform education in general and the endeavor of training clinicians in clinical hypnosis in particular. Preliminary findings derived from Porges' Polyvagal Theory (Porges, 2003, 2022) and its clinical integration (Dana, 2018) suggest that in order to facilitate all levels of the cognitive and psychomotor aspects of learning about clinical hypnosis – from gathering information to integrating and flexibly applying it – the affective dimension of learning is crucial and needs to be tended to deliberately and consistently.

Therefore, teaching is tailored to the clinical situations the trainees encounter at their places of work, so that new content is relevant and applicable (Linden & Anbar, 2017; Wark & Kohen, 1998). Joint problem-solving of trainee-generated clinical case challenges applying just-learned hypnosis concepts is part of every lecture. In order to keep interest, attention, and motivation alive, hypnosis demonstrations and experiences are offered during each lecture period to elicit a felt sense of the just presented hypnosis concepts. Gradual exposure from cognitive presentation to observed demonstration, to invitation to experience a hypnotic phenomenon (or abstain), and finally to offer it to a peer allows trainees to pace their explicit and implicit learning according to their emotional readiness to engage.

Generally, clinician-trainees, by nature and by training, are competitive high achievers who strive to follow procedures correctly with low tolerance for making mistakes. They have learned as students in highly competitive environments to hide their struggles and vulnerabilities for fear of receiving negative evaluations, not measuring up to peers, and of not being seen as competent (Devendorf & Victor, 2022; Victor et al., 2021; Willyard, 2012). In order to keep the risk of new learning manageable, undercurrents of habitual competition and anxiety about falling short and being publicly embarrassed need to be monitored during the training, so that a training experience free of shame dynamics can be accomplished (Benau, 2022).

Emphasizing a growth mindset becomes essential when developing trainees' potential to competently and collaboratively offer the benefits of clinical hypnosis (Dweck, 2008). It is equally important to offer continuous encouragement for taking educated risks and learning from what did not go as anticipated (Nicolaides & Poell, 2020). Clinical hypnosis training thus provides the opportunity to broaden and enhance the trainees' experience and perspective of themselves as learners and clinicians in an emotionally supportive, non-competitive, and non-evaluative learning environment. Clinical hypnosis can thus be experienced as a valuable personal and professional resource for growth and change (Yapko et al., 1998).

In order to offer an inclusive training, every learner deserves to be engaged by accommodating different learning styles. Information is offered visually (power point slides, videos), auditorily (verbal explanations), and experientially (demonstrations, role play, dyadic practices of hypnotic principles within the whole group and in small group practices).

Throughout the training, each individual's unique, expert contribution to the collective learning and growth experience is actively elicited. Neurodiversity is understood and welcomed as the sum of everyone's differences rather than as a collection of pathologies (Walker, 2021). Thus, clinician-trainees are encouraged to regularly attune to and take charge of their own mind-body needs throughout the training in order to allow new learning to occur comfortably (Ogden, 2015; Payne et al., 2015; Siegel, 2012).

Furthermore, inclusivity entails accommodating trainees who are not fluent in the dominant language utilized at the training and encouraging their active participation throughout (Linden & Anbar, 2017). This may include translation of words and terms as well as inviting and valuing the different perspectives and experiences of non-majority trainees, enriching everybody (Beerkens et al., 2020; Lubliner & Grisham, 2017; Prasad et al., 2022).

Similarly, the training promotes a respectful and welcoming learning environment for trainees of diverse and intersecting identities, cultures, and lived experiences. To signal that all belong equally from the get-go, name plates ask how trainees want to be addressed, including their preferred pronouns. Diversity, equity, and inclusion are central to a multiculturally oriented training. This is also reflected in the choice of visuals illustrating a concept, clinical examples, and case materials, so that all trainees can find themselves and their patients represented in the teachings (Mena, 2022).

Just as the experience of trauma in the general population is not a rare occurrence (Merians et al., 2023), clinician-trainees will bring their histories of traumatic experiences and their manifestations to the training (Van der Kolk, 2015; Victor et al., 2021). Faculty unaccustomed to working hypnotically with traumatized individuals may inadvertently display their discomfort with signs of traumatic adaptations in trainees, and reinforce shame and secrecy about such symptoms in the participants. The different adaptations to stressors experienced in the training situation need to be welcomed and normalized during the training, in order to allow these clinician-trainees to successfully negotiate their conflict between wanting to learn about hypnosis and guarding against experiencing it.

If a clinician-trainee copes with the stressor of a new and unpredictable learning situation through the autohypnotic process of dissociation (Dell, 2017, 2019, 2021), increased sympathetic nervous system activation and/or shut down can quickly ensue. Instead of dreading such an experience, it is welcomed as an important in vivo learning opportunity how to relationally and collaboratively modify unwanted autohypnotic coping within a framework of self-acceptance and self-compassion (Neff, 2011). Such witnessing prepares the clinician-trainees to effectively respond to their own dissociative patients' similar experiences.

Considerations for Faculty in Clinical Hypnosis Trainings

This model of training asks faculty to teach clinical hypnosis as the development of "a communication skill set" (Sugarman et al., 2020, p. 23), and to understand trance as a natural state of absorption (Lankton & Zeig, 2013; Lynn et al., 2010; Matthews et al., 1993), and a "dynamic process of mind-change that alters function, occurring both intentionally and unintentionally" (Sugarman et al., 2020, p. 87). It requires faculty to combine content and process of their teaching, demonstrating the science and the art of clinical hypnosis, as they work with the trainees' different states of absorption to the trainees' benefit.

Beyond the teaching of content, faculty of all professional backgrounds is tasked with monitoring and co-regulating trainees' Window of Tolerance, especially during the practice and experiential components of the training. It is hypnosis training in action, when a trainee's demonstrated vulnerability is accepted and normalized as an opportunity to learn self-regulation of an involuntary trance experience with attuned support (Azoulay et al., 2020; Clark, 2020; Modestin et al., 2002).

As faculty models how to facilitate individual learning toward self-regulation and self-knowledge collaboratively using hypnosis, they navigate the intersection of intellectual and interpersonal expertise in collaboration with their trainees (Cravens et al., 2022). This requires faculty's astute management of many parallel processes during the training, as trainees manifest in vivo what is being taught in vitro.

For example, attention needs to be paid to the effects of repeated trance experiences throughout the training in terms of loosened reality orientation, unexpected appearance of memories, thoughts, feelings, and images, and a heightened receptivity to others (e.g., in interactions with fellow trainees or instructors). If a trainee's distress becomes noticeable and is not addressed constructively, it can quickly affect the sense of safety for the entire training community (Peebles, 2018).

Anticipation and acceptance of heightened transference and countertransference situations because of the intentionally attuned interactional nature of clinical hypnosis are equally essential for maintaining a safe and successful training in clinical hypnosis (Bányai, 1998; Dalenberg, 2000; Peebles, 2018; Peebles-kleiger, 2001; Varga, 2021).

Similarly, the enactment of earlier attachment experiences during the training is possible because of the nature of human interactional neuropsychology (Schore, 2002, 2014; Siegel et al., 2021), and therefore also the experience of disruption or loss of attachment (Bowlby, 1985). Real – if unintentional – harm can be done, when faculty-trainee interactions are experienced as dismissive or shaming and are not immediately repaired. Examples of such counterproductive interactions are an instructor's rigid adherence to a particular model of teaching clinical hypnosis, an insistence of a right way of executing an invitation to enter a state of trance, and a hierarchical approach to knowing. Faculty needs to be willing and able to maintain a deeply respectful, curious, and collaborative demeanor toward any challenges to content or process of their teaching in particular, or any aspects of the training itself.

When ruptures occur during the training, constructively addressing the rupture can provide a growth opportunity for the learning community. Satisfactory repair of the rupture strengthens the overall safety of interactions and actually reduces the risk of participating in the training process, making disengagement less likely (Marmarosh, 2021; Tasca & Marmarosh, 2023). Even though it is intended and executed as a *training* in clinical hypnosis, *therapeutic, nurturing and corrective experiences* are possible!

Most faculty have decades of clinical experience with utilizing hypnosis, and their preferred methods of passing on their knowledge and experience. Adult learners also come with their acquired truths and biases, and a flexible teaching style combined with non-defensive active listening and emotional attunement goes a long way. When faculty can accept and welcome a trainee's ways of self-expression, faculty is demonstrating attunement, "pacing and leading" by example in order to create an emotionally safe environment conducive to learning clinical hypnosis while actually experiencing it.

The Relational Aspect of Training Clinicians in Clinical Hypnosis

Just as the trance begins before the first clinical encounter for those in our care, and every contact holds relatedness whether in virtual reality or face to face (Peebles, 2012), the training relationship may begin with a prospective participant's contemplating to register.

And just as clinicians begin to build the therapeutic relationship (Bordin, 1979) through their web presence, the web-based information about the hypnosis training serves as an invitation to engage. For that purpose, the chair of the training is available to clarify aspects of the training concerning to prospective participants, often related to common myths about hypnosis such as loss of one's agency or control (Green & Lynn, 2010; Milling, 2012; Montgomery et al., 2018). The acceptance and validation of concerns, actually a form of initial co-regulation and co-creation of interpersonal safety (Schore, 1996), invites the prospective participant to lower their perception of risk related to the training in hypnosis in favor of curiosity and interest in registering.

The concerns the prospective participant has shared can be considered an initial gift of trust that can be responded to relationally during the training. It increases the opportunity to collaboratively reduce avoidable stressors and maintain the trainee's Window of Tolerance for their successful cognitive, emotional, and relational engagement with clinical hypnosis as a beneficial felt experience.

A welcome letter to the registrants detailing logistics of the training further increases predictability and begins the process of forming the training's learning community. Participants learn that their participation in any informal or formal experiential aspects of the training is voluntary. This provision reduces stress and vulnerability for participants concerned about engagement in hypnotic experiences and allows for genuine, non-coercive, personalized learning about the power of hypnosis in changing the mind-body toward intended constructive goals (Pert, 2003). Participation or non-participation in the formal and informal trance experiences of the training are considered equally valuable in the trainee's individual process of taking charge of their approach to clinical hypnosis. The freedom to decide whether, when, and how to explore what hypnosis "feels like" at the trainee's own pace and level of comfort in a non-judgmental setting eliminates the stigma of non-compliance. The trainees experience unequivocal acceptance of their own autonomy in allowing an intentional and guided hypnotic experience to occur, or not. This non-coercive stance then becomes the trainees' template of how to approach offering a hypnotic experience with their own patients/clients in the future.

Often, a trainee's initial decision not to participate in any invited trance experience changes to incremental, self-directed participation as their understanding of clinical hypnosis and their experience of relational safety grows. Respect for the trainee's internal self-knowledge of what is a tolerable exposure to the novel stimulus of an intentional trance permits the trainee's voluntary and gradual desensitization of their fears of losing emotional control during a hypnotic experience. The trainee then allows the self-directed and faculty-supported process of replacing their habitual avoidance control strategies with the developing self-regulation skill of entering and exiting a voluntary and constructive trance state. Following the fundamental principle of prioritizing participants' self-knowledge over prioritizing and creating expectations for participation creates equality among the trainees. The opt-in or opt-out choice is available to everyone and is understood as good self-care, not as an admission of deficiency.

It has been the author's experience that participants who chose not to experience formal or informal hypnosis during the training were able to be excellent and skillful facilitators for their peers in the training.

In order to create a stable frame and the sense of community for the training, the group of trainees and teaching faculty attends the entirety of the training together. Teaching faculty attend their colleagues' didactic portions of the training and offer additional perspectives and approaches to the clinical issues at hand.

Each training segment begins and starts on time to maintain predictability and accountability. Segments of 90 minutes are divided into units of didactic information, videos or live demonstrations, dyadic practices, and discussion about clinical applications in order to maintain the participants' attention and motivation (Bradbury, 2016; Geri et al., 2017). Several two-hour blocks allow groups of six to seven trainees to practice formal elicitations of trance experiences. The availability of food and beverages during breaks is ensured as part of the care extended to the whole person. Faculty join and are available for conversation in order to continuously model approachability and interest in the well-being of the trainees, facilitating a climate of interactivity (Creasey et al., 2009; Martin et al., 2020).

Introductions of participants and faculty begin the process of turning strangers into better known members of the learning community. Purposefully, title, profession, and professional affiliation are excluded from the introduction in order to prevent hierarchy and biases to interfere with the process of building an egalitarian peer group of trainees. Participants and faculty share their name and how they want to be addressed, where they live, and something they enjoy – the latter a first glimpse into participants' spontaneous enjoyable trance experiences.

Faculty are asked to remember the names and pronouns of the participants within the first segment of the training, in order to acknowledge and value each person's presence. This facilitates familiarity among the group members, and counters self-disappearance and self-devaluing tendencies often encountered in more anonymous groups of learners.

All participants are reminded that their attendance and participation in the training are meaningful and essential to create safety, predictability, and group cohesion for all. Participants know to contact the chair of the training for any absence exceeding 15 minutes.

Confidentiality is stressed for the entire training and after its conclusion. Discussion of any small group process after the conclusion of the training group is strongly discouraged in order to maintain the group's boundaries and to allow all participants their undisturbed break times.

Trainees are not asked to volunteer for the demonstration of hypnotic phenomena. A video demonstration or a faculty volunteer/facilitator dyad will illustrate the hypnotic phenomenon, so that all training participants can observe and ask questions. Feedback from trainees has confirmed that this has brought relief to the group, as it eliminates the stress of deciding whether to volunteer or not. It also eliminates the observers' stress of anticipatory anxiety about what may inadvertently transpire during the volunteer's experience. No volunteer is experiencing the stress of being observed as the unknown process of an elicited hypnotic phenomenon and/or a longer trance unfolds. Any inadvertent reenactment of a participant's tendency to perform or please, or a previous demand-compliance experiences is avoided.

Implicit and Explicit Learning in Clinical Hypnosis Training

Training in clinical hypnosis guided by the fundamental tenets of interpersonal neurobiology treats each moment of interaction as meaningful communication between the embodied minds of each participant (Banks & Hirschman, 2016). Therefore, care needs to be given to intentionally facilitate the "neuroception" of safety, a frame of reference brought to clinical awareness by Porges (2003). In order to optimize learning and creativity, threat perception and disempowerment experiences need to be avoided. This means conveying information about hypnosis in implicit and explicit ways that engage the orienting system (Hope & Sugarman, 2015; Sugarman et al., 2020; Yapko, 2012, 2018). A sympathetic nervous system regulated for optimal arousal will welcome novelty with interest. From the first interaction on, the goal is to engender enough trust among all members of the learning community to further connection and a collaborative "shared mind" experience (Flemons, 2022).

Hypnosis needs to be demystified on the levels of content *and* process, in the didactic and the experiential portions of the training and experienced as accessible, user-friendly, and integratable into one's existing clinical skill set (Alter & Sugarman, 2017; Hope & Sugarman, 2015). Purposefully, the training begins with conversational invitations to focus attention on one's own body-mind and to become curious about what mindful attention can affect. Building on the experience of internal attunement, invitations for more absorptive experiences are extended, for instance, involuntary salivation, an autonomic physiological change, to demonstrate a surprising mind-body collaboration (Eccles, 1973).

Before trainees are exposed to a formal elicitation of trance via an established hypnotic ritual, they are invited into a first collaborative experience of (hypnotic) absorption, nonverbally attuning to each other in a brief dyadic practice as individuals and equals, sharing intentional space without performance requirements. Participants report increased self- and co-regulation, with breathing, posture, and facial expressions becoming synchronized – an initial recognition of the power of being seen and held during the interplay of mutual pacing/following and leading.

Here, participants are introduced to the essence of this relationally and psycho-neuro-biologically oriented training in clinical hypnosis: to co-create a shared personal space with curiosity about what may transpire and how to utilize it collaboratively and beneficially. Any experience is welcome, and its expression is respected as a guide for the next interaction (Flemons, 2022; Sugarman et al., 2020). Participants begin to recognize and hypnotically capitalize on short moments of absorption as openings for connection and change. The following lectures, demonstrations, and practices about being hypnotic build on the now directly experienced principle of mutuality and collaboration.

As trainees begin to recognize the frequency, fluidity, and plasticity of informal, everyday experiences of trance, they learn to harness the enormous potential of utilizing those absorptive moments to offer surprise engagement for constructive change (Erickson, 1959; Short et al., 2016). Participants learn to develop verbal and nonverbal, direct and indirect suggestions, and co-create images and metaphors in the context of their actual clients/patients. Rather than setting up a prescriptive hypnotic ritual as a distinct part of the therapy session, trainees begin to appreciate the hypnotic suggestion as seamlessly embedded in the ongoing conversation. They learn to expand on an already existing state of absorption to direct this moment of openness and plasticity toward novel, personally meaningful problem-solving and mind-body healing (Rossi et al., 2008; Rossi, 2003).

Increasing familiarity and safety with entering and exiting their own trance states allows trainees to own their experiences of absorption and to appreciate the internal decision-making process about how to respond to an offered direct or indirect suggestion, letting go of fear-based, rigid control, and allowing a useful trance to progress. Trainees recognize that trance is a fluid process, developed collaboratively and creatively – an intra- and interpersonal phenomenon built on developing trust and connection, and more patient-centered than clinician-centered (Baker & Spiegel, 2019). It is attuned to work with a person, not with an agenda, devoid of performance and pass-fail anxieties. Therefore, destructive dissociative attunement (the reenactment of fear-based interaction rules, for example, submission and pleasing) or co-dependency between participants can change in favor of collaborative inter-dependency between equals (Hopenwasser, 2008; Lyons-Ruth, 1999; Tronick et al., 1998).

The hypnotic skills trainees develop as a base for any formal trance elicitation consist in recognizing and creatively responding to signs of absorption/trance and offering a surprising, empowering, and sometimes delightful new perspective on how to disrupt old patterns in favor of moving forward. A non-authoritarian stance – truly not knowing where the recipient of a suggestion will/not take the process – frees both clinician-trainee and their peer-client/patient from any pressure to obtain preordained outcomes, and instead allows them to stay attuned and curious about the developing individual resources (Sugarman et al., 2020).

Teaching Formal Hypnotic Elicitations in Small Group Practices

Trainees (and patients) are interested in formal elicitations of hypnosis. A small group learning environment of 6–7 trainees allows for the practice of established formal hypnotic routines to create novelty, surprise, and wonderment about the power of the human mind-body to affect as yet unknown possibilities for desired change. They offer hope. The model of training described here approaches the formal practices within the paradigm of attuned collaboration, respect for, and curiosity about, the individual's process, a non-evaluative, non-performative, no-fail, psychologically safe environment, without any notion of predetermined outcomes.

The small practice groups, assembled randomly, stay together for all two-hour practices, while faculty moves on after the second practice, so groups can sample different teaching styles. Faculty and group members are already known to each other from previous interactions in lectures and attunement practices, noticeably reducing the number of unknowns and the degree of apprehension.

At the time trainees head to their first small group practice, they are already well-prepared to enter and exit light trance experiences (Howard, 2017). They have observed demonstrations of conversational and formal trance elicitations, and have interacted with each other in an attuned way. They have developed understanding, tolerance, and curiosity for the necessary and intentional unpredictability of a hypnotically guided trance experience, and the collaborative nature of developing a more formal trance experience. They understand that the nature of the formal trance state their fellow trainee decides to engage in is not a statement of success or failure about the facilitator or subject, but a statement about their level of attunement with each other, as the subject has full ownership and autonomy over their trance experience. They have practiced attuning to themselves in the process of offering trance as well, striving to embody readiness to co-regulate and convey a calm confidence about giving care and consideration facilitated by hypnosis (Butler & Randall, 2013). All members of the group learn together, in turn taking on the roles of facilitator, subject of the invited trance as an option, and observer, jointly creating a safe enough holding environment as a forum for joint discovery.

Faculty contributes to the holding environment by encouraging each trainee's autonomy in finding their own way of responding to each other in the process of generating a useful state of absorption. By the last small group practice, group members demonstrate their implicit relational knowing of each other's mental states, gained through time spent consciously and unconsciously attuning to each other (Tronick, 2007).

A subject's embodied or verbalized self-protection is anticipated and welcomed as an important message that guides the process of collaborative discovery of the subject's best interests. For example, a trainee, given the suggestion that an arm may feel lighter and float upward, may report that the arm instead feels weighted down and won't move at all, a response met with the same acceptance and curiosity, as if an arm levitation had occurred. Therefore, demand for compliance with a scripted procedure, a preordained outcome, or covert power struggles is avoided. All responses are equally valid. Control remains with the subject of the invited trance. The competencies demonstrated in the interaction lie solely in the attuned, flexible, and open-minded utilization of what is transpiring. This is a jointly generated success of attunement, independent of any quantifiable hypnotic phenomena.

Following this model of training, untoward abreactions during a hypnotic experience – a serious concern with standard hypnosis trainings (Kluft, 2012a, 2012b) – have been minimized. The collaborative practices in this model have led to increased cohesion of the small groups and a robust holding environment with adequate support for the processing of regularly occurring emotional experiences (Winnicott, 1991). These authentic expressions of internal processes facilitated by hypnosis are treated as valuable real-life contributions to the integration of the trainees' emerging hypnosis skills into their clinical practice.

Instead of the threat of losing control over the process of inviting and accepting trance, trainees feel empowered to trust their own process, readiness, and freedom of choice. They gain the invaluable lesson that therapeutic hypnosis is not about loss of power, undue influence, and submission to a standard protocol of expected hypnotic phenomena, but that it offers the corrective and healing experience of self-determination, autonomy, and agency in collaboration with another human being in the service of changing one's mind in a chosen beneficial direction. Negotiating the power of clinical hypnosis therefore can be experienced as therapeutic, a concept the trainees can take to their patients.

Because small group practices are intense experiences for all involved, they are scheduled early enough in the day to leave ample time for processing and sharing general reflections by the whole group before dispersing for the evening. In this way, the process moves from experiencing, to cognitive processing, to joint sharing of observations, to the internalization of new learnings. Participants are asked to ascertain their regular level of alertness and emotional comfort before leaving the training for the day. They are encouraged to seek faculty support if necessary to process any unresolved experience from the training privately in order to regain their equilibrium. This level of support and holding allows the training to proceed smoothly.

Attunement and care for each participant before, during, and after the training result in group cohesion and an interpersonally and relationally predictable and safe holding environment (Winnicott, 1960). The building of rapport throughout the training is not a checked-off technicality, but a continuously demonstrated effort, conducive to learning and experiencing the challenges and the benefits of a training in clinical hypnosis in a state of mind-body regulation (Selvam, 2022). Feeling supported, grounded, and emotionally connected enables trainees to access their creativity and flexibility in relating to each other, allowing for playfulness and delight as part of the learning process.

Reinhild Draeger-Muenke

A Vision for the Future of Training in Clinical Hypnosis

Clinical hypnosis has been called the oldest form of biopsychosocial therapy (De Benedittis, 2021). It bridges many fields and has immense applicability. Education in clinical hypnosis deserves to become a must for professionals of all backgrounds who are interested in person-centered care for their diverse patients, including those who have been traumatized. Trainees deserve to be taught how to readily and unbiasedly integrate clinical hypnosis into many different clinical settings. Training in clinical hypnosis deserves to be an empowering and joyful experience for the training faculty and the trainees. In order for this to happen, the delivery of content and process needs to respect the clinician-trainees' existing competencies in their respective fields as well as their adaptive Window of Tolerance for challenge and intensity. To achieve no-fail hypnotic interactions, it will be important to forgo strict adherence to established hypnosis protocols for the elicitation of prescribed hypnotic phenomena in favor of collaborative attunement/entrancement toward a desired mind-change – the wider opening of everybody's Window of Welcome. When the joint creation of neurobiologically felt safety in hypnosis trainings becomes the new standard of training, hypnosis will have gained an important opportunity to hold a prominent place in many trainees' clinical repertoire and practice.

References

Alter, D. S., & Sugarman, L. I. (2017). Reorienting hypnosis education. *The American Journal of Clinical Hypnosis*, *59*(3), 235–259. 10.1080/00029157.2016.1231657

Azoulay, E., Cariou, A., Bruneel, F., Demoule, A., Kouatchet, A., Reuter, D., Souppart, V., Combes, A., Klouche, K., Argaud, L., Barbier, F., Jourdain, M., Reignier, J., Papazian, L., Guidet, B., Géri, G., Resche-Rigon, M., Guisset, O., Labbé, V., ...Kentish-Barnes, N. (2020). Symptoms of anxiety, depression, and peritraumatic dissociation in critical care clinicians managing patients with COVID-19. A cross-sectional study. *American Journal of Respiratory and Critical Care Medicine*, *202*(10), 1388–1398. 10.1164/rccm.202006-2568OC

Baker, E. L., & Spiegel, E. B. (2019). Dancing in the in-between: Hypnosis, transitional space, and therapeutic action. *American Journal of Clinical Hypnosis*, *62*(1–2), 31–59. 10.1080/00029157.2019.1585328

Banks, A., & Hirschman, L. A. (2016). *Wired to connect: The surprising link between brain science and strong, healthy relationships* (First trade paperback edition). Jeremy P. Tarcher/Penguin.

Bányai, É. I. (1998). The interactive nature of hypnosis: Research evidence for a social-psychobiological model. *Contemporary Hypnosis*, *15*(1), 52–63. 10.1002/ch.116

Beere, D. B., Simon, M. J., & Welch, K. (2001). Recommendations and illustrations for combining hypnosis and EMDR in the treatment of psychological trauma. *American Journal of Clinical Hypnosis*, *43*(3–4), 217–231. 10.1080/00029157.2001.10404278

Beerkens, R., Le Pichon- Vorstman, E., Supheert, R., & Thije, J. D. ten (Eds.). (2020). *Enhancing intercultural communication in organizations: Insights from project advisers*. Routledge.

Benau, K. (2022). *Shame, pride, and relational trauma: Concepts and psychotherapy*. Routledge.

Bloom, B. S. (Ed.). (1956). *Taxonomy of educational objectives: The classification of educational goals. Handbook 1, Cognitive domain; by a committee of college and university examiners; Benjamin S. Bloom, editor [and others]* (1st ed.). Longman Group.

Bordin, E. S. (1979). The generalizability of the psychoanalytic concept of the working alliance. *Psychotherapy: Theory, Research & Practice*, *16*(3), 252–260. 10.1037/h0085885

Bowlby, J. (1985). *Attachment and loss. 2: Separation: anxiety and anger* (3. impr). Hogarth Press.

Bradbury, N. A. (2016). Attention span during lectures: 8 seconds, 10 minutes, or more? *Advances in Physiology Education*, *40*(4), 509–513. 10.1152/advan.00109.2016

Butler, E. A., & Randall, A. K. (2013). Emotional coregulation in close relationships. *Emotion Review*, *5*(2), 202–210. 10.1177/1754073912451630

Clark, T. R. (2020). *The 4 stages of psychological safety: Defining the path to inclusion and innovation* (1st ed.). Berrett-Koehler Publishers, Inc.
Craparo, G., Cocco Ortu, F., & Hart, O. van der (Eds.). (2019). *Rediscovering Pierre Janet: Trauma, dissociation, and a new context for psychoanalysis*. Routledge.
Cravens, A. E., Jones, M. S., Ngai, C., Zarestky, J., & Love, H. B. (2022). Science facilitation: Navigating the intersection of intellectual and interpersonal expertise in scientific collaboration. *Humanities and Social Sciences Communications*, *9*(1), 256. 10.1057/s41599-022-01217-1
Creasey, G., Jarvis, P., & Gadke, D. (2009). Student attachment stances, instructor immediacy, and student–instructor relationships as predictors of achievement expectancies in college students. *Journal of College Student Development*, *50*(4), 353–372. 10.1353/csd.0.0082
Dalenberg, C. J. (2000). *Countertransference and the treatment of trauma* (1st ed). American Psychological Association.
Dana, D. (2018). *The polyvagal theory in therapy: Engaging the rhythm of regulation* (1st ed.). W.W. Norton & Company.
De Benedittis, G. (2021). Neurophysiology and neuropsychology of hypnosis. *American Journal of Clinical Hypnosis*, *63*(4), 291–293. 10.1080/00029157.2021.1892411
Dell, P. F. (2017). What is the essence of hypnosis? *International Journal of Clinical and Experimental Hypnosis*, *65*(2), 162–168. 10.1080/00207144.2017.1276360
Dell, P. F. (2019). Reconsidering the autohypnotic model of the dissociative disorders. *Journal of Trauma & Dissociation: The Official Journal of the International Society for the Study of Dissociation (ISSD)*, *20*(1), 48–78. 10.1080/15299732.2018.1451806
Dell, P. F. (2021). Hypnotizability and the natural human ability to alter experience. *International Journal of Clinical and Experimental Hypnosis*, *69*(1), 7–26. 10.1080/00207144.2021.1834859
Devendorf, A., & Victor, S. E. (2022). Psychologists are starting to talk publicly about their own mental illnesses – and patients can benefit4. *The Conversation*. https://theconversation.com/psychologists-are-starting-to-talk-publicly-about-their-own-mental-illnesses-and-patients-can-benefit-177716
Doidge, N. (2015). Hypnosis, neuroplasticity, and the plastic paradox. *American Journal of Clinical Hypnosis*, *57*(3), 349–354. 10.1080/00029157.2015.985572
Dweck, C. S. (2008). *Mindset: The new psychology of success* (Ballantine Books trade pbk. ed). Ballantine Books.
Eccles, J. C. (1973). *The understanding of the brain: Based on the 33d series of lectures on the Patten Foundation delivered at the Bloomington Campus, Indiana University*. McGraw-Hill.
Elkins, G. R., & Hammond, D. C. (1998). Standards of training in clinical hypnosis: Preparing professionals for the 21st century. *American Journal of Clinical Hypnosis*, *41*(1), 55–64. 10.1080/00029157.1998.10404185
Erickson, M. H. (1959). Further clinical techniques of hypnosis: Utilization techniques. *American Journal of Clinical Hypnosis*, *2*(1), 3–21. 10.1080/00029157.1959.10401792
Fine, C. G., & Berkowitz, A. S. (2001). The wreathing protocol: The imbrication of hypnosis and EMDR in the treatment of dissociative identity disorder and other dissociative responses. *American Journal of Clinical Hypnosis*, *43*(3–4), 275–290. 10.1080/00029157.2001.10404282
Flemons, D. G. (2022). *The heart and mind of hypnotherapy: Inviting connection, inventing change* (1st ed.). W. W. Norton & Company.
Geri, N., Winer, A., & Zaks, B. (2017). Challenging the six-minute myth of online video lectures: Can interactivity expand the attention span of learners? *Online Journal of Applied Knowledge Management*, *5*(1), 101–111. 10.36965/OJAKM.2017.5(1)101-111
Gilligan, S. (2002). EMDR and hypnosis. In F. Shapiro (Ed.), *EMDR as an integrative psychotherapy approach: Experts of diverse orientations explore the paradigm prism.* (pp. 225–238). American Psychological Association. 10.1037/10512-009
Green, J. P., & Lynn, S. J. (2010). Hypnotic responsiveness: *Expectancy, attitudes, fantasy proneness, absorption, and gender. International Journal of Clinical and Experimental Hypnosis*, *59*(1), 103–121. 10.1080/00207144.2011.522914
Hawkins, J. A. (2021). The discovery and implications of neuroplasticity. In J. A. Hawkins (Ed.), *Brain plasticity and learning* (pp. 1–36). Springer International Publishing. 10.1007/978-3-030-83530-9_1

Hilgard, E. R. (1962). Motivation in learning theory. In S. Koch (Ed.), *Psychology: A study of a science. Study II: Empirical substructure and relations with other sciences. Volume 5. The process areas, the person, and some applied fields: Their place in psychology and in science.* (pp. 253–283). McGraw-Hill. 10.1037/10040-005

Hilgard, E. R., Marquis, D. G., & Kimble, G. A. (n.d.). *Conditioning and learning*. Prentice-Hall.

Hope, A. E., & Sugarman, L. I. (2015). Orienting hypnosis. *American Journal of Clinical Hypnosis*, *57*(3), 212–229. 10.1080/00029157.2014.976787

Hopenwasser, K. (2008). Being in rhythm: Dissociative attunement in therapeutic process. *Journal of Trauma & Dissociation*, *9*(3), 349–367. 10.1080/15299730802139212

Howard, H. A. (2017). Promoting safety in hypnosis: A clinical instrument for the assessment of alertness. *American Journal of Clinical Hypnosis*, *59*(4), 344–362. 10.1080/00029157.2016.1203281

Jha, A. (2021). *Peak mind: Optimizing your performance, productivity and purpose with the new science of attention: Find your focus, own your attention, invest 12 minutes a day*. Piatkus.

Kluft, R. P. (2012a). Issues in the detection of those suffering adverse effects in hypnosis training workshops. *American Journal of Clinical Hypnosis*, *54*(3), 213–232. 10.1080/00029157.2011.631228

Kluft, R. P. (2012b). Approaches to difficulties in realerting subjects from hypnosis. *American Journal of Clinical Hypnosis*, *55*(2), 140–159. 10.1080/00029157.2012.660891

Kumar, S. A., Brand, B. L., & Courtois, C. A. (2022). The need for trauma training: Clinicians' reactions to training on complex trauma. *Psychological Trauma: Theory, Research, Practice, and Policy*, *14*(8), 1387–1394. 10.1037/tra0000515

Lankton, S. R., & Zeig, J. (Eds.). (2013). *Difficult contexts for therapy Ericksonian monographs No.* (0 ed.). Routledge. 10.4324/9780203777251

Linden, J. H., & Anbar, R. (2017). Hypnosis training and education: Distinctive features of training hypnosis educators. *American Journal of Clinical Hypnosis*, *59*(3), 260–275. 10.1080/00029157.2016.1225253

Loewenstein, R. J. (1993). Dissociation, development, and the psychobiology of trauma. *Journal of the American Academy of Psychoanalysis*, *21*(4), 581–603. 10.1521/jaap.1.1993.21.4.581

Lubliner, S., & Grisham, D. L. (2017). *Translanguaging: The key to comprehension for Spanish-speaking students and their peers*. Rowman & Littlefield.

Lynn, S. J., Rhue, J. W., & Kirsch, I. (Eds.). (2010). *Handbook of clinical hypnosis*. American Psychological Association. 10.2307/j.ctv1chs5qj

Lyons-Ruth, K. (1999). The two-person unconscious: Intersubjective dialogue, enactive relational representation, and the emergence of new forms of relational organization. *Psychoanalytic Inquiry*, *19*(4), 576–617. 10.1080/07351699909534267

Marmarosh, C. L. (2021). Ruptures and repairs in group psychotherapy: From theory to practice. *International Journal of Group Psychotherapy*, *71*(2), 205–223. 10.1080/00207284.2020.1855893

Martin, F., Wang, C., & Sadaf, A. (2020). Facilitation matters: Instructor perception of helpfulness of facilitation strategies in online courses. *Online Learning*, *24*(1). 10.24059/olj.v24i1.1980

Matthews, W. J., Lankton, S., & Lankton, C. (1993). An Ericksonian model of hypnotherapy. In J. W. Rhue, S. J. Lynn, & I. Kirsch (Eds.), *Handbook of clinical hypnosis*. (pp. 187–214). American Psychological Association. 10.1037/10274-009

Mena, J. A. (2022). Social justice pedagogy: Diversity, equity, and inclusion in the teaching of psychology. *Teaching of Psychology*, 009862832211306. 10.1177/00986283221130697

Merians, A. N., Spiller, T., Harpaz-Rotem, I., Krystal, J. H., & Pietrzak, R. H. (2023). Post-traumatic stress disorder. *Medical Clinics of North America*, *107*(1), 85–99. 10.1016/j.mcna.2022.04.003

Milling, L. S. (2012). The Spanos attitudes toward hypnosis questionnaire: Psychometric characteristics and normative data. *American Journal of Clinical Hypnosis*, *54*(3), 202–212. 10.1080/00029157.2011.631229

Modestin, J., Lötscher, K., & Erni, T. (2002). Dissociative experiences and their correlates in young non-patients. *Psychology and Psychotherapy: Theory, Research and Practice*, *75*(1), 53–64. 10.1348/147608302169544

Montgomery, G. H., Sucala, M., Dillon, M. J., & Schnur, J. B. (2018). Interest and attitudes about hypnosis in a large community sample. *Psychology of Consciousness: Theory, Research, and Practice*, *5*(2), 212–220. 10.1037/cns0000141

Neff, K. D. (2011). Self-compassion, self-esteem, and well-being. *Social and Personality Psychology Compass*, *5*(1), 1–12. 10.1111/j.1751-9004.2010.00330.x
Nemeth, D., Janacsek, K., Polner, B., & Kovacs, Z. A. (2013). Boosting human learning by hypnosis. *Cerebral Cortex*, *23*(4), 801–805. 10.1093/cercor/bhs068
Nicolaides, A., & Poell, R. F. (2020). "The only option Is failure": Growing safe to fail workplaces for critical reflection. *Advances in Developing Human Resources*, *22*(3), 264–277. 10.1177/1523422320927296
Ogden, P. (2015). *Sensorimotor psychotherapy: Interventions for trauma and attachment* (1st ed.). W.W. Norton & Company.
Otani, A. (2016). Hypnosis and mindfulness: The twain finally meet. *American Journal of Clinical Hypnosis*, *58*(4), 383–398. 10.1080/00029157.2015.1085364
Payne, P., Levine, P. A., & Crane-Godreau, M. A. (2015). Somatic experiencing: Using interoception and proprioception as core elements of trauma therapy. *Frontiers in Psychology*, *6*. 10.3389/fpsyg.2015.00093
Peebles, M. J. (2012). *Beginnings, second edition*. Routledge. 10.4324/9780203846155
Peebles, M. J. (2018). Harm in hypnosis: Three understandings from psychoanalysis that can help. *American Journal of Clinical Hypnosis*, *60*(3), 239–261. 10.1080/00029157.2018.1400811
Peebles-kleiger, M. J. (2001). Contemporary psychoanalysis and hypnosis. *International Journal of Clinical and Experimental Hypnosis*, *49*(2), 146–165. 10.1080/00207140108410065
Pert, C. B. (2003). *Molecules of emotion: Why you feel the way you feel*. Scribner.
Peyton, S., & Badenoch, B. (2017). *Your resonant self: Guided meditations and exercises to engage your brain's capacity for healing* (1st ed.). W.W Norton & Company.
Porges, S. W. (2003). The polyvagal theory: Phylogenetic contributions to social behavior. *Physiology & Behavior*, *79*(3), 503–513. 10.1016/S0031-9384(03)00156-2
Porges, S. W. (2022). Polyvagal theory: A science of safety. *Frontiers in Integrative Neuroscience*, *16*, 871227. 10.3389/fnint.2022.871227
Prasad, G., Auger, N., & Le Pichon-Vorstman, E. (Eds.). (2022). *Multilingualism and education: Researchers' pathways and perspectives*. Cambridge University Press.
Putnam, F. W. (1989). Pierre Janet and modern views of dissociation. *Journal of Traumatic Stress*, *2*(4), 413–429. 10.1002/jts.2490020406
Rossi, E., Erickson-Klein, R., & Rossi, K. (2008). Novel activity-dependent approaches to therapeutic hypnosis and psychotherapy: The general waking trance. *American Journal of Clinical Hypnosis*, *51*(2), 185–200. 10.1080/00029157.2008.10401664
Rossi, E. L. (2003). Gene expression, neurogenesis, and healing: Psychosocial genomics of therapeutic hypnosis. *American Journal of Clinical Hypnosis*, *45*(3), 197–216. 10.1080/00029157.2003.10403526
Sansbury, B. S., Graves, K., & Scott, W. (2015). Managing traumatic stress responses among clinicians: Individual and organizational tools for self-care. *Trauma*, *17*(2), 114–122. 10.1177/1460408614551978
Sapp, M. (2016). Hypnosis and postmodernism: Multicultural applications. *Sleep and Hypnosis – International Journal*, 19–25. 10.5350/Sleep.Hypn.2016.180104
Schore, A. N. (1996). The experience-dependent maturation of a regulatory system in the orbital prefrontal cortex and the origin of developmental psychopathology. *Development and Psychopathology*, *8*(1), 59–87. 10.1017/S0954579400006970
Schore, A. N. (2002). Advances in neuropsychoanalysis, attachment theory, and trauma research: Implications for self psychology. *Psychoanalytic Inquiry*, 22(3), 433–484. 10.1080/07351692209348996
Schore, A. N. (2014). The right brain is dominant in psychotherapy. *Psychotherapy*, *51*(3), 388–397. 10.1037/a0037083
Selvam, R. (2022). *The practice of embodying emotions: A guide for improving cognitive, emotional, and behavioral outcomes*. North Atlantic Books.
Short, S., Erickson, B. A., & Erickson-Klein, R. (2016). *Hope & resiliency: Understanding the psychotherapeutic strategies of Milton H. Erickson, MD* (Published in paperback). Crown House Publishing.
Siegel, D. J. (1999). *The developing mind: How relationships and the brain interact to shape who we are*. Guilford Press.

Siegel, D. J. (2012). *Pocket guide to interpersonal neurobiology: An integrative handbook of the mind* (1st ed). W. W. Norton & Co.

Siegel, D. J., Schore, A. N., & Cozolino, L. J. (Eds.). (2021). *Interpersonal neurobiology and clinical practice*. W.W. Norton & Company.

Spiegel, E. B., & Baker, E. L. (2019). The generative presence of relatedness. *American Journal of Clinical Hypnosis*, *62*(1–2), 1–11. 10.1080/00029157.2019.1609840

Sugarman, L. I., Linden, J. H., & Brooks, L. W. (2020). *Changing minds with clinical hypnosis: Narratives and discourse for a new health care paradigm*. Routledge.

Tasca, G. A., & Marmarosh, C. (2023). Alliance rupture and repair in group psychotherapy. In C. F. Eubanks, L. W. Samstag, & J. C. Muran (Eds.), *Rupture and repair in psychotherapy: A critical process for change*. (pp. 53–71). American Psychological Association. 10.1037/0000306-003

Tovar-Moll, F., & Lent, R. (2016). The various forms of neuroplasticity: Biological bases of learning and teaching. *PROSPECTS*, *46*(2), 199–213. 10.1007/s11125-017-9388-7

Tronick, E. (2007). *The neurobehavioral and social-emotional development of infants and children* (1st ed). W. W. Norton & Co.

Tronick, E. Z., Bruschweiler-Stern, N., Harrison, A. M., Lyons-Ruth, K., Morgan, A. C., Nahum, J. P., Sander, L., & Stern, D. N. (1998). Dyadically expanded states of consciousness and the process of therapeutic change. *Infant Mental Health Journal*, *19*(3), 290–299. 10.1002/(SICI)1097-0355(199823)19:3<290::AID-IMHJ4>3.0.CO;2-Q

Van der Kolk, B. A. (2015). *The Body keeps the score: Brain, mind and body in the healing of trauma*. Penguin Books.

Varga, K. (2021). Possible mechanisms of hypnosis from an interactional perspective. *Brain Sciences*, *11*(7), 903. 10.3390/brainsci11070903

Victor, S. E., Devendorf, A., Lewis, S., Rottenberg, J., Muehlenkamp, J. J., Stage, D. L., & Miller, R. (2021). *Only human: Mental health difficulties among clinical, counseling, and school psychology faculty and trainees* [Preprint]. PsyArXiv. 10.31234/osf.io/xbfr6

Voss, P., Thomas, M. E., Cisneros-Franco, J. M., & de Villers-Sidani, É. (2017). Dynamic brains and the changing rules of neuroplasticity: Implications for learning and recovery. *Frontiers in Psychology*, *8*, 1657. 10.3389/fpsyg.2017.01657

Walker, N. (2021). *Neuroqueer heresies: Notes on the neurodiversity paradigm, autistic empowerment, and postnormal possibilities*. Autonomous Press.

Wark, D., & Kohen, D. P. (1998). Facilitating facilitators' facilitation: Experience with a model for teaching leaders of hypnosis practice groups. *American Journal of Clinical Hypnosis*, *41*(1), 75–83. 10.1080/00029157.1998.10404187

Watkins, J. G. (1998). Training in clinical hypnosis, a historical perspective: The Montana experience. *American Journal of Clinical Hypnosis*, *41*(1), 10–17. 10.1080/00029157.1998.10404181

Willyard, C. (2012). *Need to heal thyself?* https://www.apa.org/gradpsych/2012/01/heal

Winnicott, D. (1960). *Holding and containing*. UK Essays. https://www.ukessays.com/essays/psychology/holding-and-containing-winnicott.php?vref=1

Winnicott, D. W. (1991). *Human nature* (Reprint). Free Association Books.

Yapko, M. D. (2011). *Mindfulness and hypnosis: The power of suggestion to transform experience* (1st ed). Norton.

Yapko, M. D. (2012). *Trancework: An introduction to the practice of clinical hypnosis* (4th ed). Routledge/Taylor & Francis Group.

Yapko, M. D. (2018). *Taking hypnosis to the next level: Valuable tips for enhancing your clinical practice*. Yapko Publications.

Yapko, M. D., Barretta, N. P., & Barretta, P. F. (1998). Clinical training in Ericksonian hypnosis. *American Journal of Clinical Hypnosis*, *41*(1), 18–28. 10.1080/00029157.1998.10404182

59

PROFESSIONAL TRAINING AND DEVELOPMENT IN PEDIATRIC HYPNOSIS

What We Have Learned and How to Make It Better

Daniel P. Kohen

National Pediatric Hypnosis Training Institute, Golden Valley, MN, USA

This chapter reviews the history of and the creation of current standards for hypnosis education both in the USA and in other parts of the world. My personal background as a pediatrician and medical educator in this field spans more than 50 years. As such, it is integral to an understanding and development of the education described. Further, this introspection upon my development is a manifestation of my pediatric training and awareness. I have been successfully conditioned to give particular attention to how life experiences traversing developmental imperatives inform our work and perspective. In retracing these personal experiences, I have realized the ways in which they informed the content and style of my teaching, and, of course, my professional growth as clinician and educator. In short, this chapter is largely and necessarily autobiographical.

But a value of autobiography is in its familiarity. I expect that these reflections and connections to my work will allow the reader to similarly reflect. It is essential that our therapeutic work – and especially hypnotic work – centers upon our respective and individual paths across our lifespan (see also the chapter on Developmental Perspectives, Chapter 13 in this volume) As a general pediatrician and developmental-behavioral pediatrics specialist I learned to explain how I did what I did from those I taught. They required that introspection. That process, in turn, directed the evolution of the teaching, and so on.

Therefore, I ask the reader to please bear with the autobiographical aspects of this chapter. My intention is to clarify for myself and explicate for this chapter the ways in which experiential opportunities brought me to the hypnosis education and models described. The first one-quarter of the introduction includes an integration of this autobiographical odyssey. It includes a description of becoming aware that the word "Doctor" *means* teacher, whereas physician means healer. I wanted to be both. I learned early on that I had to teach. This is followed by becoming a teacher, what it entailed, and how it felt.

The Introduction flows into discussion and description of hypnosis learning, teaching, curricular development, and the theoretical focus underpinning our evolving 35-year curriculum. This is followed by an account of the evolution of hypnosis training curriculum

DOI: 10.4324/9781003449126-77

and its current status. The phenomenology within the curriculum is discussed and is followed by new research, perspectives, and applications. We conclude with the increasing therapeutic relevance of the future of training and education, with recommendations for how and what we hope it will become.

Introduction

All pediatric medical interns and pediatric residents teach the medical students and junior residents for whom they are responsible. For my part, I thought then that I was pretty sure that I knew what I knew, and what I didn't know. The only guides I had for teaching others were, of course, my own experiences as a learner. Those were in the categories of "good, "bad," and "I never thought about it much before." There were my own teachers and mentors. I knew and revered those that were good. Sadly, many I knew to be lousy. Thankfully some were outstanding. What made them outstanding? Besides being clearly wise and experienced clinicians, these truly wonderful mentors *listened and attended to my learning needs*. While they were conversant with the professional literature that supported and guided what we needed to know, *they tailored their teaching to my abilities to learn*.

In retrospect, I have come to honor and respectfully consider their greatest gifts to me were that they were *superior role models*. As I ponder my own development, I realize that these mentors reflected in language, deed, and clinical behavior the "do what I do and how I do it," usually without saying it *per se*, but by "just" doing it. They did it confidently, competently, kindly, efficiently, respectfully, and effectively. They did so easily, willingly, and patiently, always anticipating and answering questions that naturally arose.

Early conscious awareness of this process grew in me. As I received feedback from my mentors and my students, I came to increasingly appreciate the nuances of the educational experiences from a developing teacher's perspective. These included teaching to a small group while "making bedside rounds" and then retiring to a consultation room to discuss personal patient issues privately. They also included the nuanced differences of one-to-one review with a student-clinician or resident, and review and critique of "write-ups" of clinical cases for the patient's medical records. While this type of teaching and learning forms the background of all occupational education, especially in health care, I realize that its nuances were moving to the foreground for me.

As a U.S. Public Health Service physician in the Indian Health Service from 1971 to 1978, this experience of teaching matured in the "real life" of third-world medicine. Many visiting students and physicians-in-training came through our Navajo Nation Indian Hospital (Fort Defiance, Arizona, USA) for several months at a time, and their "on-the-job-training" from our medical staff as the teachers became the norm. As a result, I was able to attend to the conduct of our indigenous Navajo colleague nurses, X-ray technicians, lab technicians, medical records personnel, and pharmacists, notably learning from the ways they related to the nearly 100% indigenous patients.

There were also health care professionals from indigenous tribes other than Navajo. I had some measure of cross-cultural learning from these colleagues. As an Anglo (White) doctor, the language barriers and learning to understand common non-verbal behaviors were myriad. In time my indigenous colleague nurses and other interpreters helped me immeasurably to learn and manage the cross-cultural challenges. This was particularly true when patients/families spoke little to no English. Particularly challenging were the children from very traditional homes who had been taught not to speak much, if at all, with adults. Efficient use of time, sharing of knowledge, and effective, economical use of language were integral to their learning and our learning, teaching, and providing care. In the development of my own clinical and cross-cultural teaching skill development, attention to what, when, and how I said things – and when to be quiet – proved to be essential elements in the evolution of our hypnosis training program.

Especially important were the daily and often intense personal learning from very patient nurse interpreters with whom I and colleague physicians worked very closely. During interim years in the Indian Health Service, I completed my pediatric residency and was asked to be Chief Pediatric Resident at the University of Oklahoma's Oklahoma Children's Memorial Hospital in Oklahoma City, Oklahoma, USA. This opportunity and responsibility to develop, coordinate, and implement medical student, intern, and resident pediatric education was a welcome challenge. I worked closely with the Director of Education, a kind, bright, and innovative mentor and role model. This leadership role furthered my continued growth and commitment to concepts of therapeutic communication that were integral to our education programs.

In the late 1970s, I became the Associate Director of Medical Education at the Minneapolis Children's Medical Center in Minneapolis, Minnesota, with a concurrent faculty appointment in the University of Minnesota Departments of Pediatrics and Family Practice. This all-encompassing role included seeing my own patients, while developing, coordinating, and creating learning experiences (e.g., Grand Rounds) for medical students, interns, and residents in pediatrics, family medicine, and community health. Early on I participated in a three-day Workshop on "Teaching Teachers of Family Medicine How to Teach," developed and implemented by the Department of Family Practice. It was challenging and inspiring. In retrospect, I realize that this experience firmly set me on the path that I would embrace, utilize, and teach for the rest of my professional career.

Along with a foundation in learning theory, the essence of the workshop was for each participant to develop and teach a brief lesson to other participants. My recollection is that it was limited to 15 minutes and, most notably, it was to be videorecorded. After teaching a group of four or five others, each presenter then met privately with a pre-determined mentor to privately review the video of their presentation in order to discuss and critique both the content and the style. My chosen topic was "Teaching Self-Hypnosis" to a client (s)/patient(s). It was an eye-opening experience, and the mentor's feedback was immeasurably formative and influential.

In the year prior to this experience, I had participated in my first two workshops in clinical hypnosis, both while still working on the Navajo Reservation in Northeastern Arizona. Under the auspices of the American Society of Clinical Hypnosis (in 1977 and 1978), these workshops were general Introductory and general Intermediate level workshops (i.e., not pediatric); and featured the finest clinical teachers whom I came to revere, notably Dr Bob Pearson (a psychiatrist who had been a general practitioner for ten years before becoming a psychiatrist) and Dr Kay Thompson (a dentist and psychotherapist). Soon thereafter I was invited to be a sit-in-with-another faculty small-group facilitator at the annual hypnosis workshops of the Minnesota Society of Clinical Hypnosis (MSCH). The role-modeling which ensued intensified the learning in our small groups. Together we explored the language of teaching and learning hypnosis. In the months and years ahead I became a regular member of the MSCH Faculty, began giving the hour-long introduction to Pediatric Hypnosis presentation, and eventually became the Director of Education and

Training for MSCH, which position I maintained for 35 years, developing and coordinating Annual Introductory and Advanced Workshops, and monthly seminars.

Along the way my close friend and esteemed colleague, David Wark, PhD, and I developed an eight-hour training for small group leaders, titled "Facilitating Facilitators' Facilitation" (FFF), to teach the teachers how to teach the small group practice sessions during workshops (Wark & Kohen, 1998). Soon thereafter, we continued our collaboration and developed the "spiral curriculum" as a methodology for teaching, especially introductory workshops in clinical hypnosis, and implemented and regularly modified in nuanced fashion through the annual Workshops of the Minnesota Society of Clinical Hypnosis (Wark & Kohen, 2002). Later, after the emergence of the National Pediatric Hypnosis Training Institute (2010, see below), we modified the FFF training to be a good fit for training future faculty for small group leaders in *pediatric* hypnosis workshop offerings; and also adapted the spiral curriculum methodology to our National Pediatric Hypnosis Training Institute (NPHTI) hypnosis workshops.

For the last couple of decades, I have focused upon teaching child health clinicians about and "how to do" pediatric hypnosis. This grew out of considerable experience in curriculum development. It also arose from teaching both pre-professional health care students and practicing clinicians in both general pediatric health care and adult clinical hypnosis. Accordingly, the following speaks from that experience while also submitting and reinforcing that this model transfers quite readily – for reasons that I hope will become evident below to those who primarily teach and work with hypnosis with adult students, patients, and clients (see also Developmental Perspectives, Chapter 13 in this volume).

Theoretical Framework

The theoretical framework for this chapter focuses upon a belief and understanding that spontaneous hypnosis is all around us. By hypnosis we mean a state of focused attention and absorbed attention, occurring or evolving spontaneously or upon invitation and/or guidance. Some have called the latter "an induction." With decades of working with developing human beings (children, teens, parents, grandparents!), we have abandoned the word "induction." We explain to pediatric patients, families, and colleague learners that hypnosis is "a state or feeling like when you are pretending, daydreaming, imagining, or 'zoning out.'" As clinicians and teachers of our patients and their families, it is our task to recognize and acknowledge this presence of hypnosis. We facilitate its utilization by the patient and family. And, we teach our colleagues and other learners and teachers *how* to do this.

Orientation

The orientation of the subject matter which follows is within the larger established domain(s) of science and health care. It includes, for example, a focus on the *intrinsic mechanisms of hypnosis,* notably what I (and our NPHTI teaching faculty) have come to understand as a focus upon *the cultivation of imagination.* Moreover, it emphasizes the importance of the orientation of the clinician to ways of characterizing, defining, and teaching about hypnosis. In so doing the intention is to meet the wide variety of needs, misconceptions, and myths of the learners (clinicians) and their patients (children and adults alike).

Second, our focus in education is not only upon the oriented *what and how* but also upon the *applications of hypnosis.* In consideration of what we must teach, it is essential to convey the wide scope and breadth of applications of hypnosis. We can carefully tailor our approaches to the orientation and foci of our audience (clinician learners) and their desired individual learning goals and objectives. The message is that clinician learners will also help their patients/clients orient themselves in developing the goals and objectives for learning and improving with hypnosis. In short, we teach about hypnosis hypnotically.

Third, explicit in teaching about teaching hypnosis is the importance of emphasizing the natural, everyday *psychophysiology of* mind-body connections which all experience at a less-than-conscious level throughout a day. These naturally include the walking, eating, tasting, smelling, breathing, elimination, and gesturing that we all have and do. We posit, demonstrate, reinforce, model, and acknowledge an integration of these "automatic" connections between mind-body as essential to teaching the what-why-when-and how of the hypnotic experience. We emphasize the integration of the conscious and hypnotic intentional behavior (self-hypnosis) in order to effect a desired change in physiology, feelings, habits, pain, and/or whatever the patient's objective is (Kohen & Kaiser, 2014).

Contextually, we seek to consistently apply and amplify a biopsychosocial model (Engel, 1977). We do so when we consider the individual and the family within which they live. We also are mindful of the relevance to them (and us as facilitators) of the orientation of their classrooms and schools, and teachers' attitudes and behaviors. To the extent possible, we also aim to be aware of the socialization of the classroom and, for adults, the socialization/milieu of their workplace.

Hypnosis Training Curriculum

Pediatric hypnosis was really the first formal "pediatric integrative medicine" specialty. It is happily and comfortably integrated with others such as biofeedback, aromatherapy, acupuncture, and craniosacral therapy. This integration is within the context of the fundamental significance in each of these disciplines in the language used. Each intentionally focuses upon the importance of what we say, and how and when we say it *while "doing"* that discipline (Kaiser et al., 2018; Kohen, 2010).

The description of the Pediatric Hypnosis Curriculum is the product of 35 years of annual experience (excluding Webinar-only training developed during Covid years of 2020 and 2021). Initially, the Curriculum was taught by a loosely aligned but committed loyal faculty for 24 years under the auspices of the U.S. Society for Developmental and Behavioral Pediatrics. Since 2010, it has evolved into a more tightly organized teaching program. It was initially sponsored by the Developmental-Behavioral Pediatrics Program of the Department of Pediatrics, University of Minnesota, and the Minnesota Society of Clinical Hypnosis. Ultimately, it evolved into NPHTI and then a 501(c)(3) non-profit educational corporation, with a Board of Directors, and the initial and growing, committed faculty. From 2010 to 2015, NPHTI provided a carefully designed curriculum, including a faculty development component, and the aforementioned six-to-eight-hour FFF curriculum (Kohen & Wark, 1998). This was developed and designed specifically to provide hands-on training for faculty to mentor small group practice sessions. Its intended and successful focus is to provide practical, experiential learning intermittently throughout our three-day hypnosis training workshops. Participants for faculty training are recruited by the current faculty from the bright, insightful, enthusiastic learners who had participated in both Fundamental (introductory) and Utilization (intermediate level) and some Individualized Consultation (advanced) Workshops. Each are invited to consider Faculty Development training.

NPHTI has since created many ongoing innovative and nuanced curricular changes and additions which have substantially contributed to the unique quality of these training workshops. Major changes over time have included, but are not limited to the following:

- The evolution of small group training from six to eight learners per group to no more than six per group (to optimize use of time structured during small group sessions).
- The increase in the number of small group sessions over three days' time to virtually 50% of Workshop time being devoted to this essential experiential learning provided. Our Fundamentals Workshops and our Utilization and Expanded Clinical Applications Workshop (Intermediate Level) each provide seven small group practice sessions. This is compared to most other workshops (pediatric, general/adult) with which we are familiar which usually provide only three to four small groups over a three-day workshop. These small group experiences have consistently been the most highly valued by participants in informal expressions of gratitude and in end-of-workshop evaluations.
- The "requirement" that all faculty presentations include reflections of utilization skills within their respective presentations. These might be video-vignettes of their own pediatric clinical hypnosis patient encounters. Such videos should be selected to highlight use of language, pacing and leading, post-hypnotic therapeutic suggestions, and/or teaching of self-hypnosis. Additionally, faculty are expected to include brief group experiential exercise to elucidate a particular point or two about hypnotic language, feelings, metaphors, etc.
- "Mini-Intensive" presentations in the Utilization Workshop are developed to allow participants to choose 75-minute options of their choice, one in the morning and one in the afternoon on the third day.
- Integration of Ericksonian Utilization principles in each presentation and all aspects of the training curriculum.
- Integration of recommendations and contributions for training from the work of Yapko (2019), and the contributions of Kaiser (personal communication) to adapt Yapko's concepts of "goal-directed hypnosis" and "*how* to do it" to the pediatric curriculum.
- Integration of highly creative and interactive video learning for and by children has been uniquely led by the work of our colleague Jody D. Thomas, PhD. Of note particularly is her work with Stanford Children's Hospital and the creativity of the Meg Foundation and the many resources for teachers, children, and families (Thomas, 2017).

All of these curricular changes have taken place over time with the guidance and coordination of Co-Directors of Education – Pamela Kaiser, PhD and Daniel P. Kohen, MD (from 2010–2019); and with the ongoing input of our diverse, insightful, experienced, and committed faculty. An example of the detailed three-day curriculum can be found in Chapter 22, "Teaching Child Hypnosis" in *Hypnosis with Children, fifth edition* (Kohen & Olness, 2023) and on the website of NPHTI: www.nphti.org.

Workshops Overview

Our three-day workshops include interspersal of presentations with demonstrations of invitations (inductions) of hypnosis (different age groups) and intermittent small group practice opportunities representing 50% of a three-day curriculum. At the Fundamental level, limited focus is upon applications except for common problems (e.g., anxiety, sleep, pain, and/or habit problems). At the Utilization level, increased focus is placed upon language, pacing and leading, formulation of hypnotic and post-hypnotic suggestions, and added foci on specific applications for common and unusual or challenging problems. A concurrent "Individualized Consultation Workshop" is offered. Applicants submit a video of their pediatric clinical hypnosis work (30–45") – and accompanying narrative materials including learning objectives and areas where they are requesting discussion and/or guidance. Following review and acceptance by workshop coordinators, each accepted applicant is matched to a faculty mentor whose expertise is closely aligned to the applicant's work experience. Each accepted applicant is assigned a half-day for review and discussion of their video. A maximum of six individual consultations are accepted for a three-day workshop. During each half-day, the applicant's video is reviewed and discussed by the mentor, the applicant, and other individual consultation participants. Generally, the faculty mentor is different for each half-day. These advanced level workshops are typically highly valued by students and faculty alike, and some participants have gone on to become Faculty.

Some other programs are similar but may include frequent follow-up training, including "homework" by participants. Some emphasize preparation of audio-recordings for patient practice at home and all seem to be clearly focused upon careful tailoring of clinical hypnosis work to the individual and developmentally sensitive and specific nature of the patient. Some hypnosis teaching programs take place within the context of a Psychology Course or courses within a University/College program. While these programs may provide effective presentation information including video-recordings or live demonstrations, they are generally lacking in adequacy and frequency of experiential training. Even a three-hour weekly class does not afford adequate mentored in-person small group practice as in two- or three-day workshops.

We strongly endorse didactic presentations that are shorter than commonly scheduled 45–60 minutes long. We believe that they should *always* be complemented and supplemented by brief video-vignettes illustrating specific concepts and/or hypnotic phenomenology within recordings of actual encounters with children and teens. Likewise, presenters should be encouraged to creatively include/intersperse (self-) hypnotic experiences for individuals, pairs, or [the] large group of maximally 3–5 minutes long in duration.

More recently the challenges of Covid-19 demanded a switch from in-person training to "Tele-Health," often by Zoom or comparable platforms. We thought this would be an immense challenge but NPHTI, like other groups, was able to switch to a Zoom platform to provide ongoing clinical education through a monthly Webinar Program. This began in 2020–2021 and was very successful and continued through 2021–2022 and is now in the third "season" of monthly education offerings. Not intended to be a substitute for in-person "hands-on" Workshop training, it has been a successful addition to our educational offerings. In 2021, we provided a two-day "Practical Strategies Workshop" designed to continue opportunities for mentored clinical case-based small group discussions (4 to a group + a mentor) all via Zoom.

This "experiment" was purposely targeted for those who had previous training in clinical hypnosis. It was successful beyond our expectations. Other hypnosis organizations have offered introductory hypnosis workshops via Zoom. Our faculty group decided, however, that the potential problems outweighed the potential benefits. We are very gratified that as of October 13–15, 2022, we have returned to in-person workshop training.

The focus of this chapter may seem to be upon children and adolescents, and educating those of us who care for and about our youth. However, it must be emphasized that all of what has been described and repeatedly amplified is relevant and effective for all clinicians who utilize hypnosis. It is for all clinicians who have ever been a child, and for all who are a doctor of some kind or who have ever *been* to a doctor! Everything applies to patients/clients of all ages. Adults, after all, should never be considered or treated or thought of as having "finished" their development. We are all evolving, learning, creating, and neuroscience has taught us about neuroplasticity that reflects our continual developmental maturation (see also Chapter on Development).

Phenomenology

We attend especially to areas in which learners request and seek additional training or sophistication. We strive to meet these needs for more information and guidance re: treatment of "x" conditions/diagnoses. Analogously we focus on requests for additional training and experience such as guidance in phenomenological approaches such as hypnoanesthesia/analgesia, regression, utilization of metaphors, post-hypnotic suggestions, use of hypnosis along with biofeedback or other integrative approaches.

Phenomenology within our curriculum accordingly is defined by the ongoing evaluations provided by the learners, i.e., primarily adult health professionals in student learning mode in our educational offerings. Whether these are our workshops, seminars, webinars, especially individualized consultation, we welcome and utilize evaluations in review and modification of what and how we teach. Beyond this our curriculum is influenced by self-evaluation from our faculty with request that all reflect and communicate about "*How* did I *do*? *How* do *I know and measure that? What can I change?*"

We learn about the needs of learners through our meticulous review of evaluations from students, and particularly their added commentary beyond "rating scales." These include various expressions of gratitude for specific skills learned and already internalized/integrated in their practice, reinforcing some of our curricular components. They also include critiques of topics or faculty which may not have been easily understood; or suggestions for timing of various presentations within the larger structure of the program.

Kohen et al. (2017) have described the remodeling of curriculum and refining of faculty development during 35 years of producing pediatric hypnosis educational offerings in their state-of-the-art *Pediatric Hypnosis* training publication (2023). This is also described in detail in Olness and Kohen's chapter in Elkins' text (Olness & Kohen, in Elkins, 2022).

We have replaced a previous, antiquated "non-model" of small group practice, with the innovation and commitment to explicit teaching of small group facilitators on how to be excellent facilitators. The old "non-model" implicitly assumed that because some good clinicians were good with patients and could teach *them* (e.g., about how to use hypnosis for teaching pain control), they would be equally good at teaching other clinicians how to do hypnosis by leading small groups. That is not true. We changed that. Now, years after the FFF training was provided initially for MSCH and NPHTI, the ASCH now also offers analogous training and requires it for clinicians to become small group leaders in ASCH workshops.

Increasing Therapeutic Relevance

How can this subject matter focus and expand the role of hypnosis in clinical care? We believe that our continual, nuanced upgrading of curriculum content and methodology are reasons for the ongoing success of our workshop training. This is evidenced in the impact upon and reflected in over a thousand clinicians trained in our US-based NPHTI workshops, and upon the growth of child hypnosis workshop training internationally in the past 10–15 years. This growth has direct links to the leadership by clinicians who have trained with NPHTI and/or have provided invited workshop training in their home countries by NPHTI faculty. This is notable particularly in the training which has been provided throughout Canada and Europe by our colleague, Dr Leora Kuttner and her exquisite videos (Kuttner, 1985, 1998, 2003, 2013) and many writings including 1988 and 2018, and many others. (Kuttner, 1988, 2018). It is also notable in the extensive teaching by our colleague Dr Laurence Sugarman for his memorable video "Hypnosis in Pediatric Practice Imaginative Medicine in action" (Sugarman, 1997/2007), his decade-long teaching in Norway, and his many writings (Sugarman, 2000; Sugarman & Wester, 2014; Sugarman et al., 2018, 2020).

Within the Swiss Pediatric Hypnosis group, Dr Camilla Ceppi as a former NPHTI trainee and now faculty has been instrumental along with other Swiss pediatricians who have trained with NPHTI, in creating and growing a network of pediatricians skilled in pediatric hypnosis (Ceppi, 2019, 2021).

Likewise, former NPHTI trainees and now NPHTI faculty, Carla Frankenhuis and Dr Arine Vlieger have created a large network of pediatric hypnosis workshops offered in Amsterdam and teaching throughout the Netherlands (Frankenhuis, 2022, Vlieger et al., 2007).

The growth of pediatric hypnosis training in Norway (Kohen & Olness, 2023; Lindheim & Helgeland, 2017; Sugarman, personal communication), in Italy (Fasciana, 2009, 2014), and especially in Germany (Mrochen, 2014; Signer-Fischer, 2019) is significant. Of particular note is the longevity of the "Kindertagung" Child Hypnosis Workshops developed and presented every 2–3 years since the 1990s in Heidelberg, Germany, and more recently Wurzburg, Germany under the leadership of Bernhard Trenkle, Psychologist and past-pesident of ISH (Kohen & Olness, 2023, Chapter 19 Applications of Hypnosis with Children Globally). The regular year-long curriculum "Kid-Hyp" has been an essential ingredient of psychology training in the Berlin program of Psychologist Hiltrud Beerbaum-Luttermann (Kohen & Olness, 2023) for many years.

We have been especially excited and gratified by the aforementioned recent and continued growth of pediatric-specific hypnosis education programs around the world. We have found this to be an ever-evolving process. While we recognize that change can be difficult and challenging, to be sure, it must be considered not just possible, but likely. Like a new pair of shoes, changes in what we teach and how we teach it may take some "using and getting used to" before those shoes become as familiar and comfortable as old slippers.

The Future of Training and Education

What can, might, and should be the future of teaching hypnosis, and for whom? Those of us in professional hypnosis organizations have strongly held beliefs about who should be teaching about clinical hypnosis and who the learners should be. I believe that the components we have outlined should have an increased prominence – even pre-eminence in all hypnosis training. How we do that remains to be discussed, debated, "tried-on-for-size," and "goodness-of-fit." We do know for certain that in teaching and in clinical care, therapy, and medication prescribing by no means does "one size fit all." By "fit" we mean both utilizing innate abilities and effective at expanding those abilities. That said, I believe that we know the components and ingredients of future *even more excellence* in training.

How, when, where, and by whom these are to be integrated and woven into different fabrics for clinical use remain our shared challenge.

Recently, I was interviewed by a curriculum coordinator as one of several to be part of a "Legacy Series" being developed by the Department of Pediatrics. I consented and recently had the opportunity to review the hour-long interview. I was asked to indicate my thoughts about it, and whether any editing would be necessary. Having forgotten precisely how the interview had flowed, I watched it in two sittings and was amused and bothered by how often I did not look at the camera. Toward the end of the interview, I was asked what advice I had for future students/doctors given all of the different experiences I had as a physician educator over 50 years. My response? "Three words come to mind: 'Be present' and 'Listen.'" As I think further about our shared future in hypnosis education, I would add "Pay attention" and "Watch."

As we talked about this briefly, I was reminded that long before there were internships, residencies, and graduate fellowships, learning in medicine and mental health was via an apprenticeship. I vote for some semblance of return to such a model, with attention to the best components thereof, and leaving out whatever negative aspects we may perceive. So, perhaps beginning from a "serial apprenticeships" perspective is better. Within this apprenticeship we imagine:

- Faculty "presentations" are less didactic and shorter. They model verbal and non-verbal approaches and strategies, with careful attention to active listening, and presence. Demonstration and discussion of these skills are routinely developed into and shown as videos of actual patient encounters and followed by discussion, demonstration, and practice.
- Modeling of all clinical and teaching interactions highlights language, non-verbal communication, mirroring, pacing, and leading.
- Training in self-hypnosis is regularly demonstrated and practiced in small groups. NPHTI incorporates this as one of seven small group practices over three days.
- Group hypnotic experiences are valued opportunities to observe personal changes and note the nature of one's own experience. These are often valuable learning for the individual sharing a question or observation and for all present in the present moment(s).
- "Mini-Intensive" presentations in a Utilization Workshop allow participants to choose an extended learning option of their choice. Expanding these options during a three-day Utilization (Level II) training allows learners a selection of a more personalized learning experience.
- Ericksonian Utilization principles become increasingly frequent and integrated components of each of these recommendations.
- Special attention is given to the growing universe of creative, imaginative, and interactive videos for and by children. Discerning the best of these allows for their selective integration with the uniquely personalized learning afforded by evolving training opportunities of the not-so-distant future. As described, the creativity of the Meg Foundation and their many resources for teachers, children, and families (Thomas, 2017) serve as a great model for the vast array of possibilities before us to "run with the ball."

Conclusion

Recent publications have thoughtfully challenged older and more "traditional" models of training in clinical hypnosis, many of which nonetheless persist. These colleagues refer to these traditional approaches as "the more dominant, ritualistic, hierarchical, inductions" and methodologies based upon the "Standards of Training in Clinical Hypnosis" (Alter & Sugarman, 2017; Hope & Sugarman, 2015; Sugarman et al., 2018, 2020). We hope you will be curious and intrigued as you review and consider the significant messages of these publications. Many have some foundational elements of Ericksonian hypnosis and the signature component of tailored utilization – noticing, evoking, and intensifying the client/patient's understanding of their stated issues to help them refine their goals and grow toward solutions. The work of Yapko (2019), Gilligan (2012), Lankton (1989), and many others who studied with Milton Erickson has taught us a great deal about utilization and its implicit, ubiquitous role in identifying hypnosis and hypnotic behaviors and helping patients cultivate their own skills toward desired solutions. In the references noted above, Sugarman, Alter, Hope, Linden, and Brooks all challenge us to move further into new territory, including new ways of teaching. We welcome readers to appreciate and be open to these new ideas and challenges, and those yet to come.

References

Alter, D. S., & Sugarman, L. I. (2017). Reorienting hypnosis education. *American Journal of Clinical Hypnosis*, *59*(3), 253–259. PMID: 27982786 DOI: 10.1080/00029157.2016.1231657

Ceppi Cozzio, C. (2019). Hypnose in der kinderärztlichen Sprechstunde. *Paediatrica.* Dossier Entwicklungspädiatrie 30-1/2019; www.paediatrica.swiss-paediatrics.org/hypnose-in-der-kinderaerztlichen-sprechstunde

Engel, G. L. (1977). The need for a new medical model: A challenge for biomedicine. *Science*, *196*(4286), 192–236. doi:10.1126/science.847460. PMID: 847460 DOI: 10.1126/science.847460

Fasciana, L. M. (a cura di) (2009). L'ipnosis con I bbini e gli adolescent – teniche psicotherapeuttiche in et evolutive Franco Angeli s.r.l. Milano, Italy.

Fasciana, L. M. (a cura di) (2014). Storytelling-Storie terapeitischje b per aiutare bambini e genitori ad aituarsi. Franco Angeli s.r.l. Milano, Italy.

Frankenhuis, C. (2022). Personal communication. www.skills4comfort.nl

Gilligan, S. (2012). *Generative trance the experience of creative flow.* Carmarthen: Crown House Publishing Ltd.

Hope, A. E., & Sugarman, L. I. (2015). Orienting hypnosis. *American Journal of Clinical Hypnosis*, *57*(3), 212–229. doi:10.1080/00029157.2014.976787

Kaiser, P., Kohen, D., Brown, M. Kajander, B., & Barnes, A. (2018). Integrating pediatric hypnosis with complementary modalities: Clinical perspectives on personalized treatment. *Children*, *5*(8), 108; 10.3390/children5080108

Kohen, D. P. (2010). Pediatric perspective on mind-body medicine. In T. P. Culbert, & K. O. Olness, (Eds.), Integrative pediatrics (pp. 267–301). New York, NY: Oxford University Press.

Kohen, D., & Kaiser, P. (2014). Clinical hypnosis with children and adolescents—What? Why? How?: Origins, applications, and efficacy. *Children*, *1*, 74–98. 10.3390/children1020074

Kohen, D. P., Kaiser, P., & Olness, K. (2017). State-of-the-art pediatric hypnosis training: Remodeling curriculum and refining faculty development. *American Journal of Clinical Hypnosis*, *59*(3), 292–310, DOI: 10.1080/00029157.2016.1233859

Kohen, D. P., & Olness, K. (2022) Hypnosis with children. In G. R. Elkins, (Ed.), *Introduction to clinical hypnosis: The basics and beyond.* Waco, TX: Mountain Pine Publishing.

Kohen, D. P. , & Olness, K. (2023). *Hypnosis with children* – 5th edition. New York: Taylor & Francis Group.

Kuttner, L. (1985). "*No fears, no tears" (29mins).* DVD available from http://bookstore.cw.bc.ca email: bookstore@cw.bc.ca US or Canada: 1-800-331-1533 x 3 or Crown House Publishing at http://www.chpus.com

Kuttner, L. (1998). "*No fears, no tears 13 years later: Children coping with pain" (46 mins).* DVD available: http://bookstore.cw.bc.ca email: bookstore@cw.bc.ca; or, Crown House Publishing at http://www.chpus.com

Kuttner, L. (1988). Favourite stories. A hypnotic pain reduction technique for children in acute pain. *American Journal of Clinical Hypnosis*, 30, 289–295. PMID: 3364392 DOI: 10.1080/00029157.1988.10402752

Kuttner, L. (2003). Making every moment count documentary (38 min.) Co-production with The National Film Board of Canada. www.nfb.ca. 1-800-267-7710

Kuttner, L. (2013). *Dancing with pain.* DVD. *Youth with chronic pain* (20 min). www.bookstore@bc.cw.ca

Kuttner, L. (2018). The pain switch for teens with complex pain. In M. Jensen (Ed.) (2018). *Hypnosis for chronic pain management: Favorite methods of master clinicians* (pp. 256–276). Kirkland, WA: Denny Creek Press.

Lankton, C. H., & Lankton, S. R. (1989). *Tales of enchantment – Goal oriented metaphors for adults and children in therapy*. New York, NY: Brunner/Mazel.

Lindheim, M., & Helgeland, H. (2017). Hypnosis training and education: experiences with a Norwegian one-year education course in clinical hypnosis for children and adolescents. *American Journal of Clinical Hypnosis*, *59*, 282–291. PMID: 27982780 DOI: 10.1080/00029157.2016.1230728

Mrochen, M., Holtz, K. L., & Trenkle, B. (2014). *Die Pupille des Bettnässers, hypnotherapeutische Arbeit mit Kindern und Jugendlichen. (8. Aufl.)*. Heidelberg: Carl-Auer-Verlag.

National Pediatric Hypnosis Training Institute (NPHTI) (2010). www.nphti.org

Olness, K., & Kohen, D. P. (2022) Hypnosis with children. In G. R. Elkins (Ed.), *Introduction to clinical hypnosis: The basics and beyond.* Waco, TX: Mountain Pine Publishing.

Signer-Fischer, S. (2019). *Hypnotherapie – effizient und kreativ.* Heidelberg: Carl-Auer-Verlag

Sugarman, L. I. (2000). Hypnosis and biofeedback. In R. A. Hoekelman, S. R. Friedman, N. M. Nelson, H. M. Seidel, & M. L. Weitzman, (Eds.), *Primary pediatric care (4th ed.)*. St. Louis, MO: Mosby Year Book.

Sugarman, L. I. (1997/2007). *Hypnosis in pediatric practice: Imaginative medicine in action [video and instructional manual]*. Bethel, CT: Crown House Publishing.

Sugarman, L. I., & Wester, W. C. (Eds.). (2014). *Therapeutic hypnosis with children and adolescents* (2nd ed.). Carmarthen: Crown House Publishing.

Sugarman, L. I., Schafer, P. M., Alter, D. S., & Reid, D. B. (2018). Learning clinical hypnosis wide awake: Can we teach hypnosis hypnotically. *American Journal of Clinical Hypnosis*, *61*, 140–158 MID: 30260302 DOI: 10.1080/00029157.2018.1437710

Sugarman, L. I., Linden, J. H., & Brooks, L. W. (2020). *Changing minds with clinical hypnosis – Narratives and discourse for a new health care paradigm.* New York, NY: Taylor and Francis, Routledge.

Thomas, J. (2017). Project Director, Primary Consultant: "You are the boss of your brain: Learning how to manage pain during medical procedures" (13 min.) Produced by Stanford Children's Health and Lucile Packard Children's Hospital. Free: https://www.youtube.com/watch?v=UbK9FFoAcvs

Vlieger, A. M., Menko-Frankenhuis, C., Wolfkamp, S. C., Tromp E., & Benninga, M. A. (2007) Hypnotherapy for children with functional abdominal pain or irritable bowel syndrome: A randomized controlled trial. *Gastroenterology*, *133*(5), 1430–1436. PMID: 17919634 DOI: 10.1053/j.gastro.2007.08.072

Wark, D., & Kohen, D. P. (1998). Facilitating facilitators' facilitation: Experience with a model for teaching leaders of hypnosis Practice Groups. *American Journal of Clinical Hypnosis*, *41*, 75–83.

Wark, D., & Kohen, D. P. (2002). The Spiral Curriculum for Hypnosis Workshop Training: The Minnesota Experience. *American Journal of Clinical Hypnosis*, *45*(2), 119–128.

Yapko, M. D. (2019). *Trancework – fifth edition – An introduction to the practice of clinical hypnosis.* New York, NY: Routledge Publishers.

Frontiers

60

PLACEBO AND NOCEBO EFFECTS

Implications for Hypnosis

Fabrizio Benedetti

Neuroscience Department, University of Turin Medical School, Turin, Italy; Program in Medicine & Physiology of Hypoxia, Plateau Rosà, Switzerland

Definitions

Early biological investigations of the placebo effect were performed in the 1960s in animals (Herrnstein, 1962) and in the late 1970s in humans (Levine et al., 1978). Today placebo research has become a complex field of investigation which ranges from psychology to psychophysiology, from pharmacology to neurophysiology, and from cellular/molecular analysis to modern neuroimaging techniques. A placebo effect is a change in the body-mind unit that occurs as a result of the symbolic significance which one attributes to an event or an object in the healing environment (Brody & Brody, 2011). Therefore, whereas in the clinical trial setting the conceptualization of placebo focuses on distal and external factors, such as inert treatments (e.g., sham surgery) and inert substances (e.g., saline solutions or water), in the context of psychology the concept of placebo focuses on proximal and internal factors, namely a set of psychosocial stimuli surrounding the patient and the therapy (Moerman, 2002; Moerman & Jonas, 2002; Price et al., 2008). When a treatment is given to a patient, it is administered within a context, which includes the physical properties of the medication (color, shape, taste, and smell), the characteristics of the healthcare setting (hospital or home, and room layout), the sight of health professionals (words, attitudes, behaviors) and medical instruments, the interaction between patient and doctors (Balint, 1955; Di Blasi et al., 2001).

The nocebo effect is opposite to the placebo effect, for it involves the pathogenic consequences of placebo administration within a negative psychosocial context (Amanzio et al., 2009; Rief et al., 2009). Unwanted effects and adverse events may occur as a result of negative expectations about some treatments (Barsky et al., 2002; Flaten et al., 1999; Rief et al., 2009; Amanzio et al., 2009; Mora et al., 2011). Since inducing negative expectations poses many ethical questions, due to the anxiogenic nature of the procedure (Benedetti et al., 2007; Colloca & Benedetti, 2007), our knowledge about the nocebo effect is still limited.

One of the main points is that there is not a single placebo or nocebo effect but many, and each one can be triggered by a variety of psychological mechanisms, such as conditioning, expectation, anxiety modulation, and reward, which in turn can be modulated by other factors like desire, motivation, and memory. There are however many confounding factors,

DOI: 10.4324/9781003449126-79

such as spontaneous remission, patient's or experimenter's biases, regression to the mean, or the effect of unidentified co-interventions, that need to be ruled out through the appropriate experimental approach in order to identify the real psychobiological placebo effect. Many neurobiological mechanisms of placebo and nocebo effects have been identified in conditions such as pain and Parkinson's disease (Carlino et al., 2014; Frisaldi et al., 2014), whereas other conditions, like anxiety, hormone secretion, and immune responses, are less understood (Benedetti, 2020). In this chapter, a concise overview of the main mechanisms that may contribute to placebo or nocebo effects is presented. A much more detailed description can be found in Benedetti (2020) and Benedetti et al. (2022).

Psychological Studies

The most common explanation of placebo and nocebo effects centers on expectation, generated as the product of cognitive engagement involving the subjectively experienced likelihood of a future effect, and often induced by verbal suggestions (Kirsch et al., 1999; Price et al., 2008). During a medical treatment, the patient has different expectations about the therapeutic outcome. The patient anticipates possible positive or negative effects of the therapy using different cues from the environment, the emotional arousal, and the interaction with care providers. This anticipatory process, in turn, triggers internal changes such as pain reduction (Amanzio & Benedetti, 1999; Benedetti et al., 1999; Wager et al., 2004). The same holds true for pain increase, but in the opposite direction (Benedetti et al., 2007; Pollo et al., 2011).

Different levels of expectations are capable of inducing different levels of placebo responses. Price et al. (1999) showed that the same placebo cream applied onto three adjacent skin areas induces a progressively stronger analgesia according to the strength of the accompanying words (strong analgesic, weak analgesic, and control agent). This has also been found in the clinical setting, where changing the symbolic meaning of a basal physiological infusion in postoperative patients resulted in different intakes of additional painkillers (Pollo et al., 2001). Similarly, different degrees of dopamine activation were found in Parkinson patients who were told that they had a specific probability (25%, 50%, 75%, or 100%) of receiving active medication, when in fact they always received a placebo. Only when patients were informed that they had a 75% probability of receiving active medication, a significant dopamine release occurred, suggesting a tight relationship between the strength of expectation of improvement and the clinical outcome (Lidstone et al., 2010).

Expectations are unlikely to work alone, as they can be modulated by other factors such as desire, self-efficacy, and reinforcing feedback (Price et al., 2008). Desire is represented by the experiential feeling of wanting a future event to happen or the opposite feeling of wanting to avoid a future situation. Self-efficacy and outcome expectancy (Brown et al., 2014) are the personal beliefs to be capable of managing an adverse event, performing the right actions to induce positive changes. Self-reinforcing, often called "somatic-focus", is a cognitive process where a subject waits for any sign of improvement during a therapy and takes these signs as positive evidence that the treatment is successful, meanwhile discarding the opposite negative evidences. These cognitive processes are likely to work together with emotional states like anxiety. A study with patients suffering from irritable bowel syndrome showed that decreased anxiety levels correlated with pain relief perception when patients received a placebo treatment (Vase et al., 2005). Whereas anxiety is linked to the anticipation of a negative event, expecting a positive event may involve the activation of the reward system through the activation of the mesolimbic and mesocortical dopaminergic reward pathways (Benedetti, 2020). Placebos have reward properties, since the expected clinical benefit is itself a form of reward (Lidstone & Stoessl, 2007).

There is compelling experimental evidence that patients can learn, based on previous experiences, that a certain pill or a certain treatment is associated with a specific therapeutic outcome (Colloca & Miller, 2011). This mechanism can involve classical conditioning, a process whereby the repeated association of an unconditioned response (e.g., salivation after food presentation) with a conditioned stimulus (e.g., the ringing bell accompanying the food), that usually would not have an effect, will lead to a conditioned response (e.g., salivation after the ringing bell without the food presence). This mechanism may occur in the clinical context, where different contextual stimuli, such as the presence of a doctor and the shape and color of a pill, can be considered conditioned stimuli in all respects (Ader, 1997; Wickramasekera, 1980; Siegel, 2002). Classical conditioning seems to be the key mechanism especially when unconscious physiological functions, such as endocrine secretion or immune responses, are involved. For example, after repeated administrations of sumatriptan, which stimulates growth hormone (GH), a placebo can mimic the effects of the drug, regardless of what the subjects expect (either decrease or increase of GH) (Benedetti et al., 2003b). Therefore, cognitive factors, such as expectations, do not seem to affect these unconscious physiological functions. Conditioned hormonal responses have also been observed in humans for insulin and glucose (Stockhorst et al., 2000) and for dexamethasone and cortisol as well (Sabbioni et al., 1997).

Behaviorally conditioned changes in peripheral immune functions have also been demonstrated in experimental animals, healthy subjects, and patients (Schedlowski & Pacheco-López, 2010; Vits et al., 2011). In patients with multiple sclerosis, the repeated association of a flavored beverage with the immunosuppressive drug cyclophosphamide led to a decrease in peripheral leukocytes after the administration of the flavored drink alone (Giang, et al., 1996). A similar paradigm was reproduced in healthy participants, in whom conditioned immunosuppression, as assessed by lymphocyte proliferation, interleukin-2, and interferon-gamma, was observed after repeated association of a conditioned stimulus with cyclosporine A (Goebel, et al., 2002).

According to more recent cognitive theories of classical conditioning, the mechanism can be based on the cognitive information implicitly contained in the conditioned stimulus. In other words, the information contained in the conditioned stimulus would lead to the specific expectation that a given event will follow another event (Reiss, 1980; Rescorla, 1988; Voudouris et al., 1990; Montgomery & Kirsch, 1996). This means that expectation and conditioning mechanisms are not mutually exclusive in the generation of placebo and nocebo effects.

Neurobiological Studies

Levine and colleagues first showed that the opiate antagonist naloxone was capable of reducing the placebo response in dental postoperative pain (Levine et al., 1978). Subsequent works in the 1980s and 1990s left little doubts that specific biochemical events were taking place after placebo administration. For example, placebo responders were found to have levels of β-endorphin in the cerebrospinal fluid (Lipman et al., 1990) and opioids released by a placebo procedure displayed the same side effects as exogenous opioids (Benedetti et al., 1999). Likewise, naloxone-sensitive cardiac effects could be observed during placebo analgesia (Pollo et al., 2003) and indirect support also came from the placebo-potentiating role of the colecystokinin (CCK) antagonist proglumide (Benedetti et al., 1995, 2011b).

Knowledge of systems other than endogenous opioids is scarce, but their existence emerges from the fact that, in some situations, a placebo effect can still occur after blockade of opioid mechanisms by naloxone (Gracely et al., 1983; Grevert et al., 1983; Vase et al., 2005). For example, with a morphine conditioning and/or expectation-inducing protocol, Amanzio and Benedetti could completely reverse placebo analgesia induced in experimental ischemic arm pain by using naloxone. However, in the same protocol, the non-opioid analgesic ketorolac induced only a partial blockade (Amanzio & Benedetti, 1999). Recently, an important non-opioid component of placebo analgesia has been identified, and this is represented by the endocannabinoid system (Benedetti et al., 2011a).

The placebo effect was first linked to dopamine in Parkinson's disease. Here, it is mediated by dopamine release in the *dorsal* striatum, a key structure in the motor circuit affected by the disease (de la Fuente-Fernández et al., 2001; de la Fuente-Fernández & Stoessl, 2002). However, it must be noted that dopamine is also released in the *ventral* striatum, notably in the nucleus accumbens, involved in the reward circuit. Contrary to the dorsal striatum, release in ventral striatum was not correlated with the experienced clinical benefit, leading the authors to suggest that this release might be related to the expectation of reward, rather than to reward itself (de la Fuente-Fernández et al., 2002; de la Fuente-Fernández & Stoessl, 2002). Indeed, in a study combining placebo analgesia and a monetary reward task, it was demonstrated that the healthy subjects with stronger nucleus accumbens synaptic activation (as measured by functional magnetic resonance imaging, fMRI) during the monetary reward anticipation also showed more robust placebo responses and greater dopamine activity in the same nucleus (as measured with dopamine-agonist [^{11}C]raclopride positron emission tomography, PET) (Scott et al., 2007). Moreover, in a subsequent PET study using the μ-opioid receptor-selective radiotracer [^{11}C] carfentanil and [^{11}C]raclopride, both opioid and dopamine neurotransmission were found to be involved (Scott et al., 2008).

PET, fMRI, magneto-electroencephalography, and electro-encephalography have all been usefully employed to characterize the spatial and temporal domains of placebo analgesia (Rainville & Duncan, 2006; Kong et al., 2007; Colloca et al., 2008), with both activations and deactivations. For example, activations of the prefrontal and anterior cingulate cortex have been identified. Reduced pain-related brain activation during placebo analgesia has been repeatedly and independently reported in many studies, often with strict correlation with psychophysical pain measures, supporting the view that during placebo analgesia what is altered is not the evaluation of unchanged incoming pain information, but rather a direct modulation of nociceptive afferent signals (Wager et al., 2004; Lieberman et al., 2004; Koyama et al., 2005; Bingel et al., 2006; Kong et al., 2006; Price et al., 2007; Watson et al., 2009). Areas of the pain matrix showing decreased activation include thalamus, insula, rostral anterior cingulate cortex (rACC), primary somatosensory cortex, supramarginal gyrus, and left inferior parietal lobule (Zunhammer et al., 2018; Zunhammer et al., 2021).

Scalp laser-evoked potentials amplitude was also found to be reduced during placebo analgesia, namely in the N2-P2 components, thought to be originated in the bilateral insula and the cingulate gyrus (Wager et al., 2006; Watson et al., 2007; Colloca et al., 2008). Modulation of pain-related neural activity by placebo has been shown to extend down to the spinal cord level (Eippert et al., 2009b).

Data from imaging and neuropharmachological studies support the model of the recruitment of the descending pain inhibitory system (Petrovic et al., 2002; Zubieta et al., 2005; Wager et al., 2007). Focusing on the pain anticipatory phase, Wager and coworkers observed an increase in dorsolateral prefrontal cortex (DLPFC) activity, negatively correlated with the signal reduction in thalamus, ACC, and insula, and with reported pain intensity, but positively correlated with increase in a midbrain region containing the periaqueductal gray (PAG) (Wager et al., 2004). Further support for a link between limbic areas and the PAG came from a connectivity analysis showing correlation between the activation of rACC and that of PAG and bilateral amygdala (Bingel et al., 2006), and these effects were abolished by naloxone (Eippert et al., 2009a).

By considering the above-mentioned studies, the prefrontal regions seem to play a key role in placebo analgesia. In Alzheimer patients, loss of placebo responses on one hand and reduction of connectivity between the prefrontal lobes and the rest of the brain on the other progress in parallel (Benedetti et al., 2006). In addition, deactivation of the prefrontal cortex by means of repetitive transcranial magnetic stimulation has been shown to be equally effective in producing abolition of placebo analgesia (Krummenacher et al., 2010).

Genetic mechanisms could also be involved in placebo responsiveness, and these may account for the differences between placebo responders and non-responders, for example in social anxiety (Furmark et al., 2008), depression (Leuchter et al., 2009), irritable bowel syndrome (Hall et al., 2012), and pain (Colloca et al., 2019). In light of the numerous neurotransmitters that are involved in placebo effects, this is not surprising, and a genetic screening could be considered in the near future in order to test the interindividual differences in placebo responsiveness. For example, the serotonin transporter-linked polymorphic region (5-HTTLPR) and the G-703T polymorphism in the tryptophan hydroxylase-2 (TPH2) gene promoter have been identified for social anxiety disorder (Furmark et al., 2008), and catechol-O-methyltransferase (COMT) for major depressive disorder (Leuchter et al., 2009). In addition, the COMT functional val158met polymorphism has been found to be associated with the placebo effect in irritable bowel syndrome, with the strongest placebo effect in met/met homozygotes (Hall et al., 2012). In a more recent study (Colloca et al., 2019), the interaction among the opioid receptor *mu* subunit (OPRM1 rs1799971), catechol-O-methyltransferase (COMT rs4680), and fatty acid amide hydrolase (FAAH rs324420) has been found to modulate placebo analgesia.

Differently from placebo, to design experiments aimed at gathering information on nocebo is not an easy task, as ethical limitations forbid inflicting deliberate harm, and many studies are carried out on healthy volunteers rather than patients. Therefore, it is not surprising that our knowledge on nocebo hyperalgesia still lags behind the more detailed understanding of placebo analgesia (Benedetti et al., 2007; Colloca & Benedetti, 2007). An early study showed that nocebo pain responses induced in postoperative patients by negative expectation regarding a saline infusion could be prevented by the CCK antagonist proglumide, a nonspecific CCK-1 and CCK-2 antagonist, in a dose-dependent manner (Benedetti et al., 1997). As the expectation of pain increase is a highly anxiogenic process, and both anxiety and anxiety-induced hyperalgesia have been shown to be enhanced by CCK and attenuated by CCK antagonists in animal models (Lydiard, 1994; Andre et al., 2005; Hebb et al., 2005), it was assumed that anxiolytic drugs could interfere with nocebo hyperalgesia. Indeed, it has been shown that nocebo hyperalgesia can be regarded as a stress response as it is accompanied by increased levels of adrenocorticotropic hormone and cortisol, which indicates hyperactivity of the hypothalamic-pituitary-adrenal (HPA) axis. After administration of the benzodiazepine anxiolytic drug diazepam, both HPA hyperactivity and nocebo hyperalgesia were blocked. When proglumide was given together with nocebo suggestions, only hyperalgesia was completely prevented. There was no effect on the HPA axis (Benedetti et al., 2006). This suggests that CCK does not act on the general process of nocebo-induced anxiety, but rather specifically on nocebo/anxiety-induced hyperalgesia. In other words, nocebo suggestions induce anxiety, which in turn induces both HPA and pain enhancement. While diazepam acts on anxiety, thus blocking both effects, proglumide acts only on the pain pathway, downstream of the nocebo-induced anxiety.

Inducing negative expectations results in both amplified unpleasantness of innocuous thermal stimuli as assessed by psychophysical pain measures (verbal subject report) and increased fMRI responses in ACC and in a region including parietal operculum and posterior insula (Sawamoto et al., 2000). Together with the hippocampus and the prefrontal cortex, these are regions also involved in pain anticipation (Koyama et al., 1998; Chua et al., 1999; Hsieh et al., 1999; Ploghaus et al., 2001; Porro et al., 2002; Porro et al., 2003; Koyama et al., 2005; Lorenz et al., 2005; Keltner et al., 2006). In some cases, the same study has addressed both positive (placebo) and negative (nocebo) expectations, with opposite modulation of pain-related brain areas (Koyama et al., 2005; Lorenz et al., 2005; Keltner et al., 2006). Kong et al. (2008) emphasized the effect of negative expectations about pain perception following sham acupuncture: increased pain reports for the nocebo sites paralleled increased activity in several areas of the medial pain matrix, including bilateral dorsal ACC, insula, left frontal and parietal operculum, orbitofrontal cortex, and hippocampus. Of particular interest is the involvement of the hippocampus, as its activity is also anxiety-driven (Ploghaus et al., 2001).

From all these studies, the circuitry underlying nocebo hyperalgesia is likely to involve, with opposite modulation, the same areas engaged by placebo analgesia. The current model suggests that the DLPFC here too might exert active control on pain perception, by modulating cortico-subcortical and cortico-cortical pathways.

Clinical Implications and Their Relevance to Hypnosis

Hidden administration of therapies provides some of the most compelling evidence that expectation is a key element in the therapeutic outcome (Benedetti et al., 2011c; Colloca et al., 2004). A hidden treatment is given without information, so that the patient is unaware that a therapy is being performed. In this situation, there are no expectations about any clinical improvement, and this leads to a reduced efficacy of the therapy. In terms of medical practice, this has profound implications because the information delivered by health professionals may make a big difference in the therapeutic outcome. This approach is quite difficult from a methodological point of view, and it is at the borderline between the experimental setting and clinical practice. Whereas the open administration is carried out by a doctor, who tells his/her patient that the injection is a powerful analgesic and that the pain is going to subside in a few minutes, a hidden injection of the same analgesic at the same dose is performed by a computer-controlled infusion machine that starts the painkilling infusion without any doctor or nurse in the room; these patients are completely unaware that an analgesic therapy has been started. The effectiveness of diazepam, one of the most frequently used benzodiazepines for treating anxiety, is reduced or completely abolished when diazepam is administered unbeknownst to the patient (Benedetti et al., 2003a, 2011c; Colloca et al., 2004). The same effects are present in other conditions such as pain and Parkinson's disease (Benedetti et al., 2003a, 2011c; Colloca et al., 2004). In postoperative pain after the extraction of the third molar (Levine et al., 1981; Levine & Gordon, 1984), a hidden intravenous injection of 6–8 mg morphine corresponds to an open intravenous injection of saline solution in full view of the patient (placebo). In other words, telling the patient that a painkiller is being injected (with what is actually a saline solution) is as potent as 6–8 mg of morphine. This holds true for a variety of painkillers such as morphine, buprenorphine, tramadol, ketorolac, and metamizole (Amanzio et al., 2001; Benedetti et al., 2003a; Colloca et al., 2004).

Expectation of remifentanil (told remifentanil, gets remifentanil) produces more pronounced analgesic effects compared to no-expectation (told saline, gets remifentanil). Moreover, expectation of interruption (told interruption, gets remifentanil) abolishes the overall analgesic effect. Functional magnetic resonance responses show that the enhancement of analgesia in the positive expectation condition is associated with activity in the DLPFC and pregenual ACC, whereas negative expectation of interruption is associated with activity in the hippocampus (Bingel et al., 2011). All these studies emphasize how the knowledge about the treatment affects the therapeutic outcome. This may have profound implications in medical practice, whereby the doctor–patient interaction and communication may have a crucial role.

Placebo and hypnosis are deeply linked by their phenomenology since hypnosis can be regarded as a non-deceptive expectation manipulation where hypnotic suggestions can produce therapeutic effects that do not require deception. In other words, hypnosis is a means of eliciting placebo effects without the use of placebos (Kirsch, 1994). The essence of this approach is to create with the patient a context in which any expectation for change will occur (Matthews et al., 1993). A number of studies have compared placebo and hypnosis effects in different clinical and experimental settings. For example, in the treatment of headache, both hypnosis induction and placebo administration were found to produce a significant decrease in headache pain compared to a control condition (Spanos et al., 1993). Likewise, in a study designed to assess the placebo component in hypnosis, participants were asked to rate experimentally induced ischemic pain. Changes in pain threshold and tolerance were evaluated following the induction of hypnotic and placebo analgesia, and compared to an initial baseline performance (McGlashan et al., 1969). As summarized in Hilgard and Hilgard (1975), the results showed that those participants who were not susceptible to hypnosis reported similar pain reductions in both placebo and hypnosis conditions, whereas those participants who were highly susceptible to hypnosis reported far greater pain reductions after hypnotically suggested analgesia compared to placebo-induced analgesia. Interestingly, although it is possible to find specific characteristics that define a participant as highly susceptible to hypnosis, it is still difficult to find a personal characteristic that can define a good placebo responder (Frischholz, 2007). Indeed, some individuals can be classified as good "placebo responders", whereas others cannot (Benedetti & Frisaldi, 2014), but a validated operational method for identifying these differences does not exist to date.

Despite the general opinion that the relationship between hypnotizability and placebo-response is "weak" (Fritscholz, 2007, 2015), recent studies found a possible correlation. For example, De Pascalis et al. (2002) found that individual differences in suggestibility contribute significantly to the magnitude of placebo analgesia. The highest placebo effect was found in highly suggestible subjects who received suggestions that were presumed to elicit high expectations for drug efficacy. A specific relation between suggestibility, hypnotic susceptibility, and placebo analgesia has been described in other studies, which favor a possible shared mechanism in hypnosis and placebo response (Derbyshire & Oakley, 2013; Huber et al., 2013).

McGeown et al. (2009) found that hypnotic inductions produce a unique pattern of brain activation in highly suggestible subjects that consist in decreased brain activity in the anterior part of the "default mode" network, a set of midline brain structures that include the anterior cingulate, ventral and dorsal medial prefrontal cortex, posterior cingulate, and precuneus (Raichle et al., 2001; Fox & Raichle, 2007; Mason et al., 2007), which are also crucially involved in placebo and nocebo effects. The default mode network refers to those areas of the brain which are activated when people are not engaged in any specific cognitive task, but rather are letting their minds wander at rest. These findings support the hypothesis that high suggestible people approach hypnosis as an active task in which attention is focused on the anticipated upcoming suggestions, rather than a fundamental shift in the functioning of consciousness (Mazzoni et al., 2013).

By translating all these considerations into routine medical practice, special attention should be paid to those psychological factors that either improve or worsen the effectiveness of hypnosis, first and foremost the promotion of positive expectations (Kirsch, 1994). Understanding placebo and nocebo effects in hypnotic treatments is certainly a challenge which will lead to a better knowledge of both clinical practice and the neurobiological underpinnings of hypnosis. Since one of the main purposes of hypnosis is to understand and gain control of our emotions with beneficial effects for stress reduction, it will be interesting to explore the possible effects of the combined use of hypnosis and placebo treatments in order to boost their positive outcomes. Likewise, it will be interesting to explore the possible interconnection between placebo, hypnosis, and meditation in order to further understand similarities and differences across these interventions (Raz, 2007; De Benedittis, 2021).

References

Ader, R. (1997). The role of conditioning in pharmacotherapy. In A. Harrington (Ed.), *The placebo effect: An interdisciplinary exploration*. Cambridge, MA: Harvard University Press.

Amanzio, M., & Benedetti, F. (1999). Neuropharmacological dissection of placebo analgesia: Expectation-activated opioid systems versus conditioning-activated specific subsystems. *The Journal of Neuroscience: The Official Journal of the Society for Neuroscience*, *19*(1), 484–494. 10.1523/jneurosci.19-01-00484.1999

Amanzio, M., Corazzini, L. L., Vase, L., & Benedetti, F. (2009). A systematic review of adverse events in placebo groups of anti-migraine clinical trials. *Pain*, *146*(3), 261–269. 10.1016/j.pain.2009.07.010

Amanzio, M., Pollo, A., Maggi, G., & Benedetti, F. (2001). Response variability to analgesics: A role for non-specific activation of endogenous opioids. *Pain*, *90*(3), 205–215. DOI: 10.1016/s0304-3959(00)00486-3

Andre, J., Zeau, B., Pohl, M., Cesselin, F., Benoliel, J.-J., & Becker, C. (2005). Involvement of cholecystokininergic systems in anxiety-induced hyperalgesia in male rats: Behavioral and biochemical studies. *The Journal of Neuroscience: The Official Journal of the Society for Neuroscience*, *25*(35), 7896–7904. 10.1523/jneurosci.0743-05.2005

Balint, M. (1955). The doctor, his patient, and the illness. *Lancet*, *268*(6866), 683–688. 10.1016/s0140-6736(55)91061-8

Barsky, A. J., Saintfort, R., Rogers, M. P., & Borus, J. F. (2002). Nonspecific medication side effects and the nocebo phenomenon. *JAMA: The Journal of the American Medical Association*, *287*(5), 622–627. 10.1001/jama.287.5.622

Benedetti, F. (2020). *Placebo effects* (3rd ed.). Oxford University Press.
Benedetti, F., Amanzio, M., Baldi, S., Casadio, C., & Maggi, G. (1999). Inducing placebo respiratory depressant responses in humans via opioid receptors. *The European Journal of Neuroscience*, *11*(2), 625–631. 10.1046/j.1460-9568.1999.00465.x
Benedetti, F., Amanzio, M., Casadio, C., Oliaro, A., & Maggi, G. (1997). Blockade of nocebo hyperalgesia by the cholecystokinin antagonist proglumide. *Pain*, *71*(2), 135–140. 10.1016/s0304-3959(97)03346-0
Benedetti, F., Amanzio, M., & Maggi, G. (1995). Potentiation of placebo analgesia by proglumide. *Lancet*, *346*(8984), 1231. 10.1016/s0140-6736(95)92938-x
Benedetti, F., Amanzio, M., Rosato, R., & Blanchard, C. (2011a). Nonopioid placebo analgesia is mediated by CB1 cannabinoid receptors. *Nature Medicine*, *17*(10), 1228–1230. 10.1038/nm.2435
Benedetti, F., Amanzio, M., & Thoen, W. (2011b). Disruption of opioid-induced placebo responses by activation of cholecystokinin type-2 receptors. *Psychopharmacology*, *213*(4), 791–797. 10.1007/s00213-010-2037-y
Benedetti, F., Carlino, E., & Pollo, A. (2011c). Hidden administration of drugs. *Clinical Pharmacology and Therapeutics*, *90*(5), 651–661. 10.1038/clpt.2011.206
Benedetti, F., Amanzio, M., Vighetti, S., & Asteggiano, G. (2006). The biochemical and neuroendocrine bases of the hyperalgesic nocebo effect. *The Journal of Neuroscience: The Official Journal of the Society for Neuroscience*, *26*(46), 12014–12022. 10.1523/jneurosci.2947-06.2006
Benedetti, F., Arduino, C., & Amanzio, M. (1999). Somatotopic activation of opioid systems by target-directed expectations of analgesia. *The Journal of Neuroscience: The Official Journal of the Society for Neuroscience*, *19*(9), 3639–3648. 10.1523/jneurosci.19-09-03639.1999
Benedetti, F., Arduino, C., Costa, S., Vighetti, S., Tarenzi, L., Rainero, I., & Asteggiano, G. (2006). Loss of expectation-related mechanisms in Alzheimer's disease makes analgesic therapies less effective. *Pain*, *121*(1–2), 133–144. 10.1016/j.pain.2005.12.016
Benedetti, F., & Frisaldi, E. (2014). Creating placebo responders and nonresponders in the laboratory: Boons and banes. *Pain Management*, *4*(3), 165–167. 10.2217/pmt.14.11
Benedetti, F., Frisaldi, E., & Shaibani, A. (2022). Thirty years of neuroscientific investigation of placebo and nocebo: The interesting, the good, and the bad. *Annual Review of Pharmacology and Toxicology*, *62*, 323–340. 10.1146/annurev-pharmtox-052120-104536
Benedetti, F., Maggi, G., Lopiano, L., Lanotte, M., Rainero, I., Vighetti, S., & Pollo, A. (2003a). Open versus hidden medical treatments: The patient's knowledge about a therapy affects the therapy outcome. *Prevention & Treatment*, *6*(1), No Pagination Specified.
Benedetti, F., Lanotte, M., Lopiano, L., & Colloca, L. (2007). When words are painful: Unraveling the mechanisms of the nocebo effect. *Neuroscience*, *147*(2), 260–271. 10.1016/j.neuroscience.2007.02.020
Benedetti, F., Pollo, A., Lopiano, L., Lanotte, M., Vighetti, S., & Rainero, I. (2003b). Conscious expectation and unconscious conditioning in analgesic, motor, and hormonal placebo/nocebo responses. *The Journal of Neuroscience: The Official Journal of the Society for Neuroscience*, *23*(10), 4315–4323. 10.1523/jneurosci.23-10-04315.2003
Bingel, U., Lorenz, J., Schoell, E., Weiller, C., & Büchel, C. (2006). Mechanisms of placebo analgesia: rACC recruitment of a subcortical antinociceptive network. *Pain*, *120*(1-2), 8–15. 10.1016/j.pain.2005.08.027
Bingel, U., Wanigasekera, V., Wiech, K., Ni Mhuircheartaigh, R., Lee, M. C., Ploner, M., & Tracey, I. (2011). The effect of treatment expectation on drug efficacy: Imaging the analgesic benefit of the opioid remifentanil. *Science Translational Medicine*, *3*(70), 70ra14. 10.1126/scitranslmed.3001244
Brody, H., & Brody, D. (2011). *The placebo response: How you can release the body's inner pharmacy for better health*. Harper.
Brown, L. A., Wiley, J. F., Wolitzky-Taylor, K., Roy-Byrne, P., Sherbourne, C., Stein, M. B., Sullivan, G., Rose, R. D., Bystritsky, A., & Craske, M. G. (2014). Changes in self-efficacy and outcome expectancy as predictors of anxiety outcomes from the CALM study. *Depression and Anxiety*, *31*(8), 678–689. 10.1002/da.22256
Carlino, E., Frisaldi, E., & Benedetti, F. (2014). Pain and the context. *Nature Reviews. Rheumatology*, *10*(6), 348–355. 10.1038/nrrheum.2014.17
Chua, P., Krams, M., Toni, I., Passingham, R., & Dolan, R. (1999). A functional anatomy of anticipatory anxiety. *NeuroImage*, *9*(6 Pt 1), 563–571. 10.1006/nimg.1999.0407

Colloca, L., & Benedetti, F. (2007). Nocebo hyperalgesia: How anxiety is turned into pain. *Current Opinion in Anaesthesiology*, *20*(5), 435–439. 10.1097/aco.0b013e3282b972fb

Colloca, L., Lopiano, L., Lanotte, M., & Benedetti, F. (2004). Overt versus covert treatment for pain, anxiety, and Parkinson's disease. *The Lancet. Neurology*, *3*(11), 679–684. 10.1016/s1474-4422(04)00908-1

Colloca, L., & Miller, F. G. (2011). How placebo responses are formed: A learning perspective. *Philosophical Transactions of the Royal Society of London. Series B, Biological Sciences*, *366*(1572), 1859–1869. 10.1098/rstb.2010.0398

Colloca, L., Tinazzi, M., Recchia, S., Le Pera, D., Fiaschi, A., Benedetti, F., & Valeriani, M. (2008). Learning potentiates neurophysiological and behavioral placebo analgesic responses. *Pain*, *139*(2), 306–314. 10.1016/j.pain.2008.04.021

Colloca, L., Wang, Y., Martinez, P. E., Chang, Y. C., Ryan, K. A., et al. (2019). OPRM1 rs1799971, COMT rs4680, and FAAH rs324420 genes interact with placebo procedures to induce hypoalgesia. *Pain*, *160*, 1824–1834. 10.1097/j.pain.0000000000001578

De Benedittis, G. (2021). Neural mechanisms of hypnosis and meditation-induced analgesia: A narrative review. *International Journal of Clinical and Experimental Hypnosis*, *69*(3), 363–382. 10.1080/00207144.2021.1917294

De la Fuente-Fernández, R., Phillips, A. G., Zamburlini, M., Sossi, V., Calne, D. B., Ruth, T. J., & Stoessl, A. J. (2002). Dopamine release in human ventral striatum and expectation of reward. *Behavioural Brain Research*, *136*(2), 359–363. 10.1016/s0166-4328(02)00130-4

De la Fuente-Fernández, R., Ruth, T. J., Sossi, V., Schulzer, M., Calne, D. B., & Stoessl, A. J. (2001). Expectation and dopamine release: Mechanism of the placebo effect in Parkinson's disease. *Science (New York, N.Y.)*, *293*(5532), 1164–1166. 10.1126/science.1060937

De la Fuente-Fernández, R., & Stoessl, A. J. (2002). The placebo effect in Parkinson's disease. *Trends in Neurosciences*, *25*(6), 302–306. 10.1016/s0166-2236(02)02181-1

De Pascalis, V., Chiaradia, C., & Carotenuto, E. (2002). The contribution of suggestibility and expectation to placebo analgesia phenomenon in an experimental setting. *Pain*, *96*(3), 393–402. 10.1016/s0304-3959(01)00485-7

Derbyshire, S. W. G., & Oakley, D. A. (2013). Role for suggestion in differences in brain responses after placebo conditioning in high and low hypnotizable subjects. *Pain*, *154*, 1487–1488. 10.1016/j.pain.2013.05.045

Di Blasi, Z., Harkness, E., Ernst, E., Georgiou, A., & Kleijnen, J. (2001). Influence of context effects on health outcomes: A systematic review. *Lancet*, *357*(9258), 757–762. 10.1016/s0140-6736(00)04169-6

Eippert, F., Bingel, U., Schoell, E. D., Yacubian, J., Klinger, R., Lorenz, J., & Büchel, C. (2009a). Activation of the opioidergic descending pain control system underlies placebo analgesia. *Neuron*, *63*(4), 533–543. 10.1016/j.neuron.2009.07.014

Eippert, F., Finsterbusch, J., Bingel, U., & Büchel, C. (2009b). Direct evidence for spinal cord involvement in placebo analgesia. *Science (New York, N.Y.)*, *326*(5951), 404. 10.1126/science.1180142

Flaten, M. A., Simonsen, T., & Olsen, H. (1999). Drug-related information generates placebo and nocebo responses that modify the drug response. *Psychosomatic Medicine*, *61*(2), 250–255. 10.1097/00006842-199903000-00018

Fox, M. D., & Raichle, M. E. (2007). Spontaneous fluctuations in brain activity observed with functional magnetic resonance imaging. *Nature Reviews. Neuroscience*, *8*(9), 700–711. 10.1038/nrn2201

Frisaldi, E., Carlino, E., Lanotte, M., Lopiano, L., & Benedetti, F. (2014). Characterization of the thalamic-subthalamic circuit involved in the placebo response through single-neuron recording in Parkinson patients. *Cortex; a Journal Devoted to the Study of the Nervous System and Behavior*, *60*, 3–9. 10.1016/j.cortex.2013.12.003

Frischholz, E. J. (2007). Hypnosis, hynotizability, and placebo. *American Journal of Clinical Hypnosis*, *50*(1), 49–58. 10.1080/00029157.2007.10401597

Frischholz, E. J. (2015). Hypnosis, hypnotizability, and placebo. *American Journal of Clinical Hypnosis*, *57*(2), 165–174. 10.1080/00029157.2015.967088

Furmark, T., Appel, L., Henningsson, S., Ahs, F., Faria, V., et al. (2008) A link between serotonin-related gene polymorphisms, amygdala activity, and placebo-induced relief from social anxiety. *Journal of Neuroscience*, *28*, 13066–13074. 10.1523/jneurosci.2534-08.2008

Giang, D. W., Goodman, A. D., Schiffer, R. B., Mattson, D. H., Petrie, M., Cohen, N., & Ader, R. (1996). Conditioning of cyclophosphamide-induced leukopenia in humans. *Journal of Neuropsychiatry and Clinical Neurosciences*, *8*(2), 194–201. 10.1176/jnp.8.2.194

Goebel, M. U., Trebst, A. E., Steiner, J., Xie, Y. F., Exton, M. S., Frede, S., Canbay, A. E., Michel, M. C., Heemann, U., & Schedlowski, M. (2002). Behavioral conditioning of immunosuppression is possible in humans. *FASEB Journal: Official Publication of the Federation of American Societies for Experimental Biology*, *16*(14), 1869–1873. 10.1096/fj.02-0389com

Gracely, R. H., Dubner, R., Wolskee, P. J., & Deeter, W. R. (1983). Placebo and naloxone can alter post-surgical pain by separate mechanisms. *Nature*, *306*(5940), 264–265. 10.1038/306264a0

Grevert, P., Albert, L. H., & Goldstein, A. (1983). Partial antagonism of placebo analgesia by naloxone. *Pain*, *16*(2), 129–143. 10.1016/0304-3959(83)90203-8

Hall, K. T., Lembo, A. J., Kirsch, I., Ziogas, D. C., Douaiher, J., et al. (2012) Catechol-O-methyltransferase val158met polymorphism predicts placebo effect in irritable bowel syndrome. *PLoS One* 7, e48135. 10.1371/journal.pone.0048135

Hebb, A. L. O., Poulin, J.-F., Roach, S. P., Zacharko, R. M., & Drolet, G. (2005). Cholecystokinin and endogenous opioid peptides: Interactive influence on pain, cognition, and emotion. *Progress in Neuro-Psychopharmacology & Biological Psychiatry*, *29*(8), 1225–1238. 10.1016/j.pnpbp.2005.08.008

Herrnstein, R. J. (1962). Placebo effect in the rat. *Science (New York, N.Y.)*, *138*(3541), 677–678. 10.1126/science.138.3541.677

Hilgard, E. R., & Hilgard, J. R. (1975). *Hypnosis in the relief of pain*. Los Altos, CA: William Kaufmann.

Hsieh, J. C., Stone-Elander, S., & Ingvar, M. (1999). Anticipatory coping of pain expressed in the human anterior cingulate cortex: A positron emission tomography study. *Neuroscience Letters*, *262*(1), 61–64. 10.1016/s0304-3940(99)00060-9

Huber, A., Lui, F., & Porro, C. A. (2013). Hypnotic susceptibility modulates brain activity related to experimental placebo analgesia. *Pain*, *154*, 1509– 1518. 10.1016/j.pain.2013.03.031

Keltner, J. R., Furst, A., Fan, C., Redfern, R., Inglis, B., & Fields, H. L. (2006). Isolating the modulatory effect of expectation on pain transmission: A functional magnetic resonance imaging study. *The Journal of Neuroscience: The Official Journal of the Society for Neuroscience*, *26*(16), 4437–4443. 10.1523/jneurosci.4463-05.2006

Kirsch, I. (1994). Clinical hypnosis as a nondeceptive placebo: Empirically derived techniques. *The American Journal of Clinical Hypnosis*, *37*(2), 95–106. 10.1080/00029157.1994.10403122

Kirsch, I., Wickless, C., & Moffitt, K. H. (1999). Expectancy and suggestibility: Are the effects of environmental enhancement due to detection? *International Journal of Clinical and Experimental Hypnosis*, *47*(1), 40–45. 10.1080/00207149908410021

Kong, J., Gollub, R. L., Polich, G., Kirsch, I., Laviolette, P., Vangel, M., Rosen, B., & Kaptchuk, T. J. (2008). A functional magnetic resonance imaging study on the neural mechanisms of hyperalgesic nocebo effect. *The Journal of Neuroscience: The Official Journal of the Society for Neuroscience*, *28*(49), 13354–13362. 10.1523/jneurosci.2944-08.2008

Kong, J., Gollub, R. L., Rosman, I. S., Webb, J. M., Vangel, M. G., Kirsch, I., & Kaptchuk, T. J. (2006). Brain activity associated with expectancy-enhanced placebo analgesia as measured by functional magnetic resonance imaging. *The Journal of Neuroscience: The Official Journal of the Society for Neuroscience*, *26*(2), 381–388. 10.1523/jneurosci.3556-05.2006

Kong, J., Kaptchuk, T. J., Polich, G., Kirsch, I., & Gollub, R. L. (2007). Placebo analgesia: Findings from brain imaging studies and emerging hypotheses. *Reviews in the Neurosciences*, *18*(3–4), 173–190. 10.1515/revneuro.2007.18.3-4.173

Koyama, T., McHaffie, J. G., Laurienti, P. J., & Coghill, R. C. (2005). The subjective experience of pain: Where expectations become reality. *Proceedings of the National Academy of Sciences of the United States of America*, *102*(36), 12950–12955. 10.1073/pnas.0408576102

Koyama, T., Tanaka, Y. Z., & Mikami, A. (1998). Nociceptive neurons in the macaque anterior cingulate activate during anticipation of pain. *Neuroreport*, *9*(11), 2663–2667. 10.1097/00001756-199808030-00044

Krummenacher, P., Candia, V., Folkers, G., Schedlowski, M., & Schönbächler, G. (2010). Prefrontal cortex modulates placebo analgesia. *Pain*, *148*(3), 368–374. 10.1016/j.pain.2009.09.033

Leuchter, A. F., McCracken, J. T., Hunter, A. M., Cook, I. A., & Alpert, J. E. (2009). Monoamine oxidase a and catechol-o-methyltransferase functional polymorphisms and the placebo response in major depressive disorder. *Journal of Clinical Psychopharmacology*, *29*, 372–377. 10.1097/jcp.0b013e3181ac4aaf

Levine, J. D., & Gordon, N. C. (1984). Influence of the method of drug administration on analgesic response. *Nature*, *312*(5996), 755–756. 10.1038/312755a0

Levine, J. D., Gordon, N. C., & Fields, H. L. (1978). The mechanism of placebo analgesia. *Lancet*, *2*(8091), 654–657. 10.1016/s0140-6736(78)92762-9

Levine, J. D., Gordon, N. C., Smith, R., & Fields, H. L. (1981). Analgesic responses to morphine and placebo in individuals with postoperative pain. *Pain*, *10*(3), 379–389. 10.1016/0304-3959(81)90099-3

Lidstone, S. C. C., & Stoessl, A. J. (2007). Understanding the placebo effect: Contributions from neuroimaging. *Molecular Imaging and Biology: MIB: The Official Publication of the Academy of Molecular Imaging*, *9*(4), 176–185. 10.1007/s11307-007-0086-3

Lidstone, S. C., Schulzer, M., Dinelle, K., Mak, E., Sossi, V., Ruth, T. J., de la Fuente-Fernández, R., Phillips, A. G., & Stoessl, A. J. (2010). Effects of expectation on placebo-induced dopamine release in Parkinson disease. *Archives of General Psychiatry*, *67*(8), 857. 10.1001/archgenpsychiatry.2010.88

Lieberman, M. D., Jarcho, J. M., Berman, S., Naliboff, B. D., Suyenobu, B. Y., Mandelkern, M., & Mayer, E. A. (2004). The neural correlates of placebo effects: A disruption account. *NeuroImage*, *22*(1), 447–455. 10.1016/j.neuroimage.2004.01.037

Lipman, J. J., Miller, B. E., Mays, K. S., Miller, M. N., North, W. C., & Byrne, W. L. (1990). Peak B endorphin concentration in cerebrospinal fluid: Reduced in chronic pain patients and increased during the placebo response. *Psychopharmacology*, *102*(1), 112–116. 10.1007/bf02245754

Lorenz, J., Hauck, M., Paur, R. C., Nakamura, Y., Zimmermann, R., Bromm, B., & Engel, A. K. (2005). Cortical correlates of false expectations during pain intensity judgments – A possible manifestation of placebo/nocebo cognitions. *Brain, Behavior, and Immunity*, *19*(4), 283–295. 10.1016/j.bbi.2005.03.010

Lydiard, R. B. (1994). Neuropeptides and anxiety: Focus on cholecystokinin. *Clinical Chemistry*, *40*(2), 315–318. 10.1093/clinchem/40.2.315

Mason, M. F., Norton, M. I., Van Horn, J. D., Wegner, D. M., Grafton, S. T., & Macrae, C. N. (2007). Wandering minds: The default network and stimulus-independent thought. *Science (New York, N.Y.)*, *315*(5810), 393–395. 10.1126/science.1131295

Matthews, W. J., Lankton, S., & Lankton, C. (1993). An Ericksonian model of hypnotherapy. In J. W. Rhue, S. J. Lynn, & I. Kirsch (Eds.), *Handbook of clinical hypnosis* (pp. 187–214). Washington, DC: American Psychological Association.

Mazzoni, G., Venneri, A., McGeown, W. J., & Kirsch, I. (2013). Neuroimaging resolution of the altered state hypothesis. *Cortex; a Journal Devoted to the Study of the Nervous System and Behavior*, *49*(2), 400–410. 10.1016/j.cortex.2012.08.005

McGeown, W. J., Mazzoni, G., Venneri, A., & Kirsch, I. (2009). Hypnotic induction decreases anterior default mode activity. *Consciousness and Cognition*, *18*(4), 848–855. 10.1016/j.concog.2009.09.001

McGlashan, T. H., Evans, F. J., & Orne, M. T. (1969). The nature of hypnotic analgesia and placebo response to experimental pain. *Psychosomatic Medicine*, *31*(3), 227–246. 10.1097/00006842-196905000-00003

Moerman, D. E. (2002). *Meaning, medicine and the "placebo effect"*. Cambridge; New York, NY: Cambridge University Press. 10.1017/CBO9780511810855

Moerman, D. E., & Jonas, W. B. (2002). Deconstructing the placebo effect and finding the meaning response. *Annals of Internal Medicine*, *136*(6), 471–476. 10.7326/0003-4819-136-6-200203190-00011

Montgomery, G., & Kirsch, I. (1996). Mechanisms of placebo pain reduction: An empirical investigation. *Psychological Science*, *7*(3), 174–176. 10.1111/j.1467-9280.1996.tb00352.x

Mora, M. S., Nestoriuc, Y., & Rief, W. (2011). Lessons learned from placebo groups in antidepressant trials. *Philosophical Transactions of the Royal Society of London. Series B, Biological Sciences*, *366*(1572), 1879–1888. 10.1098/rstb.2010.0394

Petrovic, P., Kalso, E., Petersson, K. M., & Ingvar, M. (2002). Placebo and opioid analgesia – imaging a shared neuronal network. *Science (New York, N.Y.)*, *295*(5560), 1737–1740. 10.1126/science.1067176

Ploghaus, A., Narain, C., Beckmann, C. F., Clare, S., Bantick, S., Wise, R., Matthews, P. M., Rawlins, J. N., & Tracey, I. (2001). Exacerbation of pain by anxiety is associated with activity in a hippocampal network. *The Journal of Neuroscience: The Official Journal of the Society for Neuroscience*, *21*(24), 9896–9903. 10.1523/jneurosci.21-24-09896.2001

Pollo, A., Amanzio, M., Arslanian, A., Casadio, C., Maggi, G., & Benedetti, F. (2001). Response expectancies in placebo analgesia and their clinical relevance. *Pain*, *93*(1), 77–84. 10.1016/s0304-3959(01)00296-2

Pollo, A., Carlino, E., & Benedetti F. (2011). Placebo mechanisms across different conditions: From the clinical setting to physical performance. *Philosophical Transactions of the Royal Society of London. Series B, Biological Sciences*, 366(1572), 1790–1798. 10.1098/rstb.2010.0381

Pollo, A., Vighetti, S., Rainero, I., & Benedetti, F. (2003). Placebo analgesia and the heart. *Pain*, *102*(1–2), 125–133. 10.1016/s0304-3959(02)00345-7

Porro, C. A., Baraldi, P., Pagnoni, G., Serafini, M., Facchin, P., Maieron, M., & Nichelli, P. (2002). Does anticipation of pain affect cortical nociceptive systems? *The Journal of Neuroscience: The Official Journal of the Society for Neuroscience*, *22*(8), 3206–3214. 10.1523/jneurosci.22-08-03206.2002

Porro, C. A., Cettolo, V., Francescato, M. P., & Baraldi, P. (2003). Functional activity mapping of the mesial hemispheric wall during anticipation of pain. *NeuroImage*, *19*(4), 1738–1747. 10.1016/s1053-8119(03)00184-8

Price, D. D., Craggs, J., Verne, G. N., Perlstein, W. M., & Robinson, M. E. (2007). Placebo analgesia is accompanied by large reductions in pain-related brain activity in irritable bowel syndrome patients. *Pain*, *127*(1–2), 63–72. 10.1016/j.pain.2006.08.001

Price, D. D., Finniss, D. G., & Benedetti, F. (2008). A comprehensive review of the placebo effect: Recent advances and current thought. *Annual Review of Psychology*, *59*, 565–590. 10.1146/annurev.psych.59.113006.095941

Price, D. D., Milling, L. S., Kirsch, I., Duff, A., Montgomery, G. H., & Nicholls, S. S. (1999). An analysis of factors that contribute to the magnitude of placebo analgesia in an experimental paradigm. *Pain*, *83*(2), 147–156. 10.1016/s0304-3959(99)00081-0

Raichle, M. E., MacLeod, A. M., Snyder, A. Z., Powers, W. J., Gusnard, D. A., & Shulman, G. L. (2001). A default mode of brain function. *Proceedings of the National Academy of Sciences*, *98*(2), 676–682. 10.1073/pnas.98.2.676

Rainville, P., & Duncan, G. H. (2006). Functional brain imaging of placebo analgesia: Methodological challenges and recommendations. *Pain*, *121*(3), 177–180. 10.1016/j.pain.2006.01.011

Raz, A. (2007). Hypnobo: Perspectives on hypnosis and placebo. *American Journal of Clinical Hypnosis*, *50*(1), 29–36. 10.1080/00029157.2007.10401595

Reiss, S. (1980). Pavlovian conditioning and human fear: An expectancy model. *Behavior Therapy*, *11*(3), 380–396. 10.1016/S0005-7894(80)80054-2

Rescorla, R. A. (1988). Pavlovian conditioning. It's not what you think it is. *The American Psychologist*, *43*(3), 151–160. 10.1037//0003-066x.43.3.151

Rief, W., Nestoriuc, Y., von Lilienfeld-Toal, A., Dogan, I., Schreiber, F., Hofmann, S. G., Barsky, A. J., & Avorn, J. (2009). Differences in adverse effect reporting in placebo groups in SSRI and tricyclic antidepressant trials: A systematic review and meta-analysis. *Drug Safety: An International Journal of Medical Toxicology and Drug Experience*, *32*(11), 1041–1056. 10.2165/11316580-000000000-00000

Sabbioni, M. E., Bovbjerg, D. H., Mathew, S., Sikes, C., Lasley, B., & Stokes, P. E. (1997). Classically conditioned changes in plasma cortisol levels induced by dexamethasone in healthy men. *FASEB Journal: Official Publication of the Federation of American Societies for Experimental Biology*, *11*(14), 1291–1296. 10.1096/fasebj.11.14.9409548

Sawamoto, N., Honda, M., Okada, T., Hanakawa, T., Kanda, M., Fukuyama, H., Konishi, J., & Shibasaki, H. (2000). Expectation of pain enhances responses to nonpainful somatosensory stimulation in the anterior cingulate cortex and parietal operculum/posterior insula: An event-related functional magnetic resonance imaging study. *The Journal of Neuroscience: The Official Journal of the Society for Neuroscience*, *20*(19), 7438–7445. 10.1523/jneurosci.20-19-07438.2000

Schedlowski, M., & Pacheco-López, G. (2010). The learned immune response: Pavlov and beyond. *Brain, Behavior, and Immunity*, *24*(2), 176–185. 10.1016/j.bbi.2009.08.007

Scott, D. J., Stohler, C. S., Egnatuk, C. M., Wang, H., Koeppe, R. A., & Zubieta, J.-K. (2007). Individual differences in reward responding explain placebo-induced expectations and effects. *Neuron*, *55*(2), 325–336. 10.1016/j.neuron.2007.06.028

Scott, D. J., Stohler, C. S., Egnatuk, C. M., Wang, H., Koeppe, R. A., & Zubieta, J.-K. (2008). Placebo and nocebo effects are defined by opposite opioid and dopaminergic responses. *Archives of General Psychiatry*, *65*(2), 220–231. 10.1001/archgenpsychiatry.2007.34

Siegel, S. (2002). Explanatory mechanisms for placebo effects: Pavlovian conditioning. In H. A. Guess, A. Kleinman, J. W. Kusek, & L. W. Engel (Eds.), *The science of the placebo: Toward an interdisciplinary research agenda*. London: BMJ Books.

Spanos, N. P., Liddy, S. J., Scott, H., Garrard, C., Sine, J., Tirabasso, A., & Hayward, A. (1993). Hypnotic suggestion and placebo for the treatment of chronic headache in a university volunteer sample. *Cognitive Therapy and Research*, *17*(2), 191–205. 10.1007/BF01172965

Stockhorst, U., Steingrüber, H. J., & Scherbaum, W. A. (2000). Classically conditioned responses following repeated insulin and glucose administration in humans. *Behavioural Brain Research*, *110*(1–2), 143–159. 10.1016/s0166-4328(99)00192-8

Vase, L., Robinson, M. E., Verne, G. N., & Price, D. D. (2005). Increased placebo analgesia over time in irritable bowel syndrome (IBS) patients is associated with desire and expectation but not endogenous opioid mechanisms. *Pain*, *115*(3), 338–347. 10.1016/j.pain.2005.03.014

Vits, S., Cesko, E., Enck, P., Hillen, U., Schadendorf, D., & Schedlowski, M. (2011). Behavioural conditioning as the mediator of placebo responses in the immune system. *Philosophical Transactions of the Royal Society of London. Series B, Biological Sciences*, *366*(1572), 1799–1807. 10.1098/rstb.2010.0392

Voudouris, N. J., Peck, C. L., & Coleman, G. (1990). The role of conditioning and verbal expectancy in the placebo response. *Pain*, *43*(1), 121–128. 10.1016/0304-3959(90)90057-k

Wager, T. D., Matre, D., & Casey, K. L. (2006). Placebo effects in laser-evoked pain potentials. *Brain, Behavior, and Immunity*, *20*(3), 219–230. 10.1016/j.bbi.2006.01.007

Wager, T. D., Rilling, J. K., Smith, E. E., Sokolik, A., Casey, K. L., Davidson, R. J., Kosslyn, S. M., Rose, R. M., & Cohen, J. D. (2004). Placebo-induced changes in FMRI in the anticipation and experience of pain. *Science (New York, N.Y.)*, *303*(5661), 1162–1167. 10.1126/science.1093065

Wager, T. D., Scott, D. J., & Zubieta, J.-K. (2007). Placebo effects on human mu-opioid activity during pain. *Proceedings of the National Academy of Sciences of the United States of America*, *104*(26), 11056–11061. 10.1073/pnas.0702413104

Watson, A., El-Deredy, W., Iannetti, G. D., Lloyd, D., Tracey, I., Vogt, B. A., Nadeau, V., & Jones, A. K. P. (2009). Placebo conditioning and placebo analgesia modulate a common brain network during pain anticipation and perception. *Pain*, *145*(1–2), 24–30. 10.1016/j.pain.2009.04.003

Watson, A., El-Deredy, W., Vogt, B. A., & Jones, A. K. P. (2007). Placebo analgesia is not due to compliance or habituation: EEG and behavioural evidence. *Neuroreport*, *18*(8), 771–775. 10.1097/wnr.0b013e3280c1e2a8

Wickramasekera, D. I. (1980). A conditioned response model of the placebo effect predictions from the model. *Biofeedback and Self-Regulation*, *5*(1), 5–18. 10.1007/bf00999060

Zubieta, J.-K., Bueller, J. A., Jackson, L. R., Scott, D. J., Xu, Y., Koeppe, R. A., Nichols, T. E., & Stohler, C. S. (2005). Placebo effects mediated by endogenous opioid activity on mu-opioid receptors. *The Journal of Neuroscience: The Official Journal of the Society for Neuroscience*, *25*(34), 7754–7762. 10.1523/jneurosci.0439-05.2005

Zunhammer, M., Bingel, U., Wager, T. D., & Placebo Imaging Consortium. (2018). Placebo effects on the neurologic pain signature: A meta-analysis of individual participant functional magnetic resonance imaging data. *Journal of the American Medical Association Neurology*, *75*, 1321–1330. 10.1001/jamaneurol.2018.2017

Zunhammer, M., Spisák, T., Wager, T. D., Bingel, U., & Placebo Imaging Consortium. (2021). Meta-analysis of neural systems underlying placebo analgesia from individual participant fMRI data. *Nature Communications*, *12*, 1391. 10.1038/s41467-021-21179-3

61

HYPNOSIS AND THE FUTURE OF THE WORLD'S CHILDREN

Karen Olness

Professor Emerita of Pediatrics, Global Health and Diseases, Case Western Reserve University, Cleveland, Ohio, USA

The Dream for All Children

I dream of child development that includes opportunities for all children to recognize their own abilities for self-regulation, including autonomic and voluntary controls, and to have coping abilities that mitigate the problems that come along in life.

My Early Experiences with Hypnosis

During medical school, I had a job in the laboratory of a famous immunologist, Dr Robert A. Good. I studied the transport of labeled protein through the glomeruli of rats and the electron microscope was my main tool. One day I heard that Dr Good was doing a new study and many of the trainees were subjects in the study. He was studying the question of whether or not delayed cutaneous hypersensitivity might be impacted by hypnosis. At that time what little knowledge of hypnosis I had was negative. I was troubled by the idea of what I thought such a silly research study by someone whom I admired so much.

Dr Good's hypnosis study demonstrated that delayed cutaneous hypersensitivity could be changed via hypnosis. However, Dr Good did not describe this work in any publication until, in 1991, when he wrote the foreword to the first edition of *Psychoneuroimmunology* by Robert Ader. I remained in communication with Dr Good throughout the rest of his life and we laughed together about my early skepticism regarding his reluctance to publish about his hypnosis research.

About a decade later, I was working in Laos where my husband was a diplomat. We were being transferred to Kenya so my job was being taken by Walter Majewski, an American family physician. One day he said, "I want to give you a gift before you leave. I want to teach you self-hypnosis". Once again, I was dubious but I respected him. He explained how helpful hypnosis had been in his medical practice. I had a conditioned epigastric pain response to stress. I told him I would be willing to learn for myself. If I found that self-hypnosis helped me overcome this pain, then I would take the workshops he suggested. He taught me an arm levitation technique. I practiced diligently and, after two

DOI: 10.4324/9781003449126-80

months, the psychophysiologic stress response disappeared. It has never recurred. I began reading about hypnosis. When we returned to the US a few years later, I began attending workshops.

The Current Demographic Situation for Children and Adolescents

In 2021, the world had 2.53 billion children under 18 years (UNICEF, 2022). Five hundred million lived in low-income countries (less than 1,046 dollars per capita per year) (World Bank, 2021). These are areas where infant and pre-school mortality remains high, where more children are orphans, and where more children suffer abuse. Children in resource-poor areas are more likely to experience early cognitive impairment from malnutrition, micronutrient deficiencies, infectious diseases, or exposure to toxins such as organophosphates (Olness, 2003). An estimated 15% of children have cognitive limitations that may impact educational programs for them. Twenty-two million children in low-income countries are not able to attend primary school. There are an estimated 147 million children who have lost one or both parents (UNICEF, 2022). About 10% of parent losses are HIV-related, and most of those orphans are in Africa. Population projections indicate that child populations will grow in resource-poor areas but not in middle-and high-income countries. In the next 35 years, it is estimated that 1.8 billion infants will be born in Africa and that the under 18 population will increase to nearly one billion (Population Pyramid, 2022). The latest global burden of disease data from 2019 indicates that chronic diseases, including disabilities and mental health issues, have increased steadily through this century (Institute for Health Metrics and Evaluation, 2022). Nearly 240 million children have some type of disability (UNICEF, 2022). UNICEF estimates that more than 13% of adolescents in the world live with a mental disorder.

Disasters and Children

Throughout the world, the number of man-made and natural disasters is escalating, increasing the likelihood that more children in disasters will suffer both emotional and physical trauma (Harkensee et al., 2021). In 2021, approximately 89 million persons were displaced by man-made disasters (UNHCR, 2021). Half were children. Some of these displacements were for a few weeks; others were for years and many resulted in moves to new countries and environments. Long-term mental health effects of such displacements include PTSD, depression, anxiety, intellectual disabilities, weather phobias, sleep disorders, and anti-social disorders (Olness, 2021). Studies vary in the frequencies reported for PTSD (Lewis et al., 2019). Children in nearly all countries are at risk of being trafficked, including those displaced by disasters. "Toxic stress" affecting young children occurs in all countries and may impact their physical and emotional health throughout life. The American Academy of Pediatrics Policy *Statement on Preventing Childhood Toxic Stress* defines toxic stress as "The biological response to frequent, prolonged, or severe adversities in the absence of at least one safe, stable and nurturing relationship" (Garner & Yogman, 2021, p. 16). There is great concern about how best to facilitate resilience in those who have been traumatized by disasters (Underwood, 2018).

Health Facilities in Resource-Poor Areas

In resource-poor areas, hospitals and clinics remain generally insufficient and there is also a shortage of trained professionals who know how to help children who experience any of the mentioned problems. Medications are often in short supply and, in some countries, they are fake. It is rare for a hospital or clinic to have a pain management program focused on children. Palliative care programs for children are also insufficient.

How Might Training in Self-Regulation via Self-Hypnosis Help Children Throughout the World?

Ideally, opportunities to learn self-hypnosis or equivalents for the purpose of recognizing one's ability to be in control should be provided to all children and to their parents while the children are in pre-school or early grade school. Such training might be offered when children see health care providers for routine care or when they are in school (Bothe et al., 2014). Achieving this ideal also requires that training in hypnosis communication skills be added to training of all child health professionals. At present the world is far from having enough child health professionals to provide the option of hypnosis training to all children.

Child health professionals familiar with language and nonverbal communication skills from training in hypnosis are likely to also have experience in using a trauma-informed approach to communicate with displaced children (Brown et al., 2017). They can contribute a great deal to the child's comfort and resilience. They are sensitive to how the child's developmental state contributes to what the child remembers, how he/she describes it. and how it might be manifested in play activities. They can use their knowledge and skills to help parents and other caretakers as well as relief workers to communicate appropriately with children. They have the capacity to be attentive to and intervene to help unaccompanied minors who are displaced. A recent American Academy of Pediatrics policy statement describes resilience as "The capacity to respond to adversity in a healthy, adaptive manner" and notes that the impacts of toxic stress can be reversed and even prevented with resilience skills (Garner & Yogman, 2021, p. 16). Dr Heather Forkey has written that the skills of resilience include a thinking and learning brain, regulation or self-control, efficacy, hope, and developmental skill mastery (Forkey et al., 2021). Training in hypnosis can enhance the skills of resilience for children who have experienced various types of trauma.

There is a great need for child health professionals who work in hospitals and clinics to learn approaches that facilitate the capacity of children to self regulate and believe that they can cope up with difficult circumstances. Training in self-regulation skills is a special gift for children with many chronic conditions such as physical disabilities, diabetes, sickle-cell disease, thalassemia, RAP, Crohn Disease, cancer, rheumatoid arthritis, asthma, congenital blindness or deafness (Kohen & Olness, 2022; Rutten et al., 2014; Tome-Pires & Miro, 2012). Non-pharmacologic pain management is helpful to children undergoing many types of procedures, including immunizations, vena punctures, burn treatment, and wound care (Chester et al., 2018; Kohen & Olness, 2022; Vagnoli, 2019).

The Current Situation for Work Force Expertise in Child and Adolescent Hypnosis

Many countries have health professionals who belong to the International Society of Hypnosis or other professional hypnosis societies. This implies that the populations of these countries have access to clinical hypnosis and also to health professionals who can teach hypnosis. Nonetheless, there is still a huge shortage of this expertise, especially for children in resource-poor areas. The majority of the world's citizens have probably never heard of hypnosis or, if they know about it, do not understand that it facilitates self-control and self-regulation. Germany perhaps leads in the number of child health professionals who have attended workshops on hypnosis.

Norway has a well-organized training program in child hypnosis. The Norwegian Association for Clinical and Experimental Hypnosis was founded in 1979, 14 years after the Swedish Hypnosis Association was formed (Nielsen & Vandvik, 1981). The Psychology Faculty at the University of Bergen offers an elective course in hypnosis for its graduate students. Workshops on Hypnosis with Children began in the early 1980s and continue to the present. In 2008, the Regional Center for Child and Adolescent Health in Norway developed a one-year training program on hypnosis for children and adolescents. This was designed for physicians and psychologists, the two professional groups allowed to use hypnosis in Norway. The program includes four 2-day seminars, four group meetings with supervisors and meetings with mentors, and a requirement for a paper describing two clinical cases (Lindheim & Helgeland, 2017).

There also have been well-organized training programs on pediatric hypnosis in Belgium, the Netherlands, Sweden, Switzerland Australia, Canada, and the US. Countries including Thailand, India, Singapore, Turkey, China, and Mexico have had occasional workshops focused on children. There remains a huge need for more training in most countries.

Ideally, experienced faculty from nearby countries should organize training in resource-poor areas and provide basic or fundamentals hypnosis training to a cohort of enthusiastic child health professionals. This group should be willing to continue meeting to share experiences and share information. Given the ease of webinar training, they should be provided opportunities to continue their hypnosis education via these webinars and also to participate in the active NPHTI listserv. They should also be provided subscriptions to hypnosis journals in either print or electronically.

Examples of Specific Efforts to Provide Training on Hypnosis with Children in Resource-Poor Areas

Thailand

The University of Khon Kaen is in the poorest province in Thailand. Children are referred from the largely rural area to Srinagarind Hospital at the University for treatment of complex problems such as cancer, hemoglobinopathies, and developmental disabilities. Prior to 2003, children with cancer were subjected to outpatient procedures such as bone marrow aspiration or chemotherapy without local anesthesia, sedation, or psychological preparation. Injectable narcotics were available for hospitalized children but oral narcotics were not available for children in rural areas. It was recognized that children who experienced repeated painful procedures sometimes developed PTSD.

Two members of the pediatric faculty and one nursing faculty had been trained in hypnosis in the US. They organized three hypnosis training workshops for 68 child health professionals who worked in the hospital. These workshops focused on nonpharmacologic pain management. In 2005, they organized a national workshop on pain management for children after a survey revealed that 81% of hospitalized children in NE Thailand experienced severe pain and received little or no treatment (Forgeron et al., 2009). Hospital guidelines were established that included both pharmacologic and nonpharmacologic management, including training in self-hypnosis. A few years later, the Thai faculty provided pediatric hypnosis training workshops in neighboring Laos.

Malawi

A few Malawian child health professionals expressed interest in learning about child hypnosis. Two of them traveled to the US and completed a three-day workshop in pediatric hypnosis. This occurred before the internet availability in Malawi. Long distance telephone service was slow and unreliable as were postal services. This made ongoing communication with the US faculty slow and irregular. Although the Malawian child health professionals were positive about the potential benefits for hospitalized children in their city, they encountered skepticism from colleagues about hypnosis. They did not continue to offer hypnosis training to Malawian children. This program might have been more successful if a group of faculty had traveled to Malawi to teach a larger group and to insure some type of practical follow-up training.

UMMEED Child Development Center, Mumbai, India

This center focuses on children with learning problems, speech issues, mental health problems, autism, and physical limitations. It provides care for children of all socio-economic levels. In 2014, Drs Kohen and Olness went to Mumbai to teach a workshop on child hypnosis for the UMMEED Center. The director of the center had herself taken the National Pediatric Hypnosis Training Institute (NPHTI) workshop in the US and used the NPHTI listserv. She was eager for the staff of UMMEED Center to learn how to teach hypnosis to children as well as how to use self-hypnosis themselves. Since then, the staff have continued to offer hypnosis training to children and families and to use self-hypnosis for themselves.

Examples of Resources to Help Traumatized Children in Areas with Little Access to Mental Health Professionals

Comfort Kits

Tim Culbert, Maura Fitzgerald, and Lynda Richtsmeier designed comfort kits initially for hospitalized children who had chronic illnesses. Culbert later adapted them to facilitate resilience in children displaced by disasters (Pairojkul et al., 2010). Small fabric or plastic bags contain finger puppets, crayons, stress squeeze balls, bubbles, pinwheels, biodots, and small toys. Items may vary somewhat on what is available and the preferences of children in different areas of the world. Culbert included instructions for parents and caretakers of children on how these items might be used. Adolescents can be taught how to use comfort kits with young children in disaster settings. The following is an example of instructions in using a pinwheel.

> Imagine you have a balloon in your belly. Breathe in slowly through your nose. Feel your belly get big like a balloon blowing up as you breathe in. Blow out against the pinwheel – slowly- and your belly gets flat. Each time you blow out you can breathe out any thing that bothers you.

Comfort kits, including translated instructions, have been made available to children in both natural and man-made disasters. These have included Thailand after the tsunami, Haiti after the 2010 earthquake, Laos after flood disasters, and Ukraine during the 2022 war.

The Meg Foundation

The Meg Foundation provides online resources to help children tolerate pain (Meg Foundation, 2022. These include several videos that appeal to children. The video on "Be the Boss of Your Brain" has multicultural appeal and is available in English, Spanish, Arabic, Chinese, Thai, and Laos (Thomas, 2017). In charming format, it explains pain signals and encourages children to focus on their own control. After the COVID-19 pandemic began, the Meg Foundation focused on teaching videos to help children tolerate immunizations.

Return to Happiness and Child to Child Programs

Other programs that can help large numbers of children in situations lacking mental health professionals include the Return to Happiness program (Herran, 2021), developed by UNICEF, and the Child to Child program first developed by Morley for use in Africa (www.childtochild.org.uk 2022).

Cultural Considerations

Culture is defined as a way of life for a group of people. It includes how people work, how they relax, their values, their senses of humor, their biases, and how they interact with other humans. Cultural norms are the ethical, moral, or traditional principles of a given society and include unwritten definitions about what is considered usual or normal. Cultures and cultural norms may change over generations of families and in different environments. Equivalent ethnicity does not mean equivalent culture. Consider the cultural differences between a man of Kikuyo ethnicity (Kenya) whose parents immigrated from Kenya and who works as an attorney in the Midwestern US and a farmer of Kikuyu ethnicity who lives in a rural village in Kenya.

There are also mini-cultures and most individuals belong to more than one. Mini-cultures also change over time, e.g., the mini-culture of the child, the adolescent, and the elderly person. Most child health professionals become quite expert at understanding the mini-cultures of children of different ages and can communicate in the language of several mini-cultures. When working in a different country, however, they may need to study the overall culture and current mini-cultures of children and adolescents.

What Questions Should Expatriate Hypnosis Faculty Ask Themselves Before Teaching in Another Country? (See Table 61.1)

Careful planning is important to increase the likelihood that hypnosis training will lead to training of children and that the educational effort will continue. The planning takes time and includes frequent communication with colleagues who coordinate the training in the resource-poor country. It must carefully consider matters such as local holidays, usual

Table 61.1 Questions Expatriate Faculty Should Ask Themselves Before Teaching in Other Countries

1	Is there a group of child health professionals in this country who are interested in and willing to study hypnosis?
2	Have I had conversations with colleagues who have taught hypnosis previously in this country?
3	Have I studied the culture of this country?
4	How might cultural factors impact understanding of hypnosis or responses to my teaching?
5	Do I understand what is appropriate in terms of sharing meals, touching colleagues, giving or accepting gifts, and participating in recreational activities?
6	What do I know about educational systems for children and adolescents in this country?
7	What are favorite games and activities of children and adolescents?
8	Who are cultural heroes?
9	Have I examined existing CME courses in this country?
10	Are learners comfortable asking questions of speakers?
11	What type of evaluation plans are appropriate in this country?
12	What regular follow-up can I arrange to help trainees after I leave this country?
13	Am I able to return on a regular basis?
14	Have I reviewed CDC guidelines with respect to the preventive health measures I should take before visiting this country?

times for beginning and ending meetings, expected tea or coffee breaks, internet accessibility, and certificates of attendance.

If previous efforts have been made to share hypnosis training in a country, it is useful to speak with faculty who have taught there previously? Where did they teach and how long was the teaching? Did trainees then teach hypnosis to children in their practice? Was there regular follow-up? It is essential to be certain that there is a group of child health professionals who are interested in and willing to learn about hypnosis. This involves substantial communication and sharing of workshop plans with emphasis on follow-up.

Faculty who are willing to share their knowledge and skills in another country benefit by devoting substantial time to studying the culture. It is important to assess how cultural factors might impact understanding of hypnosis and impact teaching. It is also important to be socially appropriate in terms of cultural norms such as behavior at meals, giving or accepting gifts, and participating in recreational activities. Faculty should assess their personal level of comfort with and tolerance of cultural differences. Ask questions about recreational activities of children, e.g., what are favorite games, tv shows, and sports? Who are child heroes? Do some children begin working at an early age?

It is also important to learn about education systems in the country. What is the general level of education? Are schools public or private? Are learners encouraged to ask questions or is this a culture in which the teacher is never challenged? What type of evaluation systems are acceptable? In some countries, learners are afraid to write any comments that might be interpreted as negative.

It is necessary to identify child health professionals who are citizens of and live in the country who are willing to take training to become faculty in future hypnosis workshops. Efforts should be made to provide special training for future faculty in subsequent workshops. This is essential for sustainability.

Before travel the faculty member should read health guidelines related to the area that will be visited. Are there requirements for specific immunizations or prophylactic medications? Are there climate or other risk factors that might impact negatively on one's health?

Consideration to follow-up training should be made before the workshop is held. Are there mentors willing to maintain communication with the trainees? Will trainees have access to a useful list serve or to webinars on hypnosis? Will trainees be able to take additional training in other countries or to join hypnosis societies?

Summary

There is a huge need for more training in hypnosis in all areas of the world, including resource-poor areas. Ideally, this should be provided by child health professionals who are native to the culture and language in a country and should emphasize the importance of providing children with a sense of coping ability. Children who are displaced by disasters and children with chronic diseases benefit especially from developing personal skills in self-hypnosis. Provision of training in Western countries for a few individuals who then return to countries has failed because of the lack of interested peers and sufficient faculty to make the efforts sustainable. Child health professionals willing to teach in other countries should pay careful attention to planning, educational systems, culture, and plans for mentorship and replication of workshops.

References

Bothe, D., Grignon, J., & Olness, K. (2014). The effects of a stress management intervention in elementary school children. *Journal of Developmental and Behavioral Pediatrics*, *35*, 62–67.

Brown, J. D., King, M. A., & Wissow, L. S. (2017). The central role of relationships with trauma-informed integrated care for children and youth. *Academic Pediatrics*, *17*, S94–S101.

Chester, S. J., Tyack, Z., DeYoung, A. et al. (2018). Efficacy of hypnosis on pain, wound-healing, anxiety and stress in children with acute burn injuries: A randomized controlled trial. *Pain*, *159*(9), 1790–1801.

Forgeron, P. A., Jongudornkarn, D., Evans, J., Finley, G. A., Thienthong, S., Sirpul, P., Pairojkul, S., Sriraj, W., & Boonyawatanangkool, K. (2009). Children's pain assessment in northeastern Thailand: Perspectives of health professionals. *Qualitative Health Research 19*(1): 71–81.

Forkey, H. C., Szilagyi, M., Kelly, E. T., & Duffee, J. (2021). Trauma-informed care. *Pediatrics 148*(2): e2021052580.doi: 10.1542/peds.2021-052580.

Garner, A., & Yogman, M. (2021). Committee on Psychosocial Aspects of Child and Family Health Section on Developmental and Behavioral Pediatrics, Council on Early Childhood. Preventing Toxic Stress: Partnering with Families and Communities to Promote Relational Health. *Pediatrics*, *148*(2), e2021052582.

Harkensee, C., Olness, K., & Esmaili, B. E., eds. (2021). *Child refugee and migrant health*, Cham: Springer.

Herran, M. (2021). Return to happiness. In C. Harkensee, K. Olness, & B. E. Esmaili, (Eds.), *Child refugee and migrant health*. Cham: Springer.

Institute for Health Metrics and Evaluation Seattle, Chronic Diseases (2022). ihme@healthdata.org

Kohen, D. P., & Olness, K. (2022). Hypnosis for pediatric medical problems, Chapter 13, In D. P. Kohen & K. Olness (Eds.), *Hypnosis with children 5th edition*. London: Taylor and Francis, Routledge Publications.

Lewis, S. J., Arseneault, L., Caspi, A. et al. (2019). The epidemiology of trauma and post-traumatic stress disorder in a representative cohort of young people in England and Wales. *Lancet Psychiatry*, *6*, 247.

Lindheim, M. O., & Helgeland, H. (2017). Hypnosis training and education: Experiences with a Norwegian one-year education course in clinical hypnosis for children and adolescents. *American Journal of Clinical Hypnosis*, *59*, 282–291.

Meg Foundation . (2022). https://www.megfoundationforpain.org (accessed September 27, 2023).

Nielsen, G. , & Vandvik, I. H. (1981). Hypnose anno 1980. *Tidsskrift for Den Norske Lægeforening*, 4, 101.

Olness, K. (2003). Effects on brain development leading to cognitive impairment: A worldwide epidemic. *Journal of Developmental and Behavioral Pediatrics*, *24*, 120–130.
Olness, K. (2021). Children's mental health at times of disasters: A narrative review. *Pediatric Medicine*. 10.21037/pm20-85.
Pairojkul, S., Siripul, P., Prateepchaikul, L., Kusol, K., & Puytrakul, T. (2010). Psychosocial first aid: Support for the child survivors of the Asian Tsunami. *Journal of Developmental and Behavioral Pediatrics*, *31*, 723–727.
Population Pyramid (2022). https://www.populationpyramid.net/world/2022 (accessed September 16, 2022).
Rutten, M., Vlieger, A., Frankenhuis, C., George, E., Groeneweg, M., Norbruis, O., Walther, T., Van Wering, H., Djikgraaf, M., Merkus, M., & Benninga, M. (2014). Gut-directed hypnotherapy in children with irritable bowel syndrome or functional abdominal pain (syndrome): A randomized controlled trial on self exercises at home using CD versus individual therapy by qualified therapists. *BMC Pediatrics*, *14*, 140.
Thomas, J. (2017). Project Director: "You are the boss of your brain: Learning how to manage pain during medical procedures" (13 min.) Produced by Stanford Children's Health and Lucile Packard Children's Hospital. FREE. https://www.youtube.com
Tome-Pires, C., & Miro, J. (2012). Hypnosis for the management of chronic and cancer procedure-related pain in children. *International Journal of Clinical and Experimental Hypnosis*, *60*, 432–457.
Underwood, E. (2018). Lessons in resilience. *Science*, *359*, 976–979. www.ummeed.org (accessed October 22, 2022), https://www.populationpyramid.net/world/2022 (accessed September 16, 2022)
UNHCR. Data: Global Report 2021. www.unhcr.org
UNICEF. (2021). Child orphans. www.unicef.org
UNICEF. (2022). Children with disabilities: Overview. www.unicef.org
Vagnoli, L., Bettini, A., Amore, E., DeMasi, S., & Messeri, A. (2019). Relaxation-guided imagery reduces perioperative anxiety and pain in children: A randomized study. *European Journal of Pediatrics*, *178*, 913–921.
World Bank (2021). New World Bank Country Classification by income level: 2021–22. www.worldbank.org

62
ACTUAL FAVORITE PLACES

Maren Østvold Lindheim
Department of Child and Adolescent Mental Health in Hospital, Oslo University Hospital, Oslo, Norway

Would You Like to Join Me on a Trip to a Cabin?

Scene 1: When Too Afraid

The boy in front of me is six years old. He is holding his mother's hand tightly and his back is against the white hospital wall as if he tries to protect himself from attacks from behind. I know that he knows that he needs to give a blood sample today. I know that he knows that I am there to make this happen. We only have this time to get to know each other, build trust, and, eventually, help him believe in his own capacity to help himself. I imagine how the smells, sounds, and colors of the hospital remind him of other times in this place. Painful memories. Times he does not remember, but that his body remembers all too well. I can see it in his watchful eyes, white cheeks, and in the tension in his little body. He is ready to run, fight, or even give up. The increasing tension and physical arousal will soon make it even harder for him to cope. It will intensify the sensation of pain. Then, I witness how everything changes the moment I say, "Hi, would you like to visit a cabin with me? It´s outside in the forest by the stream." He seems a bit puzzled, looks up into my eyes and nods. As we walk outside his body starts to relax, he breaths deeply, let's go of her mother's hand, walks with lighter steps, color returns to his cheeks. He looks around and asks, "Where is it? Is it that way?" He leads the way up the small hill, listening to the birds and feeling the wind against his cheek. He says with excitement in his voice "Is that the place? Can we go inside?" He has discovered a strange cabin with crooked walls almost like a tree hut a child would have made. Curious. Inside it smells of wood and he can see the forest through the windows and the sky through a window in the ceiling. His mother lets out a sigh "Aah!" and sits down on one of the colorful cushions. Maybe it reminds her of a cabin she used to visit in the summers as a child. Good memories. The boy starts to explore and find a fishing rod. And as we walk down to the water, he takes my hand.

Children in a Hospital Setting and the Meaning of Nature

In the Department of Child and Adolescent Mental Health in Hospital at Oslo University Hospital, we prepare children, adolescents, and their families for medical procedures and

DOI: 10.4324/9781003449126-81
This chapter has been made available under a CC BY-NC-ND 4.0 license.

support them through challenging hospitalizations. Meeting children in a hospital setting always makes me aware of how unfamiliar and scary this place must seem to them. Imagine being five years old, holding your mother's hand, and going through those huge doors for the first time: white halls with people dressed in white walking hurriedly with serious faces. You may feel how your mother`s grip changes, her hand feels a bit strange, and tense, and it is as if she is not really listening. When you are a little child, the body is sacred; nothing should enter or be taken from it. Imagine how much energy you must spend on protecting your body from "painful stuff that might happen here." For some children (and parents), the high level of bodily arousal caused by such a stressful situation makes it impossible for them to find and use good coping strategies.

We know that children and adolescents with serious and chronic diseases have a higher risk of developing mental, psychosocial, and family-related difficulties compared to somatically healthy children and adolescents, and that this group is at greater risk of developing symptoms of post-traumatic stress (Diseth, 2014; Diseth & Christie, 2005; Gjems & Diseth, 2011). Therefore, children and adolescents who must undergo frightening and painful procedures in the hospital need help to find strategies to get through the procedures and effects that accompany life-protecting treatment.

Helping medically ill children and adolescents to find ways to reduce sympathetic nervous system arousal is an important intervention in preventing and managing pain, anxiety, and stress/trauma-related conditions (Gjems & Diseth, 2011). Psychosocial factors may also affect medical conditions, for example, modulating the impact of stress and inflammatory responses in cases of cancer (Cole, 2013). In these conditions, both relational and contextual factors may influence the outcome (Hauge et al., 2023). Over the years, researchers have tried to define common factors in therapy (e.g., Lambert & Bergin, 1994; Wampold, 2015) mainly studying qualities in the therapist, the client, and the relationship between them (e.g., therapist empathy, patient expectations, agreement about goals). According to Finsrud and colleagues, confidence in the therapist and confidence in the treatment (e.g., positive expectation) are essential factors (Finsrud, 2021). Much less is known about the effect of the qualities in the surroundings and how to facilitate desired change by inviting clients to be in their preferred environment (Hauge et al., 2023). There is little research on how different indoor interior and architecture may affect therapy (Jackson, 2018) although some studies suggest that environments in which the interior looks like someone's home may help patients feel safer (Jones, 2020) and a safe setting might heighten positive expectation (Frank, 1982; Frank & Frank, 1991). Over the years there has also been a growing interest in the field of nature-based therapy and the positive effects of bringing patients out into nature (e.g., Fernee et al., 2020). To reduce stress and facilitate beneficial coping and empowerment, we should consider all aspects of a child's hospital experience, using communication skills to imbue each encounter with accumulating safety and acceptance. This can start with the admission letter, the hospital milieu, and the way we greet each young person. When faced with a scared child or adolescent, we could start by asking them, "Where would you rather be than here?" Sometimes they can travel there in their mind and other times it works better to actually go there.

This chapter is about how we may enhance absorption, interconnectedness, and creativity through the environment and thereby evoke malleability and flexibility that can be brought back into the hospital (see Sugarman et al., 2020). We will look at the concepts of relational and contextual hypnosis, favorite places imagined (inscapes) and actual favorite places (landscapes), attachment/place attachment, and the meaning of natural surroundings in therapy and hypnotic work. We will explore through stories from practice at the Outdoor Care Retreat, how we, by taking in the environmental landscape and making it an intensely memorable inscape, can encourage a memorable presence.

Clinical Hypnosis

Clinical hypnosis may be understood as an interpersonal communication method that aims to cultivate change in the embodied mind (Sugarman et al., 2020). I find it helpful to think of trance as a creative inner process rather than a state. Working with children, I find that trance happens naturally without the need for induction. However, if I am to think in terms of induction, I like to think of it as similar to a parent`s soothing humming to a child (Gerge, 2009). Hypnotic nonverbal communication such as tone of voice, pacing, and utilization have qualities that can be seen as parallel to the healthy primary attachment relationship (Linden, 2020; Spiegel, 2016; Zelinka et al., 2014). In this way, clinical hypnosis "speaks" to the child within and offers new healthy attachment experiences that facilitate beneficial learning (plasticity). When attending a child bedside, I aim to create – through focused shared attention – a secure "bubble" surrounding me and the child/family. The bubble shields us from disturbing sounds, people, and light. Through helpful suggestions (i.e., what is communicated verbally or nonverbally in trance), the child/family is invited to experience themselves or the world in a new way (Helgeland et al., 2021). In my experience, clinical hypnosis may be used together with a range of different therapeutic approaches as it involves biopsychosocial factors (e.g., facilitating subjective experiences, psychobiological change, hope, and positive expectancy) that might be of importance for a positive treatment outcome (Jensen et al., 2015). In this way, hypnotic communication may facilitate and strengthen therapy in general.

"Inscapes" and "Landscapes"

Safe-place inductions are considered important in stabilizing, self-regulation, and resource installation in trauma-informed psychotherapy (Diseth & Christie, 2005; Gerge, 2018; Shapiro, 2001). "Safe place" may be thought of as an emotional sanctuary where a person can go in their mind to recover stability when feeling stressed (Shapiro, 2001). Imagined favorite or special places (inscapes) can be remembered or projected into the future. These can induce processes of safety and belongingness because, "when clients feel sufficiently secure in the moment, they can begin to change their patterns and learn in depth" (Gerge, 2018). I often prefer to introduce the concept of a "good place" rather than a "safe place" as some patients do not have a safe place and the word "safe" also lead to associations with something being "unsafe." With children, I often find it useful to talk of good "experiences" or "activities" rather than good "places" and even make the conversation into a good experience of empowerment:

> "You are here to have a vaccine. I imagine that this is not your favorite activity. So, if I ask you how you feel right now ... ? Not so great? Right. I wonder where you would rather be than here? Right. That's the place – and you feel just great! Would it help you to tell me where you are? What do you do there? Maybe we could draw a picture of it with your favorite colors? Look at this wonderful picture ... How do you feel right now? Great? How did you do that? Change from "not so good" to "great"?

You did it "just" by drawing a picture of things you like to do and places you like to be and kind of "just" go there in your mind? Isn't that interesting? I wonder if this may be a picture of some of your superpowers?"

Asking patients "Where would you rather be than here," carefully listening to the words chosen and repeating them back to the patients to help them be more and more there, is a way to invite them to dissociate from the situation they are in for a while. Dissociation, disorientating from the physical environment and even one's body, is an innate response to protect oneself in a challenging or traumatic situation. In therapeutic hypnosis, dissociation is utilized to create a sensation of control, safety, and beneficial associations. Inspired by Milton Erickson's (1985) concept of utilization, we can use what the person is already doing and help them use it for something good. Thus, creating an inscape is not only about distraction but also about finding one's own "superpowers."

When asked about good or favorite places, many patients (and people in general) refer to places connected to natural environments and activities that occur within them (Korpela 2003; Korpela & Hartig, 1996). For an environment to be categorized as natural, it might be sufficient that it includes some natural elements (Korpela, 2003). However, for many of us, the concept of nature is associated with a place different from an urban environment, a place that is dominated by natural elements and large enough for us to feel some level of absorption in the element (Johnsen, 2011). Natures' positive effect on psychological well-being is documented across cultures (Hartig et al., 1991; Hartig et al., 2003; Kaplan, 1995; Park et al., 2010; Ulrich et al., 1991). We know that spending time in nature can have a regulating effect on the body and that exposure to daylight and images of real or simulated nature influences perceived pain, stress, and the length of hospitalizations (Kaplan, 1995; Malenbaum et al., 2008; Ulrich, 1984; Ulrich, 2008; Walch et al., 2005). Spending time in forest areas has been shown to lower cortisol levels, heart rate, and blood pressure, increase parasympathetic activity, and decrease sympathetic activity to a greater extent than time spent in urban areas (Kaplan, 1995). Even just sitting in a room with a view of the natural surroundings reduces blood pressure more than sitting in a room without a view (Hartig et al., 2003). In many illnesses, physical activity can help to improve a patient's physical and mental health, and physical activity in nature can have an additional positive impact (Martinsen, 2004; Ryan et al., 2010). Several studies show that nature has characteristics that can have a restorative effect on people's temporarily reduced mental resources (Kaplan, 1995; Park et al., 2010). Furthermore, several studies suggest that spending time in nature can reduce physiological arousal, enhance positive emotions, and minimize negative emotions (Hartig et al., 2003; Hartig et al., 1991; Ulrich et al., 1991). As a result, time spent in nature proves to be significant for emotion regulation, and some people deliberately use nature to create more comfortable mindsets (Hartig et al., 2003; Korpela, 2003; Johnsen, 2011; Johnsen, 2013). People may experience a long-term positively affected bond to a place and seek comfort by visiting specific places or places associated with positively affected experiences in childhood (e.g., "place attachment," Korpela & Hartig, 1996; Morgan, 2010). With this knowledge, it is tempting to ask the question, why is so much therapy conducted indoors and in a setting decided by the clinician?

In our daily lives, our attention is effortfully directed toward different objects (mobile phones, computer screens, persons, toys in a therapy playroom) in service of specific goals. Nature, on the other hand, offers an undemanding setting where attention can be directed more effortlessly toward whatever is experienced as fascinating at that moment (e.g.,

Attention Restoration Theory; Kaplan, 1995). Helping patients to experience an actual good place that stimulates all senses (sounds, smells, colors, feels) in an open and undirected way may start a trance process, thereby strengthening their experience of being able to help themselves feel good (e.g., self-soothing capacity). This may also make it easier for the person to find the way "back" to that place in their mind's imagination when in the hospital in a challenging situation. The landscape trance can become an inscape when in the hospital.

Where Would You Rather Be Than Here?

Scene 2 When Words Are Not Enough

The first time I really understood the impact of nature in therapy was in 2010. I was attending a teenager with a heart disease who was referred to us because she had stopped talking and responding to the hospital staff. The nurses were worried that she was depressed. I remember entering her room. She was laying with her head under the blanket. She had been in the hospital for a long time. I imagine she was fed up with treatment, giving blood and giving answers. I imagined that the last thing she wanted to do was to talk with yet another new person, a psychologist. As I struggled to get in touch with the girl under the blanked her father said, to excuse her behavior, "I think she is just so tired of being inside this place. Back home she is always outside in our garden or in the forest." I remember asking; "Would you rather be outside in the forest?" Then there was a nod from under the blanket. What surprised me then was the fact that she had been in the hospital for such a long time, and no one had thought of bringing her outside. We got her into a wheelchair, tucked in a warm blanket, and went outside, over a small bridge and into the forest that borders the hospital ground. We sat down by the stream. The girl gazed out on the water as her father and I talked about the smell of grass, the sound of the stream, and the activities of the birds and animals we have seen in the forest. And as we sat there, I could see how her face relaxed and how relieved her father was to see her like this. After a while, she whispered to her father, and he told me that she loved horses and used to ride a horse back home. And when I asked her if she would like to visit the horses that lived close by, she looked at me for the first time and said in a clear voice "Yes." When we later returned to the hospital, I could remind her of the sounds of the forest, the softness of the horse`s muzzle, and how good it smelled. And in this way I help her get through painful treatment. I remember thinking "We have to do more of this."

Life within the four walls of a hospital entails a considerable loss of perspective, predictability, and control. This can result in emotional and physiological strain and a feeling of hopelessness. Seriously and/or chronically ill children and adolescents might experience life as unfair, feel different from their peers, find interaction with their parents challenging, and develop an illness identity: "I am ill and weak, I cannot trust my body, I always make things worse." They may have few and "thin" life stories of mastery (e.g., narrative therapy; White, 1990). Facilitating hope and positive expectations is a critical intervention (Helgeland et al., 2021; Lindheim & Helgeland, 2017). We attempt to help children and adolescents in ways that help them feel empowered, using play, externalization, fantasy, storytelling, and hypnotic communication. But in some situations, this is just not enough.

Over the last 12 years, we have made many positive clinical experiences incorporating nature into our therapeutic work. We experience how nature and enjoyable activities bring spontaneous joy, provide a break from difficult hospital experiences, and promote relaxation (Lindheim et al., 2020). For some patients, regular trips outside in nature have been a motivating factor in their treatment and have given them positive associations with the hospital. Patients tell us that what they remember best from all the time they have spent in the hospital are our trips outside in the forest. Families have reported that it feels good to get out of the hospital, see what their children can manage to do, be a "normal" family again, spend quality time together, take part in meaningful activities, and learn new things. These experiences might contribute to "thicker" life stories of mastery (White, 1990). We are witnesses to these experiences; we can retell the stories (to doctors, nurses, and family members) and in this way make these positive life stories even more robust. "You actually managed to make a bonfire together even though it rained so hard. You are a family who really won't give up."

Furthermore, shared nature experiences might also change the relationship between therapist/clinicians and patient. I will never forget a young girl who saw a nurse she had known for years suddenly wearing a rain jacket as we were going outside together. It was as if her eyes were asking, "Are you a normal person?" I like to think of trance as a set of parameters for processing inputs. As novelty drives trance, new important experiences of this sort may create opportunities for change.

We experience how nature profoundly expands the child and family's frames of references and their resources for managing uncertainty. Just as the hospital setting evokes a sense of externalized and human-design control where, even though we try to escape by dissociating from it, the smells, sounds, and sensations impinge on us. Nature provides us with an infinitely expansive environment. Here we can be both effective (in discovery, collecting things, making bonfires) and part of something growing, healing, changing, and decaying (seasons changing, flowers growing and withering). Nature provides a literal landscape of possibilities and metaphors that might drive trance. When the hospital environment may not be a creative environment, nature is endlessly so.

These positive experiences created in me a desire to establish a therapeutic space in nature close to the hospital so that patients, who for various reasons cannot leave the hospital area, can spend time in nature. A physical cabin provides a sheltered space and can be used by patients who cannot be outdoors for long periods.

The Meaning of the Outdoor Care Retreat

The Outdoor Care Retreat ("Friluftssykehuset") was built in 2018. The cabin was developed in cooperation with the father of a patient and an architectural firm (Snøhetta). The collaboration arose from a common desire to create a positive place in nature for patients and their families. The cabin has a "biophilic" design. The goal of biophilic design is to connect the satisfying elements of nature to a built environment through organic forms, natural elements, and vegetation (Kellert & Calabrese, 2015). What we came to realize after inviting patients and relatives out to the cabin was that the architectural design and location of the Outdoor Care Retreat provided a unique therapeutic space that in itself facilitated therapeutic work (Lindheim et al., 2020). The feedback from both clinicians and patients tells us that the surroundings at the Outdoor Care Retreat stimulate curiosity and creativity, give access to positive associations, and facilitate belief in their coping abilities and positive expectations for change and development. All of these are important factors in driving trance and facilitating positive change.

Therapists using the Outdoor Care Retreat report that the playful architecture and natural materials in the cabin and surrounding nature are actively used in therapy for relationship building, in narrative therapy, metaphors, and restorative effects (Lindheim et al., 2020). To look more closely at the meaning of the Outdoor Care Retreat, we conducted a study comparing the Outdoor Care Retreat to traditional hospital environments interviewing hospital leaders, therapists, and parents of children. We found that the setting influenced therapy through affordance (the natural setting gave more flexibility and diversity in activities, positive distractions, and easier access to many favorite places), natural bodily reactions (more active body, more relaxed and open body language, more energy level in line with the form of the day), identity and role (therapist and child seeing themselves as more equal, the child focused more on normal healthy sides), emotions (more positive emotions of joy, safety, and restoration), stronger alliance (attachment and contact between the therapist and patient was quicker built, the child was more in control), therapeutic flow in a holding environment (easier to motivate, regulate emotions; easier to open up to more playful creative therapy using nature metaphors), and valuable expectations (more positive memories and more positive expectations regarding future treatment) (Hauge et al., 2023).

Finding "Superpowers"

When "Not Suited" for Therapy

I remember meeting a girl who taught me a lot about therapy. She was referred to us because she needed medical care that she resisted because of previous traumatic hospital experiences. She was also defined as "not suitable for therapy" (by previous therapists) due to different challenges. I do not think she would ever have agreed to meet me inside the hospital. But as she was told of the cabin, she agreed to meet me there once and then decide whether she would come back again. The first time we met she was sitting inside our play tent, with her legs sticking out, as I spoke with her mother and father. The same happened the next session. Eventually she started to peek out and join us in our conversations about favorite places and favorite activities. I learned then that she had a dog that she loved. The next time she brought the dog, and we went for a walk up the stream. I told her she and the dog could lead the way and I would try to follow in her footsteps. She liked that. We spent many sessions exploring the steam. Later I learned that she was very brave when it came to insects and worms. She showed me how to handle the creatures and, as I do not like worms, she had to expose me gradually to them to help me feel safe. Later we used worms as actors to re-tell her experiences in the hospital: what had happened and what she would prefer to imagine happened instead. We sat inside the cabin in the small room and looked out into the forest as she told her story. She was the director, I acted through the worms and her parents were the audience. Eventually we could also practice the medical procedure she needed done. After practicing inside the cabin, we went outside and into the forest to "get it all out of our body." Now that she was in an actual good place we could also explore the effect of deep breathing, progressive relaxation, and good place exercises. She liked to imagine being outside with her dog. This helped her relax, but she found it difficult to bring herself to this place when she was in the hospital. Her brilliant solution in the end was to bring her dog with her and have the dog on her lap as the treatment was performed the practitioner could see when she was ready by observing the dog's bodily reactions. When the dog was calm, she was in her favorite place and ready. After the procedure was done, we had a celebration at the cabin and invited the practitioners and her family. We celebrated all she had managed to do and told stories of our journey together.

The positive experiences of being in a favorite place, feeling safe, and having the time to find her own "superpowers" bring up the question of whether this girl was unsuited for therapy or not suited for the limited type of therapy offered. It also questions whether the therapy we tend to offer children is more suited for adults (who like to talk) than children (who like to do).

Bringing It Together

A good place: In our clinical work, we experience inviting patients and their families to the Outdoor Care Retreat has a positive impact on their perceived level of stress and anxiety. Patients and family members who visit the Outdoor Care Retreat often say that they find it easier to relax and feel good inside the cabin than within the four walls of the hospital. Many talk spontaneously about other places and experiences in which they feel or have felt good. In this way, the surroundings can facilitate access to positive sensory experiences and memories. Moreover, the therapists can help the patients recapture the feelings of peace and joy from the forest when they are in challenging hospital situations: "Do you remember when we were out by the stream, and your bark boat went over the rapids?" In this way, the cabin becomes an *actual* favorite or safe place. For patients who find it hard to imagine, concentrate, verbalize, or are too afraid, it can be easier to establish a good bodily sensation when exposed to a physical landscape that then, in turn, becomes an inscape. Further, some might find it easier to bring the experience back in to mind when they have used their senses (smell, touch, sound, colors, shape) together with a therapist that can help them bring the experience back to live, especially if the situation is challenging having an operation, experiencing postoperational pain, or undergoing needle insertions. Sharing good activities and places may also influence relationships. In a therapy group with adolescents, we invited the participants to bring the group members to their local favorite place in nature. The intimate gesture of sharing these places strengthened the relationships and feelings of worth.

A place for journeying together: "Where would you rather be?" Patients often spontaneously choose to sit inside the cabin by the window in the small room looking down toward the stream when they need to concentrate or talk about challenging subjects. Then many suddenly get up and walk into the bigger room with cushions when they want to be more active, play, and feel joy. They might even open the doors and move out into the forest to get a break from it all. The cabin gives flexibility and opportunities to move between qualitatively different therapeutic settings inside and outside and thereby regulate bodily sensations and feelings. We experience that patients who are given the opportunity to do this are better able to tolerate strong emotions and find more effective ways to stabilize (Lindheim et al., 2020). Also, by asking the young person: where would you prefer to be? Where do you find your strength and superpowers? Where would you like to talk about this? In a therapy room? Outside in the forest? In the cabin? Where? And *follow them there* we strongly communicate that we trust their ability to help themselves. In addition, when they are *there* – we can give a suggestion that will stick: "You really know how to take care of yourself."

A place for making life stories of mastery thicker: which stories from the hospital will a child remember? What will be their story? Diseases and hospitalizations affect the entire family. Patients can feel different from their peers, find it hard to cope in different situations, and interaction within the family can be challenging. To encourage families to have a good experience out in nature is a therapeutic intervention in itself. Furthermore, the Outdoor Care Retreat invites patients and their family to be in a protected, homely, and private surrounding where they might feel like a normal family. The surrounding nature often makes it easier to experience a feeling of dignity and equality. Nature also gives many opportunities for positive experiences such as caring for yourself and for others (making a bonfire together to stay warm, making food together when feeling hungry), mastery (shooting with a bow and an arrow), and seeing new sides (a father's warmth toward his son as compared to anxious and distant behavior when inside the hospital). After a child has completed a "big job" in the hospital (such as an operation), we invite family and hospital staff to a celebration at the Outdoor Care Retreat and retell stories of everything they have done. In this way, we may think of ourselves as storytellers contributing to positive life stories and good memories.

A place of metaphors, symbolism, and creativity: Remember the story about the girl and the horse? I left out an important part of the tale; *On our quest to find a horse, it turned out that there were no horses in the stable. However, as we had set out to find a horse, we agreed not to give up. We continued to search for a horse, and I became increasingly worried that we would not find any. Then suddenly the most beautiful horse appeared on the road. The rider stopped and the horse bowed its head as the girl touched its muzzle.* The synchronicity of this event may have added to her natural hypnotic experience. Nature provides many opportunities for metaphors (seasons changing, bumblebees ability to fly even though they supposedly are too heavy to do so), co-therapists (worms, dogs, and horses), and symbolic actions (following the child up the stream), and invitations to hypnotic surroundings that may strengthen our suggestions. The therapeutic symbols and metaphors we find in surrounding nature are also especially strong because they are experienced with *all* senses. This bodily experience of the metaphor creates a learning process that is more robust and remembered in another way than words are (Corazon et al., 2011; Naor & Mayseless, 2021). *There lives a heron by the stream close to the cabin. I remember sitting with a young boy looking out the window as he told of his illness and how he coped. Suddenly, the heron came flying through the wood landing by the stream. The boy was amazed. The majestic bird stood still as if it was listening, and I said, "The heron only comes when someone says something important. Say that again? Can you see how he listens?"*

A place where anything is possible: The Outdoor Care Retreat is a place where anything is possible. A place of novelty and adventure. It is a place for creativity, possibilities, and discovery of superpowers. The therapist's ability to create an interest and belief in the therapeutic project is a crucial factor in therapy (e.g., Finsrud et al., 2021). The invitation to visit a strange looking cabin with crooked walls by the stream usually makes children curious and interested. This curiosity may drive trance and thereby help them get access to their own recourses. Being in the cabin allows the child to become more open to suggestions of the sort: "Being so afraid of a future needle poke tells me that you have a good imagination. Do you know why I know that? Because you can imagine stuff so life-like that you become afraid now—even in this comfortable place. This imagination is exactly what you can use to solve the problem. It is a superpower. I wonder how you will use it."

Bringing Clinical Hypnosis Further

Patients have started their journey of change long before they meet us (Sugarman et al., 2020). They come to our first meeting with expectations, worries, earlier experiences, and a focused attention. Awareness of this, detecting naturally occurring trance, strengthening this process (through how we meet people), communicating positive suggestions to strengthen their belief in their own capacity to help themselves ("superpowers" and positive expectation regarding wanted change), and then continuing a journey together to explore what works best for that person are what therapeutic hypnosis is for. In this way, hypnotic skills may facilitate and strengthen all other therapeutic methods. An important aspect of effective hypnotic communication is a deep attunement with the patient's embodied mind (following a patient's breath, bodily communication, manifestations of their autonomic balance, intensifying focus) that may have qualities in common with safe attachment (Spiegel, 2016; Zelinka et al., 2014). We facilitate relational experiences that might give comfort to the other person and create an environment for positive change (Linden, 2020). A less explored, but important, way people seek comfort is by seeking out specific places, "place attachment" (Korpela & Hartig, 1996; Morgan, 2010). These specific places, and even nature in itself, might be understood as a secure base (Jordan, 2009). Bringing into awareness the importance of a person's connectedness to special places and surroundings might strengthen our ability to help people heal. Therefore, combining hypnotic relational and communicational skills with hypnotic surroundings and activities strengthens our therapeutic work. Imagine all the possibilities! I wonder how you will use them?

Acknowledgment

The author gratefully acknowledges Trond H. Diseth, colleagues at the Department of Child and Adolescent Mental Health in Hospital, Håvard Hernes, Åshild Hauge, and Svein Åge Johnsen for their support and inspiration in the development of the Outdoor Care Retreat. I also thank Laurence Sugarman and Julie Linden for valuable comments on the manuscript.

References

Cole, S. W. (2013). Nervous system regulation of the cancer genome. *Brain Behavior and Immunity*, *30*, 10–18. doi: 10.1016/j.bbi.2012.11.008.

Corazon, S. S., Schilhab, T. S., & Stigsdotter, U. K. (2011). Developing the therapeutic potential of embodied cognition and metaphors in nature-based therapy: Lessons from theory to practice. *Journal of Adventure Education & Outdoor Learning*, *11*(2), 161–171. 10.1080/14729679.2011.633389

Diseth, T. H. (2014). Kronisk somatisk sykdom og symptomatologi hos barn og unge. In A. A. Dahl, J. H. Loge, & T. F. Aarre (Eds.), *Psykiske reaksjoner ved somatisk sykdom*. (pp. 674–694). Oslo: Cappelen Damm Akademisk.

Diseth, T. H., & Christie, H. J. (2005). Trauma-related dissociative (conversion) disorders in children and adolescents – An overview of assessment tools and treatment principles. *Nordic Journal of Psychiatry*, *59*, 278–292. 10.1080/08039480500213683

Erickson, M. H. (1985). *Life reframing in hypnosis* Rossi, E. L., & Ryan M. O. (Eds). (Vol 2). New York: Irvington Publishers.

Fernee, C. R., Gabrielsen, L. E., Andersen, A. J. W., & Mesel, T. (2020). Emerging stories of self: Long-term outcomes of wilderness therapy in Norway. *Journal of Adventure Education and Outdoor Learning*, *21*, 1–15. 10.1080/14729679.2020.1730205

Finsrud, I., Nissen-Lie, H. A., Vrabel, K., Høstmælingen, A., Wampold, B. E., & Ulvenes, P. G. (2021). It's the therapist and the treatment: The structure of common therapeutic relationship factors. *Psychotherapy Research*, *32*(2), 139–150. 10.1080/10503307.2021.1916640

Frank, J. D. (1982). Therapeutic components shared by all psychotherapies. In J. H. Harvey, M. M. Park (Eds.), *The master lecture series. Psychotherapy research and behavior change*. (pp. 9–37). (Vol. 1). Washington: Am Psychol.Assoc. 10.1037/10083-001

Frank, J. D., & Frank, J. B. (1991). *Persuasion and healing: A comparative study of psychotherapy* (3rd ed.). Baltimore: Johns Hopkins University Press.

Gerge, A. (2009). *Hypnos i psykoterapeutiskt arbete – ett integrativt perspektiv*. Stockholm: Insidan.

Gerge, A. (2018). Revisiting the safe place: Method and regulatory aspects in psychotherapy when easing allostatic overload in traumatized patients. *International Journal of Clinical and Experimental Hypnosis*, *66*(2), 147–173. doi: 10.1080/00207144.2018.1421356.

Gjems, S., & Diseth, T. H. (2011). Somatic illness and psychological trauma in children. Prevention and treatment strategies. *Tidsskrift for Norsk psykologforening*, *48*, 857–862.

Hartig, T., Mang, M., & Evans, G. (1991). Restorative effects of natural environment experiences. *Environment and Behavior*, *23*, 3–26. doi:10.1177/0013916591231001

Hartig, T., Evans, G. W., Jamner, L. J., Davis, D. S., & Garling, T. (2003). Tracking restoration in natural and urban field settings. *Journal of Environmental Psychology*, *23*, 109–123. 10.1016/S0272-4944(02)00109-3

Hauge, Å. L., Lindheim, M. Ø., Røtting, K., & Johnsen, S. Å. K. (2023). The meaning of the physical environment in child and adolescent therapy – A qualitative study of the outdoor care retreat (in press).

Helgeland, H., Lindheim, M. Ø., Diseth, T. H., & Brodal, P. A. (2021). Clinical hypnosis – A re-vitalisation of the art of medicine. *Tidsskrift for Den Norske Legeforening*. (7), 21. doi: 10.4045

Jackson, D. (2018). Aesthetics and the psychotherapist`s office. *Journal of Clinical Psychology*, *74*(2), 233–238. 10.1002/jclp.22576

Jensen, M. P., Adachi, T., Tomé-Pires, C., Lee, J., Osman, Z. J., & Miró, J. (2015). Mechanisms of hypnosis: Toward the development of a biopsychosocial model. *International Journal of Clinical and Experimental Hypnosis*, *63*, 34–75.

Johnsen, S.Å.K. (2011). The use of nature for emotion regulation: Toward a conceptual framework. *Ecopsychology*, *3*, 175–185.

Johnsen, S.Å.K. (2013). Exploring the use of nature for emotion regulation: Associations with personality, perceived stress, and restorative outcomes. *Nordic Psychology*, 306–321.

Jones, J. K. (2020). A place for therapy: Clients reflect on their experience in psychotherapists offices. *Qualitative Social Work*, *19* (3), 406–423. 10.1177/1473325020911676

Jordan, M. (2009). Nature and self – An ambivalent attachment? *Ecopsychology*, *1*(1), 26–31. doi: 10.1089/ECO.2008.0003.

Kaplan, S. (1995). The restorative benefits of nature: Towards an integrative framework. *Journal of Environmental Psychology*, *15*, 169–182. 10.1016/0272-4944(95)90001-2

Kellert, S. R., & Calabrese, E. (2015). *The practice of biophilic design*. www.biophilic-design.com.

Korpela, K. (2003). Negative mood and adult place preferences. *Environment & Behaviour*, *35*, 331–346. doi: 10.1177/0013916503035003002.

Korpela, K., & Hartig, T. (1996). Restorative qualities of favorite places. *Journal of Environmental Psychology*, *16*, 221–233. 10.1006/jevp.1996.0018

Lambert, M. J., & Bergin, A. E. (1994). The effectiveness of psychotherapy. In A. E. Bergin & S. L. Gardfield (Eds.), *Handbook of psychotherapy and behavior change* (pp. 143–189). John Wiley & Sons.

Linden, J. H. (2020). Relationship factors in the theatre of the imagination: Hypnosis with children and adolescents. *American Journal of Clinical Hypnosis*, *62*, 60–73.

Lindheim, M. Ø., & Helgeland, H. (2017). Hypnosis training and education: Experiences with a Norwegian one-year education course in clinical hypnosis for children and adolescents. *American Journal of Clinical Hypnosis*, *59*, 3, *Exploring, Evolving, and Refining Hypnosis Education*.

Lindheim, Ø.M., Johnsen, S.Å.K., Hauge, Å.L., & Diseth, T. H. (2020). The outdoor care retreat. *Tidsskrift for Den Norske Legeforening*. doi:10.4045.

Malenbaum, S., Keefe, F. J., Williams, A. C. C., Ulrich, R., & Somers, J. T. (2008). Pain in its environmental context: Implications for designing environments to enhance pain control. *Pain*, *134*, 241–244. doi: 10.1016

Martinsen, E. W. (2004). *Kropp og sinn: fysisk aktivitet og psykisk helse*. Bergen: Fagbokforlaget.

Morgan, P. (2010). Toward a developmental theory of place attachment. *Journal of Environmental Psychology*, *30*, 11–22.

Naor, L., & Mayseless, O. (2021). The art of working with nature in nature-based therapies. *Journal of Experiential Education*, *44*(2), 184–202. 10.1177/1053825920933639

Park, B. J., Tsunetsugu, Y., Kasetani, T., Kagawa, T., & Miyazaki, Y. (2010). The physiological effects of Shinrin-yoku (taking in the forest atmosphere or forest bathing): Evidence from field experiments in 24 forests across Japan. *Environmental Health and Preventive Medicine*, *15*(1), 18–26. doi: 10.1007/s12199-009-0086-9.

Ryan, R. M., Weinstein, N., Bernstein, J., Brown, K. W., Mistretta, L., & Gagne, M. (2010). Vitalizing effects of being outdoors and in nature. *Journal of Environmental Psychology*, *30*, 159–168.

Shapiro, F. (2001). *Eye movement desensitization and reprocessing: Basic principles, protocols, and procedures*, (2nd ed.). New York: The Guilford Press.

Spiegel, E. (2016). Attachment – Focused hypnosis in psychotherapy for complex trauma: Attachment, representation, and mentalization. *International Journal of Clinical and Experimental Hypnosis*, *64*(1), 45–74.

Sugarman L., Linden, J. H., & Brooks, L. W. (2020). *Changing minds with clinical hypnosis*. Taylor and Francis, Routledge.

Ulrich, R. S. (1984). View through a window may influence recovery from surgery. *Science*, *224*, 420–421.

Ulrich, R. S. (2008). Biophilic design of healthcare environments. I Kellert S., Heerwagen J., Madpr M., (Eds.) *Biophilic design for better buildings and communities*. New York: John Wiley, 87–106.

Ulrich, R. S., Simons, R. F., Losito, B. D., Fiorito, E., Miles.M. A., & Zelson, M. (1991). Stress recovery during exposure to natural and urban environments. *Journal of Environmental Psychology*, *11*, 201–230.

Walch, J. M., Rabin, B. S., Day, R., Williams, J. N., Choi, K., & Kang, J. D. (2005). The effect of sunlight on postoperative analgesic medication use: A prospective study of patients undergoing spinal surgery. *Psychosomatic Medicine*, *67*, 156–163. doi:10.1097/01.psy.0000149258.42508.70.

Wampold, B. E. (2015). How important are the common factors in psychotherapy? An update. *World Psychiatry*, *14*(3), 270–277. doi: 10.1002/wps.20238.

White, M., & Epston, D. (1990). *Narrative means to therapeutic ends*. New York: Norton.

Zelinka, V., Cojan, Y., Desseilles, M. (2014). Hypnosis, attachment, and oxytocin: An integrative perspective. *International Journal of Clinical and Experimental Hypnosis*, 62(1), 29–49. doi: 10. 1080/00207144.2013.841473

63
HYPNOTIC HORIZONS

Richard Hill[1], *Daniel Short*[2], *Kathryn Lane Rossi*[3], *Roxanna Erickson-Klein*[4], *and Laurence Irwin Sugarman*[5]

[1]Clinical Science Director, The Science of Psychotherapy; [2]Sonoran University of Health Sciences; [3]PsychoSocial Genomics Institute; [4]Milton H. Erickson Foundation; [5]Rochester Institute of Technology

Hypnotic Horizons

Hypnosis has a long, fabled history of turning out to be something other than what it first seems. The earliest forms of what we now call hypnosis can be traced back to shamanic/spiritual healing rituals in nearly every culture since the beginning of recorded history. With unlimited ritualistic variations, practices have in common the power to convey extraordinary, therapeutic mind-body changes and beneficial social outcomes. In early Western medicine, through emphasizing suggestion effects, hypnosis focused on obedience to and compliance with an authority figure. Increasingly over the last half-century, this focus has shifted to individual empowerment, personal growth, and the interactional/relational aspects of such encounters (Erickson & Rossi, 1976/2010; Diamond, 1987; Varga, 2021). As we seek to learn more about hypnosis and consider its future trajectory, we need to consider how hypnosis is fundamentally distinct from other therapeutic methodologies and how distinctions drive science and society to continually update and redefine the phenomenological experiences of hypnosis.

Unlike hard sciences, hypnosis scholars continue to debate its precise definition. Accordingly, hypnosis keeps evading consensual boundaries. Despite contentions, the clear practical value of hypnosis is its power as a shared idea to serve specific, individual needs, while keeping pace with the zeitgeist of a changing society. Hence, as the conditions and intentions of hypnosis evolve, so does the significance of its phenomena and therapeutic applications. As with any other social construct (such as health or justice), perceptions and performance of hypnosis continue to evolve both publicly and professionally.

From the earliest history of hypnosis, a key feature of fascination, investigation, and identification is the concept of non-volition – a perceived lack of free individual choice (Fromm & Nash, 1992). The authors contend that this issue of "agency" – the attributed source of ideas and suggestions – in hypnotic interactions is a critical factor in the evolution of hypnosis. Over the last decade, a shift in published definitions now places lesser emphasis on the element of suggestibility and more on the evocation of self-direction, self-efficacy, and mastery within a problem-solving contexts (Hope & Sugarman, 2015; Short, 2022a; Sugarman, 2021).

DOI: 10.4324/9781003449126-82
This chapter has been made available under a CC-BY-NC-ND 4.0 license.

Despite this shift toward evocation, a lingering public perception of hypnosis is one in which verbal communication is used by one individual to manipulate another. This perspective has contributed to a great deal of misunderstanding about the nature and limitations of hypnosis. Such misunderstandings, and in many instances, misrepresentations, have attributed special hypnotic powers to the hypnotist such as the capacity to override another individual's facility for decision-making or physical control of one's own body. The seductive appeal of such power has spread hypnosis to non-therapeutic settings including ambitions in romance, marketing, workforce productivity, war interrogation, cults, and undue influence (see Scheflin & Hassan and Hassan & Scheflin in this volume). We contend that this deep fascination has to do with how the relational power of hypnosis permeates boundaries of self.

Hypnosis is solidly based on an incumbent human ability to be unconsciously susceptible to social influence. That is why it is possible to elicit behaviors that, while consistent with naturally developed capacities, may seem novel or even contrary to existing patterns of behavior. As with all hyper-social animals, human society has evolved so that a majority comply automatically with acts of leadership. This is why phylogenetic behaviors – eye-contact, mimicry, certain gestures – are utilized in hypnosis. However, pluralistic models of hypnosis indicate that other beneficial, person-centered, and individually empowering operations of influence can serve as a vital nexus for heath and care (see Short, 2020 for a conceptual overview).

From its conception, hypnosis was meant to be an extraordinary, unexpected, and somehow spectacular experience. The practical benefit of this construction of hypnosis is that participation in novelty can often lead individuals to activate beneficial growth-oriented mindsets and behavioral potentials that were previously unrecognized or under-utilized (Rossi, 2004; Sugarman, 2021). However, as societies and individuals change so does the realization of what constitutes an extraordinary experience, thus hypnosis's ongoing metamorphosis.

In this final chapter, we consider hypnosis as both a social construct and a methodology. First, we look inward toward the hypnotic processes that occur between and within us. Next, we look outward toward how those subjective processes can be measured and studied. Finally, we look forward, projecting a potential future in which hypnosis takes its place at the heart of health and care.

Looking Inward

Having progressed from spiritual forces, to magnetic energies, to nervous system pathology, and then to sleep and suggestion, we can see how hypnosis has been enacted and reified as if it is immutable. This clearly is not the case. Rather, we see the invisible hand of shared belief, expectancy effects, psychobiological reflexes (e.g., dissociation), and social mimicry. Speaking to a broader class of social phenomena, Jaynes (1976) introduced the term "collective cognitive imperative" to describe culturally agreed on behavioral constraints and roles to be acted-out in the absence of conscious intention. Interestingly, as far back as 1852, James Braid came to the realization that hypnosis is not an altered state of consciousness but rather the result of expectancy effects and imitation (social mimicry). However, Braid lacked the language needed to translate his insights into a compelling paradigm shift (see Short, 2022b).

History and cultural comparisons show that the methodology of hypnosis is much more diverse than the directive, stepwise, problem-centered rituals employed in research, coached in professional training, and, consequently, enacted in clinical practice. Many chapters of this book have outlined the parameters of a more capacious domain for hypnotic interaction that includes idiosyncratic and multilevel conversations *as well as* scripted protocols (for a conceptual overview see also Teleska & Roffman, 2004). As complexity theory starts to replace Immanual Kant's notion of an entirely conscious empirical self (see Smith, 2021), a more complex and less determinate ecology of interactions (e.g., embodied cognition and an adaptive unconscious) will continue to emerge across the social sciences. Similarly, hypnosis further develops its own empiric research and teachable skills.

Validating Hypnosis

The practical value of hypnosis is that it is uniquely different from other psychotherapies and medico-surgical interventions. This distinction can be made using universally meaningful terminology, without recourse to unconventional jargon. Milton Erickson described hypnosis simply as:

> … a special but normal type of behavior encountered when attention is directed to the body of experiential learnings acquired from or achieved in the experiences of living. In the special state of awareness called hypnosis, the various forms of behavior of everyday life may be found differing in relationships and degrees, but always within normal limits. There can be achieved no transcendence of abilities, no implantations of new abilities, but only the potentiation of the expression of abilities which may have gone unrecognized or not fully recognized. Hypnosis cannot create new abilities within a person, but it can assist in a greater and better utilization of abilities already possessed, even if these abilities were not previously recognized.
>
> *(Erickson, 2021, p. 85)*

While some techniques of persuasion may have some similarities with hypnosis, and while some misconceptions that the hypnotizer possesses some sort of exceptional power may have some therapeutic applications, we invite a more expansive view of therapeutic hypnosis, which includes active states (Bányai, 2018), collaborative dialog (Short, 2018), as well as other measurable interactional aspects of hypnotic relationship (Varga et al., 2006).

Today's hypnosis, particularly when utilized for clinical or therapeutic outcomes, is *a dynamic relational process enriched by experiential communication wherein the participant's attention is drawn inward with the intention of accessing personal internal experiential resources to generate adaptive adjustments*. Insights, understandings, and behavioral changes that accompany adaptive adjustments are problem-solving in nature and contribute to enhanced well-being and clarity.

Here, we differ slightly but significantly from Erickson's "special state of awareness" (Erickson, 2021; Short, 2019). We refer to hypnosis as the *process*, not a state and not its effects. Non-consciously derived experiential processes such as insights, inspirations, and decisions to change one's behavior can and do occur without hypnotic interactions. We identify hypnosis as that *dynamic relational process* that purposefully facilitates the utilization of embodied emotions, cognitions, and conditioned learnings as resources.

Further, because hypnosis operates within a complex system of dynamic and embodied networks that underlie and join our consciousness and our biology (from thought to genome), it fills what has traditionally been a "mind-body gap." That gap has existed primarily in the therapeutics and practice of Western biomedicine, but not within the integrated systems of the human organism. Hypnosis contrasts with most psychotherapies and medical/surgical approaches by deliberately leveraging the resources of the embodied mind. Thus, the effects of *problem-solving* are not, and cannot be limited to decisions about behavior or emotions – as if the domain of psychology is disembodied – but necessarily apply to embodied functions such as inflammation, metabolism, cellular-repair, and genomics. In this way, hypnosis is an essential relational interaction for ongoing adaptability and homeostasis.

It is important to distinguish "therapeutic hypnosis" as distinct within the broader social construct and methodology called hypnosis. As Scheflin and Hassan (*chapters referenced in this book*) have demonstrated, any given individual's innate abilities are the qualities that respond to suggestion and influence. This sets parameters that define an individual's "suggestibility," something which can be, and sometimes is, effectively evoked to harm. However, many didactic interactions in the process of providing medico-surgical care – such as giving risk information, sharing findings that evidence disease, preparing for procedures, and obtaining informed consent – inadvertently harm (Lang et al., 2005; Zech et al., 2019). As a higher standard, therapeutic hypnosis points to practical outcomes that are evocative, effective, and beneficial. Briefly speaking, therapeutic hypnosis helps people help themselves.

Responsiveness Versus Suggestibility

Hypnosis is distinct in that it seeks to evoke change through activation of innate resources. It is not about what answers are sought; rather it is a process of stimulating an internal search, thus accessing the individuals' embodied resources and talents. As a dynamic relational process, hypnosis is at least as much about what questioning *does* than what an answer *is*.

When academically framed as a linear, cause-effect, monistic ritual, hypnosis has been validated in terms of compliance with specific directives or "suggestions" and correlated with quantitative measures of "suggestibility" as well as "hypnotizability." However, there is circular logic in this construction. It restricts the definition of hypnosis to overt responses to influence and then tests one's ability to respond as expected. In short, hypnosis is compliance with behavior that the operator deems to be hypnotic. However, as argued by Short (2018), suggestibility is not equivalent to "responsivity," let alone plasticity. There is always incongruity – and sometimes discontinuity – between the hypnotic directive and innate abilities.

Teleska and Sugarman (2014) argue that most known "hypnotic phenomena" do not correlate closely with an individual's "hypnotic abilities." To move hypnosis toward further effective benefit, the current trajectory needs to shift toward tailoring the hypnotic interaction such that it evokes and activates innate resources rather than proxies for compliance. This paradigm shift is not optional if practitioners of hypnosis wish to maintain credibility within the context of 21st-century health care, and beyond.

As declared in standards set by the American Psychological Association guidelines for evidence-based therapy and cited by Cook et al. (2017) "Psychotherapists must prioritize understanding their patients, recognizing them as agents of change within sessions, supporting them as self-healers, and intentionally shaping their interventions based on being attuned to the patients' experiences of psychotherapy" (p. 540). (Cook et al., 2017, p. 540).

This principle applies just as much to medicine when "psychotherapist" is replaced by "clinician" and "psychotherapy" is replaced by "medical and surgical care." For therapeutic hypnosis – in both psychology and medicine – this means that the utilization of responsivity is merely a *first step* in a greater process of mental activation that ultimately results in what interpersonal neurobiology terms *self-organizing processes*, an evolutionary imperative recognized across the broad disciplines of mental health, medicine, and organizational functioning (Siegel, 2019).

Future "looking inward" research will need to include those signals or common denominators that correlate with an individual's responsive behaviors and signify plasticity and reorganization within the embodied mind and beneath conscious awareness.

Self-Hypnosis and Hetero-Hypnosis

The aforementioned issues of influence and agency that are inherent in hypnosis arise in the questions of whether self-hypnosis is as effective or different from hetero-hypnosis (i.e., hypnosis induced in one person by another) and whether self-hypnosis represents the variant of the same phenomenon or if it is a separate phenomenon (De Benedittis, 2022). Some claim that hetero-hypnosis is a pre-cursor of self-hypnosis (Laidlaw et al., 2005; Naito et al., 2003). Others identify self-hypnosis as a self-administered hetero-hypnosis or as a by-product of the same (Crasilneck et al., 1985; Erickson, 2022a; Ruch, 1975; Werner, 2013). Fromm and Khan (1990) consider hetero and self-hypnosis as completely distinct entities. Diametrically opposed is the widespread conception that the vast majority of hetero-hypnotic procedures can be recognized as self-hypnosis (Barber, 1985; Orne & McConkey, 1981; Sanders, 1991). These questions are all parsed from a larger discussion about the notion of "self" and its elusive boundaries (Wickramasekera, 2015, see also Nyiri & Lynn in this volume).

Conceptually, self-hypnosis can include negative self-talk. This adverse self-influence is accumulated from life experience and formative relationships. In that sense, one might call all hypnosis hetero-hypnosis, which we internalize as self-hypnosis. It follows then that hetero-hypnosis, when therapeutic, can be understood as cultivating more beneficial self-hypnosis. Future studies should consider how to develop hetero-hypnotic interactions that are less inhibitory and more facilitative of beneficial self-hypnosis.

Future research into the question of whether hetero-hypnosis is, in effect, guided self-hypnosis, or the reverse, is likely to yield the answer that it depends on the persons involved. This is another hypnotic horizon.

Agents of Change

The difficulties specific to the ethical practice of hypnosis are that a significant part of the process of change occurs outside of conscious awareness within the embodied mind. This includes a sense of involuntariness or automaticity as change occurs. These phenomena can lead to attribution errors (see Weinberger et al., 2022). The ethical questions that are specific to hypnosis are associated with changing perspectives of suggestibility and attribution of agency within the hypnotic interaction.

Hypnosis is one of a variety of unorthodox treatment modalities affected by drifting cultural attitudes according to Scheflin (2019). Hypnosis endures periods of public favor and scorn, including, in the therapeutic context, innovation and stagnation. At the heart of these waves of acceptance and rejection is the ethical question: does hypnosis cause harm? Scheflin (2019) and Hammond (1995) have identified the formidable challenges for both clinicians and researchers to generate a legal parameter that does not stifle or smother therapeutic innovation. Again, we require methods to assess innovative treatments that work outside of conscious awareness, within the adaptive unconscious and embodied mind (Smith, 2021). The concept of therapeutic responsibility becomes even more complex when it is recognized that hypnotic suggestion can be influential whether or not formal trance induction/awakening is used and regardless of whether the hypnotic process is hetero- or self-hypnotic in nature (Short, 2018). This leads to practical procedural questions. Should antiquated, domineering terminology (such as "induction") be discarded in favor of more modern, relationship-oriented language (such as "invitation" or "hypnotic conversation") that more accurately describes a process of voluntary participation, personal empowerment, and shared responsibility? More fundamentally, should all health care interactions include explicit education, awareness, and advocacy on the part of both clinicians and people in care that we share relational influences on healing? How might this change the process of obtaining pre-operative consent forms or informing about prognosis? Answering such questions will require parameters for determining responsivity and plasticity that do not depend on technique, but on how a given person in care changes their embodied mind.

Looking Outward

As can be seen in the shift away from direct suggestion toward the growing use of open-ended exploratory processes, including hypnotherapeutic imagery (Short, 2022a), the basic accessing questions (Rossi & Rossi, 1996/2024), metaphor (Fabre, 2022), and story (Casula, 2022), self-directed learning and unconscious deliberation will eventually supersede the emphasis on suggestibility that we know today. Already it is generally accepted that suggestibility is not a therapeutic end unto itself but rather a means of enhancing responsiveness to positive treatment expectancies; focusing attention; engaging imagination; strengthening rapport; bolstering personal resources; stimulating spontaneous psychobiological activity with novel associations; and facilitating self-regulation (Lynn et al., 2022).

Today, therapeutic hypnosis often involves ongoing feedback as the process unfolds. This interaction empowers a person in care with the opportunity to either endorse or reject various elements of the experience. As the experience of choice and spontaneity is elicited, and further developed at every turn, the client's sense of responsibility for treatment outcomes is greatly enhanced, presumably along with the experience of self-efficacy (Bandura, 2000). Furthermore, when procedural dogma is replaced with emergent co-creative processes, both client and therapist are free to explore. This variability, and what might be described as inconsistency, in a co-created experience presents a challenge to traditional forms of research that look for reproducible and consistent protocols "done to" a passive and hypnotizable client. With this complexity, research is challenged to explore and document the nature and effectiveness of this type of more dynamic and idiosyncratic hypnosis.

Two critical but generally undervalued aspects of the progressive evolution of hypnosis are hypnosis with children and the role of development. From Erickson's (Erickson & Rossi, 2010) initial advice to "go with the child" (p. 149) to the compelling research showing the enduring effectiveness of hypnotic interventions with children (Kohen & Olness, 2022), it is clear that not only are we most innately adept at changing our embodied minds when we are young, but also such conditioning during our first two decades significantly affects all those subsequent. Further, if hypnosis cultivates and influences plasticity, developmental tasks – especially when we are young – can be understood as a "governing influence in trance. It determines how and why we 'go plastic'" (Sugarman et al., 2020, p. 151). Research and application of developmentally oriented hypnosis with young people have far-reaching and very practical implications for addressing chronic disease, trauma, and the development of resilience throughout the lifespan.

Creativity Markers

Hypnosis research has by and large aligned with the biomedical model in which consistent and replicable allopathic intervention is introduced in an otherwise controlled context. However, to extend the definition, operation, and creativity of hypnosis beyond a prescribed linear procedure requires a shift in our research paradigm. Allowance must be made for a more person-centered evocation of an array of individual abilities – even indeterminate and idiosyncratic ones. This shift entails *moving the nexus from between the hypnotic act and the person's response to the interpretive responses of the participant.*

For example, Ernest Rossi and others have attempted to correlate dependent variables of immediate early gene expression (through RNA micro-arrays) and inflammatory markers (Cozzolino & Celia, 2021) as biomarkers of plasticity within the embodied mind. Notably, the independent variable in these experiments is a relatively non-directive set of invitations for inner exploration using the Mind Body Therapy Transformation Scale (Cozzolino & Celia, 2021). This approach allows for a more individualized and heuristic search compared to compliance with specific directives.

Although this research is still preliminary, expensive, and currently lacking controls, it moves us in the direction of finding common denominators of plasticity that originate within a person's innate resources.

Subjectivity and Observation

Responses to hypnosis are highly subjective and personal, yet indicators of hypnosis have traditionally relied on outside observation of specific hypnotic phenomena. It is common for subjects to offer fanciful dream-like narratives in response to hypnotic sessions. While it is possible that such internal journeys may be an indicator to help us better appreciate the nature of hypnosis, no methodology has yet been reported that correlates subjective reports of creative autonomy, expansive self-awareness, and growing self-trust. Though logic suggests these elements are associated with adaptive growth, they are not yet concretely measurable hypnotic phenomena.

Further, the way expectancy contributes to therapeutic outcome cannot be overlooked. The integration of hypnosis into a therapeutic alliance brings with it a multitude of useful assets including mobilization of the subjects' own internal hope and positive expectancy. Therapeutic alliance affects the potential for placebo or nocebo effects on individuals. Studies by Carlino and colleagues (2014) using brain imaging have shown that capitalizing on the placebo effect has a dramatic effect on patient response to treatment and subsequently to clinical outcome. In the ideal therapeutic context, hypnosis mobilizes internal experiential associations, enhances internal capacity to problem solve, and may even result in a sensation that problems magically self-resolve.

Exploration and applications of hypnosis within the clinical context bring with it agreements between the professional and client seeking treatment. In 1964, Erickson (2022b) first wrote that the burden of effective responsibility for psychotherapy is primarily to be borne by the client. Ernest Rossi later expanded this principle by adding that it was the task of the therapist to let go of this responsibility, return it to the client, and make all effort to not interfere with the client's natural problem-solving activity. The professional provides guidance and encouragement to facilitate awareness of the client's internal curiosity and personal search. These discoveries and new associations can directly and positively impact the client's decisions and actions without resistance (Hill and Rossi, 2018). The client bears the burden to discover their ever-growing ability of self-agency within the process of creative adaptive adjustments.

Clinical hypnosis is both a science and an art. Researchers have forged the evolving process of seeking concrete identifiers to verify and better understand the nature of hypnosis. The therapeutic practice of hypnosis involves the cooperative process of assessment and adaptive adjustments to an ever-changing perspective of mind-body healing. While professional roles of the researcher and clinician differ, they are united in the commitment to advance understanding, efficacy, and the reliability of hypnosis.

Therapeutic hypnosis embraces the concept that both clinicians and clients can learn to use a variety of hypnotic techniques for the purpose of enhancing health. Hypnotic techniques involve recognition and engagement of biological energy cycles, novelty, participation, broadening of perspective, and suggestive inferences to promote problem resolution and beneficially adaptive adjustments (Rossi, 1993).

Expanding Hypnosis Through Evolving Scientific Studies

As mentioned earlier, the construct that we currently refer to as therapeutic hypnosis has progressed from shamanic rituals toward scientifically studied medical procedures. As we seek to provide ethical guidelines and better understand the nature of hypnosis, there are growing opportunities to explore some of the ritualistic traditions that bear similarities to the hypnotic process. Given the variety of ways that the social construct of hypnosis can be integrated into care, recognizing, studying their effects, and integrating such practices within a hypnotic frame improves cultural competency in health and care, and perhaps outcomes.

Current trends are leaning in the direction of integrated care as medical professionals seek to unite wholistic experiences of the mind and body. This orientation opens doors for treatments in which a psychotherapeutic approach can enhance desired physiological responses (Hartman & Zimberoff, 2011). Throughout the history of medicine, hypnosis has been consistently contributing to stress reduction, pain management, and other therapeutic outcomes (NIH, 1996). Today, a recognition for honoring the bio-psycho-social integrity of an individual requires integration of qualitative methodology, which is becoming more widely accepted in academia. Several significant works, such as Erika Fromm's Chicago Paradigm (Fromm & Kahn, 1990) and Dan Short's (2021) Core Competencies, seek to bridge the gap of bringing together qualitative research and individual experiences while providing a scientific platform. These essential individual perceptual experiences are clearly fundamental to hypnosis and the healing process.

An integral part of investigating the nature and efficacy of hypnosis is incorporating developing technological resources and identifying significant biomarkers correlated to the hypnotic process. Current methods include fMRIs, brain wave assessment, and activity-dependent and RNA gene expression sequences. These and other quantitative indicators provide documentation of changes mediated by the hypnotic process.

Numerous functional neuroimaging studies (fMRIs) show how hypnosis affects brain attention by modulating the conflict monitoring and cognitive control functions in the anterior cingulate cortex (Terhune et al., 2017). Hypnosis-induced altered reality perception and the central role of mental imagery in hypnosis are associated with activation of the occipital and temporal brain cortices, precuneus, and other extrastriate visual areas. In contrast, non-hypnotically delivered motor commands are processed differently. Functional neuroimaging also shows that posthypnotic suggestions alter cognitive processes. Further research should investigate the effects of hypnosis on other executive functions and personality measures (Casale et al., 2012).

Jensen and colleagues (2017) succinctly summarize the discussions among a group of contemporary hypnosis researchers on two decades of ongoing neurophysiological exploration on the nature of hypnosis. Chief among their recommendations, they urge sharing data and tighter collaboration.

Looking Forward

Our future orientation to research requires a shift to the systemic study of how each unique individual generates recognized (behavioral and technological) signals of their own (person-based) plasticity and away from signals derived from hypnotic rituals (procedure-based). Such study will help illuminate how to reliably reproduce those phenomena in a variety of ways (new, progressive rituals) and toward recognition of interpersonal factors to best promote beneficial use of hypnosis across the continuum of health and care. In one sense, this type of interpersonal and contextual tailoring of therapy can be viewed as amplifying the placebo effect (see also Benedetti in this volume). Because we are cultivating one's innate plasticity in the service of healing, Moerman's and Jonas's (2002) term "meaning effect" may be more apt. This research trajectory also aims to expose the interface between the intervention, its meaning to the individual in care, and what makes it therapeutic.

While we expect treatment technology to continually evolve, *it is important to recognize that the phenomenology used to define hypnosis is also evolving.* Thus, throughout this chapter, as well as across the broader science of hypnosis, we see new lines of inquiry, from systems theory, gene expression, and electrodynamics adding new dimensionality to the social construct collectively known as hypnosis. More specifically, the domineering hypnotherapist directing the thoughts and actions of a groggy hypnotic subject, who uncritically responds with compliance, is an image of the past. This pre-systemic, unilateral model of influence is being replaced with more dynamic forms of interpersonal engagement that prioritize connectedness and collaboration along with individual resources and co-creation (BoVee-Akyurek, 2017; Hasan et al., 2014; Short, 2021). For the duration of this chapter, we will speculate on what might be on the horizon for hypnosis.

Professional Education: Thinking in a Systems Context

Engel's (1977) revolutionary biopsychosocial paradigm was derived from an attempt to provide a method of training young physicians that includes a person's lived experiences and critical relationships in their care. Because therapeutic hypnosis operates intentionally within the embodied mind – where biology and experience are one – education and training in therapeutic hypnosis necessitates a conceptualization of such a complex evolving system. It must progress from the teaching of linear, stepwise inductions, deepening-suggestions, etc. (all based upon diagnosis and condition-based directions and protocols) toward teaching an expanding array of conversational skills that tailor to individual abilities and responses. One can foresee experiential learning that is focused on developing both relational skills and the evocation of plasticity guided by real-time data provided by a combination of autonomic, brain-based, and even genomic sensors.

Instead of learning inductions and suggestions for given types of problems, in given types of people, in specified clinical contexts, hypnosis training can be a series of interpersonal exercises that teach how to safely explore and evoke the behaviors and underlying mechanisms that correlate with how a given individual changes their mind.

Given our understanding of the psychobiology of meaning, modern hypnotic practice can entail that clinicians are sensitive to the fit of the cultural narrative of peoples' own understandings of health or of identified problems.

From a technological perspective, we can foresee a future in which the power of artificial intelligence and quantum computing enhances individual tailoring, and thus effectiveness of care. Interpersonal communication is required to evoke and cultivate each individual's capacities for altering those most germane immune, genomic, neural, cardiovascular, and autonomic responses in beneficial ways. Embedding hypnosis within care can be integrated into digital therapeutics that construct and render holographic, virtual realities, tailored to depict those components that best evoke an individual's healing potentials.

We can anticipate hypnosis contributing to an individual thriving in ways that go far beyond the "diagnose and treat" model to more wholistic paradigms such as the "risks and resources" model (Sugarman et al., 2020). In this lifespan-based developmental model, everyone is born with and accumulates biological, environmental, behavioral, and relational risk factors for health conditions. Eventually we all meet criteria for several diagnoses. But we are also each born with, and can accrue, a variety of lived experiences that can be evoked, cultivated, and utilized to modify and ameliorate those risk factors. Not too long from now, those health risks might be routinely cataloged and well known to both clinician and the person in care. Traditionally, treatment begins when diagnostic criteria are met. But the challenge of wholistic health is not on this allopathic front. In these emerging models, therapeutic interaction is focused on the ongoing cultivation and agency of bringing individual resources to bear – something that hypnosis does very well.

The future of hypnotherapy will likely be shaped by clinicians and researchers who expand their own capacity for curious exploration. To fully find its place in the science of health and care, hypnosis must be personalized and operationalized for sufficient continuity that allows meaningful research. The ongoing development of core competency principles is one way of providing a framework in which individual clinicians, regardless of their cultural orientation, can give individual qualitative and quantitative information to join the quest to work together to contribute to a shared body of knowledge (Short, 2021).

Building Tomorrow on Yesterday

In modern medicine, clinicians and researchers are challenged to find indicators that identify the effects of hypnosis on the individual. Leonard Ravitz discovered a valuable electronic signature of hypnosis in experiments done with Milton H. Erickson in the 1940s (Ravitz, 1950). Ernest Rossi further explored electrodynamics with Ravitz (Rossi & Ravitz, 1980) and then in private practice research with Kathryn Rossi (Rossi & Rossi, 2016). Recognizing this uniqueness of the individual has ushered in a future of gene-expression-based personalized medicine where pharmacotherapy is tailored to individual needs and abilities. The same can be true with hypnosis.

Seminal work initiated by Ernest Rossi indicates that gene expression might provide biomarkers for hypnosis. Chronobiological rhythm patterns, particularly ~90–120-minute ultradian cycles, are significant variables that enhance effects of hypnotic work and underpin all life processes (Rossi, 1993). These chronobiological discoveries were further advanced with groundbreaking pilot studies done by Ernest Rossi and colleagues to form the field of psychosocial genomics (e.g., Cozzolino et al., 2014; Rossi et al., 2008; Rossi & Rossi, 2014) that demonstrate activation of gene expression responsiveness by hypnosis immediately following a hypnotherapy session and with many more health generating genes expressed 24 hours later. While this work is preliminary, uncontrolled, and requires replication by others, it holds exciting possibilities for uniting the scientific and experiential worlds of hypnosis.

Each of these discoveries brings us forward not only in the direction of understanding the process of hypnosis but also in the direction of new discoveries waiting to be conceptualized. The future of therapeutic hypnosis is to develop research protocols where individual clinicians can participate. Ideal statistics for this are Bayesian, wherein the individual subject acts as their own baseline (Rossi et al., 2015). Future research will use case-by-case measures to make inferences that can collectively contribute to longitudinal studies.

What Can We Imagine into Reality?

The challenge for the idealized future clinician-trainee reporting to their interdisciplinary team about a given person in their care is not whether they have all the diagnosis-related clinical data together but how they have learned about and helped the person in care activate their embodied abilities. We can imagine that the feared question on rounds in a professional peer group is not, "Do you have the diagnosis?" but is instead, "What do you know of their relevant innate resources?" Not, "What is the pain level?" but, "How did you inquire about their pain?"

Finally, we can imagine that this future trajectory of hypnosis in health and care drives a shift from exemplifying the power and agency of the clinician/shaman/hypnotherapist to more egalitarian, mutually beneficial relationship in health and care. As we use hypnosis to recognize and amplify the capacities of individuals for changing their embodied minds, *the role of clinician changes from an operator working on a subject to a creative evocateur exploring the outer margins of human potential.*

Clinicians Become the Sorcerers' Apprentices

The traditional wisdom that dominated the field in the last century was that hypnosis is a technique, rather than a full-fledged approach to treatment. Therefore, it must always be embedded within some other healing tradition, such as hypnoanalysis, cognitive behavioral hypnotherapy, or as an adjunct to pain management or anesthesia. However, as the growing integration of various methodologies replaces strict adherence to theoretical dogma, and as the individualization of treatment becomes more common across the field, the segregation of hypnotic treatments from general psychotherapy and biomedicine has become more difficult to justify. Furthermore, hypnosis has been shown to enhance other treatments (Kirsch et al., 1995), flipping the current delivery model upside down. If this trend continues, we could see hypnosis develop into an umbrella approach that encapsulates many different treatment methodologies. If we begin to recognize the importance of acknowledging and utilizing unconscious processes during every problem-solving endeavor – from anxiety to wound-healing – then we see that hypnosis is not *less than* (merely a technique) but rather *more than* – an approach to problem-solving that adds unexpected possibility to all other methods of treatment.

Can you imagine that?

References

Bandura, A. (2000). Exercise of human agency through collective efficacy. *Current Directions in Psychological Science*, *9*(3), 75–78. 10.1111/1467-8721.00064

Bányai, É. I. (2018). Active-alert hypnosis: History, research, and applications. *American Journal of Clinical Hypnosis*, *61*(2), 88–107. 10.1080/00029157.2018.1496318

Barber, T. X. (1985). Hypnosuggestive procedures as catalysts for psychotherapies. In S. J. Lynn & J. P. Garske (Eds.), *Contemporary psychotherapies: Models and methods* (pp. 333–376). Charles E. Merrill.

BoVee-Akyurek, A. (2017). *The delicate process and relational style of solution focused brief therapy: Ericksonian hypnotherapy resemblances in SFBT*. ProQuest Dissertations Publishing. https://www.proquest.com/openview/44b5eb237c1ec1a85e4fd4d5b27b0cc1/1?pq-origsite=gscholar&cbl=51922&diss=y

Carlino, E., Benedetti, F., & Pollo, A. (2014). The effects of manipulating verbal suggestions on physical performance. *Zeitschrift Für Psychologie*, *222*(3), 154–164. 10.1027/2151-2604/a000178

Casale, A. D., Ferracuti, S., Rapinesi, C., Serata, D., Sani, G., Savoja, V., Kotzalidis, G. D., Tatarelli, R., & Girardi, P. (2012). Neurocognition under hypnosis: Findings from recent functional neuroimaging studies. *International Journal of Clinical and Experimental Hypnosis*, *60*(3), 286–317. 10.1080/00207144.2012.675295

Casula, C. C. (2022). Stimulating unconscious processes with metaphors and narrative. *American Journal of Clinical Hypnosis*, *64*(4), 339–354. 10.1080/00029157.2021.2019670

Cook, S. C., Schwartz, A. C., & Kaslow, N. J. (2017). Evidence-based psychotherapy: Advantages and challenges. *Neurotherapeutics*, 14(3), 537–545. 10.1007/s13311-017-0549-4

Cozzolino, M., Iannotti, S., Castiglione, S., Cicatelli, A., Rossi, K., & Rossi, E. (2014). A bioinformatic analysis of the molecular-genomic signature of therapeutic hypnosis. *The International Journal of Psychosocial and Cultural Genomics, Consciousness & Health Research*, *1*(1), 6–11.

Cozzolino, M., & Celia, G. (2021). The psychosocial genomics paradigm of hypnosis and mind-body integrated psychotherapy: Scientific evolution and experimental evidence. *American Journal of Clinical Hypnosis*, *64*(2), doi: 10.1080/00029157.2021.1947767

Crasilneck, H. B., & Hall, J. A. (1985). *Clinical hypnosis: Principles and applications*. (2nd ed.). Grune & Stratton.

De Benedittis, G. (2022). Auto-Ipnosi. Alla ricerca della risorsa interiore (eng. *Self hypnosis. In search of your inner resource*) *Ipnosi*, *2*, 5–20.

Diamond, M. J. (1987). The interactional basis of hypnotic experience: On the relational dimensions of hypnosis. *International Journal of Clinical and Experimental Hypnosis*, *35*(2), 95–115. doi: 10.1080/00207148708416046.

Engel, G. L. (1977). The need for a new medical model: A challenge for biomedicine. *Science*, *196*(4286), 192–236. doi:10.1126/science.847460.

Erickson, M. H. (2021). Hypnosis: Its renascence as a treatment modality. (Original work published 1966) In E. L. Rossi, R. Erickson-Klein & K. L. Rossi (Eds.), *Basic hypnotic induction and therapeutic suggestion, Volume 2 of the collected works of Milton H. Erickson, M.D.* (p. 85). www.Erickson-Rossi.com

Erickson, M. H. (2022a). Self-exploration in hypnosis. (Original work published 1955). In E. L. Rossi, R. Erickson-Klein & K. L. Rossi (Eds.), *Opening the Mind, Volume 3 of The Collected Works of Milton H. Erickson, M.D.* (pp. 358–375). www.Erickson-Rossi.com

Erickson, M. H. (2022b). The burden of responsibility in effective psychotherapy. (Original work published 1964). In E. L. Rossi, R. Erickson-Klein & K. L. Rossi (Eds.), *Opening the mind, Volume 3 of the collected works of Milton H. Erickson, M.D.* (pp. 97–112). www.Erickson-Rossi.com

Erickson, M. H., & Rossi, E. L. (2010). Hypnotic realities: The induction of clinical hypnosis and forms of indirect suggestion. (Original work published 1976). In E. L. Rossi, R. Erickson-Klein, & K. Rossi (Eds.), *The collected works of Milton H. Erickson – Volume 10*. Milton H. Erickson Foundation Press.

Fabre, C. (2022). Indirect work with hypnosis using metaphorical objects. *American Journal of Clinical Hypnosis*, *64*(4), 355–372.

Fromm, E., & Kahn, S. (1990). *Self-hypnosis: The Chicago paradigm* (pp. xiii, 254). Guilford Press.

Fromm, E., & Nash, M. R. (1992). *Contemporary hypnosis research*. Guilford Press.

Hammond, D. C. (1995). *Clinical hypnosis and memory: Guidelines for clinicians and for forensic hypnosis*. American Society of Clinical Hypnosis Press.

Hartman, D., & Zimberoff, D. (2011). *Hypnosis and hypnotherapy in the milieu of integrative medicine: Healing the mind/body/spirit. Journal of Heart-Centered Therapies*, *14*(1), 41–75.

Hasan, F. M., Zagarins, S. E., Pischke, K. M., Saiyed, S., Bettencourt, A. M., Beal, L., Macys, D., Aurora, S., & McCleary, N. (2014). Hypnotherapy is more effective than nicotine replacement therapy for smoking cessation: Results of a randomized controlled trial. *Complementary Therapies in Medicine*, *22*(1), 1–8. 10.1016/j.ctim.2013.12.012

Hill, R., & Rossi, E. L. (2018). *The practitioner's guide to mirroring hands: A client-responsive therapy that facilitates natural problem-solving and mind-body healing*. Crown House Publishing Ltd.

Hope, A. E., & Sugarman, L. I. (2015). Orienting hypnosis. *American Journal of Clinical Hypnosis*, *57*(3), 212–229. 10.1080/00029157.2014.976787

Jaynes, J. (1976). *The origin of consciousness in the breakdown of the bicameral mind*. Houghton-Mifflin.

Jensen, M. P., Jamieson, G. A., Lutz, A., Mazzoni, G., McGeown, W. J., Santarcangelo, E. L., Demertzi, A., De Pascalis, V., Bányai, É. I., Rominger, C., Vuilleumier, P., Faymonville, M.-E., & Terhune, D. B. (2017). New directions in hypnosis research: Strategies for advancing the cognitive and clinical neuroscience of hypnosis. *Neuroscience of Consciousness*, *2017*(1), nix004. 10.1093/nc/nix004

Kirsch, I., Montgomery, G., & Sapirstein, G. (1995). Hypnosis as an adjunct to cognitive-behavioral psychotherapy: A meta-analysis. *Journal of Consulting and Clinical Psychology*, *63*(2), 214–220. 10.1037/0022-006X.63.2.214

Kohen, D. P., & Olness, K. N. (2022). *Hypnosis with children*. Routledge.

Laidlaw, T., Bennett, B. M., Dwivedi, P., Naito, A., & Gruzelier, J. (2005). Quality of life and mood changes in metastatic breast cancer after training in self-hypnosis or Johrei: A short report. *Contemporary Hypnosis*, *22*(2), 84–93.

Lang, E. V., Hatsiopoulou, O., Koch, T., Berbaum, K., Lutgendorf, S., Kettenmann, E., Logan, H., & Kaptchuk, T. J. (2005). Can words hurt? Patient-provider interactions during invasive procedures. *Pain*, *114*(1–2):303–309. doi: 10.1016/j.pain.2004.12.028.

Lynn, S. J., Cardeña, E., Green, J. P., & Laurence, J.-R. (2022). The case for clinical hypnosis: Theory and research-based do's and don'ts for clinical practice. *Psychology of Consciousness: Theory, Research, and Practice*, 9(2), 187–200. 10.1037/cns0000257

Moerman, D. E., & Jonas, W. B. (2002). Deconstructing the placebo effect and finding the meaning response. *Annal of Internal Medicine*, *136*(6), 471–476.

Naito, A., Laidlaw, T. M., Henderson, D. C., Farahani, L., Dwivedi, P., & Gruzelier, J. H. (2003). The impact of self-hypnosis and Johrei on lymphocyte subpopulations at exam time: A controlled study. *Brain Research Bulletin*, 62(3), 241–253.

NIH. (1996). Integration of behavioral and relaxation approaches into the treatment of chronic pain and insomnia: NIH Technology Assessment Panel on Integration of Behavioral and Relaxation Approaches Into the Treatment of Chronic Pain and Insomnia. *JAMA*, *276*(4), 313–318. 10.1001/jama.1996.03540040057033

Orne, M. T., & McConkey, K. M. (1981). Toward convergent inquiry into self-hypnosis. *International Journal of Clinical and Experimental Hypnosis*, *29*(3), 313–323. doi:10.1080/00207148108409164

Ravitz, L. J. (1950). Electrometric correlates of the hypnotic state. *Science*, *112*(2908), 341–342. 10.1126/science.112.2908.341

Rossi, E. L. (1993). *Psychobiology of mind body healing revised edition*. W. W. Norton & Company.

Rossi, E. L. (2004). Gene expression and brain plasticity in stoke rehabilitation: A personal memoir of mind-body healing dreams. *American Journal of Clinical Hypnosis*, *46*(3), 215–227. doi: 10.1080/00029157.2004.10403601

Rossi E., Rossi K., Cozzolino M., & Joly, J. (2015). The quantum field theory of psychosocial genomics: Quantum Bayesian notation for therapeutic consciousness and cognition. *International Journal of Psychosocial and Cultural Genomics: Consciousness and Health Research*, *1*(4), 11–25.

Rossi E., Iannotti S., Cozzolino M., Castiglione S., Cicatelli A., & Rossi K. (2008). A pilot study of positive expectations and focused attention via a new protocol for therapeutic hypnosis assessed with DNA microarrays: The creative psychosocial genomic healing experience. *Sleep and Hypnosis: An International Journal of Sleep, Dream, and Hypnosis*, 10(2), 39–44.

Rossi, E. L., & Ravitz, L. (1980). *Electromagnetic field measurements in altered states of consciousness?* The First International Congress of Ericksonian Approaches to Hypnosis and Psychotherapy, Phoenix, AZ.

Rossi, E. L., Rossi, K. L. (1996/2024). *The symptom path to enlightenment: The new dynamics of self organization in hypnotherapy*. Palisades Gateway Press.

Rossi, E. L., & Rossi, K. L. (2014). An evolutionary RNA/DNA psychogenomic theory of the transformations of consciousness: The quest for therapeutic mind/gene search algorithms. *The International Journal of Psychosocial and Cultural Genomics, Consciousness & Health Research*, *1*(1), 1–20.

Rossi, E. L., & Rossi, K. L. (2016). A quantum field theory of neuropsychotherapy. *The Science of Psychotherapy*. https://www.thescienceofpsychotherapy.com/a-quantum-field-theory-of-neuropsychotherapy/

Ruch, J. C. (1975). Self-hypnosis: The result of heterohypnosis or vice versa? *International Journal of Clinical and Experimental Hypnosis*, 23(4), 282–304. 10.1080/00207147508415952

Sanders, S. (1991). *Clinical self-hypnosis: The power of words and images*. Guilford Press.

Scheflin, A. (2019). Ethics and hypnosis: Unorthodox or innovative therapies and the legal standard of care. In W. Matthews & J. Edgette (Eds.), *Current thinking and research in brief therapy* (pp. 41–55). Routledge.

Short, D. (2018). Conversational hypnosis: Conceptual and technical differences relative to traditional hypnosis. *American Journal of Clinical Hypnosis*, *61*(2), 125–139. 10.1080/00029157.2018.1441802

Short, D. (2019). *Principles and core competencies of Ericksonian therapy: 2019 edition* [PDF]. The Milton H. Erickson Institute of Phoenix. http://www.iamdrshort.com/PDF/Papers/Core%20Competencies%20Manual.pdf

Short, D. (2020). Whispering hypnosis: Phylogenetically programmed behavior and a pluralistic understanding of hypnosis. *American Journal of Clinical Hypnosis*, *62*(3), 178–197. 10.1080/00029157.2019.1640180

Short, D. (2021). What is Ericksonian therapy: The use of core competencies to operationally define a nonstandardized approach to psychotherapy. *Clinical Psychology: Science and Practice*, *28*(3), 282–292. 10.1037/cps0000014

Short, D. (2022a). Beyond words: A conceptual framework for the study and practice of hypnotherapeutic imagery. *American Journal of Clinical Hypnosis*, *64*(4), xx. 10.1080/00029157.2021.2020709

Short, D. (2022b). La plus importante des leçons de James Braid. *La Revue de l'hypnose et de la santé*, *19*(2), 85–89. English version: http://www.iamdrshort.com/New_Papers/Braid's%20razor.pdf.

Siegel, D. J. (2019). The mind in psychotherapy: An interpersonal neurobiology framework for understanding and cultivating mental health. *Psychology and Psychotherapy: Theory, Research and Practice*, *92*(2), 224–237. 10.1111/papt.12228

Smith, J. A. (2021). *Emotions, embodied cognition and the adaptive unconscious: A complex topography of the social making of things*. Routledge.

Sugarman, L. I. (2021). Leaving hypnosis behind? *American Journal of Clinical Hypnosis*, *64*(2), 139–156. doi: 10.1080/00029157.2021.1935686

Sugarman, L. I., Linden, J. H., & Brooks, L. W. (2020). *Changing minds with clinical hypnosis: Narratives and discourse for a new health care paradigm*. Routledge.

Teleska, J., & Roffman, A. (2004). A continuum of hypnotherapeutic interactions: From formal hypnosis to hypnotic conversation. *American Journal of Clinical Hypnosis*, *47*(2), 103–115. doi: 10.1080/00029157.2004.10403629

Teleska, J. A., & Sugarman, L. (2014). Hypnotic abilities. In L. L. Sugarman & W. Wester (Eds.), *Therapeutic hypnosis with children and adolescents: Second edition*. Crown House Publishing.

Terhune, D. B., Cleeremans, A., Raz, A., Lynn, S. J. (2017). Hypnosis and top-down regulation of consciousness. *Neuroscience and Biobehavioral Reviews*, *81*(A), 59–74.

Varga, K. (2021). Possible mechanisms of hypnosis from an interactional perspective. *Brain Science*, *11*(7), 903. doi: 10.3390/brainsci11070903.

Varga, K., Józsa, E., Bányai, É. I., & Gősi-Greguss, A. C. (2006). A new way of characterizing hypnotic interactions: Dyadic Interactional Harmony (DIH) questionnaire. *Contemporary Hypnosis*, *23*(4), 151–166. 10.1002/ch.320

Weinberger, J., Brigante, M., & Nissen, K. (2022). Conscious intelligence is overrated: The normative unconscious and hypnosis. *American Journal of Clinical Hypnosis*, *54*(4), 290–305. 10.1080/00029157.2021.2025032

Werner, A., Uldbjerg, N., Zachariae, R., & Nohr, E. A. (2013). Effect of self-hypnosis on duration of labor and maternal and neonatal outcomes: A randomized controlled trial. *Acta Obstetricia Et Gynecologica Scandinavica*, *92*(7), 816–823.

Wickramasekera, E. (2015). Mysteries of hypnosis and the self are revealed by the psychology and neuroscience of empathy. *American Journal of Clinical Hypnosis*, *57*(3), 330–348.

Zech, N., Seemann, M., Grzesiek, M., Breu, A., Seyfried, T. F., Hansen, E. (2019). Nocebo effects on muscular performance – An experimental study about clinical situations. *Frontiers in Pharmacology*, *10*, 219. doi: 10.3389/fphar.2019.00219.

INDEX

Pages in *italics* refer to figures and pages in **bold** refer to tables.

For Product Safety Concerns and Information please contact our EU representative GPSR@taylorandfrancis.com
Taylor & Francis Verlag GmbH, Kaufingerstraße 24, 80331 München, Germany

www.ingramcontent.com/pod-product-compliance
Lightning Source LLC
Chambersburg PA
CBHW081206220326
41598CB00037B/6693